Practical
Gastroenterology

Practical Gastroenterology

edited by Stuart Bloom

Department of Gastroenterology, University College London Hospitals, London, UK

MARTIN DUNITZ

First published in the United Kingdom in 2002
by Martin Dunitz Ltd, The Livery House, 7–9 Pratt Street, London
NW1 0AE

Tel.:   +44 (0) 20 7482 2202
Fax.:   +44 (0) 20 7267 0159
E-mail: info.dunitz@tandf.co.uk
Website: http://www.dunitz.co.uk

A CIP record for this book is available from the British Library.

ISBN 1-84184-121-8

Distributed in the USA by
Fulfilment Center
Taylor & Francis
7625 Empire Drive
Florence, KY 41042, USA
Toll Free Tel.: +1 800 634 7064
E-mail: cserve@routledge_ny.com

Distributed in Canada by
Taylor & Francis
74 Rolark Drive
Scarborough, Ontario M1R 4G2, Canada
Toll Free Tel.: +1 877 226 2237
E-mail: tal_fran@istar.ca

Distributed in the rest of the world by
ITPS Limited
Cheriton House
North Way
Andover, Hampshire SP10 5BE, UK
Tel.: +44 (0)1264 332424
E-mail: reception@itps.co.uk

Composition by Scientifik Graphics (Singapore) Pte Ltd

Printed and bound in Spain by Grafos SA Arte sobre papel

Practical
Gastroenterology

Contents

Preface   ix

Contributors   xi

PART I: Gastroenterology Trainee's Survival Guide

A: Refresher course in basic gastroenterology

1.   Eliciting the Gastrointestinal History   3
     Robin Vicary

2.   Examination of the Gastrointestinal System   9
     Robin Vicary

3.   Clinical Anatomy of the Gastrointestinal Tract
     3.1   Macroscopic   15
            Paul Boulos
     3.2   Microscopic   25
            Marco Novelli

B: Dealing with inpatient consultations/referrals

4.   Gastrointestinal Problems in Patients with Metabolic and Endocrine Disorders   41
     Anne Ballinger

5.   Gastrointestinal Problems in Haematology Patients   55
     Brian J. Hennessy and Atul B. Mehta

6.   Gastrointestinal Problems in Patients with Rheumatological and Connective Tissue Diseases   71
     Alastair Forbes

7.   Gastrointestinal Problems in the Immunocompromised   85
     Ross D. Cranston, Peter Anton and Ian McGowan

8.   Gastrointestinal Problems in Neurological Patients   103
     Helen Fidler and Julian Fearnley

9.   Gastrointestinal Problems on the Obstetric Unit   115
     Elspeth Alstead and Catherine Nelson-Piercy

C: Selected procedures

10.   Endoscopy for Gastrointestinal Emergencies   127
      Paul Swain

PART II: Managing Gastroenterology Inpatients

11.   Upper Gastrointestinal Bleeding
      11.1   Peptic Ulcers   139
              Tim Rockall
      11.2   Management of Variceal Bleeding   149
              Lucy Dagher, Andrew K. Burroughs and David Patch

12.   Lower Gastrointestinal and Occult Bleeding   167
      Tim Rockall

13.   Acute Abdominal Pain   171
      Marc Winslett

14.   Oesophageal Problems   177
      Anthony Watson

15.   Intestinal Obstruction   197
      Marc Winslett

16.   Management of Severe Inflammatory Bowel Disease   205
      David Rampton

17.   Biliary Colic and Cholangitis   221
      Adrian Hatfield

18.   Gastrointestinal Malignancy
      18.1   Oncology   225
              Pauline Leonard & Jonathan Ledermann
      18.2   Diagnosis and Treatment of Hepatocellular Carcinoma   241
              Stephen M. Riordan

19.   Ascites and Spontaneous Bacterial Peritonitis   251
      Stephen M. Riordan

20.   Intestinal Failure and Enterocutaneous Fistulae   267
      Jeremy Nightingale

21.   Nutritional Support   273
      Jeremy Powell-Tuck

22.   Liver Failure:
      22.1   Acute Liver Failure   287
              David Mutimer
      22.2   Chronic Liver Disease   297
              David Mutimer and Andrew Douds

23.   Acute Alcoholic Hepatitis   305
      Geoffrey Haydon and Peter Hayes

PART III: A Problem-Based Approach to Gastroenterology Outpatients

24.   Nausea and Vomiting   315
      Robin Vicary

25.   Anaemia   321
      Atul B. Mehta

26. Dyspepsia and Gastroesophageal Reflux 331
    Magda Newton

27. The Irritable Bowel Syndrome 343
    David Gertner

28. Diarrhoea 351
    Stuart Bloom

29. Problems with Swallowing 357
    Stephen Kane

30. Postgastrectomy Disorders 367
    Marc Winslet

31. Malabsorption amd Weight Loss 371
    Parveen J. Kumar and Michael L. Clark

32. Constipation 383
    Anton Emmanuel

33. Faecal Incontinence 393
    Carolynne Vaizey

34. Colorectal Cancer Screening and Surveillance 399
    Isis Dove-Edwin and Huw Thomas

35. Infectious Diarrhoea 409
    Michael Farthing

36. Managing Inflammatory Bowel Disease in Outpatients 425
    Simon Travis

37. Motility Disorders of the Oesophagus and Stomach 445
    Owen Epstein

38. Gastrointestinal Aspects of Excess Alcohol Consumption 455
    Peter Hayes

39. Gallstones 461
    Stephen P. Pereira

40. Helicobacter pylori: Diagnosis and Management 471
    Anne E. Duggan and Robert P.H. Logan

41. Viral Hepatitis 485
    Simon Whalley, George Webster, Ellie Barnes and Geoffrey Dusheiko

42. Abnormal Liver Function Test in an Asyptomatic Patient 503
    Lucy Dagher and Andrew K. Burroughs

43. Perianal Problems 507
    Carolynne Vaizey

PART IV: Procedures and Investigations in Gastroenterology

44. The Gastrointestinal Endoscopy Unit: Information for Users 517
    Russell Cowan

45. Laser Therapy and Photodynamic Therapy 535
    Stephen Bown

46. Endoscopic Retrograde Cholangiopancreatography 545
    Adrian Hatfield

47. Liver Biopsy Indications and Procedure
   Lucy Dagher and Andrew K Burroughs
   549

48. Ultrasound for Gastroenterologists
   Kate Walmsley
   553

49. Radiological and Magnetic Resonance Imaging of the Gastrointestinal Tract
   Alice Gillams
   581

50. Investigation of Gastrointestinal Motility
   Owen Epstein
   591

51. Tests for Malabsorbtion
   Parveen J. Kumar and Michael L. Clark
   595

52. Nuclear Medicine in Gastroenterology
   N.K. Gupta and Jamshed B. Bomanji
   601

Appendix: Gastroenterology Training in Europe
   Alistair D. Beattie
   615

Index
   625

Preface

This book is intended as a practical guide to gastroenterology for trainees and specialists. The introduction of the specialist registrar grade into the United Kingdom in 1996–7 has resulted in a more structured training in the specialty, and this text was commissioned in an attempt to complement this trend. There are many weighty and worthy textbooks on the market which, although good for detail and reference, are somewhat impractical as guides, and there are no books which combine the evidence base for key aspects of the specialty with a practical handbook-type approach.

The aims and principles of the book are:

- To provide a practical guide to clinical gastroenterology with enough basic science and pathophysiology to allow appreciation of current issues in clinical management.
- To comprise essential reading for the Specialist Registrar, but also to appeal to the practising gastroenterologist.

- To use, wherever possible, a clinical, problem-based approach.
- To incorporate the key evidence in support of important management points (whether basic science or clinical trials) without making the whole text referenced.
- To incorporate annotated references, giving some idea of those references regarded as seminal by the authors in particular areas.

We hope this has resulted in an original and useful book which will appeal to both trainees and experienced gastroenterologists.

The editor would like to thank staff at Harwood Academic Publishers for their interest and commitment to the project. Many of them displayed stamina and confidence in the eventual outcome when sometimes the editor wavered. Thanks are also due to the many authors for their patience through a long gestation period.

Stuart Bloom
London, February 2001

Contributors

Elspeth Alstead
Department of Gastroenterology
Whipps Cross Hospital
London, UK

Anne Ballinger
Department of Gastroenterology
Royal London Hospital
London, UK

Alistair D. Beattie
Gastro-intestinal Unit
Southern General Hospital
Glasgow, UK

Paul Boulos
Department of Surgery
University College London Hospitals
London, UK

Andrew K. Burroughs
Department of Gastroenterology
Royal Free Hospital
London, UK

Russell Cowan
Department of Gastroenterology
Colchester Hospital
Colchester, UK

Lucy Dagher
Department of Gastroenterology
Royal Free Hospital
London, UK

Peter Anton
Division of Gastroenterology
UCLA Medical School
Los Angeles, USA

Ellie Barnes
Department of Gastroenterology
Royal Free Hospital
London UK

Stuart Bloom
Department of Gastroenterology
University College London Hospitals
London, UK

Jamshed B. Bomanji
Institute of Nuclear Medicine
Middlesex Hospital
London, UK

Stephen Bown
Department of Surgery
University College London Hospitals
London, UK

Michael L. Clark
Digestive Disease Research Centre
St Bartholomews & The Royal London
    School of Medicine and Dentistry
London, UK

Ross D. Cranston
Department of Microbiology and Immunology
University of California, San Francisco
San Francisco, USA

Isis Dove-Edwin
ICRF Family Cancer Clinic
St Mark's Hospital at Northwick Park
Harrow, UK

Anne E. Duggan
Department of Gastroenterology
John Hunter Hospital
Australia

Anton Emmanuel
Department of Physiology
St Mark's Hospital at Northwick Park
Harrow, UK

Michael Farthing
Dean, Faculty of Medicine
University of Glasgow
Glasgow, UK

Helen Fidler
Department of Gastroenterology
University Hospital Lewisham
London, UK

David Gertner
Department of Gastroenterology
Basildon Hospital
Basildon, UK

Narainder K. Gupta
Department of Nuclear Medicine
Manchester Royal Infirmary
Manchester, UK

Geoffrey Haydon
Liver and Hepatobiliary Unit
Queen Elizabeth Hospital
Birmingham, UK

Geoffrey Dusheiko
Department of Gastroenterology
Royal Free Hospital
London, UK

Owen Epstein
Department of Gastroenterology
Royal Free Hospital
London, UK

Julian Fearnley
Consultant Neurologist
Royal London Hospital
London, UK

Alastair Forbes
St Mark's Hospital and Imperial College
    School of Medicine
Harrow, UK

Alice Gillams
Department of Radiology
Middlesex Hospital
London, UK

Adrian Hatfield
Department of Gastroenterology
Middlesex Hospital
London, UK

Peter Hayes
Department of Medicine
Edinburgh Royal Infirmary
Edinburgh, UK

Brian Hennessy
Department of Haematology
Royal Free Hospital
London, UK

Parveen J. Kumar
Department of Gastroenterology
Homerton Hospital
London, UK

Pauline Leonard
CRC Viral Oncology Group
The Wolfson Institute for Biomedical Research
University College London
London, UK

Ian McGowan
UCSF Medical School
San Francisco, USA

David Mutimer
The Liver and Hepatobiliary Unit
The Queen Elizabeth Hospital
Birmingham, UK

Magda Newton
Department of Gastroenterology
Oldchurch Hospital
Romford, UK

Marco Novelli
Department of Pathology
University College London Hospitals
London, UK

Stephen Kane
Department of Gastroenterology
West Middlesex Hospital
Isleworth, UK

Jonathan Ledermann
Department of Oncology
University College, London
London, UK

Robert P.H. Logan
Department of Gastroenterology
Queen's Medical Centre
Nottingham, UK

Atul B. Mehta
Department of Haematology
Royal Free and University College
   School of Medicine
London, UK

Catherine Nelson-Piercy
St Thomas's Hospital
London, UK

Jeremy Nightingale
Department of Gastroenterology
Leicester Royal Infirmary
Leicester, UK

David Patch
Department of Gastroenterology
Royal Free Hospital
London, UK

Steve Pereira
Department of Gastroenterology
The Middlesex Hospital
London, UK

Jeremy Powell-Tuck
Department of Gastroenterology
Royal London Hospital
London, UK

Stephen M. Riordan
Department of Gastroenterology
The Prince of Wales Hospital
Randwick, NSW
Australia

Paul Swain
Department of Gastroenterology
Royal London Hospital
London, UK

Huw J.W. Thomas
Department of Gastroenterology
St Mary's Hospital
London, UK

Carolynne Vaizey
Department of Surgery
University College London Hospitals
London, UK

Kate Walmsley
Department of Radiology
Middlesex Hospital
London, UK

George Webster
Department of Gastroenterology
Royal Free Hospital
London, UK

David Rampton
Department of Gastroenterology
Royal London Hospital
London, UK

Tim Rockall
Division of Surgical Oncology and Technology
Department of Surgery
Imperial College School of Medicine
London, UK

Simon Travis
Department of Gastroenterology
John Radcliffe Hospital
Oxford, UK

Robin Vicary
Department of Gastroenterology
Whittington Hospital
London, UK

Anthony Watson
Department of Surgery
Royal Free Hospital
London, UK

Simon Whalley
Department of Gastroenterology
Royal Free Hospital
London, UK

Mark Winslet
Department of Surgery
Royal Free Hospital
London, UK

Part I: Gastroenterology Trainee's Survival Guide

A: Refresher Course in Basic Gastroenterology

1. Eliciting the Gastrointestinal History

ROBIN VICARY

Patients are usually apprehensive of doctors. If the doctor fails to help the patient relax, the patient will fail to tell the doctor important aspects of the history. An example is given by the study by Lucas *et al.* (1), showing that patients admitted greater alcohol consumption to a computer than to doctors.

Many trainees un-learn their social, family-based skills by watching a consultant do a ward round without once introducing himself. A handshake, a smile and some eye-contact are reassuring features of a doctor's possible humanity, and giving one's name is, one would hope, part of a doctor's normal social skill training.

In clinic, consider sitting the patient at the side of the desk. Confrontational positions hinder relationships, whereas too intimate a physical presence can be threatening.

LISTENING

Obtaining an accurate history will enable diagnosis in the majority of patients, but doing so depends on the listening skills of the doctor. Listening is an active process in which the listener takes part in a two-way exchange. Contrary to the views of many, complete silence, rather than interruption, is the best way to stop a garrulous historian. The opening statement of a patient should, however, be heard in silence on the part of the gastroenterologist. The patient will often have prepared their opening statement and will not thank you for interrupting. All consultations have a time limit, however, and the doctor will need to interrupt if the opening statement appears to be taking over that time-slot.

Kagan (2) described four levels of listening:

1. *Exploratory response*: When a patient is trying to tell the doctor their concern, often they do not know how to put that concern into words. Exploratory responses encourage patients to use language and get more deeply involved in communication with you. An exploratory response prompts the patient to assume greater responsibility for the direction of the history. Responses may be simple, for example "Go on" or "Tell me more", or more complex, for example "How did that make you feel?" or "Any idea about what had occurred?"

2. *Listening response*: Patients want to feel that the doctor is actively and carefully listening. A good listener will periodically paraphrase or "check out" with the patient that they have truly understood the history. For instance "What you are saying is .... have I got that right?", or similar words.

3. *Affective response*: This refers to the patient's feelings – for example "What about your symptoms worries you most?"

4. *Honest labelling response*: These are unusually frank responses, to encourage a patient to be honest and direct with themselves and with you.

FACTORS AFFECTING THE HISTORY

Family and culture

In Fildes' "The Doctor", the child suffers (?diphtheria), the doctor observes, but the father (often ignored in accounts of the painting) has an experience of disease. In the late 20th century, most people with serious disease are removed from the community, taken to a hospital or nursing home, and rarely die in their own home. Experience of disease is thus often limited to a person's experience of disease in intimate family members.

The **family history** is important for various reasons. Often, drawing a good family tree is more helpful than a long written history:

1. It helps us to understand the patient's response to their disease or symptoms. The importance of the fact that the mother of a patient presenting with dyspepsia died of carcinoma of the stomach lies, not in the possibility that this gives us a clue to the diagnosis (although this occasionally is a factor), but rather in that the patient's experience of disease suggests to them that some of their symptoms are akin to their mother's, contributing to their anxiety.

2. Many gastroenterological complaints have a strong genetic component. For example, Sarin *et al.* (3) have shown that, within a given population, first degree relatives of index cases of persons with gallstones have been shown to be 4.5 times more likely to develop stones than are matched controls. (In taking a family history, it is rare, in my experience, for a patient to volunteer information of another family member with gallstones. A question needs to be asked specifically to jog the patient's memory, for example "Did your mother or other relative have her gallbladder removed?" This is not an area for subtlety or open questions!)

3. Responses to adversity are learnt through family and culture. A child has to learn that eating has to occur at meal times and that defecating occurs in the toilet. As the child is in control of these activities, conflict can occur with the parent. If these issues are not handled well within the family, disorder can occur, lasting into adult life. Patients with functional constipation, psychogenic vomiting and anorexia nervosa may represent examples of dysfunctional early learning (4–6). The family is of course important, not only to enable understanding of the context in which the patient has learnt his response to disease, but also to gain understanding of his experience of disease and, most importantly, to be able to assess the probability for the disease in this patient. Doctors need an understanding of differing cultural responses, in order to understand the individual's response in illness.

Psychological factors

The symptoms of functional gastrointestinal disease may also be precipitated by unresolved psychosocial upset, such as the loss of a parent or some other traumatic major life event. Functional symptoms may also relate to the anniversary of such events (8). Physical or sexual abuse may also affect a patient's response to their symptoms; for example, such patients often have higher pain scores and more surgical procedures (9).

Other factors

1. *Sex*: In one study grading pain from various tumours, men rated their pain as more severe (10).
2. *Age*: There is some evidence (11) that pain diminishes in old age.
3. *Personality*: Introverts appear to have lower pain thresholds than extroverts, but the former complain less readily than the latter (12).

THE PROCESS OF DIAGNOSIS

The process of diagnosis is rarely taught in medical schools, where rote learning of a myriad of facts and lists of causes is often emphasized without an explanation of their relevance to the diagnostic process. Diagnostic ideas come to mind after the first few items of the history, and from then the consultation is strongly influenced by the examination of these ideas (13). The process has been compared to the analytical pattern of working of the great detectives (14).

Bayes' theorem and clinical diagnosis

Thomas Bayes was a parish priest from Tonbridge Wells whose work on probability has been used continuously over the past two centuries, with minor modifications, as a statistical technique. His theorem sets out the probability of the validity of a proposition on the basis of a prior estimate of its probability. In other words, because we know there have been more sparrows than golden eagles in the park in the last year, the probability is greater that a bird seen tomorrow in the park will be a sparrow, rather than a golden eagle.

In a medical context, Bayes' theorem is used to calculate the probability of a patient presenting with a particular clinical complex. In order for us to understand and apply Bayes' Theorem to making a diagnosis, we need to know two sets of probabilities about our patient:

1. the **prior probability** of a patient presenting with a particular disease, and
2. the probability of occurrence of any clinical complex in any disease — the **likelihood** of the complex

The **prior probability** is the incidence of the disease in the population. This factor needs to be adjusted for the individual; for example, a 40-year-old female will have a much smaller prior probability of carcinoma of the stomach than a 60-year-old male. Then, further to this, the trainee should look at the **likelihood**. For example, as a presenting feature, weight loss with anorexia is common in carcinoma of the stomach and in depression, but is not common in carcinoma of the colon (15). Most trainees use only the **likelihood** and fail to use **prior probability**. Many diagnostic computer programs in gastroenterology have been written using modifications of Bayes' Theorem (16,17).

TRUTH AND MYTH IN THE CLINICAL COMPLEX

The trainee needs to recognize real clinical complexes as opposed to mythical ones. Some myths come about as a result of forceful clinical personalities; others from past lack of evidence. Nowhere is this better illustrated than in the field of gallstone disease.

Myths

The two great myths are:

1. *"Gallstones occur in females who are fair, fat, fertile, and forty"*

Biliary disease is more common in women than in men (18) and in severely obese patients (19), although rapid weight loss is also an associated factor in the development of gallstones (20). Being "fertile" does not in itself relate to gallstones but, during pregnancy, bile does become more lithogenic (probably as a result of increased oestrogen concentrations) (21). Women who have gallstones before they become pregnant are more likely to develop biliary pain during pregnancy than they are when not pregnant (22). There is no evidence that "fairness" of hair or skin is important, although there is a high incidence in Scandinavians. This is balanced by the dark hair and skin of Pima Indians, most Chileans, and the Amerindians in Alaska (23), all of whom have a high incidence of gallstones. As for "forty", it is quite clear that the prevalence of gallstones increases relatively linearly with age (24, Table 1.1).

2. *"The pain of biliary colic occurs in the right hypochondrium and radiates to the back"*

Gunn & Keddie (25) looked at the pain of patients presenting with biliary pain, whose pain was cured by cholecystectomy, with follow-up for 2 years. The sites of pain and sites of radiation of pain are shown in Figures 1.1 and 1.2 (26).

Truth

The true symptom complex in biliary colic is (25):

Table 1.1. Gallstone prevalence by age in women by country.

Population	Prevalence (%)				
	21–30 yr	31–40 yr	41–50 yr	51–60 yr	60+ yr
Mexico	11	13	20	22	27
Norway	6	15	25	29	41
Italy	3	9	17	21	28

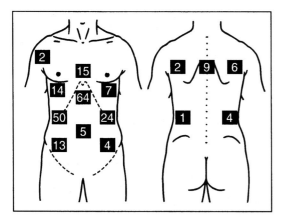

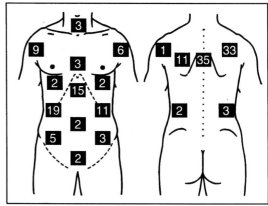

Figure 1.1. Sites of most severe pain (%) in 107 patients with gallstones. Adapted with permission (26).

Figure 1.2. Sites of pain radiation (%) in 107 patients with gallstones. Adapted with permission (26).

- severe pain that is *not* colicky, but a steady un-remitting, boring pain
- vomiting
- duration normally a few hours, with complete lack of pain before and after
- periodicity (with pain-free intervals of from 1 week to more than 1 year)
- localization as illustrated above

The trainee's dilemma

There is a converse to the problem of clinical complexes that trainees find hard to deal with, usually in the outpatient setting. A trainee will often come into my room and tell me the history of a patient with a totally unrecognizable pattern of symptoms. The trainee is anxious, usually because they feel they must be "missing something" — that is, that this is a clinical complex they have not yet learnt about. This is rarely so, most trainees being extremely well read. My response to their anxiety is to tell them that there are two possibilities from the story they have told me — either they have discovered a new disease or clinical complex in my clinic (a comparatively rare event), or this is a functional problem. It is important to understand that functional disease presents in a myriad of individual clinical complexes and that, until we clone the human, this will continue to represent the joy of the diversity of mankind. Even with improved understanding of all these factors, the immense complexity of the human organism means that no rules will govern all individuals. Recognizing the major clini-

cal complexes is the first step and should not be disregarded just because the clinical profile of a particular patient does not adhere to these complexes.

COMMUNICATION

Telling the likely diagnosis

All patients visiting a doctor will have thoughts on their own possible diagnosis. Patients visiting a gastroenterologist may well have more inaccurate thoughts than normal, mainly because most patients' knowledge of the anatomy and physiology of the gastrointestinal tract is so lacking. Most patients have no idea of the position of the liver, stomach, or colon in their abdomen, let alone the function of these organs. Lucas (26) found that words such as "midline" were only understood by 38% of his population. For this reason, the symptoms will be more frightening than, for example, a pain in the arm (which most patients will know to contain bone and muscle). In my experience, considerably more than 50% of all gastroenterology outpatients fear that they have cancer. In order for the doctor to deal with this fear, he needs to ask an open question such as "What did you imagine was wrong?" or, slightly less open, "Were you worried there was something serious wrong?" These questions should be asked after the doctor has given his diagnosis, as it will be easier for the patient to express their fears at that point.

Ending the consultation

Many trainees find this difficult, and do it abruptly. A terminating question may be used; for example, "Was there anything else you wished to say/ask?" Then, having explained to the patient where to go (for tests etc.), the doctor should rise and open the door for the patient, and shake their hand on leaving. Small social skills such as this considerably enhance a patient's views of the consultation and the doctor.

References

1. Lucas RW, Mullin PJ, Luna CBX *et al*. Psychiatrists and a computer as interrogators of patients with alcohol related illnesses: a comparison. *Br J Psych* 1977; **131**: 60–167.
2. Kagan N. *The Medical Teacher*. Eds. KR Cox and CE Ewen. UK: Churchill Livingstone, 1990; 125–131.
3. Sarin SK, Negi VS, Dewan R *et al*. High familial prevalence of gallstones in the first degree relatives of gallstone patient. *Hepatology* 1995; **22**: 138–142.
4. Broxboum E, Sodergren SS. A disturbance of elimination and motor development: The mother's role in the development of the infant. *Child* 1977; **32**: 195–198.
5. Hill OW. Psychogenic vomiting. *Gut* 1968; **9**: 348–354.
6. Drossman DA, Ontjes DA, Heizer WH. Clinical conference: anorexia nervosa. *Gastroenterology* 1979; **77**: 1115–1119.
7. Almy TP. Experimental studies on the irritable colon. *Am J Med* 1951; **10**: 60–66.
8. Stermer E, Bar H, Levy N. Chronic functional gastrointestinal symptoms in Holocaust survivors. *Am J Gastroenterol* 1991; **86**: 417–421.
9. Drossman DA, Li Z, Lesermann J *et al*. Health status by gastrointestinal diagnosis and abuse history. *Gastroenterology* 1996; **110**: 999–1006.
10. Fairley P. *The Conquest of Pain*. London: M. Joseph, 1978; p. 63.
11. Fairley P. *The Conquest of Pain*. London: M. Joseph, 1978; p. 127
12. Editorial: Understanding pain. *Lancet* 1971; **(7712)**: 1284.
13. Campbell EJM. The diagnosing mind. *Lancet* 1987; **i**: 849–851.
14. Howell M, Ford P. *The Ghost Disease and Twelve Other Stories of Detectives Work in the Medical Field*. London: Penguin Books, 1985.
15. Wanebo H, Kennedy BJ, Chmiel J *et al*. Cancer of the stomach. *Ann Surg* 1993; **218**: 583–592.
16. Knill-Jones RP, Stern RB, Grimes DH *et al*. Use of sequential Bayesian Model in diagnosis of jaundice by computer. *BMJ* 1973; **1**: 530–533.
17. Alton EW, Newman N, Vicary FR. Solubile-decision making in the diagnosis of jaundice. *Int J Biomed Comput* 1991; **27**: 47–57.
18. Jensen KH, Jorgensen T. Incidence of gallstones in a Danish population. *Gastroenterology* 1991; **100**: 790–797.
19. Stampfer MJ, Maclure KM, Colditz GA *et al*. Risk of symptomatic gallstones in women with severe obesity. *Am J Clin Nutr* 1992; **55**: 652–657.
20. Shiffman ML, Sugerman HJ, Kellam JM *et al*. Gallstone formation after rapid weight loss. *Am J Gastroenterol* 1991; **86**: 1000–1007.
21. Lynn J, Williams L, O'Brien J *et al*. Effects of oestrogen upon bile. *Ann Surg* 1973; **178**: 514–521.
22. Maringhini A, Ciambra M, Bacelliere P *et al*. Biliary sludge and gallstones in pregnancy: Incidence risk factors and natural history. *Ann Intern Med* 1993; **119**: 116–121.
23. Egbert AM. Gallstone symptoms: myth and reality. *Postgrad Med J* 1991; **90**: 119–128.
24. Bihart LE, Horton JD. Gall-stone disease and its complications. In: *Sleisenger and Fordtran's Gastrointestinal and Liver Disease*, 6th edn. Eds. Feldman *et al*. London: WB Saunders, 1998; p. 949.
25. Gunn H and Keddie N. Some clinical observations on patients with gallstones. *Lancet* 1972; **2**: 239–244.
26. Lucas RW. Computer based system of patient interrogation. PhD Thesis University of Glasgow, 1974.

2. Examination of the Gastrointestinal System

ROBIN VICARY

"Physical examination rather than ancillary investigations helps to complete a diagnosis"
Hamilton Bailey, 1960 (1)

Recent advances in imaging highlight the limitations of the above statement, in terms of both the amount of information produced, and the accuracy of the physical examination. An ultrasonic study of patients said clinically to have a mass in the abdomen found that 39% of the masses were not present on scanning (2).

Nevertheless, a systematic approach to clinical examination is essential. The natural tendency after a succession of normal physical examinations is to reduce the examination to a rather casual affair and to rely on investigations. This must be guarded against; failure to find an abnormal physical sign will lead to a misleading clinical complex (see Chapter 1) and, in turn, this will lead to a mistaken diagnosis and investigation.

The pressures of time put upon today's gastroenterologist, however, mean that a full examination is not possible in all patients. The history must inevitably point the doctor towards what to examine. This chapter aims, therefore, to guide the trainee to perform a thorough and relevant examination, and to clarify signs poorly taught or explained at undergraduate level.

THE PRELIMINARIES

The **handshake** may reveal Dupuytren's contracture, excess sweating, and a tremor (clues to alcohol withdrawal or thyroid disease). **Eye contact** allows the clinician to observe jaundice and eye signs of thyroid disease, and a quick glance at the face simultaneously with the eye contact will reveal the "grog blossoms" (dilated and telangectatic malar capillaries) of alcoholism, and the "hamster pouches" of pseudo-Cushing's disease of the alcoholic. The trained eye will also quickly pick up the enlarged parotids of alcoholic or auto-immune liver disease.

Looking at the skin

Although jaundice is best determined by looking at the sclera, a small degree of jaundice — for example, serum bilirubin less than 50 mmol/l — can be difficult to detect. The best way to detect it if in doubt, is to hold a white sheet next to the skin — minor degrees of yellow discoloration of the skin become more apparent in contrast with white. **Carotenaemia** is an increasingly common cause of skin colour change in patients presenting to the outpatient department. The colour differs from jaundice in being a more orange hue of yellow, and is usually most prominent on the palms of the hands and soles of the feet. In itself, carotenaemia is not harmful, as carotene is not toxic (although hypervitaminosis A, characterized by hepatosplenomegaly and encephalopathy, is extremely dangerous). The diagnosis of carotenaemia does not need to be confirmed biochemically. Many patients with this condition will be aware that their skin is a strange colour, and may even have noticed a lightening of hair colour, which occurs in many. They will not usually link this to their heavy consumption of carrots, carrot juice, tomato juice, or other vegetables.

The skin in haemochromatosis is described in medical text books and to medical students as being a grey-brown colour, or "deep pigmentation". In my experience, there is a wide range of hue, and the skin discoloration is usually picked up upon receipt of the serum ferritin result!

Anaemia

Usually, the inspection of the lachrymal surface of the lower eyelid is reliable, but it is not invariably so. Koilonychia is a much touted, but unreliable physical sign. I see koilonychia about once every 2 years — that is to say, in fewer than 1% of the iron-deficient patients presenting to my clinic.

THE MOUTH

Inspect the surface and sides of the tongue for signs of human immunodeficiency virus infection, which is regularly seen in gastrointestinal clinics. The tongue should be elevated and the floor of the mouth and under-surface of the tongue inspected for the ulceration that gives the clue to chronic inflammatory bowel disease. The sides of the cheek should then be retracted with a spatula, to inspect not only the sides of the oral cavity for more ulcers, but also the greater part of the lateral border of the tongue, which can only then be seen. Each lip should then be retracted to permit full inspection of the dentition and gums and, finally, the fauces, tonsillar bed, uvula, and hard and soft palates viewed. Examination concludes with palpation of the salivary glands (and especially the parotids). I normally feel for enlargement of both the cervical and the supraclavicular lymph glands from behind, with the patient seated, at this time.

NUTRITIONAL STATUS (see chapter 21)

A rapid assessment of nutritional status is easy and important. I look at four things.

1. *Facial appearance*: Are the malar fat pads absent (ie. does the patient have a "high cheek

bone" appearance)? This is a sign of low stores of body fat, and is found in malignant disease, anorexia nervosa and the malabsorption of chronic pancreatitis (but not usually in malabsorption from coeliac disease as the quantitative malabsorption of fat is never as great).
2. *The ribs*: Are the ribs prominently visible?
3. *Fat*: Estimate the skin fold thickness by picking up the skin over the forearm (not the back of the hand, which is misleading) and moving it gently back and forward between thumb and forefinger. This gives a rough index of body fat content.
4. *Protein*: Finally, I estimate muscle (and protein) bulk by attempting to approximate the thumb and third finger of my right hand around the middle of the patient's right upper arm.

OBSERVATIONS OF THE ABDOMEN

The abdomen should be observed both from above in the normal way, but also from a point level with the abdomen and from the foot of the bed. Asymmetry (from a mass or other cause) is often obvious from the foot of the bed and not apparent from above. Use of light that can be moved — for example the patient's reading light in a hospital bed — will help enormously to detect asymmetry by casting shadows. Nowhere is this better demonstrated than in the "visible" gallbladder. Courvoisier forgot, in his famous statement on the aetiology of obstructive jaundice, to mention that a gallbladder is often visible in addition to palpable. If the light is set to shine from the right side, the distended gallbladder can often be seen because of the shadow cast on the immediate left of the protuberance.

Visible peristalsis (gastric outlet obstruction) is one of those signs that should be looked for either carefully or not at all. Do not waste time looking for it in the patient presenting with diarrhoea etc. Do it correctly in the patient with vomiting, upper abdominal pain, and weight loss. The sign is frequently missed, either because the doctor looks at the wrong place (visible peristalsis occurs above the umbilicus in patients with carcinoma of the stomach, but below the umbilicus in patients with benign disease, as the stomach has had a much greater time to distend), or because the doctor does not observe the abdomen for long enough. The abdomen must be observed for as long as it takes for a peristaltic wave to occur—normally three to five minutes. Testing for a **gastric splash** has, rightly to my mind, gone out of fashion, because of its lack of reliability. Even Hamilton Bailey had doubts about it, 50 years ago!

PHYSICAL SIGNS OF LIVER DISEASE

Spider naevi

Malchow-Miller *et al.* (3) looked at 22 clinical features in more than 1000 jaundiced patients. Spider naevi emerged as the second most useful parameter (after the age of the patient) in diagnosing chronic liver disease, most other stigmata being of much less use. However, in two series of otherwise apparently well-matched patients with chronic liver disease spider naevi were present in 95% (4) and 45% (5). To complicate matters further, spider naevi have been observed, over a period of time, to appear and regress with evidence of no clinical or biochemical changes (6).

Palmar erythema

A strict restriction of the observation of "palmar erythema" to those patients with blotchy reddening of thenar and hypothenar eminences and the tips of the fingers, and not those with generally red palms, is important. Pedal erythema, with a similar distribution on the soles of the feet, is sometimes also found. The incidence in large series is variable (7,8).

Leuconychia

This is another much disputed sign. An early series found "white nails" in 82 of 100 patients with cirrhosis (9). In most large series, the numbers are fewer than 10%.

Clubbing

I believe clubbing to be of little use in diagnosing cirrhosis or chronic inflammatory bowel disease. Most large clinical series do not even mention clubbing in lists of prevalence of various clinical signs.

Dupuytren's contracture

Dupuytren's contracture is associated with alcoholic cirrhosis in between 4.6 and 66% of cases (10,11). Some authors say that it is "uncommon" in patients with chronic active hepatitis and primary biliary cirrhosis (7,8). Recently, the question has been asked whether the linkage is to cirrhosis or to consumption of alcohol. Bradlow & Mowat (12) compared the drinking habits of patients attending for surgery on Dupuytren's contracture with those of patients attending for other types of hand surgery, and found statistical correlation between alcohol consumption and Dupuytren's contracture. There was also correlation with γ-glutamyltransferase and mean cell volume. None of their patients apparently had clinical evidence of cirrhosis, but liver biopsies were not available. This study suggests that it may be the alcohol *per se*, and not the cirrhosis, that is the linkage. The hypothesized mechanism is that alcohol alters both palmar and liver fat composition, and that the altered fat acts as an irritant, precipitating fibrosis both in the liver and in the hand.

Gynaecomastia

It is important to distinguish between true gynaecomastia — that is, mammary tissue that is clearly well circumscribed — and fat that is commonly deposited in the male in the mammary area, and has no distinct edge. The reported incidence varies from rare, up to 80% in one large survey of haemochromatosis. The condition is said to occur more commonly in alcoholic cirrhosis than in other forms of liver disease (5), although the findings of some studies dispute this (13). Recently, one group have even suggested that it is no more common in patients with cirrhosis than in the rest of the population (14). This group found that the prevalence of gynaecomastia in patients with cirrhosis did not differ from that in men admitted to hospital for other reasons. By measuring oestrogen and free testosterone, they also showed that factors other than the ratio of these hormones caused gynaecomastia. They suggest that the impression that palpable gynaecomastia occurs more frequently in cirrhotic patients than in controls may have developed because gynaecomastia is sought more assiduously in the cirrhotic groups.

Ascites

The presence of ascites can be accurately assessed by ultrasound, which can detect as little as 100 ml of fluid in the abdominal cavity. In an interesting study (15), three gastroenterologists in Bethesda, Maryland, conducted a clinical examination of 21 patients suspected of having ascites and compared the results with ultrasonic findings. Each patient was examined independently by these three experienced clinicians, none of whom was given any clinical information. The methodology of examination for five common physical signs was agreed beforehand, as was a definition of positivity of the sign. For example "bulging of the flanks" was positive only if it was bilateral; "flank dullness" was also required to be bilateral with the patient lying supine, and positive shifting dullness occurred when the patient was turned to lie both on the right and on the left lateral decubitus positions, and the dullness had moved. After the clinicians had completed their clinical assessments, all patients were assessed ultrasonically and, where clinically relevant, fluid was aspirated. Six of the 21 patients had ascites ultrasonically and 15 did not. The clinicians' clinical ability thus revealed is presented in Table 2.1.

Three important facts emerged from this study. First, none of the gastroenterologists achieved better than 85% accuracy with any sign, and some of them achieved only around 50%. Second, no one sign was much better than any other. Third, one physician was better than the other two! Interestingly, flank dullness was the most sensitive of the signs, but had poor specificity. The trainee gastroenterologist will not do better than these figures and should remember them with due humility.

Hepatomegaly

There is no standard for normality for the clinical size of the liver. An estimate of liver volume should be made by assessing liver span by percussion. Sir William Osler, in 1890, described the method of examining the lower edge by inching the fingers upwards from the right iliac fossa to the right subcostal region, and Sir James Cantlie described the scraping auscultation method in 1901. I use the latter method in patients who are fat, or in whom the abdomen is difficult to examine. The stethoscope is placed anteriorly over the right lower ribs and scraping movements are made sequentially,

Table 2.1. Accuracy of individual physical signs in the detection of ascites: number correct/total assessed.

Clinical sign	Physicain		
	A	B	C
Bulging at the flanks	10/21	11/21	13/21
Flank dullness	8/21	12/21	10/21
Shifting dullness	12/21	11/21	17/21
Fluid "wave" detected	14/21	14/21	17/21
The puddle sign	9/19	5/18	15/19

parallel to the edge of the ribs, from the lower chest to the abdominal wall. The pitch of the sound becomes lower and quieter as the liver edge is passed.

CONCLUDING THE EXAMINATION

The **rectal** examination has been regarded over the last century as an essential feature of the examination. Trainees often ask whether it is reasonable to omit it in a patient whose symptoms are clearly not related (e.g. a patient with dyspepsia). Furthermore, many clinicians regard a rectal examination as unnecessarily stressful (even dangerous (16)) in a patient presenting with chest pain. Many would still regard as negligent the failure to perform a rectal examination in a patient with abdominal pain.

Performing the rectal examination is often poorly taught and results in pain to the patient. The patient should lie on the left side with the right hip flexed and the left leg straight (1) (not, as is taught, with both hips flexed, as this increases anal tone). The examiner should then press posteriorly on the anal skin with the gloved lubricated finger of the second right finger. The initial posterior pressure will help relaxation of anal tone and the finger can usually then slide into the anus. Sticking the finger straight in at right angles to the anus (as is often taught) will cause contracture of the sphincter and pain to the patient.

References
1. Bailey H. *Physical Signs in Clinical Surgery.* Eds. Bristol: John Wright & Sons Ltd, 1960; p. 398
2. Barker CS and Lindsell DR. Ultrasound of the palpable abdominal mass. *Clin Radiol* 1990; **41**: 98–99.
3. Malchow–Muller A and Thomson C. Computer diagnosis of jaundice. *Scand J of Gastroenterology* 1987; 162–168.

4. Read A, Sherlock S, Harrison CV. Active juvenile cirrhosis as part of systemic disease and the effect of corticosteroid therapy. *Gut* 1963; **4**: 378–393.

5. Mistilis SP, Skyring AP & Blackburn CRB. Natural history of active chronic hepatitis — clinical features, course, diagnostic criteria. *Austr Ann Med* 1968; **17**: 214–223.

6. Baker HWG, Burger HG, de Kretser DM. A study of the endocrine manifestations of hepatic cirrhosis. *Q J Med* 1976; **45**: 145–178.

7. Powell LW, Mortimer R, Harris OD. Cirrhosis of the liver. A comparative study of the four major aetiological groups. *Med J Austr* 1971; **1**: 941–950.

8. Hallen J, Krook H. Studies on 360 patients with cirrhosis in one community. *Acta Med Scand* 1963; **173**: 479–493.

9. Lloyd CW, Williams RH. Endocrine changes in Laennec's cirrhosis. *Am J Med* 1948; **48**: 315–318.

10. Powell WJ, Klatskin G. Duration of survival in patients with cirrhosis. *Am J Med* 1968; **44**: 406–420.

11. Wolfe SJ, Summerskill WH, Davidson CS. Dupuytren's Contracture associated with alcoholism and hepatic cirrhosis. *N Engl J Med* 1956; **255**: 559–562.

12. Bradlow A and Mowat AG. Dupuytren's contracture and alcohol. *Ann Rheum Dis* 1986; **45**: 304–307.

13. Mowat NAG, Edwards CRW, Fisher R *et al*. Hypothalmic-pituitary-gonadal function in men with cirrhosis of the liver. *Gut* 1976; **17**: 345–350.

14. Cavanaugh J, Niewoehner CB, Nutall FQ. Gynaecomastia and cirrhosis of the liver. *Arch Int Med* 1990; **150**: 563–568.

15. Cattau EL, Benjamin SB, Knuff TE. The accuracy of the physical exam in the diagnosis of suspected ascites. *JAMA* 1982; **24**: 1164–1168.

16. Lee, JR, Fred HL. Digital rectal examination during early acute MI. *Hosp Pract* 1997; **32**: 15–16.

3.1.   Clinical Anatomy of the Gastrointestinal Tract: Macroscopic

PAUL BOULOS

INTRODUCTION

This chapter covers those aspects of clinical anatomy of the abdomen and gastrointestinal tract that are relevant to gastroenterologists, especially those involved in procedures in which a knowledge of the relevant surface anatomy is extremely important in avoiding complications.

THE ABDOMINAL WALL

Skin

Nerve supply

T7–T12 and L1. The surface markings of help are:

*   Xiphoid process   T7
*   Umbilicus   T10
*   Pubis   L1

Blood supply

The superior epigastric artery (a terminal branch of the internal thoracic artery) and the inferior epigastric artery (a branch of the external iliac artery) run behind the rectus abdominus. When performing a paracentesis, the needle puncture should either be sited in the midline or well lateral to the inferior epigastric artery.

Lymphatic drainage

Above the umbilicus, cutaneous lymph vessels drain into the anterior axillary lymph nodes; below the umbilicus, lymph drains into the superficial inguinal lymph nodes.

THE ABDOMINAL CAVITY

The **parietal peritoneum** is richly innervated segmentally by the spinal nerves. When irritated, it causes pain localized to the area and to others supplied by the same nerve roots — for example, pain from the diaphragmatic peritoneum referred to the tip of the shoulder, which is supplied by the same nerve roots via the phrenic nerve. The **visceral peritoneum** is poorly supplied with nerves, therefore pain is vague and not localized; however, **midgut pain** (jejunum to transverse colon) tends to localize to the umbilicus, whereas **hindgut pain** (transverse colon to anal canal) is more suprapubic. In the female, the peritoneal sac is not closed: through the free end of the uterine tube it communicates with the uterus and vagina. This is the reason for peritonitis complicating puerperal sepsis and *Staphylococcus aureus* infection associated with intravaginal tampons.

THE OESOPHAGUS

The oesophagus has three sites of anatomical and physiological constriction. The first is where the pharynx joins the upper end; the second is where the aortic arch and the left bronchus cross anteriorly; and the third is where the oesophagus passes through the diaphragm into the stomach. These sites are the most common sites for strictures caused by caustic damage, and are also the most common sites for carcinoma. The respective distances from the upper incisor teeth are 15 cm, 25 cm and 41 cm. The lower oesophageal sphincter is usually situated within the diaphragmatic hiatus, and the diaphragmatic fibres that impinge on the lower oesophageal sphincter contribute to the pressure profile of the sphincter. The inner lining of the organ comprises stratified squamous epithelium which, at the lower end, forms the junction with the gastric mucosa at the dentate line.

Nerve supply

The vagus nerve provides the oesophagus with its major neural input. The fibres that innervate the striated muscle are lower motor neurones, with cell bodies originating in the nucleus ambiguus; the dorsal motor nucleus of the vagus nerve innervates the smooth muscle of the oesophagus. The vagus nerve provides sensory fibres to the cervical oesophagus, whereas sensory fibres to the remainder of the organ are carried by the recurrent laryngeal nerve. In the mucosa, submucosa, and muscular layers, free nerve endings can be identified. It is believed that these are vagal afferents that are stimulated by distension of the organ. Between the longitudinal and circular muscle layers, there is a network of nerves known as the myenteric plexus (Auerbach's plexus). These function as relay neurones between the vagus and smooth muscle and also provide sensory and integrative elements. There is also a plexus of nerves in the submucosa; this is known as Meissner's plexus and is situated between the circular muscle layer and the muscularis mucosa. The myenteric and submucosal plexus constitutes the enteric nervous system, which is important in integrating movements throughout the gastrointesinal tract.

There are two types of neurones within the myenteric plexus. Excitatory cholinergic neurones mediate contraction of both the circular and longitudinal muscle layers. Inhibitory neurones relax the circular muscle layer, nitric oxide acting as the neurotransmitter. Both sets of neurones impinge on the lower oesophageal sphincter.

THE STOMACH

The **fundus** is that part of the stomach above the cardiac orifice. Below the fundus lies the body or **corpus** of the stomach, which extends to the level of the **incisura**, a notch in the lower part of the lesser curvature. The pyloric **antrum** extends from this level,

narrowing gradually towards the **pylorus** which is a sphincter of smooth muscle and derives its thickness mainly from thickening of the circular muscle; its canal is closed, but its duodenal aspect is open. The pylorus lies in the **transpyloric plane**, which bisects the body where the lateral margin of the rectus abdominis crosses the costal margin (tip of the 9th costal cartilage). This plane also passes through the duodenol-jejunal junction, neck of pancreas, and hila of both kidneys.

The fundus and upper part of the corpus lie in contact with the diaphragm and the left lobe of the liver. The lower part of the body and the pyloric antrum project beyond the costal margin, are in contact with the anterior abdominal wall, and can therefore be percussed. The greater curve lies slightly below the level of the umbilicus, but is higher when the body is supine and the stomach is empty.

These anatomical landmarks are particularly important when **percutaneous endoscopic gastrostomy** is performed. The anatomical demarcations of the stomach are clear at endoscopy and it is essential that, when a lesion is viewed, its site is precisely defined, particularly when surgery is planned.

Posteriorly, the stomach, interposed by the lesser sac, lies on the **stomach bed**, which includes the pancreas, the upper half of the left kidney and the left suprarenal gland, the left crus of the diaphragm, the left coeliac ganglion, and the spleen. Tumour or ulcers of the stomach often penetrate posteriorly to involve these structures, and diseases of these structures may involve the stomach.

Blood supply

The blood supply is derived from branches of the coeliac artery (Figure 3.1.1). The left gastric artery supplies the lower third of the oesophagus and the upper right part of the stomach. The right gastric artery (from the hepatic artery) supplies the lower right portion of the stomach. The short gastrics from the splenic artery supply the fundus. The greater curve of the stomach is supplied by the left gastroepiploic (arising from the splenic artery) and the right gastroepiploic (from the gastroduodenal) artery.

Lymph drainage

Four main groups of vessels all drain ultimately into the celiac lymph nodes.

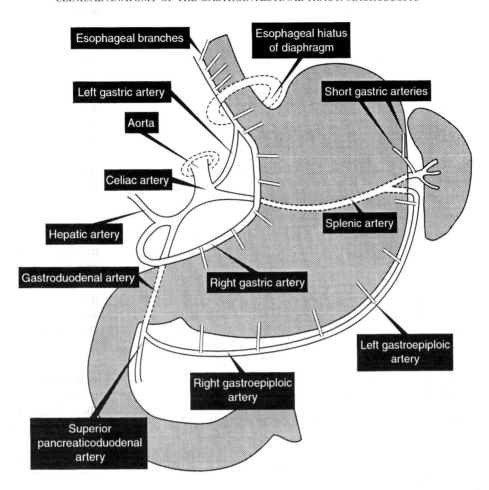

Figure 3.1.1. Blood supply of the stomach. (Adapted from Snell RS. *Clinical Anatomy for Medical Students*, 1st Edition. Boston: Little, Brown & Co., 1973.)

THE SMALL INTESTINE

Duodenum

The duodenum is named for its length: 12 fingers, or 25 cm. The respective lengths of its four parts are 5, 7.5, 7.5, and 5 cm. It is a C-shaped tube that encloses within it the head of the pancreas. The first 2.5 cm is within the peritoneum and is mobile, but its remaining parts are entirely retroperitoneal and are fixed. This anatomical arrangement limits the leakage from a posterior duodenal wall perforation at the site of the duodenal papilla (see later) at endoscopic sphincterotomy; a retroperitoneal perforation can usually be managed conservatively. Appreciation of the directions of the various parts of the duodenum is helpful in the interpretation of a barium meal.

The **first part** runs upwards, to the right, and backwards to come in close contact with the undersurface of the right lobe of the liver and the fundus of the gallbladder; duodenal or pyloric ulcers may therefore penetrate the liver, as a gallstone may erode into the duodenum. Running posterior to the first part is the **common bile duct** as it runs to the second part of the duodenum, the **portal vein**, and the **gastroduodenal artery**. The last of these is a large branch of the hepatic artery; it produces brisk bleeding when a posterior duodenal ulcer erodes through it. Such bleeding often is not controlled by endoscopic haemostatic procedures; surgical ligation is often required.

The **second part** of the duodenum curves downwards over the hilum of the right kidney. It is crossed by the transverse colon and may be involved in inflammation or malignancy of this segment of the colon. The **ampulla of Vater** is situated about halfway down the second part, about 10 cm from the pylorus on the posteromedial wall. The small opening of the **accessory pancreatic duct** lies 2.5 cm proximal to the papilla. Thus presence or absence of bile in the vomitus is a clinical indication of the level of obstruction.

The **third part** of the duodenum runs transversely across the abdomen and passes over the **inferior vena cava** and **aorta**. This is an important relationship: aneurysms of the aorta may rupture into the duodenum, although this is more likely to occur when the aneurysm has been repaired with a prosthetic graft. Anteriorly, the third part of the duodenum is crossed by the **superior mesenteric vessels** as they enter the small bowel mesentry, which may compress the duodenum, causing its occlusion — "superior mesenteric artery syndrome" — believed to occur in thin patients, in whom loss of mesenteric fat results in visceroptosis.

The **fourth part** of the duodenum ascends upwards to the left of the aorta, then curves forwards and to the right as the duodenojejunal flexure, which is supported by the suspensory **ligament of Treitz**; a fibromuscular band that runs from the right crus of the diaphragm and blends with the outer muscle coat of the flexure.

Blood supply

The blood supply of the duodenum is via the superior and inferior pancreaticoduodenal arteries, arising from the gastroduodenal artery and the superior mesenteric artery, respectively.

Jejunum and ileum

Together, the jejunum and ileum are 6 m long, the jejunum comprising the proximal two-fifths, and the ileum the distal three-fifths. The jejunum is much thicker than the ileum, because of the accumulation of the circular folds, and the calibre decreases towards the terminal ileum, which is the narrowest part of the small intestine. The circular folds are numerous in the upper small bowel and diminish distally in the ileum; this feature becomes relevant when one interprets the gas shadow on a plain film or the appearances in a small-bowel enema. The lymphoid tissue is more abundant distally, where it aggregates to form large patches — Peyer's patches — which are most numerous in the terminal ileum and lie on the antimesenteric border. The distribution of the lymphoid follicles explains the site predilection in typhoid, tuberculosis, and lymphomas.

Blood supply

The blood supply of the jejunum and most of the ileum is via branches of the superior mesenteric artery; the lowest part of the ileum is supplied by the ileocolic artery.

LARGE INTESTINE

This has a larger calibre than the small intestine: the longitudinal muscle coat is condensed into three distinct bundles, called **taenia coli**, which can be seen through the serosa. Because the taenia coli are shorter than the length of the bowel, the colon has a sacculated appearance. The **caecum** is the widest and the **distal sigmoid** the narrowest segment of the large bowel. Contents of the former being fluid and the latter solid, obstructive symptoms are more common in lesions of the sigmoid colon.

The caecum

The caecum lies in the right iliac fossa and projects downwards from the commencement of the ascending colon as a blind diverticulum from the point where the ileum joins. It is the segment of colon with the thinnest walls, and is vulnerable to perforation at endoscopy. It is completely invested by the peritoneum but, from its posterior surface, the peritoneum is reflected downwards to the floor of the iliac fossa, creating a retrocaecal fossa in which the appendix may lie; with this anatomical arrangement, tenderness of an inflamed appendix is not evident, as it is protected by the overlying caecum.

When distended, the caecum may come into contact with the anterior abdominal wall; when it is collapsed, coils of the small intestine are interposed. Posteriorly, it is related to the iliac vessels and the psoas fascia. Medially, the vermiform appendix arises from the caecum 2.5 cm below the ileal termination.

The ileocaecal valve lies at the orifice of the ileum into the colon and consists of upper and lower lips, which are prolapsed into two folds for a short distance round the gut as the frenula of the valve. At the lower end of the ileum, the circular muscle coat is thickened to form a true sphincter. It is normally in a state of tonic contraction by sympathetic control, and relaxes in response to the vagal stimulation that coincides with the arrival of a peristaltic wave. A caecal tumour at the ileocacal valve causes symptoms of acute or subacute small bowel obstruction. When the caecum is distended, the frenula are distracted, the valve narrows and the influx of ileal contents is prevented (**ileal intubation** at colonoscopy usually requires a decompressed caecum). Forming a blind end, the caecum is, therefore, the site of perforation in large bowel obstruction, except when the valve is incompetent and allows the large bowel contents to drain into the small bowel.

The colon

Above the ileocaecal valve, the caecum becomes the **ascending colon** and extends retroperitoneally to the undersurface of the liver, where it bends forward and to the left, forming the **hepatic flexure**. It is 10–13 cm long and lies on the muscles of the posterior abdominal wall and, nearer the liver, the lower pole of the right kidney. From the right colic flexure, the colon extends with a wide U-shaped curve of 35–50 cm to form the **transverse colon** before reaching the **splenic flexure**. It is slung from the posterior abdominal wall by the transverse mesocolon, which separates the abdominal cavity into an upper **supracolic compartment**, containing the stomach, spleen, liver, and pancreas, and a lower **infracolic compartment** containing the small intestine.

The **splenic flexure** lies at a higher level than the hepatic flexure, under cover of the left costal margin, and is held to the diaphragm by a peritoneal fold, the **phrenicocolic ligament**. It turns downwards and backwards to become the descending colon. The descending colon, it is less than 30 cm long, and extends from the splenic flexure to the pelvic brim; like the ascending colon, it is fixed to the posterior abdominal wall by the overlying peritoneum. On reaching the pelvic brim, the colon turns medially to pick up mesentry and form the **sigmoid colon**, which extends to the commencement of the rectum in front of the third piece of the sacrum. The sigmoid colon is completely invested in the peritoneum and hangs free on a mesentry, which allows mobility and enables the colon to twist as a volvulus.

The rectum

The rectum commences in the hollow of the sacrum at the level of its third piece, and curves forward over the coccyx and anococcygeal raphe to pass through the pelvic floor into the anal canal. The angle at this anorectal junction is maintained by the sling of the puborectalis muscle as it pulls the rectum forward towards its attachment to the pubic bone, which is a mechanism for continence. The upper and lower thirds are straight, but the middle third curves to the left, which produces indentations into the rectum: two lie on the left, with one between them on the right. These are known as the rectal valves of Houston, easily identifiable at endoscopy. The taenia coli become a single layer as they spread out around the wall of the rectum. The rectum is never involved in diverticular disease, as hypertrophy of the taenia coli is an aetiological factor in intraluminal segmentation and high pressure associated with diverticulosis.

The pelvic peritoneum is reflected onto the rectum except for its lower third; except for this part of the rectum, instrumental injury will result in peritonitis. Rectal biopsies above 8 cm should be performed with care.

THE BLOOD SUPPLY OF THE ALIMENTARY CANAL

Arteries

The abdominal aorta gives rise to three large vessels: the **coeliac artery**, which supplies the foregut (oesophagus to ampulla of Vater), the **superior mesenteric**, supplying the midgut (ampulla to the junction of the middle and left-thirds of the transverse colon), and the **inferior mesenteric**, supplying the hindgut (from the left third of the transverse colon to halfway down the anal canal).

The **superior rectal artery** over the pelvic brim is a continuation of the inferior mesenteric artery and runs in the pelvic mesocolon to the commencement of the rectum, where it divides into right and left branches and the former divides into anterior and posterior branches. These three main branches sink into the muscle walls in the line of the three primary haemorrhoids — 4, 7 and 11 o'clock at the anal margin when the patient is viewed in the lithotomy position.

The **marginal artery** commences with the ileal branches of the superior mesenteric artery, and its lower part is between the lowest sigmoid branch and the upper rectal branch from the superior mesenteric artery. The anastomosis of the arterial branches from the superior and inferior mesenteric arteries, along the mesenteric border of the large intestine from the ileocolic junction to the pelvirectal junction, forms this single arterial trunk named the **marginal artery** (of Drummond). The artery supplies the colon by vessels that sink into the walls. The marginal artery is deficient where the superior and inferior mesenteric branches anastomose in the region of the splenic flexure, which becomes vulnerable to ischaemia when blood perfusion is low, as in atherosclerosis.

Portal circulation

The venous drainage of the alimentary canal is similar to the arterial supply — a venous tributary accompanies each arterial branch. The **inferior mesenteric vein** draining the hindgut joins the **splenic vein** deep to the body of the pancreas. The splenic vein runs in contact with the posterior surface of the pancreas and is joined with the **superior mesenteric vein**, draining the midgut to form the **portal vein** behind the neck of the pancreas. A pancreatic mass may occlude the splenic vein, resulting in back flow with distension of the splenic vein and the veins in the cardia, predisposing to gastric varices. This is described as "segmental hypertension". The portal vein runs with the **hepatic artery** and the **common bile duct** to the liver hilum, where it divides into left and right branches. The left branch is joined by the obliterated *umbilical vein* (ligamentum teres), which can be cannulated to allow cytotoxic liver infusion, and which opens up in portal hypertension. The sluggishness of the stream from the main tributaries of the portal vein allows little mixing, so that the right branch receives mostly superior mesenteric blood and the left branch mostly splenic (and inferior mesenteric) blood. This explains some differences in disease distribution: substances absorbed in the small intestine, when toxic, will cause more damage in the right lobe, whereas deficiencies of substances such as choline or methionine will lead to cirrhosis in the depleted left lobe of the liver.

Although the portal vein blood is deoxygenated, its larger blood flow relative to the hepatic artery provides a larger oxygen supply to the liver parenchyma. As it is the major source of blood supply of liver tumours, it has been occluded by embolization and ligation in the treatment of liver tumours, without adverse effect.

The portal circulation communicates with the systemic circulation, and this is pronounced and is clinically manifest when the portal vein is obstructed.

Sites of portal–systemic anastomosis

The portal vein receives tributaries from the systemic circulation. Its occlusion results in an increased back pressure into the systemic veins resulting in opening up normally insignificant anastomotic channels, with distension and dilatation of the veins. The main site of communications are (Figure 3.1.2):

1. In the lower third of the oesophagus, tributaries of the **azygous vein** (systemic circulation) anastomose with oesophageal tributaries of the left gastric vein, which drains into the portal vein.
2. The **paraumbilical veins** accompanying the ligamentum teres in the falciform ligament connect the left branch of the portal vein with the superficial veins of the anterior abdominal wall. When distended, this system produces a characteristic dilatation of the paraumbilical veins, described as **caput medusae**.
3. The **superior haemorrhoidal** vein drains into the inferior mesenteric vein and communicates, via the middle and inferior haemorrhoidal veins, with the **iliac vein**. Its distension results in rectal varices, which may be mistaken for haemorrhoids.
4. The veins of the ascending colon, descending colon, duodenum, pancreas, and liver (portal tributaries) anastomose with renal, lumbar, and phrenic veins (systemic tributaries).

LYMPH DRAINAGE OF THE ALIMENTARY CANAL

The lymph vessels pass from the **lymphoid follicles** in the mucosa to glands that lie at the margin of the gut. The next group of glands lie along the arteries between the gut wall and the aorta, in the mesentery of the bowel. From there, lymph drains to the next group of glands that lie in front of the aorta, which receive lymph from the hindgut, midgut, and foregut. These are the **coeliac, superior mesenteric** and **inferior mesenteric** groups. They drain into each other from below upwards, the coeliac group draining by two or three lymph channels into the **cisterna chylae**, which is a thin-walled sac that lies in front of the bodies of L1 and L2 and leads directly into the **thoracic duct**. This duct drains into the internal jugular vein in the neck, after receiving lymphatic trunks that drain the head and neck and the upper limbs. Hence, the presence of palpable lymph nodes

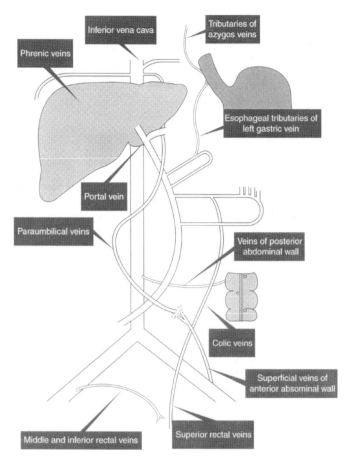

Figure 3.1.2.   Portal–systemic anastomoses. (Adapted from Snell RS. *Clinical Anatomy for Medical Students*, 1st Edition. Boston: Little, Brown & Co., 1973.)

in the neck in malignancy of the alimentary canal is a sign of advanced metastatic disease. In curative surgery for malignancy of the alimentary tract, the lymphatics and lymph nodes are cleared with the tumour, by removing *en bloc* the mesentry that contains the lymphovascular tissues.

THE LIVER

Segments of the liver

The surgical anatomy of the liver is based on the segmental nature of its vascular and bile duct distribution. The liver receives a dual blood supply from both the portal vein and the hepatic artery. The portal pedicle divides into right and left branches and then supplies the liver in a segmental fashion. Venous drainage is via the hepatic veins, which

drain directly into the inferior vena cava. A detailed description and diagram of liver segmentation can be seen in Figure 3.1.3.

Segmental anatomy becomes important in considering surgical resection, when essentially any segment or combination of segments can be resected if attention is paid to maintaining vascular and biliary continuity to remaining segments.

THE EXTRAHEPATIC BILIARY SYSTEM

The **common bile duct** is about 8 cm long and lies in the right free edge of the lesser omentum in the first part of its course, behind the first part of the duodenum in the second part of its course, and in a groove on the posterior surface of the head of the pancreas in the third part of its course. The final intraduodenal segment of the duct is about 2 cm

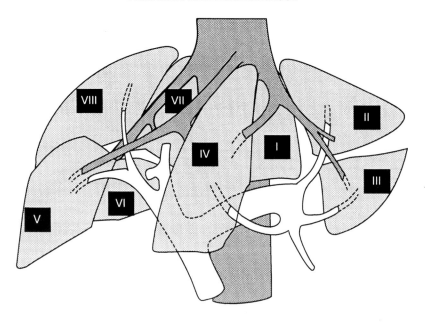

Figure 3.1.3.   Schematic representation of the functional anatomy of the liver. Hepatic segmentation is based on the distribution of the portal pedicles and their relation to the hepatic veins. The three hepatic veins run in the portal scissurae and divide the liver into four sectors, which are in turn divided by the portal pedicles running in the hepatic scissurae. The liver is divided into right and left hemilivers by the middle hepatic vein. The right hemiliver is divided by the right hepatic vein into anterior and posterior sectors. The anterior sector is divided by the plan of the portal pedicle into an inferior segment (V) and a superior segment (VIII). The posterior sector is similarly divided by the plan of the portal pedicle into an inferior segment (VI) and a superior segment (VII).

The left hemiliver lies to the left of the middle hepatic vein and is divided into anterior and posterior sectors by the left hepatic vein. The anterior sector is divided by the umbilical fissure into segment IV medially and segment III laterally. The segment posterior of the left hepatic vein is segment II. Segment I is the caudate lobe, which lies between the inferior vena cava and the date lobe, which lies between the inferior vena cava and the hepatic veins. The caudate lobe has variable portal venous, hepatic arterial and biliary anatomy, and is essentially independent of the portal pedicle divisions and hepatic venous drainage. (Adapted from Sherlock S. *Diseases of the Liver and Biliary System*, 8th Edition. Oxford: Blackwell Scientific Publication, 1989.)

long. In 30% of patients, a septum persists between the common bile duct and the pancreatic duct, and the two ducts empty on the papilla as separate ostia.

The **cystic duct** usually (in 70% of individuals) joins the common hepatic duct directly, but the point of joining can vary from the right hepatic duct down to the ampulla (Figure 3.1.4).

Common structural anomalies of the gallbladder, biliary tree, and vascular supply

Gallbladder

Duplication of the gallbladder occurs in 1 every 4000 humans and may be complete or incomplete. An absent gallbladder is usually associated with extrahepatic biliary atresia. Left-sided gallbladders can occur in association with situs inversus.

Hepatic ducts

Accessory hepatic ducts occur in about 10% of people. Biliary atresia has an incidence of 1 in 15 000 live births.

Choledochal cysts

Advances in imaging have resulted in increased identification of these lesions. They have been classified into five types (Figure 3.1.5). Sixty percent of affected patients present before the age of 10 years, but 25% of patients are older than 20 years at the time of presentation. Complications include pancreatitis, cholangitis, cholecystitis, cyst rupture, cirrhosis, portal hypertension, and cholangiocarcinoma. The last of these has an incidence of 3–28%.

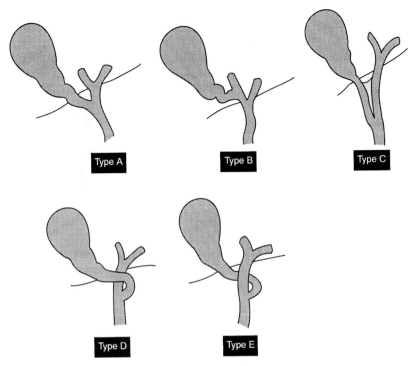

Figure 3.1.4. Cystic Duct anatomy. Cystic duct joins A: common hepatic duct; B: the right hepatic duct; C: low junction with common hepatic duct; D: anterior spiral of cystic duct before joining common hepatic duct; E: posterior spiral of cystic duct before joining common hepatic duct. (Adapted from Yamada *et al. Textbook of Gastroenterology*, 3rd Edition. Philadelphia: Lippincott Williams and Wilkins, 1999.)

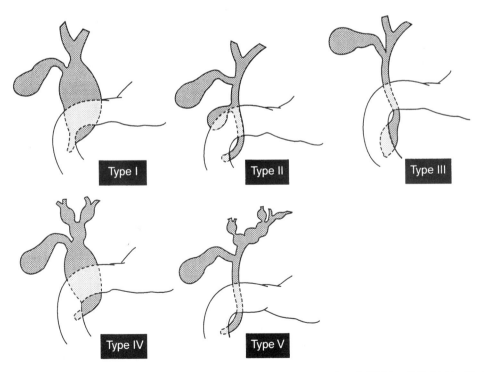

Figure 3.1.5. Choledochal cysts. (Adapted from Yamada *et al. Textbook of Gastroenterology*, 3rd Edition. Philadelphia: Lippincott Williams and Wilkins, 1999.)

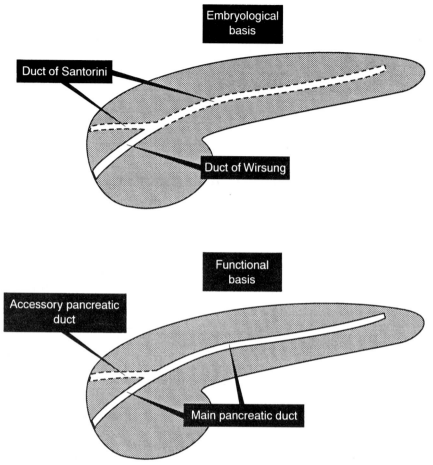

Figure 3.1.6.   The pancreatic duct system. (Adapted from Yamada *et al. Textbook of Gastroenterology*, 3rd Edition. Philadelphia: Lippincott Williams and Wilkins, 1999.)

Variations in the cystic artery

The blood supply to the gallbladder is usually from a single cystic artery arising from the right hepatic artery, which then divides into two branches. Occasionally (20% of individuals), the two branches leave the right hepatic artery independently. The cystic artery may also come off the left hepatic artery or, more rarely, directly off the coeliac axis.

THE PANCREAS

The pancreas is divided into the head, neck, body, and tail. The **head** lies within the concavity of the duodenum; part of it, the **uncinate process**, extends to the left behind the superior mesenteric vessels. The **neck** lies in front of the beginning of the portal vein and origin of the superior mesenteric artery from the aorta. The **body** runs up and to the left across the midline. The **tail** comes into contact with the hilum of the spleen.

Pancreatic ducts

The typical duct anatomy (Figure 3.1.6) is subject to important variations. These include non-patency of the accessory duct (8% of individuals), and independent openings of the common bile duct and the main pancreatic duct (6%). Non-communication between the main duct and the accessory duct, resulting in pancreas divisum, occurs in 2–6% of people. In a series of patients with pancreatitis, the incidence of pancreas divisum was 16%, and it appears, therefore, that pancreas divisum is associated with pancreatitis.

3.2. Clinical Anatomy of the Gastrointestinal Tract: Microscopic

MARCO NOVELLI

INTRODUCTION

The aim of this chapter is to review the basic histology and histopathology commonly seen in clinical practice, and to highlight the features important to the interpretation of their pathology. This information should not only aid the trainee gastroenterologist faced with the prospect of the dreaded histopathology meeting, but also highlight some of the needs of the histopathologist who is faced with reporting biopsies and larger surgical specimens. For more detailed information regarding both gastrointestinal histology (1,2) and histopathology (3,4,5) the reader is directed to more specialized texts.

BIOPSIES

Taking a biopsy

For routine histological analysis, the biopsy should be rapidly immersed in a reasonable volume of a formaldehyde-based fixative before drying occurs (a minimum of 10 times the biopsy volume of formalin should be used). In special cases, different conditions of tissue preservation may be required and suitable preparations made before taking the biopsy — for example, glutaraldehyde fixation for electron microscopy, snap freezing in liquid nitrogen for enzyme assays, and some antibody staining.

How many biopsies?

The more tissue sent, the more likely an accurate diagnosis will be reached. In most instances, several well-prepared biopsies from a single site of macroscopic pathology (e.g. a suspected colonic carcinoma) should suffice. If repeated negative biopsies are obtained despite strong clinical suspicion, alternative methods of biopsy/investigation should be considered. In cases in which more diffuse pathology is suspected (e.g. chronic idiopathic inflammatory bowel disease), many more biopsies may be required, both to make a correct diagnosis and to assess disease extent. Published guidelines suggesting the number and sites of biopsies are now available for the assessment of gastritis and Barrett's metaplasia.

- Gastritis: five biopsies — two from the middle antrum, two from the body and one from the incisura (6).
- Barrett's metaplasia: quadrant biopsies at 2 cm intervals within the Barrett's segment (7).

THE HISTOPATHOLOGY REPORT

Histopathology reports are expressions of opinions, and as such are only as good as the tissue sample, the clinical information provided, and the diagnostic ability of the individual histopathologist reporting the histology. Interpretation of histology is dependent upon basic clinical information (age, sex, relevant previous medical history, medication, etc.). Pathologists need to know what has been found clinically and the clinical question that needs to be answered. If the colon looks microscopically normal, but pathology needs to be excluded, this should be stated. This will save the pathologist's time, and may prevent him/her agonizing over a small collection of inflammatory cells of dubious significance in an otherwise normal biopsy. Similarly, if the activity of liver disease in a patient with hepatitis C needs to be assessed, this should be stated on the request form; if the typical generic clinical history "liver biopsy" is provided, the report may concentrate upon hepatitis C and the other differential diagnoses of the histological picture, with less emphasis on assessment of disease activity. Finally, in complicated situations, the histopathologist is usually more than grateful to discuss the case either over the telephone or at clinicopathological review meetings. It is always helpful to include on the request form the bleep or telephone numbers of a clinician who knows about an individual case.

BASIC GASTROINTESTINAL HISTOLOGY AND PATHOLOGICAL PROCESSES

At the junction with the skin surface (oral cavity, oesophagus, and anus), the gastrointestinal tract is lined by squamous epithelium. The gut lying between these structures is lined by glandular epithelium. This variation in epithelial morphology is reflected in the common tumour types seen at these sites (e.g. squamous carcinoma in the upper oesophagus, adenocarcinoma in the colon).

The structure of the gut is broadly similar throughout its length, being composed of mucosa, submucosa, muscularis propria, and serosa (Figure 3.2.1). The vast majority of pathology is mucosal, reflecting the fact that the epithelium acts as the interface between the body and the environment. Three main processes need to be considered when the pathology of the gastrointestinal tract is being examined: inflammation, metaplasia, and neoplasia.

Inflammation

The number of inflammatory cells normally present varies markedly in different areas of the gastrointestinal tract. This largely reflects the type of mucosa and type of microbiological flora to which the mucosa is exposed. An idea of the normal content of mucosal inflammatory cells is necessary to allow interpretation of inflammatory cell infiltrates.

Inflammation arises in the gastrointestinal tract in response to a large variety of stimuli, ranging from infectious organisms to idiopathic inflammatory disorders (e.g. Crohn's disease). Generally, inflammation is classified as **acute** (inflammatory infiltrate composed predominantly of neutrophils), **chronic** (inflammatory infiltrate composed of lymphocytes, macrophages, plasma cells, and eosinophils), or **active chronic** (acute inflammation superimposed upon chronic inflammation). Further more specific subtypes of chronic inflammation occur including granulomatous, eosinophilic, and lymphocytic inflammation.

Metaplasia

Metaplasia is a conversion of one type of differentiated tissue into another type of differentiated tissue. This is most commonly seen affecting epithelium, usually as an adaptive change in response to alterations in the local environment. Typical examples in the gastrointestinal tract are gastric metaplasia in the lower oesophagus as a result of acid reflux (Barrett's oesophagus), gastric metaplasia in the duodenum possibly resulting from local hyperacidity, and intestinal metaplasia in the stomach, largely caused by *Helicobacter pylori* infection. Metaplasia is important, not only in that it acts as a histological marker of the underlying pathological process, but more importantly in that, in some situations there is believed to be an associated increased risk of malignant transformation (e.g. in Barrett's oesophagus and gastric intestinal metaplasia).

Neoplasia

As with other forms of pathology in the gut, neoplasia predominantly effects the epithelium. This bias is further exaggerated by the fact that many stromal tumours are asymptomatic and are, therefore, not detected clinically. The gut is unusual in that a number of its epithelial malignancies pass through a readily detectable clinically benign "premalignant" phase. These premalignant lesions provide the potential for the future development of screening programmes.

In the past there have been marked discrepancies between Western and Japanese pathologists in the diagnosis of gastrointestinal neoplasia. These discrepancies are thought to account for some of the differences seen between these countries in both the incidence and clinical outcome of neoplasia. In an attempt to unify the diagnostic criteria used to

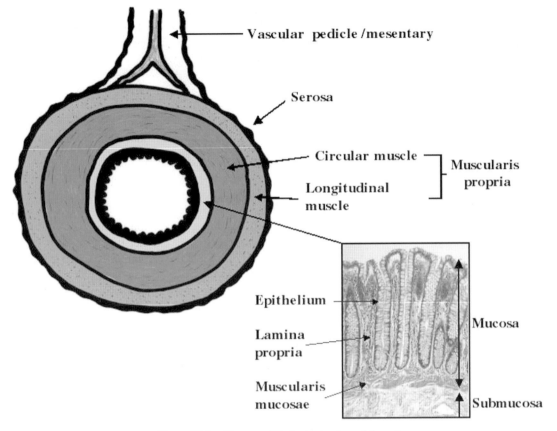

Figure 3.2.1. Diagram of the basic structure of the gut.

classify neoplasia an international group of gastrointestinal pathologists has recently developed the Vienna classification of gastrointestinal epithelial neoplasia (8).

Dysplasia

Dysplasia is a combination of morphological changes that are associated with malignancy. By definition, these changes are not invasive; however, they may precede malignancy, and are commonly seen adjacent to invasive carcinoma. The term "dysplasia", can be used to describe changes in a variety of tissues, but is commonly used to describe changes in epithelia. Dysplasia involves changes at both an architectural and a cellular level. At the cellular level, there is an increase in the size of cell nuclei relative to the volume of cytoplasm (increase in nuclear:cytoplasmic ratio) and an irregular nuclear outline, with a coarse nuclear chromatin pattern. There is loss of cellular differentiation (e.g. a loss

of mucin production), and loss of nuclear polarity. In glandular epithelia, cells may become piled up on top of each other (pseudostratification) and there are architectural changes, with glandular irregularity and glands lying close together without intervening stroma ("back-to-backing" of glands).

In the UK dysplasia has traditionally been graded depending on the severity of these changes into either low and high grade dysplasia (e.g. in Barrett's oesophagus) or mild, moderate and severe dysplasia (e.g. in intestinal adenomas). Following the recent publication of the Vienna classification (8), the exact categorization of dysplasia may change but this new grading system depends upon similar histological criteria (cytology, architecture and absence/presence of invasion) (Table 3.2.1).

Invasive malignancy

In epithelial tumours, the diagnosis of malignancy depends upon the demonstration of tissue invasion

Table 3.2.1. The Vienna classification of gastrointestinal epithelial neoplasia.

Category	Histological assessment
1	Negative for neoplasia/dysplasia
2	Indefinite for neoplasia/dysplasia
3	Non-invasive low grade neoplasia (low grade adenoma/dysplasia)
4	Non-invasive high grade neoplasia
	4.1 High grade adenoma/dysplasia
	4.2 Non-invasive carcinoma (carcinoma in situ)*
	4.3 Suspicion of invasive carcinoma
5	Invasive neoplasia
	5.1 Intramucosal carcinoma[†]
	5.2 Submucosal carcinoma or beyond

*Non-invasive indicates absence of evident invasion.
[†]Intramucosal indicates invasion into the lamina propria or muscularis mucosae.
(Adapted from Ref 8)

by tumour cells. Tumour cells must be seen to have **broken through the basement membrane into the lamina propria**. Typically, there is a stromal response to tumour cells, producing fibrosis around them (a "desmoplastic reaction").

OESOPHAGUS

The normal oesphageal mucosa is composed of muscularis mucosae, and lamina propria covered by non-keratizing stratified squamous epithelium (Figure 3.2.2A). There are scattered mucosal and submucosal mucous glands throughout the length of the oesophagus, which drain through ducts into the oesophageal lumen.

Pathology

There is a limited spectrum of pathology seen commonly affecting the oesophagus.

Non-malignant ulceration

The main causes of ulceration are the topical effects of drugs (e.g. non-steroidal anti-inflammatory drugs and potassium preparations) and infections in the immunocompromised patient (candidiasis, cytomegalovirus, and herpes simplex infection). The typical histological features are those of epithelial loss with replacement by necrotic slough, and acute and chronic inflammation of the underlying tissues. In cases of infection, herpetic multinucleated giant cells, cytomegalovirus inclusions and candidal hyphae may be seen. In the case of candidal infection, a careful search for malignancy is required, as candida often colonizes malignant ulcers.

Barrett's oesophagus (columnar-lined esophagus, CLO)

This metaplastic condition is thought to result from gastro-oesophageal reflux disease (GORD). The local squamous epithelium may be replaced by the full spectrum of epithelial types seen in the normal and metaplastic stomach (see below). To make a definite diagnosis of Barrett's metaplasia the pathologist needs to know that the biopsy has certainly been taken from above the oesophagogastric junction (9). Some pathologists also require the presence of intestinal metaplasia to make a diagnosis of Barrett's oesophagus but this remains a contentious issue.

Neoplasia

Dysplasia may be seen to arise in both squamous- and glandular-type epithelium. Most commonly, it is seen in Barrett's epithelium, where it is graded as low-grade or high-grade dysplasia. The presence of high-grade dysplasia is an indication for further treatment, as concomitant invasive adenocarcinoma is present in 38–64% of patients with Barrett's oesophagus (9,10). Carcinomas arising in the upper two-thirds of the oesophagus tend to be of invasive squamous cell type, whereas those arising in the lower one-third are commonly adenocarcinoma. Other malignant oesophageal tumour types (small cell carcinoma, lymphoma, etc.) and benign tumours are uncommon in routine clinical practice.

STOMACH

Histology

The stomach is divided anatomically into cardia, fundus, body, antrum, and pylorus (Figure 3.2.2D). The surface epithelium covering the mucosa (foveolar epithelium) is similar throughout the stomach, but there is marked variation of the glandular content of the mucosa. Gastric epithelium stem cells are present at the base of gastric foveolae (pits), probably residing among cells known as mucous neck cells. From this stem cell zone, cells migrate

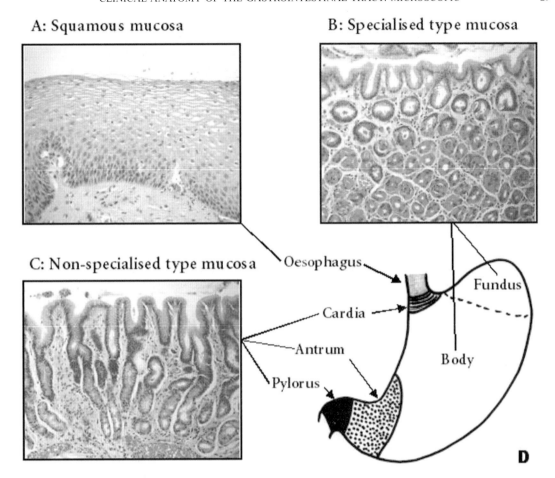

Figure 3.2.2. Mucosal histology. A: Normal squamous mucosa of the oesophagus. B: "Specialized type" mucosa of the stomach. C: "Non-specialized type" mucosa of the stomach. D: Diagrams of the regions of the stomach in which these mucosae are located.

upwards into the gastric pits as foveolar epithelium, or down into the gastric glands.

At the **cardia**, **antrum** and **pylorus**, the gastric glands are of the relatively simple "nonspecialized type", occupying approximately half of the width of the mucosa, and secreting neutral mucin only (Figure 3.2.2C). In the **body** and **fundus**, the mucosal glands are of the more complicated "specialized type", occupying approximately three-quarters of the mucosal thickness, (Figure 3.2.2B). These glands are composed of two main cell types:

1. *Chief cells*: These are small, basophilic cells that are localized principally to the base of the glands. These cells produce pepsinogen.

2. *Parietal cells*: These are larger, pale cells with a central nucleus and copious eosinophilic cytoplasm (sometimes described as "fried egg" cells). These cells produce hydrochloric acid and intrinsic factor.

Neuroendocrine cells are scattered in the gastric glands throughout the stomach. They produce a variety of hormones, but in the antrum more than 50% of these cells produce gastrin.

The lamina propria of the stomach is populated by **fibroblasts** and **histiocytes**. Scarce **plasma cells** and **lymphocytes** may be seen, but the presence of an obvious inflammatory cell infiltrate suggests pathology.

Pathology

Inflammation

Gastritis is commonly classified and graded using the Sydney classification, which was devised by an international working group on the pathology of gastritis (5). Unlike most other classifications of gastritis, this classification combines topographical, morphological, and aetiological information. The revised classification incorporates a visual analogue scale that allows biopsies to be graded reproducibly on a range of features:

1. Glandular atrophy — loss of glands.
2. Acute inflammation.
3. Chronic inflammation.
4. Intestinal metaplasia — replacement of gastric epithelium by either small-intestine type epithelium (complete intestinal metaplasia) or large-intestine type epithelium (incomplete intestinal metaplasia).
5. Presence of helicobacter organisms.

Polyps

A variety of polyps occur in the stomach, including regenerative (hyperplastic) polyps, adenomas, hamartomas, and fundic glandular cysts. Gastric polyps are relatively uncommon, regenerative polyps being seen most frequently. These are composed of hyperplastic foveolar epithelium and cystically dilated glands, with chronically inflamed, oedematous lamina propria. Gastric adenomas are similar to colonic adenomas in appearence and, as in the colon, have an associated risk of malignant transformation.

Gastric carcinoma

Gastric carcinomas are adenocarcinomas that arise from the gastric epithelium. They can be classified according to the stage of disease (early or late) or to histological type (intestinal or diffuse). Early gastric cancer is defined as an invasive tumour that is restricted to the gastric mucosa. At the present time, such tumours are rarely seen in the West, but are commonly found in Japan, where endoscopic screening for gastric carcinoma is performed. Histopathologically, the tumours are classified as two types:

1. *Intestinal*: Malignant tumour cells form invasive glandular structures. These tumours are thought to commonly arise upon a background of incomplete intestinal metaplasia.
2. *Diffuse*: These tumours are composed of discohesive malignant cells, often demonstrating an intracellular mucin globule (signet ring carcinoma). Cells diffusely invade throughout the local tissues and may produce a shrunken, contracted stomach ("leather bottle stomach" or linitis plastica). Because of their extensive local invasion and propensity to metastasize, these tumours are associated with a poor prognosis.

Gastrointestinal stromal tumours

These tumours are thought to arise from stromal tissue in the stomach and at other sites in the gastrointestinal tract. They are typically composed of solid sheets of spindle cells. The clinical behaviour of these tumours is notoriously unpredictable, but the likely behaviour is assessed using a combination of criteria, a small tumour size (less than 5 cm), a low mitotic count, and the absence of haemorrhage or necrosis being associated with a benign clinical course. Immunocytological staining shows that these tumours may stain for smooth muscle markers (desmin and smooth muscle actin), neural markers (NSE, S100), CD34 and for CD117 (c-kit).

SMALL INTESTINE

Histology

The small intestinal epithelium is organized into crypts and villi (Figure 3.2.3A). The crypt is a pouch-shaped infolding, and the villi are finger-like extensions of the mucosa. The villi have the effect of massively increasing the surface area of the small intestine, to increase the absorptive capacity. The crypt acts as a cell production unit, cells originating from near the base of each crypt from a stem cell zone; cells differentiate as they migrate up out of the crypts onto surrounding villi. Each crypt supplies several villi and each villus is supplied by a number of crypts. Cells constantly migrate out of the crypts, up the villi, and die at the villus tips, probably through the process of apoptosis.

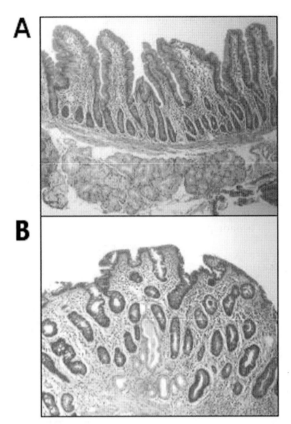

Figure 3.2.3. Photomicrograph of duodenal mucosa. A: Normal duodenal mucosa. B: A case of coeliac disease showing subtotal villous atrophy and crypt hyperplasia.

The small intestinal epithelium is composed of four resident cell types, all of which derive from a common stem cell. A variable number of intraepithelial T lymphocytes are also normally present.

1. *Paneth cells*: These are found clustered at the very base of the crypts, and can be recognized by their cytoplasmic content of refractile eosinophilic granules. Their function is not fully understood, but they have been implicated in the regulation of the crypt microflora.
2. *Goblet cells*: These cells are so named because of their wineglass-shaped cytoplasmic vacuoles of mucus. Their function is to excrete mucus.
3. *Enterocytes*: These are the most frequent cells in the epithelium. They are responsible for membrane digestion (proteins and carbohydrates) and absorption.

4. *Neuroendocrine cells*: These are scattered within the crypt epithelium, and are responsible for the secretion of a variety of peptide hormones.

Pathology

Small intestinal biopsy is most commonly performed to exclude coeliac disease (Figure 3.2.3B) and infections such as giardiasis. Initially, the overall architecture of the mucosa is assessed, looking for the presence of well-formed villi. The mucosal inflammatory cell infiltrate is then assessed. Large numbers of chronic inflammatory cells are normally present in the lamina propria of the small intestine, making the assessment of chronic inflammation difficult. The presence of acute inflammatory cells, particularly in the epithelium, is suggestive of acute inflammation. Intraepithelial lymphocytes are normally present, but should be no more frequent than one lymphocyte for every five epithelial cells. Careful inspection of the surface epithelium and ulcer slough for intracellular or attached microorganisms is also made.

Coeliac disease

The classical features of coeliac disease are **total or subtotal villous atrophy** (flattening of villi), **crypt hyperplasia** (increase in crypt length, with an increase in the size of the proliferative compartment as the crypt increases cell output), and an **increase in intraepithelial lymphocytes** (Figure 3.2.3B). These features are not specific for coeliac disease, being present in other enteropathies (e.g. tropical sprue). Individual biopsies may show pathology consistent with coeliac disease, but are not diagnostic. A diagnosis of the condition strictly requires histopathological demonstration of disease, amelioration in response to institution of a gluten-free diet and (possibly) recurrence of pathology after reintroduction of dietary gluten.

Giardiasis

The histopathological features of intestinal infection with the protozoan *Giardia lamblia*, are nonspecific, a histological diagnosis requiring demonstration of classical "kite-shaped" trophozoites in small intestinal biopsies.

Crohn's disease

This disease can involve any part of the gut from the mouth to the perianal skin, but it most commonly affects the terminal ileum and colon (40% of cases), or terminal ileum alone (30%). The macroscopic and microscopic features are similar in both the small intestine and the colon (see below).

Tumours

Tumours of the small intestine are uncommon. This is despite the fact that the epithelium of the small intestine has a markedly larger surface area and a greater rate of proliferation than the large intestine, in which carcinomas are relatively common. Tumours occurring in the small intestine include:

1. adenocarcinomas (the most frequent malignant small intestinal tumours)
2. carcinoid tumours
3. lymphomas
4 stromal tumours
5. metastases

LARGE INTESTINE

Histology

The epithelium of the large intestine is organized into crypts in a fashion similar to that seen in the small intestine, although no villi are present (Figure 3.2.4). Cells originate in a stem cell zone near the base of the crypt and migrate up to reach the surface epithelium, where they eventually die and are sloughed into the lumen. The large intestinal epithelium consists of four main resident cell types: **absorptive cells, goblet cells, neuroendocrine cells** and **Paneth cells**, although Paneth cells are normally restricted to the proximal colon in humans. **Intraepithelial lymphocytes** are present in the large intestine, but are fewer in number than in the small intestine (a maximum of one lymphocyte for every 20 epithelial cells).

Pathology

The following features need to be considered when the histology of large intestinal biopsies is being interpreted (11):

1. *Crypt architecture*: Depending upon the plane of tissue section, crypts are seen as regular circles or ovals (transverse section) or as finger-shaped inpouchings of the epithelium (longitudinal section). The crypts should be closely packed in regular arrays. In longitudinal section, occasional bifid or budding crypts are allowed but, if present in large numbers, these suggest pathology.
2. *Inflammatory cell infiltrate*: In the normal colon there is a gradient of chronic inflammatory cells in the lamina propria, with more cells at the luminal aspect (where the majority of antigens are located). Loss of this gradient is one of the first signs of chronic inflammation. Occasional lymphoid aggregates are seen in the lamina propria. Very occasional neutrophils scattered in the lamina propria are allowed but, otherwise, acute inflammatory cells are not a normal feature.

Colonic biopsies are most commonly performed to determine if inflammation is present, to distinguish infective from chronic idiopathic inflammatory bowel disease, and in the screening for and investigation of malignancy (Table 3.2.2).

Irritable bowel syndrome

In this condition the large intestine shows no pathological changes.

Infective colitis

In infective-type colitis, the crypt architecture is well preserved. There is an increase in both acute

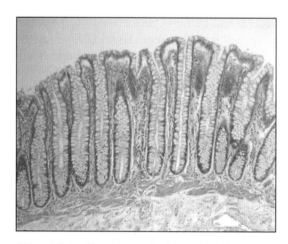

Figure 3.2.4. Photomicrograph of normal colonic mucosa.

Table 3.2.2.   Histological features of inflammatory bowel disease, infective colitis, and ischaemic colitis biopsies.

	Crypt architecture	Lamina propria	Acute inflamation
Chronic inflammatory bowel disease	Crypt distortion present, particularly in ulcerative colitis	Increased chronic inflammatory cells across full thickness of mucosa	Cryptitis affecting whole of crypt, with crypt abscess formation
Infective colitis	Normal crypt architecture. Scattered "withered" crypts	Increase in cellularity with mixed infiltrate, predominantly affecting the luminal aspect of the mucosa	Cryptitis predominantly affecting the luminal aspect of the crypt, with occasional crypt abscesses
Ischaemic colitis	Overall crypt architecture often maintained, but necrosis of luminal aspect of mucosa. In regenerated cases there may be marked crypt distortion	Oedema and vascular congestion in acute cases. Fibrosis in chronic cases	Inflammation related to acute mucosal necrosis

and chronic inflammatory cells, but they tend to be concentrated towards the luminal aspect of the mucosa. In most cases, no infective organisms will be identified, although a careful search for amoebae should be made, particularly in patients with a history of foreign travel.

Chronic idiopathic inflammatory bowel disease

The recognition, diagnosis, and monitoring of chronic idiopathic inflammatory bowel disease is an important aspect of gastrointestinal histopathology. The disease should be considered as a spectrum, with classical Crohn's disease at one extreme, classical ulcerative colitis at the other, and indeterminate colitis in between. Although histological assessment of mucosal biopsies may readily distinguish classical Crohn's disease from classical ulcerative colitis, away from these extremes such assessment is often more difficult. Differentiation of these conditions requires consideration of their macroscopic features, in addition to their clinical and histological features.

Crohn's disease

Macroscopically, there are skip lesions with fat wrapping (extension of fat from the mesentary over the serosal surface of the intestine), thickening of the bowel wall, stenoses, mucosal ulceration, mucosal cobblestoning, fissuring, and fistula formation. **Microscopically**, there is transmural inflammation, predominantly in the form of lym-

phoid aggregates, mucosal crypt abscesses, mucosal ulceration, fissuring, and granuloma formation. Granulomas are seen in about 50% of cases, found lying in any layer of the bowel wall or in local lymph nodes. In addition to the inflammation, there is a marked increase in the stromal tissues of the bowel wall — "neuromuscular hyperplasia".

Ulcerative colitis

Macroscopically, the bowel wall is of normal thickness or thinned. The mucosa shows continuous disease, with ulceration and **pseudopolyp** formation (islands of surviving mucosa in a sea of ulceration) starting in the rectum. Disease severity is usually most advanced distally, although the use of rectal steroids may produce apparent rectal sparing. Disease is limited to the large intestine, although there may be involvement of the terminal ileum (backwash ileitis) in association with pancolitis. **Microscopically**, there is diffuse chronic inflammation, which is limited to the mucosa, except in areas of ulceration, where inflammation may extend into the tissues directly beneath the ulcer base. There is acute inflammation of the crypt epithelium (cryptitis), with formation of crypt abscesses. The crypts are depleted of goblet cells (mucin depletion), and Paneth cells may be found in the crypt bases throughout the large intestine (Paneth cell metaplasia). There are changes in crypt architecture, with crypt budding and bifurcation, and loss of crypts (crypt atrophy). Long-standing ulcerative colitis may also lead to the development of epithelial dysplasia.

Colorectal tumours

In the western world, colorectal carcinoma is the third most common cause of cancer-related mortality. Colorectal adenocarcinoma accounts for the vast majority of malignant colorectal tumours. There is a well-defined adenoma—carcinoma sequence, and many of the genetic events associated with this progression have been outlined (12). Morphologically, there is a spectrum of adenoma types, ranging from small tubular adenomas, through larger tubulovillous adenomas to villous adenomas. The malignant potential of adenomas is believed to increase as the adenoma increases in size and becomes more villous (13).

Colorectal adenocarcinoma is believed to arise commonly from a pre-existing adenoma. Tumours are graded according to their morphological resemblance to normal colonic epithelium:

1. *Well differentiated*: The tumour forms glands composed of regular tumour cells.
2. *Moderately differentiated*: The tumour forms irregular glands composed of tumour cells of varying size.
3. *Poorly differentiated*: The tumour cells show marked variation in size and shape, and show few signs of gland formation.

In practice, the vast majority of tumours (approx 80%) are graded as moderately differentiated.

Colorectal tumours can be staged using a variety of different systems (e.g. Dukes', the Astler–Coller system, and tumour–nodes–metastasis (TNM) staging). At present, the oldest and simplest of these systems, Dukes' staging, is favoured in the UK. Tumours are classified according to the extent of their invasion of the bowel wall, and the presence or absence of lymph node metastases. Tumours that invade any proportion of the bowel wall, but fall short of breaching the muscularis propria, are classified as Dukes' A, tumours that have invaded the full thickness of the muscularis propria (main muscle coat) are Dukes' B, and tumours with lymph node involvement are Dukes' C (Figure 3.2.5). In the UK guidelines on the grading and staging of colorectal cancer have recently been published (14).

ANUS

Histology

In the anus, there is a rapid transition from the glandular epithelium of the rectum, through an intermediate mucosa at the anal transition zone, to the keratinizing stratified squamous mucosa of the lower anus. The transition from squamous to transitional epithelium occus at the dentate line, with the anal transitional zone typically extending for approximately 1 cm proximal to this. Submucosal anal glands producing acidic and neutral mucin are present in the anal transitional zone.

Pathology

Anal biopsy is commonly performed for a limited range of pathology including condyloma accuminata (anal warts), Crohns's disease, and anal carcinoma.

Anal carcinoma

Anal carcinoma is a rare tumour accounting for less than 2% of large intestinal malignancies. Squamous cell carcinomas are the most frequent type, although both primary adenocarcinoma and small cell carcinoma can also occur. Squamous cell carcinoma of the anus can show a variety of morphological patterns of differentiation, including keratinizing squamous, basaloid, and ductal differentiation (15).

LIVER

Histology

The liver is an epithelial organ, composed of sheets of hepatocytes organized around portal tracts and central veins. The portal tract contains three vessels: a portal vein, a hepatic artery, and a bile duct. The liver receives a dual blood supply, from the hepatic artery (30%) and portal vein (70%). Blood percolates from the portal tracts between the liver cell plates in hepatic sinusoids to the central vein, from where blood returns to the systemic circulation. Bile is produced by hepatocytes and released into small tubules called canaliculi, which are located within the liver cell plates between individual hepatocytes. Bile flows in a direction opposite to

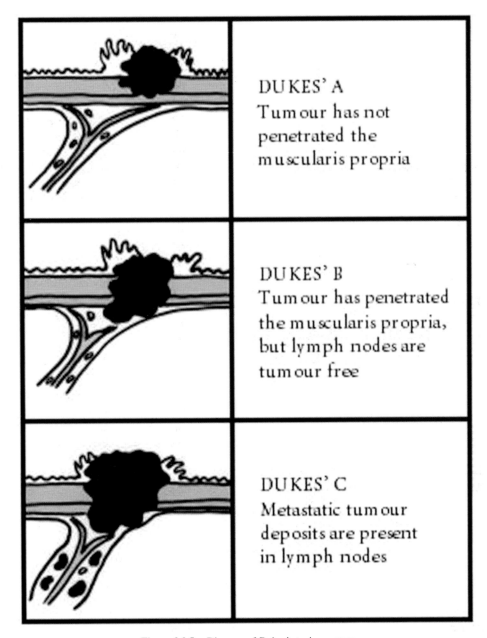

Figure 3.2.5. Diagram of Dukes' staging system.

that of the blood (from the central veins towards the portal tracts), into the bile ducts.

The structure of the liver can be considered in two dimensions (the hepatic lobule), or in three dimensions the (hepatic acinus):

1. *Hepatic lobule*: This model is centred upon the central vein. Cords of hepatocytes radiate out to portal tracts, six of which are arranged in a hexagonal fashion around each central vein. For functional and descriptive purposes, the lobule is then divided into **centilobular** (around the central vein), **midzonal**, and **periportal** areas.

2. *Rappaport's hepatic acinus*: The acinus is considered to be an ellipsoid centred upon a portal tract. It is divided into three zones depending

upon distance from the portal tract: zone 1, closest (equivalent of periportal); zone 3, furthest (equivalent of centrilobular); zone 2, between zones 1 and 3 (equivalent of midzonal).

Current opinion favours the hepatic acinus model, as this represents the smallest functional unit in the liver.

There are marked variations in oxygenation, nutrition, and enzyme activity in different parts of the lobule/acinus. This has an important bearing upon the distribution of pathology that is seen (e.g. the centrilobular area/zone 3 receives the least-oxygenated blood, and is therefore more prone to ischaemic damage).

The normal human adult hepatocytes are arranged in sheets, which are one cell in thickness and are supported by a delicate reticulin scaffold. Between the plates lie the hepatic sinusoids, so that both sides of the hepatocyte plates are bathed in blood. The sinusoids are partially lined by a mixed population of endothelial cells and macrophage-like cells called Kupffer cells. Between these cells and the hepatic plates, a potential space is formed known as the space of Disse. Within this space, two further cell types are seen: Ito cells (interstitial fat storing cells) and pit cells (large, granular lymphocyte-like cells with natural killer activity). Hepatocytes retain the ability to re-enter the cell cycle and proliferate in response to cell injury. Whether there are true stem cells in the adult liver, and where they reside, remain controversial topics.

Pathology

The liver is a complicated organ containing a variety of cell types, and showing a spectrum of pathological change, even within the same cell type, between different zones of the hepatic lobule. The liver demonstrates a limited range of pathological changes, with the consequence that determination of disease aetiology can be difficult. This is especially the case in established cirrhosis, which is the endstage of a broad spectrum of liver disease. The situation is not helped by the fact that xenobiotics can produce a pathological picture that mimics most other major liver pathologies. A good clinical history, including a drug history and serological results is, therefore, a prerequisite when a liver biopsy is being reported.

Because of this complexity, most pathologists use a systematic approach to examine and describe liver pathology. Currently, there are a variety of classification systems in routine use, many of which grade the activity (inflammation and necrosis) and stage (extent of fibrosis) of liver disease (e.g. (16)).

1. *Architecture*: The architecture of the liver is usually examined by using a special stain for reticulin fibres and collagen (Figure 3.2.6). This highlights the thickness of the hepatocyte plates (normally one cell in adults), the arrangement of portal tracts and central veins, and shows any areas of fibrosis. If fibrosis runs between portal tracts or joins portal tracts and central veins it is called "bridging fibrosis". Cirrhosis is the endstage of chronic liver disease. It can result from a wide range of different aetiologies. By definition, cirrhosis is a diffuse process affecting the whole liver, showing a combination of regeneration nodules and bands of fibrosis.

2. *Portal tracts*: Every portal tract should contain a portal triad (hepatic artery, portal vein, and bile duct). The bile duct should be of approximately the same size as the hepatic artery. The portal tracts are assessed for the presence of **bile ducts**, for inflammation (acute and chronic) and for **interface hepatitis** (inflammation spilling from the portal tract into the liver parenchyma)

3. *Lobules*: The lobules are examined to look for inflammation (lobulitis), necrosis, Councillman bodies (apoptotic hepatocytes), steatosis (fatty change classified as either macrovesicular or microvesicular), and bile stasis (build up of bile in the canaliculi). Further histochemical staining is routinely performed in most histopathology departments, to highlight a variety of substances including iron, copper, α_1-antitrypsin globules, and HBV surface antigen.

Interpretation of liver pathology can be extremely difficult and, as already emphasized, dependent upon a good clinical history. There are, however, classical features associated with certain pathologies, such as the following.

Alcoholic liver disease

Architectural changes include perivenular fibrosis, pericellular fibrosis, and bridging fibrosis leading to cirrhosis in advanced disease. In the lobules,

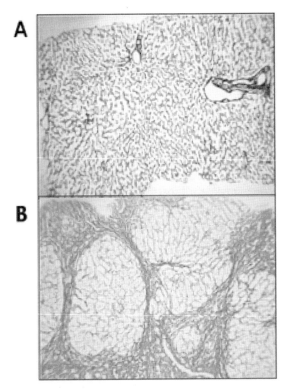

A

B

Figure 3.2.6. Photomicrographs of reticulin-stained normal (A) and cirrhotic (B) liver.

there may be marked macrovesicular steatosis and lobular inflammation, with a prominent infiltrate of neutrophils and necrotic hepatocytes. Hepatocytes containing aggregates of eosinophilic amorphous material known as "Mallory's hyaline" are also commonly seen.

Chronic viral hepatitis

Chronic HBV infection is typified by a moderate portal chronic inflammatory cell infiltrate with marked interface hepatitis. Scattered Councillman bodies are often seen in the lobules, in addition to "ground glass" hepatocytes (hepatocytes with their cytoplasm distended with HBV surface antigen). Periportal fibrosis leads to bridging fibrosis and eventually, to full-blown cirrhosis.

Chronic hepatitis C virus (HCV) inflammation classically has a mild portal chronic inflammatory cell infiltrate, with bile duct damage and prominent portal lymphoid aggregates. There is usually mild to minimal interface hepatitis and mild macrovesicular steatosis.

Primary biliary cirrhosis and primary sclerosing cholangitis

Both these diseases typically show focal pathology, so may be difficult to diagnose, particularly early in the disease history. Their pathology is centred upon the bile ducts in such a way that the fibrotic damage is concentrated in the portal tracts, producing biliary cirrhosis as the endstage of both diseases. In biliary cirrhosis there is fibrotic expansion of the portal tracts, with sparing of the centrilobular zone. This produces a cirrhotic liver, but the nodules may contain a central vein.

In primary biliary cirrhosis there is, typically, lymphocytic infiltration and destruction of small to medium sized bile ducts, leading to complete loss of bile ducts and proliferation of small bile ductules around the perimeter of the portal tracts. Epithelioid granulomas centred upon bile ducts are characteristic of this condition. In primary sclerosing cholangitis there is concentric fibrosis around bile ducts, leading to an "onion skin" appearance. Eventually, the bile ducts completely disappear, leaving a fibrous "tombstone".

Primary liver tumours

The most common primary liver tumours are hepatocellular carcinoma and cholangiocarcinoma (see Chapter 18.2). These tumours may both appear multifocal and prove difficult to distinguish histologically. Pointers useful in separating them are that, unlike cholangiocarcinoma, hepatocellular carcinoma usually arises on a background of cirrhosis (in Western countries), tumour cells commonly produce bile, and tumour cells may immunostain for α-fetoprotein.

PANCREAS

Histology

The pancreas is formed of two main elements: the **exocrine pancreas**, composed of serous acini and ducts, and the **endocrine pancreas**, comprising the islets of Langerhans (Figure 3.2.7).

Pathology

Pancreatic biopsy is commonly performed to differentiate chronic pancreatitis from pancreatic adeno-

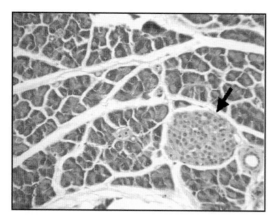

Figure 3.2.7. Photomicrograph of mouse pancreas showing both exocrine and endocrine components. Arrow shows islet of Langerhans.

carcinoma. Differentiating between these two conditions can be notoriously difficult, particularly in small trephine biopsies and on frozen sections. In chronic pancreatitis, there is chronic inflammation and fibrosis, typically with loss of glandular tissue but retention of islets. Ductal and acinar tissue that remains tends to retain the lobular organization of the normal pancreas. In contrast, in pancreatic adenocarcinoma, a dense **desmoplastic (fibrous) stroma** containing scattered tumour cells, lying in clusters and forming ducts, effaces the normal pancreatic architecture.

References

*Of interest; ** of exceptional interest

1   Young B, Barbara JW. Wheater's *Functional Histology*. Fourth Edition. Edinburgh. Churchill Livingstone, 2000.

2. *Histology for Pathologists*. Second Edition. Ed Sternberg S, Philadelphia. Lippincott-Raven, 1997.

3. *Gastrointestinal and Oesophageal Pathology*. Second edition. Ed Whitehead R: London. Churchill Livingstone, 1995.

4. *Pathology of the Gastrointestinal Tract*. Second edition. Eds Ming S, Goldman H. Baltimore. Williams and Wilkins 1998.

5. Morson B, Dawson I, Day D, Jass J, Price A, Williams G. *Morson and Dawson's Gastrointestinal Pathology*. Third edition. Oxford. Blackwell Scientific Publications, 1990.

6. *Dixon M, Genta R, Yardley J, Correa P. Classification and grading of gastritis. The updated Sydney System. *Am J Surg Pathol* 1996; **20**(10): 1161–1181.
    Guidelines for reporting gastric biopsies together with suggestions on biopsy site and numbers.

7. Levine D, Haggitt R, Blount P, Rabinovitch P, Rusch V, Reid B. An endoscopic biopsy protocol can differentiate high-grade dysplasia from early adenocarcinoma in Barrett's esophagus. *Gastroenterology* 1993; **105**: 40–50.

8. Schlemper R, Riddell R, Kato Y, Borchard F, Cooper S, Dawsey S, Dixon M, Fenoglio-Preiser C, Flejou J, Geboes K *et al*. The Vienna classification of gastrointestinal epithelial neoplasia. *Gut* 2000; **47**: 251–255.

9. *Shepherd N, Biddlestone L. The histopathology and cytopathology of Barrett's oesophagus. *CPD Bulletin Cellular Pathology* 1999, 1(2): 39–43.
    A useful review article covering all aspects of Barrett's.

10. Heitmiller R, Redmond M, Hamilton S. Barrett's esophagus with high-grade dysplasia. An indication for prophylactic esophagectomy. *Ann Surg* 1996; **224**(1): 66–71.

11. *Jenkins D, Balsitis M, Gallivan S, Dixon M, Gilmour M, Shepherd N, Williams G, Theodossi A. A structured approach to colorectal biopsy assessment. Guidelines in Gastroenterology 9. *British Society of Gastroenterology*, 1997. (Available electronically at www.bsg.org.uk/guidelines). Simply explained and well-illustrated guidelines to reporting of colorectal biopsies.

12. Ilyas M, Tomlinson I. Genetic pathways in colorectal cancer. *Histopathology* 1996; **28**: 389–399.

13. Muto T, Bussey H, Morson B. The evolution of cancer of the colon and rectum. *Cancer* 1975; **36**: 2251–2257.

14. *Quirke P, Williams GT. Minimum dataset for colorectal cancer histopathology reports. Standards and Minimum datasets for Reporting Common Cancers. The Royal College of Pathologists, London, 1998. (Available electronically at www.rcpath.org). Guidelines for reporting colorectal cancer specimens including illustrated explanations of Dukes' and TNM staging systems.

15. Williams G, Talbot I. Anal carcinoma—a histological review. *Histopathology* 1994; **25**(6): 507–16.

16. Ishak K, Baptista A, Bianchi L, Callea F, De Groote J, Gudat F, Denk H, Desmet V, Korb G, MacSween RN, *et al*. Histological grading and staging of chronic hepatitis. *J Hepatol* 1995; **22**(6): 696–699.

B: Dealing with Inpatient Consultative/Referrals

4. Gastrointestinal Problems In Patients With Metabolic And Endocrine Disorders

ANNE BALLINGER

DIABETES MELLITUS

Abnormal gastrointestinal function is common in patients with long-standing diabetes mellitus (1). Damage to the autonomic nervous system and denervation of gastrointestinal smooth muscle explain many of the clinical features; diffuse damage to both parasympathetic and sympathetic nerves is common in diabetic patients with peripheral neuropathy. Patients with gastrointestinal symptoms resulting from autonomic neuropathy will often, but not always, have involvement of other systems (Table 4.1). Conversely, impaired glucose tolerance or diabetes mellitus may be a presenting feature or subsequent manifestation of a range of gastrointestinal and liver conditions (Table 4.2).

Diabetic gastroparesis

Clinical features and diagnosis

Delayed gastric emptying causes nausea, vomiting, anorexia, epigastric fullness or discomfort, and heartburn. Poor blood sugar control and impaired absorption of orally administered drugs may also be related to delayed gastric emptying. The reported prevalence of gastric motor abnormalities varies enormously, depending on the patients selected for study (e.g. duration of diabetic history) and the methods used to evaluate gastric emptying (e.g. barium studies or scintigraphy). Approximately 25% of patients with long-standing insulin-dependent diabetes mellitus

Table 4.1. Clinical features of autonomic neuropathy.

Gastrointestinal	Diarrhoea
	Gastroparesis
	Faecal incontinence
Cardiovascular	Postural hypotension
	Resting tachycardia
	Warm foot with bounding pulses (as a result of vasodilation)
Genitourinary	Impotence
	Neurogenic bladder
Sweating	Gustatory sweating (facial sweating occuring while eating)
	Dry feet
Ventilatory	Susceptibility to ventilatory arrest with drugs that depress depression

complicated with peripheral neuropathy reported early satiety, nausea, and vomiting (2). However, in unselected patients, the prevalence of upper gastrointestinal symptoms was similar to that in a non-diabetic control population (3). In a separate study, 50% of unselected patients had a delay in gastric emptying of solids, suggesting that many patients with gastroparesis are asymptomatic (4).

A **diagnosis** of diabetic gastroparesis is strongly suspected in a patient with suggestive symptoms and absence of a structural lesion on upper gastrointestinal endoscopy or barium meal exami-

Table 4.2. Gastrointestinal conditions causing or associated with diabetes mellitus.

Conditions	Comments
Coeliac disease	Increased frequency of Type I diabetes in coeliac disease. 1–7.8% of patients with Type I diabetes have coeliac disease
Pancreatic disease	
Hereditary HHC	Diabetes occurs in 40–50% of haemochromatosis patients. 0.3–1.0% of unselected diabetics patients have HHC
Chronic pancreatitis	Diabetes occurs late (>20 years after disease onset) in 30–70% of patients
Pancreatic cancer	New onset diabetes in 15% of patients
Pancreatic resection	
Glucagonoma	Diabetes presenting symptom in 38%, eventually develops in 76–91% of patients. Diabetes may develop years before other symptons.
Liver disease	
Chronic liver disease and cirrhosis	Glucose intolerance is common, less frequently diabetes mellitus
Autoimmune liver disease	Increased frequency of Type I diabetes

HHC, haemochromatosis.

nation. Grossly delayed gastric emptying of barium during radiographic examination, or the presence of residual food in the stomach after an overnight fast support the diagnosis. Measurement of gastric emptying of solids and liquids is determined separately by scintigraphy, using different isotopes. However, this technique is not widely available and may be of limited practical value because of the poor correlation between symptoms and laboratory abnormalities.

Pathophysiology

The pathophysiology of diabetic gastric motor dysfunction is probably multifactorial.

1. Manometric studies in diabetic patients have shown increased frequency of postcibal antral dysrhythmias, reduced frequency or absence of gastric phase III of the interdigestive migrating motor complex that normally stimulates antral contractions, and prolonged pyloric contractions that may cause functional outflow obstruction. The antral motility disturbance is particularly implicated in the accumulation of undigestible solid particles and eventual formation of a gastric bezoar.
2. Recent studies have shown evidence of gastric smooth muscle degeneration, which may occur in the absence of major vagal nerve degeneration, suggesting that a gastromyopathic process

may also be a cause for gastroparesis in some diabetic patients (5).
3. Morphometric and functional abnormalities of the gastric vagus nerve have been demonstrated in diabetic patients with and without dyspeptic symptoms. Some investigators have suggested that patients with diabetes also have abnormalities in visceral perception of gut activity.
4. Acute hyperglycaemia reduces antral contraction, stimulates pyloric contractions and delays gastric emptying, both in healthy controls and in diabetic patients (6,7). However, the exact role of chronic hyperglycaemia in the pathogenesis of diabetic gastroparesis is not known.
5. Finally, altered secretion of gut hormones (including motilin, pancreatic polypeptide, and somatostatin) that affect gastric emptying have been reported in diabetic patients. However, these abnormalities may be secondary to the disordered motor activity, rather than a primary event.

Management

In practice, most diabetic patients with symptomatic gastroparesis are managed by introduction of small, frequent meals, tight control of blood glucose concentrations and treatment with a prokinetic agent (Table 4.3). Gastric emptying studies are usually reserved for patients with symptoms that persist despite these measures. Rarely, patients with severe resistant symptoms will require endoscopic

Table 4.3. Prokinetic drugs used in the treatment of diabetic gastroparesis.

Drug and pharmacological effect	Clinical effect	Oral dose	Comments
Metoclopramide Dopamine antagonist	Inhibits dopamine-induced gastric smooth muscle relaxation. Inhibits central chemoreceptor triger zone for vominting.	10 mg 30 min before each meal and at bedtime	Acute efffects on gastric emptying no longer demonstrable after chronic (1 month) dosing. Symptomatic improvement continues
Stimulates ACh release from myenteric plexus	Stimulates fundic and antral smooth mucle contractions		
Domperidone Dopamine antagonist	Inhibits dopamine-induced gastric smooth muscle relaxation	10—20 mg four times daily	Acute effects on gastric emptying no longer demonstrable after chronic (1 month) dosing. Symptomatic improvement continues
Cisapride Stimulates ACh release from postganglionic neurons	Increases antral motility, stimulates duodenal motility, increases antroduodenal coordination	10–20 mg before each meal and at bedtime	Improved gastric emptying and symptomatic improvement persists after 4 weeks of dosing. Withdrawn in the UK.
Erythromycin Motilin agonist	Induces phase III contractions	500 mg three times daily	No sustained improvement in gastric emptying

ACh, acetylcholine.

placement of a jejunostomy feeding tube for long-term enteral nutrition. Recently, there has been renewed interest in the use of electrical pacing to improve gastric emptying and ameliorate symptoms in severe gastroparesis. Pacing wires are placed along the greater curvature of the stomach and embedded in the seromuscular layer of the stomach. The wires are brought out through the abdominal wall and a constant electrical current delivered in order to achieve entrainment of the gastric slow-wave. Pacing improved the symptoms of gastroparesis and gastric emptying in the five diabetic patients who were included in the study (8).

Diabetic diarrhoea

Chronic diarrhoea associated with diabetes mellitus is an uncommon finding in population-based studies, but is reported in up to 22% of patients in tertiary referral centres. Diarrhoea occurs most commonly in patients with a long history of Type I diabetes. There appears to be a strong association with autonomic neuropathy: patients commonly suffer from concomitant impotence, postural hypotension, and bladder dysfunction. The clinical features are non-specific. The diarrhoea may occur at any time, but is often nocturnal, and may alternate with normal bowel habits, or even with constipation. Diarrhoea is often watery, and may be associated with anal incontinence. In other patients, faecal incontinence occurs without true diarrhoea — that is to say, stool volumes are not increased.

Pathophysiology

The pathogenesis of chronic diabetic diarrhoea is incompletely understood, but a number of diverse mechanisms are believed to contribute (Table 4.4). In one tertiary referral practice, the most common causes included small-bowel bacterial overgrowth and coeliac disease (9).

1. Diabetic autonomic neuropathy may result in abnormalities of small-bowel motor function and bacterial overgrowth. Small-bowel bacteria

Table 4.4. Mechanisms of chronic diarrhoea in patients with diabetes mellitus.

Causes associated with autonomic neuropathy	Abnormal motility with stasis and small-bowel bacterial growth
	Abnormal motility with rapid transit
	Impaired intestinal fluid reabsorption
	Exocrine pancreatic insufficiency
Associated conditions	Ingestion of artificial sweeteners
	Coeliac disease
	Thyrotoxicosis
	Bile acid malabsorption
	Collagenous colitis
Unrelated conditions	

deconjugate bile salts, resulting in fat malabsorption and steatorrhoea. Increased bile acid concentrations in the colon induce colonic secretion and contribute to diarrhoea. Adrenergic nerves normally stimulate sodium chloride and water absorption via α_2-adrenergic receptors in the small and large intestine. In diabetic rats, impaired adrenergic regulation of mucosal transport of ions resulted in decreased fluid and electrolyte absorption in the small intestine and colon (10). Thus, autonomic neuropathy may cause diarrhoea as a result of bacterial overgrowth, and as a result of alterations in transport of water and electrolytes with decreased rate of fluid absorption.

2. There is some evidence that exocrine pancreatic insufficiency may contribute to the pathogenesis of diabetic diarrhoea and steatorrhoea. Pancreatic amylase output is subnormal in response to a stimulus of intravenous cholecystokinin or intraduodenal amino acids. Furthermore, some patients with steatorrhoea improve with pancreatic enzyme supplements. Pancreatic insufficiency may be a further manifestation of autonomic neuropathy, with disruption of cholinergic enteropancreatic reflexes — the major physiological regulator of postprandial exocrine pancreatic secretion.

3. Sorbitol, used as a sweetener in dietetic foods, may produce diarrhoea in diabetic patients and healthy individuals. Sorbitol is a sugar that is neither digested nor absorbed, and therefore passes into the distal small intestine and colon, where it drives an osmotic purge. As little as 10 g has been shown to produce diarrhoea in healthy volunteers. Many individuals consuming sorbitol are unaware of its presence in the diet and its ability to cause diarrhoea. Diarrhoea is significantly more common in diabetic individuals who regularly consume sorbitol than in those not consuming it (11).

4. In some diabetic patients, diarrhoea is attributable to an associated gastrointestinal condition that occurs with increased frequency in the diabetic population. As discussed previously, the prevalence of coeliac disease in patients with Type I diabetes is greater than expected, with rates of 1.0–7.8% (12), and one small study has suggested an increased prevalance of collagenous colitis (13).

Diagnostic approach and management of diabetic diarrhoea

The approach to the diabetic patient with diarrhoea begins with a full history and examination, with emphasis on ingestion of sorbitol-containing foods, and symptoms and signs of autonomic neuropathy. All patients must be asked directly about the presence of faecal incontinence. Stool volumes should be measured, to differentiate true diarrhoea from faecal incontinence. The diagnosis of diarrhoea associated with autonomic neuropathy is made by demonstration of abnormalities on autonomic function tests (Table 4.5) and exclusion of other causes of diarrhoea. Patients with autonomic neuropathy invariably have evidence of peripheral neuropathy (at least absent ankle jerks) and this should be sought on clinical examination. An algorithm for the investigation of chronic diabetic diarrhoea is shown in Figure 4.1.

Management

Specific treatment should be directed at the cause of diarrhoea, together with tight control of blood glucose concentrations.

Patients with **no identified cause of diarrhoea** fall into the group with so-called idiopathic diarrhoea. Clonidine (0.1–0.6 mg twice daily), an α_2-adrenergic agonist, increases enteral fluid absorption in diabetic rats, and has been shown to

Table 4.5. Simple test of autonomic function.

Test	Normal	Abnormal

Heart rate variation during deep breathing (beats/min)
    The heart rate difference (maximum during deep, 5-s, inspiration minus minimum
    during 5-s expiration) measured on ECG
	>15	<10

Increased in heart rate on standing (at 15 s) (beats/min)	>15	<12
Ratio of maximum to minimum heart rate during Valsalva manoeuvre	>1.21	<1.20

The patient blows hard through the empty barrel of a 20-ml syringe to maintain the
    column of a sphygmomanometer at 40 mm for 10 s. Maximum heart rate
    during blowing, followed by minimum heart rate after cessation, are recorded		

Postural decrease systolic blood pressure at 2 min (mmHg)	<10	>30

ECG, electrocardiogram

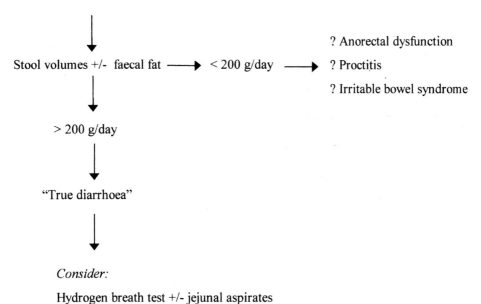

Figure 4.1. Evaluation of the diabetic patient who complains of diarrhoea.

reduce stool number and volume in uncontrolled studies of human diabetic diarrhoea. However, it can cause orthostatic hypotension and sedation.

Diarrhoea associated with autonomic neuropathy and rapid intestinal transit may respond to antidiarrhoeal agents such as loperamide, codeine, or diphenoxylate. Octreotide (50–75 µg two to three times daily) has been used in a few patients with severe diarrhoea resistant to other treatments. The mechanism of action is not entirely clear, but may be related to reduced small-bowel motility. Side effects included hypoglycaemia with reduced insulin requirements and ileus in one patient.

Faecal incontinence

The prevalence of faecal incontinence amongst diabetic patients has probably been underestimated, because of a reluctance by patients to volunteer this symptom, and the failure of physicians to ask patients directly about this problem. Recent studies have found an incidence of 4–20% of unselected diabetic outpatients. Most, but not all, patients with faecal incontinence have chronic diarrhoea and evidence of autonomic neuropathy. Diabetic patients with faecal incontinence have impaired anorectal sensory and motor function, which results from a combination of sensory neuropathy, autonomic denervation, and defects in the smooth muscle itself. In healthy individuals, acute hyperglycaemia to 12 mmol/l inhibits internal and external anal sphincter function and increases rectal sensitivity (14). However, it is not known if chronic hyperglycaemia contributes to anorectal dysfunction in diabetic patients. Management of faecal incontinence involves strict control of blood glucose concentrations, treatment of associated diarrhoea, and biofeedback techniques to modify abnormalities of motor and sensory function.

Liver and biliary function

Gallstones

Diabetic patients have impaired gallbladder contraction and an increase in bile lithogenicity. However, contrary to earlier findings, recent studies have failed to demonstrate an increase in gallstone formation in diabetic patients when results were adjusted for obesity (15). Diabetic patients with acute cholecystitis have a significantly increased morbidity and mortality rate, although this seems to be restricted to those patients with concomitant heart, kidney, and peripheral vascular disease.

"Fatty liver"

Diabetes mellitus is associated with an increased frequency of glycogen deposition within hepatocytes, fatty liver (steatosis), fibrosis, and cirrhosis. The increase in glycogen is believed to be stimulated by excessive exogenous insulin. Accumulation of triglycerides in the cytoplasm of hepatocytes occurs most frequently in patients with Type II diabetes and is related to obesity and excessive ingestion of dietary fat and carbohydrate. In patients with Type I diabetes, fat deposition correlates with poor blood sugar control. Liver biochemistry is usually normal or values are minimally increased in patients with fatty liver. Previously, steatosis was believed to be a benign process, but recent studies suggest that it may progress to fibrosis and, rarely, cirrhosis. Finally, the sulphonylurea drugs may cause cholestasis and, rarely, granulomatous hepatitis.

ADDISON'S DISEASE

Gastrointestinal symptoms are common in patients with adrenocortical insufficiency (Addison's disease) and occur in almost all advanced cases. Nausea, vomiting, abdominal pain, diarrhoea, and constipation occur in about 50% of patients in most series. Anorexia and weight loss are almost invariable. There have been reports of steatorrhoea in Addison's disease, and studies in the adrenalectomized rat have shown a functional defect in enterocytes, which returns to normal after treatment with corticosteroids (16, 17). The diagnosis may be overlooked, particularly when pigmentation or biochemical abnormalities are absent — a feature of about 8% of cases (18). Patients with Addison's disease may also present with an abnormal liver biochemistry. Three patients who underwent investigation for an isolated increase in serum transaminases were found to have Addison's disease; the enzyme concentrations returned to normal in response to corticosteroid treatment (19).

THYROID DISEASE

Thyroid hormones affect the structure or function of most of the gastrointestinal tract and not surprisingly patients with thyroid dysfunction may present with gastrointestinal symptoms.

Hyperthyroidism

Gastrointestinal symptoms and signs in hyperthyroidism include weight loss, change in bowel habit, and steatorrhoea. In addition, there are isolated case reports of patients with thyrotoxicosis presenting with severe abdominal pain and vomiting. Contrary to popular belief, constipation may be more common than diarrhoea in patients with hyperthyroidism (20,21). However, diarrhoea is more frequently reported as a clinical problem. Diarrhoea is believed to be, at least in part, the result of rapid intestinal transit, which reduces the contact time of intestinal contents with absorptive epithelial cells. Intestinal secretion may be another mechanism producing diarrhoea. *In vitro* triiodothyronine binds to erythrocyte membranes, producing an increase in intracellular cyclic adenosine monophosphate. It is possible that triiodothyronine has a similar physiological effect on the intestinal mucosa, and thus acts like other intestinal secretagogues such as vasoactive intestinal polypeptide. Severe watery diarrhoea with stool volumes up to 3 litres a day and unaffected by fasting (suggesting a secretory mechanism) has been described as a presenting feature of thyrotoxicosis; other causes of secretory diarrhoea were excluded, and the diarrhoea resolved when the patient was treated with propylthyrouracil (22). Steatorrhoea is believed to result from a combination of increased intestinal motility and excessive ingestion of dietary fat. There is no evidence that it is due to a primary defect of small intestinal absorptive function or biliary/pancreatic function. In normal individuals, excessive ingestion of dietary fat (300 g/day) may result in steatorrhoea (about 11 g/day). Fat intake in excess of 300 g/day in hyperthyroid patients has been documented, and this may be a major mechanism producing steatorrhoea. However, fat excretion does not always return to normal values with institution of a 100-g fat diet, suggesting that hyperphagia is not the only cause of steatorrhoea. Steatorrhoea is usually mild but, rarely, faecal fat excretion as great as 47 g/day has been documented (23).

Treatment with antithyroid drugs that render the patient euthyroid is associated with normalization of intestinal transit and resolution of diarrhoea and steatorrhoea.

Hypothyroidism

Hypothyroidism is most often attributable to autoimmune thyroiditis, which may be associated with pernicious anaemia, coeliac disease, and autoimmune hepatitis. Impaired gastrointestinal motility may result in constipation, faecal impaction, rectal prolapse and, rarely, intestinal pseudo-obstruction. Mild increases in serum liver enzymes, which return to normal in response to treatment, have been described and are believed to represent altered metabolism of the enzymes, rather than liver damage.

ACROMEGALY

Complications of excessive growth hormone secretion

The major gastrointestinal complication of acromegaly is an increased risk of developing colorectal cancer and adenomatous polyps. Among patients undergoing colonoscopic screening, colonic adenomas were found in 22–26% and colonic cancer in 5% (24,25). Compared with a control population, the odds ratio for colorectal cancer is increased, at 13.5, in those with acromegaly. On the basis of these observations, it has been suggested that surveillance colonoscopy is indicated in this group of patients. Acromegalic patients do not appear to have an increased incidence of gastric tumours.

Complications of octreotide treatment

Patients with acromegaly may have macroglossia, but clinical organomegaly of the liver, spleen, and kidneys is unusual and should warrant further investigations. Other gastrointestinal problems in acromegalic patients usually arise as a complication of treatment with octreotide (a long-acting somatostatin analogue). Octreotide suppresses growth hormone secretion and, in some acromegalic patients, will shrink the pituitary tumour by virtue of the fact that growth hormone-secreting pituitary tumours have a high density of somatostatin receptors. Octreotide is used in the long term in patients who have undergone an unsuccessful transsphenoidal operation or those who are awaiting the therapeutic effect of external pituitary irradiation, or as primary treatment in elderly patients.

Adverse effects of treatment include nausea, abdominal cramps, diarrhoea, fat malabsorption, and flatulence. These symptoms begin within hours of the first subcutaneous injection, but often subside despite continuing treatment. The adverse effects of octreotide can be explained on the basis of the physiological role that endogenous somatostatin plays in normal gastrointestinal tract function, including inhibition of exocrine pancreatic secretion, prolongation of intestinal transit, and inhibition of glucose and amino acid absorption. Cholesterol gallstones develop in 20–30% of patients receiving long-term treatment with octreotide (26). However, prophylactic cholecystectomy is not indicated because, in most cases, gallstones remain asymptomatic and the risks of operation are considered to outweigh any potential benefit. The formation of gallstones during octreotide treatment probably involves inhibition of cholecystokinin secretion and impaired gallbladder emptying, increased cholesterol saturation of bile, and prolongation of intestinal transit, which contributes to the lithogenic changes in bile composition (27). Finally, there are two case reports of acute liver injury developing in acromegalic patients treated with octreotide. In one, abnormalities of serum liver enzymes were noted after the patient received two doses of octreotide, and drug causality was confirmed by re-challenge (28).

Lanreotide is a long-acting form of octreotide that is administered by intramuscular injection every 2 weeks. Treatment is well tolerated, but further studies will be needed to obtain accurate assessments of long-term complications such as gallstone formation.

PARATHYROID DISEASE AND HYPERCALCAEMIA

Primary hyperparathyroidism is usually caused by a single adenoma of the chief cells of the parathyroid. Less commonly, it is due to diffuse hyperplasia or multiple adenomata. Since the introduction of multiple-channel autoanalysers in clinical practice, the most common presentation, in 50–70% of patients, is asymptomatic hypercalcaemia found on blood testing for an unrelated complaint or routine medical examination. The gastrointestinal complications of hyperparathyroidism are due to the associated hypercalcaemia and include nausea, vomiting, constipation, and peptic ulceration. Acute pancreatitis is an uncommon complication of hyperparathyroidism. Many of the earlier studies that suggested a high incidence of acute pancreatitis failed to control for other aetiological factors, such as gallstones and alcohol abuse. Animal experiments suggest that hypercalcaemia causes pancreatitis by activation of pancreatic enzymes.

Hypoparathyroidism most commonly results from damage or removal of the glands during parathyroid or thyroid surgery. Rarely, hypoparathyrodism may result from infiltration of the glands by iron in haemochromatosis, or copper in Wilson's disease. Gastrointestinal manifestations include malabsorption, mild steatorrhoea, constipation and, rarely, pseudo-obstruction. Some patients have gastric atrophy and hypochlorhydria, and oral and oesophageal candidiasis.

MULTIPLE ENDOCRINE NEOPLASIA

Multiple endocrine neoplasia (MEN) is the name given to the synchronous or metachronous (occurring at different times) occurrence of tumours involving a number of endocrine glands (Table 4.6). It is subdivided into MEN types 1, 2A and 2B.

Multiple endocrine neoplasia type 1

MEN1 comprises the association of tumours in the pituitary, and parathyroids, and the pancreatic and intestinal islets. There may also be tumours in the adrenals and thyroid gland. There is an autosomal dominant mode of transmission, with a high degree of penetrance. Occasional sporadic cases arise, suggesting a new mutation. MEN type 1 is caused by a mutation in the *menin* gene on chromosome 11 (29); the normal protein product of this gene may act as a tumour suppressor. Clinical evidence of the disease is not usually manifest until the patient is aged in the early 20s, and presentation may be many years later. One, two, or all three endocrine

Table 4.6.   Multiple endocrine neoplasia (MEN) syndrome.

Organ	Frequency (%)	Tumours/clinical manifestations
Type 1		
Functioning adenomas in:		
Parathyroid	95	Hypercalcaemia
Islets (pancreas and	50	Insulinoma, VIPoma, glucagonoma, gastrinoma
duodenum)		
Pituitary	40	Prolactinoma, acromegaly, Cushing's disease
Adrenal	40	Non-functional adenomas
Thyroid	20	Adenomas — multiple or single
Type 2A		
Medullary thyroid	Most	Thyroid mass, diarrhoea, increased plasma calcitonin
carcinoma		
Adrenal	50	Phaeochromocytoma, Cushing's syndrome
Parathyroid hyperplasia	10	Hypercalcaemia
Type 2B		Like type 2A (but parathyroid disease does not occur),with a typical phenotypic appearance: slim body habitus, cutaneous ganglioneuromas around the lips, tongue, eyelids, and throughout the gastrointestinal tract,especially the large bowel.

VIP, Vasoactive intestinal polypeptide.

sites may be affected. Primary hyperparathyroidism is the most common endocrine abnormality and usually the first to present. Problems associated with islet cell tumours are usually identified in the fourth and fifth decades, and pituitary tumours present in the fifth and sixth decades (30). The diagnosis should be considered in a patient with hyperparathyroidism, islet cell or pituitary tumour who presents at a young age or has a family history of relevant disorders.

Initial treatment of MEN1 is either surgical resection or, sometimes, appropriate medical treatment in the case of multiple tumours of one type — for example, gastrinomas associated with MEN are frequently multiple submucosal tumours within the duodenum, and complete surgical resection may not be possible. In a patient known to have MEN, life-long surveillance for additional features of the disease is required. Depending on the initial presentation and treatment, follow-up would include yearly measurement of serum calcium and prolactin, with 2-yearly magnetic resonance imaging of the pituitary. First-degree relatives should be offered counselling and screening (as for follow-up of affected patients), beginning in early adult life (30). Definitive genetic testing may soon be widely available.

Multiple endocrine neoplasia type 2

The genetic abnormality in MEN2 lies within the *RET* proto-oncogene on chromosome 10. The gene encodes a tyrosine kinase receptor. The most common presentation is with a medullary thyroid carcinoma. Genetic testing is offered to relatives of patients in order to identify affected family members. MEN2B often results from a new mutation and, typically, presents in childhood with locally metastatic thyroid disease or with gastrointestinal symptoms similar to Hirschsprung's disease.

MEASUREMENT OF GASTROINTESTINAL HORMONES

The clinical indications for measurement of circulating hormones include patients with unexplained secretory diarrhoea and patients known or suspected to have MEN. In addition, serum gastrin is measured in patients suspected of having a gastrinoma. The usual hormone screen in a patient with unexplained diarrhoea includes measurement of serum concentrations of vasoactive intestinal polypeptide, glucagon, calcitonin, gastrin, and somatostatin.

Concentrations of one more of these hormones will be increased in patients with diarrhoea resulting from a neuroendocrine tumour. Patients with suspected carcinoid syndrome are investigated with a 24-h urine collection for measurement of 5-hydroxyindole acetic acid, the breakdown product of serotonin. Gastrointestinal hormones, such as gastrin, can usually be detected in small concentrations in peripheral blood of healthy individuals, and concentrations increase in response to eating. Therefore, patients are asked to fast for 10–12 h before blood sampling. Gastric acid antisecretory drugs — for example, proton pump inhibitors and H_2 antagonists, induce a release of gastrin into the circulation and serum gastrin values may increase to values approaching those usually associated with gastrinomas. The more potent the antisecretory drug, the greater the increase in serum gastrin concentration. Patients who are found to have increased fasting gastrin concentrations while taking antisecretory drugs will need to be re-tested after stopping treatment for 2–4 weeks.

Many gastrointestinal hormones are rapidly degraded in serum; therefore, after collection, the serum should be separated as soon as possible (within minutes) by centrifugation, and frozen immediately. A telephone call to the laboratory to warn of the arrival of samples is a sensible precaution. Collected blood should be stored on ice until centrifugation if a delay is expected.

In healthy individuals, average fasting serum gastrin concentrations are usually less than 60 pg/ml. Patients with gastrinoma almost always have markedly increased fasting serum gastrin concentrations (>1000 pg/ml); however, a few patients with gastrinoma do not exhibit such high values. Patients in whom a gastrinoma is strongly suspected, but who do not have greatly increased plasma concentrations (<1000 pg/ml) should undergo a secretin test. Patients with gastrinoma have a paradoxical increase in serum gastrin after intravenous injection of secretin; in healthy persons and patients with a straightforward duodenal ulcer, the gastrin response is decreased, unchanged, or slightly increased. Blood for measurement of serum gastrin is taken 5 min before an intravenous injection of secretin (Pure porcine secretin, 2 units/kg over 30 s) and then at 5 min intervals after injection for 30 min. In patients with gastrinoma, serum gastrin increases promptly, by at least 200 pg/ml.

DISORDERS OF BODY WEIGHT REGULATION

Under stable conditions, most adults maintain a relatively narrow range of body weight, despite psychological and environmental influences. Energy intake and body weight are regulated precisely by chemical, endocrine, and neuroregulatory pathways (31) acting both peripherally and centrally, and appear to be governed by a combination of short-term mechanisms originating in the gastrointestinal tract and long-term processes that monitor fat mass, integration of these signals occurring predominantly in the hypothalamus of the brain.

Self-reported food intake in obese persons would suggest that obesity results entirely from a reduction in energy expenditure, because they invariably report low levels of energy intake. However, total energy expenditure is, in reality, substantially increased (presumably affecting the higher energy cost of weight-bearing activities) in obese adults and children. At the other end of the spectrum, weight loss is an integral feature of anorexia nervosa, and wasting is a common accompaniment to many chronic inflammatory conditions, cancer, and advanced human immunodeficiency virus infection. Weight loss is believed to be due to loss of appetite and reduced energy intake, because total energy expenditure (when measured) has not been shown to be increased.

In summary, in virtually all cases, **obesity and various weight losing conditions are explained entirely by an increase or decrease in energy intake**. The metabolism is not to blame; total energy expenditure is appropriate for the body weight.

Obesity

Obesity, defined as an excess of body fat contributing to comorbidity, is a common problem in developed countries. A body mass index (BMI: body weight/(height)^2, measured as kg/m^2) of 25 kg/m^2 or greater is a standard commonly used to define obesity. The acceptable range of BMI is 20–25 kg/m^2 for men and 19—24 kg/m^2 for women. Several conditions and complications are associated with obesity (32):

* Ischaemic heart disease
* Hypertension

- Diabetes mellitus
- Hyperlipidaemia
- Obstructive sleep apnoea
- Symptomatic heartburn, but 24-h pH monitoring similar to controls
- Fatty liver
- Gallstones
- Abdominal wall hernias
- Postoperative problems
- Osteoarthritis
- Increase incidence of malignancy
  — Colon, oesophagus, breast, endometrium, ovary, prostate
- Depression and psychiatric problems

Histological **liver abnormalities** are a common finding in obese patients. Liver biopsy specimens taken from morbidly obese patients undergoing Roux-en-Y gastric bypass revealed histological abnormalities in almost all patients, ranging from mild fatty infiltration, through inflammatory changes, to fibrosis and cirrhosis (33). The fat deposits comprise triglycerides, fatty acids, and mono- and diglycerides. The mechanism of fatty change in obese individuals is not clear, but may be related to their diet, which tends to be low in protein and high in carbohydrate and fat. Fatty liver may be associated with hepatomegaly and slight increases in the serum liver enzymes, but jaundice or features of hepatic cell failure should not be ascribed to fatty liver in this group of patients. Diagnosis of fatty liver is by ultrasound examination. The fat content in obese patients is reduced by weight loss and near-normal liver histology is observed in obese subjects who lose weight and subsequently maintain a near normal weight.

The risk of **gallstone** formation is increased about three-fold over that of a control population. This increased risk is believed to result from impaired gallbladder motility and changes in biliary lipid composition. Obese subjects are also at increased risk of gallstone formation during dieting, particularly with very low calorie diets (800 kcal/day). This is related to increased cholesterol saturation of bile, and gallbladder stasis as a result of a decrease in meal-stimulated release of cholecystokinin. Gallstone formation can be prevented during dieting by prophylactic use of ursodeoxycholic acid (10–15 mg/kg), which decreases bile lithogenicity, or diets that contain a minimum of 15–25 g fat in order to stimulate gallbladder contraction. Acute gallstone pancreatitis tends to have a worse outcome in obese patients. Hypertriglyceridaemia is also a risk factor for acute pancreatitis, but the serum concentrations of triglycerides in obesity do not usually attain the very high values associated with pancreatitis.

Epidemiological studies suggest an increased incidence of some malignancies, including colon cancer, in obese individuals. However, obesity may merely be a surrogate marker for other risk factors, including a high-fat, energy-dense diet, reduced consumption of fruit and vegetables, and lack of physical activity, all of which have been associated with an increased risk of colon cancer (34). No studies have adequately examined these confounding influences.

Anorexia nervosa

Anorexia nervosa is a psychological illness, predominantly affecting young females and characterized by marked weight loss (BMI <17.5 kg/m^2), intense fear of gaining weight, a distorted body image, and amennorhoea. Patients with anorexia nervosa control their body weight by a process of semi-starvation and may develop complications as a result of this. Gastrointestinal symptoms are common in patients with anorexia nervosa and include abdominal pain, vomiting, and bloating. These may be related to an antral motility disturbance and delay in gastric emptying. Slow colonic transit and severe constipation are also common in patients with anorexia nervosa (35). These abnormalities are corrected by improved nutrition and weight gain.

Refeeding severely malnourished patients can be associated with complications, particularly during the first week of therapy (36). Refeeding with carbohydrates stimulates insulin release and uptake of phosphate into cells, with a decrease in serum phosphate concentrations. Severe hypophosphataemia is associated with muscle weakness, paresthesias, fits, coma, and cardiac arrhythmias. Serum magnesium and potassium concentrations may also decrease, as a result of hyperinsulinaemia, stimulation of protein synthesis, and an increase in body cell mass. Other complications include hyperglycaemia and renal retention of sodium and water, which may result in congestive cardiac failure. Individual requirements vary, but during the first week of feeding a reasonable daily regimen includes 800 ml water plus insensible losses, 60 mmol sodium, 1.2–1.5 g/kg protein and 150 g carbohydrate, contributing to a total calorie intake of 20 kcal/kg. Phosphate, potassium, and magnesium supplements should be commenced early, and intake of vitamin and mineral adjusted to meet normal daily requirements.

Gastrointestinal diseases such as coeliac disease, pancreatic insufficiency, and inflammatory bowel disease may also present with abdominal pain, bloating, and extreme weight loss. However, unlike the patient with an eating disorder, in these patients there is no morbid preoccupation with food, and laboratory investigations may be abnormal — for example, the presence of anaemia, leucocytosis, hypoalbuminaemia, and increased erythrocyte sedimentation rate.

In contrast to the patient with anorexia nervosa, patients with bulimia nervosa have repeated episodes of binge eating and, in an attempt to control their weight, they induce vomiting and ingest diuretics and laxatives. The complications of bulimia arise as a result of the physical and metabolic derangements of binging and purging. These include dental caries, gum disease, parotid enlargement, oesophagitis, Mallory–Weiss tear, and oesophageal rupture. Metabolic abnormalities include hypokalaemia, hypochloraemic metabolic alkalosis, and hypophosphataemia.

HYPERLIPIDAEMIA

Gastrointestinal complaints in the patient with hyperlipidaemia are usually a complication of drug treatment. The exception is acute pancreatitis, which is an uncommon complication in patients with hypertriglyceridaemia (usually >10 mmol/l) and is believed to be due to small-vessel damage and pancreatic ischaemia secondary to the release of free fatty acids from triglycerides caused by lipase in the pancreatic microcirculation (37).

Gastrointestinal side effects of lipid-decreasing drugs

Three classes of drug are in common use in the UK: bile-acid sequestrating agents, 3-hydroxy-3-methylglutaryl coenzyme A (HMG CoA), reductase inhibitors, and the fibrate drugs.

Bile-acid sequestrating agents

Agents such as cholestyramine and colestipol are indicated in the treatment of hypercholesterolaemia in the absence of hypertriglyceridaemia, which they may exacerbate. Gastrointestinal side effects are the most commonly reported side effects and include nausea, flatulence, heartburn, abdominal bloating, and alteration in bowel habit.

Statins

Statins (e.g. simvastatin, pravastatin, and atorvastatin) competitively inhibit HMG CoA, an enzyme involved in cholesterol synthesis, especially in the liver. They are very effective in decreasing low-density lipoprotein cholesterol and total plasma cholesterol. The most common gastrointestinal side effects in patients taking statins are nausea, abdominal pain, flatulence, constipation, and diarrhoea. These are often mild and self-limiting. The most worrisome side effects associated with statin treatment have been hepatic toxicity and myopathy. Liver inflammation, indicated by increases in serum transaminase concentrations to greater than three times the upper limit of normal, occurs in fewer than 1% of patients receiving starting doses of statins, and in up to 2% who receive a maximum dose. In some of the trials, these figures are no greater than those in the placebo treated group. However, when these effects occur they are reversible either spontaneously, by a reduction in dose, or after discontinuation of treatment. No permanent liver damage has been reported as a result of statin treatment. It is recommended that the patient's liver biochemistry is checked before they start treatment, after 4–8 weeks, and then at 1 year unless the dose is increased. The dose should be reduced if there is an increase in serum liver enzymes. In preclinical studies, lovastatin produced hepatocellular adenomas and carcinomas when given in very high doses (38). However, results from several randomized clinical trials with simvastatin and pravastatin have not shown any increase in malignant neoplasms during treatment periods of from 5 to 6 years (39,40).

Fibrates

The fibrates include benzafibrate, ciprofibrate, fenofibrate, gemfibrozil, and clofibrate. Their exact mechanism of action is unknown, but their main effect is to decrease serum triglycerides. Clofibrate is associated with an increased risk of causing gallstones and is now only used in patients who have had a cholecystectomy. Gastrointestinal problems in patients treated with this class of drug include nausea, abdominal discomfort, and a change in bowel habit. As with the statins, liver changes in rodents have included the development of hepatic adenomas and carcinomas in association with very high doses of fibrates (38), but there appears to be no increased risk to patients treated with fibrates. Hepatitis, which resolved with discontinuation of the drug, has been described during treatment with clofibrate. The hepatitis recurred when the patient was re-challenged with fenofibrate (41).

References
*Of interest; **of exceptional interest
1. Falchuk KR, Conlin D. The intestinal and liver complications of diabetes mellitus. *Adv Int Med* 1993; **38**: 269–287.
    One of the very few relatively recent reviews of the gut and diabetes mellitus. Provides a comprehensive review of complications and an approach to the management.
2. Iber FL, Parveen S, Vandrunen M *et al.* Relation of symptoms to impaired stomach, small bowel, and colon motility in long-standing diabetes. *Dig Dis Sci* 1993; **38**: 45–50.
3. Janatuinen E, Pikkarainen P, Laakso M *et al.* Gastrointestinal symptoms in middle-aged diabetic patients. *Scand J Gastroenterol* 1993; **28**: 427–432.
4. Horowitz M, Maddox AF, Wishart JM *et al.* Relationships between oesophageal transit and solid and liquid gastric emptying in diabetes mellitus. *Eur J Nucl Med* 1991; **18**: 229–234.
5. Mosoco GJ, Driver M, Guy RJ. A form of necrobiosis and atrophy of smooth muscle in diabetic autonomic neuropathy. *Pathol Res Pract* 1996; **181**: 188–194.
6. *Fraser R, Horowitz M, Dent J. Hyperglycaemia stimulates pyloric motility in normal subjects. *Gut* 1991; **32**: 475–478.
    Fasting gastroduodenal manometry was performed during euglycaemia and hyperglycaemia (12–16 mmol/l) induced by intravenous dextrose in healthy volunteers. During hyperglycaemia, there was stimulation of pyloric contractions and inhibition of antral contractions.
7. *Samsom M, Akkermans LM, Jebbink RJ *et al.* Gastrointestinal motor mechanisms in hyperglycaemia induced delayed gastric emptying in type 1 diabetes mellitus. *Gut* 1997; **40**: 641–646.
    Antroduodenal manometry and scintigraphic measurement of gastric emptying of a mixed solid–liquid meal was measured during euglycaemia and induced hyperglycaemia in diabetic patients with autonomic neuropathy. Hyperglycaemia reduced antral motility and delayed gastric emptying of the solid, but not the liquid meal.
8. McCallum RW, Chen J, Lin Z *et al.* Gastric pacing improves emptying and symptoms in patients with gastroparesis. *Gastroenterology* 1998; **114**: 456–461.
9. Valdovinos MA, Camilleri M, Zimmerman BR. Chronic diarrhoea in diabetes mellitus: mechanisms and an approach to diagnosis and treatment. *Mayo Clin Proc* 1993; **68**: 691–702.
    Causes of diarrhoea were assessed retrospectively in 33 patients with diabetes at a tertiary referral centre. Small bowel bacterial overgrowth was identified as a definite or possible cause of diarrhoea in 24% of patients, and coeliac disease as a definite or possible cause in 12%.
10. Chang EB, Bergenstal RM, Field M. Diarrhoea in streptozotocin-treated rats: loss of adrenergic regulation of intestinal fluid and electrolyte transport. *J Clin Invest* 1985; **75**: 1666–1670.
11. Badiga MS, Jain NK, Casanova C *et al.* Diarrhoea in diabetics: the role of sorbitol. *J Am Coll Nutr* 1990; **9**: 578–582.
12. Cronin CC, Fergus S. Insulin-dependent diabetes mellitus and coeliac disease. *Lancet* 1997; **349**: 1096–1097.
13. Kandemir O, Utas C, Gonen O *et al.* Colonic subepithelial collagenous thickening in diabetic patients. *Dis Colon Rectum* 1995; **38**: 1097–1100.
14. Russo A, Sun WM, Sattawatthamrong Y *et al.* Acute hyperglycaemia affects anorectal motor and sensory function in normal subjects. *Gut* 1997; **41**: 944–949.
15. Ikard R. Gallstones, cholecystitis and diabetes. *Surg Gynecol Obstet* 1990; **171**: 528–532.
16. Guarini G, Macaluso M. Steatorrhoea in Addison's disease. *Lancet* 1963; **2**: 955–956.
17. Bavetta L, Hallman L, Deuel HJ *et al.* The effect of adrenalectomy on fat absorption. *Am J Physiol* 1941; **134**: 619–622.
18. Brosnan CM, Gowing NFC. Lesson of the week: Addison's disease. *BMJ* 1996; **312**: 1085–1087.
19. Olsson RG, Lindgren A, Zettergren L. Liver involvement in Addison's disease. *Am J Gastroenterol* 1990; **85**: 435–8.
20. Scarf M. Gastrointestinal manifesations of hyperthyroidism. *J Lab Clin Med* 1936; **21**: 1253–1258.
21. Shirer JW. Hypermotility of the gastrointestinal tract in hyperthyroidism. *Am J Med Sci* 1933; **186**: 73–78.
22. Culp KS, Piziak VK. Thyrotoxicosis presenting with secretory diarrhoea. *Ann Intern Med* 1986; **105**: 216–217.
23. Sheehy TW, Allison TM. Apathetic thyrotoxicosis causing gastrointestinal malabsorption. *JAMA* 1974; **230**: 69–71.
24. Jenkins PJ, Fairclough PD, Richards T *et al.* Acromegaly, colonic polyps and carcinoma. *Clin Endocrinol* 1997; **47**: 17–22.
    A prospective study of 129 patients with acromegaly who underwent colonosocpic screening by a single skilled endoscopist. Colon cancer was present in six (5%) patients, only two of whom had symptoms. One or more tubulovillous adenomas was found in 26% of patients. There was no difference in disease duration or growth hormone concentrations in patients with and without tumours.
25. Delhougne B, Deneux C, Abs R *et al.* The prevalence of colonic polyps in acromegaly: a colonoscopic and pathological study in 103 patients. *J Clin Endocrinol Metab* 1995; **80**: 3223–3226.
26. Acromegaly Therapy Consensus Development Panel. Benefits versus risks of medical therapy for acromegaly. *Am J Med* 1994; **97**: 468–473.
27. *Hussaini SH, Pereira SP, Veysey MJ *et al.* Role of gallbladder emptying and intestinal transit in the pathogenesis of octreotide induced gallbladder stones. *Gut* 1996; **38**: 775–783.

A single dose of octreotide inhibited meal-stimulated gall-bladder emptying in healthy controls, untreated acromegalics, and acromegalic patients receiving long-term octreotide treatment. Single-dose octreotide also prolonged small-bowel transit time in controls individuals, untreated acromegalics, and acromegalics receiving long-term treatment with octreotide. In the last group, single-dose octreotide prolonged mouth-to-caecum transit time from 170 to 247 min.

28. Gonzalez-Martin JA, Donnay S, Morillas J *et al.* Acute liver injury and octreotide. *Am J Gastroenterol* 1996; **91**: 2434–2435.

29. Chandrasekharappa SC, Guru SC, Manickam P *et al.* Positional cloning of the gene for multiple endocrine neoplasia – type 1. *Science* 1997; **267**: 404–407.

30. Franklyn J, Stewart PM. Multiple endocrine neoplasia. *J R Coll Physicians Lond* 1998; **32**: 98–101.

31. Ballinger AB, Clark ML. Nutrition, appetite control and disease. In: J Payne-James, G Grimble, D Silk. *Artificial Nutrition Support in Clinical Practice*, 2nd edn. Greenwich Medical Media Ltd., in press.

32. Jung RT. Obesity as a disease. *Br Med Bull* 1997; **53**: 307–321.

33. Klain J, Fraser D, Goldstein J *et al.* Liver histology abnormalities in the morbid obese. *Hepatology* 1989; **10**: 873–876.

34. Shike M. Body weight and colon cancer. *Am J Clin Nutr* 1996; **63**: 442S–444S.

35. Chun AB, Sokol MS, Kaye WH *et al.* Colonic and anorectal function in constipated patients with anorexia nervosa. *Am J Gastroenterol* 1997; **92**: 1879–1883.

36. Kohn MR, Golden NH, Shenker IR. Cardiac arrest and delerium: presentations of the refeeding syndrome in severely malnourished adolescents with anorexia nervosa. *J Adolesc Health* 1998; **22**: 239–243.

37. Havel RJ. Pathogenesis, differentiation and management of hypertriglyceridaemia. *Adv Intern Med* 1969; **15**: 117–154.

38. Newman TB, Hulley SB. Carcinogenicity of lipid lowering agents. *JAMA* 1996; **275**: 55–60.

39. Scandinavian Simvastatin Survival Study Group. Randomised trial of cholesterol lowering in 4444 patients with coronary heart disease: the Scandinavian Simvastatin Survival Study (4S). *Lancet* 1994; **344**: 1383–1389.

40. Shepherd J, Cobbe SM, Ford I *et al.* Prevention of coronary heart disease with pravastatin in men with hypercholesterolaemia. *N Engl J Med* 1995; **333**: 1301–1307.

41. Migneco G, Mascarella A, La Ferla A *et al.* Clofibrate hepatitis. A case report. *Minerva Med* 1986; **77**: 799–800.

5. Gastrointestinal Problems in Haematology Patients

BRIAN J. HENNESSY and ATUL B. MEHTA

GASTROINTESTINAL TOXICITY RELATED TO THE TREATMENT OF HAEMATOLOGICAL MALIGNANCY

Gastrointestinal toxicity associated with intensive treatment regimens for haematological malignancies is second in frequency and severity only to bone marrow suppression caused by such treatments. The high turnover of gut epithelium renders it exquisitely sensitive to acute toxicity from chemoradiotherapy. The resultant mucositis can affect the whole gastrointestinal tract, to cause pain, vomiting, diarrhoea, bleeding, and infection. Some forms of treatment for haematology patients (e.g. allogeneic bone marrow transplantation) can cause chronic gastrointestinal toxicity (e.g. hepatitis, graft versus host disease (GVHD), malabsorption).

Pathological processes

Mucositis

Chemotherapeutic agents vary in the degree of mucositis they cause. Etoposide, melphalan, busulphan, high-dose cyclophosphamide, and total body irradiation (particularly single fraction) are prone to cause mucositis; combination treatment increases the risk and severity of mucositis. The whole gastrointestinal tract can be affected. **Neutrophils** have a key role in healing mucositis, as indicated by its rapid resolution once neutrophils reappear in the peripheral blood. Shortening the duration of neutro-

penia by the use of granulocyte-colony stimulating factor (G-CSF) also results in more rapid healing of mucositis.

Oropharyngeal mucositis caused by chemoradiotherapy can be exacerbated by other factors such as minor trauma, infection (caused by normal commensal organisms and acquired pathogens), GVHD, and xerostomia (resulting from salivary gland dysfunction). Gum infiltration at presentation (Figure 5.1) occurs in monocytic varieties of acute leukaemia (FAB subtype M4 and M5). Prophylactic management consists of good oral hygiene such as dental review before high-dose treatment, rinses with chlorhexidine mouthwash, fungal prophylaxis with topical nystatin or mycostatin or systemic fluconazole, and shortening

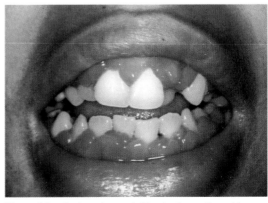

Figure 5.1. Leukaemic gum infiltration in a patient with acute monoblastic leukaemia.

the duration of neutropenia. In severe cases, oral therapy with mucosal coating agents such as sucralfate, alginate sodium, and antacid solutions may give added protection and symptomatic relief. Cryotherapy with fine ice chips held in the mouth during, for example, methotrexate administration will induce local vasoconstriction and decrease access of methotrexate to the mucosa. Topical analgesia of established mucositis with anaesthetics such as lignocaine gel, cocaine mouthwash, or benzydamine hydrochloride (Difflam) mouthrinse is frequently sufficient in mild to moderate cases; continuous systemic narcotic analgesia may be required. Specific approaches used in GVHD of the mouth include mouthwashes with cyclosporin or G-CSF, or systemic treatment with thalidomide. Mucositis of the oesophagus and the stomach causes ulceration, pain, dysphagia, and blood loss. Antacids provide symptomatic relief but, by decreasing the pH, can promote fungal colonization predisposing to potential systemic infection. Mucositis of the small and large bowel causes malabsorption and diarrhoea.

Colitis

Neutropenic enterocolitis (typhlitis) is a caecitis that often presents with pain and tenderness in the right iliac fossa, mimicking appendicitis. Signs of peritonism may be present, but do not necessarily indicate perforation. It is probably the result of direct bacterial invasion of the colon, with local release of enterotoxin and direct toxic mucosal necrosis. A combination of mucositis, neutropenia, and local infection is the likely triad of causative factors. *Clostridium septicum* has been implicated, but other bacteria, fungal, or viral infection may be causative. Plain X-ray of the abdomen may show a right-sided soft tissue density attributable to caecal dilatation. Endoscopy will reveal multiple ulcerated lesions, with necrosis and haemorrhage. Awareness of this clinical diagnosis is essential so that antibiotic treatment can be instituted and life-threatening surgery can be avoided. Intensive antibiotic treatment with aminoglycosides and metronidazole is sufficient, particularly if neutrophil recovery is impending, but the use of G-CSF and neutrophil transfusion should be considered in severe cases. Close clinical review is required to detect progressive signs, and a daily erect chest X-ray is advised, to obtain evidence of pneumoperitoneum. However, surgery may be required, with subtotal colectomy and ileostomy formation.

Gas-forming clostridial species often supervene in neutropenic colitis, producing an intense acute necrotizing fasciitis through adjacent tissue planes. Wide surgical debridement of necrotic fascia may be required, with high-dose penicillin and hyperbaric oxygen treatment. Mortality is high.

Pseudomembranous colitis is relatively common because of the intense antibiotic treatment of neutropenic patients. Diagnosis is based on the presence of profuse, often bloody diarrhoea and isolation of *Clostridium difficile* toxin. Endoscopy, if performed, will show characteristic endoscopic and histological features.

Cytomegalovirus (CMV) colitis is uncommon except in allograft recipients, and presents as abdominal pain and diarrhoea. Endoscopy may reveal inflammation and often deep ulceration, but may be macroscopically normal. There is a risk of procedure-related or spontaneous perforation. Biopsy should be taken from the ulcer edge and random tissue, and may reveal CMV-infected cells.

Graft versus host disease of the bowel

Both acute and, to a lesser extent chronic GVHD are associated with colitis and severe, high-volume diarrhoea — often more than 1.5 litre per day. Acute GVHD may present as haemorrhagic colitis. The presence of crypt cell apoptosis on biopsy will help to distinguish between this condition and infarction. CMV infection causes similar histological appearances. Lymphocyte marker studies show an increase in CD57[+] and CD8[+] lymphoid cells and a decrease in CD4[+] T cells (1). Acute GVHD of the bowel generally resolves with immunosuppression. Extensive chronic GVHD can involve the bowel with segmental focal fibrosis of the lamina propria and submucosa, with stricture formation. Oesophageal involvement occurs in 6% of patients with chronic GVHD and presents with dysphagia, oesophageal reflux, and substernal pain. Histological changes in the colon can also resemble quiescent chronic inflammatory bowel disease. Colonic involvement causes diarrhoea, abdominal pain, and malabsortion. Management includes immunosuppression, nutritional support, and, occasionally, endoscopic dilatation of strictures, although there is a risk of rupture with this last approach. Treatment with anti-Tumor Necrosis Factor (TNF) antibodies may be of benefit.

Pancreatitis

Pancreatitis is uncommon after bone marrow transplantation, with a reported incidence of less than 5%. However, at post-morten examination, pancreatitis was found in 28% of patients in a recent series (2). The aetiology is likely to be multifactorial, with toxicity of the conditioning regimen, immunosuppressive drugs, lipids in total parental nutrition (TPN), infection, and possibly GVHD as contributing factors. Gallbladder sludge is frequently seen on ultrasound, and may be causative in pancreatitis and cholecystitis. Viral pancreatitis is rare; CMV, adenovirus, and varicella zoster are the main viruses implicated. Pancreatitis should be included in the differential diagnosis of abdominal pain and serum amylase concentrations should be checked; they are high after conditioning radiotherapy, because of the salivary gland isoenzyme. Management is conservative with gut rest, TPN, analgesia, maintenance of a strict fluid balance, and glucose monitoring.

Exocrine pancreatic insufficiency occurs in Schwachman—Diamond syndrome along with somatic abnormalities and bone marrow dysfunction. It is an inherited (autosomal recessive) syndrome of bone marrow failure, which manifests early in infancy with signs of pancreatic insufficiency. There is a high incidence of transformation to myelodysplasia and acute myeloid leukaemia.

Symptoms

Nausea and Vomiting

Nausea and vomiting are multifactorial and contributory factors include chemoradiotherapy, other medications (e.g. antimicrobials, analgesics, and immunosuppressive agents), GVHD of liver and gut, and infections.

The **emetogenic potential of chemotherapeutic agents** varies according to the drug combination, dose, schedule, patient characteristics, and effectiveness of the antiemetic treatment. Emesis can be severe, acute, anticipatory, or delayed. High doses of cyclophosphamide, melphalan, and cytosine arabinoside are highly emetogenic, as are standard doses of anthracyclines, platinums, and lomustine. In contrast, vinca alkaloids, etoposide, and chlorambucil are of low emetogenic potential.

Antiemetics such as serotonin $5HT_3$ receptor (5-hydroxytryptamine) antagonists (ondansetron, granisetron, and tropisetron) have significantly improved the quality of life of cancer patients. Other useful antiemetic agents include standard agents such as domperidone, metoclopromide, lorazepam, and dexamethasone. They may be used alone or as part of combination therapy, tailored according to the emetogenic potential of the chemotherapy regimen. Lorazepam is useful in anticipatory vomiting, whereas dexamethasone is effective in delayed emesis. Side effects of antiemetic treatment include constipation and headache ($5HT_3$ antagonists), extrapyramidal reactions (metoclopromide, domperidone), increased risk of fungal infections and hyperglycaemia (dexamethasone), and drowsiness (lorazepam).

Mucosal trauma to the midbody of the stomach is the most common cause of **coffee-ground vomitus**. Mallory–Weiss tears at the gastrooesophageal junction result in more severe bleeding, especially in severely thrombocytopenic patients. Persistent nausea and vomiting post transplantation is usually due to acute GVHD, herpes simplex virus (HSV), or CMV infection of the gastrointestinal tract, or certain medications (e.g. antimicrobial agents).

Constipation

Vincristine-induced autonomic neuropathy and gut hypomotility can result in severe constipation and ileus. Constipation frequently complicates the use of opiate analagesics particularly in myeloma patients. Attentive, and sometimes aggressive, laxative treatment is required. Combination laxative regimens such as a stimulant and an osmotic laxative are frequently effective. No patient should begin to take a long-term slow release morphine preparation without appropriate laxative cover.

Diarrhoea

Diarrhoea after chemotherapy or transplant conditioning can be particularly severe. Judicious management of fluid balance and electrolytes is required. The principal cause is mucosal damage. Contributory factors include pseudomembranous colitis or other infection, medication (e.g. nonabsorbable antibiotics), and acute or chronic GVHD. Stool culture is mandatory, and antidiarrhoeal compounds should be withheld until culture results are available. Severe secretory diarrhoea has a limited response to loperamide. Octreotide may be useful in refractory, persistent cases.

Bleeding

Contributory factors in bleeding include mucosal trauma from retching, mucositis, thrombocytopenia, coagulopathy, infection, and GVHD. Correction of thrombocytopenia and coagulopathy is generally sufficient. Appropriate endoscopic investigation is important in severe cases.

Gastric antral vascular ectasia is a recently recognised cause of severe upper intestinal bleeding in transplant recipients. Diffuse areas of haemorrhage in the gastric antrum and proximal duodenum with intact underlying mucosa may be present at endoscopy. Mucosal biopsy is diagnostic with thrombosis in abnormal dilated capillaries and fibromuscular hyperplasia in the lamina propria. Treatment is with endoscopic laser therapy. Iatrogenic causes of bleeding include endoscopic biopsy of duodenal mucosa. The incidence of significant bleeding including intramural duodenal hematomas is unacceptably high. Platelet counts should be $>50 \times 10^9$/dl and maintained at this level for at least three days.

Abdominal pain (Table 5.1)

Specific causes of abdominal pain in haematology patients are outlined in Table 5.1. Surgical intervention in the cytopenic patient is associated with greater morbidity and mortality. Radiological investigation and conservative management are, fortunately, frequently sufficient. Dysphagia in a neutropenic patient warrants investigation if it does not settle with simple measures. Important causes include mucositis, acid/peptic oesophagitis, GVHD, and infections (fungal, especially candida (Figures 5.2 and 5.3) and viral (HSV, CMV)).

Ileus

Ileus frequently develops in patients treated with high dose chemotherapy. It is commonly iatrogenic and causes significant morbidity in neutropenic patients. The **causes of ileus in haematology patients** include:

* medication — opiate anagesics, vinca alkaloids
* severe sepsis
* acute GVHD of gut
* electrolyte imbalance, especially hypokalemia
* intestinal infection, including CMV enteritis and candida enteritis
* pancreatitis

Perianal problems

Approximately 6% of patients with leukemia will develop perianal problems at some point in their treatment (3). A history of previous anorectal problems is the single biggest risk factor. Constipation, often induced by narcotic analgesics, may lead to the development of hemorrhoids. Use of suppositories may lead to bacteremia. Perianal sepsis may be an initial presenting complaint of acute leukemia. Subepithelial leukemic infiltrates, often after an initiating event such as a small tear, are well documented, but biopsy is rarely indicated, as risks of infection and poor healing generally outweigh benefits. Neutropenia predisposes to poor localization of infection, absence of pus, local tissue destruction, necrotizing fasciitis, fistula formation, ulceration, and even systemic infection. Recovery of neutrophils can result in extensive local inflammation and abscess formation.

Organisms responsible are those present in stool, *Escherichia coli, Pseudomonas spp.* and *Enterobacter cloacae* being the most common. Candida and HSV infection are less common. Conservative treatment is

Table 5.1. Causes of abdominal pain in haematology patients, classified as causes in transplant/chemotherapy patients and in non-transplantation groups.

Transplant groups	Peptic ulceration
	Intestinal infection
	Visceral varicella zoster
	Neutropenic typhlitis
	Liver disease (VOD — veno-occlusive disease)
	Pancreatitis
	Gallbladder disease
	GVHD (graft-versus-host disease)
	Hemorrhagic cystitis
	Bleeding into retroperitoneum or rectus sheath
Non-transplant groups	Mesenteric thrombosis with bowel infarction e.g. thrombophilia, thrombocytosis, paroxysysmal nocturnal hemoglobinuria
	Abdominal crisis in sickle-cell anemia
	Splenic infarction (e.g. sickle-cell anemia, thrombocytosis)
	Acute intermittent porphyria
	Lead poisoning
	Lymphomas
	Hemochromatosis
	Familial mediterranean fever (recurrent polyserositis)

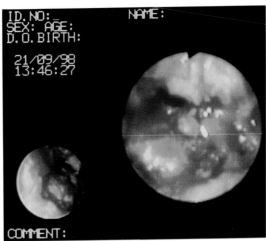

Figure 5.3. Endoscopic picture of fungal oesophagitis (*Candida glabrata*).

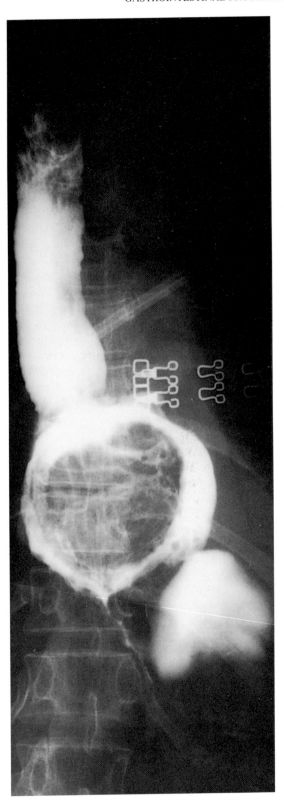

Figure 5.2. Barium swallow in a patient with a fungal ball (*Candida glabrata*) in the oesophagus.

sufficient in the majority of patients. Appropriate systemic antibiotic cover usually includes an aminoglycoside combined with an antipseudomonal agent, and anaerobic cover includes a third-generation cephalosporin (ceftazadime) or piperacillin derivative (piperacillin, tazobactam).

Careful local cleaning, stool softeners if appropriate, and analgesia aid comfort and healing. Haemopoietic growth factors (G-CSF or granulocyte macrophage-colony stimulating factor (GM-CSF)) to accelerate neutrophil recovery should be considered, as the theoretical risk of stimulating the leukaemic clone is small and unproven compared with the definite benefit of shortening the duration of neutropenia. Neutrophil transfusion therapy may be of short-term benefit. Surgery is best withheld until recovery of bone marrow function, but may be required in the case of fluctuance, development of necrotic tissue, progression of infection, and failed medical treatment. Colostomy is necessary in more severe cases, to divert faeces, facilitate healing, and prevent recurrence.

Management

Endoscopy in neutropenic patients

Endoscopic procedures can be safely carried out in neutropenic patients by an experienced operator. Prophylactic antibiotics are unproven, but advisable. Severe thrombocytopenia should be corrected, aiming for a platelet count greater than 50×10^9/dl, particularly if biopsy is required. Endoscopy should not be deferred pending recovery of neutropenia, as it provides rapid macroscopic and tissue diagnosis of infection (Figure 5.3) and GVHD. Oesophageal mucosa can be friable, and care should be taken at intubation, to prevent laryngopharyngeal bleeding and oedema. Patients are often too unwell to tolerate large-volume oral bowel preparation; in sick patients with diarrhoea, the procedure can usually be performed without bowel preparation. The colonic wall can be ulcerated and very thin, particularly in viral colitis, severe GVHD, and neutropenic colitis (4). As little air as possible should be instilled, as overdistension can lead to perforation.

Gastrointestinal problems before treatment

Diseases of the gastrointestinal tract and liver may cause problems after high-dose treatment, and should be investigated and treated, if possible, before chemotherapy and transplant conditioning. Upper gastrointestinal dyspepsia and symptoms characteristic of peptic ulceration or inflammation should be investigated. In immunocompromised patients, these symptoms may have an infectious aetiology. Two rare conditions, basophilic leukaemia and systemic mastocytosis, have a greater association with peptic ulceration, as a result of the increased concentrations of histamine. *Helicobacter pylori*, if present, should be treated, although there is no evidence that this infection can disseminate during the neutropenic phase.

Inflammatory bowel disease should, if possible, be in remission before treatment is instituted to reduce the risk of bleeding from ulcerated lesions. Both Crohn's disease and ulcerative colitis improve in the period immediately after chemotherapy and transplant, as a result of intensive immunosuppression. In patients with a history of severe recurrent perianal sepsis, serious consideration should be given to performing a colostomy before the commencement of high-dose treatment, with a view to reversing the colostomy on recovery.

Patients with lymphoma, relapsed leukaemia, or breast cancer can have bowel involvement. Cytotoxic treatment leading to tumour cell necrosis can, rarely, lead to bowel perforation.

Patients with chronic diarrhoea should be investigated for organisms that can disseminate during immunosuppression. Intestinal parasites such as *Enterobacter histolytica* and *Strongyloides* can cause death in immunocompromised hosts.

GASTROINTESTINAL INFECTION IN HAEMATOLOGY PATIENTS

Patients receiving high-dose chemotherapy frequently develop bacteraemia or septicaemia caused by a bacterium from their gastrointestinal tract. The spectrum of infection seen in haematology patients differs from that seen in patients with acquired immunodeficiency syndrome (AIDS), in whom decreased cellular immunity is the main risk factor. Neutropenia and disruption of the anatomical barrier of mucosal surfaces are the principal contributory factors in haematology patients; dysfunction of cellular and humoral immunity and hyposplenism are also important. The severity and duration of neutropenia are equally significant. Furthermore indwelling intravenous catheters form convenient sites for colonization by both Gram-negative and Gram-positive organisms. The most common sites for localized infections in the gut are the perianal area, distal oesophagus, colon, and oropharynx.

Common organisms that cross the mucosal barrier to cause infection are Gram-negative organisms: *Pseudomonas aeruginosa*; *Ps. cloacae*; *E. coli*, and *Klebsiella sp*. Gram-positive organisms such as *staphylococci* and *streptococci* can also gain access via the mucosa. Fungi such as *Aspergilli sp*, and *Candida sp* now pose the greatest risk to neutropenic patients. Vancomycin-resistant enterococci are resistant to most currently available antibiotics.

Localized fungal infection in the gut is caused mainly by *Candida sp*, which predominantly involve the oropharynx and oesophagus. Mucositis, achlorhydria resulting from the use of prophylactic antacids, and loss of normal gut flora as a result of the use of antibiotics encourage growth of candida. Phagocytosis by neutrophils and monocytes are the most important mechanisms for preventing dissemination of fungal infection. Aspergillus, the most feared infection in neutropenic patients, mainly infects the lungs and is inhaled, but may also cross the disrupted mucosal gut barrier.

Decontamination of the gut with either a combination of a non-absorbable antibiotic or a quinolone such as ciprofloxacin with an antifungal agent such as fluconazole or itraconazole are now widely used prophylactically. In combination with sterile food and laminar air flow facilities, there is clear reduction in bacterial and fungal infections. However, this may not necessarily result in improved survival. Development of resistant organisms is a constant risk.

Infection of the liver

Hepatic infections are relatively common in haematology patients. Transfusion-transmitted hepatitis is discussed later in this chapter. In patients undergoing bone marrow transplantation, liver infection is difficult to diagnose becuase of the high prevalence of other liver disease such as veno-occlusive disease (VOD) and GVHD (5). Viral infection usually occurs 6–10 weeks after bone marrow transplantation, because of the long periods of incubation for primary infection. Biochemically, there is usually a mild to moderate increase in concentrations of serum alanine (ALT) and aspartate (AST) transaminases, with variable degrees of hyperbilirubinaemia. The clinical course may vary from asymptomatic or mild disease to fulminant hepatic necrosis and death.

CMV hepatitis is usually seen only in disseminated CMV infection. Clinically, symptoms are mild; ALT and AST concentrations may be 10 times the upper limit. Massive hepatic necrosis is rare. Treatment is with ganciclovir, foscarnet, or both. Adenovirus, HSV and varicella zoster virus can, rarely, cause fulminant viral hepatitis in patients undergoing bone marrow transplantation. The clinical presentation is that of a non-specific viral prodrome, accompanied by a rapid increase in ALT and AST concentrations beyond 400–600 IU/l.

Epstein–Barr virus (EBV) infection usually presents as a mild clinical hepatitis, but can also lead to a malignant B-cell proliferative syndrome caused by EBV-transformed immunoblasts that infiltrate the liver and intestine. It is usually seen in immunosuppressed patients with GVHD or after monoclonal anti-T cell antibody treatment. It presents with jaundice, rapidly progressive painful hepatomegaly, and infiltration of other viscera. Histologically, there is portal infiltration with B-cell immunoblastic lymphocytes. In the early stages, this lymphoma may respond to withdrawal of immunosuppression and donor lymphocyte infusions.

Fungal infection develops in severe neutropenia either early after transplant or in patients with poor engraftment. Candida sp are the most frequently involved, although other organisms such as aspergillus, trichosporon, rhizopus, and fusarium are occasionally isolated. Fungal liver disease usually develops in patients with disseminated fungal disease; up to one third of all patients with disseminated visceral candidiasis have liver involvement. Most patients with proven fungal liver disease will have positive surveillance cultures. Clinically, fungal hepatitis presents with fever, tender hepatomegaly, and increased serum alkaline phosphatase concentrations. Hepatosplenic candidiasis is diagnosed when, coincident on restoration of the neutrophil count to normal, microabscesses form in the liver and spleen and are visualized by ultrasound or computed tomography (CT) scanning. Definitive diagnosis can be made by CT scan, guided fine-needle aspiration, or biopsy of the lesion. Treatment is with intravenous amphotericin or liposomal amphotericin.

SPECIFIC HEPATIC AND SPLENIC PROBLEMS IN HAEMATOLOGICAL PATIENTS

Hepatic complications

Veno-occlusive disease

Hepatic VOD is a non-thrombotic obliteration of the lumina of small intrahepatic veins. Its reported incidence varies widely, with rates of 0–70%. The two largest series quote an incidence of 21–22% (6,7). The pathogenesis of VOD after bone marrow transplantion is probably multifactorial. Pre-existing liver disease, high-dose conditioning regimens, previous vancomycin treatment, involvement of the liver by haematological malignancy, advanced age, and positive CMV serology all increase the risk of VOD. Endothelial injury to the sinusoids and small hepatic veins is considered to be the initial pathogenetic event. This injury is followed by deposition of fibrin-related aggregates in the subendothelial zone. These aggregates, and the intramural entrapment of fluid and cellular debris, progressively occlude the hepatic venous outflow and generate a postsinusoidal intrahepatic hypertension.

Clinically, VOD is characterized by jaundice, weight gain, ascites, painful hepatomegaly, and platelet refractoriness, usually within the first 20 days after transplantation (7). Severe VOD can present as a progressive confusional state resulting in severe encephalopathy and coma. Changes in liver size and liver tenderness are usually the first signs, occurring 8–10 days after the beginning of cytoreductive treatment. Occasionally, liver pain is severe and acute because the liver capsule is abruptly stretched, and it may mimic an acute abdominal crisis. Fluid retention and ascites are frequent. The extent of the disease can vary from mild, reversible disease to fatal disease associated with multiorgan failure. Serum bilirubin in excess of 400 mmol/l is associated with extensive hepatocellular damage and an extremely poor prognosis. More than 50% of affected patients develop renal impairment; 25% require dialysis.

Liver histology gives the most accurate **diagnosis** of VOD, but is often contraindicated because of refractoriness to platelet transfusion. Liver biopsy can give a false negative result, because of the patchy nature of the disease. Transjugular liver biopsy and measurement of the gradient between wedged and free hepatic venous pressure is a safer and more accurate alternative. Doppler ultrasound is useful, as it shows hepatomegaly and abnormal hepatoportal blood flow.

Treatment of VOD is primarily supportive, with careful management of fluid overload and its attendant complications. Prophylaxis with continuous infusion of a low dose of heparin appears to be useful. Prostaglandin E_1, oxpentifylline and ursodeoxycholic acid have also been used, with varying success rates. Recombinant tissue plasminogen activator with heparin is an effective combination in some patients. However, there is a risk of fatal bleeding which is reduced by maintaining platelet counts greater than 50×10^9/litre. Recently, defibrotide — a polydeoxy-ribonucleotide with activity in vascular disorders — has shown greater response rates, with fewer side effects than previous treatments (8). Defibrotide is a large, single-stranded polydeoxy-ribonucleotide that is derived from porcine mucosa and has been found to have antithrombotic, anti-ischaemic, anti-inflammatory, and thrombolytic properties, without significant systemic anticoagulant effects. It has a complex mechanism of action, including acting as an adenosine receptor agonist, increasing the concentrations of endogenous prostaglandins, reducing the concentrations of leukotriene B_4, and modulating anticoagulant and antifibrinolytic activity. The technique of transjugular intrahepatic portosystemic shunting is currently being evaluated. Liver transplantation has been performed successfully in a small number of cases.

VOD improves in 50–80% of patients, the remaining 20–50% die with complications.

Acute GVHD of the liver

Acute GVHD usually develops from 15 days after transplantation, as marrow engraftment appears, although a hyperacute form may develop if prophylaxis is not given. Immunological mechanisms mediate the injury, which is predominantly to biliary epithelial cells. The incidence increases with the degree of marrow incompatibility (range 35–90%). Presentation is with jaundice, hepatomegaly, and alkaline phosphatase and bilirubin concentrations increased by up to 20 times the normal values. Hepatocellular enzymes are also increased, although seldom to greater than 10 times normal. A maculopapular skin rash involving the palms, soles, ears, and eventually the trunk, and gastrointestinal involvement with nausea, vomiting, and diarrhoea usually preceed liver involvement.

Liver biopsy is not necessary in all patients with GVHD of the liver, but is considered in those in whom there is persistent liver dysfunction despite improvement in the other manifestations of GVHD, to exclude other causes of liver disease. The histological pattern is variable, and depends on when the biopsy is taken. In the early stages, hepatic necrosis may be present, with changes similar to those in acute viral hepatitis. Later, portal tract changes with cytological changes in the biliary epithelial cells develop.

Treatment consists of increasing immunosuppression — which, unfortunately, may increase susceptibility to opportunistic and bacterial infection.

Chronic GVHD of the liver

Chronic GVHD may progress from acute GVHD that has not responded to treatment; in 25% of patients it may develop *de novo*, without preceding clinical manifestations of acute GVHD. A chronic cholestatic liver disease sometimes develops, with obliteration of interlobular bile ducts (vanishing bile duct syndrome). Serum liver function tests reveal a cholestatic picture with elevation of alkaline phosphate and GGT (gamma glutamyl transferase) followed by bilirubin. Rarely, progression to biliary cirrhosis may occur, and intercurrent hepatitis C virus (HCV) infection may be implicated. Histological findings are confined to the portal tracts, with an intense portal infiltration of lymphocytes and plasma cells, disorganized or absent bile ductules, and inflammatory piecemeal necrosis. Immunosuppression and ursodeoxycholic acid are the main treatments.

Drug-induced liver disease

Drug hepatotoxicity is common in association with high-dose chemotherapy and bone marrow transplantation. Drugs used in the period after transplant for prophylaxis against infection and GVHD may induce hepatitis or cholestasis; cylosporin commonly causes cholestasis. Antifungal agents used prophlactically, such as fluconazole and itraconazole, or therapeutically, such as amphotericin or its liposomal derivatives, can also cause abnormalities of liver function. Total parenteral nutrition (TPN) is commonly implicated in causing mild elevations of bilirubin, transaminases and alkaline phosphatase after transplantation. Methotrexate and 6-mercaptopurine used in the maintenance treatment of acute lymphoblastic leukemia frequently cause abnormal liver function tests.

Iron overload

Refractory anaemias such as thalassaemias, congenital dyserythropoeitic anaemias, sideroblastic anaemia, and myelodysplasia lead to iron overload as a result of repeated transfusions and ineffective erythropoiesis: each 500 ml of blood contains 250 mg of iron.

Serum liver enzyme concentrations are not an accurate indicator of liver damage resulting from iron overload, and liver biopsy remains the best method of assessing liver damage and iron loading. Magnetic resonance imaging and magnetic susceptometry offer non-invasive methods of assessing the concentration of iron in the liver. HCV infection and iron overload commonly occur together, and then lead to more rapid development of fibrosis than when they occur in isolation.

Chelation is generally started when the serum ferritin concentration is greater than 1000 µg/litre, with the aim of keeping the ferritin concentration below this value. Serum ferritin, however, provides a very imprecise measurement of body iron stores as it is also influenced by factors such as haemolysis, ineffective erythropoiesis, ascorbate deficiency, and liver disease — all of which are common in chelated patients. The average iron intake in chronically transfused patients is 0.5 mg/kg per day. Desferrioxamine 20–40 mg/kg given subcutaneously by continuous infusion over 8–12 h daily for 5–7 days per week, plus ascorbic acid 200 mg/day orally will lead to excretion of up to 200 mg of iron per day. Side effects include ototoxicity, retinal damage, and growth inhibition. The oral iron chelator, L1 (deferiprone), is associated with agranulocytosis, arthropathy, zinc deficiency, and fluctuations in plasma concentrations of liver enzymes. It is not as effective as desferrioxamine, but compliance is better.

Venesection is often practised in bone marrow transplantion patients who have hepatitis C and iron overload as a result of multiple transfusions before and directly after transplantation, to reduce the rate of progression to fibrotic liver disease.

Hepatomegaly in haematology patients

Haematology patients frequently develop hepatomegaly at some point in their illness, and this can be due to infiltration with malignant cells, iron overload, storage disorders, extramedullary haemopoiesis, infection, or clotting disorders. Extramedullary haemopoiesis in myelofibrosis may worsen or appear *de novo* after splenectomy.

Specific *haematological causes of hepatomegaly* include:

- Leukemia
- Lymphoma
- Myeloprofilerative disorders
- Storage disorders
- Extramedullary hemopoiesis
  - — myelofibrosis
  - — thalassaemia major
- Portal vein thrombosis
  - — thrombophilias
  - — paroxsysmal nocturnal hemoglobinuria
- Veno-occlusive disease
- Infection
  - — fungal
  - — viral

Splenic complications

Hyposplenism (Table 5.2)

Characteristic blood film appearances are seen in hyposplenism (Figure 5.4). A greater incidence of bacterial and protozoal infection is observed post-splenectomy, particularly with capsulated microorganisms (pneumococcus, *Haemophilus influenzae* type b, and meningococcus) and protozoa infecting the red blood cells (malaria and babesiosis) (9). Pneumococcal infection is most common, and carries a mortality of up to 60%. Table 5.2 outlines the main causes of functional hyposplenism.

There is a 10% risk of infection if splenectomy is performed in children younger than 5 years, therefore splenectomy is deferred, when possible, until after this age. The risk in adults is approximately 1% per year, with a maximum risk in the first 2 years after splenectomy. The risk is increased in patients on immunosuppressive treatment. Vaccination with pneumovax and haemophilus vaccines 2 weeks

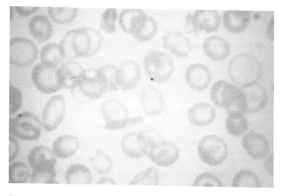

Figure 5.4. Blood film appearance in hyposplenism: red cell poikilocytosis, Howell–Jolly body, basophilic stippling, and bite cell.

before splenectomy is recommended. Re-vaccination every 5 years is recommended, but it may be necessary to re-vaccinate more frequently, particularly if there is an underlying disease causing immunosuppression (9). Meningococcal vaccine covers groups A and C, but group B is the most common in the UK. Therefore, until an appropriate vaccine is developed, use of meninogoccal vaccine should be restricted to individuals who frequently travel to high-risk regions. Influenza vaccine on a yearly basis may be of benefit in asplenic patients.

Lifelong prophylactic antibiotics should be offered to all patients, especially in the first 2 years after splenectomy, for all children up to 16 years, and when there is underlying impaired immune function. In addition, patients not allergic to penicillin, should keep a supply of amoxycillin at home (and take it on holiday), for use immediately should they develop infective symptoms of increased temperature, malaise, or shivering. In such a situation, the patient should seek immediate medical help. Antibiotic prophylactic regimens currently recommended for adults are either penicillin V 250 mg twice daily, amoxycillin 500 mg daily, or erythromycin 250–500 mg daily. Precaution is also recommended if a hyposplenic individual is bitten by a dog as they are particularly susceptible to *Capnocytophagia canimorsus* (DF-2 bacillus), which is associated with dog bites.

Splenomegaly in haematological disease

In the adult, the length of the normal spleen is 8–13 cm; a spleen enlarged to more than 14 cm is palpable. The normal spleen weighs about

Table 5.2. Causes of functional hyposplenism.

Congenital aplasia	
Haematological disorders	Chronic lymphocytic leukaemia
	Sickle-cell disease
	Thalassaemia major
	Essential thrombocythaemia
	Lymphoma
	Malaria
	Myelofibrosis
Autoimmune diseases	Systemic lupus erythematosus
	Rheumatoid arthritis
	Hyperthyroidism
	Sarcoidosis
	Chronic GVHD
	Combined immunodeficiency
Gastrointestinal	Coeliac disease
	Dermatitis herpetiformis
	Crohn's disease
	Ulcerative colitis
	Tropical sprue
Infiltrations	Lymphoma
	Sezary syndrome
	Myeloma
	Amyloidosis
	Secondary carcinoma
	Cysts
Miscellaneous	Splenic arterial/venous thrombosis
	Nephrotic syndrome
	Drugs: methyldopa, intravenous gammaglobulin
	Irradiation
	Bone-marrow transplantation

150–250 mg, but can increase up to a massive 2 kg in some blood disorders. The cause of splenomegaly is subject to geographical variation: malaria is the most common cause of massive splenomegaly in the tropics, whereas in Western countries the leukaemias (particularly chronic myeloid leukaemia) and the myeloproliferative disorders, (particularly myelofibrosis) are the most common causes. The various **haematological causes of splenomegaly** are:

- chronic myeloid leukemia
- myelofibrosis
- polycythaemia rubra vera
- hairy cell leukemia
- lymphoma
- chronic lymphocytic leukemia
- Gaucher's disease, Niemann–Pick disease
- Langerhans' cell histiocytosis X
- haemoglobinopathies; sickle-cell sequestration crisis in children
- haemolytic anaemia

Intra-abdominal thrombosis

Mesenteric artery and venous thrombosis leading to mesenteric infarction and Budd–Chiari syndrome are frequently caused by an underlying haematological or thrombophilic disorder. Essential thrombocythaemia and paroxsysmal nocturnal haemoglobinuria are two acquired clonal disorders that are associated with intra-abdominal thrombosis. Inherited thrombophilia is associated with an increased risk of thrombosis at many sites (10), and is likely to have a role in mesenteric thrombosis. Thrombosis is often multifactorial in aetiology; smoking and use of the oral contraceptive pill contribute to expression of the underlying thrombophilic tendency.

The current established thrombophilic conditions are:

- protein C deficiency
- protein S deficiency
- antithrombin III deficiency
- lupus anticoagulant
- factor V Leiden (activated protein C resistance)
- hyperhomocysteinemia (eg. thermolabile methylenetetrahydratefolate reductase variant)
- prothrombin polymorphism (eg. prothrombin 3' UTR polymorphism)
- dysfibrinogenemias
- increased factor VIII

Conditions with less certain thrombophilic tendencies are not within the scope of this discussion.

Assays currently in use for screening for thrombophilia include those based on blood clotting, enzyme-linked immunosorbent assays that measure protein concentrations, and molecular methods using polymerase chain reactions (PCR). The disadvantage of the clotting-based assays is that they are sensitive to the effects of anticoagulants, and are best done before the commencement or after the discontinuation of anticoagulants.

HAEMATOLOGICAL MALIGNANCY AFFECTING THE GASTROINTESTINAL TRACT

Lymphoma

Lymphoma affecting the gastrointestinal tract account for only 4–9% of all non-Hodgkin's lymphoma, but gastrointestinal lymphomas represent about one-third of all extranodal lymphomas, two-thirds of these occurring in the stomach (11). Enteropathy-associated T-cell lymphoma of the gut is a complication of coeliac disease and, typically, presents with small-bowel ulceration. Histological changes of coeliac disease may not be present, because of latency. Presentation with lymphoma may be the first manifestation of coeliac disease, whereas other patients may have a long-standing history of coeliac disease. Histology is highly variable. The neoplastic cells express pan-T cell markers and, in most cases, the CD103 integrin molecule (found on normal intestinal T lymphocytes). The prognosis is generally poor.

Mucosa-associated lymphoid tissue of the gut (MALT) may be a normal tissue component, as in the small intestine, or occur as a consequence of an autoimmune or inflammatory condition or infection with *H. pylori*, as in the stomach. Tumours arising in this tissue may be multifocal in distribution and of low-, or high-grade histology, depending on the predominant cell type. Recent data from the British National Lymphoma Investigation group describe 175 patients with gut lymphomas, approximately 50% of which were in the stomach and 50% in the intestine (12). Of the gastric lymphomas, 50% were believed to have arisen from MALT, compared with 27% of the intestinal lymphomas. MALT lymphomas may spread to other parts of the body but rarely spread to the bone marrow. The association of *H. pylori* with more than 90% of gastric lymphomas is of particular interest, especially as the lymphoma may regress with anti-helicobacter treatment (13). There is a greater incidence of gastric MALT lymphoma where there is a greater incidence of *H. pylori*.

Histologically, it is important to distinguish low-grade lymphoma from follicular gastritis, and to exclude a hidden high-grade lymphoma or carcinoma before diagnosing low-grade gastric MALT lymphoma. There is a high incidence of additional tumours, 21% of patients showing second or even third tumours — either other haematological malignancies or solid tumours. The majority of patients are at stage IE, although 20% are at stage IIE at presentation. All patients should have a course of anti-helicobacter treatment, regardless of whether they are to receive additional treatment. In low-grade disease anti-helicobacter treatment with endoscopic follow-up should be given as first line treatment. The response may take from 6 to 18 months. In refractory cases, single-agent alkylating chemotherapy such as chlorambucil, local radiotherapy, or combination chemotherapy for high-grade disease and gastrectomy are other therapeutic options, depending on the age of patient, performance status, and the stage and grade of disease.

Previously, gastric MALT lymphoma was treated with gastrectomy. Good lymphoma-free survival was obtained, but with significant morbidity, mortality, and impairment of quality of life. In one-third of patients, disease is multifocal, therefore partial gastrectomy is unlikely to be effective. High-grade gastric lymphoma (diffuse large-cell), with or without a low-grade MALT lymphoma component, and with aggressive clinicopathological features, has a poorer prognosis than pure low-grade MALT lymphoma. This disease entity may evolve from low-grade MALT lymphoma and be aetiologically linked to *H. pylori*. Cure can be effected with combination chemotherapy with or without radiotherapy, obviating the need for resection.

Immunoproliferative small intestinal disease (IPSID) or Mediterranean lymphoma is a rare lymphoproliferative disorder of the upper small intestine. It is considered a special form of MALT lymphoma that has a propensity to malignant transformation. This disease occurs almost exclusively in countries with low socioeconomic status and may present as chronic malabsorption. IPSID is frequently misdiagnosed as intestinal tuberculosis. Histologically, there is diffuse infiltration of small intestinal mucosa by neoplastic lymphoid cells in the early stages, with features of high-grade lymphoma in advanced disease with masses in the gut wall, abdominal lymphadenopathy, and involvement of other organs, including bone marrow. A paraprotein consisting of the heavy chain of immunoglobulin A (α-heavy chain) is present in the serum, urine, or jejunal juice in 65% of patients. The disease is believed to be triggered by a chronic infectious antigenic stimulus. Therefore, in early disease, long-term antibiotic therapy (tetracycline) is the treatment of choice. Regression of disease has been reported after eradication of *H. pylori*. Combination chemotherapy is required in more advanced disease, using anthracycline-containing regimens.

Mantle-cell lymphoma (MCL) commonly involves the liver with atypical lymphoid infiltrates. The gastrointestinal tract is involved in 20% of cases; multiple lymphomatous polyposis, often accompanied by a large localized mass, has been reported, but this is not entirely specific for MCL.

AIDS – related non-Hodgkin's' lymphoma has a greater tendency to involve the gastrointestinal tract (15%) and liver (13%) than non-Hodgkin's lymphoma of similar histology arising in the general population. Histologically, lymphomas are of the high-grade B cell variety, usually of small, non-cleaved cells, and immunoblastic. Lymphoma may exclusively involve the gastrointestinal tract or liver. Pathogenetic factors in AIDS-related lymphomagenesis include disrupted immuno-surveillance, chronic antigen stimulation, cytokine deregulation, and EBV/CMV viral infection.

In children abdominal non-Hodgkin's lymphoma localised to the gastrointestinal tract generally involves the distal ileum, caecum, and mesenteric nodes, and often leads to intussusception. Histologically, the lymphoma is usually of small, non-cleaved cells.

Plasmacytoma

Extramedullary plasmacytoma is a plasma cell tumour that arises outside the bone marrow. Extramedullary plasmacytomas in the gastrointestinal tract can occur as a solitary lesion or in multiple myeloma (particulary in patients who have suffered relapse). Treatment consists of radiotherapy and chemotherapy for selected patients. The prognosis for solitary lesions involving the gastrointestinal tract is favourable; however, progression to myeloma occurs in approximately 20% of patients.

Heavy-chain disease

Heavy-chain diseases (HCD) comprise a group of lymphoproliferative disorders characterized by variant paraproteins (M proteins) consisting of defective immunoglobin heavy chains (14). The anomalous proteins formed are incomplete versions of four major heavy-chain moieties: γ, α, ν and δ. α-HCD is the most common form and occurs primarily in older children and young adults. Enteric disease is endemic in the Mediterranean, Middle East, Asia, Africa, and South America where intestinal infections are common. The disease progresses in three stages. Initially the lamina propria (duodenum, jejunum) and regional lymph nodes (mesenteric, retroperitoneal) are diffusely infiltrated by plasma cells and lymphocytes. Next, the lamina propria becomes heavily infiltrated by α-chain-secreting plasma cells extending deeply into the submucosa and muscularis, with eventual obliteration of the villous architecture. If diagnosed at this stage, the disease is premalignant and complete remission can be achieved by the administration of oral antibiotics. Further progression is characterized by the appearance of overt immunoblastic tumours of the small bowel and mesenteric nodes, dissemination outside the abdomen being a rare, late event. Patients present with chronic painful diarrhoea, severe malabsortion syndrome, and cachexia.

Amyloidosis

Amyloidosis is characterized by the deposition of a homogenous eosinophilic protein material in body tissues. Classification can be according to the clinical syndrome it causes, or by the chemical nature of the amyloid protein. The most common form is systemic amyloidosis (either primary or in association with B-lymphocyte neoplasm), which is characterized by immunoglobulin light-chain deposition. Primary amyloidosis is best considered and treated as a variant of myeloma and is a B-cell malignancy. Reactive (secondary) amyloidosis can occur in inflammatory bowel disease. Diagnosis depends on identification of amyloid in tissue biopsy, by means of Congo Red stain and birefrigence with polarized light. Aspiration of abdominal fat and rectal or gingival biopsy are positive in 80% of cases. Gastrointestinal tract involvement occurs in 50–80% of cases. Clinical manifestations include macroglossia (Figure 5.5), malabsorption, diarrhoea,

protein-losing enteropathy, hepatomegaly and splenomegaly. There is an increased susceptibility to gastrointestinal haemorrhage in patients who received autografts for amyloidosis. Liver and splenic infiltration is common.

GASTROINTESTINAL AND HEPATIC COMPLICATIONS OF BLOOD TRANSFUSION

Infections

Bacterial contamination of blood products, either at the time of collection or during storage, have now replaced viral contamination as the single most important cause of transfusion-transmitted infections. In the past, transfusion-transmitted hepatitis, initially from hepatitis B virus (HBV) and then from non-A non-B hepatitis (mainly HCV), was a frequent and serious complication of transfusion. Currently, rigorous screening of blood donors and sensitive tests for HBV and

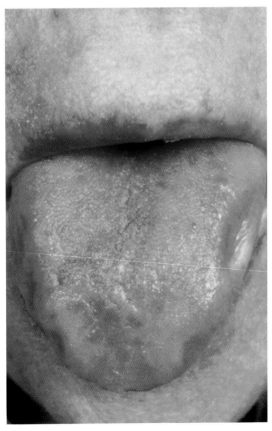

Figure 5.5. Amyloid infiltration of the tongue.

HCV have eliminated well over 90% of cases of post-transfusion hepatitis. Separation of donor blood into various constituents means that a virally contaminated unit of donated blood can potentially infect many recipients, as part of a platelet pool, fresh frozen plasma, or cryoprecipitate, or as part of pooled lyophilized factor concentrate. Fortunately, this is now a rarity, thanks to donor selection, screening, viral inactivation steps in the processing of factor concentrates and, more recently, the availability of single-unit fresh frozen plasma. As 50% of recipients of all blood transfused have died of their underlying disease after 1 year, most transfusion-transmitted viruses will not produce clinically significant disease.

Risk of contamination remains, from individuals donating blood during the seronegative window period immediately after exposure, when they have yet to mount an antibody response (75 days for HCV, 35 days for HBV and 21 days for human immunodeficiency virus (HIV)) that can be detected by conventional antibody-based assays. Donor education and rigorous selection criteria are aimed at discouraging individuals in high-risk categories from donating blood. The present risk for transfusion transmitted HBV and HCV is estimated at less than 1 in 20 000 donations for each virus. Future implementation of nucleic acid testing by PCR analysis of pooled products is likely to reduce further the transmission of viruses by transfusion. In 1996 in the UK and Ireland, one case each of HCV, HBV and HIV were reported to the Serious Hazards of Transfusion scheme (15), all of which were attributable to donors who were in the marker-negative window period of infection. Expansion of autologous donation programmes will further reduce, but not totally eliminate, transfusion hazards. Potential risk also remains from newer viruses and viruses as yet unknown. According to current knowledge, the so-called hepatitis G virus or GBV-C virus does not in fact cause liver disease or any significant post-transfusion infection.

As the number of cases of viral infections continues to decrease, more emphasis is being focused on bacterial contamination of blood products. Unlike viral diseases, this is also a potential problem in autologous units. Of interest to the gastroenterologist are the roles of *Yersinia enterocolitica* and *Clostridium perfringens*. *Y. enterocolitica* is a cyrophilic bacterium that grows well in red-cell concentrates stored at 4°C and forms a potent endotoxin. Interestingly, patients receiving iron chelation therapy are particulary susceptible to infection

with this organism, because of the high concentrations of iron excreted in the stools. As this organism is transmitted in leucocytes, prestorage leuco-depletion of donated blood will substantially reduce this as a transfusion-transmitted infection. *C. perfringens* has been implicated as a causative agent in severe septic reactions after transfusions of platelets, which are stored at 22°C.

Hepatitis in bone marrow transplantation

Until 1990, the prevalence of viral hepatitis among candidates for bone marrow transplantation was 15–25%, largely as a result of prior exposure to blood products contaminated with HCV. The introduction of sensitive screening assays has significantly reduced infection with HCV.

The presence of hepatitis before transplantation carries three risks:

– an increased frequency of liver toxicity (VOD increased to 38% compared with 14%) (8) after cytoreductive therapy
– fulminant viral hepatitis after transplantation
– progressive liver disease after recovery from bone marrow transplantation.

Fatal reactivation of HCV infection has been reported in two recipients of bone marrow transplantation after withdrawal of immunosuppressive treatment (8).

Hepatitis viruses in aplastic anaemia

Acute viral hepatitis, in common with other viral infections, may cause a mild transient pancytopenia. Viral hepatitis, however, precedes aplastic anaemia in about 5–10% of affected patients in the West, and up to 25% in the Far East (16). No specific virus can be identified in the majority of patients, and the association is based on clinical grounds and the presence of abnormal liver function tests. The delay between the clinical hepatitis and the onset of pancytopenia is of the order of 6–12 weeks. Males appear more likely to develop aplasia than females, and the condition tends to affect younger persons. The bone marrow aplasia is probably immunologically mediated. Further evidence to support the association is a finding that 28% of patients who underwent liver transplantation for fulminant liver failure after viral hepatitis developed aplastic anaemia, whereas patients transplanted for other reasons had no marrow failure (17). The prognosis in these patients is poor, and depends on the severity of the marrow depression, not that of the hepatitis. The aplastic anaemia may resolve spontaneously, therefore initial supportive treatment with antibiotics and blood products is appropriate. Immunosuppressive treatment with either antithymocyte globulin or high-dose methylprednisolone is effective in some patients. However, in severely affected patients allogeneic stem cell transplantation is the treatment of choice if a histocompatible donor is available.

Hepatitis in patients with hemophilia

Nearly all hemophiliac patients treated with clotting factor concentrates before 1985 have been exposed to HCV; almost 100% of these are HCV antibody-positive. New cases of hepatatis C in the developed world are now rare as a result of the introduction of effective screening methods and decontamination of factor concentrates. Hepatitis C is discussed in detail in Chapter 41.

In hemophiliac patients, the rate of sustained response to α-interferon and ribavirin is lower than that in non-hemophiliac individuals. In patients with thrombocytopenia, leucopenia, ascites, variceal hemorrhage, or hepatic encephalopathy, α-interferon is of little therapeutic value and may be hazardous. The role of liver biopsy in the management of HCV in patients with hemophilia is controversial; however, most would agree that a biopsy is indicated in patients with focal lesions. The risk of hemorrhage in patients adequately treated with factor concentrate replacement is low. Such procedures should be carried out only in an expert unit and by an experienced operator. Coinfection with HIV and CMV is common, particularly in severe hemophilia and this may lead to an acceleration of the liver disease. Liver transplantation is of proven value in endstage liver disease caused by HCV, and indications for transplantation in hemophiliac patients are the same as other clinical groups. An added benefit in those with hemophilia is cure of their underlying hemophilia, with a rapid normalization of their deficient clotting factor.

In several countries, hepatitis A virus (HAV) infection recently has been reported in non-immune patients with haemophilia who are receiving solvent detergent-treated factor concentrates. This process of viral inactivation does not destroy viruses that lack a lipid envelope, such as HAV and parvovirus B19. Superinfection with HAV in patients with HCV hepatitis can lead to liver failure. Non-immune hemophiliac patients are currently vaccinated for hepatitis A and B. Approximately 3–5% of UK hemophiliac patients are Hepatitis B surface antigen (HbsAg) positive, indicating continuing infection; 50% have evidence of past exposure. Screening of donors, treatment of factor concentrates and vaccination of non-immune individuals has substantially reduced new cases of hepatitis B in hemophiliac patients.

Immunological complications

Immunomodulatory effects of blood transfusion are mediated by white cells. Lymphocytes are implicated in transfusion-associated GVHD, which presents as an acute fulminant pancytopenia, hepatitis and skin rash in individuals transfused with blood from donors of a similar human leucocyte antigen (HLA) type — such as family members — in populations with limited HLA polymorphisms, such as the Japanese.

Postoperative infections may be increased in individuals who are transfused perioperatively. A prospective, randomized study comparing autologous with homologous donation in colorectal surgery found significantly fewer infections in the autologous group. Suppression of a variety of lymphocyte subsets and of natural killer cells after transfusion has been demonstrated in human and animal models; this may form the basis of the proposed increased recurrence of colorectal cancer after transfusion. However, this effect is not proven, many published studies presenting contradictory results. All blood donated in the UK after April 1999 is subjected to leucodepletion, in an effort to reduce the risk of transmission of new-variant Creutzfeld—Jacob disease.

References
1. Weisdorf SA, Salati JA, Weisdorf SA, Salats JA, Longsdorf NKC *et al.* Graft-versus-host disease of the intestine: a protein losing enteropathy characterised by fecal alpha 1-antitrypsin. *Gastroenterology* 1993; **85**: 1076–1081.
2. Ko CW, Gooley T, Schoch HG *et al.* Acute Pancreatitis in marrow transplant patients: prevalence at autopsy and risk factor analysis. *Bone Marrow Transplantation* 1997; **20**: 1081–1086.
3. O'Connor T. Perianal Complications. In: *Clinical Bone Marrow and Blood Stem Cell Transplantation 2nd Ed*. K. Atkinson, Cambridge: Cambridge University Press, 2000; pp. 925–929.

4. Vickers CR. In: *Clinical Bone Marrow Transplantation.* Ed K. Atkinson. Cambridge: Cambridge University Press, 1994; pp. 903–911.

5. Strasser SI, McDonald GB. Gastrointestinal and hepatic complications. In: *Bone Marrow Transplantation.* Eds SJ Forman KG, Blume ED, Thomas. Boston: Blackwell Scientific Publications, 1994; pp. 454–481.

6. Bearman SI. The syndrome of hepatic veno-occlusive disease after bone marrow transplantation. *Blood* 1995; **85**: 3005–3020.

7. Carreras A, Granena A, Rozman C. Hepatic veno-occlusive disease after bone marrow transplantation. *Blood Reviews* 1993; **7**: 43–51.

8. Richardson PG, Elias AD, Krishnan A *et al.* Treatment of severe veno-occlusive disease with defibrotide: compassionate use results in response without significant toxicity in a high risk population [review]. *Blood* 1998; **92**: 737–744.

9. Working Party of the British Committee for Standards in Haematology Clinical Haematology Taskforce. Guidelines for the prevention and treatment of infection in patients with an absent or dysfunctional spleen. *BMJ* 1996; **312**: 430–434.

10. Laffan M, Tuddenham E. Science, medicine and the future: assessing thrombotic risk. *BMJ* 1998; **317**: 520–523.

11. Linch DC, Goldstone AH, Mason DY. Malignant Lymphomas. In: *Postgraduate Haematology.* Eds AV Hoffbrand, SM Lewis, EGD Tuddenham. Oxford: Butterworth Heineman, 1999; pp. 479–504.

12. Morton JE, Leyland MJ, Vaughan Hudson G *et al.* Primary gastrointestinal non-Hodgkins lymphoma: a review of 175 British National Lymphoma Investigation Cases. *Br J Cancer* 1993; **67**: 776–782.

13. Witherspoon AC, Dogliani C, Diss TC *et al.* Regression of primary low grade gastric lymphoma of mucosa-associated lymphoid tissue after eradication of Helicobacter pylori. *Lancet* 1993; **342**: 575–577.

14. Durie BGM, Giles F. In: *Postgraduate Haematology.* Eds AV Hoffbrand, SM Lewis, EGD Tuddenham. Oxford: Butterworth Heineman, 1999, pp. 462–478.

15. Serious Hazards of Transfusion (SHOT). *Summary of Annual Report 1996–1997.* Manchester: Manchester Blood Centre, 1998.

16. Mehta AB, McIntyre N. Haematological disorders in liver disease. *Trends Exp Clin Med* 1998; **8**; 8–25.

17. United Kingdom Haemophilia Centre Directors' Organisation Executive Committee: Guidelines on the Diagnosis and Management of Chronic Liver Disease in Haemophilia.

6. Gastrointestinal Problems in Patients with Rheumatological and Connective Tissue Diseases

ALASTAIR FORBES

INTRODUCTION

There are a number of conditions peculiar to the gut and liver of the rheumatology patient, and the limited mobility of the patient with advanced arthritis may itself have implications when gastrointestinal investigation is considered. Most referrals will be of those with upper gastrointestinal bleeding as a direct complication of the use of non-steroidal anti-inflammatory drugs (NSAIDs). The nature and management of this complication is not fundamentally different from the general management of upper gastrointestinal bleeding, which is dealt with elsewhere in this volume. Nevertheless, the future pharmacological approach in the patient with a continuing rheumatological condition deserves attention.

NON-STEROIDAL ANTI-INFLAMMATORY DRUGS AT THE RHEUMATOLOGY/ GASTROENTEROLOGY INTERFACE

Upper gastrointestinal tract

NSAID gastropathy is typified by focal subepithelial haemorrhage, erosions, and ulcers. Although up to 50% of those taking NSAIDs regularly have these lesions at endoscopy (especially if the procedure is performed after only a few weeks of treatment), clinically significant problems are uncommon. Probably no more than 0.75% of patients develop major morbidity — rather more in the elderly, those receiv-ing anticoagulants and steroids, and those with a previous peptic ulcer. However, because these are very widely used drugs, the relatively low individual risk translates to approximately 12 000 ulcer bleeding episodes and 1200 deaths each year in the UK (1). Aspirin is generally more toxic to the upper gastrointestinal tract than are non-aspirin NSAIDs, but neither seems to cause a diffuse gastritis, and there is no obvious and consistent effect on the consequences of infection with *Helicobacter pylori* (2).

Rheumatologists are now very conscious of the potential hazards of NSAIDs, and do their best to avoid inappropriate use, not least through the earlier use of disease-modifying treatments such as sulphasalazine and gold preparations, and a greater emphasis on paracetamol-based analgesia. Despite this, there will clearly remain patients for whom the indication for a NSAID is strong, or suitable alternatives lacking. Prodrugs such as etodolac or nabumetone, which are less active until after absorption and metabolism, or the combination of an NSAID with a prostaglandin analogue such as misoprostol may be considered. There is good evidence that the combination of misoprostol with NSAIDs reduces the risk of future gastric ulceration (2,3), and less compelling, but still statistically significant, evidence that duodenal lesions also will be reduced. Acid suppression also can be of benefit in the prevention of NSAID-related damage, exemplified by studies of H_2-blockers and proton pump inhibitors (which tend to procure similar or better protection of the duodenum, and less protection of the stomach than prostaglandin analogues) (1). Sucralfate — more specifically a mucosal protectant — has been less studied in this context, but is probably of similar value (3).

Steroids as contributory risk factors for gastrointestinal bleeding

Steroids alone seem to have a minor effect on the incidence of gastrointestinal bleeding, although reliable data on which to base this conclusion are lacking. When combined with non-steroidal agents however, the risks associated with steroids do seem to be considerably greater than those from non-steroidal agents alone (4,5).

COX-1 and COX-2 pathways

It is probable that that most NSAID-induced damage is caused by inhibition of the constitutive type 1 cyclo-oxygenase (COX-1) pathway, which has a "housekeeper" role in cell integrity — for example, in the maintenance of normal expression of prostaglandins in the kidney and in the suppression of gastric acid secretion. Conversely, the benefits of NSAIDs arise predominantly from inhibition of the (inducible) COX-2 system, which generates proinflammatory prostaglandins, and which is expressed almost entirely at sites of active inflammation. Much effort has accordingly gone into development of selective COX-2 inhibitors, and a small number are available for clinical use. The data are becoming compelling, and it is likely that their introduction will diminish gastrointestinal injury to a clinically valuable extent.

Best studied of the selective COX-2 inhibitors is meloxicam, a drug that has been generally available for prescription in the UK for some months, and which has a more selective mechanism of action than older drugs. Meloxicam preferentially inhibits inducible COX-2 and, in animal models, is an especially potent inhibitor of prostaglandin synthesis in sites of inflammatory exudate, but relatively weak in the stomach and kidney, with a low rate of upper gastrointestinal ulceration (6).

In a 4-week volunteer study, meloxicam 7.5 and 15 mg caused less endoscopic abnormality and a little less gastrointestinal bleeding than piroxicam 20 mg (7). Interest has subsequently and correctly focused on rheumatological patients rather than animals or healthy controls and in a "global safety analysis", Distel et al. (8) have reviewed the data from several clinical studies. Meloxicam 7.5 and 15 mg (n = 893 and 3282, respectively) were compared with piroxicam 20 mg (n = 906), diclofenac 100 mg slow release (n = 324) and, naproxen 750–1000 mg (n = 243). From the point of view of gastrointestinal toxicity, meloxicam proved better (always numerically and sometimes significantly) than the other drugs, both in rheumatoid arthritis and in osteoarthritis. Critically, it does not appear to be an inferior anti-inflammatory agent. There must be a little concern that there has been a heavy influence of the sponsoring pharmaceutical company in these studies, however.

NSAIDs and intestinal injury

Despite the natural historic emphasis on the upper gastrointestinal tract, it is increasingly clear that NSAIDs damage the more distal gut also. It is possible that chronic low-volume bleeding from widespread small-bowel lesions is a more common cause of anaemia than is gastric pathology, and the rarely seen but dramatic obstructive strictures may represent one end of a spectrum of inflammatory and fibrotic disease caused to the small intestine. The seminal paper in this field was that from Levi et al. (9), in which they described four patients with strictures of the small bowel. Each had received NSAIDs for at least 18 months, and all presented with subacute small bowel obstruction. Barium studies showed multiple discrete strictures, some of which were similar to those of Crohn's disease, but others were the narrow "diaphragm-like" septae encroaching on and narrowing the lumen, shown histologically to be caused by submucosal fibrosis, and which are now considered the classic features of late NSAID injury to the small bowel.

Subsequent animal work indicated that NSAIDs cause a prostaglandin-dependent increase in intestinal permeability and direct inflammatory changes, which may be prevented or reversed by steroids or thromboxane inhibitors (10). The increased small intestinal permeability appears to be a prerequisite for the development of NSAID enteropathy in man also (11).

Enteroscopy reveals a high prevalence of jejunal pathology in patients taking NSAIDs who have chronic occult gastrointestinal bleeding. Among a series of patients in Glasgow who underwent extended small-bowel examination with a Sonde enteroscope, 47% were found to have pertinent jejunal or ileal ulceration (12) which was taken by these authors as good justification for use of the technique when conventional endoscopy has failed to reveal a cause of blood loss. The magnitude of the background prevalence of clinically significant small-bowel damage remains unclear, and it is uncertain whether COX-1 inhibition is critical — although this seems likely. There is an impression that patients with rheumatoid arthritis are especially at risk. Bjarnason & Macpherson (13) estimated that NSAIDs cause small intestinal inflammation in 65% of patients receiving the drugs in the long term. They attributed substantial hypoalbuminaemia to this enteropathy, in addition to iron deficiency and the less frequent frank ulcers and strictures.

More distal parts of the intestine are also susceptible to adverse effects from NSAIDs, as exemplified by a patient with the now characteristic diaphragm, but in the ascending colon (14). However, NSAID-related colitis is well recognized — and is, indeed, the basis of several animal models of idiopathic inflammatory bowel disease. It is not common when NSAIDs are used therapeutically (13), but NSAIDs may be an important contributor to complications of diverticulosis and the relapse (or mimicry of) inflammatory bowel disease (15). There is also an association between NSAID intake and appendicitis in the elderly.

OTHER DRUGS OF POTENTIAL GASTROINTESTINAL RELEVANCE USED BY RHEUMATOLOGISTS

Sulphasalazine

With the recognition that most, if not all, of its effect in colitis resulted from the 5-aminosalicylic acid (5-ASA) moiety, and the majority of the toxicity from the sulphonamide component, gastroenterologists have increasingly moved away from the use of sulphasalazine towards alternative pharmaceutical or pharmacological packagings of 5-ASA. Rheumatologists, however, find that the intact parent drug is necessary for full benefit in rheumatoid arthritis, a disease in which sulphasalazine has a true disease-modifying effect. For reasons that are not clear, leucopenia, and thrombocytopenia (especially in the first 3–6 months of treatment) — reversible but potentially severe — are much more frequent in patients with rheumatoid arthritis than in other groups of patients who are similarly treated (16). Although the degree of haematological wariness with which rheumatologists utilize sulphasalazine may appear exaggerated to gastroenterologists, it is warranted.

Gold

Gold salts in various formulations have a well-established place in the disease-modifying treatment of rheumatological disorders. The toxicity is well described in standard texts and proteinuria-associated nephritis, haematological problems, pulmonary fibrosis, alopecia, and itchy rashes are unlikely to present to the gastroenterologist. Diarrhoea, however, is reported to affect 50% of treated patients. Increased dietary fibre is advocated as sufficient treatment, but until recently neither aspect had been well tested. In a large and well-conducted placebo-controlled trial of psyllium in oral gold treatment for rheumatoid arthritis, the frequency of diarrhoea proved to be only 15% in the control group. A total of 7% of this control group had troublesome watery stools. The group receiving psyllium had no watery diarrhoea, but as 14% had some degree of diarrhoea it was not considered necessary to advise fibre supplements prophylactically (17).

Frank colitis of a nature similar to ulcerative colitis has also been described as a consequence of treatment with gold, and can be severe and extensive enough to necessitate colectomy (18). The same authors reviewed the literature, which at that time included reports of 29 other cases of intestinal inflammation, ranging in severity from limited ileal involvement to fulminant pan-enteritis. Disease usually began whilst active gold administration was continuing, but was also observed to follow its cessation by several weeks. A response to withdrawal of gold, intravenous fluids, steroids, and antibiotics was usual, but four patients also required surgery. The mechanism of injury remains unknown, but it seems wise to consider this possible complication in patients taking gold who develop inflammatory bowel-disease-like symptoms. Coexistence of severe gold colitis and intrahepatic cholestasis (19) suggests that there is a subgroup of patients with a propensity to gastrointestinal complications of gold therapy. It is possible that this is determined by genetic factors (20).

Gold therapy may also produce mouth ulcers of such severity that cessation of treatment is required. Mild hepatic toxicity, with a predominantly cholestatic picture, may also be a problem.

Azathioprine and cyclosporin

Azathioprine and, to a lesser extent, cyclosporin are familiar to gastroenterologists through their use in inflammatory bowel disease. There are no particular differences in the problems seen or expected when they are used rheumatologically, other than an apparently greater risk of drug-related malignancy with prolonged administration.

Methotrexate

Methotrexate is becoming more familiar to gastroenterologists, but is much more widely used by rheumatologists. Short-term toxicity is uncommon with the regimens used. Occasional patients describe minor upper gastrointestinal symptoms, but stomatitis and mucositis are not seen with doses used for non-chemotherapeutic purposes. Concurrent administration of aspirin and NSAIDs may, however, increase the toxicity profile. Myelosuppression is relatively predictable, and unlikely to present with gastrointestinal manifestations.

Hepatic fibrosis and progression to clinical liver disease have been described in association with methotrexate treatment when total doses of 2 g or more have been given, but are rarely seen with contemporary use of the drug for non-malignant conditions. Only when the cumulative dose substantially exceeds 1 g is monitoring likely to contribute usefully, and liver biopsy very rarely needs to be considered before a total dose of 1.5 g. There is now general agreement that liver biopsy before institution of methotrexate is not indicated in patients with normal standard liver function tests (21), or even on a routine basis in surveillance, unless there are other risk factors for chronic liver disease such as alcohol excess. In a review of 14 patients who had received more than 3 g methotrexate for juvenile rheumatoid arthritis (22), there were occasional abnormalities in liver function tests (enzyme concentrations more than three times normal) in five and, minor histological changes in 13, but significant fibrosis in none.

Cyclophosphamide

By far the most common gastrointestinal side effect of cyclophosphamide treatment is the nausea and vomiting most characteristic of its use in chemotherapy for malignancy. This is often a problem, even with the lower doses used in rheumatological practice, occurring in 68% of patients in one series (23). Oral pulse therapy (5 mg/kg per day for 3 days at a time) is suggested to be less emetogenic than more continuous regimens or those given intravenously. Ondansetron or granisetron may nevertheless be required if nausea is severe and the indication for the drug is strong.

Veno-occlusive disease of the liver is normally a problem only with the high doses used in chemotherapy, and perhaps particularly when cyclophosphamide has been used in preparation for bone marrow transplantation. Nevertheless veno-occlusive disease, hepatotoxicity, and acute liver failure have been described in association with doses as low as 100 mg daily used for rheumatoid arthritis, vasculitis, and Wegener's granulomatosis (24,25). A link between the poor-metabolizer phenotype for debrisoquine, which occurs in 7% of white populations, and severe hepatic dysfunction provides one plausible explanation for this apparently idiosyncratic response (26). The ability of cyclophosphamide to reactivate chronic viral infections such as hepatitis C is real, but probably no greater than that of other immunosuppressants.

Penicillamine

Penicillamine is not often associated with major gastrointestinal problems, but hepatotoxicity has been reported, and there has been at least one death from progressive cholestatic liver failure in a patient with rheumatoid arthritis (27). Aphthoid ulcers in the oesophagus are also known to occur (28). It should also be noted that gastroenterologists may, here, have the opportunity to provoke a rheumatological problem, as penicillamine used in management of primary biliary cirrhosis has provoked polymyositis (29)!

Colchicine

Colchicine can damage the small bowel, causing hyperplasia of the crypts and villous atrophy. There is consequent enhanced intestinal permeability, and associated lactase deficiency, with acquired lactose intolerance (30,31). The abdominal pain and diarrhoea sometimes seen in patients taking colchicine are probably direct results of this, and a lactose-free diet can be helpful.

Antimalarial agents

Antimalarial drugs such as chloroquine, hydroxychloroquine, and mepacrine are occasionally used in rheumatoid arthritis and systemic lupus, and more frequently for discoid lupus. In addition to the concerns about ophthalmic toxicity, non-specific gastrointestinal toxicity is common, but usually minor. These drugs are actively taken up into lysosomes and delivered as such to the liver, where occasional severe damage may ensue, including granulomatous hepatitis and fulminant hepatic failure (32–34). Damage may also be caused to the upper gastrointestinal mucosa (35). A protective effect may, however, be induced in the pancreas (36,37).

SPECIFIC RHEUMATOLOGICAL AND CONNECTIVE TISSUE DISEASES

There are a number of rheumatological and connective tissue diseases that warrant specific consideration. It should be understood that this chapter concentrates on the gastrointestinal aspects of these conditions. The more common conditions, rheumatoid arthritis and osteoarthritis, do not figure largely in the gastrointestinal literature. Apart from the considerable relevance of these diseases to drug-induced problems, involvement of the gastrointestinal tract is essentially limited to the occasional patient with rheumatoid vasculitis or with amyloidosis (see below).

Rheumatoid arthritis

Rheumatoid arthritis is associated with hepatitis C virus (HCV) infection, and there is evidence that the virus itself has a tropism for the synovial membrane, such that some of these cases are in fact HCV arthritis (38). The broader issue of chronic liver disease in rheumatoid arthritis has been examined in a postmortem series of 182 patients (39). In the absence of exposure to methotrexate or other recognized hepatotoxic drugs, histology demonstrated diffuse hepatic fibrosis in 15 patients, but was severe only in two, in whom alcohol excess and prior viral hepatitis were previously suspected. Rheumatoid arthritis has a protective effect against colorectal carcinoma (directly or through the presumed beneficial effects of aspirin and NSAID use). In a large Finnish study (9469 rheumatoid arthritis patients: 65 400 person-years follow-up), the incidence of colonic and all colorectal carcinomas was significantly lower than in the general population (standardized incidence ratios and 95% confidence intervals: 0.57 and 0.33 to 0.93, compared with 0.62 and 0.42 to 0.88, respectively), whereas the combined incidence for all malignancies was marginally greater than that in the general population (40).

Osteoarthritis

Osteoarthritis is loosely linked to gastrointestinal practice through the positive correlation with obesity, but more specifically in respect of haemochromatosis, in which iron deposition in joints produces a distinctive arthropathy tending to affect predominantly the second and third metacarpophalangeal joints of the hand, with more general evidence for degenerative osteoarthritis and chondrocalcinosis (41). Management of the hepatic and pancreatic manifestations is not especially influenced by the presence or absence of rheumatological features.

Spondarthritides

The spondarthritides and the reactive arthritides have a special relationship with gastroenterology, given that there is a high frequency of (often semi-occult) inflammatory bowel disease in these patients. Human leucocyte antigen B27 is associated weakly with ulcerative colitis and strongly with ankylosing spondylitis, and there is evidence for a number of crossreacting, bacterially derived antibodies in both groups of conditions (in particular antibodies to *Chlamydia*, *Klebsiella*, *Proteus*, and *Escherichia coli*) (42–44). There are no clinical therapeutic implications of these observations at present.

Reiter's syndrome

Reiter's syndrome is a particular variant of the reactive arthritides linked to infection, often, but not exclusively, sexually acquired. It was originally defined from the triad of arthritis, urethritis, and conjunctivitis, but is now applied to those with peripheral arthritis of more than 1 month duration, in association with urethritis, cervicitis, or both, with or without mucocutaneous lesions. It occurs in human immunodeficiency virus infection, in which it runs a more severe and progressive course. *Chlamydia*, *Campylobacter*, *Clostridia*, and *Cryptosporidia* are among the most common microorganisms involved. Overt gastrointestinal problems are unusual once the initiating infection is overcome. In the occasional patient with continuing diarrhoea, mesalazine may be helpful, for both the joint and the gastrointestinal manifestations.

Inflammatory bowel-disease-related arthropathy

Patients with ulcerative colitis and Crohn's disease are susceptible to the generally non-erosive condition of inflammatory bowel disease-related arthropathy (45). This is not easy to manage, as the drugs best suited to its treatment (NSAIDs) tend to aggravate the intestinal symptoms. Often this becomes more tractable to treatment as the inflammatory bowel disease comes under control; this should be the gastroenterologist's contribution, but injection of steroid to single affected joints can also be efficacious.

Scleroderma

Scleroderma (progressive systemic sclerosis) (46–49) is characterized by the pathological laying-down of normal collagen in a wide range of connective tissues. In its simplest and most benign form there is skin thickening alone, but the disease may cause not only generalized and profound skin thickening, but also visceral involvement, which sometimes progresses rapidly. The entire gastrointestinal tract may then become involved, and almost all patients will have some symptomatic gastrointestinal problems during the course of their disease. It is convenient to consider the manifestations of scleroderma in terms of their predominant focus, but it should be borne in mind that multiple sites may be affected concurrently or sequentially. Unfortunately, treatment is symptomatic and supportive only.

A general feature of scleroderma that may pose clinical difficulty is the vasculopathy and poor healing quality of the abnormal connective tissue. For example, the relatively trivial wound of a removed gastrostomy tube (which will normally close in a matter of hours) can be expected to take several weeks to heal. Similarly, a cuffed "Hickman-type" central venous catheter will require to be *in situ* for 3 or 4 weeks before the collagen response around the cuff is sufficient to preclude accidental displacement; this is in contrast to the requirement in normal patients, in whom confidence in the response will exist after 5–7 days. Although apparently trivial, these examples are representative of the additional difficulties with which patients with scleroderma have to contend.

Oesophagus

Scleroderma commonly affects the smooth muscle of the oesophagus. Evidence for its involvement can be established in 90% of patients if investigation is thorough, but fortunately it is less often a clinical problem. Nonetheless, about 60% of patients complain of at least intermittent dysphagia, and reflux symptoms are similarly prevalent (well in excess of those in control populations of similar age). Conventional barium radiology is abnormal in 75% of unselected patients with scleroderma. Characteristically, there is evidence of abnormal peristaltic activity, which may include free gastrooesophageal reflux and a dilated oesophagus, but sliding hiatus hernia or stricture are also seen. Formal manometric studies are almost invariably abnormal in the patient with established scleroderma, the usual manifestations including lack of propagation and a generally low amplitude of contractions. This is particularly apparent in the lower two-thirds of the oesophagus, and is associated with diminished lower oesophageal sphincter pressure, which presumably contributes to the prominence of reflux in these patients.

It is common for patients to fail to respond adequately to H_2-blockade, and to need doses of proton pump inhibitors that are greatly in excess of those known to achieve complete acid suppression. This phenomenon suggests that there is another mechanism at work, but one currently of unknown nature. Pragmatically, patients should be prescribed the minimum dose of a proton pump inhibitor that seems effective, but with the recognition that this may be two to three times greater than is usual in reflux practice. Prevention of oesophageal stricturing is an important corollary goal, as this complication poses a particular hazard in the scleroderma patient. Unfortunately, the good results otherwise to be expected with pro-motility agents such as domperidone are not always replicated in scleroderma-related oesophageal symptoms. It is always worth trying one or more of this group of drugs, but it is common to find that unacceptable levels of abdominal discomfort or frank pain result. Again, a clear mechanism is yet to be established.

Stomach

Gastric atony, hypomotility, and megagastria are common and add to the difficulties experienced from oesophageal involvement. Prokinetic agents should be tried, but are often insufficient or poorly tolerated. Low-rate, modest-volume overnight feeding by nasogastric tube or gastrostomy may permit the maintenance of adequate nutrition in patients with intractable early satiety.

Small bowel

Bloating, cramps, or alterations of bowel habit are the most common symptom of small bowel involvement in scleroderma. Many patients go on to develop significant problems from malabsorption, and a few proceed to formal intestinal failure. There are almost always elements associated both with small-bowel bacterial overgrowth and with motility disorder. Barium studies characteristically reveal features of hypomotility, with proximal dilatation and retention of barium, and with evidence of atony on screening. More distally in the small bowel, the "stack of coins" sign results from the combination of atony and continuing close apposition of the valvulae conniventes; this is almost pathognemonic of scleroderma.

Management

Management of the intestinal manifestations and complications of scleroderma can be difficult. It is, however, unusual for a patient with scleroderma to present with gastrointestinal symptoms before the confirmation of the underlying diagnosis, so the clinician has, at least, the opportunity to be aware of likely problems. The most informative data come from confirmation or refutation of small-bowel bacterial overgrowth. Any of the standard breath-test techniques, or culture of endoscopically obtained aspirates from the distal duodenum can confirm the

diagnosis. Barium studies (as above) are graphic, but do not usually contribute usefully, beyond helping to exclude pathology unrelated to scleroderma. Isotopic methods of assessing gastric emptying and small-bowel transit, available in specialist centres, may demonstrate a variety of abnormalities. The combination of delayed gastric emptying and slow small-bowel transit is common in those with predominant reflux-like symptoms — a picture that changes to one of dominant rapid small-bowel transit when intestinal bacterial overgrowth supervenes. It is unusual for such investigation to influence management greatly, as the prevailing problem will usually be obvious from the patient's symptoms.

Bacterial overgrowth in scleroderma responds well to a wide range of antibiotics when first recognized. Unfortunately, there is little prospect of long-term resolution, as the underlying motility disorder is irreversible, and re-colonization soon occurs. Further courses of increasingly broad-spectrum antibiotics, and for increasing durations, yield progressively less benefit. Periods of no antibiotic treatment are advised, to permit recovery of the commensal flora, but many patients find this intolerable and prefer instead to take antibiotics continuously. In this event, it is preferable to alternate two or more different drugs at 2–4-week intervals. Agents that are relatively broad spectrum and cheap (such as tetracycline, amoxycillin, and metronidazole) are popular, but drugs that are poorly absorbed or rarely used in oral formulations (such as neomycin) have an advantage from the point of view of minimizing the development of resistant strains in the bacterial pool. It is usually possible to obtain benefit from low-dose regimens (e.g. tetracycline or amoxycillin 250 mg twice daily or metronidazole 200–400 mg twice daily), but there are no reliable controlled data. There is nothing to be gained from re-investigation of the patient with scleroderma in whom a diagnosis of bacterial overgrowth has previously been made. The condition almost always recurs, and bacterial cultures and sensitivities have a limited and always very transient applicability. It is better to permit patients to determine the anti-biotic cocktails that suit them best, recognizing that these may change with time.

Small-bowel motility disorders are difficult to manipulate positively in patients with scleroderma. Although delayed transit may respond to pro-motility agents (metoclopramide, domperidone, or erythromycin) and rapid transit may be helped by opioids (loperamide, codeine, etc.), many patients find that these agent provoke cramping abdominal pain, even in the absence of demonstrable intestinal hold-up. It is nevertheless worth trying these drugs, in the hope of finding a regimen that suits. Global intestinal pseudo-obstruction, with pain and constipation, is also seen. In its most advanced stages, pseudo-obstruction necessitates intravenous feeding if adequate nutrition is to be maintained; this itself present extra difficulties in the patient with scleroderma, as the digital mobility and general dexterity needed to perform intravenous nutrition in the home may be severely impeded by the joint and skin manifestations of the disease. Some patients with pseudo-obstruction are said to gain from "venting" of the most obstructed segments of the intestine. Our experience with surgical intervention has, however, been very disappointing. There is, nevertheless, a place for a percutaneous venting gastrostomy in carefully selected patients with intractable vomiting associated with intestinal pseudo-obstruction from scleroderma.

Large bowel

Patchy atrophy of the muscularis of the large bowel leads to the development of characteristic wide-mouthed sacculations, usually located along the antimesenteric border of the transverse and descending colon. These are possibly unique to scleroderma. The entire colon tends to become atonic, and may be subject to sigmoid or caecal volvulus. Severe constipation has been described, but seems to be less common than in the past — perhaps because of the frequent coexistence of bacterial overgrowth and small-bowel malabsorption.

A more recent observation provides an explanation for the passive faecal incontinence that troubles a significant minority of patients with scleroderma (50). Physiological tests show low resting pressure (internal anal sphincter) and endosonography shows marked thinning of the internal anal sphincter, with changed reflectivity suggestive of fibrosis (which may be confirmed histologically). Surgical or electrical measures, or both, to achieve continence may have to be considered.

Scleroderma is also complicated by pneumatosis (51). Management of the pneumatosis is not greatly influenced by the association of the two conditions, but it tends to occur only at a late stage in scleroderma, when the prognosis is already poor.

Mixed connective tissue disease

Mixed connective tissue disease (52,53) is a catch-all term for a syndrome in which there is multisystem involvement with features of a number of connective tissue diseases. There are subdiagnostic, but usually overlapping, features of systemic lupus erythematosus, scleroderma, polymyositis, or rheumatoid arthritis. Patients typically have a high circulating titre of antibody to extractable nuclear antigen. In around 85% of these patients, radiographic and manometric studies have revealed evidence of oesophageal dysfunction that is or becomes symptomatic in at least 50%. The characteristic abnormalities are essentially those of scleroderma (see above) and similar management strategies are required. Most of the other literature relating mixed connective tissue disease to gastroenterology is in the form of case reports, of which some dramatic examples exist, ranging through atrophy of the tongue, pneumatosis, mesenteric panniculitis, protein-losing enteropathy, pancreatitis, and otherwise idiopathic portal hypertension, to fulminant hepatic failure secondary to cardiac tamponade. Autoimmune hepatitis does seem more generally over-represented, however (54).

VASCULITIDES

Polyarteritis nodosa

Polyarteritis nodosa (55–58) involves the gastrointestinal tract in about two-thirds of patients, to a clinically important extent in about half of these; in 10–15% gastrointestinal involvement will be the presenting feature that leads to the diagnosis of polyarteritis. Most often, the underlying vascular problem is aneurysmal and affects moderately sized vessels such as the superior and inferior mesenteric and the hepatic arteries. The clinical presentation is accordingly with bleeding or with an acute abdomen, with or without intestinal ischaemia. More chronic ischaemia, with substantial weight loss and pain, also occurs. Dramatic bleeds from hepatic vessels producing the classic triad of pain, jaundice, and melaena will be recognized, although not always so easily treated. Less often, pancreatic vessels are involved and death from exsanguination from a pancreatic pseudocyst has been reported. Bleeding may also result from ischaemic gastric ulcers — another relatively common gastrointestinal complication of polyarteritis. Ischaemic colitis from involvement of mesenteric vessels is effectively indistinguishable from other causes of ischaemic colitis. Ischaemic pain in polyarteritis may be responsive to nitrates.

Patients with polyarteritis who have gastrointestinal manifestations probably represent a subgroup with a younger age of onset and a generally worse prognosis than those without. The outlook may be especially poor if haemorrhage, intestinal perforation, or other need for digestive tract surgery occur. Survival curves for those with severe gastrointestinal manifestations suggest a 10-year survival of less than 50%, compared with about 80% in those without these complications.

It is still not clear why there is such a strong link between hepatitis B and polyarteritis, but the link is undeniable, and is stronger in those with other gastrointestinal manifestations. Its significance is diminishing with the declining prevalence of hepatitis B since vaccination was introduced. Idiopathic nodular regenerative hyperplasia of the liver is also described in association with polyarteritis. Again of uncertain provenance is the rare but real association between polyarteritis and gastric carcinoma; stronger links with marrow-derived neoplasms also exist, suggesting that there may be an underlying deficit in immune regulation.

Wegener's granulomatosis

Wegener's granulomatosis (59) is characterized by a granulomatous vasculitis of the upper and lower respiratory tract and kidneys that responds to immunosuppression (particularly cyclophosphamide), but it is not unduly unusual for other organs to become involved. Most of the literature consists of, or is derived from, case reports.

Erosive granulomatous oesophagitis with resulting odynophagia and tracheo–oesophageal fistula is well described, but not always recognized before death. Granulomatous gastritis may be responsible for haemorrhagic ulcers and, as with granulomatous inflammation elsewhere in the gastrointestinal tract, may best be differentiated from Crohn's disease by the associated circulating cytoplasmic anti-neutrophil cytoplasmic antibodies. Involvement of the small bowel may lead to ulceration, perforation and late stenotic stricturing, while lower bowel disease presents with a patchy granulomatous colitis, sometimes associated with perianal ulceration.

There are occasional patients in whom primary biliary cirrhosis overlaps Wegener's granulomatosis; as with polyarteritis nodosa there may be aneurysmal involvement of the hepatic artery. Pancreatic Wegener's granulomatosis is especially perplexing, as it may be responsible for relapsing pancreatitis and may mimic pancreatic carcinoma.

Confusion has resulted from pulmonary toxicity caused by sulphasalazine (given for colitis) being incorrectly attributed to Wegener's granulomatosis.

Churg–Strauss syndrome — Allergic granulomatous angiitis

Allergic granulomatous angiitis (Churg–Strauss syndrome) (60) is an unusual idiopathic hypereosinophilic vasculitis associated with asthma, and both tissue and circulating eosinophilia. Gastrointestinal involvement is not rare. Presentation is mostly with acalculous cholecystitis or with infarction of the small bowel, with ulceration or fistula formation in cases less catastrophic than those which lead to major intestinal resection. Colorectal involvement seems less frequent than with Wegener's granulomatosis or polyarteritis. The extragastrointestinal features help to differentiate Churg–Strauss syndrome from eosinophilic gastritis/enteritis. The condition is often responsive to steroids.

Other systemic vasculitides

Systemic vasculitis involves the gastrointestinal tract relatively rarely other than in polyarteritis nodosa, Wegener's granulomatosis and Churg–Strauss syndrome. In systemic lupus erythematosus (SLE), and in rheumatoid vasculitis (61), abdominal symptoms are usually less severe, and generally occur in association with other evidence of disease activity. The associations and pathogenesis of gastrointestinal involvement in these conditions are similar to those of polyarteritis nodosa, and together account for most remaining cases of arteritis affecting the gut and biliary tree. Symptoms include abdominal pain, diarrhoea, and gastrointestinal bleeding. Ileus and protein-losing enteropathy also occur, especially with the serositis of the bowel that is associated with SLE. Ileal and colonic ulcers may both bleed and perforate, and the fatality rate from infarction consequent on mesenteric arteritis or aneurysm remains high.

The diagnosis of gastrointestinal involvement in systemic vasculitis is essentially a clinical one, aided by awareness of the underlying condition if there is a prior diagnosis. Endoscopic biopsies may show vasculitis, but are unlikely to be sufficiently deep to show arteritis. In one series of 63 patients with localized gastrointestinal vasculitis (62), there were 35 intestinal infarcts requiring resection, 14 cholecystectomies, five partial pancreatectomies, six appendicectomies, one omentectomy, one gastrectomy, and one oesophagectomy. Vasculitis was classified histologically as polyarteritis nodosa ($n = 33$), phlebitis ($n = 12$), Churg–Strauss ($n = 8$), small-vessel vasculitis ($n = 6$), Buerger's disease ($n = 2$), and giant-cell arteritis ($n = 1$). Eight of the cases of phlebitis involved the right colon, where there were often giant cells, and there was a history of NSAID use in seven of the eight, without evidence of systemic disease. Follow-up to a mean of 5 years demonstrated other systemic disease in 25% of the polyarteritis patients, and in patients with giant-cell arteritis or Buerger's disease. Systemic vasculitis did not develop in patients with gastrointestinal phlebitis, polyarteritis without serum autoantibodies, or small-vessel vasculitis.

OTHER RHEUMATOLOGICAL CONDITIONS

Behçet's syndrome

Behçet's syndrome (63,64) includes oral and genital ulceration, uveitis, cutaneous vasculitis, synovitis, and meningoencephalitis; associated lesions similar to erythema nodosum may also occur. More than 50% of affected Scottish (but not Turkish) patients have gastrointestinal involvement at sites distinct from the mouth and perineum; the differential diagnosis is usually Crohn's disease, as the intestinal disease includes skip lesions and linear ulcers macroscopically indistinguishable from those in Crohn's. Radiological features can nevertheless be diagnostic, especially in the presence of large, ovoid or geographic, deep ulcers with persistent surrounding deformity, localized to the ileocaecal area (65). Diarrhoea and features suggestive of inflammatory bowel disease affect only about 15% of patients in Turkey, where Behçet's syndrome is most common — perhaps reflecting a

greater awareness of the condition and the recognition of milder cases.

Thrombosis of major vessels occurs in around 10% of all cases of Behçet's syndrome, leading especially to Budd–Chiari syndrome (about 25% of all thromboses) (66). Less common gastrointestinal problems include those of acute pancreatitis, gastrointestinal bleeding from superior mesenteric artery aneurysm and from Dieulafoy's lesions in the stomach, and intestinal perforation. Lesions similar to primary sclerosing cholangitis have been described, as has cavernous transformation of the portal vein. Underlying vasculitis, thrombosis or both, is probably implicated in each of these. Perhaps for this reason, the rates of recurrence after excisional surgery for intestinal perforation are high (67).

Amyloidosis

Amyloidosis (68,69) represents a group of disorders characterized by the accumulation of abnormal extracellular fibrillar protein in the connective tissues of the body. It may be hereditary or acquired, focal or generalized, but the systemic forms are usually progressive and ultimately fatal. The amyloidoses are characterized by the immunochemical analysis of their specific amyloid protein (serum amyloid A, monoclonal immunoglobulin light chains, transthyretin, β_2-microglobulin, β-protein, or islet amyloid polypeptide), but all deposits include a serum amyloid P component, which is most helpful in diagnosis as it permits the specific use of isotopic scanning of high sensitivity.

Reactive systemic amyloid (AA amyloid) affects no more than 2% of patients with Crohn's disease (and is very rare in ulcerative colitis). It is seen in a considerably greater proportion of those with rheumatoid arthritis. The presentation is usually with nephrotic syndrome, and its management nephrological. The joints themselves are not involved.

AL amyloid (with associated immunocyte dyscrasia) complicates overt myeloma, but may occur in apparent isolation and can then be responsible for macroglossia, diffuse gastrointestinal bleeding, an ulcerative colitis-like colitis, and motility problems. Cholestatic liver disease or malnutrition are poor prognostic signs. When abnormal light chains are deposited in the joints, a rheumatoid-like symmetrical arthritis of the wrists and small joints of the hands occurs, sometimes with carpal tunnel syndrome or subcutaneous nodules. Management is with haematological chemotherapy and is moderately successful.

Familial amyloid polyneuropathy may present to the rheumatologist because of the unusual pains that result; the visceral involvement and secondary malnutrition that follow are ultimately fatal in the absence of liver transplantation to restore normal transthyretin gene function. Otherwise, the gastroenterologist is best placed to help in the management of amyloid, through supervision of intensive nutritional support by whatever route is necessary.

Lyme disease

Lyme disease (tick-borne Borreliosis) typically causes intermittent attacks of oligoarticular arthritis in a few large joints, especially the knee, and, less often, a chronic arthritis, again affecting primarily the knee. The diagnosis is usually prompted by knowledge that the patient has been exposed to deer in an endemic area, and is confirmed by antibodies to *Borrelia burgdorferi*. The gastroenterologist is most often involved because of concern about the two-thirds of patients with Lyme disease who have substantially abnormal liver function tests (70), and the occasional patient in whom diarrhoea forms part of the presentation. A 4–8 week course of appropriate antibiotics is usually curative once the diagnosis has been made (71).

Whipple's disease — *Tropheryma whippelii* infection

Whipple's disease — *Tropheryma whippelii* infection — may present to either gastroenterologist or rheumatologist, given its multiorgan nature; in the early phases joint manifestations are more common (67%) than digestive ones (15%), but at later stages up to 80% of affected patients have arthropathy (usually a spondarthritis) and as many as 85% have diarrhoea, weight loss, and malabsorption. Only around 15% fail to exhibit gastrointestinal features (72). If the diagnosis is made promptly, a good response can be expected from trimethoprim—sulphamethoxazole, or penicillin with streptomycin. The diagnosis is difficult until it is considered and satisfactory histological specimens obtained: biopsy of intestinal mucosa reveals infiltration of the lamina propria with periodic acid Schiff-positive macrophages. Molecular techniques to identify

T. whippelii without need for culture should soon be possible and permit development of a sensitive, non-invasive diagnostic test (73).

Familial Mediterranean fever — hereditary recurrent polyserositis — periodic disease

Familial Mediterranean fever (74,75), also known (in the USA) as periodic disease, and now more helpfully as hereditary recurrent polyserositis, is an inherited disorder characterized by recurrent self-limiting attacks of the joints, and chest, and abdominal pain associated with fever. It occurs almost exclusively in Arabs, Jews, and Turks, hence its geographical appellation, but the recessive gene presumed to be responsible has now been identified on chromosome 16. The gastrointestinal problem is in the differential diagnosis of pain, given that (despite claims to the contrary) there is no diagnostic test. A high index of suspicion and increased concentrations of C-reactive protein will lead to the therapeutic test of a trial of colchicine, which is usually effective. Laparotomy is clearly to be avoided whenever possible, and units around the Mediterranean where the diagnosis is more common find that laparoscopic assessment of those with a differential diagnosis of appendicitis or other surgical emergency is most helpful (76). Presumably, now that the genetic basis is clearer, we can expect a diagnostic test within a year or two. Around 2% of all affected patients go on to develop amyloidosis; idiopathic hepatitis and an increased incidence of lymphoma are also reported.

CONCLUSIONS

Gastrointestinal assessment of the rheumatological patient is usually interesting, often rewarding, and yields unexpected gains, such as improved understanding of the anaemia of chronic disease, because in addition to non-specific effects from overexpression of cytokines and the depression of renal erythropoietin secretion, there is now evidence from sequential duodenal biopsies (77) that there is a disease-associated decrease in intestinal iron absorption (and increased intestinal mucosal ferritin), which is reversed by successful immunosuppressive treatment. The continuing close collaboration between practitioners of the two disciplines is to be encouraged, spurred on, perhaps by the current friendly rivalry in the assessment and implementation of the new molecular technology-based treatments (such as interleukins and tumour necrosis factor antibodies) for the inflammatory conditions common to both rheumatology and gastroenterology.

References

1. Hawkey CJ. Non-steroidal anti-inflammator, drug gastropathy: causes and treatment. *Scand J Gastroenterol Suppl* 1996; **220**: 124–127.
   Useful review article.
2. Laine L. Nonsteroidal anti-inflammatory drug gastropathy. *Gastrointest Endosc Clin North Am* 1996; **6**: 489–504.
   Useful review article.
3. Ballinger A. Cytoprotection with misoprostol: use in the treatment and prevention of ulcers. *Dig Dis* 1994; **12**: 375.
   Useful review article.
4. Ellershaw JE, Kelly MJ. Corticosteroids and peptic ulceration. *Palliat Med* 1994; **8**: 313–319.
   Useful review, but slanted to terminal neoplasia.
5. Mueller X, Rothenbuehler JM, Amery A *et al.* Factors predisposing to further hemorrhage and mortality after peptic ulcer bleeding. *J Am Coll Surg* 1994; **179**: 457–61.
   Useful review–steroids only one of several risk factors.
6. Engelhardt G. Pharmacology of meloxicam, a new nonsteroidal anti-inflammatory drug with an improved safety profile through preferential inhibition of COX-2. *Br J Rheumatol* 1996; **35 (suppl 1)**: 4–12.
7. Patoia L, Santucci L, Furno P *et al.* A 4-week, double-blind, parallel-group study to compare the gastrointestinal effects of meloxicam 7.5 mg, meloxicam 15 mg, piroxicam 20 mg and placebo by means of faecal blood loss, endoscopynd symptom evaluation in healthy volunteers. *Br J Rheumatol* 1996; **35 (suppl 1)**: 61–67.
8. Distel M, Mueller C, Bluhmki E *et al.* Safety of meloxicam: a global analysis of clinical trials. *Br J Rheumatol* 1996; **35 (suppl 1)**: 68–77.
   Not a meta-analysis, but a useful review of clinical trial data for the drug.
9. Levi S, de Lacey G, Price AB *et al.* "Diaphragm-like" strictures of the small bowel in patient, treated with non-steroidal anti-inflammatory drugs. *Br J Radiol* 1990; **63**: 186–189.
   Seminal paper on NSAID membrane disease.
10. Banerjee AK, Peters TJ. Experimental non-steroidal anti-inflammatory drug-induced enteropathy in the rat: similarities to inflammatory bowel disease and effect of thromboxane synthetase inhibitors. *Gut* 1990; **31**: 1358–1364.
11. Bjarnason I, Smethurst P, Levi AJ *et al.* The effect of polyacrylic acid polymers on small-intestinal function and permeability changes caused by indomethacin. *Scand J Gastroenterol* 1991; **26**: 685–688.
12. Morris AJ, Madhok R, Sturrock RD *et al.* Enteroscopic diagnosis of small bowel ulceration in patients receiving non-steroidal anti-inflammatory drugs. *Lancet* 1991; **337**: 520.
13. Bjarnason I, Macpherson AJ. Intestinal toxicity of non-steroidal anti-inflammatory drugs. *Pharmacol Ther* 1994; **62**: 145–157.
    Useful review article.
14. Fellows IW, Clarke JM, Roberts PF. Non-steroidal anti-inflammatory drug-induced jejunal and colonic diaphragm disease: a report of two cases. *Gut* 1992; **33**: 1424–1426.
15. Gleeson MH, Lim SH, Spencer D. Non-steroidal anti-inflammatory drugs, salicylates, and colitis. *Lancet* 1996; **347**: 904–905.
16. Wijnands MJ, Van 'T Hof MA, Van De Putte LB *et al.* Rheumatoid arthritis: a risk factor for sulphasalazine toxicity? A meta-analysis. *Br J Rheumatol* 1993; **32**: 313–318.
17. van Beusekom HJ, van de Laar MA, Franssen MJ *et al.* The moderate intestinal side effects of auranofin do not resuire prophylactic therapy with a bulk-forming agent. *Clin Rheumatol* 1997; **16**: 471–476.
18. Teodorescu V, Bauer J, Lichtiger S *et al.* Gold-induced colitis: a case report and review of the literature. *Mt Sinai J Med* 1993; **60**: 238–241.
    Useful review article.
19. Nisar M, Winfield J. Gold induced colitis and hepatic toxicity in a patient with rheumatoid arthritis. *J Rheumatol* 1994; **21**: 938–939.
20. Evron E, Brautbar C, Becker S *et al.* Correlation between gold-induced enterocplitis and the presence of the HLA-DRB1*0404 allele. *Arthritis Rheum* 1995; **38**: 755–759.
21. West SG. Methotrexate hepatotoxicity. *Rheum Dis Clin North Am* 1997; **23**: 883–915.
    Useful review article.
22. Hashkes PJ, Balistreri WF, Bove KE *et al.* The long-term effect of methotrexate therapy on the liver in patients with juvenile rheumatoid arthritis. *Arthritis Rheum* 1997; **40**: 2226–2234.
23. Omdal R, Husby G, Koldingsnes W. Intravenous and oral cyclophosphamide pulse therapy in rheumatic diseases: side effects and complications. *Clin Exp Rheumatol* 1993; **11**: 283–288.
    Useful review article.
24. Snyder LS, Heigh RI, Anderson ML. Cyclophosphamide-induced hepattoxicity in a patient with Wegener's granulomatosis. *Mayo Clin Proc* 1993; **68**: 1203–1204.
25. Modzelewski JR Jr, Daeschner C, Joshi VV *et al.* Veno-occlusive disease of the liver induced by low-dose cyclophosphamide. *Mod Pathol* 1994; **7**: 967-972.
26. Gustafsson LL, Eriksson LS, Dahl ML *et al.* Cyclophosphamide-induced acute liver failure requiring transplantation in a patient with genetically deficient debrisoquine metabolism: a causal relationship? *J Intern Med* 1996; **240**: 311–314.
27. Jacobs JW, Van der Weide FR, Kruijsen MW. Fatal cholestatic hepatitis caused by D-penicillamine. *Br J Rheumatol* 1994; **33**: 770–773.
28. Ramboer C, Verhamme M. D-penicillamine-induced oesophageal ulcers. *Acta Clin Belg* 1989; **44**: 189–191.
29. Ahn JH, Kim TH, Peck KR *et al.* A case of polymyositis in a patient with primary biliary cirrhosis treated with D-penicillamine. *Korean J Intern Med* 1993; **8**: 46–50.
30. Fradkin A, Yahav J, Diver Haber A *et al.* Colchicine enhances intestinal permeabity in patients with familial Mediterranean fever. *Eur J Clin Pharmacol* 1996; **51**: 241–245.
31. Hart J, Lewin KJ, Peters RS *et al.* Effect of long-term colchicine therapy on jejunal mucosa. *Dig Dis Sci* 1993; **38**: 2017–2021.

32. Schneider P, Korolenko TA, Busch U. A review of drug-induced lysosomal disorders of the liver in man and laboratory animals. *Microsc Res Tech* 1997; **36**: 253–275.

33. van Everdingen-Bongers JJ, Janssen P, Lammens M *et al.* Granulomatous hepatitis attributed to the combination pyrimethamine-chloroquine. *Ned Tijdschr Geneeskd* 1996; **140**: 320–322.

34. Makin AJ, Wendon J, Fitt S *et al.* Fulmnant hepatic failure secondary to hydroxychloroquine. *Gut* 1994; **35**: 569–570.

35. Bhasin DK, Chhina RS, Sachdeva JR. Endoscopic assessment of chloroquine phosphate-induced damage oesophageal, gastric, and duodenal mucosa. *Am J Gastroenterol* 1991; **86**: 434–437.

36. Leach SD, Bilchik AJ, Karapetian O *et al.* Influence of chloroquine on diet-induced pancreatitis. *Pancreas* 1993; **8**: 64–69.

37. Zeilhofer HU, Mollenhauer J, Brune K. Selective growth inhibition of ductal pancreatic adenoarcinoma cells by the lysosomotropic agent chloroquine. *Cancer Lett* 1989; **44**: 61–66.

38. Lovy MR, Starkebaum G, Uberoi S. Hepatitis C infection presenting with rheumatic manifestations: a mimic of rheumatoid arthritis. *J Rheumatol* 1996; **23**: 979–983.
    Case report with useful background on rheumatoid arthritis and HCV.

39. Ruderman EM, Crawford JM, Maier A *et al.* Histologic liver abnormalities in an autopsy series of patients with rheumatoid arthritis. *Br J Rheumatol* 1997; **36**: 210–213.

40. Kauppi M, Pukkala E, Isomaki H. Low incidence of colorectal cancer in patients with rheumatoid arthritis. *Clin Exp Rheumatol* 1996; **14**: 551–553.

41. Jager HJ, Mehring U, Gotz GF *et al.* Radiological features of the visceral and skeletal involvement of hemochromatosis. *Eur Radiol* 1997; **7**: 1199–1206.
    Useful review article on radiology.

42. Keat A. ABC of rheumatology. Spondyloarthropathies. *BMJ* 1995; **310**: 1321–1324.
    Useful review article.

43. De Vos M, Mielants H, Cuvelier C *et al.* Long-term evolution of gut inflammation in patients with spondyloar-thropathy. *Gastroenterology* 1996; **110**: 1696–1703.

44. Tiwana H, Wilson C, Walmsley RS *et al.* Antibody responses to gut bacteria in ankylosing spondylitis, rheymatoid arthritis, Crohn's disease and ulcerative colitis. *Rheumatol Int* 1997; **17**: 11–16.

45. Orchard TR, Wordsworth BP, Jewell DP. Peripheral arthropathies in inflammatory bowel disease: their articular distribution and natural history. *Gut* 1998; **42**: 387–391.
    New classification (uncertain validity), but very useful review.

46. Lock G, Holstege A, Lang B *et al.* Gastrointestinal manifestations of progressive systemic sclerosis. *Am J Gastroenterol* 1997; **92**: 763–771.
    Useful review article.

47. Sjogren RW. Gastrointestinal features of scleroderma. *Curr Opin Rheumatol* 1996; **8**: 569–575.
    Useful review article.

48. Abu-Shakra M, Guillemin F, Lee P. Gastrointestinal manifestations of systemic sclerosis. *Semin Arthritis Rheum* 1994; **24**: 29–39.

49. Sjogren RW. Gastrointestinal motility disorders in scleroderma. *Arthritis Rheum* 1994; **37**: 1265–1282.

50. Engel AF, Kamm MA, Talbot IC. Progressive systemic sclerosis of the internal anal sphincter leading to passive faecal incontinence. *Gut* 1994; **35**: 857–859.
    Novel observation of clinical significance — several cases.

51. Quiroz ES, Flannery MT, Martinez EJ *et al.* Pneumatosis cystoides intestinalis in progressive syptemic sclerosis: a case report and literature review. *Am J Med Sci* 1995; **310**: 252–255.

52. Doria A, Bonavina L, Anselmino M *et al.* Esophageal involvement in mixed connective tissue disease. *J Rheumatol* 1991; **18**: 685–690.

53. Marshall JB, Kretschmar JM, Gerhardt DC *et al.* Gastrointestinal manifestations of mixed connective tissue disease. *Gastroenterology* 1990; **98**: 1232–1238.
    Useful review article.

54. Tomsic M, Ferlan-Marolt V, Kveder T *et al.* Mixed connective tissue disease associated with autoimmune hepatitis and thyroiditis. *Ann Rheum Dis* 1992; **51**: 544–546.

55. Choy CW, Smith PA, Frazer C *et al.* Ruptured hepatic artery aneurysm in polyarteritis nodosa: a case report and literature review. *Aust N Z J Surg* 1997; **67**: 904–906.
    Useful review article.

56. Guillevin L, Lhote F, Gayraud M *et al.* Prognostic factors in polyarteritis nodosa and Chur-Strauss syndrome. A prospective study in 342 patients. *Medicine (Baltimore)* 1996; **75**: 17–28.
    A major series and a useful review in one article.

57. Guillevin L, Lhote F, Cohen P *et al.* Polyarteritis nodosa related to hepatitis B virus. A prospective stdy with long-term observation of 41 patients. *Medicine (Baltimore)* 1995; **74**: 238–253.

58. Guillevin L, Lhote F, Gallais V *et al.* Gastrointestinal tract involvement in polyarteritis nodosa and Churg–Strauss syndrome. *Ann Med Interne (Paris)* 1995; **146**: 260–267.

59. Leavitt RY, Fauci AS. Less common manifestations and presentations of Wegener's granulomatosis. *Curr Opin Rheumatol* 1992; **4**: 16–22.

60. Shimamoto C, Hirata I, Ohshiba S *et al.* Churgi–Strauss syndrome (allergic granulomatous angiitis) with peculiar multiple colonic ulcers. *Am J Gastroenterol* 1990; **85**: 316–319.

61. Babian M, Nasef S, Soloway G. Gastrointestinal infarction as a manifestation of rheumatoid vasculitis. *Am J Gastroenterol* 1998; **93**: 119–120.

62. Burke AP, Sobin LH, Virmani R. Localized vasculitis of the gastrointestinal tract. *Am J Surg Pathol* 1995; **19**: 338–349.

63. Yurdakul S, Tuzuner N, Yurdakul I *et al.* Gastrointestinal in,volvement in Behçet's syndrome: a controlled study. *Ann Rheum Dis* 1996; **55**: 208–210.
    A major controlled series from the Mecca for the disease.

64. Jankowski J, Crombie I, Jankowski R. Behcet's syndrome in Scotland. *Postgrad Med J* 1992; **68**: 566–570.
    An interesting contrast to the Turkish data.

65. Kim JH, Choi BI, Han JK *et al.* Colitis in Behçet's disease: characteristics on double contrast barium enema examination in 20 patients. *Abdom Imaging* 1994; **19**: 132–136.

66. Bayraktar Y, Balkanci F, Bayraktar M *et al.* Budd–Chiari syndrome: a common complication of Behçet's disease. *Am J Gastroenterol* 1997; **92**: 858–862.

67. Iida M, Kobayashi H, Matsumoto T *et al.* Postoperative recurrence in patients with intestinal Behçet's disease. *Dis Colon Rectum* 1994; **37**: 16–21.

68. Lee JG, Wilson JA, Gottfried MR. Gastrointestinal manifestation of amyloidosis. *South Med J* 1994; **87**: 243–247.

69. Lovat LB. Amyloidosis for the gastroenterologist. *CME J Gastroenterol Hepatol Nutr* 1998; **1**: 68–73.
Useful review article.

70. Horowitz HW, Dworkin B, Forseter G *et al.* Liver function in early Lyme disease. *Hepatology* 1996; **23**: 1412–1427.

71. Steere AC. Diagnosis and treatment of Lyme arthritis. *Med Clin North Am* 1997; **81**: 179–194.

72. Durand DV, Lecomte C, Cathebras P, for the Société Nationale Française de Médecine Interne (SNFMI) Research Group on Whipple Disease. Whipple disease. Clinical review of 52 cases. *Medicine (Baltimore)* 1997; **76**: 170–184.
Major series with useful commentary.

73. Fantry GT, James SP. Whipple's disease. *Dig Dis* 1995; **13**: 108–118.

74. Majeed HA, Barakat M. Familial Mediterranean fever (recurrent hereditary polyserositis) in children: analysis of 88 cases. *Eur J Pediatr* 1989; **148**: 636–641.
Useful review article, but obviously with a paediatric slant.

75. Babior BM, Matzner Y. The familial Mediterranean fever gene – cloned at last. *N Engl J Med* 1997; **337**: 1548–1549.
Not in this report itself; nevertheless a useful paper, as it provides data, and analysis of the clinical significance of the genetic work.

76. Reissman P, Durst AL, Rivkind A *et al.* Elective laparoscopic appendectomy in patients with familial Mediterranean fever. *World J Surg* 1994; **18**: 139–141.

77. O'Toole PA, Sykes H, Phelan M *et al.* Duodenal mucosal ferritin in rheumatoid arthritis: implications for anaemia of chronic disease. *Q J Med* 1996; **89**: 509–514.

7. Gastrointestinal Problems in the Immunocompromised

ROSS D. CRANSTON, PETER ANTON and IAN MCGOWAN

INTRODUCTION

Gastrointestinal disease secondary to immunosuppression that is not associated with human immunodeficiency virus (HIV) remains relatively uncommon outside transplantation medicine, therefore the majority of this chapter will review the clinical presentation, diagnosis, and treatment of HIV-associated gastrointestinal disease. Gastrointestinal disease caused by iatrogenic and familial immunosuppression will be discussed briefly at the end of the chapter.

HIV-ASSOCIATED GASTROINTESTINAL DISEASE

The differential diagnosis of HIV-associated gastrointestinal disease is similar for all anatomical sites and symptoms and is summarized in Table 7.1

Treatment options are summarized in Table 7.2. **Gastrointestinal endoscopy** is central to the diagnosis of many HIV-associated gastrointestinal diseases. The procedure is discussed in depth in Chapter 44.

As with all other clinical investigation, attempts should be made to construct algorithms that maximize diagnostic information whilst minimizing inconvenience to the patient and the use of resources. In patients with advanced HIV disease, a multifactorial aetiology is not uncommon. In addition, as the natural history of opportunistic infection (in the absence of effective antiretroviral treatment) is one

Table 7.1. The differential diagnosis of HIV-associated gastrointestinal disease.

Opportunistic infection	Bacterial
	Protozoal
	Viral
	Fungal
Opportunistic malignancy	Kaposi's sarcoma
	Lymphoma
Drug toxicity	
Motility disorder	
Psychological	

of relapse, many conditions will require the use of maintenance therapy. The immune restoration seen with "highly active antiretroviral therapy" (HAART) may obviate the need for continued maintenance therapy for opportunistic infections.

Oral and oesophageal disease

Inspection of the oral mucosa should be a routine component of the examination of the patient as it may allow a clinician to diagnose HIV infection in an otherwise asymptomatic individual.

Oral candidiasis

Oral candidiasis is a common initial manifestation of HIV infection; characteristically seen as immune function that is declining, it may also be seen in the setting of primary HIV infection. Four clinical presentations have been described:

Table 7.2. Treatment of HIV-associated gastrointestinal disease.

Problem	Cause	Treatment	Dose	Comment
Oral or oesophageal disease	*Candida albicans*	Topical		
		Nystatin suspension	500 000 U 4 × daily	7 days
		Systemic		
		Fluconazole	50–100 mg 1 × daily	14–30 days
		Ketoconazole	200–400 mg 1 × daily	14 days
		Itraconazole	200 mg 1 × daily	14 days
		Amphotericin	0.3–0.5 mg/kg per day IV (after test dose)	2nd-line therapy for resistant strains
	Oral hairy leucoplakia	*Acyclovir	400 mg 5 x daily	5 days
	Herpes simplex	Acyclovir	400 mg 5 × daily	5 days
		Valaciclovir	0.5–1.0 g 2 × daily	5 days
		Foscarnet	40 mg/kg IV 3 × daily	14–21 days
	CMV	Ganciclovir (induction)	5 mg/kg IV 2 × daily	14–21 days
		Ganciclovir (maintenance)	5 mg/kg IV 1 × daily	
		Foscarnet (induction)	60 mg/kg IV 3 × daily	14–21 days
		Foscarnet (maintenance)	60 mg/kg IV 1 × daily	
	Kaposi's sarcoma	HAART		
	Periodontitis	Dental care		
		Metronidazole	200 mg 3 × daily	3 days
	Apthous ulceration	Antiseptic mouthwash		
		*Thalidomide	200 mg 1 × daily	1–2 weeks
Acute diarrhoea	*Salmonella*	Ciprofloxacin	500–750 mg 2 × daily	2–4 weeks
	Shigella	Ciprofloxacin	500–750 mg 2 × daily	5 days
	Campylobacter jejuni	Ciprofloxacin	500–750 mg 2 × daily	5 days
	Clostridium difficile	Metronidazole	250–500 mg 3 × daily	7 days
		Vancomycin	125 mg 4 × daily	7–10 days
Chronic diarrhoea	Enterocytozoon bienusi	HAART		
		*Atovaquone		
		*Thalidomide	200 mg 1 × daily	
	Encephalitozoon intestinalis	*Albendazole	400–800 mg 2 × daily	21–28 days
	Cryptosporidium	HAART		
		*Paromomycin	500 mg 4 × daily	21 days
		*Nitazoxanide	1000 mg 1 × daily	21–28 days
	CMV	See above		
	Mycobacterium avium/intracellulare	Clarithromycin + ethambutol + rifabutin	500 mg 2 × daily 15 mg/kg 1 × daily 300 mg 1 × daily	Indefinitely unless immune status improves on HAART
	Isospora	*Co-trimoxazole	960 mg 3 × daily	7 days
	Entamoeba histolytica	Metronidazole	800 mg 3 × daily	5 days
	Giardia	Metronidazole	2 g 1 × daily	3 days
	Cyclospora	*Co-trimoxazole	960 mg 2 × daily	7 days
	Small–bowel overgrowth	Doxycycline	100 mg 2 × daily	7 days
	Idiopathic	HAART		
		Loperamide	4 mg initially then 2 mg after each loose stool. Max. 16 mg/day	5 days
Wasting		*Megestrol acetate	400–800 mg 1 × daily	Depends on response
		Cyproheptadine	4 mg 3 × daily	Depends on response
		*Growth hormone		Depends on response
		*Thalidomide	100–200 mg 1 × daily	Depends on response
		Testosterone	100–400 mg IM 2-weekly	Depends on response
		Testosterone patch	5 mg patch 1 × daily	Depends on response

*Drugs that are available on a named-patient basis, or as part of clinical trials, or are being used outside their licensed indication.

1. The typical **pseudomembranous** variety (thrush) is unlikely to cause any diagnostic difficulty.
2. The **erythematous** form (smooth red patches on the hard or soft palate, buccal mucosa or tongue, sometimes with depapillation of the tongue) may be less obvious.
3. The **hyperplastic** form (white plaques that can not be scraped away, usually found on the buccal mucosa) also may be less obvious.
4. The fourth presentation is **angular cheilitis**. Oral culture can be confusing, as **Candida albicans** is a common oral commensal.

Treatment of oral candidiasis is usually with topical antifungal agents, such as nystatin suspension or lozenges. In more severe cases, systemic antifungals such as fluconazole or ketoconazole are indicated. Symptoms and signs usually disappear within 1–2 weeks of treatment, but it may be necessary to offer maintenance antifungal therapy to prevent recurrence of oral candidiasis.

Oral hairy leucoplakia

In its most characteristic form, oral hairy leucoplakia (OHL) presents as vertical white folds on the lateral margins and dorsal surface of the tongue. It is believed to represent epithelial hyperplasia secondary to persistent Epstein—Barr virus (EBV) or human papilloma virus (HPV) infection (1). Patients are usually asymptomatic and no specific treatment is necessary. In rare cases of discomfort, the lesions may respond to oral acyclovir.

Periodontal disease

HIV-associated periodontitis involves rapid loss of periodontal attachment and destruction of underlying bone, and may be associated with features of acute necrotizing ulcerative gingivitis or necrotizing stomatitis (2). Treatment is empirical and includes improved dental hygiene, antiseptic mouthwashes such as chlorhexidine, and short courses of metronidazole.

Mucosal ulceration

This may be caused by herpes simplex infection, apthous ulceration or cytomegalovirus (CMV) infection. Management is directed at excluding specific causes of mucosal ulceration. Herpes simplex can be treated with acyclovir. Apthous ulceration can often be controlled with antiseptic mouthwashes and local steroid preparations. In severe cases, treatment with thalidomide may be of benefit (3). More unusual causes of oral ulceration include lymphoma, EBV, atypical *Mycobacterium spp.*, *M. tuberculosis*, *Histoplasma spp.* and *Cryptococcus* (4).

Kaposi's sarcoma

This is commonly found in the mouth. Its characteristic violaceous colour usually makes diagnosis straightforward, but confusion may arise with macular lesions and when the tumour infiltrates the gums. Oral Kaposi's sarcoma is often associated with visceral involvement.

Oesophageal syndrome

Although *Candida* is the most common cause of oesophageal symptoms such as retrosternal discomfort or dysphagia, the differential diagnosis of oesophageal disease in HIV infection is wide (Table 7.3).

Treatment is directed at the underlying cause of the symptoms, but while a specific therapeutic response is awaited, symptomatic relief may be obtained, with a liquidized diet in combination with antacid preparations, particularly those containing a local anaesthetic such as mucaine suspension.

Many centres advocate empirical systemic antifungal treatment, reserving endoscopy for patients who fail to respond to initial treatment or for those patients who relapse after treatment (5). Subse-

Table 7.3. The differential diagnosis of oesophageal symptoms in HIV infection.

Candida albicans	
Herpes simplex	
CMV	
Apthous ulceration	
Lymphoma	
Drug induced	Doxycycline
	NSAIDs
	Zidovudine
	Zalcitabine
Dysmotility	
Reflux disease	

NSAIDs, non-steroidal anti-inflammatory drugs.

quent endoscopic investigation should be directed at finding the specific cause of the patient's symptoms. This may require careful examination of the oesophageal mucosa, as plaques of *Candida* may obscure other additional pathogens such as CMV. In addition, multiple endoscopic biopsies may be required to identify mucosal CMV infection. Biopsy specimens should be collected from the base of ulcers, to exclude CMV infection, and from the ulcer margins, to exclude other agents associated with squamous cells, including herpes simplex. Endoscopy, combined with appropriate microbiological and histological sampling, can offer a diagnostic rate of 95.5% in patients with oesophageal symptoms (6).

Table 7.4. The differential diagnosis of HIV-associated diarrhoea.

Protozoa	Microsporidia
	Cryptosporidium
	Isospora
	Giardia
	Cyclospora
	Entamoeba
Viral	CMV
	Adenovirus
	HIV
Bacterial	*Salmonella*
	Shigella
	Campylobacter
	Escherichia coli
	Clostridium difficile
	Mycobacterium avium/intracellulare
Fungal	*Histoplasma capsulatum*
Drugs	Protease inhibitors
Lactose intolerance	
Small-bowel overgrowth	
Kaposi's sarcoma/lymphoma	
Fat malabsorption	

Diarrhoea

Up to 50% of patients with HIV will have diarrhoea during the course of their illness (7). The differential diagnosis is broad (Table 7.4). Diarrhoea may result from opportunistic infection or be secondary to the use of medications such as protease inhibitors.

The organisms associated with diarrhoea can be divided into three main groups: **protozoal**, **viral**, and **bacterial**.

Protozoal infections

Cryptosporidium

This organism affects both immunocompetent and immunosuppressed individuals. Its increased recognition has been a consequence of improved laboratory diagnostic tests. Prevalence rates for immunocompetent individuals with diarrhoea range from 0.6–10% in developed countries to 4–20% in developing countries. In the United States, 3–4% of patients with acquired immunodeficiency syndrome (AIDS) have cryptosporidiosis, whereas a study from Uganda showed that 48% of patients with AIDS-related diarrhoea had evidence of cryptosporidiosis (8).

Histologically, *Cryptosporidium* is a small (2–8 µm), single-celled round body. It has a characteristic intracellular extracytoplasmic location in the gut mucosa. In immunocompetent individuals, after an incubation period of 3–8 days, *Cryptosporidium* produces diarrhoea with symptoms lasting 2–4 weeks. Oocyst excretion stops shortly after the cessation of symptoms, and an asymptomatic carrier state appears unusual. How-

ever, one study from New York demonstrated oocysts in the duodenal aspirate in 12.7% of patients undergoing endoscopic examination; none of them had diarrhoea or was immunosuppressed (9).

There are several different **modes of transmission**, including occupational exposure, person-to-person (particularly children in day-care centres), nosocomial infection, travellers' diarrhoea and environmental water supplies. Pollution of the domestic water supply with *Cryptosporidium* is a difficult problem to treat, as cryptosporidial oocysts are remarkably resistant to conventional chemical treatment; 1 µm domestic filtration units may be helpful. Patients with CD4 counts of less than 200/mm³ should be advised to boil drinking water, to minimize the acquisition of enteric pathogens, including Cryptosporidium.

In immunocompromized individuals, cryptosporidiosis is a more persistent and sometimes life-threatening illness. The organism is most commonly found in the small intestine, but can disseminate throughout the gastrointestinal tract and hepatobiliary tree. Very occasionally, the organism is found in extraintestinal sites such as the lung. Patients present with a variety of symptoms including nausea, vomiting, anorexia and, most importantly, diarrhoea of varying severity.

Diagnosis is based on identification of oocysts of *Cryptosporidium* in faecal smears. A variety of techniques are available; most involve modified acid-fast stains (10). Concentration techniques may be helpful when small quantities of oocysts are present. Monoclonal antibodies directed against oocyst antigens are available (11). In patients who are persistently stool-negative, endoscopy with duodenal aspiration and distal duodenal biopsy may be helpful.

Specific antimicrobial **treatment** for cryptosporidial diarrhoea has been uniformly disappointing, although HAART may alleviate symptoms. Transient improvement in symptoms has been attributed to a wide range of pharmaceutical agents, including paromomycin, azithromycin, and nitazoxanide. A placebo-controlled trial of nitazoxanide is under way and results are awaited. Meanwhile, symptoms should be palliated with conventional antidiarrhoeal treatments. A placebo-controlled study of the somatostatin analogue, octreotide, was unable to demonstrate efficacy in the treatment of cryptosporidial diarrhoea (12).

Microsporidia

Although the clinical manifestations of HIV-associated microsporidial infection have been characterized (13), the prevalence of microsporidial infection as a cause of HIV-associated diarrhoea is uncertain. Estimates range from 7 to 50%, and may reflect local expertise in diagnosis, true geographical variation, or both. The two principal species of Microsporidia in HIV infection are *Enterocytozoon bienusi* and *Encephalitozoon intestinalis*; *E. bienusi* accounts for 80–90% of microsporidial disease and *E. intestinalis* the remainder. Infection with *E. bienusi* is usually localized to the intestinal and hepatobiliary tracts (14,15), but *E. intestinalis* disseminates to the renal and respiratory tracts (16). Hepatitis, peritonitis, keratopathy, conjunctivitis, glomerulonephritis, nasal obstruction, and sclerosing cholangitis have all been reported in association with microsporidial infection.

The small size of microsporidial organisms, particularly *E. bienusi* (1–2 μm in diameter) presents a significant diagnostic challenge. Transmission electron microscopy has been the definitive method for diagnosing human microsporidial infection and remains useful for ultrastructural speciation. Recent advances in the diagnosis of microsporidial infection have included demonstration of microsporidial

spores in stool specimens using chemoflourescent agents that bind to the chitinous walls of the microsporidial spores (17) and, most recently, molecular diagnosis, which allows the amplification of microsporidial DNA (18,19). Despite this, many centres still rely on the use of standard histological examination of tissue, augmented by a range of specific stains.

Treatment is difficult, apart from initiating HAART. Albendazole has shown promise in patients with AIDS who are infected with *E. intestinalis*, but has no effect on *E. bienusi* (16,20). Recently, atovaquone and thalidomide have shown promise against *E. bienusi* (21,22). In the case of thalidomide, the benefit may be mediated by downregulation of intestinal mucosal production of tumour necrosis factor α.

Isospora belli

Infection with *Isospora belli* presents in manner similar to cryptosporidiosis. The organism is usually detected in faeces using a modified acid-fast staining proceedure. Oocysts of *Isospora* are 10 times larger than those of *Cryptosporidium*. Successful treatment has been reported with oral co-trimoxazole. Approximately 50% of affected patients will suffer relapse unless they receive maintenance treatment (23).

Other protozoal infections

Entamoeba histolytica is a common parasite found in homosexual men, and was initially believed to be a potential pathogen in AIDS-related diarrhoea. Isolates of *E. histolytica* have been classified into zymodemes on the basis of their isoenzyme pattern on electrophoresis. The zymodemes found commonly in both HIV-negative and HIV-positive homosexual men are non-pathogenic types. If *E. histolytica* is found in an HIV-positive patient with diarrhoea, there is usually some other cause for the symptoms. However, invasive amoebic dysentery should be excluded in patients with an appropriate exposure when travelling abroad.

Giardia lamblia may also cause diarrhoea. Some studies have shown a greater prevalence of infection in homosexual controls, others have not. There is no evidence that HIV-positive patients are at greater risk, although the duration and severity of the diarrhoea may be increased.

Cyclospora cayetanensis is a coccidian parasite, previously described as blue-green algae or cyanobacterium-like bodies, which has been described as an important cause of prolonged diarrhoea in travellers returning from the tropics (24). These organisms may also affect patients with HIV infection and produce a prolonged illness characterized by watery diarrhoea and weight loss. Treatment is with cotrimoxazole.

Blastocystis hominis is often isolated from the gastrointestinal tract, but is not considered pathogenic in either immunocompetent or immunosuppressed patients (25).

Viral infections

Cytomegalovirus

Approximately 50% of adults in developing countries are seropositive for CMV, but up to 100% of homosexual men may have antibodies to CMV. After primary infection, the virus usually remains dormant throughout life. With severe immunosuppression, CMV has been shown to reactivate, causing a variety of clinical problems including retinitis, oesophagitis, colitis, pneumonia, encephalitis, and adrenalitis (26).

CMV colitis occurs in 5–10% of patients with AIDS and symptoms include diarrhoea, abdominal pain, weight loss, anorexia, and fever (27). Toxic dilatation, perforation, and haemorrhage have also been described. Sigmoidoscopy often reveals diffuse erythema with mucosal ulceration. **Diagnosis** requires tissue biopsy and demonstration of inflammation and cytopathic effects. Isolation alone of CMV does not indicate that it is the cause of the patient's symptoms. Histological changes include vasculitis, neutrophil infiltration, and non-specific inflammation. Characteristic 'owl's eye' inclusions may also be seen; these inclusions are often seen most readily in the vascular endothelium of inflamed areas, suggesting that the colitis is caused by a virally induced vasculitis. Monoclonal antibodies are also available to demonstrate CMV antigens in tissues, by immunofluorescence (28).

The drug most commonly used in the **treatment** of CMV infections is ganciclovir, an acyclic nucleoside analogue of acyclovir that has been shown to produce significant inhibition of CMV replication *in vitro*. Ganciclovir only has a 4% oral bioavailability, and so is usually given as an intravenous preparation, although an oral formulation is available for patients requiring prophylaxis. Treatment of CMV disease varies: some centres use ganciclovir for a 2–3 week period, followed by

withdrawal of the drug, whereas other centres prefer an induction course followed by indefinite maintenance therapy. Response rates of up to 75% have been reported. The main problem with treatment is the associated neutropenia, which can occur particularly when ganciclovir is combined with antiretroviral therapy. Alternative antiviral agents include foscarnet and cidofovir. Both agents have to be given intravenously; foscarnet can cause hypocalcaemia, renal insufficiency, and genital ulceration, and cidofovir is nephrotoxic.

Herpes simplex

Herpes simplex causes mucocutaneous lesions at the upper and lower end of the gastrointestinal tract. The most common clinical problem associated with herpes simplex is recurrent, chronic perianal ulceration. Pain is often a very prominent symptom, and herpes simplex proctitis may be associated with urinary retention. **Diagnosis** is usually straightforward, by culture of the virus from ulcer sites. Treatment is with acyclovir, famciclovir, or valaciclovir; often it is necessary to give maintenance therapy to prevent relapses.

Patients have been described with ulcerative mucocutaneous herpes infection that failed to heal even with high-dose intravenous acyclovir (Figure 7.1). Isolates showed a 7–80-fold decrease in sensitivity and the resistant strains were found to be deficient in thymidine kinase (29). Foscarnet has been found to be helpful in this situation, as it does not require phosphorylation to achieve antiviral activity (30).

Human papilloma virus

HPV infection is common in homosexual men. Perianal warts tend to be more resistant to ablative treatment in patients with HIV infection. More worrying is the association between HPV infection, anal intraepithelial neoplasia, and HIV infection (Figures 7.2).

Bacterial infections

The most common presentation of infection of *Salmonella*, *Shigella* and *Campylobacter* in HIV-positive patients is with diarrhoea. However, they may also present with isolated pyrexia secondary to bacteraemia, or with complications such as toxic megacolon.

Diagnosis is made on the basis of faecal and blood cultures. **Treatment** is with appropriate antibiotics,

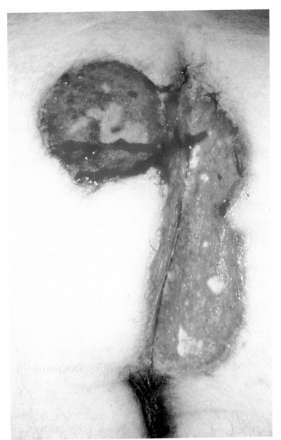

Figure 7.1. Aciclovir-resistant perianal herpes simplex ulceration.

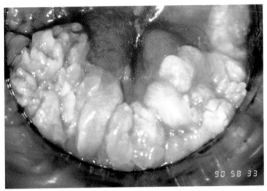

Figure 7.2. (A) Anal condylomata secondary to human papilloma virus infection.

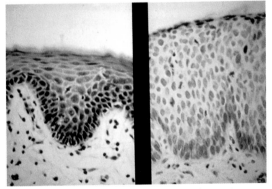

Figure 7.2. (B) Anal biopsy, showing features of intraepithelial dysplasia

particularly when there is evidence of bacteraemia. Treatment should be guided by the results of *in vitro* susceptibility data, and maintenence therapy may be needed to prevent relapses.

Atypical *Mycobacteria* of the *Mycobacterium avium/intracellulare* complex are ubiquitous organisms with little virulence for the immunocompetent host. Disseminated infection occurs in patients with AIDS who have multiorgan involvement. Patients usually have advanced disease with CD4 counts of less than 50/mm^3. Gastrointestinal infection is associated with anaemia, fever, weight loss, diarrhoea, and malabsorption. **Diagnosis** is suggested by finding acid-fast staining organisms in the stool, although a definitive diagnosis requires identification of *M. avium* complex in intestinal tissue biopsies.

Gut involvement may mimic Whipple's disease in appearance (31). The small intestine shows prominent folds, with periodic acid Schiff-positive foamy macrophages containing the organisms and filling the lamina propria. The bacteria are acid-fast, unlike those of Whipple's disease. They are sensitive *in vitro* to a variety of antituberculosis agents, and current initial treatment is with three agents — for example, rifabutin, ethambutol, and clarithromycin — in association with HAART (32).

Infection with *Clostridium difficile* is common in patients with AIDS, probably secondary to multiple exposures to antibiotic therapy. **Diagnosis** is by identifying *C. difficile* toxin in stool, and **treatment** is with oral metronidazole or vancomycin. Persistent carriage of *C. difficile* may respond to treatment with cholestyramine, which binds the toxin (33).

Management of HIV-associated diarrhoea

This is a controversial area (for reviews see (34–36)), but nevertheless it is possible to make

certain recommendations. Patients who are stable
on HAART are unlikely to have an opportunistic
enteric infection, but may be at risk of acquiring
pathogens such as *Salmonella* or toxogenic
C. difficile. Diarrhoea in patients receiving HAART
is more likely to be a consequence of the HAART
per se than one of enteric infection. Aggressive
investigation of diarrhoea, including endoscopy,
should be reserved for patients with chronic diarrhoea (at least two loose stools daily over a period
of at least 1 month) and CD4 counts of less than
200/mm^3.

The most useful, cost-effective, and often the least-
used tests in the diagnostic investigation of diarrhoea
are repeated examination of stool samples by experienced microbiologists and parasitologists. A minimum of three stool samples should be examined
for: *Salmonella, Shigella, Campylobacter, E. coli,
C. difficile* toxin, *Mycobacterium, Cryptosporidium,
Microsporidiua, Giardia* and *Isospora*.

In patients who have negative stool examinations, the next logical step is to perform
gastrointestinal endoscopy, with the collection of
small or large intestinal tissue. The decision to
perform upper or lower gastrointestinal endoscopy
(unless both are scheduled) should reflect the nature of the patient's symptoms: central abdominal
pain, large-volume diarrhoea, and malabsorption
suggest small intestinal pathology: frequent, small-
volume, bloody diarrhoea suggests large intestinal
disease. Intestinal tissue biopsies should be processed and reviewed by experienced pathologists
who are aware of the patient's HIV infection. Histological examination should include haematoxylin, and eosin acid-fast stain, Giemsa, and fluorescent
stains for CMV and Microsporidia.

Management of an HIV-infected patient with
diarrhoea is a challenge. Initially, it is necessary to
try to find specific, potentially treatable causes for
symptoms, which may then be treated with appropriate medication. In approximately 20% of cases,
no cause will be found, despite intensive investigation (37), and even specific causes may fail to respond to appropriate treatment or may relapse after
initial improvement. In these circumstances it is
very important to try to provide symptomatic treatment with antidiarrhoeal medication. Fluid depletion should be corrected by oral or intravenous
fluids. Many patients will also have nausea and
vomiting, which should be treated in a conventional
manner.

Malabsorption and weight loss

In the pre-HAART era, AIDS was associated with
profound weight loss, which arose from a combination of factors, including opportunistic infections,
anorexia, malabsorption, and chronic diarrhoea.
Fortunately, this problem is now seldom seen in
patients in developed countries with access to
antiretroviral medication. Indeed, many patients are
developing a 'protease paunch' as part of the poorly
defined lipodystrophy syndrome. However,
enteropathic AIDS is still seen in Africa in an extreme form, where it is known as 'slim disease' (38)
and appears to be closely associated with the presence of disseminated mycobacterial disease (39).

In the small number of patients who experience
weight loss, opportunistic infection should be excluded, and dietary assessment and advice, together
with dietary supplements, may be beneficial. A
variety of agents have been used to treat HIV-associated wasting, including recombinant human growth
hormone (40), thalidomide (41), megestrol acetate
(42), and testosterone (43). Many of these agents
produce modest increases in weight that may be of
fat rather than lean body mass, or, in the case of
human growth hormone, are extremely expensive.
Enteral and parenteral feeding are useful adjuncts
to nutritional support, but their timing and duration
are controversial.

AIDS and the liver

Abnormal liver function occurs commonly in AIDS,
but is seldom a cause of significant morbidity or
mortality. Factors contributing to liver disease in
HIV include pre-existing disease such as viral hepatitis, transfusion-related abnormalities, the effects
of systemic disease, malnutrition, AIDS-related
opportunistic infection or neoplasm, and the side
effects of multiple-drug treatment.

Hepatic opportunistic infection usually occurs in
the setting of disseminated infection with multiple
visceral involvement. Numerous viral, bacterial, fungal, and protozoal organisms have been identified,
including *M. avium/intracellulare, Cryptococcus
neoformans* and *Histoplasma spp*. Infection is usually
associated with a granulomatous hepatitis, with biochemistry suggesting cholestasis. Peliosis hepatitis may
present with fever, weight loss, abdominal pain, and
hepatosplenomegaly as a result of infection with
Bartonella henselae — the organism associated with

bacillary angiomatosis (cat scratch disease) (44). Abdominal computed tomography (CT) scanning reveals multiple small lesions throughout the liver parenchyma, and the Gram-negative organism can be detected on liver biopsy using the Warthin–Starry stain. Treatment is with erythromycin or doxycycline.

Interaction between HIV and hepatitis B/C virus

Many of the routes of transmission of HIV are shared by the hepatotropic viruses that can cause chronic hepatitis: hepatitis B virus (HBV), HCV and hepatitis D virus (HDV/delta virus). HIV infection may alter the natural history of HBV in a number of ways. Pre-existing HIV infection with quantitative or qualitative T4 lymphocyte defects may favour the establishment of chronic infection (45,46). After HBV vaccination, there is a lower response rate and faster rate of loss of antibody to HBV surface antigen in responders in the presence of HIV (47,48). HBV replication may be increased in the presence of HIV infection (49). Furthermore, the spontaneous loss of 'e' antigen with time may be reduced, and reactivation of viral replication may occur. Conversely, co-incident HIV infection in the chronic HBV carrier may decrease hepatic inflammatory activity as measured by transaminase concentrations and histology (49). Finally, HIV may diminish the response to treatment in chronic HBV infection.

In those who are co-infected with HIV and HCV, the results of immunoblot assays may be indeterminate, and molecular diagnostic techniques such as the polymerase chain reaction (PCR) may be required to provide an accurate diagnosis of HCV infection (50,51). HIV infection does not predispose to an increased incidence of fulminant or symptomatic HCV infection, but does appear to increase the progression of HCV-associated chronic liver disease (52); conversely, HCV does not increase the progression of HIV disease (52). As more patients have their disease stabilized with HAART, the amount of co-infection with HCV is likely to increase. Treatment remains empirical, but it seems that patients with CD4 counts greater than $350/mm^3$ respond to interferon in a manner similar to HIV-negative HCV-positive patients (53). Unfortunately, current antiretroviral therapy has no effect on HCV replication.

Investigation of abnormal liver function

The differential diagnosis of abnormal liver function in HIV infection is summarized in Table 7.5.

The criticial investigations in determining the aetiology of abnormal liver function are a CD4 count, liver enzyme profiles, viral hepatitis serology; consideration should be given to the use of ultrasonography and liver biopsy importantly, concurrent medications should be reviewed for hepatotoxicity. The many **hepatotoxic drugs used in HIV medicine** include:

- albendazole
- amphotericin B
- azithromycin
- carbamazepine
- co-trimoxazole
- didanosine
- erythromycin
- ethionamide
- ganciclovir
- isoniazid
- ketoconazole
- metronidazole
- penicillins
- pentamidine
- phenytoin
- prochlorperazine
- pyrazinamide
- rifampin
- tetracyclines
- valproic acid
- zidovudine

As with so many other complications of HIV infection, opportunistic liver infection is unusual in patients with a CD4 count greater than $200/mm^3$.

Table 7.5. The differential diagnosis of liver disease in HIV infection.

Disease	Causes	Specific organisms
Hepatitis	HBV, HCV, HDV	
	CMV	
	Epstein–Barr virus	
	Herpes simplex	
	Adenovirus	
	Varicella zoster	
	HIV	
	Hepatotoxic drugs	
	Alcohol	
Granulomatous inflammation	Mycobacteria	*Mycobacterium avium*
		M. tuberculosis
	Fungal	*Histoplasma capsulatum*
		Cryptococcus neoformans
		Coccidioides immitis
		Candida albicans
	Protozoa	*Pneumocystis carinii*
		Toxoplasma gondii
		Microsporidia
		Schistosoma
		Cryptosporidium parvum
Mass lesions	Kaposi's sarcoma	
	Lymphoma	
Vascular lesions	Peliosis hepatis	
	Kaposi's sarcoma	

Classification of liver disease into cholestatic or hepatitic disease on the basis of increases in liver enzymes can be useful, but in many cases the enzyme profile is mixed, with increases in transaminases and alkaline phosphatase. Most patients under clinic review will have had viral hepatitis serology analyses performed at baseline; if the result were seronegative for hepatitis A/B, vaccination will have been offered. Acquisition of new infection in seronegative patients, or reactivation of latent hepatitis B infection may subsequently occur. When the diagnostic profile is unclear, ultrasonography or endoscopic retrograde cholangiopancreatography (ERCP), or both, may be used to exclude abnormalities of the biliary tree or to demonstrate mass lesions within the liver.

Liver biopsy is necessary for definitive diagnosis of liver disease in patients in whom other investigations have failed to provide an adequate diagnosis. Biopsy can provide a specific diagnosis in 30–80% of patients with AIDS (54). In immunocompetent patients, the procedure is safe, with a morbidity of 0.1–0.6% and a mortality of 0–0.12% (55). In a recent study in New York that reviewed the results of 501 liver biopsies, 64% had specific diagnoses, mycobacterial disease being the most common finding (56).

Treatment

Treatment of liver disease is directed towards specific pathologies. Hepatotoxic medication should be stopped and systemic infections such as *Mycobacterium avium/intracellulare* treated where possible. Peliosis hepatitis may be treated with erythromycin or doxycycline. The response of chronic hepatitis B/C infection to interferon is disappointing, but the use of antiretroviral agents such as adefovir and lamivudine, which have activity against hepatitis B and HIV, is currently being studied. The treatment of visceral Kaposi's sarcoma is discussed below.

Pancreatic disease

Although a variety of post-mortem pancreatic abnormalities have been described in patients with AIDS, clinical pancreatitis with increased amylase appears to be less common. A differential diagnosis of HIV-associated pancreatitis is provided in Table 7.6.

It should be remembered that patients with AIDS are at risk of pancreatitis secondary to non-HIV associated causes, including alcohol. Pancreatitis severity should be scored using the Apache 2 method, which takes account of immunosuppression (57) and patients treated in the conventional manner. Patients with AIDS may have pre-existing hyperamylasaemia, and this should be fractionated into salivary and pancreatic components before pancreatitis is diagnosed. Alternatively, pancreatic lipase may be used to diagnose pancreatitis.

The prognosis for acute pancreatitis in patients with AIDS may be worsened by the presence of immunosuppression, or opportunistic infection.

AIDS sclerosing cholangitis

Acalculous cholecystitis has been described in association with infection with CMV, *Cryptosporidium* and *Campylobacter* in patients with AIDS (58,59).

AIDS sclerosing cholangitis is characterized by intermittent right upper-quadrant abdominal pain and increased concentrations of alkaline phosphatase, usually without increased bilirubin. Abdominal ultrasound and CT scans are effective in identifying biliary disease in patients, but do not display precise anatomical details. The intrahepatic cholangiographic changes seen at ERCP are suggestive of primary sclerosing cholangitis combined with an irregularly dilated common bile duct (Figures 7.3). Dilatation and irregularity of the pancreatic duct have also been reported.

The pathogenesis of AIDS sclerosing cholangitis remains unclear. Histologically, there is a non-spe-

Table 7.6. The dfferential diagnosis of pancreatitis in HIV infection.

Alcohol	
Cholelithiasis	
Hyperlipidaemia	
Hypercalcaemia	
HIV medications	Pentamidine
	Co-trimoxazole
	Didanosine
	Zalcitabine
Opportunistic infections	CMV
	Toxoplasma gondii
	Cryptococcus neoformans
	Candida albicans
	Cryptosporidium
	Mycobacterium tuberculosis
	M. avium/intracellulare

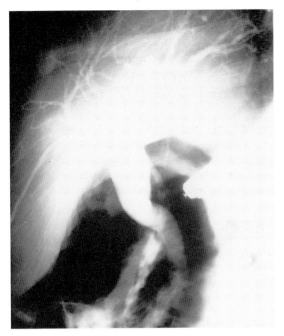

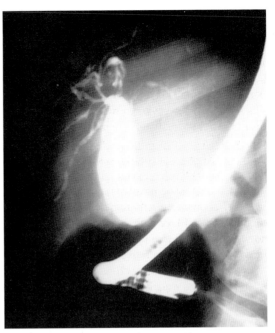

Figure 7.3. (A) ERCP performed on patient with HIV-1, who had right upper-quadrant pain and increased alkaline phosphatase.

Figure 7.3. (B) ERCP performed 6 months later demonstrates AIDS sclerosing cholangitis with papillary stenosis and intrahepatic sclerosis of the biliary tree. The patient was known to have cryptosporidial intestinal infection.

cific inflammation and ulceration. *Cryptosporidium* and CMV have been demonstrated in the majority of patients with AIDS sclerosing cholangitis, and implicated as a cause of this syndrome, but gram-negative bacteria and *Candida spp.* have also been cultured. There is no specific treatment, although treatment of associated infections, such as cryptosporidiosis or CMV, has been tried. Some patients with right upper-quadrant pain and stenosis of the papillary region may benefit from endoscopic sphincterotomy (60,61), with relief of pain, but liver function usually fails to improve.

Tumours

Kaposi's sarcoma

Before the use of HAART, Kaposi's sarcoma was the presenting feature in 26% of patients with AIDS in the United States, and the second most common AIDS diagnosis at presentation. Before the AIDS epidemic, this was a rare tumour, with an annual incidence of 0.02–0.06 per 100 000. It occurred mainly in men older than 50 years of age and of Jewish or Mediterranean ancestry. This classical form was usually confined to the lower limbs, ran an indolent course, and responded well to radiotherapy or chemotherapy. Kaposi's sarcoma was also a common tumour in Central Africa, where, in some areas, it accounted for 9% of all malignancies. AIDS-associated KS occurs in a younger age group, and has a much more aggressive natural history. The disease is more common in HIV-infected homosexual/ bisexual men than in other groups of patients. In one study, it was found in 19.8% of homosexual/bisexual men, compared with 2.7% of men who were users of injected drugs, suggesting that the condition might be associated with a sexually transmitted organism (62).

In 1994, Chang *et al.* (63) identified unique DNA sequences in Kaposi's sarcoma tumours that were related to EBV and herpes saimiri. The new virus acquired the name human herpes virus 8 (HHV8) and has been identified in the majority of Kaposi's sarcoma tissue samples, irrespective of the type of Kaposi's sarcoma. It is also found in body-cavity B cell lymphomas and Castleman's disease. Seroepidemiological studies have demonstrated a high level of antibodies to HHV8 in patients with Kaposi's sarcoma, although there is a background level of 1–25% in the general population, depending on which assay is used.

Clinically, Kaposi's sarcoma presents as violaceous lesions scattered on the skin. With the passage of time, these become more widespread, and mucous membrane, visceral, and lymph node involvement occurs. If upper and lower gastrointestinal endoscopy is performed at presentation, lesions will be demonstrated in about 40% of patients. At postmortem examination, they are present in more than 70%. Involvement of the hard palate and alveolar ridges, oropharynx, oesophagus, stomach, duodenum, colon, and rectum have been demonstrated. Lesions resemble the range seen in the skin: from small, flat telangiectatic lesions, not well demonstrated by contrast studies and only seen at endoscopy, to larger nodular or polypoid lesions. Endoscopic biopsy has a high false-negative rate, with only 23% of suspicious lesions being confirmed histologically, because of their deep position in the submucosa (64). Endoscopy is not routinely required to demonstrate visceral involvement if the diagnosis is made on the basis of mucocutaneous lesions.

Complications from the involvement of the gut are unusual. Haemorrhage from lesions, either acute or chronic, leading to iron deficiency anaemia may occur. Several cases of Kaposi's sarcoma presenting as an acute inflammatory-bowel-like syndrome, with diarrhoea and ulceration on barium enema, have also been described (65). Protein-losing enteropathy may also occur. The median survival from the time of diagnosis for patients with Kaposi's Sarcoma alone is substantially better than for those with opportunistic infections.

The first line **treatment** of Kaposi's sarcoma is to initiate or maximize HAART (66,67). Clinical resolution of the lesions in response to HAART may take 2–3 months. If a more rapid response is required, radiotherapy or combination chemotherapy may be used.

Treatment of gastrointestinal Kaposi's sarcoma is indicated if there are major symptoms. Local lesions in the mouth may respond to radiotherapy, but chemotherapy is the main modality of treatment. A variety of chemotherapeutic regimens have been used. Complex combination chemotherapy has the disadvantage of causing increased immunosuppression and increased risk of opportunistic infection. Simple regimens using vincristine and bleomycin alone or in combination produce a response in up to 75% of patients, with a low risk of bone marrow suppression. Alpha interferon may be used to induce remission of Kaposi's sarcoma in patients with CD4 counts of 200/mm^3 or more, but high doses are needed, and side effects such as fatigue, fever, and alopecia are common. This form of treatment is not beneficial in more immunosuppressed patients.

Lymphoma

Early studies identified homosexual men in whom non-Hodgkin's lymphoma was developing in a setting of persistent generalized lymphadenopathy, opportunistic infections, and Kaposi's sarcoma. The tumours are of B cell origin and may present *de novo*. B cell lymphomas are 60–100 times more common in patients with AIDS than in the general population (68). The majority of patients present with extranodal involvement, predominantly in the central nervous system, bone marrow, and gut. These features are similar to those of the generalized and aggressive Kaposi's sarcoma of AIDS. Non-Hodgkin's lymphomas, including Burkitt's, are now recognized as other manifestation of AIDS. The mechanisms involved in the transition from the follicular hyperplasia and polyclonal B cell activation of persistent generalized lymphadenopathy through to B cell lymphoma have yet to be fully determined. EBV co-infection and release of cytokines such as interleukins IL-6 and IL-10 may be important factors in the pathogenesis of HIV-associated lymphoma (69). HHV8 has been demonstrated in effusions from patients with body-cavity lymphomas. Interestingly, the reduced incidence of Kaposi's sarcoma that is observed in patients receiving HAART is not seen with lymphoma.

The outlook with lymphoma is generally poor, but depends on the histological characteristics of the tumour, large, non-cleaved cell tumours having the best prognosis. Treatment with modified combination chemotherapy regimens containing agents such as methotrexate, bleomycin, doxorubicin, cyclophosphamide, vincristine, and dexamethasone may produce a clinical response, although colony stimulating factors such as granulocyte macrophage-colony stimulating factor are often required.

Anal cancer

As the AIDS epidemic developed, the incidence of anal cancer began to increase (70). It is clear that there is a close association between the acquisition of HPV–HIV dual infection and the subsequent development of anal dysplasia/cancer (71). The dynamics of this relationship are the focus of active research. The absolute risk of developing anal cancer is not yet known, although HPV types 16/18 have the greatest oncogenic potential (72). Also, there is clear evidence that HIV-positive men are more likely than HIV-negative men to develop anal dysplasia (73). The clinical implications of this observation have resulted in certain centres advocating a screening programme analogous to that of cervical cytology screening. Screening is performed by anal cytology or anal canal inspection and biopsy or both (73). Early identification of high-grade dysplasia allows local ablative therapy by surgery or laser therapy before the patient develops invasive disease.

Gastrointestinal endoscopy in HIV-positive patients

In 1988, a British Society of Gastroenterology Working Party published recommendations for cleaning and disinfection of endoscopy equipment. These guidelines have recently been revised (1) and the key points for clinical practice with respect to HIV-positive patients are given below:

1. When 2% glutaraldehyde is used for manual and automated disinfection, 10 min of immersion is recommended for endoscopes before the session and between patients. This will destroy vegetative bacteria and viruses (including HBV and HIV). A 5-min contact period is recommended for 0.35% peracetic acid and for chlorine dioxide (average concentration 1100 p.p.m.), but if immersion is for 10 min, sporicidal activity will also be achieved. At the end of each session, 20 min of immersion in glutaraldehyde or 5 min in paracetic acid or chlorine dioxide is recommended.

2. Microbiological studies show that 20 min of exposure to 2% glutaraldehyde destroys most organisms, including *Mycobacterium tuberculosis*. The Working Party concludes, therefore, that immersion of the endoscope in 2% glutaraldehyde for 20 min is sufficient for endoscopy involving patients with acquired immunodeficiency syndrome (AIDS) and other immunodeficiency states or pulmonary tuberculosis. Similarly, 20 min of immersion is recommended at the start of the session and between patients undergoing ERCP when high-level disinfection is required.

3. Cleaning and disinfection of endoscopes should be undertaken by trained staff in a dedicated room. Thorough cleaning with detergent remains the most important first step in the process.

4. Automated washer/disinfector machines have become an essential part of the endoscopy unit. They must be reliable, effective, easy to use, and should prevent atmospheric pollution by the disinfectant if an irritating agent is used. Troughs of disinfectant should not be used unless containment or exhaust ventilation facilities are provided.

5. Whenever possible, "single use" or autoclavable accessories should be used. The risk of transfer of infection from inadequately decontaminated re-useable items must be weighed against the cost. The re-use of accessories labelled for single use will transfer legal liability for the safe performance of the product to the user or his/her employers and should be avoided unless Department of Health criteria are met. Manufacturers are encouraged to produce more reusable items that are readily accessible for cleaning and are autoclavable.

6. Health surveillance of staff is mandatory and should include a pre-employment enquiry regarding asthma, skin and mucosal sensitivity problems, and lung function by spirometry. Occupational health records must be kept for 30 years.

7. Those involved in endoscopic practice should be vaccinated against HBV, should wear gloves and appropriate protective clothing, and should cover wounds and abrasions.

Summary

The introduction of HAART has produced a profound change in the spectrum of diseases currently referred for gastroenterological investigation. Patients are more likely to present with complications of HAART than with microsporidial diarrhoea or oesophageal ulceration. However, some patients will

Table 7.7. Primary immunodeficiency disorders with gastrointestinal symptoms.

Type of immunodeficiency	Type of GI disease
Antibody deficiency	
Infantile X-linked agammaglobulinaemia	Malabsorption / diarrhoea
Selective IgA deficiency	Coeliac disease, pernicious anaemia, giardiasis
Secretory IgA deficiency	Intestinal candidiasis
Transient hypogammaglobulinaemia of infancy	Diarrhoea
X-linked immune deficiency with increased IgM	GI malignancy, diarrhoea, candidiasis
T cell deficiency	
Thymic aplasia (Di George syndrome)	Diarrhoea, failure to thrive, candiasis, oral ulceration
Combined B/T-cell deficiency	
Variable immune deficiency	Coeliac disease, nodular lymphoid hyperplasia, giardiasis, pernicious anaemia, gastric carcinoma
Ataxia telangiectasia	Vitamin B_{12} malabsorption, gastric carcinoma
Wiskott-Aldrich syndrome	Diarrhoea/malbsorption
Severe combined immune deficiency	Diarrhoea, candidiasis, CMV infection

GI, gastrointestinal; IgA, IgM, immunglobulins A and M.

be unable to tolerate or will fail to respond to HAART, and it is likely that these individuals will develop the gastrointestinal complications seen in the pre-HAART era.

GASTROINTESTINAL DISEASE IN THE NON-HIV INFECTED IMMUNOSUPPRESSED PATIENT

A number of primary immunodeficiency states may present with gastrointestinal symptoms (Table 7.7). The immune defects may involve T-cell or B-cell function, or present with a mixed pattern with defects of both T- and B-cell function. These diseases are generally rare, and the only types likely to be seen by gastroenterologists are selective immunglobin A deficiency and common variable hypogammaglobulinaemia.

Immunodeficiency states may also occur as the result of immunosuppressive treatments used in transplantation or cancer medicine. The timing and nature of the gastrointestinal sequelae of this form of immunodeficiency are well recognized and result either from the acquisition of opportunistic infection or from the development of immunolgical complications such as graft-versus-host disease seen in the setting of bone marrow transplanation. More detailed management of these complications can be found in Chapter 5.

References

*Of interest; **of exceptional interest

1. Courtade M, Brousset P, Delsol M *et al.* Simultaneous detection by non isotopic in situ hybridization of human papilloma viruses and Epstein Barr virus during the lytic cycle in oral hairy leukoplakia lesions. *Ann Pathol* 1992; **12**: 353–357.

2. Winkler JR, Murray PA, Grassi M *et al.* Diagnosis and management of HIV associated periodontal lesions. *J Am Dent Assoc* 1989; **(Suppl)**: 25S–34S.

3. Jacobson JM, Greenspan JS, Spritzler J *et al.* Thalidomide for the treatment of oral apthous ulcers in patients with human immunodeficiency virus infection. National Institute of Allergy and Infectious Disease AIDS Clinical Trials Group. *N Eng J Med* 1997; **336**: 1487–1493.

4. Lynch DP, Naftolin LZ. Oral Cryptococcus neoformans infection in AIDS. *Oral Surg Oral Med Oral Pathol* 1987; **64**: 449–453.

5. Wilcox CM, Alexander LN, Clark WS *et al.* Fluconazole compared with endoscopy for human immunodeficiency virus-infected patients with esophageal symptoms. *Gastroenterology* 1996; **110**: 1803–1809.

6. Connolly GM, Forbes A, Gleeson JA *et al.* Investigation of upper gastrointestinal symptoms in patients with AIDS. *AIDS* 1989; **3**: 453–456.

7. Connolly GM, Shanson D, Hawkins D *et al.* Non-cryptosporidial diarrhoea in human immunodeficiency virus (HIV) infected patients. *Gut* 1989; **30**: 195–200.

8. Sewankambo N, Mugerwa RD, Goodgame R *et al.* Enteropathic AIDS in Uganda. An endoscopic, histological and microbiological study. *AIDS* 1987; **1**: 9–13.

9. Roberts WG, Green PH, Ma J *et al.* Prevalence of cryptosporidiosis in patients undergoing endoscopy: Evidence for an asymptomatic carrier state. *Am J Med* 1989; **87**: 537–539.

10. Ma P, Soave R. Three step stool examination for cryptosporidiosis in 10 homosexual men with protracted watery diarrhoea. *J Infect Dis* 1983; **147**: 824–828.

11. Stibbs HH, Ongerth JE. Immunofluorescence detection of Cryptosporidium oocysts in faecal smears. *J Clin Microbiol* 1986; **24**: 517–521.

12. *Simon D, Cello JP, Valenzuela J *et al.* Multicenter trial of octreotide in patients with refractory acquired immunodeficiency syndrome-associated diarrhea. *Gastroenterology* 1995; **108**: 1753–1760.
    Refractory HIV-1-associated diarrhoea was a significant clinical problem in the early, pre-HAART, years of the AIDS epidemic. Empirical treatment with a range of anti-diarrhoeal agents produced variable results. This study was unique in that it investigated the use of octreotide in a multicentre, placebo-controlled, fashion. Unfortunately, in the doses studied, octreotide was not more effective than placebo in patients with diarrhoea.

13. Eeftinck Schattenkerk JK, van Gool T, Van Ketel RJ *et al.* Clinical significance of small-intestinal microsporidiosis in HIV-1-infected individuals. *Lancet* 1991; **337**: 895-898.

14. Orenstein JM, Tenner M, Kotler DP. Localization of infection by the microsporidian Enterocytozoon bienusi in the gastrointestinal tract of AIDS patients with diarrhea. *AIDS* 1992; **6**: 195–197.

15. Orenstein JM, Zierdt W, Zierdt C *et al.* Identification of spores of Enterocytoooon bienusi in stool and duodenal fluid from AIDS patients. *Lancet* 1990; **336**: 1127–1128.

16. Molina JM, Oksenhendler E, Beauvais B *et al.* Disseminated microsporidiosis due to Septata intestinalis in patients with AIDS: clinical features and response to albendazole therapy. *J Infect Dis* 1995; **171**: 245–249.

17. DeGirolami PC, Ezratty CR, Desai G *et al.* Diagnosis of intestinal microsporidiosis by examination of stool and duodenal aspirate with Weber's modified trichrome and Uvitex 2B stains. *J Clin Microbiol* 1995; **33**: 805–810.

18. *Talal AH, Kotler DP, Orenstein JM *et al.* Detection of Enterocytozoon bienusi in fecal specimens by polymerase chain reaction analysis with primers to the small-subunit rRNA. *Clin Infect Dis* 1998; **26**: 673–675.
    Microsporidia are associated with diarrhoea in up to 30% of immunocompromised patients with AIDS. Definitive identification may require small-bowel biopsy and transmission electron microscopy to confirm the species of microsporidia involved. This paper describes a method for the detection of microsporidia in stool specimens that utilizes polymerase chain reaction analysis with use of primers based on the small-subunit *rRNA* gene of *Enterocytozoon bienusi*.

19. Coyle CM, Wittner M, Kotler DP *et al.* Prevalence of microsporidiosis due to Enterocytozoon bienusi and Encephalitozoon (Septata) intestinalis among patients with AIDS-related diarrhea: determination by polymerase chain reaction to the microsporidian small-subunit rRNA gene. *Clin Infect Dis* 1996; **23**: 1002–1006.

20. Blanshard C, Ellis DS, Tovey DG *et al.* Treatment of intestinal microsporidiosis with albendazole in patients with AIDS. *AIDS* 1992; **6**: 311–313.

21. Anwar-Bruni DM, Hogan SE, Schwartz DA *et al.* Atovaquone is effective treatment for the symptoms of gastrointestinal microsporidiosis in HIV-1-infected patients. *AIDS* 1996; **10**: 619–623.

22. Sharpstone D, Rowbottom A, Nelson M *et al.* The treatment of microsporidial diarrhoea with thalidomide. *AIDS* 1995; **9**: 658–659.

23. DeHovitz JA, Pape JW, Boncy M *et al.* Clinical manifestations and therapy of Isospora belli infection in patients with the acquired immune deficiency syndrome. *N. Engl J Med* 1986; **315**: 87–90.

24. Ortega YR, Sterling CR, Gilman RH *et al.* Cyclospora species – a new protozoan pathogen of humans. *N. Engl J Med* 1993; **328**: 1308–1312.

25. Albrecht H, Stellbrink HJ, Koperski K *et al.* Blastocystis hominis in human immunodeficiency virus-related diarrhea. *Scand J Gastroenterol* 1995; **30**: 909–914.

26. Drew WL. Cytomegalovirus infection in patients with AIDS. *J Infect Dis* 1988; **158**: 449–456.

27. Dieterich DT. Cytomegalovirus: a new gastrointestinal pathogen in immunocompromised patients. *Am J Gastroenterol* 1987; **82**: 764–765.

28. Hackman RC, Myerson D, Meyers JD *et al.* Rapid diagnosis of cytomegalovirus pneumonia by tissue immunofluorescence with a murine monoclonal antibody. *J Infect Dis* 1985; **151**: 325–329.

29. Erlich KS, Mills J, Chatis P *et al.* Acyclovir-resistant herpes simplex virus infections in patients with the acquired immune deficiency syndrome. *N. Engl J Med* 1989; **320**: 293–296.

30. Safrin S, Crumpacker C, Chatis P *et al.* A controlled trial comparing foscarnet with vidaribine for acyclovir-resistant mucocutaneous herpes simplex in the acquired immundeficiency syndrome. *N Engl J Med* 1991; **325**: 551–555.

31. Rotterdam J, Sommers SC. Alimentary tract biopsy lesions in the aquired immune deficiency syndrome. *Pathology* 1985; **17**: 181–192.

32. Shafran SD, Singer J, Zarowny DP. A comparison of two regimens for the treatment of Mycobacterium avium complex bacteremia in AIDS: rifabutin, ethambutol and clarithromycin versus rifampin, ethambutol, clofazimine and ciprofloxacin. Canadian HIV Trials Network Protocol 010 Study Group. *N Engl J Med* 1996; **335**: 377–383.

33. Lew EA, Poles MA, Dieterich DT. Diarrheal diseases associated with HIV infection. *Gastroenterol Clin N Am* 1997; **26**: 259–290.

34. Crotty B, Smallwood RA. Investigating diarrhea in patients with acquired immunodeficiency syndrome. *Gastroenterology* 1996; **110**: 296–310.

35. Simon D, Kotler DP, Brandt LJ. Chronic unexplained diarrhea in human immunodeficiency infection: determination of the best diagnostic approach. *Gastroenterology* 1996; **111**: 269–270.

36. Wilcox CM, Schwartz DA, Cotsonis G *et al.* Chronic unexplained diarrhea in human immunodeficiency virus infection: determination of the best diagnostic approach. *Gastroenterology* 1996; **110**: 30–37.

37. Smith PD, Lane HC, Gill VJ *et al.* Intestinal infections in patients with the acquired immunodeficiency syndrome (AIDS): Etiology and response to therapy. *Ann Intern Med* 1988; **108**: 328–333.

38. Serwadda D, Mugerwa RD, Sewankambo KN *et al.* Slim disease: a new disease in Uganda and its associations with HTLV-III infection. *Lancet* 1985; **2**: 849–852.

39. Lucas SB, De Cock KM, Hounnou A *et al.* Contribution of tuberculosis to slim disease in Africa. *BMJ* 1994; **308**: 1531–1533.

40. Ellis KJ, Lee PD, Pivarnik JM *et al*. Changes in body composition of human immunodeficiency virus-infected males receiving insulin-like growth factor 1 and growth hormone. *J Clin Endocrinil Metab* 1996; **81**: 3033–3038.

41. Reyes-Teran G, Sierra MJG, Martinez DCV *et al*. Effects of thalidomide on HIV-associated wasting syndrome: A randomized double-blind, placebo-controlled clinical trial. *AIDS* 1996; **10**: 1501–1507.

42. Summerbell CD, Youle M, McDonald V *et al*. Megestrol acetate vs cyproheptadine in the treatment of weight loss associated with HIV infection. *Int J STD AIDS* 1992; **3**: 278–280.

43. Coodley GO, Coodley MK. A trial of testosterone therapy for HIV-associated weight loss. *AIDS* 1997; **11**: 1347–1352.

44. Mohle-Boetani JC, Koehler JE, Berger TG *et al*. Bacillary angiomatis and bacillary peliosis in patients infected with human immunodeficiency virus: Clinical characteristcis in a case-control study. *Clin Infect Dis* 1996; **22**: 794–800.

45. Horvath J, Raffanti SP. Clinical aspects of the interactions between human immunodeficiency virus and the hepatotrophic viruses. *Clin Infect Dis* 1994; **18**: 339–347.

46. Hadler SC, Judson FN, O'Malley PM *et al*. Outcome of hepatitis B virus infection in homosexual men and its relation to prior human immunodeficiency virus infection. *J Infect Dis* 1991; **163**: 454–459.

47. Carne CA, Weller IVD, Waite J *et al*. Impaired responsiveness of homosexual men with HIV antibodies to plasma derived hepatitis B vaccine. *BMJ* 1987; **294**: 866–868.

48. Biggar RJ, Goedert JJ, Hoofnagle J. Accelerated loss of antibody to hepatitis B surface antigen among immunodeficient homosexual males infected with HIV. *New Engl J Med* 1987; **316**: 630–631.

49. McDonald JA, Harris S, Waters JA *et al*. Effect of human immunodeficiency virus (HIV) infection on chronic hepatitis B viral antigen display. *J Hepatol* 1987; **4**: 337–342.

50. Cribier B, Rey D, Schmitt C *et al*. High hepatitis C viremia and impaired antibody response in patients co-infected with HIV. *AIDS* 1995; **9**: 1131–1136.

51. Sherman KE, O'Brien J, Gutierrez AG *et al*. Quantitative evaluation of hepatitis C virus RNA in patients with concurrent human immunodeficiency virus infections. *J Clin Microbiol* 1993; **31**: 2679–2682.

52. Zylberg H, Pol S. Reciprocal interactions between human immunodeficiency virus and hepatitis C virus infections. *Clin Infect Dis* 1996; **23**: 1117–1125.

53. Causse X. Chronic hepatitis C should be treated even among HIV patients: a prospective, multicenter study conducted in France [abstract]. *Hepatology* 1997; **26**: 312A.

54. Poles MA, Lew EA, Dieterich DT. Diagnosis and treatment of hepatic disease in patients with HIV. *Gastroenterol Clin North Am* 1997; **26**: 291–321.

55. Piccinino F, Sagnelli E, Pasquale G *et al*. Complications following percutaneous liver biopsy: A multicentre retrospective study on 68,276 biopsies. *J Hepatol* 1986; **2**: 165–173.

56. *Poles MA, Dieterich DT, Schwarz ED *et al*. Liver biopsy findings in 501 patients infected with human immunodeficiency virus (HIV). *J Acquir Immune Defic Syndr Hum Retrovir* 1996; **11**: 170–177.
    This paper describes a retrospective study of 501 HIV-1 infected patients to assess the yield of percutaneous liver biopsy. The most common indications for liver biopsy were abnormal liver biochemistry (89.5%), fever for 2 weeks (71.9%), and hepatomegaly (52.0%). The most common biopsy-derived diagnosis was *Mycobacterium avium* complex, seen in 87 biopsies (17.4%). Among patients with fever for 2 weeks after an extensive negative investigation including bone marrow biopsy, 58.2% had a diagnosis by liver biopsy. Liver biopsy may be a helpful diagnostic tool in patients with fever, biochemical abnormalities, or hepatomegaly.

57. Larvin M, McMahon MJ. APACHE-II score for assessment and monitoring of acute pancreatitis. *Lancet* 1989; **2**: 201–205.

58. Blumberg RS, Kelsey P, Perrone T *et al*. Cytomegalovirus and Cryptosporidium associated acalculous gangrenous cholecystitis. *Am J Med* 1984; **76**: 1118–1123.

59. Kavin H, Jonas RB, Chowdhury L *et al*. Acalculous cholecystitis and cytomegalovirus infection in the acquired immune deficiency syndrome. *Ann Intern Med* 1986; **104**: 53–54.

60. Benhamou Y, Caumes E, Gerosa Y *et al*. AIDS-related cholangiopathy: Critical analysis of a prospective series of 26 patients. *Dig Dis Sci* 1993; **38**: 1113–1118.

61. Cello JP. Acquired immunodeficiency syndrome cholangiopathy: spectrum of disease. *Am J Med* 1989; **86**: 539–546.

62. Peterman TA, Jaffe HW, Beral V. Epidemiological clues to the etiology of Kaposi's sarcoma. *AIDS* 1993; **7**: 605–611.

63. **Chang Y, Cesarman E, Pessin MS *et al*. Identification of herpesvirus-like DNA sequences in AIDS-associated Kaposi's sarcoma. *Science* 1994; **266**: 1865–1869.
    Representational difference analysis was used to isolate unique sequences in Kaposi's sarcoma tissues obtained from patients with AIDS. These sequences were not present in tissue DNA from, non-AIDS patients, but were present in 15% of non-Kaposi's sarcoma tissue DNA samples from AIDS patients. The sequences were homologous to, but distinct from herpesvirus saimiri and Epstein–Barr virus. The authors concluded that these Kaposi's sarcoma-associated herpesvirus-like sequences appear to define a new human herpesvirus. This virus has become known as HHV8.

64. Friedman SL, Wright TL, Altman DF. Gastrointestinal Kaposi's sarcoma in patients with acquired immune deficiency syndrome. Endoscopic and autopsy findings. *Gastroenterology* 1985; **89**: 102–108.

65. Weber JN, Carmichael DJ, Boylston A, *et al*. Kaposi's sarcoma of the bowel presenting as apparent ulcerative colitis. *Gut* 1985; **26**: 295–300.

66. Aboulafia DM. Regression of acquired immunodeficiency syndrome related pulmonary Kaposi's sarcoma after highly active antiretroviral therapy. *Mayo Clin Proc* 1998; **73**: 439–443.

67. Conant MA, Opp KM, Poretz D *et al*. Reduction of Kaposi's sarcoma lesions following treatment of AIDS with ritonavir. *AIDS* 1997; **11**: 1300–1301.

68. Beral V, Peterman T, Berkelman R *et al*. AIDS-associated non-Hodgkin lymphoma. *Lancet* 1991; **337**: 805–809.

69. Marsh JW, Herndier B, Tsuzuki A *et al*. Cytokine expression in large cell lymphoma associated with acquired immunodeficiency syndrome. *J Interferon Cytokine Res* 1995; **15**: 261–268.

70. Crombleholme T, Schecter WP, Wilson W. Anal carcinoma: changes in incidence, natural history, and treatment: a 25 year review of the UCSF–SFGH experience [Abstract]. *Proc Soc Clin Oncol* 1989; **8**: 4.

71. Palefsky JM, Gonzales J, Greenblatt RM *et al.* Anal intraepithelial neoplasia and anal papilloma virus infection among homosexual males with group 4 HIV disease. *JAMA* 1990; **263**: 2911–2916.

72. Zaki SR, Judd R, Coffield LM *et al.* Human papillomavirus infection and anal carcinoma. *Am J Path* 1992; **140**: 1345–1355.

73. **Palefsky JM, Holly EA, Ralston ML *et al.* High incidence of anal high-grade squamous intra-epithelial lesions among HIV-positive and HIV-negative homosexual and bisexual men. *AIDS* 1998; **12**: 495–503.

The incidence of anal cancer in homosexual men exceeds that of cervical cancer in women. This prospective cohort study determined the incidence of high-grade squamous intra-epithelial lesions (HSIL) in 623 HIV-1 positive and 483 HIV-1 negative homosexual men. The 4-year incidence of HSIL was 49% and 17% respectively in the HIV-1 positive and negative men. If further studies clearly link HSIL with anal cancer, patients may need to receive routine anal screening.

8. Gastrointestinal Problems in Neurological Patients

HELEN FIDLER and JULIAN FEARNLEY

INTRODUCTION

Neurological complications of gastrointestinal diseases such as inflammatory bowel disease, coeliac disease, Whipple's disease and other malabsorptive states have been extensively reviewed (1, 2). Rarely, primary tumours of the gastrointestinal tract can present with neurological symptoms (3).

This chapter will review five fields in which gastroenterologists are frequently called on to help manage a gastrointestinal manifestation of a neurological disease:

- Neurogenic dysphagia
- Use of percutaneous endoscopic gastrostomy in stroke patients
- Gastrointestinal problems in Parkinsons's disease, particularly constipation
- Autonomic neuropathy
- Gastrointestinal side effects of common antiepileptic and antiparkinsonian medications

NEUROGENIC DYSPHAGIA

Dysphagia may be the presenting symptom of underlying neurological pathology. The aim in this situation is to avoid unnecessary investigation and management that will predispose toward aspiration pneumonia, which carries a high mortality (4–6). Fluids commonly present more problem to the patient than does more solid food. Normal people may aspirate small amounts of saliva, but do not develop problems; the risk of aspiration pneumonia in neurological patients results from a combination of factors (7):

- failure to protect the airway
- large volumes of aspirate
- a cough that is inadequate to expel the aspirate once it has entered the airway
- nasogastric tubes
- oesophageal reflux
- vomiting
- lying horizontal
- poor swallowing technique
- altered consciousness

The common causes of neurogenic dysphagia can be categorized anatomically and are shown in Table 8.1. All these may present with symptoms of oropharyngeal dysphagia, which is a transfer problem caused by the inability to manipulate food or liquid efficiently down from the mouth through the cricopharynx whilst safely protecting the airway. A careful history and examination can usually detect this, and may avoid potentially hazardous and inappropriate investigations. The extent to which dysphagia can safely be attributed to the neurological disease and endoscopy avoided is highly individual for each patient. The decision should be a joint one between the gastroenterologist and the neurologist.

A standard barium swallow should never be performed in a patient suspected of having neurogenic dysphagia, as high-density barium can cause fatal aspiration pneumonia (8). The endoscopic investigation of heartburn might be appropriate in a young patient with well-controlled myasthenia gravis, but it may be safer to defer investigation and give empirical treatment in an elderly victim of stroke who is too debilitated to protect their airway during the procedure. Similarly, detecting an oesophageal tumour in a patient with endstage motor neurone disease (MND) will not lead to any change of management.

Clinical features of neurogenic dysphagia

The index of suspicion should obviously be high in a patient with known neurological disease, in whom bulbar involvement is a possibility (see Table 8.1). Early on, the patient may not volunteer that they have dysphagia, but when asked they may say that it is more difficult to swallow or that it takes two swallows rather than one. Another useful guide is whether they take more than 30 min to consume a meal or are unable to consume more than half of the meal (9).

Occasionally, the gastroenterologist will be asked to see a patient with neurogenic dysphagia in whom a structural cause is being considered. In this type of patient there are four stages to their assessment: recognition that the dysphagia is neurogenic, detection of aspiration, assessment of any neurogenic respiratory failure and, if possible, diagnosis of underlying illness. The two illnesses that are most likely to present in this way are MND and myasthenia gravis, both of which can be difficult to diagnose in their early stages, especially if the diagnoses are not considered. It is important to pay attention to features in the history and examination that indicate that the dysphagia is neurogenic (Table 8.2).

Symptoms

The patient should be asked whether they cough during or after swallowing. This stongly suggests aspiration, and this occurs particularly with liquids, which are a more stringent test of laryngeal closure (10). This is the cardinal symptom of neurogenic dysphagia and is highly predictive of the risk of aspiration, with a sensitivity and specificity of 74% (11). Less frequently, the patient may regurgitate liquids through the nose on swallowing, as a result of palatal weakness failing to close off the nasopharynx. Difficulty chewing is another pointer, and it is important to note whether it is fatiguable, being relatively normal at the beginning of the meal and

Table 8.1. Causes of neurogenic dysphagia.

Cerebral	Cerebrovascular disease
	Multiple sclerosis
	Bingswanger's (hypertensive)
Basal ganglia disease	Parkinson's disease (late complication)
	Multiple system atrophy
	Steele–Richardson–Olszewski syndrome
	Huntington's disease
	Wilson's disease
Brainstem	Motor neurone disease
	Cerebrovascular disease
	Multiple sclerosis
	Post-polio syndrome
	Tumour
	Syringobulbia
	Spinocerebellar degenerations
	— Friedreich's ataxia
	— spinocerebellar ataxias (genetic)
Cranial neuropathy	Basal meningitis
	— bacterial, fungal, tuberculous
	— malignant (carcinoma, lymphoma)
	Guillain–Barré syndrome
	Connective tissue disease (especially Sjögren's syndrome)
	Tumour
	— nasopharyngeal carcinoma
	— chordoma
Neuromuscular junction	Myasthenia gravis
	Lambert–Eaton myasthenic syndrome (rarely)
Muscle	Polymyositis, dermatomyositis
	Inclusion body myositis
	Hypothyroidism
	Dystrophic
	— myotonic dystrophy
	— oculopharyngeal dystrophy

becoming virtually impossible at the end. If there is facial weakness, the patient may say that food collects inside the cheek and liquids dribble out of the mouth when swallowing. Eliciting a history of double vision or eyelid drooping is also important. When asked, patients often say that they have double vision; but this is normal if it lasts only a few seconds.

Signs (Table 8.2)

Examination of the patient should start while the history is being taken. Does the voice have a nasal quality (nasal dysarthria) because of palatal weakness with a quality similar to a cleft palate? Is the voice low-volumed (dysphonic) — the result of laryngeal weakness — or is it bubbly, because swal-

Table 8.2. Clinical pointers towards a neurogenic cause of dysphagia.

History	Known neurological illness and prolonged time in feeding
	Diplopia
	Difficulty chewing
	Aspiration: coughing or choking on swallowing liquids
	Palatal palsy: nasal regurgitation with liquids
	Dyspnoea
Examination	Voice: dysphonia, pharyngeal pooling, and dysarthria
	Eyes: ptosis or ophthalmoplegia
	Facial or jaw opening weakness and jaw jerk
	Tongue wasting or fasciculation
	Palatal weakness: nasal dysarthria
	Neck flexion weakness
	Cough: weak or bovine
	Ventilation: vital capacity and diaphragmatic movement
	Swallow: 3-oz water-swallow test

lowing fails to clear the pharynx (pharyngeal pooling)? Is there an obvious ptosis or deviation of the eyes or facial asymmetry?

Once the history has been taken, the cranial nerves should be formally tested, and this should be tailored to what has been elicited so far. Clearly, if there is at this point no indication of a neurogenic dysphagia, then it is not necessary to carry out a formal examination. If there is any doubt then, at the very least, a 3 oz **water-swallow test** should be performed as described below. Otherwise, the cranial nerves should be examined, starting from the optic nerves and looking for specific signs (Table 8.2). Swelling of the optic discs may point to a brainstem lesion, such as a basal meningitis or a tumour, that is causing hydrocephalus. Apparent swelling can also occur as a result of malignant infiltration of the optic nerves in a malignant meningitis. Always look for a **ptosis**, otherwise it will be missed, and test the eye movements. Remember that the pupils are not involved in myasthenia gravis. **Facial weakness** can be assessed by how well the patient buries their eyelashes and resists eye opening, and lower facial weakness by whether they can keep their lips pursed against the examiner trying to prise them open. **Pterygoids** (motor Vth nerve) should be tested by asking the patient to open their mouth against resistance; and certainly, once the jaw is partially open, the examiner should not be

able to close it. A brisk jaw jerk is very important in the context of an upper motor neurone lesion and MND. If the patient has a **bulbar palsy**, then it may be worthwhile checking for VIIIth nerve involvement, by simply seeing whether they can repeat a whispered number while masking the opposite ear by waggling the tragus. Very rarely, a bulbar palsy can be caused by a glomus tumour, which may be seen on otoscopy as a red mass behind the tympanic membrane.

The lower cranial nerves are tested by asking the patient to open their mouth and observing the **tongue** at rest. Is it wasted, with a crinkled appearance, and is it fasiculating? If there is a unilateral XIIth nerve palsy, then the tongue will deviate to the affected side on protrusion. Remember that the tongue will also deviate to one side with a facial nerve palsy in the absence of XIIth nerve involvement; furthermore, fasiculations present on protrusion but not at rest are not pathological. Next, move to the **palate**, observe its movement (Xth nerve), and test sensation using an orange-stick (IXth nerve). The **gag reflex** is not a good predictor of aspiration (12), in that it may be present even when the patient is aspirating and is absent in many normal elderly patients. You will already have noted the voice, and you will need to check whether the **cough** (Xth nerve) is bovine in vocal cord paralysis or has reduced explosiveness with laryngeal weakness, respiratory impairment, or a reduced level of consciousness (10). The **sternomastoids** (XIth nerve) should be tested by gentle forceful rotation of the neck. Here, one is looking at muscle contraction rather than power, as there are some very powerful rotators at the back of the neck. If the sternomastoid fails to come up on rotation, you will know that it is either paralysed or wasted. Weakness of neck flexion testing both sternomastoids together is a crucial sign; the four main causes are myotonic dystrophy, polymyositis, myasthenia gravis, and MND.

Water-swallow test

Swallow should be tested formally by using the 3-oz water-swallow test (13,14). Three fluid ounces is equivalent to half a cup or 90 ml. In order that the test be safe, the patient must be:

- alert
- able to sit up

- able to phonate
- able to cough

the patient must not:

- have a clear history of aspiration
- significant ventilatory compromise

The patient should repeat their address before and after the test, to assess their voice "bubbliness" and pharyngeal pooling. The test is abnormal if the patient coughs either during the swallow or during a period of 1 min after the swallow, or if there is pharyngeal pooling. The test should start with the patient taking a sip of water; if they pass this, then they may proceed to the full test by drinking the entire volume without interruption.

The 3-oz water-swallow test is highly sensitive in detecting significant aspiration. Aspiration is defined as significant when associated with an increased risk of pneumonia, which equates with greater than 10% of the bolus being aspirated (15). The test has been validated in 44 patients with stroke (11,14).

If the patient fails the test, they should be assigned to a "nil by mouth" regimen, and fluids given by subcutaneous or intravenous infusion, or by nasogastric tube.

Ventilation

In patients with neurogenic dysphagia, there is a high chance of neurogenic ventilatory failure; patients are at risk of ventilatory arrest and may require elective intubation and ventilation of the lungs. Clearly, for those patients with a terminal illness such as MND, a definitive diagnosis should be made as soon as possible, to avoid inappropriate ventilation. Unlike cardiogenic and pulmonary causes of ventilatory failure, the neurological patient rarely complains of dyspnoea, despite severe restrictions of ventilatory reserve; they may say they become breathless on talking or swallowing. If there is diaphragmatic weakness, the patient will suffer orthopnoea as the abdominal contents force the diaphragm upwards on lying down. In subacute illnesses such as Guillain–Barré syndrome and myasthenia gravis, complaints of tiredness, or agitation, are ominous signs that ventilatory arrest is imminent.

At the bedside, ventilation can be assessed by chest expansion, checking for paradoxical abdominal movement indicative of diaphragmatic weakness. On sniffing, the abdominal wall should move outwards as the diaphragm forces the abdominal contents down and outwards. The vital capacity should be measured, and regularly so in critical cases, as peak expiratory flow rates and measurements of arterial blood-gases are not helpful. It is not only the vital capacity, but also its rate of decline, that is helpful in assessing the need for ventilation. If the patient has nasal escape as a result of palatal weakness, the nose should be pinched closed during measurements: if there is facial weakness stopping the patient from making a seal around the tube, a mask should be used.

Videofluoroscopy modified barium swallow

Forty percent or more of all patients with neurogenic dysphagia will have aspiration on video swallow that is missed on clinical examination (16). Video modified barium swallow is the gold-standard investigation for aspiration and is highly sensitive, allowing the radiologist and speech therapist to look specifically at the oral and pharyngeal phases of swallowing. The patient is placed in their side and given food and liquid boluses of variable consistency and impregnated with barium, in sequential aliquots starting with a teaspoonful only. The risk of large quantities of barium being suddenly aspirated is thus reduced and assessment of hypopharyngeal spillage, pharyngeal pooling, laryngeal penetration, and aspiration into the trachea can be made dynamically under fluoroscopy (7).

However, video modified barium swallow may be overly sensitive in predicting clinically significant swallowing impairment, as aspirates of less than 10% of the bolus are not associated with increased risk of complication (15). It may also underestimate problems, as it assesses only one point in time, when the patient may be at their optimum. In assessing the risk of oral feeding, it is better to base the decision on bedside assessments — preferably by a speech therapist — repeated over time, and observation of the ability to take an oral diet, than to rely on a single video swallow. Finally, in practical terms, the procedure may not be immediately available when needed, and it requires trained personnel and expensive equipment.

Dysphagia in stroke

This is the most common cause of neurogenic dysphagia, occurring in 30–45% of acute strokes (7,17), but persistent dysphagia is rare. This is because either the majority of patients recover their swallow after 2–4 weeks (18) or the stroke is so severe that the patient dies. It is important to remember that dysphagia is a poor prognostic indicator, occurring in the most severe strokes, and it is the severity of the stroke, and not the dysphagia *per se* that carries the high mortality of around 50% and the ultimate poor functional recovery (17). Patients at greatest risk are those with large cerebral hemisphere strokes, brainstem strokes, and those with a reduced level of consciousness. Transcranial magnetic resonance stimulation has established that the pharyngeal phase of swallowing tends to receive its innervation principally from one hemisphere; however, this has no relation to speech dominance, and there does not yet appear to be much evidence for particular stroke sites correlating with specific deficits in oropharyngeal transit (19). Bilateral hemispheric strokes are associated with a greater incidence and severity of dysphagia, and may result from sequential strokes caused by carotid artery disease, diffuse cerebral small vessel disease with deep cerebral small-lacunar infarcts, or multiple cortical infarcts caused by cardiac emboli.

Symptoms specific for a vertebrobasilar stroke (posterior circulation) as opposed to a carotid stroke (anterior circulation) are diplopia, bilateral perioral numbness (pontine), vertigo, and bilateral field loss or scintillations and amnesia (bilateral mesial temporal lobes) caused by ischaemia in the territory of the posterior cerebral arteries.

Video swallow has identified abnormalities of the oral or pharyngeal phase of swallowing in more than 90% of stroke patients, and frank aspiration in up to 50% within the first month (19). Silent aspiration in stroke is associated with an approximately sixfold risk of pneumonia (15). The most frequent problem is in the oral phase, with delayed triggering of the swallow reflex allowing part of the bolus to seep into the pharynx and then into the airway before the swallow is activated. Failure to form a proper bolus in the oral phase may also lead to difficulties if mastication is affected because of reduced level of consciousness or orolingual weakness or apraxia. Aspiration may also occur because of impaired laryngeal adduction. Failure of pharyngeal peristalsis will result in an incomplete swallow and collections of food and drink and aspiration after the swallow. Of those attending a stroke unit more than 5 weeks after the event, only 20% showed aspiration on video swallow (20) and of these 12% developed aspiration pneumonia, compared with only 6% in the non-aspiration group.

Management

Every patient with stroke should have their swallowing tested at the bedside, including the 3-oz water-swallow test. If the patient fails the bedside testing, they should be assigned to a "nil by mouth" regimen and hydrated through an alternative route. Failing the water-swallow test increases by a factor of 2.3 the risk of developing pneumonia, upper airway obstruction, and death (9). It is most likely that the swallow will recover spontaneously within 1–2 weeks. It will be aided by correct posture (upright), chin tuck (swallowing with the neck flexed) or head turn, and using a thickener for fluids. The services of a speech therapist are invaluable for continuing assessment and advice, but it is imperative that the hospital ward staff identify the problem in the first place.

Dysphagia in Parkinsonism

Drooling correlates with the severity of the Parkinson's disease, starting at night with wetting the pillow and, later during the day, sometimes causing major problems with wetting the clothes. It is the result of reduced swallowing rather than of hypersecretion (21). Chewing gum can both trigger and improve swallowing. Anticholinergic drugs, including tricyclic antidepressants, will dry the mouth, but may lead to confusion. As a last resort, irradiation of the salivary glands can be carried out, but will lead to excessive dryness of the mouth.

Symptomatic dysphagia is common in Parkinson's disease, occurring in 50% of sufferers compared with 6% of age-matched controls (22). However, it is rarely a problem until very late in the illness. The occurrence of significant dysphagia, especially early in the disease, suggests that the patient does not have Parkinson's disease, but an alternative diagnosis such as multiple system atrophy, Steele–Richardson–Olszewski syndrome, or corticobasal degeneration. A review of any clinical study of Parkinson's disease, will reveal that 15%

of cases diagnosed in life by a neurologist are found to have an alternative diagnosis at post-mortem examination (23).

Dysphagia in Parkinson's disease is usually caused by problems in the oropharyngeal phase of swallowing, but may also result from oesophageal dysmotility (24). Unfortunately, treatment with levodopa does not result in any improvement in swallowing (25), underlining the fact that Parkinson's disease affects more than the dopaminergic system. Silent aspiration is also common in Parkinson's disease and Alzheimer's disease (5). Intriguingly, in a pathological series of achalasia, two of eight patients had Lewy bodies in the ganglion cells of the myenteric plexus of the oesophagus (26); one of them had Lewy bodies in the central nervous system that were compatible with a diagnosis of presymptomatic Parkinson's disease. In the same study, 22 patients with Parkinson's disease were reviewed and three had significant dysphagia; of these, two had Lewy bodies in the myenteric plexus. Another feature of oesophageal dysmotility is "off-period" belching (27).

Dysphagia should not be attributed solely to the disease itself as there may be an alternative explanation that can be effectively managed. Heartburn is more common in Parkinson's disease (28,29), occurring in up to 25% of patients. In fact, documented gastrooesophageal reflux occurs in 26% of parkinsonian patients compared with 6% of controls (30). Endoscopy has a high yield for detecting oesophagitis or duodenal ulceration that respond to conventional treatment (28). Standard barium meals should be avoided if constipation is severe, as the barium may precipitate a paralytic ileus (31).

Dysphagia and MND (amyotrophic lateral sclerosis)

More than 70% of patients with MND have difficulty swallowing and more than 50% have difficulty chewing (4). Swallowing may be painful, and solids and liquids equally difficult. MND may present with dysphagia if the onset is predominantly bulbar. This will usually be accompanied by dysarthria, which should immediately point the clinician towards neurogenic dysphagia. The prognosis for MND is very poor, and it is a general principle that a diagnosis is made only when there are definite clinical features and other treatable conditions have been excluded. In the case of a bulbar onset, myasthenia gravis should be considered. Polymyositis can cause dysphagia, but the limb symptoms are predominant.

Dysphagia and myasthenia gravis

Dysphagia has been estimated to be a prominent symptom in at least 30% of patients with myasthenia gravis (1). Diagnosis may be difficult in the early stages, and it is not unusual for it to be misdiagnosed as being psychogenic or myalgic encephalomyelitis or chronic fatigue syndrome. This is because the symptoms may be vague, there is considerable variability during the day and from day to day, and give-way weakness bedside testing as a result of fatigue may be misinterpreted as a psychogenic sign. Apart from dysphagia, the patient may suffer from fatiguable dysphonia, difficulty chewing, double vision, eyelid drooping, and limb weakness.

It is important to remember that constipation in these patients should not be treated with magnesium salts (epsom salts, Milpar, Andrews liver salts), because these may precipitate acute weakness. The colic and diarrhoea associated with anticholinesterase treatment can be reduced by giving oral atropine 0.5 mg with each dose.

PERCUTANEOUS ENDOSCOPIC GASTROSTOMY (PEG) INSERTION

In neurogenic dysphagia, enteral feeding should be commenced in those patients for whom swallowing is either unsafe or inadequate. Swallowing is unsafe if there is significant aspiration, as discussed in the section on clinical features, that can not be corrected by an improved swallowing technique or because of liquid thickeners, supervised by a speech therapist. Swallowing is inadequate if the patient is unable to take sufficient fluids or calories and has poor hydration, weight loss, and hunger, or for those in whom mealtimes are laborious, time consuming and distressing and interfering with their daily activities. In this situation, enteral feeding is supplementary and the patient can still enjoy some oral intake. PEG feeding is invaluable in the palliative care of chronic neurological diseases such as MND, multiple sclerosis and the "Parkinson's-plus syndromes" that are associated with severe difficulties swallowing.

Once a decision has been made to start enteral feeding, the choice has to be made between using a nasogastric tube or a PEG. A nasogastric tube is a sensible option in those patients with an acute illness in whom recovery is expected. Those patients with a chronic illness are clearly more suited for a PEG, as are those patients who are confused and will pull out their nasogastric tubes. The general indications and contraindications of PEG insertion are well known and apply similarly to chronic stable neurological deficits, but certain points deserve special mention.

The most common **indication** for enteral nutrition in neurogenic dysphagia is stroke. Malnutrition in stroke is associated with an increased duration of hospital stay and greater mortality (32); early enteral feeding shortened the hospital stay in an non-controlled study (33). PEG has many advantages over nasogastric feeding (14). It enables the patient to be transferred out of hospital into long-term residential care (6) and it is more comfortable than nasogastric feeding, which is associated with greater treatment failures, is less cosmetically pleasing, can cause nasal ulceration, interferes with swallowing, and can cause aspiration. There is no convincing evidence that PEG reduces mortality compared with nasogastric feeding, although one small study revealed a reduction in the relative risk of dying of 80% (6). That trial needs to be repeated with greater numbers of participants, to ensure that both groups are comparable in the severity of their strokes.

With respect to **timing the placement** of a PEG after an acute stroke, it should be reiterated that most dysphagic stroke patients recover normal swallowing within 2–4 weeks (20). However, it is unreasonable to leave a patient with nasogastric feeding for this period of time, and most clinicians would pass a nasogastric tube within the first few days and insert a PEG after 2 weeks if clinical findings suggested significant aspiration. The decision should be made in close collaboration with the speech and language therapists. Many clinicians would not consider a PEG in those acutely ill or with rapidly worsening neurological deficit if the patient were unlikely to live beyond 4 weeks, in view of the relative risk of the procedure (14).

The **complication rate** of PEG in stroke patients may be geater than the standard 5%, and one study found it to be as high as 30% (34). This may reflect the severity of the stroke, rather than the procedure.

Most patients requiring a PEG have had a very severe stroke and in this study of 37 patients, only six were alive by 30 months, and all but one was severely disabled. Certainly, the risk of aspiration and pneumonia is increased during the procedure, but this is separate from the underlying risk. All centres inserting PEGs should, ideally, have a written procedure use for patient selection and aftercare. Leakage around the tube site after several days is an indication for further endoscopic assessment, and no attempt should be made to re-introduce the tube blindly, as fatal leakage into the abdominal wall may occur (35). Oesophageal reflux and aspiration may occur with large bolus feeding (36) during the day, or continuous feeding at night while supine.

Consent

There may be a problem obtaining patient consent for a PEG procedure, as they may be too cognitively impaired to understand the risks involved and it is not an emergency, life-saving procedure (see Chapter 44).

One common misconception is that consent from a relative is valid — this is not so, although relatives should obviously be involved with the decision. The best compromise is to have the consent form signed by two consultants, of whom both write in the notes that the PEG is in the patient's best interests. One should be the consultant actually performing the procedure, and the other the consultant in charge of the patient's care.

CONSTIPATION IN PARKINSON'S DISEASE

James Parkinson noted in his monograph on "the shaking palsy" that constipation can be severe and, in the later stages, required powerful laxatives and manual evacuation because of failure of expulsion of faeces from the rectum (37). This, in some ways, foresaw the current concept that constipation in Parkinson's disease is caused by slow intestinal transit and, in some cases, by outflow obstruction resulting from pelvic floor dystonia. Patients often complain bitterly of constipation, which can be more problematic than their neurological symptoms. About 30% of those with Parkinson's disease have bowel movements fewer than three times a week, compared with 10% of age-matched controls; defecation is difficult, with straining and incomplete evacuation in 67% compared with 28% of controls. These problems are directly related to the duration and severity of the Parkinson's disease (24). Overflow incontinence may mask constipation, which will be evident only on plain abdominal radiography and rectal examination.

Intestinal transit throughout the entire gut is slow (38) and this is probably secondary to degeneration of the myenteric plexus, which is exacerbated by anticholinergic drugs (39). One of the most useful investigations is to ask the patient to keep a stool diary, as in one study only seven of 12 patients complaining of constipation actually passed fewer than three stools per week (40). Constipation may be related to reduced physical activity and inadequate fibre and fluid intake. Fibre is the first-line treatment, resulting in increased stool weight and frequency, although the effect may last for only a few months (38,40). Quite considerable amounts of fibre may need to be taken: for example, an effect was documented with 28 g per day (normal recommended dose 18 g) of bran/pectin in tablet form. Studies with cisapride also suggest a beneficial effect of this drug (41). Constipation may be exacerbated by a low internal sphincter pressure, which is present in the majority of patients with Parkinson's disease (28).

Ineffective defecation also occurs as a result of paradoxical activation of the puborectalis muscle during straining, accentuating the flap-valve action of the anorectal angle or dystonic contraction of the anal sphincter (42–44). If this is demonstrated on proctography and anorectal manometry, subcutaneous injection of apomorphine or local injection of botulinum toxin may be beneficial. The effect of a botulinum injection can last for up to 3 months, but re-injection will then be required. Although promising in this subgroup of patients, this procedure carries a potential risk of faecal incontinence and should only be carried out in specialist centres.

AUTONOMIC NEUROPATHY

Autonomic neuropathy as a complication of diabetes mellitus is discussed elsewhere in this volume (see Chapter 4). Other causes of the condition include:

- acute pan-dysautonomia (probably a variant of the Guillan–Barré syndrom)
- pure cholinergic dysautonomia
- paraneoplastic autonomic neuropathy
- familial amyloid polyneuropathy
- Fabry's disease
- porphyria

In addition, autonomic failure (without neuropathy) occurs in pure autonomic failure (a Lewy body disease) and multiple system atrophy. Patients with these conditions do not present solely with a gastrointestinal problem, but will have other **symptoms of autonomic failure**:

- Hypotension
  — orthostatic
  — postprandial
- Sweating
  — loss of sweating
  — gustatory sweating
- Genitourinary
  — impotence
  — urinary frequency, urgency, and incontinence
  — urinary voiding difficulty
- Ocular
  — blurred near vision: failure of pupillary accommodation
  — photophobia: failure of pupillary constriction
  — dry eyes, mouth, or both

Symptoms

The most reliable symptoms are related to hypotension and genitourinary involvement. The patient feels faint on standing, similar to the normal experience of feeling "woozy" on getting up too quickly. There will be visual symptoms, with obscurations (black spots) and loss of vision. There may be an ache at the back of the neck and shoulders (coat hanger pain). If the patient has severe postural hypotension, they may suddenly lose consciousness and fall to the ground. Postprandial hypotension relates to faintness resulting from diversion of blood to the splanchnic circulation. If the patient is male, impotence and loss of morning erections are good indicators as to the diagnosis. If the patient can not "hold on" for a few minutes after they have the urge to micturate, they have urinary urgency, which can be another indication of autonomic disturbance. Voiding difficulties, with poor stream, stop-start stream, and incomplete bladder emptying — so that the bladder can be emptied again soon afterwards — are also suggestive.

Signs

In the gastrointestinal system, signs are usually normal, but a succussion splash suggestive of gastroparesis should be tested for, and rectal examination may reveal impacted faeces. Formal autonomic testing is possible (45), but impracticable during a basic ward consultation. However, at the very least the patient should be assessed for postural hypotension (sympathetic nervous system) (46). The patient lies on the bed supine in a relaxed state for 5–10 min if possible. Blood pressure is then measured immediately before and after they stand up and measurements are repeated over the next 30 s and, preferably, 2 min. The brachial pulse should be palpated, just in case the pulse becomes very weak. A decrease of 30 mmHg or more is significant. Note that the patient should not be taking any medication that might decrease the blood pressure, as this will invalidate the test. The pupils are easily tested, but rarely involved.

Other tests of autonomic function

There are several other tests of autonomic function (see also chapter 4). These include:

1. Postural changes in heart rate (vagal function).
2. Measuring the ratio of the maximum and minimum heart rate within the first 30 s of standing using an electrocardiagraph (ECG). Normal ranges of values are recognized depending on the age of the patient (45).
3. Change in heart rate during a Valsalva manoeuvre. This is a test of sympathetic and vagal function. The patient is asked to blow into the end of a syphgmomanometer, creating a pressure of 30–40 mmHg for 10–15 s. During the manoeuvre a tachycardia (sympathetic) should occur and be followed, after the manoeuvre, by a compensatory bradycardia (vagal). An ECG is used to monitor the heart rate, and the test is considered abnormal if the ratio between the maximum R–R interval after and the minimum R–R interval during the manoeuvre is less than 1.5.

4. Sinus arrhythmia (vagal) can be tested by requesting the patient to take six deep breaths per minute and measuring the minimum heart rate during inspiration and maximum heart rate during expiration, using an ECG. In autonomic neuropathy, and especially if it is diabetic, sinus arrhythmia is usually absent, in normal individuals the difference is at least 10 beats.
5. Parasympathetic function (vagal) is affected more frequently and earlier in the course of diabetes than is sympathetic function. In the cold pressor test (sympathetic), a hand is immersed in 4°C cold water and the systolic blood pressure should increase by 15 mmHg after 1 min.

Symptoms of autonomic neuropathy may also be indirectly related to the neuropathy; in this respect, it is important to recognize bacterial overgrowth secondary to gut stasis, as it is treatable. The association between diabetes and coeliac disease, and the effects of pancreatic insufficiency should be remembered, as the symptoms of autonomic neuropathy are diverse and non-specific. Thus nausea, vomiting, abdominal pain and distension, diarrhoea or constipation may be the presenting problem, and often patients complain of several of these. The most difficult to manage, because it may require inpatient care, is intractable vomiting. Using similar tests in study of 114 patients with insulin-dependent or non-insulin-dependent diabetes mellitus, Clouse *et al.* (47) found that 40% had vagal parasympathetic involvement; however, no gastrointestinal symptoms were predictive of this, and all symptoms correlated more with psychiatric illnesses such as anxiety and depression than with diabetic neuropathy. Whether some symptoms are more specific than others for objective autonomic neuropathy remains to be seen, and there is a great need for further clinical studies in this field to categorize rigorously the history, physiology, pathology, and type of investigation (48).

Autonomic involvement may even play a part in irritable bowel syndrome, but the precise nature of this remains to be seen. Some authors have found that a subgroup of patients with constipation had cholinergic abnormalities whereas a subgroup with diarrhoea had adrenergic abnormalities (49). There is even some evidence that these different patterns of involvement respond differently to motility-promoting agents, with the best effect being seen in those with intact vagal innervation and sympathetic dysfunction (50).

Physiology and further investigations

A detailed description of the physiology and investigation of autonomic neuropathy is beyond the scope of this book, but it is useful to consider briefly the underlying mechanisms causing the patient's symptoms (See also Chapters 37 and 50). Many techniques have been used to assess gut motility in patients with suspected autonomic dysfunction. The most readily available is video barium examination of the upper gastrointestinal tract and scintigraphic clearance of a radiolabelled meal from the antrum. Antral ultrasound can also be used to assess antral clearance after a standard meal. Colonic motility can be assessed using the shapes test in which clearance of ingested radioopaque shapes is measured by sequential plain abdominal radiography. Although available to most gastroenterologists, these tests are functional and do not give manometric information. For patients with a clinical diagnosis of autonomic involvement and severe intractable symptoms or weight loss, referral to a gastrointestinal physiology unit may be indicated. Before this, it is reasonable to perform endoscopy and consider a trial of antibiotics for possible bacterial overgrowth, if there is clinical suspicion for this.

Studies conducted in gastrointestinal physiology units use techniques such as electrogastrography and ambulatory antroduodenal manometry. Electrogastrography may be useful in the future, as it is non-invasive, but it is not of great clinical use at present. Ambulatory antroduodenal manometry is not yet widely available but, using this technique, it has been found that most patients with gastroparesis have a delay in emptying of solid foods from the stomach, with the rate of liquid emptying preserved. This may be because the antrum is the most affected part of the stomach in autonomic degeneration. Liquids entering the fundus trigger a vagally mediated relaxation, so the fundus has a key role in gastric emptying. In contrast, gastric emptying for digestible solids is more dependent on antral motor activity (51). Antral hypomotility is especially evident in diabetic populations after ingestion of high-calorie meals, and corresponds to dyspeptic symptoms (46,52). The latter study (52) also found prolonged migra-

tory motor complexes, with a total absence of antral phase 3 in 50% of patients. Abnormalities of small-bowel motility commonly coexist with gastroparesis, and may be due to non-propagated bursts of phasic pressure activity and reduced frequency and amplitude of contraction postprandially.

Treatment

Simple measures such as small frequent meals, and avoiding medication such as anticholinergic agents (tricyclic antidepressants), narcotics, and sympathomimetics (theophylline, β-blockers) may be beneficial. As previously stated, bacterial overgrowth should be suspected, and bloating and diarrhoea may improve with cyclical antibiotic therapy. As for constipation in Parkinson's disease, cisapride may have a role. The mechanisms for this include acetylcholine release at the myenteric plexus, increased oesophageal clearance, greater lower oesophageal sphincter tone, and increased antroduodenal motility. However, clinical studies in autonomic neuropathy affecting the upper gastrointestinal system have been disappointing. Thus the overall effect of cisapride 20 mg three times a day in a population with diabetes, previous gastric surgery, and idiopathic small-bowel motility problems was no different from that of placebo (50). Antroduodenal manometry findings did not predict the overall response to cisapride in this double-blind, placebo-controlled 12-week study. However, there is some suggestion that specific subgroups of patients may benefit from treatment with cisapride, and further studies are in progress. As discussed in the section on Parkinson's disease, this drug may also be more useful in this context. As cisapride is relatively safe and therapeutic options are limited, a 1-month trial is probably worthwhile.*

GASTROINTESTINAL SIDE EFFECTS OF COMMON ANTIEPILEPTIC AND ANTIPARKINSONIAN MEDICATIONS

Many medications used for neurological conditions can cause gastrointestinal side effects or give rise to abnormal liver blood tests. A detailed discussion

---

*EDITORS NOTE: Cisapride has been withdrawn from the market, but at the time of editing is still available in the UK on a named-patient basis.

Table 8.3. Liver and gut side effects of common antiepileptic and antiparkinsonian drugs.

	Cholestatic liver function tests	Increased transaminase concentrations	General GI upset
Antiepileptic drugs			
Carbamazepine	++	++	++
Phenytoin	+	++	++
Valproate	++	++	++
Lamotrigine	–	–/+	++ (0.1–1%)
Topiramate	–	–	++
Ethosuxamide	–	–	++
Phenobarbitone	–	++	++
Antiparkinson drugs			
Levodopa	+	++	++
Bromocriptine	–	+	++
Tolcapone	–	++ (licensed USA only)	++
Selegeline	–	–	++

GI, gastrointestinal; ++, well recognized; +, case reports; –, not documented.

of these is beyond the scope of this text, but a summary of the gastrointestinal side effects of the common antiepileptic and antiparkinsonian drugs is given in Table 8.3.

References

*Of interest; **of exceptional interest

1. Perkin G, Murray-Lyon I. Neurology and the gastrointestinal system. *J Neurol Neurosurg Psychiatry* 1998; **65**: 291–300.
2. Wills A, Hovell C. Neurological complications of enteric disease. *Gut* 1996; **39**: 501–504.
3. van de Pol M, van Aalst V, Wilmink J *et al.* Brain metastases from an unknown primary tumour: which diagnostic procedures are indicated? *J Neurol Neurosurg Psychiatry* 1996; **61**: 321–323.
4. Mayberry J, Atkinson M. Swallowing problems in patients with motor neuron disease. *J Clin Gastroenterol* 1986; **8**: 233–234.
5. Horner J, Alberts M, Dawson D *et al.* Swallowing in Alzheimer's disease. *Alzheimer Dis Assoc Disord* 1994; **8**: 177–189.
6. **Norton B, Homer–Ward M, Donnelly M *et al.* A randomised prospective comparison of percutaneous endoscopic gastrostomy and nasogastric tube feeding after acute dysphagic stroke. *BMJ* 1996; **312**: 13–16.
   A controversial paper showing dramatically better survival in stroke patients managed by PEG rather than by nasogastric feeding. When read with the ensuing correspondence, this gives a good overview of differing opinions in the field.
7. Aviv J, Sacco R, Mohr J *et al.* Laryngopharyngeal sensory testing with modified barium swallow as predictors of aspiration pneumonia after stroke. *Laryngoscope* 1997; **107**: 1254–1260.
8. Gray C, Sivalogananthan S, Simpkins K. Aspiration of high-density barium contrast medium causing acute pulmonary inflammation – report of two fatal cases in elderly women with disordered swallowing. *Clin Radiol* 1989; **40**: 397–400.
9. DePippo KL, Holas MA, Redding MJ. The Burke dysphagia screening test: validation of its use in patients with stroke. *Arch Phys Med Rehabil* 1994; **75**: 1284–1286.
10. Hughes AJ, Daniel SE, Blankson S *et al.* A clinicopathological study of 100 cases of Parkinson's disease. *Arch Neurol* 1993; **50**: 140–148.
11. Mari F, Matei M, Ceravolo MG *et al.* Predictive value of clinical indices in detecting aspiration in patients with neurological disorders. *J Neurol Neurosurg Psychiatry* 1997; **63**: 456–460.
12. Smithard D. Percutaneous endoscopic gastrostomy feeding after acute dysphagic stroke. Gag reflex has no role in ability to swallow [letter]. *BMJ* 1996; **312**: 973.
13. Castell D. Esophageal disorders in the elderly. *Gastroenterol Clin N Am* 1990; **19**: 235–254.
14. DePippo KL, Holas MA, Reding MJ. Validation of the 3-oz water swallow test for aspiration following stroke. *Arch Neurol* 1992; **49**: 1259–1261.
15. Holas MA, DePippo KL, Reding MJ. Aspiration and relative risk of medical complication following stoke. *Arch Neurol* 1994; **51**: 1051–1053.
16. Raha S, Woodhouse K. Who should have a PEG? *Age Ageing* 1993; **22**: 313–315.
17. Gordon C, Langton Hewer R, Wade D. Dysphagia in acute stroke. *BMJ* 1987; **295**: 411–412.
18. Akpunonu B, Mutgi A, Roberts C *et al.* Modified barium swallow does not affect how often PEGs are placed after stroke. *J Clin Gastroenterol* 1997; **24**: 74–78.
19. Chen M, Ott D, Peele V *et al.* Oropharynx in patients with cerebrovascular disease: evaluation with videofluoroscopy. *Radiology* 1990; **176**: 641–643.
20. Teasell R, McRae M, Marchuk Y *et al.* Pneumonia associated with aspiration following stroke. *Arch Phys Med Rehabil* 1996; **77**: 707–709.
21. Bateson MC, Gibberd FB, Wison RSE. Salivary symptoms in Parkinson's disease. *Arch Neurol* 1973; **29**: 274–275.
22. Edwards LL, Pfeiffer RF, Quigley EMM *et al.* Gastrointestinal symptoms in Parkinson's disease. *Mov Disord* 1991; **6**: 151–156.
23. Hughes TAT, Wiles CM. Neurogenic dysphagia: the role of the neurologist. *J Neurol Neurosurg Psychiatry* 1998; **64**: 569–572.
24. Edwards LL, Quigley MM, Pfeiffer RF. Gastrointestinal dysfunction in Parkinson's disease: frequency and pathophysiology. *Neurology* 1992; **42**: 726–732.
25. Bushmann M, Dobmeyer S, Leeker L *et al.* Swallowing abnormalities and their response to treatment in Parkinson's disease. *Neurology* 1989; **39**: 1309–1314.
26. Qualman SJ, Haupt HM, Yang P *et al.* Esophageal Lewy bodies associated with ganglion cell loss in achalasia. Similarity to Parkinson's disease. *Gastroenterology* 1984; **87**: 848–856.
27. Kempster PA, Lees AJ, Crichton P *et al.* Off-period belching due to a reversible disturbance of oesophageal motility in Parkinson's disease and its treatment with apomorphine. *Mov Disord* 1989; **4**: 47–52.

28. Byrne K, Pfeiffer R, Quigley E. Gastrointestinal dysfunction in Parkinson's disease. A report of clinical experience at a single center. *J Clin Gastroenterol* 1994; **19**: 11–16.

29. Eadie MJ, Tyrer JH. Alimentary disorders in Parkinsonism. *Aust Ann Med* 1965; **14**: 13–22.

30. Eadie MJ, Tyrer JH. Radiological abnormalities of the upper part of the alimentary tract in parkinsonism. *Aust Ann Med* 1965; **14**: 23–27.

31. Umeki S. Caution in uppper gastrointestinal X-ray in constipated parkinsonian patients [letter]. *South Med J* 1989; **82**: 1589.

32. Davalos A, Ricart W, Gonzalez-Huix F, Soler S, Marrugat J, Molins A, Suner R, Genis D. Effect of malnutrition after acute stroke on clinical outcome. *Stroke* 1996; **27**(6): 1028–1032.

33. Nyswonger GD, Helmchen RH. Early enteral nutrition and length of stay in stroke patients. *J Neurosci Nurs* 1992; **24**: 220–223.

34. Wanklyn P, Cox N, Belfield P. Outcome in patients who require gastrostomy after stroke. *Age Ageing* 1995; **24**: 510–514.

35. Botterill I, Miller G, Dexter S *et al.* Deaths after delayed recognition of percutaneous endoscopic gastrostomy tube migration. *BMJ* 1998; **317**: 524–525.

36. Short TP, Patel NR, Thomas E. Prevalence of gastroesophageal reflux in patients who develop pneumonia following percutaneous endoscopic gastrostomy: a 24 hour pH monitoring study. *Dysphagia* 1996; **11**: 87–89.

37. Parkinson J. *An essay on the shaking palsy.* London: Sherwood, Neely and Jones, 1817,

38. Astarloa R, Mena M, Sanchez V *et al.* Clinical and pharmacokinetic effects of a diet rich in insoluble fiber on Parkinson disease. *Clin Neuropharmacol* 1992; **15**: 375–380.

39. Jost W. Gastrointestinal motility problems in patients with Parkinson's disease. Effects of antiparkinsonian treatment and guidelines for management. *Drugs Aging* 1997; **10**: 249–258.

40. Ashraf W, Pfeiffer R, Park F *et al.* Constipation in Parkinson's disease: objective assessment and response to psyllium. *Mov Disord* 1997; **12**: 946–951.

41. Jost W, Schimrigk K. Long–term results with cisapride in Parkinson's disease. *Mov Disord* 1997; **12**: 423–425.

42. Albanese A, Maria G, Bentivoglio A *et al.* Severe constipation in Parkinson's disease relieved by botulinum toxin. *Mov Disord* 1997; **12**: 764–766.

43. Mathers S, Kempster P, Law P *et al.* Anal sphincter dysfunction in Parkinson's disease. *Arch Neurol* 1989; **46**: 1061–1064.

44. Mathers SE, Kempster PA, Swash M *et al.* Constipation and paradoxical puborectalis contraction in animus and Parkinson's disease: a dystonic phenomenon? *J Neurol Neurosurg Psychiatry* 1988; **51**: 1503–1507.

45. Bannister R, Mathias C. *Autonomic Failure*, 3rd edn. Oxford: Oxford University Press, 1992.

46. Camilleri M, Ford K. Functional gastrointestinal disease and the autonomic nervous system: a way ahead? [editorial]. *Gastroenterol* 1994; **106**: 1114–1118.

47. Clouse R, Lustman P. Gastrointestinal symptoms in diabetic patients: lack of association with neuropathy. *A J Gastroenterol* 1989; **84**: 868–872.

48. Quigley E. The clinical pharmacology of motility disorders: the perils (and pearls) of prokinesia. *Gastroenterology* 1994; **106**: 1112–1120.

49. **Aggarwal A, Cults TF, Abell TL, Cardosa S, Familoni B, Bremer J, Karas J. Predominant symptoms in irritable bowel syndrome correlate with specific autonomic nervous system abnormalities. *Gastroenterology* 1994; **106**: 945–950.
A clear study looking at patients with irritable bowel syndrome, and assessing in detail the autonomic function of cholinergic and adrenergic pathways. Understandable to non-neurologists, and includes important controls of psychological variables.

50. Camilleri M, Balm R, Zinsmeister A. Determinants of response to a prokinetic agent in neuropathic chronic intestinal motility disorder. *Gastroenterology* 1994; **106**: 916–923.

51. Chaudhuri T, Fink S. Gastric emptying in human disease states. *Am J Gastroenterol* 1991; **86**: 533–538.

52. Samsom M, Jebbink R, Akkermans L *et al.* Abnormalities of antroduodenal motility in type 1 diabetes. *Diabetes Care* 1996; **19**: 21–27.

9. Gastrointestinal Problems on the Obstetric Unit

ELSPETH ALSTEAD and CATHERINE NELSON-PIERCY

INTRODUCTION

The physiological changes of pregnancy cause a decrease in gastrointestinal motility, reduced lower oesophageal pressure, and decreased gastric emptying, resulting in nausea and constipation in the majority of normal pregnancies. There are a number of important conditions affecting the digestive system that are unique to pregnancy, and some other gastrointestinal and liver disorders are exacerbated by or more complicated in pregnancy. Unrelated gastrointestinal disease may arise at any time during pregnancy. Diagnosis and management may be difficult because of atypical symptoms, a reluctance to use invasive investigations, and concerns about treatments.

GASTROINTESTINAL SYMPTOMS

Nausea and vomiting

Nausea and vomiting are common in the first trimester of pregnancy: 70–90% of pregnant women experience nausea and 50% have at least one episode of vomiting or retching. In most women these symptoms are self-limiting and usually tolerated. They are influenced, but not completely explained, by maternal age (young), occupation, parity, smoking, infant gender (male) and mother's personality (1). In the wake of thalidomide, most doctors and pregnant women are cautious with the use of antiemetics during pregnancy and they are generally avoided, unless vomiting is very severe (see hyperemesis gravidarum). Extensive data support a lack of teratogenesis, but nevertheless antiemetics are rarely prescribed in uncomplicated pregnancies. In recent years, there has been increased interest in alternative therapies, which are perceived, at least by pregnant women, as safer. Randomized trials have demonstrated possible benefits for acupressure and definite benefit for pyridoxine and ginger (2,3). There is insufficient evidence to support the efficacy of hypnosis (4).

Hyperemesis gravidarum

Hyperemesis gravidarum occurs in about 0.1% of pregnancies and presents with severe and persistent nausea and vomiting, leading to dehydration. Onset is usually in the first trimester of pregnancy, usually around 6–8 weeks gestation. In addition to nausea and vomiting, there may be ptyalism (inability to swallow saliva) and spitting. The persistent vomiting may lead to dehydration, postural hypotension, electrolyte disturbances, ketosis, muscle wasting, and weight loss.

Hyperemesis appears to have a complex metabolic background, and a number of hormonal and psychological factors have been implicated. It is undoubtedly a severe physical illness that is life-threatening to both mother and fetus, and should be treated seriously. Maternal death can result from aspiration of vomit or from Wernicke's encephalo-pathy, and serious morbidity can result from inadequate or inappropriate treatment (5). Laboratory investigations may reveal hyponatraemia, hypokalaemia, low urea, ketosis, and a metabolic hypochloraemic alkalosis.

115

Both liver biochemistry and thyroid function tests are often also abnormal. Abnormalities of liver biochemistry will be discussed later in this chapter.

Two-thirds of patients with hyperemesis gravidarum have abnormal thyroid function tests. These patients are clinically euthyroid, but have increased concentrations of free-thyroxine (T_4), a suppressed thyroid stimulating hormone (TSH), or both. The plasma concentration of human chorionic gonadotrophin (hCG), which shares an α subunit with TSH, peaks at 6–12 weeks gestation. TSH and hCG receptors share a structural homology; hCG concentrations are directly correlated with free T_4 concentrations and the severity of vomiting, and correlate inversely with TSH concentrations (6). The relationship between hCG and the severity of vomiting explains the increased incidence of hyperemesis in multiple pregnancies and hydatidiform mole.

Important points in the **treatment of hyperemesis gravidarum** include:

1. Careful hydration with normal saline
2. Early administration of high-dose thiamine (150 mg daily orally or 100 mg weekly intravenously) to prevent Wernicke's encephalo-pathy (treatment of Wernicke's encephalopathy requires higher doses of thiamine). Wernicke's encephalopathy may be precipitated by dextrose-containing intravenous fluids and total parenteral nutrition (TPN).
3. In hyponatraemic individuals, rapid correction of the hyponatraemia with hypertonic saline can precipitate central pontine myelinolysis.
4. Attention to nutrition is vital and occasionally TPN is required. There are reports of the successful use of enteral nutrition. It is also important to address any psychological problems that may predate or be precipitated by the illness. The only definitive cure of hyperemesis gravidarum is termination of pregnancy, which may only be recommended in extreme cases. Restoration of adequate nutrition will improve liver biochemical abnormalities (7).
5. Antiemetics may play a part in the management of patients who do not respond to fluid and electrolyte replacement. Dopamine agonists (metoclopramide, domperidone), phenothiazines (chlorpromazine, proclorperazine), and antihistamines (cyclizine, promethazine) have all been shown to be safe (8). H_2-receptor antagonists

have been used occasionally, with some benefit. The use of the 5-hydroxy-tryptamine receptor 3 ($5HT_3$) receptor blocker, ondansetron, has been reported in intractable hyperemesis, although in one study it was shown to be no more effective than promethazine (9).

6. In uncontrolled studies of intractable hyperemesis, corticosteroids have produced dramatic improvement. In patients responding to steroid treatment (10), the dose must be reduced slowly and usually can not be discontinued until the gestation at which the hyperemesis would resolve spontaneously, which may be at delivery. With appropriate management, the outcome of pregnancy in hyperemesis gravidarum is comparable to that in the general population.

Heartburn and reflux symptoms

Approximately 60% of women experience heartburn at some time in the third trimester (11). Antacids are the mainstay of treatment, are safe in pregnancy, and may be used liberally. Most women will find that antacids taken before meals and at bedtime, together with avoidance of eating late at night and, sometimes, raising the head of the bed will adequately control reflux symptoms.

H_2-receptor antagonists have been used throughout pregnancy without adverse effect (12,13). Ranitidine is theoretically preferable to cimetidine because it does not affect androgen receptors. Ranitidine 150 mg twice daily was shown to be effective in a randomized controlled trial (14). Proton pump inhibitors have been used in pregnancy, and although there is some evidence of toxicity in animal studies, there are no data regarding their safety in human pregnancy. They are therefore not a first-line treatment, and they are not licensed for use in pregnancy. Metoclopramide and sucralfate are safe in pregnancy, although not very effective in the treatment of reflux symptoms. Heartburn usually resolves after delivery.

Abdominal pain

Acute abdominal conditions both related and unrelated to pregnancy can prove life-threatening for both mother and fetus. Delay in diagnosis in the pregnant woman may result from mimicry of symptoms and signs of pregnancy-related conditions, a change in the usual presentation of abdominal disease, and a reluctance to use radiological and endoscopic investigations during pregnancy. **Constipation**, **uterine contractions** and **labour pains** are the most common causes of abdominal pain, but do not usually present diagnostic difficulty. The common surgical conditions unrelated to pregnancy are **appendicitis**, **gallbladder disease** and **pancreatitis** (usually biliary). Appendicitis is the most common non-obstetric indication for laparotomy in pregnancy (15–17). There are concerns about the effect of anaesthetics and surgery on pregnancy, and there is some evidence for an increase in spontaneous abortion (up to 25%) if surgery is performed in the first few weeks of pregnancy.

Gallstone disease and pancreatitis

Asymptomatic gallstones are present in 2.5–11% of pregnant women, and cholecystitis occurs in about 0.1% of pregnancies. In studies with ultrasound, biliary sludge has been detected in up to a 33% of pregnant women, but does not usually cause symptoms. This finding probably reflects the increased cholesterol saturation and decreased gallbladder motility during pregnancy. The clinical features of gallbladder disease in pregnancy are similar to those in non-pregnant individuals. The management is as in non-pregnant patients. In those with severe symptoms of cholecystitis who do not settle, laparoscopic cholestectomy has been reported to be safe for mother and fetus in a small number of patients (18), but should be generally deferred until after delivery.

Pancreatitis is rare, complicating about 1 in 10 000 pregnancies. This is usually mild biliary pancreatitis occurring in the third trimester. Management is exactly as in a non-pregnant patient. Endoscopic retrograde cholangiopancreatography and stent drainage can, in exceptional circumstances — for example the presence of a common-bile-duct stone — be performed safely by an experienced operator with minimal or no radiation to the fetus. It is preferable to defer sphincterotomy, which may require considerable screening time, until after delivery (19,20).

Peptic ulcer disease

Peptic ulcer disease is probably less common in pregnant women, and the complications of bleeding and perforation are very rare. H_2-receptor antagonists are relatively safe with ranitidine the preferred choice (see page 116). Proton pump inhibitors have been used in pregnancy, but with caution, as there is concern about teratogenesis from animal studies, and little evidence about their prolonged use in human pregnancy (13,14). Misoprostil is contraindicated because of the risk of uterine contractions and spontaneous abortion. Antacids are safe, and can be used to control symptoms. Upper gastrointestinal endoscopy is safe if indicated (21). Eradication therapy for *Helicobacter pylori* could be used if essential, but can generally be postponed until after pregnancy, as it involves the administration of three drugs, including a proton pump inhibitor.

Constipation

Decreased colonic motility, poor fluid intake as a consequence of nausea, and iron supplements can all contribute to constipation, which is experienced by 40% of pregnant women, especially in early pregnancy. Management usually involves advice about increasing fluid and fibre intake and stopping oral iron supplements, at least temporarily. Laxatives are rarely required, but osmotic laxatives and bulking agents are safe and may be helpful in some women.

Diarrhoea

Enteric infection

Gastrointestinal infections may occur in pregnancy, but the incidence is not increased compared with that in non-pregnant individuals. There is very little literature on the severity or persistence of enteric infection in pregnancy and, in general terms, investigation and management are unchanged. *Salmonella enteritidis* and *Campylobacter jejuni* infections have been associated with fetal mortality from transplacental passage of organisms, and maternal mortality has also been reported (22,23). There are currently no treatment recommendations for these infections in pregnancy, but reports of severe, sometimes fatal infection might suggest that early use of antibiotics might be appropriate.

Infection with *Listeria monocytogenes* is a well recognized cause of intrauterine infection and perinatal death. The infection is acquired through eating foods contaminated with the organism, and appropriate dietary advice should be given to all pregnant women concerning the avoidance of foods such as soft and blue-veined cheeses and unpasteurized milk. Clinicians must maintain a high index of suspicion for this infection, which can present with 'flu-like' symptoms and premature labour. Once suspected, appropriate specimens should be sent for *Listeria* culture and empirical treatment with amoxycillin instituted (24,25).

INFLAMMATORY BOWEL DISEASE

Inflammatory bowel disease (IBD) affects young adults, and it is therefore common for affected individuals to express concerns about fertility and pregnancy. Women with ulcerative colitis do not appear to have impaired fertility. Fertility may be decreased in women with active Crohn's disease, but this is related to disease activity: in quiescent disease it is not impaired compared with the general population. Flare-up in disease activity is no more likely during pregnancy or in the puerperium than it is in any other year of a patient's life. Women with active IBD at the time of conception are more likely to continue to have disease activity during the pregnancy, and in these patients there is an increased risk of fetal loss and premature delivery. Conversely, women with quiescent disease at conception often report feeling unusually well during pregnancy. Patients presenting for the first time with a suspected diagnosis of IBD in pregnancy *must* be investigated because if the diagnosis is confirmed, treatment is essential. Flexible sigmoidoscopy or colonoscopy may be safely performed if necessary (26).

A large epidemiological study from Sweden (27) has suggested that pre-term birth (before 33 weeks) is more common in IBD (odds ratio 1.81, 95% confidence interval 1.06 to 3.07), as is low birth weight (odds ratio 2.15, 95% confidence interval 1.10 to 1.99). There are no data concerning disease activity in these women, and more recent prospective evidence suggests that preterm delivery in patients with Crohn's disease is associated with disease activity and smoking during pregnancy (28). Previous bowel resection, ileostomy or pouch surgery do not confer any increased risk in pregnancy. Some obstetricians, however, favour delivery by caesarean section in patients after ileoanal pouch surgery, and in those with perianal Crohn's disease. The issues relating to pregnancy and its outcome should certainly be discussed before conception with every patient with inflammatory bowel disease.

Treatment of IBD

Sulphasalazine, 5-aminosalicylates and steroids are safe in pregnancy and breast feeding (29,30). The use of second-line immunosuppressive agents such as azathioprine and 6-mercaptopurine is more controversial. There is extensive experience of the use of azathioprine in pregnancy in renal transplant recipients and patients with systemic lupus erythematosus, and some data concerning its use in patients with severe IBD (31). No increase in congenital abnormalities or subsequent problems such as childhood malignancy has been observed in children followed for up to 20 years. Patients with complicated IBD who require azathioprine to remain in remission may elect to continue to take the drug; however, it is not recommended to start azathioprine or 6-mercaptopurine during pregnancy. Cyclosporin has been used in pregnancy in other conditions, but should obviously be used with caution and these agents should be continued only after full discussion with the patient (and partner). Methotrexate is contraindicated in pregnancy. Metronidazole has been extensively used in other diseases in pregnancy, without evidence of teratogenesis.

In women with IBD, pregnancy outcome is usually normal. Active disease is a definite adverse factor and a more serious concern than any risk of drug therapy. This needs to be fully explained to the patient and her partner.

LIVER DISEASE

Liver disease in pregnancy is extremely important, and the liver diseases specifically associated with pregnancy may be life-threatening for mother and fetus and, subsequently, the surviving child. Some liver diseases, such as viral hepatitis, may be more severe in pregnancy and, although pregnancy is rare in patients with pre-existing severe chronic liver disease, it is increasingly common in those who have undergone liver transplantion. The pattern of liver biochemistry abnormalities may be helpful in the diagnosis, as in a non-pregnant patient, provided the physiological changes produced by pregnancy are appreciated (32).

Normal physiological changes

The physiological changes of normal pregnancy result in signs and laboratory results that mimic abnormalities usually associated with liver disease in non-pregnant individuals:

1. Up to 60% of pregnant women exhibit spider naevi or palmar erythema.
2. Serum albumin decreases from a mean of 42 g/l to 31 g/l in late pregnancy.
3. Serum alkaline phosphatase concentrations increase to two to four times the normal range after the fifth month of pregnancy. Alkaline phosphate concentrations are therefore not useful in the assessment of liver disease in pregnancy.
4. Other liver enzymes remain normal; indeed, transaminases, bilirubin, and gamma glutamyl transaminase concentrations in uncomplicated pregnancy are lower than the expected non-pregnant laboratory ranges (33). Increase in any of these markers reflect hepatobiliary pathology.

Hyperemesis gravidarum

Hyperemesis gravidarum (see above also) presents in the first trimester and, rarely, may persist throughout gestation. Abnormal liver biochemistry is found in up to 50% of women admitted to hospital with hyperemesis. The bilirubin concentration is mildly increased (<70 μmol/l), but obvious jaundice is rare. The liver biochemistry abnormalities are believed to be the result of malnutrition and impaired excretion of bilirubin, but improve dramatically when adequate nutrition is restored. Liver biopsy is not required for diagnosis in this condition but, when performed, it has been reported to be normal or show fatty change.

Acute fatty liver of pregnancy

Acute fatty liver of pregnancy (AFLP) is a condition of the 3rd trimester, presenting after 30 weeks gestation (mean 36 weeks); it has never been reported in the first trimester of pregnancy. It is rare (1 in 9000–13 000 pregnancies), but essential to recognize, as it is potentially fatal for both mother (20–30% mortality) and fetus (20–50% mortality), especially if diagnosis is delayed (33–35). AFLP is most common in first pregnancies and in multiple pregnancies, as is the case with pre-eclampsia. Early recognition and appropriate management are crucial. The initial symptoms are vague, with nausea, anorexia, and malaise. More severe vomiting (in 70%) and upper abdominal discomfort or pain

(50–80%) may develop. There are often mild coexisting features of pre-eclampsia. These symptoms should alert clinicians to the possibility of AFLP. Jaundice appears 1–2 weeks after the onset of these symptoms, and is usually associated with a three- to 10-fold increase in transaminases. Fulminant hepatic failure, with all its sequalae, can develop rapidly in this situation.

In at least some women, AFLP is a metabolic disorder, and there is a recognized association between AFLP and long-chain 3-hydroxyacyl coenzyme A dehydrogenase (LCHAD) deficiency — a disorder of mitochondrial fatty acid oxidation. A woman who is heterozygous for LCHAD deficiency may develop AFLP if carrying a fetus homozygous for the defect (34,36–38). The mechanism of hepatocellular damage remains unclear, but possibly involves the production of abnormal fatty acid metabolites by the affected fetus: the metabolites enter the mother's circulation and overwhelm the mitochondrial oxidation machinery in the heterozygous mother, who is already stressed by the increased demand for fatty acid oxidation in late pregnancy; this results in microvesicular steatosis and liver failure. AFLP appears to occur only in association with certain mutant LCHAD alleles. In affected individuals, the risk of recurrent AFLP is 25% or greater. The baby born from a pregnancy complicated by AFLP should undergo urgent metabolic screening for LCHAD deficiency, as this can result in sudden death, cardiomyopathy, skeletal myopathy, or fulminant hepatic failure in infancy (38).

The **diagnosis** of AFLP is a clinical one. Hypoglycaemia and hyperuricaemia may be prominent features. The liver is not enlarged. There is characteristically an increased white cell count (>15 × 10⁹/litre), a low albumin concentration and evidence of disseminated intravascular coagulation. Hepatic steatosis can sometimes be visualized by ultrasound, and possibly also by computed tomography or magnetic resonance imaging. The "gold standard" for diagnosis is liver biopsy, with staining for microvesicular fatty change, but this is rarely performed. The **management** of AFLP involves expeditious delivery, which usually results in dramatic recovery of the mother. Hypoglycaemia and coagulopathy must be treated aggressively before delivery, and the sick patient needs to be managed in an intensive care setting. The development of hepatic failure requires transfer of the patient to a liver unit, for assessment for transplantation.

HELLP syndrome

The HELLP syndrome (**h**aemolysis, **e**levated **l**iver enzymes, **l**ow **p**latelets) is one of several crises that can develop as a variant of severe pre-eclampsia. It appears to be caused by endothelial cell injury, and microangiopathic platelet activation and consumption. HELLP syndrome occurs in 4–20% of pre-eclamptic pregnancies, although up to 50% of women with pre-eclampsia have mildly abnormal liver biochemistry without the full-blown HELLP syndrome. There is increased maternal (1%) and perinatal morality (approximately 35%) (39). There is significant maternal morbidity from placental abruption (16%), subcapsular liver haematoma, acute renal failure, massive hepatic necrosis, and liver rupture. **Clinical features** are those of right upper-quadrant pain (65%) with nausea and vomiting (35%). The liver may be enlarged and tender. There may be features of pre-eclampsia, although HELLP may be the first manifestation of pre-eclampsia. There is a low-grade haemolysis, rarely with severe anaemia and a low platelet count (usually $< 100 \times 10^9$/litre). Serum bilirubin and transaminase concentrations are mildly increased, (mean 150 units/litre); greater values are suspicious of hepatic infarction or subcapsular haemotoma. Serum lactate dehydrogenase is also increased. In some patients, the platelet count decreases to less than 30×10^9/litre and disseminated intravascular coagulation develops. The **differential diagnosis** of HELLP syndrome includes AFLP, haemolytic uraemic syndrome, and thrombotic thrombocytopaenic purpura (40). Ultrasound may be useful in excluding other diagnoses such as AFLP, hepatic haematoma, or biliary disease. Liver biopsy has rarely been performed in this syndrome, because of the coagulopathy. Liver histology is similar to that in pre-eclampsia, with periportal and sinusoidal fibrin deposition and haemorrhage. Hepatic necrosis and subcapsular haemorrhage may occur.

Prompt delivery is indicated, especially if there is severe right upper-quadrant pain and tenderness suggesting liver capsule distension and risk of liver rupture. Aggressive correction of the coagulopathy in women with frank evidence of disseminated intravascular coagulation (about 20%) and attention to the blood pressure are important before delivery. Patients may initially deteriorate in the 48 h after delivery before improvement is seen post-partum, and 30% of cases of HELLP present postpartum. These women are at particular risk of pulmonary oedema and renal failure. Recovery is usually rapid and complete, but there is a significant risk of pre-eclampsia and its sequelae in future pregnancies. Risk of recurrent HELLP syndrome is low (39,41,42).

Obstetric cholestasis

Obstetric cholestasis, previously known as intrahepatic cholestasis of pregnancy, usually presents in the third trimester at a mean of 30 weeks. It is common in Chile (6.5%), Scandinavia, Bolivia, and China (43). It is increasingly recognized in the UK, but this may be related to increased ascertainment. The pathogenesis is unknown, but it runs in families, possibly with an autosomal dominant inheritance: 40–50% of patients may have a positive family history. These individuals may also have a history of cyclical itching during the menstrual cycle and cholestasis with the oral contraceptive pill, so a disorder of oestrogen physiology has been hypothesized; there is possibly a decrease in sulphation of bile acids in the presence of excess oestrogen.

The major **symptom** of obstetric cholestasis is pruritus affecting the limbs and trunk, and particularly the palms and soles. Insomnia as a result of nocturnal itching and malaise may be associated, but there is no rash. There may be other features of cholestasis, with dark urine, pale stools and anorexia. Liver biochemistry is abnormal. Jaundice develops in a small percentage of affected women, 1–4 weeks after the onset of pruritus. The symptoms persist until delivery and resolve quickly afterwards. Serum bilirubin concentrations may be increased (<100 μmol/litre), alkaline phosphatase concentrations are greater than that expected in pregnancy (around four times normal), and alanine transaminase concentrations — which are the most sensitive of the conventional markers — are two to 10 times normal. If measured, total serum bile acids are increased 10–100 times and may be the first or the only biochemical abnormality detected (44). This test is of limited availability, but may occasionally be useful to confirm the diagnosis. Liver biopsy is rarely performed, but shows cholestasis with minimal or no inflammatory changes. An ultrasound scan should be performed, to exclude common-bile-duct stones as a cause of the cholestasis.

Malabsorption of fat-soluble vitamins may lead to vitamin K deficiency and coagulopathy, and there is an increased risk of postpartum haemorrhage. Obstetric cholestasis is associated with an increased risk of premature labour (12–44%) and stillbirth, in addition to fetal distress, fetal passage of meconium, and fetal intracranial haemorrhage. Fetal mortality is reported as about 2–4% (45,46). The risk of adverse events to the fetus are possibly related to the maternal serum bile acid concentration, and increased concentrations of bile acids have been found in amniotic fluid and the fetal circulation. Fetal asphyxia as a result of the vasoconstrictive effects of bile acids has been postulated (47). It is however, very difficult to predict fetal compromise, and extremely close surveillance of mother and fetus is required once the diagnosis has been made. There is a strong suggestion that meconium staining of the amniotic fluid obtained at amniocentesis is the most important indicator of risk to the fetus.

Vitamin K 10 mg orally daily should be given to any woman with a prolonged prothrombin time or who is prescribed cholestyramine. Vitamin K should also be given to the neonate on delivery. Cholestyramine is generally unpalatable and poorly tolerated. Antihistamines such as chlorpheniramine, terfenidine, or promethazine may be used for itching. At least one controlled trial has confirmed the efficacy of ursodeoxycholic acid, which is a choloretic agent (48,49), but this drug is not licensed for use in pregnancy, although there is no evidence of adverse effects on the fetus. Dexamethazone has been shown, in one small observational study, to relieve pruritus and decrease serum bile acids and transaminases (50).

Obstetric cholestasis recurs in subsequent pregnancies in at least 50% of women. Those who have experienced this condition should be advised to avoid oestrogen-containing oral contraceptives, but not hormone replacement therapy, which contains a physiological dose of oestrogen and can usually be tolerated.

Liver diseases that may be more severe in pregnancy

World-wide, acute viral hepatitis is the most common cause of liver disease in pregnancy. The clinical features of these diseases are similar to those in non-pregnant individuals. There is evidence that hepatitis E, herpes simplex hepatitis and, possibly, hepatitis A are more severe in pregnancy, especially if acquired in the third trimester, and may more commonly lead to fulminant hepatic failure. The risk from hepatitis E, which seems to have a predeliction for pregnant women, and from herpes simplex is particularly high. Herpes simplex virus hepatitis is extremely rare and may be diagnosed using serology and histology from liver biopsy, which shows specific changes, with extensive focal haemorrhagic necrosis and intranuclear inclusion bodies. Acyclovir is helpful if the disease is recognized at an early stage, but the prognosis for mother and fetus is extremely poor.

Pregnancy in women with pre-existing liver disease

Pregnancy may be uncomplicated in patients with mild, treated autoimmune chronic active hepatitis. Regarding drug treatment, the same comments apply as for patients with IBD (see above). In patients with mild chronic viral hepatitis, concerns are mainly centred around prevention of transmission of the virus to the baby. Retrospective studies of small numbers of patients in pregnancy have reported both deterioration of liver function and no change in function, in primary biliary cirrhosis, autoimmune chronic active hepatitis, and primary sclerosing cholangitis (51,52). Careful monitoring is required during pregnancy, and joint care between the obstetrician and gastroenterolgist or hepatologist may be appropriate.

Cirrhotic chronic liver disease of all aetiologies is generally associated with infertility, but if conception occurs, variceal bleeding has been reported to be a common complication in patients with portal hypertension, especially in the second and third trimesters. It is actually doubtful whether variceal haemorrhage is more common during pregnancy, because pregnancy is so rare in women with cirrhosis. Patients with portal hypertension and whose condition is stabilized on propranolol should be advised not to stop their medication, as there is an increased risk of variceal bleeding on stopping the drug. The risk to mother and fetus from the mortality of variceal bleeding far outweighs the risk of continuing β-blocker therapy. There may be decompensation of the liver disease, and this has generally been reported to improve after delivery.

After liver transplantation, fertility may return to normal. Pregnancy in liver transplant recipients has been reported to be frequently complicated by preterm delivery, pre-eclampsia, and infection. Immunosuppressive drugs must be continued throughout pregnancy in these patients, with careful monitoring of drug concentrations, although there is no evidence of teratogenesis. These patients and their partners therefore require careful advice about contraception, pre-conception counselling, and monitoring in a specialized unit during their pregnancy (53).

References
* Of interest ** of exceptional interest.
1. *O'Brien B, Zhou Q. Variables related to nausea and vomiting during pregnancy. *Birth* 1995; **22**: 93–100.
2. *Vutyavanich T, Wongtra-ngan S, Ruangsri R. Pyridoxine for nausea and vomiting of pregnancy: a randomised, double-blind, placebo-controlled trial. *Am J Obstet Gynecol* 1995; **88**: 343–346.
3. **Jewell D, Young G. Treatment for nausea and vomiting in early pregnancy. (Cochrane review). In: *The Cochrane Library* 1998; Issue 2. Oxford Update Software; updated quarterly.
4. *Aikins Murphy PA. Alternative therapies for nausea and vomiting of pregnancy. *Obstet Gynaecol* 1998; **91**: 149–155.
5. *Bergin PS, Harvey P. Wernicke's encephalopathy and central pontine myelinolysis associated with hyperemesis gravidarum. *B M J* 1992; **305**: 517–518.
6. *Tareen AK, Baser A, Jaffry HF, et al. Thyroid hormone in hyperemesis gravidarum. *J Obstet Gynecol* 1995; **173**: 495–501.
7. *Hsu JJ, Clark-Glena R, Nelson DK et al. Nasogastric enteral feeding in the management of hyperemesis gravidarum. *Obstet Gynecol* 1996; **88**: 343–345.
8. Nelson-Piercy C. Hyperemesis gravidarum. *Curr Opin Obstet Gynecol* 1997; **7**: 98–103.
9. *Sullivan CA, Johnson CA, Roach H et al. A pilot study of intravenous ondansetron for hyperemesis gravidarum. *Am J Obstet Gynecol* 1996; **174**: 1565–1568.
10. *Taylor R. Successful management of hyperemesis gravidarum using steroid therapy. *Q J Med* 1996; **89**: 103–107.
11. *Knudsen A, Lebech M, Hansen M. Upper gastrointestinal symptoms in the third trimester of pregnancy. *Eur J Obstet Gynaecol Reprod Biol* 1995; **60**: 29–33.
12. *Larson JD, Patataman E, Miner PB et al. Double-blind placeo-controlled study of ranitidine for gastro-oesophageal reflux symptoms during pregnancy. *Obstet Gynecol* 1997; **90**: 83–87.
13. *Lalkin A, Magee L, Addis A et al. Acid-suppressing drugs during pregnancy. *Can Fam Physician* 1997; **43**: 12923–12926.
14. *Magee LA, Inocencion G, Kamboj J et al. Safety of first trimester exposure to histamine H_2 blockers: a prospective cohort study. *Dig Dis Sci* 1996; **41**: 1145–1149.

15. *Smoleniac JS, James DK. Gastrointestinal crises during pregnancy. *Dig Dis* 1993; **11**: 313–324.
16. *Fallon WF, Newman JS, Fallon GL et al. The surgical management of intra-abdominal inflammatory conditions during pregnancy. *Surg Clin North Am* 1995; **75**: 15–31.
17. **Nathan L, Huddleston JF. Acute abdominal pain in pregnancy. *Obstet Gynaecol Clin North Am* 1995; **22**: 55–68.
18. *Gouldman JW, Sticca RP, Rippon MB et al. Laparoscopic cholecystectomy in pregnancy. *Am Surg* 1998; **64**: 93–98.
19. *Jamidar PA et al. ERCP in pregnancy. *Am J Gastroenterol* 1995; **90**: 1263–1267.
20. *Lin TC, Steinberg S. ERCP for biliary tract disease in pregnancy. *Gastroenterology* 1998; **114**: A529.
21. *Cappell MS, Sidhom O. A multicentre, multiyear study of the safety and clinical utility of oesophageal gastroduodenoscopy in 20 consecutive pregnant females with follow-up of fetal outcome. *Am J Gastroenterol* 1993; **88**: 1900–1905.
22. *Roll C, Schmid EN, Menten U et al. Fatal Salmonella enteritidis sepsis acquired prenatally in a premature infant. *Obstet Gynecol* 1996; **88**: 692–693.
23. *Meyer A, Stallbactch T, Goldenberger D et al. Lethal maternal sepsis caused by Campylobacter jejuni: pathogen preserved in placenta and identified by molecular methods. *Mod Pathol* 1997; **19**: 1253–1256.
24. *Alstead EM. Listeria and food. *Gastroenterol in Practice* 1990; **1**: 23–24.
25. *Craig S, Permezel M, Doyle L et al. Perinatal infection with Listeria monocytogenes. *Aust N Z J Obstet Gynecol* 1996; **36**: 286–290.
26. *Cappell MS, Colon VJ, Sidhom OA. A study at ten medical centres of the safety and efficacy of 48 flexible sigmoidoscopies and 8 colonoscopies during pregnancy with follow-up of fetal outcome and with comparison to control groups. *Dig Dis Sci* 1996; **41**: 2353–2361.
27. **Kornfeld D, Crattingnuis S, Ekbom A. Pregnancy outcomes in women with IBD – a population-based cohort study. *Am J Obstet Gynaecol* 1997; **177**: 942–946.
28. *Ardizzone S, Bollani S, Moltenil P et al. Fertility and pregnancy in inflammatory bowel disease: a case-controlled study. *Gastroenterology* 1998; **114**: A922.
29. *Modigliani R. Drug therapy for ulcerative colitis during pregnancy. *Euro J Gastroenterol Hepatol* 1997; **9**: 854–857.
30. *Diavcitrin O, Park YH, Veerasuntharam G. The safety of mesalazine in human pregnancy: a prospective cohort study. *Gastroenterology* 1998; **114**: 23-28.
31. *Alstead EM, Ritchie JK, Lennard Jones JL et al. Is azathioprine safe in pregnancy in inflammatory bowel disease? *Gastroenterology* 1990; **98**: 325–328.
32. **Know TA, Olans LB. Current concepts in liver disease in pregnancy. *N Engl J Med* 1996; **335**: 569–576.
33. *Girling JC, Dow E, Smith JH. Liver function test in pre-eclampsia: importance of comparison with a reference range derived for normal pregnancy. *Br J Obstet Gynaecol* 1997; **104**: 246–250.
34. *Rinaldo P, Treem WR, Riely CA. Liver disease in pregnancy. *N Engl J Med* 1997; **336**: 377–379.
35. *Nelson-Piercy C. Liver disease in pregnancy. *Curr Opin Obstet Gynecol* 1997; **7**: 36–42.

36. **Sims HF, Brackett JC, Powell CK. The molecular basis of pediatric long chain 3-hydroxyacyl Co-A dehydrogenase deficiency associated with maternal acute fatty liver of pregnancy. *Proc Natl Acad Sci USA* 1995; **92**: 841–845.

37. *Isaacs JD, Sims HG, Powell CK *et al*. Maternal acute fatty liver of pregnancy associated with fetal trifunctional protein deficiency: molecular characterisation of a novel maternal mutant allele. *Pediatr Res* 1996; **40**: 393–398.

38. **Wilken B, Leung K-C, Hammond J *et al*. Pregnancy and fetal long chain 3-hydroxyacyl coenzyme A dehydrogenase deficiency. *Lancet* 1993; **341**: 407–408.

39. *Sibai BM, Ramadan MK, Usta I et al. Maternal morbidity and mortality in 442 pregnancies with hemolysis, elevated liver enzymes and low platelets (HELLP syndrome). *Am J Obstet Gynecol* 1993; **169**: 1000–1006.

40. *Treem WR, Shoup ME, Hale DE *et al*. Acute fatty liver of pregnancy, haemolysis, elevated liver enzymes and low platelets syndrome, and long chain 3-hydroxyacyl-coenzyme A dehydrogenase deficiency. *Am J Gastroenterol* 1996; **91**: 2293–2300.

41. *Sibai BM, Ramadan MK, Chari RS *et al*. Pregnancies complicated by HELLP syndrome (hemolysis, elevated liver enzymes and low platelets): subsequent pregnancy outcome and long-term prognosis. *Am J Obstet Gynecol* 1995; **172**: 125–129.

42. *Visser W, Wallenburg HC. Temporising management of severe pre-eclampsia with and without the HELLP syndrome. *Br J Obstet Gynaecol* 1995; **102**: 111–117.

43. *Fagan EA. Intrahepatic cholestasis of pregnancy. *BMJ* 1994; **309**: 1243–1244.

44. *Laatikainen TJ, Ikonen E. Serum bile acids in cholestasis of pregnancy. *Obstet Gynecol* 1977; **50**: 313–318.

45. *Londero F, San Marco L. Intrahepatic cholestasis of pregnancy: are we really able to predict fetal outcome? *Am J Obstet Gynecol* 1997; **177**: 1274.

46. *Davies MH, da Silva RCMA, Jones SR *et al*. Fetal mortality associated with cholestasis of pregnancy and the potential benefit of therapy with ursodeoxycholic acid. *Gut* 1995; **37**: 580–584.

47. *Sepulveda WH, Gonzalez C, Cruz MA *et al*. Vasoconstrictive effects of bile acids on isolated human placental chorionic veins. *Eur J Obstet Gynecol Reprod Biol* 1991; **42**: 211–215.

48. *Palma J, Reyes H, Ribalta J *et al*. Effects of ursodeoxycholic acid in patients with intrahepatic cholestasis of pregnancy. *Hepatology* 1992; **15**: 1043–1047.

49. **Palma J, Reyes H, Ribalta J *et al*. Ursodeoxycholic acid in the treatment of intrahepatic cholestasis of pregnancy: a randomised, double-blind study controlled with placebo. *Hepatology* 1997; **27**: 1022–1028.

50. *Hirvioja ML, Tumala R, Vuori J. The treatment of intrahepatic cholestasis of pregnancy by dexamethazone. *Br J Obstet Gynaecol* 1992; **99**: 109–111.

51. *Pajor A, Lehoczky D, Pregnancy in liver cirrhosis. Assessment of maternal and fetal risks in eleven patients and review of the management. *Gynecol Obstet Invest* 1994; **38**: 45–50.

52. *Janczewska I, Olsson R, Hultcrantz R *et al*. Pregnancy in patients with primary sclerosing cholangitis. *Liver* 1996; **16**: 326–330.

53. *Laifer SA, Guido RS. Reproductive function and outcome of pregnancy after liver transplantation in women. *Mayo Clin Proc* 1995; **70**: 388–394.

C: Selected Procedures

10. Endoscopy for Gastrointestinal Emergencies

PAUL SWAIN

Most emergency endoscopy relates to the diagnosis and treatment of patients with **upper gastro-intestinal bleeding**. This chapter is intended to give practical advice on this topic. A selected list of references reviews the evidence on which the management of this subject is based (1–7). For further details of the management of bleeding varices, particularly the technique of inserting a sengstaken tube, the reader is referred to Chapter 11.2. There are other emergency requirements for endoscopy, which include upper gastrointestinal endoscopy for foreign body removal, colonoscopy — usually for bleeding (see Chapter 12) — and emergency endoscopic retrograde cholangiopancrea-tography (ERCP), often for acute cholangitis or pancreatitis.

Endoscopy in patients with gastrointestinal emergencies is sometimes more difficult than routine diagnostic endoscopy, for the following reasons:

- the patient tends to be more frightened
- the patient is more likely to be haemodynami-cally compromised
- some patients with bleeding will have severe associated cardio-pulmonary diseases, which increases the risk of endoscopy
- patients bleeding because of liver disease may be encephalopathic; alcoholic patients may be difficult to sedate and become disinhibited during the procedure
- endoscopy may take longer because it can be more difficult to define the bleeding site and takes extra time to treat it
- the procedure may have to be performed out of

hours, with the assistance of less experienced nursing staff
- the endoscope is more likely to become blocked

EXPLANATION, CONSENT AND SEDATION

If there is a chance that therapeutic endoscopy will be used, the patient should be informed of the possible risks (increased bleeding or perforation, both with an incidence of less than 1%) and the benefits of the procedure, and a statement to this effect should probably be included in the consent form. In patients with shock and a substantial bleed, it makes sense to obtain their consent for possible operative treatment in addition to endoscopy, so that they can go quickly to theatre if necessary, without having to be recovered in order to give new consent after the endoscopy.

Greater flexibility in choice of sedation

Discriminating use of sedation is required in some groups of patients with gastrointestinal bleeding. Very elderly patients, those with cardiopulmonary disease, and patients with liver failure usually require smaller doses or no sedation. Pulse oximetry, with supplementary oxygen saturation, expert oropharyngeal suction, and careful observation of clinical condition are especially helpful during the endoscopy. Alcoholic patients tend to be poorly responsive to benzodiazepines and can become disinhibited during endoscopy. Opiates or no sedation may be a better choice and it may be helpful to have an extra member of staff present if the patient appears likely to be uncooperative. Patients who have delirium tremens, or who are "fighting drunk" are usually best left to undergo their endoscopy on the next morning, unless they are clearly bleeding substantially. In some cases, consideration should be given to asking an anaesthetist for assistance with a short general anaesthetic.

EQUIPMENT AND ANCILIARY PROCEDURES

Use of airway

Occasionally, it may be necessary to pass an **endotracheal tube**, especially for endoscopy in patients with hepatic coma. It is essential that all endoscopists are trained to be able to pass an endotracheal tube in patients with incipient aspiration or who have been over-sedated, without waiting for an anaesthetist to arrive. More commonly, it is necessary for patients to undergo endoscopy on Intensive Care Units with an airway *in situ*. Occasionally, the endotracheal tube with a well-distended balloon, combined with the fact that the patient is lying their back, can make oesophageal intubation difficult. It can be helpful to ask an anaesthetist to relax the patient and partially deflate the balloon during endoscopic intubation.

Avoidance of nasogastric tubes

Nasogastric tubes are used routinely in some countries and casualty units, to verify the presence of blood in the stomach, and to select patients requiring early endoscopy. It is usually more unpleasant for the patient to have nasogastric tube passed than to undergo endoscopy. Further more, nasogastric tubes can cause misleading erosions and oesophagitis and, rarely, precipitate bleeding from ulcers or varices. In addition, a patient may have a particularly unpleasant experience if an inexperienced member of the hospital staff attempts to pass a nasogastric tube. It is my opinion that the use of a nasogastric tube in cases of gastrointestinal bleeding constitutes cruelty to patients. I discourage the practice, believing that if a tube of some kind is necessary, an endoscope is the best choice; however, I am an avowed proponent of early endoscopy.

Should it have been necessary to use a nasogastric tube, it is usually best either to remove it before the endoscopy, or to use it as a marker for the oesophageal orifice, and remove it as soon as the oesophagus is intubated. Although it is usually possible to perform an endoscopy with a nasogastric tube *in situ*, it is important to cap the end of the tube, so that the intragastric air does not escape. Finally, even if an endoscope is well lubricated, a nasogastric tube inserted alongside it is likely to be withdrawn when the endoscope is remove.

Choice of endoscope

The choice of endoscope depends on what is available to the endoscopist.

1. *Video endoscopes*: These are useful for teaching, photography, video-recording and demonstrating therapeutic practice with bleeding patients but sometimes give poor images especially in patients with major bleeding. This is mainly due to the CCD chip quenching response to red colour of blood and the greater absorption of light by blood. If the view is inferior it is sometimes best to cut one's losses and change to a non-video fiberoptic endoscope.

2. *Large-diameter endoscopes*: With bigger light bundles and larger channels, these have some advantages. They offer a clearer, better lit view and allow more rapid suction of blood; if they have a large diameter channel they allow the passage of larger therapeutic accessories. These endoscopes are probably preferable if bipolar or heater probes are to be used optimally, as the small-diameter probes are demonstrably less effective than their larger diameter counterparts at haemostasis in experimental studies.

3. *Double-channel endoscopes*: The advantage of these is that suction can be maintained while treatment is delivered. They can be very helpful with patients who have major bleeding, but it can be difficult to pass them, especially in small, elderly ladies. Large-diameter endoscopes (>11 mm) can not be used for band ligation of varices in conjuction with some of the commercially available single- or multiple-band ligation devices as configured at present.

4. *Side-viewing duodenoscope*: A better view is obtained of the medial wall of the duodenum, especially in the second part. Occasionally, this

is useful if haemobilia is suspected or if bleeding is seen to be coming from the distal bulb or second part of duodenum.

Avoiding blockage

Endoscope blockage is more likely to occur during endoscopy of patients who are bleeding than during routine endoscopy. To avoid blockage:

- check that the scope is blowing enthusiastically, before starting by placing the endoscope tip under water and covering the blowing valve
- use inflation and washing, rather than suction, to improve visualization of an area
- avoid using the suction channel if clots are seen
- if the views are poor and you suspect that the endoscope is blocked, it is usually quickest to remove the endoscope and check that it is still blowing
- check that the blowing function is working well after the endoscopy, and flush the system and use the clearance valves, especially if the endoscope is to be cleaned by less experienced staff out of hours

The most common cause of a poor view during endoscopy for bleeding is that the blowing channel is blocked. One trick that reduces the chance of blocking the endoscope, if there is clot and blood that need to be aspirated and which might block the endoscope, is to connect the suction tubing directly to the biopsy port, rather than to the connection on the umbilical cord at its insertion into the light source. The biopsy channel is straighter, and does not have the step down in diameter in the umbilical cord that is the usual site of blockage. If the biopsy channel does become blocked, a brush can be pushed down and will unblock the endoscope, without the need to remove the endoscope from the patient's stomach.

Use of ancillary washing facility

A means to **wash blood away** is the single most useful endoscopic accessory for the diagnosis of bleeding site at endoscopy. It is useful for clearing loose blood clot away to allow a view of the mucosal or the ulcer surface. It is essential for the diagnosis of oozing, which can only be made securely by seeing a point that looks as if it might be oozing, washing the blood away and watching to see that

blood really is coming from that bleeding point. Some thermal devices, such as the bipolar probe and heater probe, have pumps that can wash the bleeding point through a small channel in the probe through the biopsy channel. These work really well, and are worth having simply for this facility alone. A hand-powered washing catheter can be readily improvised from an ERCP cannula and a syringe of water, or the ulcer can be washed by attaching a large syringe to the biopsy channel. We made a cheap endoscopic washing pump from a car windscreen wiper pump and a cannula; a teeth-cleaning device called a Waterpik has also been connected to a water cannula to provide a cheap and effective washing facility. It can help to put some silicone oil in the washing liquid to reduce bubbling.

Use of an overtube

The passage of an **orooesophageal overtube**, provided it passes the cricopharyngeus easily, can be an asset to endoscopy in patients with substantial bleeding and a stomach full of blood, as it protects the airway if the patient regurgitates large quantities of blood, allows aspiration of stomach and oral secretions separately, and facilitates the frequent removal and re-insertion of the endoscope for cleaning and attachment of therapeutic accessories — for example banding for varices. If an overtube is being used, it is helpful to soak it in hot water, which makes it more pliable and lubricates the plastic, making it easier to insert. The passage of a guidewire, with the subsequent use of a dilator that fits the overtube, is also helpful, especially if there is resistance to passage at the cricopharyngeus.

BLOOD!

What to do if there is a lot of blood

Don't panic. Tell the nurse at the patient's head to be ready with suction, and keep the patient well over in the left lateral position. Encourage the patient not to retch. Most retching settles once the endoscope is in the stomach and if the movements of the endoscope are gentle. Inflation of the stomach will lift the lesser curve of the stomach away from the dependent pool of blood; substantial bleeding from gastric ulcers is likely to derive from ulcers high on the posterior aspect of the lesser curve. The endoscope can be slipped along the lesser curve into the antrum, which is usually relatively free of blood, as it is sloping upwards when the patient is lying in the left lateral position. It is usually relatively easy to identify the pylorus and enter the duodenum, even in the presence of a considerable quantity of blood. Active bleeding in the bulb is usually cleared quickly by peristaltic duodenal activity. Endoscopic difficulty in this area is usually due to large floppy clots obscuring the ulcerated area. These can prolapse through the pylorus, cover the ulcer, and be difficult to clear.

It is unwise to try to roll the patient over with the endoscope *in situ*, as this can cause aspiration, and rarely improves the view. If you are suspicious that bleeding is coming from high on the greater curve, take the endoscope out, turn the patient carefully over, and position the patient so that the feet are at the head end of the table, with the patient lying facing the endoscopist, so that the greater curve is uppermost. Major bleeding is uncommon from sites high on the greater curve of the stomach, and is usually associated with angiodysplasia, leiomyoma, or cancers.

If the patient is shocked, or has clearly had a substantial bleed, it can be helpful to examine the stomach for a succussion splash, which will give some indication that a large volume of blood is likely to be encountered. If the patient has had aortic graft surgery, it is important to reach the third part of the duodenum, which is the common site at which grafts erode into the duodenum.

Try not to get covered with blood

Performing endoscopy in a patient with gastrointestinal bleeding can be a messy business. Wearing aprons and protective clothing is sensible. Those performing endoscopy outside normal working hours may need to know where a bucket and mop are kept. Eye protection is important, especially when an HIV-positive patient with bleeding is undergoing endoscopy. The risks of eye splash are greater with optical rather than video scopes, because the eye is closer to the biopsy channel.

Hepatitis B protection

Hepatitis B vaccination should be an essential precaution for doctors and nursing or endoscopy associate staff who are performing endoscopy on patients, who are bleeding.

DIAGNOSTIC CONSIDERATIONS

A plan of endoscopy for a patient who is bleeding

Have a check-list of diagnoses that are being excluded as the endoscopy proceeds.

Look at the **pharynx**: a lot of blood here, but little in the oesophagus or stomach, may indicate a nasal, throat, or bronchial source. In bleeding patients the **mid-oesophagus** is sometimes poorly examined by endoscopists who are in a hurry to reach the stomach and duodenum. Check for **varices** and try to see the **cardiooesophageal junction** before crossing it especially at the "1 o'clock" position, which is the common site for Mallory–Weiss tears. If an ulcer is present in the **stomach** or **duodenum** try to commit yourself to an assessment of whether stigmata are present or not, and then whether there is a vessel to be seen; if unsure, try to wash the ulcer. Check that the difficult areas have been seen, especially the **posterior duodenal bulb**, the **second part of the duodenum**, **under the angulus**, and examine the **high posterior lesser curve** and the **cardia** fully with a J manoeuvre. If one ulcer or lesion is seen do not allow this finding to prevent a full examination of the upper gastrointestinal tract for another lesion. Ask yourself if the findings fit with the clinical story and if, there has been a big bleed and the endoscopic findings are trivial, have another look around. Check that the endoscope is inflating well throughout the examination, and change it if the view is inferior.

What to do if you are sure there has been upper gastrointestinal bleeding but no source is obvious

Consider whether another endoscope would give a better view or do the job better. Ask yourself if the inflation is adequate, if the light is bright enough or a larger diameter endoscope would give a better view, and if the image is poor because the lens is fogged or has mucus attached to it. Consider scheduling a repeat endoscopy once the patient has undergone transfusion if the patient is severely anaemic. Always cross the pylorus at least twice; the endoscope commonly fails to visualize ulcers just inside the bulb positioned posteriorly, because the endoscope is usually pointing at the anterior wall as the pylorus is crossed.

Common catches

1. About 50% of Mallory–Weiss tears are missed on the first pass into the stomach. This is because the stomach may need to be inflated to open up the folds at the cardiooesophageal junction in order to allow this lesion to be well seen.
2. Multiple ulcers can cause diagnostic problems. A prepyloric ulcer can be associated with a large duodenal ulcer. Usually the duodenal ulcer will be the significant source of bleeding. Occasionally there are two or more ulcers high on the lesser curve. The bleeding is most likely to be coming from the largest — usually the most proximal — ulcer.
3. The diagnosis of early varices is more difficult than non- or inexperienced endoscopists realize. If you are uncertain, withdraw the endoscope about 3 cm from the cardiooesophageal junction and look for the cordlike appearance. Overinflating the oesophagus can flatten the varices; they do not always have a blue colour, and sometimes appear whiter or browner than the oesophageal mucosa.

Rarities cause difficulty because the endoscopist lacks experience of them. Dieulafoy's lesion or "exulceratio simplex" usually is found within 3 cm of the cardia (at the classic site for high lesser-curve gastric ulcers). The appearance is of a visible vessel high on the lesser curve, with minimal surrounding ulceration. Solitary gastric angiomas can occur at the junction of gastric body and fundus on the greater curve, and may be hidden under a pool of blood. **Watermelon stomach** is often mistaken for gastritis. **Oesophageal apoplexy**, with a huge blue haematoma dissecting the oesophageal mucosa, is puzzling when first encountered. Gastric angiomas can be mistaken for suction artefacts. Linear erosions on the edge of a hiatus hernia, called Cameron erosions, can cause anaemia and bleeding and are under-recognized.

Bleeding from angiomata or aneurysms in the duodenum require a clear endoscopic view, recognition of abnormal pulsation. The diagnosis of haematobilia (bleeding from the biliary tract) or wirsungorrhagia (bleeding from the pancreatic duct) at endoscopy requires patience, a washing facility and, sometimes, a side-viewing endoscope.

Severe anaemia makes endoscopy difficult as the pale anaemic mucosa is difficult to distinguish from superficial ulcers and erosions. Transfusing the patient and scheduling a repeat endoscopy can help in achieving a diagnosis. Repeat the endoscopy later if the first attempt is limited by the presence of a large quantity of blood in the stomach.

TECHNIQUES OF ENDOSCOPIC TREATMENT OF HAEMORRAGIC LESIONS

It is probably valuable to have training in both injection and thermal methods of endoscopic treatment, and all endoscopy units offering an emergency service should try to keep both available, if only because it is sometimes easier to use one than the other.

Preparation of the ulcer floor for treatment

Washing free blood, mucus, or clot out of the ulcer base before treatment may help identify the precise target for treatment and make delivery of injection, thermal, or mechanical methods of treatment easier. Floppy adherent clot can interfere with treatment and make assessment of the risk of further bleeding more difficult. Washing will not always remove this clot — but is very safe, in that it almost never causes bleeding. Using a snare to cut the clot off the floor of the ulcer, by closing the snare around the clot without using electrocautery, will sometimes be worth while, and may reveal whether there is a vessel visible under the clot, making endoscopic treatment easier and more likely to be effective. It may occasionally precipitate active bleeding, so should be undertaken only by an experienced endoscopist with endoscopic therapy ready to apply.

Injection treatment of bleeding peptic ulcer

If **adrenaline** is injected, a 1:10 000 solution should be used (some practitioners use more dilute solutions). It is probably not worth while to inject much more than 10 ml. Try to keep the injection cannula and needle in view close to the tip of the endoscope, as this increases the control and allows more force to be exerted if the endoscope tip and the needle are advanced simultaneously. Allowing a few drips to emerge from the tip of the needle immediately before injection can give some information on the orientation of the ulcer, because the drips will fall downwards; nonetheless, the rotation of the patient may still make it difficult to be sure if the ulcer is anterior or posterior, especially in the duodenum. It may help to try to inject just beyond the visible vessel initially. If you start by injecting proximally, this may raise a proximal bleb, which may make it more difficult to inject the far side of the ulcer floor. **Scar tissue**, which looks white in the floor of the ulcer, may make it more difficult, both to inject and to make the needle penetrate the tissue. Watch to see if the injection produces a submucosal bleb, and observe the direction in which the bleb runs. Ideally, a bleb will be seen to be raised all round the vessel. Often the bleb is asymmetrical, and will not lift scarred tissue. Sometimes the fluid simply runs backwards out of the needle track without tracking submucosally; if this happens, the needle should be pulled out of the tissue and another area tried. Injection of adrenaline can make the surrounding tissues look white with ischaemia after a couple of minutes, and after 5–10 m the tissue may turn black and look rather worrying; however, the tissues almost always recover after 12 h.

Injection of a **sclerosant** is more dangerous than injection of adrenaline or any of the thermal methods, in that it will produce tissue necrosis and can occasionally cause infarction of the stomach or duodenum. The volume should be limited to 5 ml or less of 5% ethanolamine or 1% polidocanol. If absolute alcohol — which is a potent dessicant — is being used the volume should be limited to 1 ml. It is not clear from experimental studies how the sclerosant is best applied, but most endoscopists try to inject small volumes into at least four different points as close to the vessel as possible. Injection of **fibrin glue** requires a specialized double-lumen needle. The individually prepared solutions of fibrinogen and thrombin are activated by combining the fibrinogen and factor XIII with aprotinin, and the thrombin with calcium chloride. They are injected simultaneously through the dual-lumen syringe to form a clot. It is helpful to load both lumens of the catheter with saline and then flush both channels with saline before withdrawing the syringe. At least two injections, and preferably more, are recommended, placed as close to the vessel as practicable. The entire 1 ml volume of both solutions should be injected in one bolus and the syringe flushed, before the needle is withdrawn from the tissue.

Thermal methods

The techniques of using **bipolar probes** and **heater probes** are similar. It is helpful to place a single pulse of energy on tissue away from the ulcer to be treated, to check that the settings are biologically appropriate. A white depression should be formed in the normal tissue. If the mark is difficult to spot, the setting should be increased; if the mucosa is broken, the setting should be reduced. When treating a non-bleeding visible vessel, place a series of pulses around and as close to the vessel as is possible, without touching the vessel itself if possible. Press firmly, and treat until any adherent red clot has been blackened and then treat the vessel again, pressing firmly on it. After treatment, the protruding vessel appearance should look flattened. Watch the ulcer for a couple of minutes to see that no further bleeding occurs. This time can be used to take a biopsy from the antrum to look for *Helicobacter pylori*.

The large-diameter bipolar probe and heater probe are more effective in stopping bleeding from larger diameter vessels in experimental studies. It makes sense to try to use a large-channel endoscope and these large-diameter thermal probe methods for therapeutic endoscopy in patients with major bleeding from peptic ulcer. The heater probe takes a few seconds to deliver its energy by thermal conduction, in contrast to the bipolar probe, which uses radiofrequency current and delivers its energy at the speed of light. The heater probe therefore has a greater tendency to slide around the ulcer during treatment as the patient breathes, and it may be helpful to tell the patient to hold their breath for a few seconds as the energy is going in.

If there is active bleeding or spurting, the probe should be pressed directly onto the vessel to stop bleeding, and several pulses of energy given to stop the bleeding. It may help to wash the ulcer floor, to try to get rid of blood and clot that may interfere with delivery of the treatment to the bleeding point either before or during the thermal treatment.

The NdYAG (neodymium-yttrium-aluminium-garnet) laser is usually used as a non-contact method. Several pulses are fired around the vessel and then pulses are delivered to the centre of the vessel. The fibre should be held about 1 cm from the tissue during treatment. The argon plasma coagulator is a monopolar device using radiofrequency current; argon gas carries the current to the tissue when it becomes ionized in the electrical field.

Mechanical methods

Clips can be applied to bleeding vessels. It is worth practising with the Olympus clips, which are a little fiddly to load. They are passed through the biopsy channel and fully opened with two actions: the first is to push the clip clear of the transparent retaining plastic sleeve; the second is to pull back a little on the finger grip, with the thumb through the ring on the delivery system, until the clip has opened fully. The endoscope with the clipping device should be pushed until one limb of the clip is on one side of the vessel and the other limb is on the other side of the vessel. The clip is pressed into the tissue and then closed by squeezing the finger grip and the thumb ring together to break open the metal release clasp. The clip is then deployed. It may make sense to apply the next clip in a different orientation, by rotating the clip through 90% before application, because the orientation of the vessel in the ulcer floor is difficult to appreciate.

ENDOSCOPIC TREATMENT OF OESOPHAGEAL VARICES

There is some evidence that band ligation is superior to sclerotherapy for both acute and chronic treatment of oesophageal varices. It is currently advantageous to have some experience using band ligation, sclerotherapy, and injection of cyanoacrylate, and perhaps to be familiar with the use of endoloops.

Band ligation of varices

Endoscopic variceal band ligation is generally considered preferable to sclerotherapy for variceal obliteration. Compared with sclerotherapy, ligation acheives more rapid obliteration, is associated with fewer episodes of re-bleeding, and is associated with fewer complications. Band ligation should be undertaken at 2-weekly intervals until varices are obliterated (see Chapters 11.2 and 22.2).

Currently, **multiple band ligation devices** have superceded the use of single band ligation techniques in most units. The **technique** for using multiple band ligation devices is as follows:

1. A planning endoscopy is carried out to assess the distance from the teeth at which the first band is to be applied and the orientation of the varices, and to decide which variceal column is the largest and most likely to be the source of bleeding. During this endoscopy, note should be taken of the manoeuvres that are required to intubate the patient's trachea, as it may be a little more difficult subsequently to insert the endoscope with the band ligator attached to its tip.
2. Check that the suction to be used is working really well.
3. Mount the band ligator on the endoscope after the planning endoscopy. Check that the valve is left in, and that the lens is clear before re-intubation, and twist the ligator so that the strings interfere with the view as little as possible.
4. Once the endoscope is in the oesophagus, advanced the endoscope to the distance and orientation of the first varix to be treated.
5. Apply suction and wait until the varix has completely filled the cavity and a "red-out" is observed before firing the varix.
6. Rotate the scope 1 cm away from the first band, but try to avoid coming proximally until the next varix can be ligated.

It is most effective to treat the varices as close to the cardiooesophageal junction as possible. There is a tendency when using band ligation to move proximally too quickly and place bands in the mid oesophagus. If a bleeding point is identified during the planning endoscopy, it makes sense to try to suck that varix into the ligator first, as the view often deteriorates during the treatment as blood and mucus and the odd misfired band obstructs the view. This can sometimes be cleared by squirting fluid down the biopsy channel.

Single band ligators are generally placed through an overtube; however, the overtube can cause upper oesophageal tears on insertion. The best way to place an overtube is by placing a guide-wire in the oesophagus and passing into the oesophagus a bougie-type dilator that is a smooth fit to the overtube; the overtube is then run smoothly into the oesophagus. Liberal lubrication — for example spraying the surfaces with cooking oil — helps to reduce friction. It may help to flex the patient's neck a little during insertion, as this makes the leading edge of the overtube press against the dilator and it is then less likely to catch the mucosa on insertion. Overtubes can be back-loaded onto the endoscope and the endoscope used as an insertion device, but there is then more space between the endoscope and the overtube, in which tissue can be caught, than when using a good-fit dilator in the overtube. Tissue can be caught between the distal tip of the overtube and the protruding proximal edge of the band ligation cap.

Injection sclerotherapy

Make sure that you, your assistant, and the patient are wearing goggles. Fill the cannula with the sclerosant. Some groups using 5% ethanolamine put the vials in warm water to reduce the viscosity before injection. It is worth asking the assistant who will do the injection to advance and retard the needle in its sheath before passing it through the endoscope, so that they are familiar with the movements required. The sclerosant should fill the cannula and drip from the needle before it is passed into the biopsy channel. Unambiguous simple commands such as "needle forwards", "needle back", "inject 1 ml" should elicit a verbal response from the assistant to confirm that the commands have been followed. Start the injection close to the cardiooesophageal junction and, if possible, begin with the biggest varix or the one with the most menacing stigmata. If there is active bleeding from an identifiable orifice in a varix, try to inject just below it and then just above it. Watch for tissue whitening, which indicates that the injection is submucosal rather than intravariceal (although there is evidence that both are effective). Watch when the needle is withdrawn and assess the amount of bleeding from the hole made by the needle: a small amount of bleeding is common and unimportant. My personal preference is to place an average of 2 ml per varix in 1-ml aliqots when using ethanolamine.

TREATMENT OF GASTRIC VARICES

Techniques for treatment of bleeding from gastric varices are controversial, and the outcome of bleeding from large gastric varices is less good than that of bleeding from oesophageal varices. Some practitioners use conventional sclerosants, but most obtain poor results with them and prefer to use the injection of the cyanoacrylate, enbucrilate (Histacryl), or to use band ligation. Enbucrilate is an unusual material that solidifies within a few second in contact with blood. It is exothermic — it releases heat on contact with liquid.

When enbucrilate is injected, it is usually diluted in a 1:1 solution with lipiodol. The addition of lipiodol reduces the viscosity of the glue a little and allows the site of injection to show up under screening: however, the two solutions do not mix easily, and the syringe containing both solutions should be rotated until they are reasonably mixed. The needle should be filled with sterile water before the injection and another syringe should be available, already filled with sterile water. The gastric varix should be approached usually in the recurve position. The needle should be pushed into the varix; the water in the syringe will produce a subcutaneous bleb if the needle is not in the varix. If the initial appearances seem satisfactory, the entire contents of the needle should be pushed forcefully through the needle and then flushed with sterile water. When the needle is withdrawn, a few drops of blood usually excide from the hole and then the bleeding generally stops. After a few seconds, it may be helpful to "palpate" the gastric varix that has been treated, using the injection sheath with the withdrawn needle to check that the material is solidifying within the varix. Very large gastric varices may require further injections.

It is probably unwise to use band ligation on huge gastric varices because the band may erode through part of the varix without inducing thrombosis in the entire varix.

CONCLUSION

Diagnostic endoscopy in gastrointestinal bleeding is an exciting and rewarding part of gastroenterology. The occasional technical difficulties that can make demands on the endoscopist's skill can usually be overcome with care.

References
1. National Institutes of Health Consensus Conference: therapeutic endoscopy and bleeding ulcers. *JAMA* 1989; **262**: 1369–1372
2. Cook DJ, Guyatt GH, Salena BJ *et al*. Endoscopic therapy for acute nonvariceal upper gastrointestinal haemorrhage: a meta analysis. *Gastroenterology* 1992; **102**: 139–148.

3. Gilbert DA, Silverstein FE, Tedesco FJ *et al*. The national ASGE survey in upper gastrointestinal bleeding. *Gastrointest Endosc* 1981; **94**: 94–102.

4. Rockall TA, Logan RF, Devlin HR *et al*. Incidence of mortality from acute upper gastrointestinal haemorrhage in the United Kingdom. *BMJ* 1995; **311**: 222–226.

5. Swain CP, Storey DW, Bown SG *et al*. Nature of the bleeding vessel in recurrently bleeding gastric ulcers. *Gastroenterology* 1986; **90**: 595–608.

6. Westaby D. Variceal bleeding. *Gastroint Endosc Clin North Am*. 1992, **2**:1–186.

7. Leung JW, Lee JG. Nonvariceal upper gastrointestinal bleeding. *Gastroint Endosc Clin North Am* 1997; **4**: 545–745.

Part II: Managing Gastroenterology Inpatients

11.1. Upper Gastrointestinal Bleeding: Peptic Ulcers

TIM ROCKALL

Peptic ulcer is the most common diagnosis amongst patients presenting with acute upper gastrointestinal haemorrhage: large observational studies (1) have consistently shown those with peptic ulcer to comprise approximately 50% of all cases (Table 11.1.1). The management pathway of an acute upper gastrointestinal haemorrhage is the same for all patients until a diagnosis has been made, at which point more specific management policies may be relevant, such as the injection of a bleeding vessel in peptic ulceration, or banding of oesophageal varices (see Chapter 11.2). From a practical point of view, the cause of bleeding remains obscure until upper gastrointestinal endoscopy has been undertaken. Even after oesophagogastroduodenoscopy, the source of bleeding may be obscure as a result of a missed lesion, a more distal lesion, or because a wrong diagnosis of gastrointestinal haemorrhage was made.

In this chapter, the practical issues of making the diagnosis, resuscitation, investigation, risk assessment, and treatment will be discussed.

MAKING THE DIAGNOSIS OF ACUTE UPPER GASTROINTESTINAL HAEMORRHAGE

In the majority of patients the diagnosis is obvious from the history and clinical examination. A history of **haematemesis** is rarely unreliable, and there is often evidence of blood around the mouth or on the clothing. Confusion may arise in patients who vomit swallowed blood from a bleeding lesion in the

Table 11.1.1. Diagnostic frequencies among patients with upper gastrointestinal haemorrhage.

Diagnosis	%	% of diagnoses made
None made	25	—
Peptic ulcer	35	46
Malignancy	4	5
Varices	4	6
Mallory—Weiss tear	5	7
Erosive disease	11	14
Oesophagitis	10	14
Other	6	8

nasopharynx, in patients with haemoptysis, and in patients with Munchausen's syndrome, who may give a very good history. Blood tests, including haemoglobin, are less reliable, but an **increased urea:creatinine** ratio (assuming baseline normal renal function) caused by absorption of blood in the small intestine can be helpful.

Melaena also usually results in a reliable history, as the stool is offensive, tarry, and black. Some patients, however, will not volunteer this information, so that direct questioning is necessary. Confusion sometimes arises with normal variation in stool colour as a result of diet or, in particular, oral iron supplementation. In these circumstances, however, examination always resolves the issue and there is rarely any confusion with true melaena. **Haemochezia** (passage of fresh blood per rectum) may result from brisk upper gastrointestinal haemorrhage, but is usually a sign of colonic haemorrhage.

Coffee ground vomiting is a good sign if it is witnessed, but less reliable from a history alone. It can also be confused with the faeculent vomiting of bowel obstruction, but this should not cause diagnostic difficulties. Occasionally, patients present with hypovolaemic shock before any haematemesis or melaena. The diagnosis usually reveals itself as resuscitation proceeds.

Examination of the patient with a suspected acute upper gastrointestinal haemorrhage must include a rectal examination and measurements of blood pressure with the patient both sitting and lying, in order to assess a postural decrease in blood pressure suggestive of hypovolaemia.

RESUSCITATION AND MONITORING

There is a wide range in the severity of acute upper gastrointestinal haemorrhage and, hence, the various measures for resuscitation and monitoring are not all required in all patients. However, consideration should be given to the following points.

Intravenous access and fluid replacement

Two large-bore peripheral venous canulae should be sited and immediate fluid replacement with crystalloid or colloid initiated, with regular monitoring of the pulse and blood pressure. Adequate fluid replacement should be accompanied by a decrease in heart rate, and increases in blood pressure, central venous pressure (CVP) and urine production. The physiological response to initial fluid resuscitation is a helpful guide to the degree of blood loss; however, it should be borne in mind that a relatively slow loss of blood over many hours will allow the patient to maintain intravascular volume well, and it is important not to overtransfuse these patients.

A simple guide to approximate volume depletion is shown in Table 11.1.2 (2).

In most patients with a significant upper gastrointestinal bleed, an initial resuscitation with 1–2 litre crystalloid, transfused rapidly is appropriate. After this, patients will fall into one of three categories:

1. Those that have a rapid response, become haemodynamically normal, and maintain this situation. In this case, one can surmise a less than 20% loss of blood volume.
2. Those in whom there is a transient response, with deterioration of the indices after the initial transfusion. This represents either continuing rapid blood loss or inadequate resuscitation. These patients have lost between 20 and 40% of their blood volume.
3. Those who fail to respond at all to this initial fluid replacement, as a result of severe volume depletion together with rapid continuing haemorrhage. This might be so, for example, in rare cases of aorto-duodenal fistula or torrential variceal bleeding, but would be unusual for peptic ulcer haemorrhage. This category is very rare in acute upper gastrointestinal haemorrhage, as the rate of blood loss is not usually sufficient.

Table 11.1.2. Simple guide to volume depletion.

	Class I	Class II	Class III	Class IV
Blood loss (ml)	<750	750–1500	1500–2000	>2000
Blood loss (%blood volume)	<15	15–30	30–40	>40
Heart (beats/min)	<100	>100	>120	>140
Blood pressure	Normal	Normal	Decreased	Decreased
Pulse pressure	Normal or increased	Decreased	Decreased	Decreased
Ventilatory rate (breaths/min)	14–20	20–30	30–40	>35
Urine output (ml/hour)	>30	20–30	5–15	Negligible
Mental status	Slightly anxious	Mildly anxious	Anxious and confused	Confused and lethargic
Fluid replacement	Crystalloid	Crystalloid	Crystalloid and blood	Crystalloid and blood

In patients in the second category and higher-risk patients in the first category more invasive monitoring is indicated. A central venous line should be placed, to measure and monitor the central venous pressure, and a urinary catheter to measure urine output. Adequate resuscitation is indicated by a positive CVP and a urine output of more than 30 ml/h. After the initial fluid resuscitation, further volume replacement should be with whole blood, and guided by the vital signs described, in addition to the haemoglobin once volume has been restored. CVP monitoring is particularly important in patients with cardiovascular co-morbidities, in whom overtransfusion may precipitate pulmonary oedema. A decreasing CVP, if measured with sufficient regularity and accuracy, may also give an early indication of further haemorrhage.

Initial investigations

Blood tests

At the time of initial placement of the cannula, blood should be drawn for crossmatch, in addition to full blood count, clotting screen, and urea and electrolytes. **Liver function tests** are an important investigation, but the results are not pertinent to the initial resuscitation. The **serum urea** concentration increases after an acute gastrointestinal bleed, as a result of absorbtion of the digested protein. A urea:creatinine ratio greater than 90 is said to be an indicator of blood loss from the upper gastrointestinal tract and a ratio less than 90 indicative of blood loss from the lower gastrointstinal tract.

The **haemoglobin** estimation is a very unreliable guide to blood loss in the acute stage and is not a predictor of likely re-bleeding or mortality. The haemoglobin concentration may be normal in a high-risk patient who presents with rapid haemorrhage and hypovolaemia as haemostatic mechanisms will not yet have diluted the blood from the extravascular compartments to maintain intravascular volume. Equally, a patient may present with a greatly reduced haemoglobin concentration, but a small acute haemorrhage, and with no intra-vascular volume depletion, but on a background of chronic bleeding leading to iron-deficiency anaemia.

The **haematocrit** is of value in assessing the degree of dilution.

Anomalies of clotting should be corrected as swiftly as possible, with appropriate use of vitamin K, fresh frozen plasma, or specific clotting factors where indicated. Bleeding may be associated with a platelet abnormality, and in these circumstances platelet transfusions can be given. In patients requiring more than 6 units of transfused blood, consideration should be given to giving fresh frozen plasma with subsequent units of blood, even if the initial clotting function is normal.

Endoscopy

Endoscopy should be undertaken at the earliest opportunity after resuscitation and stabilization. **The majority of patients do not require endoscopic assessment out of normal working hours, but those with suspected varices and patients who remain unstable after adequate resuscitation measures can benefit from out-of-hours endoscopy for the purposes of endoscopic therapy or for localization of the lesion and excluding varices before surgery**.

Patients undergoing endoscopy are at risk of vomiting and aspiration, and the procedure should be undertaken by experienced endoscopists with adequate support staff and in a fully equipped endoscopy unit with facilities for monitoring, suction, and oxygen delivery, and with rapid access to resuscitation equipment. The endoscopist should be capable of recognising and treating particular lesions using appropriate haemostatic modalities. Adequate visualization of the bleeding point is usually possible if determined efforts are made to remove blood from the stomach and duodenum. Ulcers with overlying clot should be washed to reveal the underlying lesion, so that accurate treatment can be directed towards any bleeding or visible vessel. Ulcers with spurting, oozing, or visible vessels (recognized as a raised red spot in the ulcer base) are all deemed appropriate for endoscopic treatment. The choice of endoscopic therapy depends on the skills of the operator and the availability of technology. The most commonly used modality is injection of adrenaline and or sclerosants. All injectable agents seem to have a similar efficacy in reducing re-bleeding rates. Alternatives are the application of heat energy using laser, heater probe, or diathermy, injection of tissue glues and, more recently, application of endoscopic clips. Two or more of these methods are sometimes used in combination.

Monitoring

For high-risk patients and those with a large initial bleed, close monitoring of vital signs — including heart rate, blood pressure, CVP, pulse oximetry and urine output — are best undertaken in a high-dependency setting. Heart rate and blood pressure should be measured at least half-hourly in the initial phase of resuscitation, until there has been a prolonged period of stability. Intensive care units, high-dependency units, or ward areas designated to the care of gastrointestinal emergencies, with an appropriately high nurse:patient ratio, may all be appropriate for individual patients. Regular assessment of haemoglobin, clotting, urea, and electrolytes are imperative and, together with close monitoring of transfusion requirements and vital signs, form the basis on which management decisions regarding endoscopy and surgery are made. Combined medical and surgical assessment from an early stage are probably beneficial in preventing delay in surgery whilst ensuring optimal care of patients with multiple co-morbidities.

There was once a vogue for placement of a **nasogastric tube** so that regular aspiration might indicate the continued loss of fresh blood from the upper gastrointestinal tract; however, in one series (3) only 53% of patients with positive aspirates were actively bleeding at endoscopy. In addition, bleeding beyond the pylorus may give a false negative and the trauma of nasogastric tube placement may give a false positive. The benefits of nasogastric tube placement are outweighed by the increased risk of aspiration, and the technique is **contraindicated**.

PROGNOSTIC FACTORS AND RISK CATEGORIZATION

The clinical factors prognostically important for re-bleeding and death are well established. The population presenting with acute upper gastrointestinal haemorrhage are increasingly aged and associated with this is an increasing number of co-morbidities; 27% of these patients are older than 80 years. Both these factors are important determinants of outcome, and are the underlying reasons why overall mortality has not declined over recent decades, despite apparent significant improvements in

management. Age-standardized mortality has declined significantly, and it is also possible to calculate risk-standardized mortality to incorporate other variables in the populations being studied.

Factors more specific to blood loss are the blood pressure at presentation, the diagnostic category, and the presence of stigmata of recent haemorrhage. The stigmata of recent haemorrage have been classified by Forrest *et al.* (4). The grading, together with the associated rebleeding rate, is shown in Table 11.1.3. The event of further haemorrhage after initial resuscitation and treatment is the most influential factor in determining risk of death. All these factors have recently been formulated into a validated *risk scoring system* that gives weighting to the various factors (5). This scoring system is presented in Table 11.1.4. The mortality associated with each risk category and for patients with and without further haemorrhage is shown in Table 11.1.5.

This scoring system has been used in comparative audit studies to assess case mix, but it can also be used clinically to define high-risk patients and identify low-risk patients (with a risk score of 2 or less) who have a minimal risk of further haemorrhage (<5%) and no mortality, and who can safely be managed with only a limited hospital stay, or even as outpatients (6).

Further haemorrhage, which encompasses both re-bleeding and continued bleeding, has itself been studied as an outcome measure, as endoscopic treatment is specifically targeted at preventing it. The most important determinants of re-bleeding are the presence of stigmata of recent haemorrhage and the nature (diagnosis, site, and size) of the bleeding lesion. A scoring system (Baylor score) for the prediction of re-bleeding has been developed that incorporates age, co-morbidity, haemodynamic status, ulcer size, ulcer location, and stigmata of recent haemorrhage (7,8) (Table 11.1.6). A duodenal ulcer positioned posteriorly is more likely to be

Table 11.1.3. Forrest classification of stigmata of recent haemorrage and associated rebleeding rates.

Class	Endoscopic observation	Rebleeding rate (%)
Ia	Spurting arterial haemorrhage	80–90
Ib	Oozing haemorrhage	10–30
IIa	Non-bleeding visible vessel	50–60
IIb	Adherent clot	25–35
IIc	Black spot in ulcer base	0–8
III	Clean ulcer base	0–12

Table 11.1.4. Acute upper gastrointestinal haemorrhage scoring system.

Variable	Score			
	0	1	2	3
Age (years)	< 60	60–79	≥ 80	
Shock	"No shock"	"Tachycardia"	"Hypotension"	
	Systolic BP ≥ 100 mmHg	Systolic BP ≥ 100 mmHg	Systolic BP <100 mmHg	
	Heart rate < 100 beats/min	Heart rate ≥ 100 beats/min		
Co-morbidity	No major co-morbidity		Cardiac failure	Renal failure
			Ischaemic heart disease	Liver failure
			Any major co-morbidity	Disseminated malignancy
Diagnosis	Mallory–Weiss tear	All other diagnoses	Malignancy of upper GI tract	
	No lesion identified and no SRH			
Major stigmata of recent haemorrhage	None, or Dark spot only		Blood in upper GI tract Adherent clot Visible or spurting vessel	

BP, blood pressure; SRH, stigmata of recent haemorrhage; GI, gastrointestinal.

Table 11.1.5. Observed rebleeding and mortality by risk score.

	Risk score								
	0	1	2	3	4	5	6	7	8+
Rebleed (%)	4.9	3.4	5.3	11.2	14.1	24.1	32.9	43.8	41.8
Deaths –									
No rebleed (%)	0	0	0.3	2.0	3.5	8.1	9.5	14.9	28.1
Deaths – Rebleed (%)	0	0	0	10.0	15.8	22.9	33.3	43.4	52.5
Deaths – Total (%)	0	0	0.2	2.9	5.3	10.8	17.3	27.0	41.1

Table 11.1.6. Baylor risk score.

Score	Pre-Endoscopy			Endoscopic	
	Age (years)	No. of co-morbidities	Status of co-morbidity	Site	Stigmata
0	<30	0	—	—	—
1	30–49	1 or 2	—	—	Clot
2	50–59	—	—	—	—
3	60–69	—	—	—	Visible vessel
4	—	3	Chronic	Posterior wall bulb	Active bleeding
5	≥ 70	≥ 5	Acute	—	—

Patients at high risk of re-bleeding are defined as those with a pre-endoscopy score >5 or a combined pre-endoscopy and endoscopy score >10.

associated with major arterial bleeding as a result of erosion of the gastroduodenal artery. The capacity for endoscopic methods such as injection or heat application is limited if the size of the bleeding vessel is large, and thus the re-bleeding rate in these patients is high. The development of mechanical clips that can be placed endoscopically may allow for the control of these larger vessels but, in the absence of such technology, early recourse to surgery is indicated if the initial treatment does not control the bleeding.

TREATMENT

The mainstay of treatment is the initial resuscitation, followed by transfusion of crossmatched whole blood. Subsequent treatment is aimed at arresting active haemorrhage and preventing recurrent haemorrhage using drugs, endoscopic techniques, and surgery.

Drug treatment

There has long been hope that the outcome of gastrointestinal bleeding and the occurrence of further haemorrhage might be improved with drug treatment. Underlying the use of all drug regimens subjected to trial has been the premise that **improving the stability of the blood clot** overlying the bleeding point would achieve this goal. It has been further surmised that endoscopic haemostasis may be more effective if a **neutral intragastric pH** is maintained. *In vitro* studies have shown both coagulation and platelet aggregation to be inhibited in an acid environment; pepsin activity, which dissolves fibrin, is also inhibited at neutral pH. There are other factors that may effect the clot in relation to haemostasis, including the activity of plasmin (which can be effected by tranexamic acid) and gastric motility. Neither of these factors is directly affected by increasing the intragastric pH.

The principal method has been to use drugs that increase the pH of the gastroduodenal contents. Simple **antacids** were superseded by **H_2-receptor antagonists**, which have been superseded by **proton pump inhibitors** (initially available only orally). Although a meta-analysis (9) of 27 randomized controlled trials of H_2-blockers, incorporating 1673 patients suggested some benefit in acute upper gastrointestinal bleeding, a subsequent large randomized placebo-controlled trial of famotidine in 1005 patients showed no benefit (10). This suggested either that pH is not important, or that the control of pH by this regimen was inadequate. The latter point is certainly supported by *in vitro* studies, but it has been shown that a bolus dose of intravenous proton pump inhibitor, followed by a continuous infusion, can achieve the goal of sustained acid suppression with stable pH values greater than 6.

There are now several published studies of **proton pump inhibitors** that give some support to their efficacy. Eight randomized trials that used different regimens of omeprazole have recently been assessed by Petersen & Cook (11). They excluded three trials either because of a lack of a discrete outcome variable or because of small size and lack of balance of cases. This left five trials (12–16) incorporating 960 patients, two of which were blinded and placebo-controlled, and three of which were comparative with H_2-antagonists. There are further major variations in the trial formats, as two studied only the pharmacological agent, whereas three also used prior endoscopic haemostasis. The individual regimens varied in dosage, administration, and duration of treatment, and the patient selection varied in terms of distribution of stigmata of recent haemorrhage.

Overall, two trials revealed a significant reduction in re-bleeding and one revealed a trend to reduction. The studies by Khuroo *et al.* (13) and Villanueva *et al.* (14) revealed the best results in the subgroups with a non-bleeding visible vessel and those with an overlying clot (Forest grades IIa and IIb). The most recent study, by Lin *et al.* (11) included only patients with Ia, Ib and IIa lesions (*n* = 100) and showed a significant reduction in rebleeding from 24 to 4% (*p* = 0.004). Analysis of the subgroups shows no benefit in the patients with active haemorrhage, although the re-bleeding rate in the control sample of these subgroups was low, presumably because of effective endoscopic treatment. There was a dramatic reduction in re-bleeding in patients with type IIa lesions, even after endoscopic treatment, but one has to be wary in analysing these subgroups because the number of patients is small. It is difficult to draw firm conclusions from these trials, as the evidence is contradictory, but there is certainly some indication that omeprazole, in an adequate intravenous dose, may benefit patients with visible vessels or overlying clot.

Two of the studies (17,18) excluded by Peterson & Cook are worth assessing. One study of 333 patients older than 60 years and with stigmata of recent haemorrhage at early endoscopy were assigned randomly to groups to receive placebo or an 80-mg bolus of omeprazole, followed by an infusion of 8 mg/h for 72 h. Endoscopic treatment was administered to patients with Forrest Ia lesions. Subsequently, both groups received omeprazole orally until day 21. At day 3, the primary endpoint of "overall outcome" was significantly in favour of the treatment group. This primary variable was judged on an ordinal scale ranked from worst to best as follows: death, surgery, need for endoscopic treatment, >3 units transfused, 0–3 units transfused.

Several of the secondary endpoints were also significantly in favour of the treatment groups: need for surgery, and degree and duration of bleeding. There was no significant difference in the number of blood transfusions, need for endoscopic treatment therapy, or mortality. At 21 days, there was a significantly lower mortality in the placebo group (0.6% compared with 6.9%), which was the rationale for stopping recruitment at that stage. It is likely, however, that this represents a chance finding of an unexpectedly low mortality in the placebo group. The mortality rates in the two groups of the parallel Nordic study were 6.2% and 5.9%.

In the second study, 274 patients older than 18 years, and with endoscopic stigmata of recent haemorrhage grades Ia, Ib, IIa and IIb were recruited. Endoscopic treatment was administered in those with grades Ia, Ib and IIa stigmata. The omeprazole and placebo treatment was identical. The primary variable was "treatment success", defined as no death, no operation, and no additional endoscopic treatment at 72 h. Treatment success was 91.0% in the treatment group and 79.7% in the placebo group; this difference is significant ($p = 0.004$), but the confidence intervals are wide (difference 11.3%; 95% confidence interval 2.3 to 20.4%). The number of blood transfusions, duration and degree of bleeding, and need for surgery and further endoscopic treatment were all significantly reduced, but deaths at 3, 21 and 35 days were similar. These studies of omeprazole do seem to support the treatment of peptic ulcers with stigmata of recent haemorrhage using an intravenous regimen for 3 days, although the overall added benefit may be small and there is no strong evidence that treatment with any antisecretory therapy reduces mortality.

Another aspect of pharmacological intervention is the treatment of *Helicobacter pylori* infection. There is no evidence that eradication of *H. pylori* affects the outcome of the acute bleed, but it is well established that recurrence of ulceration is reduced by its eradication. Studies specific to upper gastrointestinal bleeding show a reduction in further bleeding episodes after eradication of the organism (19–21). These studies were small and follow-up was short, but eradication therapy after acute upper gastrointestinal haemorrhage is to be recommended.

A drug for which there is some evidence of efficacy, but which is not widely used, is the antifibrinolytic drug tranexamic acid. No single large study of this drug has been undertaken but a meta-analysis (22) has suggested an advantage in the treatment group, both in terms of re-bleeding and mortality. Tranexamic acid probably needs to given early, so that it is incorprated in the clot, where it can inactivate plasmin. Unfortunately, the drug has side effects that include thromboembolism.

Endoscopy

Endoscopy forms part of the diagnostic and risk-assessment process. In addition to the diagnosis, the procedure reveals stigmata of recent haemorrhage (Table 11.1.3). With reference to peptic ulcers, in patients in whom lesions of Forrest grades Ia, Ib, IIa, and IIb are identified, endoscopic haemostatic therapy should be applied. Endoscopic haemostatic methods can be broadly divided into injection techniques (adrenaline, sclerosants, thrombin, tissue glues etc.), thermal techniques (laser, heater probe, diathermy) or the application of physical methods (clips, banding). These techniques are discussed in Chapter 10.

Surgery

When and on whom to operate are perennial questions. About 10% of peptic ulcer bleeds eventually require an operation to arrest active haemorrhage. The **indication** for urgent surgery for acute upper gastrointestinal haemorrhage is uncontrolled further haemorrhage. This usually becomes evident after initial resuscitation and stabilization, and is evident as further fresh haematemesis or haemochezia (passage of melaena is not necessarily associated with concurrent active haemorrhage), and periods of hypovolaemic cardiovascular instability demonstrated by tachycardia, tachypnoea, hypotension, and oliguria, and an increasing transfusion requirement associated with a decreasing haemoglobin concentration. In terms of the age of the patient and transfusion requirement as indicators for surgical intervention, there is no absolute indication and each patient should be assessed individually. However, elderly patients are less able to tolerate repeated episodes of haemorrhage and hypotension, and consideration should be given to early surgery in those in whom haemostasis is not rapidly achieved (23).

On occasion, the endoscopic view may be such

that urgent surgery is indicated, in particular in patients in whom there is a large arterial spurting vessel (often the gastroduodenal artery) that fails to stop spurting after application of haemostatic methods, or in those in whom the view is completely obscured by large quantities of fresh blood in association with haemodynamic instability but oesophageal varices have been excluded.

Re-bleeding rates after endoscopic treatment for bleeding peptic ulcer may be as high as 25%. In these patients who re-bleed after endoscopic therapy, there is an option for further endoscopic treatment, which is favoured in some units; Saeed *et al.* (24) showed a reduction of re-bleeding to 0% by planned repeated endoscopy. However, a more recent controlled trial (25) in which patients with Forrest I, IIa and IIb lesions were assigned randomly to groups to receive planned repeat endoscopy every 24 h until the lesions were graded Forrest 11c/III, or to undergo a single episode of endoscopic therapy, failed to show any significant benefit of the repeat endoscopy. The authors surmised however, that the period of 24 h may have been be too long, as most of the re-bleeds occur within this time. There is no place for a third attempt at endoscopic haemostasis; surgery is then indicated.

Patients requiring surgical intervention must be adequately resuscitated with whole blood, clotting should be optimized, and an experienced surgeon should be involved. Appropriate blood products must be immediately available and access to ITU care after operation is often necessary.

The current vogue is for a minimalist surgical approach. The surgeon is usually informed as to the site of the bleeding lesion by preoperative endoscopy. If not, endoscopy of the patient while they are on the operating table may be beneficial. Duodenal ulcers are under-run. Gastric ulcers may also be under-run, but should be subjected to biopsy. More usually, gastric ulcers are excised. If they are large, a partial gastrectomy may be necessary. Diffuse haemorrhage from multiple erosions may also require more extensive resection.

References

1. Rockall TA, Logan RFA, Devlin HB *et al.* Incidence of and mortality from acute upper gastrointestinal haemorrhage in the United Kingdom. *BMJ* 1995; **311**: 222–226.
2. Committee on Trauma–American College of Surgeons. *Advanced Trauma Life Support Student Manual*. USA, American College of Surgeons, 1993: chapter 3.
3. Cuellar RE, Gavaler JSM, Alexander JA. Gastrointestinal tract haemorrhage: the value of a nasogastric aspirate. *Arch Intern Med* 1990; **150**: 1381–1384.
4. Forrest JAH, Finlayson NDC, Shearman DJC. Endoscopy in gastrointestinal bleeding. *Lancet* 1974; **2**: 394–397.
5. Rockall TA, Logan RFA, Devlin HB *et al.* Risk assessment following acute upper gastrointestinal haemorrhage. *Gut* 1996; **38**: 316–321.
6. Rockall TA, Logan RFA, Devlin HB *et al.* Selection of patients for early discharge or outpatient care after acute upper gastrointestinal hamorrhage. *Lancet* 1995; **347**: 1138–1140.
7. Saeed ZA, Winchester CB, Michaletz PA *et al.* A scoring system to predict rebleeding after endoscopic therapy of nonvariceal upper gastrointestinal hemorrhage, with a comparison of heat probe and ethanol injection. *Am J Gastroenterol* 1993; **88**: 1842–1849.
8. Saeed ZA, Ramirez FC, Hepps KS *et al.* Prospective validation of the Baylor bleeding score for predicting the likelihood of rebleeding after endoscopic haemostasis of peptic ulcers. *Gastrointest Endosc* 1995; **41**: 561–565.
9. Collins R, Langman M. Treatment with histamine H2 antagonists in acute upper gastrointestinal haemorrhage. Implications of randomised trials. *N Engl J Med* 1985; **313**: 660–666.
10. Walt RP, Cottrell J, Mann SG *et al.* Randomised, double blind, controlled trial of intravenous famotidine infusion in 1005 patients with peptic ulcer bleeding. *Lancet* 1992; **340**: 1058–1062.
11. Peterson WL, Cook DJ. Antisecretory therapy for bleeding peptic ulcer. *JAMA* 1998; **280**: 877–879.
12. Lin H, Lo W, Lee F. A prospective randomised comparative trial showing that omeprazole prevents rebleeding in patients with bleeding peptic ulcer after successful endoscopic therapy. *Arch Intern Med* 1998; **158**: 54–58.
13. Khuroo MS, Yattoo GN, Javid G. A comparison of omeprazole and placebo for bleeding peptic ulcer. *N Engl J Med* 1997; **336**: 1054–1058.
14. Villanueva C, Balanzo J, Torras X. Omeprazole versus Ranitidine as adjunct therapy to endoscopic injection in actively bleeding ulcers. *Endoscopy* 1995; **27**: 308–312.
15. Lanas A, Artal A, Blas LM. Effect of parenteral omeprazole and ranitidine on gastric pH and the outcome of bleeding peptic ulcer. *J Clin Gastroenterol* 1995; **21**: 103–106.
16. Daneshmend TK, Hawkey CJ, Langman MJS *et al.* Omeprazole versus placebo for acute upper gastrointestinal bleeding: randomised double blind controlled trial. *BMJ* 1992; **304**: 143–147.
17. Schaffalitzky de Muckadell OB, Havelund T, Harling H *et al.* Effect of omeprazole on the outcome of endoscopically treated bleeding peptic ulcers. *Scand J Gastroenterol* 1997; **32**: 320–327.
18. Hasselgren G, Lind T, Lundell L *et al.* Continuous intravenous infusion of Omeprazole in elderly patients with peptic ulcer bleeding. *Scand J Gastroenterol* 1997; **32**: 328–333.
19. Labenz J, Borsch G. Role of Helicobacter pylori eradication in the prevention of peptic ulcer bleeding relapse. *Digestion* 1994; **55**: 19–23.
20. Graham DY, Hepps KS, Ramirez FC *et al.* Treatment of Helicobacter pylori reduces the rate of rebleeding inpeptic ulcer disease. *Scand J Gastroenterol* 1993; **28**: 939–942.

21. Rokkas T, Karameris A, Mavrogeorgis A *et al*. Eradication of Helicobacter pylori reduces the possibility of rebleeding in peptic ulcer disease. *Gastrointest Endosc* 1995; **41**: 1–4.

22. [Anthor to give ref. for meta-analysis of tranexamic acid].

23. Morris DL, Hawker PC, Brearley S *et al*. Optimal timing of operation for bleeding peptic ulcer: prospective randomised trial. *BMJ* 1984; **288**: 1277–1280.

24. Saeed ZA, Cole RA, Ramirez FC *et al*. Endoscopic retreatment after initial hemostasis prevents ulcer rebleeding: a prospective randomised trial. *Endoscopy* 1996; **28**: 288–294.

25. Ell C. Scheduled endoscopic retreatment vs. single injection therapy in bleeding gastroduodenal ulcers: results of a multicentre study [abstract]. *Dig Dis Week* 1998; **2100**: A–524.

11.2. Upper Gastrointestinal Bleeding: Management of Variceal Bleeding

LUCY DAGHER, ANDREW K. BURROUGHS and DAVID PATCH

DEFINITION OF PORTAL HYPERTENSION AND MEASUREMENT OF PORTAL VENOUS PRESSURE GRADIENT

Portal hypertension is defined as **an increase in the portal venous pressure gradient** (PVPG). The PVPG equals inferior vena cava (IVC) pressure minus portal venous pressure (PVP). The PVPG across a non-diseased liver is 2–6 mmHg. (When there is no disease of the hepatic veins, hepatic venous pressure (HVP) equals IVC pressure.) The normal PVP is 5–10 mmHg. When IVC pressure is high (as in cardiac disease), PVP must increase to maintain antegrade blood flow through the hepatic sinusoids, and PVPG remains unchanged. Under this circumstance, collateral circulation (i.e. portosystemic shunting) is not promoted, and varices do not form. Varices do not form until the PVPG is greater than 10 mmHg, and bleeding is not observed when the PVPG is less than 12 mmHg. Above this threshold value of 12 mmHg, the absolute value of the PVPG correlates poorly with risk for variceal haemorrhage.

Measurement of PVPG

Transvenous catheterization of the hepatic veins permits measurement of HVP and of the wedged hepatic venous pressure (WHVP). Just as the wedged pumonary arterial pressure gives an indirect measurement of the PVP, measuring the WHVP may provide a measure of the PVP. WHVP actually measures hepatic sinusoidal pressure, but in most forms of cirrhosis (when resistance is sinusoidal or post-sinusoidal) the sinusoidal pressure approximates the PVP. In portal vein thrombosis and in pre-sinusoidal hypertension (see Chapter 19) associated with certain liver diseases, WHVP is significantly less than PVP. The **hepatic venous pressure gradient** (HVPG) equals HVP minus WHVP, and approximates the PVPG. In other words, in most circumstances, HVPG equals PVPG, and provides a measure of portal hypertension.

In practice, few patients undergo measurement of HVP. This measurement is an important element of studies that evaluate pharmacological treatment of portal hypertension (see below). Probably, its measurement should be more routine.

NATURAL HISTORY AND PROGNOSIS OF VARICEAL BLEEDING

At the time of diagnosis of cirrhosis, varices are present in about 60% of decompensated and 30% of compensated patients (1). The minimal portal pressure gradient or its equivalent HVPG threshold for the development of varices is 10–12 mmHg ((2), and see chapter 22). In most patients, oesophageal varices enlarge over time, although regression of varices in a minority of patients has also been observed. The presence and size of oesophageal varices is associated with the severity of liver disease and continued alcohol abuse.

Although the incidence of variceal bleeding in unselected patients who have never previously bled is low (4.4/100 per year) (3), mortality of the first bleeding episode is high (25–50%) (3), and is related to failure to control haemorrhage or early re-bleeding. Hence the identification of patients with varices who will bleed is important, in order to offer effective prophylactic treatment to those who need it and avoid it in those who do not, particularly if the treatment is invasive or costly.

The **risk factors for the first episode of variceal bleeding** in cirrhotic patients are:

- the severity of liver dysfunction
- large size of varices
- the presence of endoscopic red colour signs.

The combination of these three factors is the basis of the North Italian Endoscopic Club (NIEC) index for the prediction of the first variceal bleeding (4). However, only about 30% of patients who present with variceal haemorrhage have all the above risk factors (5). Hence, there is a need to define additional predictive factors that could be combined in the NIEC index in order to improve its validity.

The main interest has been in the identification of haemodynamic factors that could more readily reflect those pathophysiological changes that lead to variceal bleeding. It is now well accepted that no bleeding occurs if HVPG decrease to less than 12 mmHg (6); in addition, the height of the HVPG has been shown to be an independent risk factor of bleeding (7). Finally, variceal pressure has been also shown, prospectively, to be an independent predictive factor for the first variceal bleeding; its addition to the NIEC index does result in a significant gain in prognostic accuracy (8), but it is difficult to use this measurement routinely.

The **risk factors for re-bleeding in patients with cirrhosis** have been little studied:

1. *Severity of liver disease*: Has been recognized as a risk factor for both early re-bleeding and short-term mortality after an episode of variceal bleeding (5).
2. *Active bleeding during emergency endoscopy* (e.g. oozing or spurting from the ruptured varix): Has been found to be a significant indicator of the risk of early re-bleeding (9).
3. *Increased portal pressure* (HVPG >16 mmHg): Has been also proposed as a prognostic factor of early re-bleeding, in an elegant study of

continuous portal pressure measurement immediately after the bleeding episode (10).
4. *Bacterial infections*: In a multivariate analysis of patients with cirrhosis admitted to hospital because of gastrointestinal bleeding who had not received antibiotic treatment in the previous 7 days, Bernard *et al.* (11) identified bacterial infections as predictive of early re-bleeding ($P < 0.02$): patients with bacterial infections had a risk of re-bleeding that was six to seven times greater than that in the remaining patients. A high **Child–Pugh score** (Table 11.2.1) was predictive of death ($P < 0.001$). These results were recently confirmed in our institution by Goulis *et al.* (12). Multivariate analysis showed that proven bacterial infection ($P < 0.0001$), antibiotic use ($P < 0.001$), active bleeding at endoscopy ($P < 0.001$), and Child–Pugh score ($P < 0.02$) were independent prognostic factors of failure to control bleeding.

The **risk factors for early death** are:

- severity of bleeding (9)
- early re-bleeding (9)
- severity of liver disease (13)
- presence of infection (15)
- presence of renal dysfunction (16)
- presence of cardiorespiratory disease

PRESENTATION AND DIAGNOSIS

Patients usually present with haematemesis or melaena. Specific features to be noted in the history are those of prolonged alcohol excess, ingestion of non-steroidal anti-inflammatory drugs or aspirin (16), previous variceal haemorrhages, previously diagnosed liver disease/portal hypertension, past abdominal sepsis/surgery or history of umbilical vein sepsis/catheterization (for portal vein thrombosis), or investigation of thrombocytopenia.

Examination must include a search for cutaneous stigmata of chronic liver disease, jaundice, hepatomegaly or splenomegaly, hepatic bruits, distended umbilical veins, ascites, and encephalopathy.

Bleeding as a result of portal hypertension may also occur in the absence of specific clinical signs of chronic liver disease. Usually, these patients have extrahepatic splanchnic vein thrombosis and other causes of non-cirrhotic portal hypertension.

Table 11.2.1. Child–Pugh grading of liver disease severity.

Clinical and biochemical measurements	Points scored for increasing abnormality		
	1	2	3
Encephalopathy grade	None	1 and 2	3 and 4
Ascites	Absent	Mild	Moderate
Bilirubin (mol/l)	17–33	34–51	>51
Albumin (g/l)	>35	28–35	<28
Prothrombin time (sec)	<17	18–20	>21
For primary biliary cirrhosis: bilirubin (mol/l)	17–67	68–170	>170

Child-Pugh Score
A < 7
B 7–9
C 10–15

The initial examination and investigations need to include an assessment of the severity of bleeding, the severity of diseases in other systems and the severity of liver disease. The latter is still most reliably obtained by using the **Child–Pugh score** (Table 11.2.1), which is based on the bilirubin and albumin concentrations, prothrombin time, ascites, and the presence of hepatic encephalopathy. The presence of portal vein thrombosis, hepatoma, or both, must be established early on, by ultrasound imaging.

Upper gastrointestinal endoscopy is essential to establish an accurate diagnosis as 26–56% of patients with portal hypertension and gastrointestinal bleeding will have a non-variceal source of their bleeding (17), particularly from peptic ulcers and portal hypertensive gastropathy. Endoscopy should be performed as soon as resuscitation is adequate, and preferably within 6 h of the patients admission to hospital. If necessary, this needs to be done under general anaesthesia when this is being performed for exsanguinating haemorrhage. Potentially inappropriate surgery is then avoided, as balloon tamponade can be used to arrest bleeding.

Definitive endoscopic diagnosis during or shortly after upper gastrointestinal bleeding can be difficult. When the view is obscured by blood, a bleeding point can not always be identified. A diagnosis of bleeding varices is accepted when a venous (non-pulsatile) spurt is seen, or if there is fresh bleeding from the oesophagogastric junction in the presence of varices, or fresh blood in the fundus when gastric varices are present.

In the absence of active bleeding (approximately 50–70% of cases), either the presence of varices in the absence of other lesions, or a "white nipple sign"

— a platelet plug on the surface of a varix (18) — suggests varices as the source of haemorrhage.

When the diagnosis is in doubt, repeat endoscopy during rebleeding is mandatory, as it will reveal a variceal source in more than 75% of patients (17). Gastric varices are particularly difficult to diagnose, because of pooling of blood in the fundus. Performing endoscopy with the patient on their right side, with the head up, may help. If the diagnosis is still not made, splanchnic angiography will establish the presence of varices, and may display the bleeding site if the patient is actively bleeding.

In the true emergency situation in which the patient is exanguinating and varices are suspected on the basis of history and examination, a Sengstaken–Blakemore (SB) tube should be passed. If control of bleeding is obtained, varices are likely to be the source of haemorrhage. If blood is still coming up the gastric aspiration port, then varices are less likely to be the cause of blood loss (however, fundal varices are not always controlled by tamponade). In practice, the position of the SB tube has to be re-checked and adequate traction applied. If there is still continued bleeding, the diagnosis of variceal bleeding should be questioned or fundal bleeding suspected, and emergency angiography performed.

MANAGEMENT OF ACUTE VARICEAL BLEEDING

Resucitation

Lung aspiration of gastric contents and blood is a particular risk, especially in encephalopathic patients who may have depressed pharyngeal reflexes; it is further exacerbated by endoscopic procedures, for which some sedation may still be required. **Endotracheal intubation** is mandatory if there is any concern about the safety of the airway.

An **internal jugular cannula** is safer than a subclavian approach, as the carotid artery can be compressed in the case of accidental puncture, but the subclavian can not. Peripheral and central venous cannulae must be inserted. The presence of coagulopathy and thrombocytopenia is not a contraindication to central venous access.

Blood should be taken for:

- full blood count
- clotting screen
- cross match (order 6 units of blood)
- urea and electrolytes, creatinine
- liver function tests, amylase
- glucose, calcium, magnesium
- blood-gases
- blood culture

Arrange for an **ascitic tap** (diagnostic, with a request for an absolute white cell count per mm³), **midstream urine specimen**, **chest radiograph**, and **electrocardiogram**.

We recommend that initial **intravascular volume replacement** should be with human albumin fraction or gelatin-based colloid, as this has no effect on clotting or bleeding times, in contrast to dextran or hydroxyethylstarch; these agents also have effects on platelet function (19).

After this, **specific treatment** can be started with a vasopressor agent, when the clinical picture is suggestive of portal hypertension. In this respect, there is evidence from a single trial that terlipressin should be instituted early (for example, in the emergency room) (20).

The patient should be **transferred to an intensive care/high dependency bed**, and preparations made for endoscopy. Early referral is important if local expertise is not available.

Cardiorespiratory monitoring

Pulse oximetry and oxygen are essential during endoscopy. There must be suitable staff available to provide suction and to ensure airway maintenance.

The **haemodynamic consequences of haemorrhage** in patients with cirrhosis may differ from normal individuals. Cirrhotic patients, particularly, may have a reduced peripheral vasoconstrictor response for several reasons:

1. The established vasodilated state of cirrhosis and portal hypertension (21)
2. A disturbed baroreceptor reflex, with an attenuated response to adrenaline (22)
3. The presence of an autonomic neuropathy, particularly in alcoholics

The presence of **covert tissue hypoxia** in decompensated cirrhosis (23) emphasizes the importance of rapid re-institution of circulating blood volume and oxygen carrying capacity in order to prevent critical deterioration of organ function.

The usual indications for **pulmonary capillary wedge pressure measurement** apply in bleeding varices: when abnormal right atrial pressures are suspected (e.g. clubbing, and hepatopulmonary syndrome), in the presence of alcoholic or ischaemic heart disease, and in the elderly. The priority of management should, however, be resuscitation first, invasive monitoring last.

Vasoconstrictor therapy (e.g. vasopressin) may reduce cardiac output, and increase right atrial pressure (24). Ascites also increases right atrial pressure measurements (25) and should be taken into account when assessing central nervous pressure readings.

All **ventilatory modes** may affect the systemic and splanchnic circulation. Positive pressure ventilation and positive end-expiratory pressure may cause a reduction in mean arterial pressure, cardiac output, and portal venous and hepatic arterial blood flows. These may be accompanied by deterioration in hepatic function (26) and reduced cardiac output (27), and consequently result in further salt and water retention. This may precipitate ascites formation.

These features help to explain why, on intensive care units, mortality of patients with combined liver and respiratory failure is more than 90% worldwide.

Transfusion

Optimal volume replacement remains controversial. After a variceal bleed, in animal models, return of arterial pressure to normal with immediate transfusion results in overshoot in PVP, with associated risk of further bleeding (28). This effect may not be relevant in clinical practice, as volume replacement is always delayed with respect to the start of bleeding.

Overtransfusion should certainly be avoided, and it is usual to aim for a haemoglobin concentration between 9 and 10 g/dl, and a right atrial pressure of 4–8 mmHg, but fluid replacement may need to be greater in the presence of oliguria, to be sure that the circulation is filled.

Large-volume transfusion may worsen the haemorrhagic state, and lead to thrombocytopenia, so that fresh frozen plasma and platelets need to be replaced. Optimal regimens for this are not known. It is reasonable to give 2 units of fresh frozen plasma after every 4 units of blood, and when the pro-thrombin time is greater than 20 s. Cryoprecipitate is indicated when the fibrinogen concentration is less than 0.2 g/litre.

Platelet transfusions are necessary to improve primary haemostasis and should be used if the baseline count is 50×10^9 or less. It is also routine to give intravenous vitamin K to patients with cir-rhosis, but no more than three doses of 10 mg are required, and it is likely to have little benefit except in biliary-type cirrhosis. Many cirrhotic patients have a background tendency to fibrinolysis. Trans-fusion of more than 15 units of blood results in prolongation of the prothrombin and partial throm-boplastin times (29) in normal individuals; in cir-rhotic individuals these effects occur with fewer units of blood transfused.

With large-volume transfusion there remains a risk of citrate toxicity, despite the low concentrations in current blood products. Changes in concentrations of ionized calcium and associated effects on the heart (prolonged Q–T interval, reduced cardiac output, changes in blood coagulation) bear witness to this (30). The associated toxicity may be enhanced by hypothermia, which also potentiates the cardiac side effects of hypocalcaemia, and further increases the affinity of haemoglobin for oxygen.

Massive transfusion may cause pulmonary microembolism, and the use of filters is recom-mended for transfusions of 5 litre or more in normal humans (31). Therefore, the routine use of filters in variceal haemorrhage could be considered, but rapid transfusions can not be administered with these, limiting their application.

Further measures in patients who continue to bleed despite balloon tamponade include the use of desmopressin (32) and antifibrinolytic factors. In cir-rhotic patients whose condition is stable, the former produces a two- to fourfold increase in factor VIII and von Willeband factor — presumably by release from storage sites — and may shorten or normalize the bleeding time (33). However, in one study of variceal bleeding, desmopressin in association with glypressin was shown to be detrimental compared with glypressin alone, and therefore its use can be recommended only when all else has failed (34).

The use of antifibrinolytic agents has not been studied in variceal bleeding, although their role has been established in liver transplantation in our unit and in others (35). Their clinical utility should be established in clinical trials, and pref-erably when increased fibrinolysis has been docu-mented. Recombinant factor VII may be useful in variceal bleeding, as it has been shown to normalize prothrombin and bleeding times in patients with cirrhosis (36).

Prevention of complications and deterioration in liver function

Infection control and treatment

Sepsis remains a major complication in patients with cirrhosis patients (37), particularly during bleed-ing episodes, when aspiration is a major risk and there may be increased translocation of gut organ-isms. Cirrhotic patients normally have defects of both humoral and cellular host defence mechanisms (38). Added to this is the well recognised suppres-sion of the immune system after simple haemor-rhage, via impaired T lymphocyte, B lymphocyte, and macrophage function (39–41). Because many of these host defenses are humorally mediated, their function is further reduced by depletion in serum factors after haemorrhage and transfusion.

In patients with cirrhosis, high concentrations of endotoxin have been detected in the portal and systemic circulation. Such high concentrations may result from the increased translocation of gut-de-rived endotoxin into the portal circulation, which — together with the impaired phagocytic function of the reticuloendothelial system and portosystemic shunting — allows endotoxin to reach the systemic circulation. In this way, endotoxin concentration progressively increases in relation to the severity of liver dysfunction. Large quantities of endotoxin are released into systemic circulation during episodes of bacterial infection. Bacterial infections have been documented into 35–66% of patients with cirrhosis who have variceal bleeding.

A recent meta-analysis (42) demonstrated that antibiotic prophylaxis significantly increased the mean survival rate (9.1% mean improvement rate, 95% confidence interval (CI) 2.9 to 15.3; $P = .004$) and also increased the mean percentage of patients who were free of infection (32% mean improvement rate, 95% CI 22 to 42, $P < .001$). On the basis of this evidence, all cirrhotic patients with upper gastrointestinal bleeding should now receive prophylactic antibiotics whether or not sepsis is suspected, using quinolones.

Spontaneous bacterial peritonitis must be suspected in any cirrhotic patient with ascites. A full discussion of this important subject is found in Chapter 19.

Ascites and renal function

Renal failure may be precipitated by a variceal bleed, usually as a result of a combination of acute tubular necrosis and hepatorenal syndrome associated with deterioration in liver function and sepsis. Hepatorenal syndrome is associated with a greater than 95% mortality (43–45). Thus any iatrogenic precipitants must be avoided.

The intravascular volume should be maintained, initially preferably with human albumin solution or blood. Dextrose solution is used for maintenance fluid, but is often not required, and there is retention of salt and water. Normal saline should be avoided, as it may cause further ascites formation. Catheterization of the bladder and hourly measurement of urine output are mandatory. Nephrotoxic drugs should be avoided, especially aminoglycosides and non-steroidal drugs.

Infusion of dopamine at a "renal" dose (2.5 µg/kg per min) has not been shown to improve survival in clinical trials, may increase gut translocation of bacterial products (46,47), and may not improve renal function. Its use can be recommended only when the urine output decreases in the presence of satisfactory filling, and it should be stopped after 24 h if no benefit is seen.

Increasing ascites may occur shortly after bleeding, but should not be the main focus of fluid and electrolyte management until bleeding has stopped and the intravascular volume is stable. If urea and creatinine are increasing, all diuretics should be stopped, and paracentesis performed if the abdomen becomes uncomfortable, with re-infusion of 8 g of albumin for every 1 litre removed.

When the patient has stopped bleeding for 24 h, nasogastric feeding can be commenced with a low-sodium feed. This avoids the need for maintenance fluid, and removes the risk of line sepsis. An unexplained increase in creatinine and urea concentrations may indicate sepsis, and is an indication for empirical antibiotic treatment on its own, after the requisite cultures have been made.

Despite these measures, patients with cirrhosis may develop increasing renal impairment, particularly after variceal haemorrhage. Unfortunately, this sequence of events has been perceived to be irreversible, as it reflects endstage liver disease, and there has been little change in the mortality of hepatorenal syndrome over many years (48,49). However, there is now increasing evidence supporting the use of vasopressin analogues in this condition (50–53), and the beneficial effect of terlipressin with respect to bleeding and survival in trials to date may be through the prevention of this catastrophic complication (54,55) although there is no documentation of this mechanism.

Portosystemic encephalopathy

Precipitant factors include haemorrhage, sepsis, sedative drugs, constipation, dehydration, and electrolyte imbalance. These should be evaluated and corrected. Any hypokalaemia, hypomagnesaemia, and hypoglycaemia that may precipitate encephalopathy should be aggressively corrected. A patient with ascites and a serum potassium concentration of 3.0 mmol/litre is likely to require in excess of 100 mmol of potassium over 24 h.

As soon as the patient is taking oral fluid, lactulose 5–10 ml four times a day is useful in clearing the bowel of blood. Once stools have returned to a normal colour, it can probably be discontinued. Phosphate enemas are used in the same way.

Nutrition

Cirrhotic patients with severe liver disease are usually malnourished (56). Most hospital diets provide a maximum of 1500 calories, even though patients with liver disease have substantially greater requirements (57). These patients often do not want to eat, are receiving "nil by mouth" because of investigations, and may find the food itself "unappealing". Thus exacerbation of malnutrition is common.

A fine-bore nasogastric tube should be passed 24 h after bleeding has ceased, and feeding should be commenced. There is no evidence that this may precipitate a variceal bleed, whereas it allows treatment of encephalopathy in comatose patients and makes fluid management easier. It is extremely rare that parenteral nutrition is required.

Vitamin replacement
All patients with a significant history of alcoholism should be assumed to be folate and thiamine deficient, and should be given at least three doses of the latter intravenously. It is easier and more practical to assume that all such patients are vitamin deficient, rather than delay treatment whilst awaiting results of red cell transketolase activity measurements.

Transfer of the patient with bleeding varices and use of balloon tamponade

Transport of these patients between hospitals should not be attempted unless their bleeding has been controlled, whether with vasopressor agents, endoscopic therapy, or tamponade. If there is any suggestion of continued blood loss, and the source is known to be variceal, then a modified Sengstaken–Blakemore (SB) tube (i.e. with an oesophageal aspiration channel such as the Minnesota tube) must be inserted before the transfer.

Prior endotracheal intubation is necessary when there is any concern about the patient's airway. This is particularly important when the SB tube is being inserted before the transfer.

The following **procedure for transfer** should be followed:

1. Ensure good suction facilities, oxygen saturation monitor, and oxygen supplies are all working. Two tamponade tubes should be kept in the freezer section of a fridge for at least 15 min. Three heavy-duty, non-serrated tubing clamps and three 60-ml bladder catheter syringes must be to hand. A modified sphygmomanometer is required to check the inflation pressure of the oesophageal balloon.

2. Three personnel are required, one of whom is responsible for airway protection and suction. Gowns, goggles, and gloves should be worn.

3. These patients are often extremely anxious. A simple, quiet explanation with reassurance will deter them from struggling. Explain to the patient that they must try to swallow, and that the airway will not be obstructed.

4. The patient should be head down, in the left lateral position, with an endoscopy mouth guard and nasal oxygen prongs in place.

5. Once ready, remove the SB tube from the fridge, and check balloon patency. Fully deflate both balloons, and lubricate them generously with lubricant jelly. Without delay, insert the tube, twisting the shaft through 180° once the balloon has passed the oropharynx, this directs the tip posteriorly towards the oesophagus. Ask the patient to swallow. If they gag, this is the time to advance the tube, as the sphincter relaxes. Occasionally one must guide the tube into the oesophagus with one's fingers — the mouth guard serves to protect from biting.

6. Push the tube down at least 60 cm, and check that it is not coiled in the pharynx. Then inflate the gastric balloon with at least 250 ml of air. If inflation is difficult or the patient is in pain, then deflate immediately, and check that the tube is in the stomach.

7. Once the gastric balloon is inflated, pull the tube back until firm resistance is encountered — usually 30–40 cm, depending on the patient's build.

8. The tube must be fixed to the face under tension. We do not recommend weights hung over the bed for traction: one simple solution is to fashion a clamp by taping two tongue depressors together, with the SB tube in between. This allows the tension to be adjusted easily.

9. The gastric and oesophageal channels should be under continuous aspiration, with the aims of detecting continued bleeding into the stomach and keeping the oesophagus clear of blood and secretions.

10. Correctly applied, the SB tube will arrest bleeding in 90% of patients (58). In the rare case of bleeding not being controlled, the oesophageal balloon should be inflated to a pressure of 40 mmHg. However, this carries a risk of pressure necrosis to the wall of the oesophagus; the oesophageal balloon should be deflated for

5 min every hour, and not left inflated for more than 12 h.

11. Check the chest X-ray.
12. Organize definitive therapy.

Nursing care

- hourly oesophageal pressure check if the oesopahgeal balloon is inflated
- change the position of the tube in mouth every 6 h.
- if continuous suction is unavailable, regular oesophageal and stomach aspiration (every 15 min)
- calming environment

There can be problems. Sometimes the SB tube will not go down. Another, cold, tube can be tried (this is more rigid); placing a set of endoscopic biopsy forceps within the lumen of the tube may also give greater rigidity. Rarely, the tube may need to be placed under direct vision, pushing it down with an endoscope. If there is continued bleeding despite the above manoeuvres, this is either from gastric fundal varices, or from a non-variceal source. Ensure that the tube is under traction. If bleeding continues, angiography is required.

All epsiodes of variceal bleeding not responding to a single session of injection sclerotherapy should be discussed with the regional or tertiary referral centre, because this group of patients are more at risk of death, and because alternative treatment modalities — such as transjugular intrahepatic portosystemic shunt (TIPS) — may be available elsewhere.

RANDOMIZED CONTROLLED TRIALS FOR THE TREATMENT OF ACUTE VARICEAL BLEEDING

Interpreting clinical trials

Effective resuscitation, accurate diagnosis, and early treatment can reduce the high mortality from variceal bleeding. The clinical aims are not only to stop bleeding as soon as possible, but also to prevent early re-bleeding. Treatment regimens should be carefully evaluated, not only in terms of immediate cessation of haemorrhage, but also in terms of providing a bleed-free interval of at least 5 days. This allows some recovery of the patient, and provides an opportunity for secondary preventative therapy to be instituted. Most clinical trials have focused on oesophageal varices, with very few designed to evaluate treatment for gastric varices. The latter may lead to more severe bleeding initially, and tend to re-bleed frequently (59). The following sections refer to oesophageal varices unless otherwise specified.

Pharmacological treatment options

Vasoactive drug treatment is the only treatment that does not require sophisticated equipment or the skills of a specialist and is immediately available, even before the patient is admitted to hospital (60). As high variceal or portal pressure is likely to cause continued bleeding or early re-bleeding, drug treatments that decrease portal pressure over days may be the optimal choice.

The vasoactive drugs that are currently used in the management of acute variceal bleeding are vasopressin, glypressin, somatostatin, and octreotide. **Vasopressin**, which is a powerful vasoconstrictor, decreases portal pressure through the induction of smooth-muscle contraction, particularly in splanchnic arterioles. However, the drug also causes systemic vasoconstriction, which leads to serious side effects such as cardiac arrhythmia, myocardial ischaemia, mesenteric ischaemia and cerebrovascular episodes, resulting in cessation of treatment in up to 25% of patients (61). **Terlipressin** is a synthetic analogue of vasopressin (triglycyl lysine vasopressin). It has an intrinsic effect in addition to being converted *in vivo* into vasopressin, by enzymatic cleavage of the triglycyl residues. This prolongs its biological half-life, so that a continuous intravenous infusion is unnecessary. **Somatostatin** has been used in the pharmacological treatment of variceal bleeding because of its reported ability to reduce splanchnic blood flow (62), portal pressure, and azygous blood flow (63) in cirrhotic patients, although only the findings regarding the reduction in azygous flow are consistent. Bolus injections of somatostatin appear to have greater haemodynamic effects than does continuous infusion (64). Finally, **octreotide** has been reported to cause a reduction in portal pressure and a transient decrease in azygous blood flow (65,66), but there are some studies — which did not confirm these data — using similar or even greater doses of the drug (67). Table 11.2.2 summarizes some of these drug treatments.

Table 11.2.2.   Drugs used in the treatment of acute bleeding varices.

Drug	Dosage and administration
Somatostin	250 µg/h intravenous infusuion for 5 days
Octreotide	50 µg/h intravenous infusuion for 5 days
Terlipressin ±	1–2-mg bolus 4–6 hourly for 48 h
Nitrates	10 mg glyceryl trinitrate patch, replaced after 24 h

Drugs compared with placebo

Vasopressin compared with placebo

Vasopressin was compared with non-active treatment or placebo in four randomized controlled trials (67–71) including only 157 patients. In two of these trials, the intra-arterial route of administration was used. There was a significant heterogeneity in the evaluation of failure to control bleeding. There was a clear trend in favour of vasopressin but the result was not statistically significant by the Der Simonian & Laird method (pooled odds ratio (POR) 0.23; 95% CI 0.05 to 1.02). Moreover, there was no difference in mortality (POR 0.98; 95% CI, 0.47 to 2.1). Complications were reported in up to 64% of patients, leading to discontinuation of treatment in 25% of them.

In order to minimize the systemic complications of vasopressin, glyceryltrimitrate has been added to the regimen. This drug is a powerful venous dilator and reduces the portal vascular resistance and improves myocardial performance. Three randomized controlled trials have compared vasopressin alone with vasopressin plus glyceryltrimitrate — transdermally (61), sublingually (72), and intravenously (73) — including 176 patients. Failure to control bleeding was significantly less common with vasopressin plus glyceryltrimitrate (POR 0.39; 95% CI 0.21 to 0.72), but there was no difference in mortality (POR 0.94; 95% CI 0.49 to 1.79). In two of the trials (72, 73) side effects were significantly reduced with the combination treatment. However, because of portocollateral shunting, glyceryltrimitrate bypasses the liver, and can cause significant systemic effects. Hence this combination treatment must be monitored very closely and thus is less applicable as an immediate therapy.

Terlipressin compared with placebo

The clinical efficacy of terlipressin has been evaluated in four placebo-controlled studies (60,74–76)

including 225 patients. In one of these studies (60), the drug was given while the patient was transferred to hospital. There was a statistically significant reduction in failure to control bleeding with terlipressin compared with placebo (POR 0.33; 95% CI 0.19 to 0.57) and, more importantly the same meta-analysis showed that terlipressin is the only vasoconstrictor that significantly reduces mortality (POR 0.38; 95% CI 0.22 to 0.69). However, there is some criticism of these studies: the sample sizes were small, allowing a large type 2 error in the first three trials, and the evidence in the early administration trial (60) of the effect of terlipressin, given only as three doses up to 8 h, does not readily explain the apparent beneficial results regarding the mortality rate (only in Child's C patients) or the control of bleeding. The causal link between early administration of terlipressin and reduction in mortality must be reproduced in other studies to establish its validity.

Somatostatin compared with placebo

Three placebo-controlled studies of somatostatin exhibited divergent results (77–79). The trials by Valenzuela et al. (77) and Gotzsche et al. (79) suggested that somatostatin was no more effective than placebo. Unfortunately, both studies had a very long recruitment period, suggesting marked patient selection. Moreover, Gotzsche et al. did not evaluate the endpoint of failure to control bleeding, and Valenzuela et al. reported an extremely high response rate (83%) in the placebo group (the highest ever reported). In contrast, the study by Burroughs et al. (78) demonstrated a statistically significant benefit for somatostatin in controlling variceal bleeding over a 5-day treatment period. These differences in the reported results caused statistically significant heterogeneity ($P = 0.006$) in the meta-analysis of the six studies that have compared somatostatin with placebo or inactive treatment (77–82). There was a trend in favour of somatostatin but the result was not statistically significant by the Der Simonian & Laird method (POR 0.6; 95% CI 0.21 to 1.65). There was no difference in mortality between the two treatment groups (POR 1.02; 95% CI 0.64 to 1.61).

Octreotide compared with placebo

There has been only one double-blind trial comparing octreotide with placebo (83). The largest-ever trial carried out to evaluate the efficacy of a vasoactive drug ($n = 262$ patients) in the management of acute variceal bleeding, it is currently available only in abstract form. In this study, the efficacy of a continuous 5-day infusion of octreotide 50 µg/h, starting as soon as possible after admission, was not different from that of placebo, whether or not injection sclerotherapy was needed for active bleeding or drug failure. Moreover, two other studies (84,85) using octreotide (100 µg 8-hourly, given subcutaneously) or placebo after the control of the initial bleeding episode failed to show any difference in early re-bleeding or mortality between the two treatment groups.

Drugs compared with balloon tamponade

There have been six trials comparing the use of vasoactive drugs and balloon tamponade. The drugs used were terlipressin (86–88), somatostatin in 2 (89,90) and octreotide (91). Meta-analysis of these six trials showed that the drugs were as effective as balloon tamponade for prevention of failure to control bleeding (POR 1.04; 95% CI 0.63 to 1.72) or death (POR 0.65; 95% CI 0.36 to 1.16). Sensitivity analysis showed that there was no difference according to the type of the drug. However, the sample sizes were small and the endpoints not very clear, indicating that these results should be interpreted with caution. Tamponade, if used properly, provides good control of bleeding: however the balloons should not be inflated for more than 12 h, and preferably less, and bleeding frequently recurs when the balloons are deflated. From the trial reports, it is not always clear at what stage the efficacy was assessed — for example, during treatment, or at the end of an interval of 24 h after termination of drug therapy or tamponade.

Drugs compared with drugs

Terlipressin compared with vasopressin
Terlipressin was compared with vasopressin in five small, unblinded studies (92–96) involving only 247 patients. In two of these studies, vasopressin was used in association with glyceryltrimitrate. Failure to control bleeding was less frequent with terlipressin, but the result was not statistically significant (POR 0.64; 95% CI 0.36 to 1.14). There was no difference in mortality between the two treatment arms (POR 1.48; 95% CI 0.85 to 2.57). More importantly, the complication rate was

significantly less with terlipressin, even when vasopressin was combined with glyceryltrimitrate.

Somatostatin compared with vasopressin
Somatostatin has been compared with vasopressin in seven studies including 301 patients (97–103). These showed that failure to control bleeding was less frequent with somatostatin, but the result was not statistically significant (POR 0.74; 95% CI 0.47 to 1.16). There was no difference in mortality between the two vasoactive agents (POR 0.93; 95% CI 0.57 to 1.5). However, a statistically significant reduction in complications was observed in the group receiving somatostatin (POR 0.11; 95% CI 0.07 to 0.19), as the mean complication rate was 51% with vasopressin and only 10% with somatostatin.

Somatostatin compared with terlipressin
Two studies have compared somatostatin with terlipressin (104,105), involving 267 patients. Both studies showed that the two drugs were similarly effective in preventing failure to control variceal bleeding and death. Moreover, in the largest of these studies (104), a significantly lower incidence of complications in the somatostatin group was reported.

Octreotide compared with other drugs
The efficacy of octreotide treatment in comparison with other vasoactive drugs, in treating for acute variceal bleeding, has not been adequately evaluated. Octreotide was found to be comparable to vasopressin in one study (106) ($n = 48$ patients) and to be comparable to terlipressin plus glyceryltrimitrate in another (107) ($n = 87$ patients). However, the sample sizes were small and the endpoints not very clear, indicating that these results should be interpreted with caution.

Emergency sclerotherapy

Injection sclerotherapy, first introduced in 1939 and "rediscovered" in the late 1970s, has, over the past two decades, rapidly become the endoscopic treatment of choice for the control of acute variceal bleeding. The best evidence for the value of sclerotherapy in the management of acute variceal bleeding has come from a recently published study by the Veterans Affairs Cooperative Variceal Sclerotherapy Group (86). In this study sclerotherapy, compared with sham sclerotherapy, stopped haemorrhage from actively bleeding oesophageal varices and significantly increased the survival of patients in hospital.

Today, it is generally accepted that sclerotherapy should be performed immediately at diagnostic endoscopy, as there is evidence that this is beneficial compared with delayed injection of sclerosants (108,109). No more than two injection sessions should be used to arrest variceal bleeding within a 5-day period. Several sclerosing agents have been used for injection — 1–3% polidocanol, 5% ethanolamine oleate, 1–2% sodium tetradecyl sulphfate, and 5% sodium morrhuate — but there is no evidence that any one sclerosant can be considered the optimal choice for acute injection. The technique used is a free-hand method, whereby a 23–25-gauge needle is advanced into the varix, and 1–4 ml of sclerosant injected. There is no reason to inject a large volume of sclerosant (10–30 ml), as this has no greater efficacy, and is much more likely to cause serious complications — some sclerotherapy ulcers never heal. After the injection, we recommend that the needle is retracted, but that the outer sheath is left up against the varix for 30 s, to tamponade the site; the alternative is to use the endoscope tip. Assuming that the patient is in the left lateral position, it is important to avoid injecting varices at "12 o'clock" first, as further bleeding will then obscure the field of vision. Paravariceal injection is probably as effective as intravariceal injection.

In patients with large oesophageal varices, in whom the bleeding site can not be identified, but in whom the duodenum is deemed "clear", we recommend blind four-quadrant sclerotherapy at the oesophagogastric junction. This procedure is probably used more frequently than is realized — textbooks may have wonderful pictures of spurting varices, but the truth is that the endoscopist may be faced with a tidal wave of red blood advancing up the oesophagus after intubation. Under these circumstances, it is paramount to avoid aspiration, and the wise endoscopist abandons the procedure, and ensures the safety of the airway before proceeding. Not all bleeding is controlled with sclerotherapy.

Sclerotherapy plus drugs/balloon tamponade compared with drugs/ballon tamponade

There have been five trials with this clinical design, comprising 410 patients; in three vasopressin was used (110–112), and in the other two, octreotide (113) and somatostatin (114). The treatment effect was evaluated within 24 h and up to 120 h. Failure to control bleeding was significantly less common with sclerotherapy plus drugs than with drugs alone (POR 2.59; 95% CI 1.59 to 4.2), without significant heterogeneity ($P = 0.24$). The number of patients required to be treated (number needed to treat, NNT) to acheive the prevention of one re-bleeding episode was seven (95% CI 4 to 13). Publication bias assessment showed that 13 null or negative studies would be needed to render the results of this meta-analysis non-significant. There were fewer deaths in the sclerotherapy-plus-drugs arm of this study than in the drugs-alone arm, but the difference was not significant (POR 1.33; 95% CI 0.78 to 2.27). The incidence of complications, when reported, varied considerably between trials, two of them stating that there were more complications in the sclerotherapy arm, and one reporting more in the control arm.

Sclerotherapy compared with drugs

Of 10 studies, including 921 patients, that compared sclerotherapy and drug treatments, vasopressin was used in one (115), terlipressin in one (116), somatostatin in three (117–119) and octreotide in five (120–124). The evaluation of the treatment effect was performed at the end of the infusion of the drug (from 48 to 120 h). The overall efficacy of sclerotherapy was 85% (range 73–94%) in studies of 12–48 h drug infusion and 74% (68–84%) in studies of 120 h drug infusion. There was significant heterogeneity ($P < 0.05$) in the evaluation of failure to control bleeding in these studies, which was mainly attributable to the different extent of benefit from sclerotherapy, rather than different outcomes in individual studies: only two of the 10 studies reported that drugs were better than sclerotherapy, but neither of them reached statistical significance. Failure to control bleeding was statistically significantly less frequent in patients receiving sclerotherapy (Der Simonian & Laird method: POR 1.68; 95% CI 1.07 to 2.63). The NNT to avoid one re-bleeding episode was 11 (95% CI 6 to 113). Publication bias assessment showed that nine null or negative studies would be needed to render the results of this meta-analysis non-significant. Sensitivity analyses including only (a) peer-reviewed articles (POR 1.3; 95% CI 0.8 to 2.1), (b) studies using only somatostatin or octreotide (POR 1.65; 95% CI 0.92 to 2.95), (c) studies with 120 h drug treatment (POR 1.42; 95% CI 0.9 to 2.26), (d) studies with cirrhotic patients (POR 1.4; 95% CI 0.99 to 1.9) always showed a strong trend in favour of sclerotherapy.

There was no significant heterogeneity in the evaluation of mortality in these studies: only two studies reported a lower mortality in the drug arm of the study, but in neither was this statistically significant. Overall there were statistically significantly fewer deaths in patients assigned randomly to groups to receive sclerotherapy (POR 1.43; 95% CI 1.05 to 1.95). The NNT to avoid one death was 15 (95% CI 8 to 69). Publication bias assessment showed that three null or negative studies are required to render the results of this meta-analysis non-significant.

Finally, the type of complications recorded in eight studies (116–123) differed considerably, resulting in a significant heterogeneity ($P = 0.04$). Four studies reported more complications in the sclerotherapy arm (117–120), whereas three (116, 121, 123) reported more complications in the drug arm and one found equal numbers in both arms (122). The meta-analysis showed a trend in favour of drug treatment, but the result was not statistically significant (Der Simonian & Laird method: POR 0.71; 95% CI 0.41 to 1.2).

Sclerotherapy plus drugs compared with sclerotherapy alone

This group comprises five studies (125–129). Two, published as abstracts (128,129), assigned patients to three treatment arms and each comparison with sclerotherapy was evaluated separately (for Signorelli's trial (129) the results 1 year later were used for the octreotide comparison). Hence, six comparisons of sclerotherapy-plus-drugs (somatostatin in two, octreotide in three and terlipressin in one) and sclerotherapy alone in five studies (125–129) including 610 patients were analysed. Only three studies were placebo controlled (125–127); two were not. In four studies the drug was administered for 120 h, and in one (128) it was given for 48 h. The efficacy of sclerotherapy was only 59% in the 48 h study (128) and 61% (range 35–75%) in the 120 h studies. Re-bleeding was statistically significantly less frequent in patients receiving sclerotherapy plus drugs (POR 0.42; 95% CI 0.29 to 0.6). The NNT to avoid one re-bleeding episode was six (95% CI 4 to 10). Publication bias

assessment showed that 29 null or negative studies would be needed to render the results of this meta-analysis statistically non-significant. However, there were equal number of deaths between the two treatment arms, and the result was not statistically significant (POR 1.02; 95% CI 0.63 to 1.64]). Moreover, in the most recently published study (126) the death rate was slightly greater in the combined treatment arm. Although it is common to find no survival-rate differences between treatments in trials of acute variceal bleeding, one might have expected a trend for lower mortality in the combined-treatment group, given the strongly significant reduction in bleeding — a very marked biological difference.

Only two studies provided data on complications (125,126). There were no significant differences between the two treatment arms in both studies.

Sclerotherapy compared with variceal ligation

There are only two studies specifically designed to compare sclerotherapy with variceal ligation for the management of the acute bleeding episode (130,131). Other data come from 10 studies comparing long-term sclerotherapy and variceal ligation (132–141). There was no statistical heterogeneity ($P = 0.21$) in the analysis of failure to control bleeding from the total of 12 studies, including a total of 419 patients. There was no difference between the two treatment modalities, although there was a trend in favour of variceal ligation (POR, 0.66; 95% CI 0.36 to 1.18). Short-term mortality was reported only in two studies (130,131): in both, there was a trend in favour of variceal ligation, but the result was not statistically significant. Finally, only the two studies specifically designed to compare emergency sclerotherapy with variceal ligation (130,131) reported the incidence of complications. Complications were less frequent in the variceal ligation arm in both studies, and the result reached statistical significance in one (131).

GASTRIC VARICES

The reported incidence of bleeding from gastric varices varied between 3 and 30%, but in most series it is less than 10% (142). Patients with gastric variceal haemorrhage bleed more profusely and require more transfusions than patients with oesophageal variceal bleeding (143). Moreover, these patients are at greater risk of re-bleeding and have a decreased survival rate compared with patients bleeding from oesophageal varices.

The optimal **treatment** of gastric variceal bleeding is not known. Limited information is available on the role of vasoactive drugs in the control of gastric fundal bleeding, and balloon tamponade has been used with little success. Use of standard sclerosants is associated with unacceptable re-bleeding, particularly from necrotic ulceration, as the gastric mucosa appears much more sensitive to this than is the oesophagus. Because of this, alternative sclerosant agents have been evaluated. The tissue glue, isobutyl-2-cyanoacrylate (Bucrylate), mixed with lipiodol to delay premature hardening, has been examined, and was found to be efficacious in a non-randomized study (144). This agent was shown to be superior to ethanolamine, in a non-randomized study (145), achieving haemostasis in 90% of 23 patients, compared with the 67% of 24 patients in whom ethanolamine was effective ($P < 0.005$). However, reports of cerebral embolism, with the tissue adhesives identified in the cerebral circulation at post-mortem examination, are worrying, and interest has therefore focused on thrombin. This is much easier to administer, and has been shown to provide good early haemostasis (146). However, in all of these studies, re-bleeding rates have remained high. Hence, in patients with re-bleeding or uncontrolled bleeding from gastric varices, devascularization surgery or portosystemic shunting has been proposed (147). We have recently shown that "salvage" TIPSS is very effective in this situation, with a more than 95% success rate for initial haemostasis, and an early re-bleeding rate of less than 20% (142).

UNCONTROLLED VARICEAL BLEEDING

There is no precise definition of uncontrolled variceal bleeding. A recent consensus meeting failed to find a suitable definition (148). Nonetheless, approximately 10–15% of patients who present with an episode of acute variceal bleeding can not have their bleeding controlled with two sessions of sclerotherapy (149) and attendance at more than two sessions is not associated with any further increase in success at stopping bleeding, but is associated with an increasing complication rate (150). The definition we use is: continued variceal bleeding,

despite two sessions of emergency endoscopic interventions and vasoactive therapy during a 5-day period, or bleeding past an SB tube, independent of the number of sclerotherapy sessions.

Bleeding gastric varices are said to be uncontrolled when haemorrhage persists despite vasoconstrictor therapy.

Once it has been decided that standard therapy has been unsuccessful in an individual patient, a salvage procedure is needed. There are no published randomized-controlled trials evaluating different "salvage" treatments in uncontrolled variceal bleeding. However, the advent of TIPSS has offered a valuable option in this condition (151—154), and it has been shown, in uncontrolled studies, that emergency TIPSS is highly effective as salvage therapy in patients with uncontrolled oesophageal or gastric variceal bleeding (155). TIPSS is an interventional radiological procedure that involves the creation of a communication between the hepatic vein and an intrahepatic branch of the portal vein, thus decompressing the portal venous system. Hence TIPSS functions in a manner similar to surgical shunts; however, the morbidity and mortality associated with the TIPSS procedure is much more favourable.

Bleeding is controlled by TIPSS in 90–95% of patients, and the procedure avoids the need for the prolonged stay in the intensive care unit, that would be required after emergency laparotomy for staple section or portocaval shunting. Indeed, the patient may be back on the ward, eating and drinking, within 6 h of the procedure. The remaining 5–10% of patients who continue to bleed are, in our experience, bleeding from sclerotherapy ulcers. Mortality after TIPSS remains high, as this group of patients is generally sick, and there are some patients in whom the procedure is futile (156). Antibiotic prophylaxis is recommended in assocation with the procedure. We use carbon dioxide as contrast medium in order to prevent contrast-induced renal dysfunction. As there may be a further reduction in systemic vascular resistance after TIPSS (157), we recommend continued use of terlipressin after the procedure, to prevent systemic hypotension.

VARICEAL BLEEDING AND PORTAL VEIN THROMBOSIS

Patients with portal vein thrombosis may bleed from oesophageal varices, ectopic varices, and — particularly in the case of sinistral portal hypertension — from gastric varices. The last may occur after splenic vein thrombosis, particularly as a result of chronic pancreatitis, or after pancreatic surgery. There are no data concerning the role of vasoconstrictors in this group of patient. Subjectively, these patients bleed in a different way, in that they tolerate the bleeding much better, with less renal dysfunction and little, if any, evidence of ascites formation. There are no evidence-based guidelines on the management of these patients. We recommend sclerotherapy, which may be performed on more than two occasions, in the event of initial failure to control bleeding and terlipressin. If bleeding continues, angiography is required to establish the venous anatomy, accurately followed by devascularization or mesenteric vein shunting, if surgically possible.

References

1. D'Amico G, Pagliaro L, Bosch J. The treatment of portal hypertension: A meta-analytic review. *Hepatology* 1995; **22**: 332–354.
2. Garcia-Tsao G, Groszmann RJ, Fisher RL *et al.* Portal pressure, presence of gastroesophageal varices and variceal bleeding. *Hepatology* 1985; **5**: 419–424.
3. Pagliaro L, D'Amico G, Pasta L *et al.* Portal hypertension in cirrhosis: natural history. In *Portal Hypertension. Pathophysiology and Treatment.* Eds J. Bosch, R. Groszmann. Cambridge, MA: Blackwell Scientific, 1994: pp. 72–92.
4. Defranchis R. Prediction of the first variceal hemorrhage in patients with cirrhosis of the liver and esophageal varices – a prospective multicenter study. *N Engl J Med* 1988; **319**: 983–989.
5. Grace ND, Groszmann RJ, Garcia-Tsao G *et al.* Portal hypertension and variceal bleeding: an AASLD single topic symposium. *Hepatology* 1998; **28**: 868–880.
6. Armonis A, Patch D, Burroughs AK. Hepatic venous pressure measurement: An old test as new prognostic marker in cirrhosis? *Hepatology* 1997; **25**: 245–248.
7. Merkel C, Gatta A. Can we predict the first variceal bleeding in the individual patient with cirrhosis and esophageal varices. *J Hepatol* 1991; **13**: 378
8. Nevens F, Bustami R, Scheys I *et al.* Variceal pressure is a factor predicting the risk of a first variceal bleeding: A prospective cohort study in cirrhotic patients. *Hepatology* 1998; **27**: 15–19.
9. Ben-Ari Z, Cardin F, Wannamethee G *et al.* Prognostic significance of endoscopic active bleeding and early rebleeding from oesophageal varices [abstract]. *J Hepatol* 1996; **20**: 92A.
10. Ready JB, Robertson AD, Goff JS *et al.* Assessment of the risk of bleeding from esophageal varices by continuous monitoring of portal pressure. *Gastroenterology* 1991; **100**: 1403–1410.
11. Bernard B, Cadranel J-F, Valla D *et al.* Prognostic significance of bacterial infection in bleeding cirrhotic patients: a prospective study. *Gastroenterology* 1995; **108**: 1828–1834.

12. Goulis J, Armonis A, Patch D *et al.* Bacterial infection is independently associated with failure to control bleeding in cirrhotic patients with gastrointestinal haemorrhage. *Hepatology* 1998; **27**: 1207–1212.
13. Dedombal FT, Clarke JR, Clamp SE *et al.* Prognostic factors in upper GI bleeding. Endoscopy 1986; **18 (suppl)**: 6–10.
14. Bleichner G, Boulanger R, Squara P *et al.* Frequency of infection in cirrhotic patients presenting with acute gastrointestinal haemorrhage. *Br J Surg* 1986; **73**: 724–726.
15. Garden OJ, Motyl H, Gilmour WH. Prediction of outcome following acute variceal haemorrhage. *Br J Surg* 1985; **72**: 91–95.
16. De Ledinghen V, Heresbach D, Fourdan O, Bernard P *et al.* Anti-inflammatory drugs and variceal bleeding: a case–control Study. *Gut* 1999; **44**: 270–273.
17. Mitchell K, Theodossi A, Williams R. Endoscopy in patients with portal hypertension and upper gastrointestinal bleeding. In: *Variceal Bleeding.* London: Pitman, 1982; pp. 62–67.
18. Siringo S, McCormick PA, Mystry P *et al.* Prognostic significance of the white nipple sign in variceal bleeding. *Gastrointest Endosc* 1991; **37**: 51–55.
19. Sarin SK, Guptan RC, Jain AK *et al.* A randomized controlled trial of endoscopic variceal band ligation for primary prophylaxis of variceal bleeding. *Eur J Gastroenterol Hepatol* 1996; **8**: 337–342.
20. Levacher S, Letoumelin P, Pateron D *et al.* Early administration of terlipressin plus glyceryl trinitrate to control active upper gastrointestinal bleeding in cirrhotic patients. *Lancet* 1995; **346**: 865–868.
21. Borizon A, Blendis L. Vascular reactivity in experimental portal hypertension. *Am J Physiol* 1987; **252**: 158–162.
22. Lunzer M, Manghani K, Newman S *et al.* Impaired cardiovascular responsiveness in disease. *Lancet* 1975; **2**: 382–385.
23. Moreau R, Lees S, Hadengue A. Relationship between oxygen transport and oxygen uptake in patients with cirrhosis: effect of vasoactive drugs. *Hepatology* 1989; **9**: 427–432.
24. Groszmann R, Kravetz D, Bosch J *et al.* Nitroglycerine improves the haemodynamic response to vasopressin in portal hypertension. *Hepatology* 1982; **2**: 757–762.
25. Panos MZ, Moore K, Vlavianos P *et al.* Sequential haemodynamic changes during single total paracentesis and right atrial size in patients with tense ascites. *Hepatology* 1991; **11**: 662–667.
26. Aruidsson D, Lindgen S, Almquise P *et al.* Role of the renin–angiotensin system in liver blood flow reduction produced by positive end expiratory pressure ventilation. *Acta Chir Scand* 1990; **156**: 353–358.
27. Mauay J, Jashie R, Hechtrain H. Abnormalities in organ blood flow and its distribution during expiratory pressure ventilation. *Surgery* 1979; **85**: 353–358.
28. Kravetz D, Bosch J, Arderiu M *et al.* Hemodynamic effects of blood volume restitution following a hemorrhage in rats with portal hypertension due to cirrhosis of the liver; influence of the extent of portal systemic shunting. *Hepatology* 1989; **9**: 808–814.
29. Bove J. What is the factual basis, in theory and in practice, for the use of fresh frozen plasma. *Vox Sang* 1978; **35**: 428.
30. Collins J. Abnormal haemoglobin–oxygen affinity and surgical haemotherapy. In: *Surgical Haemotherapy.* Eds J Collins, P Lumsgaard-Hansen. 1980. Basel: Skager.

31. Reul G, Beale A, Greenberg S. Protection of the pulmonary vasculature by fine screen blood filtration. *Chest* 1974; **44**: 6.

32. Cattaneo N, Tenconi P, Albera I *et al.* Subcutaneous desmopressin shortened the prolonged bleeding time in patients with cirrhosis. *Br J Haematol* 1981; **47**: 283–293.

33. Burroughs AK, Matthews K, Quadira M *et al.* Desmopressin and bleeding time in patients with cirrhosis. *BMJ* 1985; **291**: 1377–1381.

34. De Franchis R, Arcidiacono PG, Andreoni B *et al.* for the NIEC. Terlipressin plus desmopressin versus trelipressin alone in acute variceal haemorrhage in cirrhotics: interim analysis of a double blind multicentre placebo controlled trial [abstract]. *Gastroenterology* 1992; **102**: A799.

35. Smith O, Hazlehust G, Brozovic C *et al.* Impact of aprotonin on blood transfusion requirements in liver transplantation. *Tranfus Med* 1993; **81**: 97–102.

36. Papatheodoridis G, Chung S, Keshav S *et al.* Correction of both prothrombin time and primary haemostasis by recombinanate factor VII during therapeutic alcohol injection of hepatocellular cancer in liver cirrhosis. *J Hepatol* 1999; **31**(4): 747–750.

37. Bleichner G, Boulanger R, Squara P *et al.* Frequency of infection in cirrhotic patients presenting with acute gastrointestinal haemorrhage. *Br J Surg* 1986; **73**: 724–726.

38. Rajkovic I, Williams R. Mechanisms of abnormality in host defences against bacterial infection in liver disease. *Clin Sci* 1985; **68**: 247–253.

39. Stephan R, Kupper T, Geha A *et al.* Haemorrhage without tissue trauma produces immunosuppression and enhances susceptibility to sepsis. *Surgery* 1987; **122**: 62–68.

40. Stephan R, Conrad P, Janeway C *et al.* Decreased interleukin–2 production following simple haemorrhage. *Surg Forum* 1986; **37**: 73–75.

41. Gomez F, Schreiber A. Impaired function of macrophage Fcy receptors and bacterial infection in alcoholic cirrhosis. *N Engl J Med* 1994; **331**: 1122–1128.

42. Bernard B, Grange JD, Nguyen KE *et al.* Antibiotic prophylaxis (AbP) for the prevention of bacterial infections in cirrhotic patients with gastrointestinal bleeding (GB): a meta–analysis. *Hepatology* 1999; **29**: 1655–1661.

43. Gines A, Escorsell A, Gines P *et al.* Incidence, predictive factors, and prognosis of the hepatorenal syndrome in cirrhosis with ascites. *Gastroenterology* 1993; **105**: 229–236.

44. Badalamenti S, Graziani G, Salerno F *et al.* Hepatorenal syndrome: new perspectives in pathogenesis and treatment. *Arch Int Med* 1993; **153**: 1957–1967.

45. Batalier R, Sort P, Gines P *et al.* Hepatorenal syndrome: Definition, pathophysiology, clinical features and management. *Kidney Int (Suppl)* 1998; **66**: 547–553.

46. Segal J, Phang P, Walley K. Low dose dopamine hastens the onset of gut ischaemia in a porcine model of haemorrhagic shock. *J Appl Physiol* 1992; **73**: 1159–1164.

47. Baldwin L, Henderson A, Hickman P. Effects of low dose post opertaive dopamine on renal function after elective major vascular surgery. *Ann Int Med* 1994; **120**: 744–747.

48. Arroyo V, Gines P, Gerbes AL *et al.* Definition and diagnostic criteria of refractory ascites and hepatorenal syndrome in cirrhosis. *Hepatology* 1996; **23**: 164–76.

49. Gines A, Escorsell A, Gines P *et al.* Incidence, predictive factors, and prognosis of the hepatorenal syndrome in cirrhosis with ascites. *Gastroenterology* 1993; **105**: 229–236.

50. Cervoni J–P, Lecomte T, Cellier C *et al.* Terlipressin may influence the outcome of hepatorenal syndrome complicating alcoholic hepatitis. *Am J Gastroenterol* 1997; **92**: 2113–2114.

51. Evrard P, Ruedin P, Installe E *et al.* Low-dose ornipressin improves renal function in the hepatorenal syndrome. *Crit Care Med* 1994; **22**: 363–366.

52. Guevara M, Gines P, Fernandez-Esparrach G *et al.* Reversibility of hepatorenal syndrome by prolonged administration of ornipressin and plasma volume expansion. *Hepatology* 1998; **27**: 35–41.

53. Kaffy F, Borderie C, Chagneau C *et al.* Octreotide in the treatment of the hepatorenal syndrome in cirrhotic patients [2]. *J Hepatol* 1999; **30**: 174.

54. Hadengue A, Gadano A, Moreau R *et al.* Beneficial effects of the 2-day administration of terlipressin in patients with cirrhosis and hepatorenal syndrome. *J Hepatol* 1998; **29**: 565–570.

55. Ganne-Carri N, Hadengue A, Mathurin P *et al.* Hepatorenal syndrome: Long-term treatment with terlipressin as a bridge to liver transplantation. *Dig Dis Sci* 1996; **41**: 1054–1056.

56. Loguercio C, Sava E, Mermo R *et al.* Malnutrition in cirrhotic patients: anthropometric measurements as a method of assessing nutritional status. *Br J Clin Pharmacol* 1990; **44**: 98–101.

57. McCullough A, Tavill A. Disordered energy and protein metabolism in liver disease. *Semin Liver Dis* 1991; **11**(4): 265–277.

58. Panes J, Teres J, Bosch J *et al.* Efficacy of ballon tamponade in treatment of bleeding gastric and oesophageal varices. results in 151 consecutive episodes. *Dig Dis Sci* 1988; **33**: 454–459

59. Sarin SK. Long-term follow-up of gastric variceal sclerotherapy: an eleven-year experience. *Gastrointest Endosc* 1997; **46**: 8–14.

60. Levacher S, Letoumelin P, Pateron D *et al.* Early administration of terlipressin plus glyceryl trinitrate to control active upper gastrointestinal bleeding in cirrhotic patients. *Lancet* 1995; **346**: 865–868.

61. Bosch J, Groszmann RJ, Garcia-Pagan JC *et al.* Association of transdermal nitroglycerin to vasopressin infusion in the treatment of variceal hemorrhage: a placebo-controlled clinical trial. *Hepatology* 1989; **10**: 962–968.

62. Sonnenburg GE, Keller U, Perruchud A *et al.* Effect of somatostatin on splanchnic haemodynamics. *Gastroenterology* 1981; **80**: 5226–5232.

63. Bosch J, Kravetz D, Rodes J. Effects of somatostatin on hepatic and systemic haemodynamics inpatients with cirrhosis of the liver: comparison with vasopressin. *Gastroenterology* 1981; **80**: 518–525.

64. Variceal Bleeding Study Group. A muticenter randomized controlled trial comparing different schedules of somatostatin administration in the treatment of acute variceal bleeding [abstract]. *Hepatology* 1998; **28**: 770A.

65. Jenkins SA, Baxter JN, Snowden S. The effects of somatostatin and SMS 201–995 on hepatic haemodynamics inpatients with cirrhosis and portal hypertension. *Fibrinolysis* 1988; **2**: 48–50.

66. McCormick PA, Dick R, Siringo S *et al.* Octreotide reduces azygous blood flow in cirrhotic patients with portal hypertension. *Eur J Gastroenterol Hepatol* 1990; **2**: 489–492.

67. Escorsell A, Bandi JC, Francosis E *et al.* Desensitization to the effects of intravenous octreotide in cirrhotic patients with portal hypertension [abstract]. *Hepatology* 1996; **24**: 207A

68. Conn HO, Ramsby GR, Storer EH *et al.* Intraarterial vasopressin in the treatment of upper gastrointestinal hemorrhage: a prospective, controlled clinical trial. *Gastroenterology* 1975; **68**: 211–221.

69. Merigan TCJ, Poltkin JR, Davidson CS. Effect of intravenously administered posterior pituitary extract on haemorrhage from bleeding esophageal varices. *N Engl J Med* 1962; **266**: 134–135.

70. Mallory A, Schaefer JW, Cohen JR *et al.* Selective intraarterial vasopressin infusion for upper gastrointestinal tract hemorrhage. A controlled trial. *Arch Surg* 1980; **115**: 30–32.

71. Fogel RM, Knauer CM, Andress LL. Continuous intravenous vasopressin in active upper gastrointestinal bleeding. A placebo controlled trial. *Ann Intern Med* 1982; **96**: 565–569.

72. Tsai YT, Lay CS, Lai KH *et al.* Controlled trial of vasopressin plus nitroglycerin vs. vasopressin alone in the treatment of bleeding esophageal varices. *Hepatology* 1986; **6**: 406–409.

73. Gimson AE, Westaby D, Hegarty J *et al.* A randomized trial of vasopressin and vasopressin plus nitroglycerin in the control of acute variceal hemorrhage. *Hepatology* 1986; **6**: 410–413.

74. Walker S, Stiehl A, Raedsch R *et al.* Terlipressin in bleeding esophageal varices: a placebo-controlled, double-blind study. *Hepatology* 1986; **6**: 112–115.

75. Freeman JG, Cobden MD, Record CO: Placebo-controlled trial of terlipressin (glypressin) in the management of acute variceal bleeding. *J Clin Gastroenterol* 1989; **11**: 58–60.

76. Soderlund C, Magnusson I, Torngren S *et al.* Terlipressin (triglycyl-lysine vasopressin) controls acute bleeding oesophageal varices. A double-blind, randomized, placebo-controlled trial. *Scand J Gastroenterol* 1990; **25**: 622–630.

77. Valenzuela JE, Schubert T, Fogel RM *et al.* A multicenter, randomized, double-blind trial of somatostatin in the management of acute hemorrhage from esophageal varices. *Hepatology* 1989; **10**: 958–961.

78. Burroughs AK, McCormick PA, Hughes MD *et al.* Randomised, double-blind, placebo-controlled trial of somatostatin for variceal bleeding. *Gastroenterology* 1990; **99**: 1388–1395.

79. Gotzsche PC, Gjorup I, Bonnen H *et al.* Somatostatin v placebo in bleeding esophageal varices – randomized trial and metaanalysis. *BMJ* 1995; **310**: 1495–1498.

80. Loperfido S, Godena F, Tosolini G *et al.* Somatostatin in the treatment of bleeding oesophagogastric varices. Controlled clinical trial in comparison with ranitidine [in Italian]. *Recenti Prog Med* 1987; **78**: 82–86.

81. Flati G, Negro P, Flati D *et al.* Somatostatin. Massive upper digestive hemorrhage in portal hypertension. Results of a controlled study [in Spanish]. *Rev Esp Enferm Dig* 1986; **70**: 411–414.

82. Testoni PA, Masci E, Passaretti S *et al.* Comparison of somatostatin and cimetidine in the treratment of acute esophageal variceal bleeding. *Curr Ther Res* 1986; **39**: 759–766.

83. Burroughs AK, for the International Octreotide Varices Study Group. Double blind RCT of 5 day octreotide versus placebo, associated with sclerotherapy for trial failures [abstract]. *Hepatology* 1996; **24**: 352A.

84. Primignani M, Andreoni B, Carpinelli L *et al.* Sclerotherapy plus octreotide versus sclerotherapy alone in the prevention of early rebleeding from esophageal varices – a randomized, double-blind, placebo-controlled, multicenter trial. *Hepatology* 1995; **21**: 1322–1327.

85. D'Amico G, Politi F, Morabito A *et al.* Octreotide compared with placebo in a treatment strategy for early rebleeding in cirrhosis. A double blind, randomized pragmatic trial. *Hepatology* 1998; **28**: 1206–1214.

86. Colin R, Giuli N, Czernichow P *et al.* Prospective comparison of glypressin, tamponade and their association in the treatment of bleeding esophageal varices. In *Vasopressin Analogs and Portal Hypertension.* Eds D Lebrec, AT Blei. Paris, John Libbey Eurotext, 1987: 149–153.

87. Fort E, Sauterau D, Silvaine C *et al.* A randomized trial of terlipressin plus nitroglycerin vs balloon tamponade in the control of acute variceal haemorrhage. *Hepatology* 1990; **11**: 678–681.

88. Blanc P, Bories J, Desprez D *et al.* Balloon tamponade with Linton–Michel tube versus terlipressin in the treatment of acute oesophageal and gastric variceal bleeding [abstract]. *J Hepatol* 1994; **21**: 133S.

89. Jaramillo JL, de la Mata M, Mino G *et al.* Somatostatin versus Sengstaken tube balloon tamponade for primary haemostasis of bleeding esophageal varices: a randomized pilot study. *J Hepatol* 1991; **12**: 100–105.

90. Avgerinos A, Klonis C, Rekoumis G *et al.* A prospective randomized trial comparing somatostatin, balloon tamponade and the combination of both methods in the management of acute variceal haemorrhage. *J Hepatol* 1991; **13**: 78–83.

91. McKee R. A study of octreotide in oesophageal varices. *Digestion* 1990; **45 (Suppl 1)**: 60–64.

92. Freeman JG, Cobden MD, Lishaman AH *et al.* Controlled trial of terlipressin ("glypressin") versus vasopressin in the early treatment of esophageal varices. *Lancet* 1989; **2**: 62–68.

93. Desaint B, Florent C, Levy VG. A randomized trial of triglycyl-lysine vasopressin versus lysine vasopressin in active cirrhotic variceal hemorrhage. In *Vasopressin Analogs and Portal Hypertension.* Eds D Lebrec, AT Blei AT. Paris, John Libbey Eurotext, 1987: 155–157.

94. Lee FY, Tsai YT, Lai KH *et al.* A randomized controlled study of triglycyl–vasopressin and vasopressi plus nitroglycerin in the control of acute esophageal variceal hemorrhage. *Chin J Gastroenterol* 1988; **5**: 131–138.

95. Chiu WK, Sheen IS, Liaw YF. A controlled study of glypressin versus vasopressin in the control of bleeding from esophageal varices. *J Gastroenterol Hepatol* 1988; **5**: 549–553.

96. D'Amico G, Traina M, Vizzini G *et al.* Teripressin or vasopressin plus transdermal nitroglycerin in a treatment strategy for digestive bleeding in cirrhosis. A randomized clinical trial. *J Hepatol* 1994; **20**: 206–212.

97. Kravetz D, Bosch J, Teres J *et al.* Comparison of intravenous somatostatin and vasopressin infusion in treatment of acute variceal hemorrhage. *Hepatology* 1984; **4**: 442–446.

98. Jenkins SA, Baxter JN, Corbett W *et al.* A prospective randomised controlled clinical trial comparing somatostatin and vasopressin in controlling acute variceal haemorrhage. *BMJ* 1985; **290**: 275–278.

99. Bagarani M, Albertini V, Anza M *et al.* Effect of somatostatin in controlling bleeding from esophageal varices. *Ital J Surg Sci* 1987; **17**: 21–26.

100. Cardona C, Vida F, Balanzo J *et al.* Efficacia terapeutica de la somatostatina versus vasopressina mas nitroglycerina en la hemorragia activa por varices esofagogastrica. *Gastroenterol Hepatol* 1989; **12**: 30–34.

101. Hsia HC, Lee FY, Tsai YT *et al.* Comparison of somatostatin and vasopressin in the control of acute esophageal variceal hemorrhage. A randomized, controlled study. *Chin J Gastroenterol* 1990; **7**: 71–78.

102. Saari A, Klvilaasko E, Inberg M *et al.* Comparison of somatostatin and vasopressin in bleeding esophageal varices. *Am J Gastroenterol* 1990; **85**: 804–807.

103. Rodriguez-Moreno F, Santolaria F, Gles-Reimers E *et al.* A randomized trial of somatostatin vs vasopressin plus nitroglycerin in the treatment of acute variceal bleeding [abstract]. *J Hepatol* 1991; **13**: S162.

104. Feu F, DelArbol LR, Banares R *et al.* Double-blind randomized controlled trial comparing terlipressin and somatostatin for acute variceal hemorrhage. *Gastroenterology* 1996; **111**: 1291–1299.

105. Walker S, Kreichgauer HP, Bode JC. Terlipressin (glypressin) versus somatostatin in the treatment of bleeding esophageal varices – Final report of a placebo-controlled, double-blind study. *Z Gastroenterol* 1996; **34**: 692–698.

106. Hwang SJ, Lin HC, Chang CF *et al.* A randomized controlled trial comparing octreotide and vasopressin in the control of acute esophageal variceal bleeding. *J Hepatol* 1992; **16**: 320–325.

107. Silvain C, Carpentier S, Sautereau D *et al.* Terlipressin plus transdermal nitroglycerin vs octreotide in the control of acute bleeding from esophageal varices – a multicenter randomized trial. *Hepatology* 1993; **18**: 61–65.

108. Prindiville T, Trudeau W. A comparison of immediate versus delayed endoscopic injection sclerosis of bleeding esophageal varices. *Gastrointest Endosc* 1986; **32**: 385–388.

109. Shemesh E, Czerniac A, Klein E *et al.* A comparison between emergency and delayed endoscopic injection sclerotherapy of bleeding esophageal varices in non-alcoholic portal hypertension. *J Clin Gastroenterol* 1990; **12**: 5–9.

110. Soderlund C, Ihre T. Endoscopic sclerotherapy v conservative management of bleeding oesophageal varices. A 5-year prospective controlled trial of emergency and long-term treatment. *Acta Chir Scand* 1985; **151**: 449–456.

111. Larson AW, Cohen H, Zweiban B *et al.* Acute esophageal variceal sclerotherapy. Results of a prospective randomized controlled trial. *JAMA* 1996; **255**: 497–500.

112. Alexandrino P, Alves MM, Fidalgo P *et al.* Is sclerotherapy the first choice treatment for active oesophageal variceal bleeding in cirrhotic patients? Final report of a randomized controlled trial [abstract]. *J Hepatol* 1990; **11 (Suppl)**: S1.

113. Novella MT, Villanueva C, Ortiz J *et al.* Octreotide vs sclerotherapy and octreotide for acute variceal bleeding. A pilot study (abstract). *Hepatology* 1996; **24**: 207A.

114. Ortiz J, Villanueva C, Sabat M *et al.* Somatostatin alone or combined with emergency sclerotherapy for acute variceal bleeding [abstract]. *Gastrointest Endosc* 1997; **45**: 77A

115. Westaby D, Hayes P, Gimson AES *et al.* Controlled trial of injection sclerotherapy for active variceal bleeding. *Hepatology* 1989; **9**: 274–277.

116. Cooperative Spanish–French Group for the Treatment of Bleeding Esophageal Varices: Randomized controlled trial comparing terlipressin vs endoscopic injection sclerotherapy in the treatment of acute variceal bleeding and prevention of early rebleeding (abstract). *Hepatology* 1997; **26**: 249A

117. Shields R, Jenkins SA, Baxter JN *et al.* A prospective randomized controlled trial comparing the efficacy of somatostatin with injection sclerotherapy in the control of bleeding esophageal-varices. *J Hepatol* 1992; **16**: 128–137.

118. Planas R, Quer JC, Boix J *et al.* A prospective randomized trial comparing somatostatin and sclerotherapy in the treatment of acute variceal bleeding. *Hepatology* 1994; **20**: 370–375.

119. Di Febo G, Siringo S, Vacirca M *et al.* Somatostatin (SMS) and urgent sclerotherapy (US) in active oesophageal variceal bleeding (abstract). *Gastroenterology* 1990; **98**: 583A

120. Sung JJ, Chung SS, Lai CW *et al.* Octreotide infusion or emergency sclerotherapy for variceal hemorrhage. *Lancet* 1993; **342**: 637–641.

121. Jenkins SA, Shields R, Davies M *et al.* A multicentre randomised trial comparing octreotide and injection sclerotherapyin the management and outcome of acute variceal haemorrhage. *Gut* 1997; **41**: 526–533.

122. Poo JL, Bosques F, Garduno R *et al.* Octreotide versus emergency sclerotherapy in acute variceal hemorrhage in liver cirrhosis [abstract]. *Gastroenterology* 1996; **110**: 1297A.

123. Kravetz D, and Group for the Study of Portal Hypertension. Octreotide vs sclerotherapy in the treatment of acute variceal bleeding [abstract]. *Hepatology* 1996; **24**: 206A

124. El-Jackie A, Rowaisha I, Waked I *et al.* Octreotide vs. sclerotherapy in the control of acute variceal bleeding in schistosomal portal hypertension: a randomized trial (abstract). *Hepatology* 1998; **28**: 533A.

125. Besson I, Ingrand P, Person B *et al.* Sclerotherapy with or without octreotide for acute variceal bleeding. *N Engl J Med* 1995; **333**: 555–560.

126. Avgerinos A, Nevens F, Raptis S *et al.*for the ABOVE Study Group. Early administration of somatostatin and efficacy of sclerotherapy in acute oesophageal variceal bleeds: the European Acute Bleeding Oesophageal Variceal Episodes (ABOVE) randomised trial. *Lancet* 1997; **350**: 1495–1499.

127. Signorelli S, Negrini F, Paris B *et al.* Sclerotherapy with or without somatostatin or octreotide in the treatment of acute variceal haemorrhage: our experience [abstract]. *Gastroenterology* 1996; **110**: 1326A.

128. Brunati S, Ceriani R, Curioni R *et al.* Sclerotherapy alone vs sclerotherapy plus terlipressin vs sclerotherapy plus octreotide in the treatment of acute variceal haemorrhage [abstract]. *Hepatology* 1996; **24**: 207A.

129. Signorelli S, Paris B, Negrini F *et al.* Esophageal varices bleeding: comparison between treatment with sclerotherapy alone vs sclerotherapy plus octreotide [abstract]. *Hepatology* 1997; **26**: 137A.

130. Jensen DM, Kovacs TOG, Randall GM *et al.* Initial results of a randomized prospective study of emergency banding vs sclerotherapy for bleeding gastric or esophageal varices [abstract]. *Gastrointest Endosc* 1993; **39**: 128A.

131. Lo GH, Lai KH, Cheng JS *et al.* Emergency banding ligation versus sclerotherapy for the control of active bleeding from esophageal varices. *Hepatology* 1997; **25**: 1101–1104.

132. Stiegmann GV, Goff JS, Michaletz-Onody PA *et al.* Endoscopic sclerotherapy as compared with endoscopic ligation for bleeding esophageal varices. *N Engl J Med* 1992; **326**: 1527–1532.

133. Laine L, El-Newihi HM, Migikovsky B *et al.* Endoscopic ligation compared with sclerotherapy for the treatment of bleeding esophageal varices. *Ann Intern Med* 1993; **119**: 1–7.

134. Gimson AES, Ramage JK, Panos MZ *et al.* Randomised trial of variceal banding ligation versus injection sclerotherapy for bleeding esophageal varices. *Lancet* 1993; **342**: 391–394.

135. Lo GH, Lai KH, Cheng JS *et al.* A prospective, randomized trial of sclerotherapy versus ligation in the management of bleeding esophageal varices. *Hepatology* 1995; **22**: 466–471.

136. Hou MC, Lin HC, Kuo BIT *et al.* Comparison of endoscopic variceal injection sclerotherapy and ligation for the treatment of esophageal variceal hemorrhage: a prospective randomized trial. *Hepatology* 1995; **21**: 1517–1522.

137. Jain AK, Ray RP, Gupta JP. Management of acute variceal bleed: Randomized trial of variceal ligation and sclerotherapy [abstract]. *Hepatology* 1996; **23**: 138P.

138. Mostafa I, Omar MM, Fakhry S *et al.* Prospective randomized comparative study of injection sclerotherapy and band ligation for bleeding esophageal varices [abstract]. *Hepatology* 1996; **23**: 185P

139. Sarin SK, Govil A, Jain AK *et al.* Prospective randomized trial of endoscopic sclerotherapy versus variceal band ligation for esophageal varices: influence on gastropathy, gastric varices and variceal recurrence. *J Hepatol* 1997; **26**: 826–832.

140. Shiha GE, Farag FM. Endoscopic variceal ligation versus endoscopic sclerotherapy for the management of bleeding varices: A prospective randomized trial [abstract]. *Hepatology* 1997; **26**: 136A.

141. Fakhry S, Omar MM, Mustafa I *et al.* Endoscopic sclerotherapy versus endoscopic variceal ligation in the management of bleeding esophageal varices: a final report of a prospective randomized study in schistisomal hepatic fibrosis [abstract]. *Hepatology* 1997; **26**: 137A.

142. Chau TN, Patch D, Chan YW *et al.* "Salvage" transjugular intrahepatic portosystemic shunts: Gastric fundal compared with esophageal variceal bleeding. *Gastroenterology* 1998; **114**: 981–987.

143. Sarin SK, Lahoti D, Saxena SP *et al.* Prevalence, classification and natural-history of gastric varices — a long-term follow-up-study in 568 portal-hypertension patients. *Hepatology* 1992; **16**: 1343–1349.

144. Ramond MJ, Valla D, Mosnier JF *et al.* Successful endoscopic obturation of gastric varices with butyl cyanoacrylate. *Hepatology* 1989; **10**: 488–493.

145. Oho K, Iwao T, Sumino M *et al.* Ethanolamine oleate versus butyl cyanoacrylate for bleeding gastric varices — a nonrandomized study. *Endoscopy* 1995; **27**: 349–354.

146. Williams SGJ, Peters RA, Westaby D. Thrombin – an effective treatment for gastric variceal hemorrhage. *Gut* 1994; **35**: 1287–1289.

147. Merican I, Burroughs AK. Gastric varices. *Eur J Gastroenterol Hepatol* 1992; **4**: 511–520.

148. De Franchis R. Developing consensus in portal hypertension. *J Hepatol* 1996; **25**: 390–394.

149. Burroughs AK, Hamilton G, Phillips A *et al.* A comparison of sclerotherapy with staple transection of the oesophagus for the emergency control of bleeding from oesophageal varices. *N Engl J Med* 1989; **321**, 857–862.

150. Bornman P, Terblanche J, Kahn D *et al.* Limitations of multiple injection sclerotherapy sessions for acute variceal bleeding. *S Afr Med J* 1986; **70**, 34–36.

151. Cabrera J, Maynar M, Granados R *et al.* Transjugular intrahepatic portosystemic shunt versus sclerotherapy in the elective treatment of variceal hemorrhage. *Gastroenterology* 1996; **110**: 832–839.

152. Chau TN, Patch D, Chan YW *et al.* Salvage transjugular intrahepatic portosystemic shunt: fundal compared to oesophageal variceal bleeding. *Gastroenterology* 1998; **114**, 981–987.

153. Richter GM, Noeldge G, Palmaz JC *et al.* The transjugular intrahepatic portosystemic stent-shunt (TIPSS): results of a pilot study. *Cardiovasc Intervent Radiol* 1990; **13**: 200–207.

154. LaBerge JM, Somberg KA, Lake JR *et al.* Two-year outcome following transjugular intrahepatic portosystemic shunt for variceal bleeding: results in 90 patients. *Gastroenterology* 1995; **108**: 1143–1151.

155. Sanyal AJ, Freedman AM, Luketic VA *et al.* Transjugular intrahepatic portosystemic shunts for patients with active variceal hemorrhage unresponsive to sclerotherapy. *Gastroenterology* 1996; **111**: 138–146.

156. Patch D, Nikolopoulou VN, McCormick PA *et al.* Factors related to early mortality after transjugular intrahepatic portosystemic shunts (TIPS) for uncontrolled variceal haemorrhage. *J Hepatol* 1998; **28**: 454–460.

157. Wong F, Sniderman KW, Liu P *et al.* Transjugular intrahepatic portosystemic stent shunt. Effects on haemodynamics and sodium homeostasis in cirrhosis and refractory ascites. *Ann Int Med* 1995; **122**: 816–822.

12. Lower Gastrointestinal and Occult Bleeding

TIM ROCKALL

LOWER GASTROINTESTINAL BLEEDING

Lower gastrointestinal haemorrhage encompasses bleeding distal to the ligament of Treitz. Bleeding from the small bowel is however, rare and represents only about 3% of all cases. The incidence of lower gastrointestinal haemorrhage has not been well defined, but the condition is common. The majority (90%) of acute lower gastrointestinal bleeds will stop spontaneously, although 35% will require blood transfusion, and 5% will require urgent surgical intervention. There is also now an important role for endoscopic and radiological intervention in acute haemorrhage.

Making the diagnosis

As in upper gastrointestinal haemorrhage, a variety of different pathologies are involved. In the Western world, diverticular disease represents the largest proportion of cases (40%), followed by inflammatory bowel disease (20%) (including Crohn's disease, ulcerative colitis, infectious colitis, and ischaemic colitis), neoplasia (15%), benign anorectal disease (10%), and arteriovenous malformations (2%). This last group includes lesions variously described as vascular ectasias, angiomas, and angiodysplasias. Other lesions are rare and include radiation injury, Meckel's diverticulum and other small-bowel pathology and varices (1).

Bleeding is commonly associated with coagulopathy, but studies have shown the distribution of causative lesions in these cases to be the same (2). In severe cases, however, generalized mucosal bleeding may be seen.

Iatrogenic causes such as post polypectomy bleeding and anastomotic bleeding should not be forgotten. The risk of haemorrhage after polypectomy is estimated between 0.2 and 3%. Haemorrhage is usually immediate, but may be delayed. When haemorrhage is recognized, endoscopic haemostatic techniques are usually successful (injection of adrenaline, re-snaring, re-coagulating, placement of a ligature or clip).

Diverticular bleeding is common. The estimated risk of bleeding with this disease is about 15%. After a single bleed, the risk of recurrence is 25%; after two bleeds, it is 50%. Eighty per cent of all bleeds stop spontaneously and no therapy is indicated. Operative intervention should be considered after two major bleeds, as the risk of further recurrence is high. However, many of these patients are frail and elderly, and continuation of conservative treatment for multiple self-limiting episodes may be appropriate.

Inflammatory bowel disease often manifests itself as bloody diarrhoea, but more rarely may present with profuse haemorrhage. This is more common in Crohn's disease than in ulcerative colitis, because the inflammation involves the entire thickness of the bowel wall. Up to 6% of patients with this disease may sustain a major haemorrhage. About 50% stop bleeding spontaneously but, of these, 35% will re-bleed. For this reason, urgent surgery is usually indicated for patients with a life-threatening haemorrhage as a result of inflammatory colitis. The operation usually required is a total colectomy. The rectum is usually preserved at this stage, unless it is the site of major haemorrhage.

Ischaemic colitis rarely causes major haemorrhage. Bloody diarrhoea is more usual, and may be accompanied by pain.

Both **benign** and **malignant neoplasia** may present as profuse bleeding, although occult blood loss and minor fresh bleeding are more common. Rarely is urgent surgical intervention required.

Vascular anomalies occur with increasing frequency with age. They may originate from chronic partial venous obstruction of submucosal veins caused by muscle contraction that results in incompetence of the precapillary sphincters and arteriovenous malformations. These lesions are usually multiple, and are most frequent in the caecum and ascending colon. Bleeding is usually slow, intermittent and recurrent although it is occasionally massive (2–15%). In 90% of patients the bleeding stops spontaneously, but in 25–85% it will recur. The treatment of choice is endoscopic coagulation, if the lesions can be identified. Colectomy is reserved for those with repeated major haemorrhage.

Benign anorectal disease does present as lower gastrointestinal haemorrhage and a careful examination of the anorectum is imperative before initiating more invasive examinations. However, anorectal lesions are common, and complete colonic evaluation is usually required, even after an anorectal source such as haemorrhoids has been identified.

Management

A good history from the patient may give clues as to the cause of the haemorrhage. Important points include a prior history of bleeding, the presence of liver disease, and drug usage (aspirin, non-steroidal anti-inflammatory drugs, and warfarin), in addition to the exact nature of the bleeding — specifically, the duration, the colour of the blood, the relationship to defecation, whether the blood is mixed with or separate from the stool, an associated change in bowel habit, or mucous discharge. Bright red blood separate from the stool suggests an anorectal cause. Diarrhoea and mucous associated with darker blood mixed in with the stool suggests colitis or neoplasm. None of the specific features, however, is absolutely diagnostic.

Resuscitation measures are as for bleeding from the upper gastrointestinal tract (see Chapters 11.1

and 11.2). However, the vast majority of lower gastrointestinal bleeds stop spontaneously and initial management should be conservative, with transfusion and correction of clotting abnormalities. Once haemorrhage has ceased, then bowel preparation and colonoscopy can be undertaken in a patient whose conditions is stable, with a much greater chance of detecting the pathological lesion (85–90%).

In the small proportion of patients in whom active bleeding continues, **investigation** to localize the source of the haemorrhage is indicated, so that directed treatment can be administered, in the form of endoscopic therapy, interventional radiology, or surgery. **Colonoscopy** is favoured by many clinicians, but the method of bowel preparation is still debated. Some favour the use of a purgative together with distal colonic washouts before endoscopy, whereas other authors have argued that this is unnecessary because of the cathartic effect of blood in the colon. Good results have been obtained with routine use of a polyethylene glycol (Golytely, Kleenprep) as a purgative (3) but, equally, the causative lesion was identified in 76% of patients without preparation in one study (4). Colonoscopy should always be undertaken in a stable patient in an adequately equipped and staffed endoscopy suite. If the patient's condition becomes unstable during the procedure, the colonoscopy should be abandoned. Colonoscopy should also be abandoned if massive haemorrhage obscures the diagnosis or severe mucosal or ischaemic colitis is encountered, as the risk of perforation in these patients is high.

Nuclear scintigraphy can be used to detect active haemorrhage. It is very sensitive, and can detect bleeding rates of less than 0.1 ml/min. Technetium-99m (^{99m}Tc)-labelled sulphur colloid can be used, which has the advantage of no preparation, but the half-life is very short and its rapid enhancement of the liver and spleen can obscure the diagnosis. A better method is the use of ^{99m}Tc-labelled red cells. Unfortunately, although sensitive, this method is also very non-specific, and localizes the lesion very poorly. For these reasons many authors do not advocate its use. It may be useful just before angiography, to confirm active haemorrhage before undertaking the more invasive procedure. Whenever there is massive active haemorrhage, however, this is unnecessary, and the patient should proceed direct to angiography.

Selective mesenteric angiography can detect a rate of bleeding of 0.5–1.0 ml/min. The sensitivity reported in various studies ranges from 40 to 86%

(1). Once the site of haemorrhage is identified, the patient can proceed directly to surgery; alternatively, there is the therapeutic possibility of arterial infusion of vasopressin or selective embolization. The choice of technique depends on the expertise available. Vasopressin infusion has considerable side effects, including mesenteric thrombosis, intestinal infarction, myocardial ischaemia, hypertension, arrhythmias, and death. Glyceryl trinitrate may be infused simultaneously to counteract the systemic effects of the drug. A wide range of initial control of the haemorrhage is reported in the literature, and the re-bleeding rate is high (22–71%). Selective embolization using coil springs or gelfoam into the most distal vessel can be effective. Initial rates of haemostasis are high, and the rate of intestinal infarction is low. It is a good technique in patients with a predicted very high operative mortality.

OCCULT GASTROINTESTINAL BLEEDING

About 5% of all gastrointestinal bleeds are occult. Occult haemorrhage can be divided into three groups: acute, chronic recurrent, and chronic persistent. Here, we will deal with the occult acute haemorrhage. A haemorrhage is occult when the source is not evident on first-line investigation of upper and lower gastrointestinal endoscopy. It is presumed to be of small-bowel origin; however, in at least 10% of patients there is a missed upper gastrointestinal lesion, and so repeat endoscopy is of value.

Subsequent investigation is based upon the fact that small-bowel radiology has a very high "miss" rate; with labelled red cell scanning, 85% of investigations fail to localize the haemorrhage and the technique is therefore of no benefit in directing angiography or surgery.

Superior mesenteric artery angiography, however, has a yield approaching 50%. Angiography localizes the lesion and dye can be injected for the benefit of the surgeon. The ability to embolize can also be a useful temporizing measure.

Small-bowel endoscopy is available in only a few centres, and so is not widely practised. It is certainly of benefit in the group of patients with chronic bleeding, among whom there is a yield of 30–40% and for whom it represents the gold standard of investigation. When surgery is required and the source of the bleeding has not been identified, an initial laparotomy (or laparoscopy) may reveal an obvious causative lesion such as a small-bowel tumour, Meckel's diverticulum, or inflammatory bowel disease. If there are no palpable or visible lesions, enteroscopy should be performed while the patient is on the operating table. The endoscope can be inserted via the oral route (which allows the upper tract to be inspected again) and through into the small bowel. The surgeon then guides the small bowel over the end of the endoscope, allowing both direct vision and transillumination. The entire small-bowel can be viewed in this manner, and the surgeon can mark lesions such as angiodysplasias or small-bowel ulcers with a suture in order to define the area for resection. The viewing should all be performed as the endoscope is passed from proximal to distal tract, and not on removal of the endoscope, as traumatic lesions are commonly created and may be falsely identified as the cause of the underlying bleeding. Colonoscopy while the patient is on the operating table can be performed in the same manner. An alternative is to place an endoscope via an enterostomy, but it is more difficult to maintain a sterile field with this procedure.

There is rarely any place for blind resection.

References
1. Vernava AM, Moore BA, Longo WE *et al.* Lower gastrointestinal bleeding. *Dis Colon Rectum* 1997; **40**: 846–858.
2. Coon WW, Willis PW. Hemorrhagic complication of anticoagulant therapy. *Arch Int Med* 1974; **133**: 386–392.
3. Caos A, Benner KD, Manier J *et al.* Colonoscopy after Golytely preparation in acute rectal bleeding. *J Clin Gastroenterol* 1986; **8**: 46–49.
4. Rossini FP, Ferrari A, Spandre M *et al.* Emergency colonoscopy. *World J Surg* 1989; **13**: 190–192.

13. Acute Abdominal Pain

MARC WINSLET

DIAGNOSIS

The initial diagnosis of acute abdominal pain is dependent on a detailed history and meticulous clinical examination. Failure to make a correct diagnosis in the emergency situation may result in increased morbidity and mortality, and unnecessary surgical intervention.

In women, a detailed gynaecological history is required; details of urinary symptoms are essential in both sexes. The physical examination must be complete as extra-abdominal surgical pathology such as tonsillitis, pyelonephritis, salpingitis, strangulated femoral hernia, and torsion of the testis may all present with abdominal pain — as may many non-surgical conditions. **Medical causes of abdominal pain** include:

- myocardial infarction
- porphyria
- lobar pneumonia
- herpes zoster
- diabetic ketoacidosis
- lead poisoning
- acute hepatitis
- *Campylobacter/Yersinia*
- sickle-cell disease/spherocytosis
- Henoch–Schoenlein purpura

The presence of associated cardiovascular disease, including congestive cardiac failure, atrial fibrillation, or known atherosclerosis, may give a clue as to the diagnosis of mesenteric ischaemia,

particularly in the elderly. Rectal and vaginal examination should not be omitted.

The **important abdominal findings indicative of significant disease** include:

- tenderness/rebound
- guarding/rigidity
- mass
- hernia
- absent, tinkling or hyperactive bowel sounds
- rectal mass/tenderness

As a result of history and examination, three clinical situations may result. First, a specific diagnosis can be made on clinical grounds alone. Second, the presence of significant acute intra-abdominal pathology is established, but only a differential diagnosis is possible and further investigation is required. Third, initial assessment is inconclusive, and further clinical reassessment and investigation are required.

INVESTIGATION

The routine investigation performed in patients with acute abdomen include a **full blood count**, **urea and electrolyte estimation**, and **urinalysis**. Serum amylase should be assessed if acute pancreatitis can not be excluded. **Arterial blood-gas analysis** will reveal a metabolic acidosis if it is present. All women of child-bearing age should undergo a pregnancy test.

An **erect chest radiograph** should be performed in patients with respiratory symptoms and possible perforation or pancreatitis. A supine abdominal film should be assessed for relevant features. **Abnormal radiological features** in **acute abdominal pain** include:

- dilatation of hollow organ, plus or minus fluid levels
- calcification
- free gas/fluid/blood in the peritoneal cavity
- distortion of gastric bubble
- obliteration of the psoas or renal outline

Contrast radiology may be useful to confirm the presence of obstruction or perforation in selected patients. Gastrograffin is commonly used, although, unlike barium, it will not cause a granulomatous reaction in the presence of perforation, it has problems associated with its hypertonicity and may cause significant fluid shifts and increased intraluminal pressure. **Intravenous urography** may be used as an alternative to ultrasound for patients with renal colic.

Ultrasonography is useful **in acute abdominal pain** in several instances:

- acute cholecystitis and obstructive jaundice
- detection of intra-abdominal collections
- pseudocyst/ascites/abscess
- assessment of abdominal masses
- abdominal aortic aneurysms

Computed tomography has a greater sensitivity than ultrasonography in most circumstances, except in the diagnosis of gallstones. It is particularly useful in the assessment of acute pancreatitis.

The role of **upper gastrointestinal endoscopy** in the assessment of acute abdominal pain is limited in the emergency situation, but is frequently used in semi-urgent situations as part of further investigation. **Colonoscopy** may have a role in the diagnosis of large-bowel obstruction, pseudo-obstruction, and sigmoid volvulus. Its use is contraindicated in the presence of peritoneal inflammation such as acute diverticulitis or toxic megacolon, in which there is a significant risk of perforation.

The role of **peritoneal lavage** in the diagnosis of acute abdominal pain is extremely limited in the absence of a history of trauma. Diagnostic laparoscopy is becoming more commonplace in selected situations, particularly mini-laparoscopy under local anaesthesia with nitrous oxide insuffla-

tion. It may facilitate the diagnostic process, avoid unnecessary surgical intervention, and provide a therapeutic modality. However, it is not appropriate in certain clinical situations. The various **indications and contraindications to diagnostic laparoscopy** include:

- Indications
  - abdominal trauma
  - differential diagnosis of right iliac fossa pain in females
  - diagnostic uncertainty
  - possible mesenteric ischaemia
- Contraindications
  - peritonitis
  - obstruction
  - abdominal wall sepsis
  - multiple abdominal scars
  - known intra-abdominal adhesions

PERITONITIS

Inflammation of the peritoneal cavity may be infective or chemical in nature, and may be classified thus:

- primary bacterial peritonitis
- acute secondary bacterial peritonitis
- acute chemical peritonitis
- chronic bacterial peritonitis
- chronic non-bacterial peritonitis

Primary bacterial peritonitis

In this condition there is no intra-abdominal focus. The usual routes of infection are retrograde from the genital tract or haematogenous in young females. Other high-risk groups include the immunosuppressed and those with chronic liver and renal disease.

The onset is frequently insidious initially, progressing to full-blown septicaemia. If primary bacterial peritonitis is suspected, a peritoneal tap may be diagnostic. Laparoscopy may be helpful, but if differentiation from secondary peritonitis is difficult, laparotomy is required. Intravenous antibiotic therapy should be dictated by the clinical picture and urgent Gram stain. In the severely ill patient, intraperitoneal administration may be warranted.

Acute secondary bacterial peritonitis

In the great majority of patients, generalized peritonitis is secondary to perforation of an intra-abdominal viscus secondary to inflammatory, ischaemic, or neoplastic disease.

Pathophysiology

Presentation depends on the site of perforation and underlying pathology. The initial insult results in a profound inflammatory reaction, with the production of copious fibrinous and purulent exudate. This results in a paralytic ileus with loss of extracellular fluid, which is further compounded by bacteraemia. Fibrinous adhesions result, which may help to localize the infection. The infection is usually mixed with Gram-negative aerobes and anaerobes in addition to Gram-positive bacteria. *Escherichia coli* and *Bacteroides fragilis* are predominant.

Clinical picture

Symptoms and signs of the underlying disease may precede the onset of peritonitis, except in the presence of a perforated duodenal ulcer or mesenteric ischaemia. Otherwise, the clinical picture will vary with the cause. Apart from the intra-abdominal signs, changes in vital signs are of significant prognostic importance and help to identify the most seriously affected group of patients — those with faecal peritonitis.

Treatment

Supportive

It is vital initially to restore water and electrolyte balance. Supportive measures include intravenous rehydration with crystalloid or Hartmann's solution, with colloid for those who are severely shocked, and nasogastric suction. The fluid balance is monitored by vital signs (1), hourly urine output, and central venous pressure. Oxygen therapy via a mask at 5 litre/min is usual. **Pain relief should not be delayed for fear of masking vital signs; indeed, it may actually facilitate their detection**.

Definitive

In light of the polymicrobial nature of acute secondary bacterial peritonitis, treatment with broad-spectrum antibiotics based on aminoglycoside, third-generation cephalosporin, and metronidazole is usual (2). Initially, all appropriate cultures should be taken.

Surgical management of the underlying disease is usually performed via a laparotomy. A specimen of pus is taken for culture, and all purulent and fibrinous exudate removed. Peritoneal lavage with copious normal saline is commonly performed. Drainage of the peritoneal cavity is determined by the clinical situation.

For acute appendicitis, the appendix is removed and, for a perforated duodenal ulcer, an oversew is undertaken (3). The management of many other intra-abdominal diseases is more controversial, particularly with regard to the colon. Decision making is determined by the underlying disease, the condition of the patient, and experience of the surgeon (4–6). The safest procedure usually comprises resection and exteriorization of the affected segment. In a few patients, exteriorization alone may suffice, but primary resection and anastomosis are rarely justified, as the results achieved by experts are not usually generally applicable.

The abdominal wall should be closed with a monofilament suture; in the presence of contamination, secondary closure of the skin is advised.

Acute chemical peritonitis

The most common non-infective agents are gastric and pancreatic juice, bile, and urine, although all will consequently evolve to secondary acute bacterial peritonitis.

Primary biliary peritonitis is probably the most life threatening, frequently presenting with septicaemic shock and with an associated mortality of 30%. This may occur with or without the presence of gallstones. The emergency management consists of cholecystotomy.

Acute pancreatitis exists in two forms: an oedematous, self-limiting, mild form, and a severe necrotizing fulminant form. The initial diagnosis is usually based on suspicion, with confirmatory serum or urinary amylase or lipase concentrations, but it is difficult to distinguish between the two forms at presentation. The considerable variety of **aetiological factors in acute pancreatitis** include:

- Alcohol
- Biliary tract disease/gallstones
- Trauma
- Drugs

— thiazides
— steroids
• Metabolic
— hyperparathyroidism
— hyperlipidaemia
• Infection
— mumps
— Coxsackie B
• Congenital
• Periampullary carcinoma
• Hereditary
• Vascular

For practical purposes the two most common underlying conditions are alcohol and gallstones.

The clinical manifestation of acute pancreatitis is variable, and can mimic any other intra-abdominal emergency. Physical findings vary from minimal to profound shock. Marked abnormalities of a full blood count and profile are commonplace, but the key to diagnosis remains a markedly increased amylase concentration (at least three times above normal). Hyperamylasaemia can occur with extrapancreatic disease, but normal concentrations also may be found in late presentation or in the presence of massive gland destruction. Persistently increased values suggest the onset of local complications. Assessment of urinary values, in addition to serum lipase, elastase, trypsin, and ribonuclease, has been advocated for diagnosis, but all remain fallible. Further investigations that may prove helpful include serum concentrations of glucose, calcium and albumin, coagulation studies, and lipid profile. An electrocardiogram may show changes similar to those of myocardial ischaemia. Radiographic changes include sentinel loops or paralytic ileus, loss of gas shadow, intraperitoneal fluid, and pleural effusion.

Identification of those in the poor prognostic group may be aided by use of the Ranson criteria (Table 13.1) with mortality ranging from 1% for those with less than three criteria, to 90% for those with more than six criteria (7,8).

The mainstay of medical treatment consists of intense supportive therapy, with serial clinical examination, amylase assessment, and early contrast-enhanced computed tomography (CT) scanning for the poor prognostic cases (9). There is some evidence to support the use of antibiotic therapy and early enteral feeding (10,11).

Surgical intervention may be considered in the early or late phase of the disease. Early indications

include a diagnosis that is in doubt and another intra-abdominal catastrophy can not be excluded, known biliary disease that does not resolve within 48 h, and failure of medical management, indicating necrotizing disease. Indications for later intervention include pseudocyst or abscess formation, and haemorrhage from left-sided portal hypertension.

Chronic bacterial or non-bacterial peritonitis

Chronic bacterial peritonitis may occur in association with tuberculosis or actinomycosis. Granulomatous peritonitis is commonly associated with a starch contamination. Neither commonly presents with acute abdominal pain.

PNEUMOPERITONEUM

The most common non-iatrogenic causes of pneumoperitoneum are perforated peptic ulcer disease or diverticular disease.

Perforated peptic ulcer disease

Free perforation of the upper gastrointestinal tract is normally associated with peptic ulcer disease and ingestion of steroidal or non-steroidal drugs, but may also occur in patients with burns, multiple injuries, and sepsis. The symptoms and signs do not usually cause diagnostic confusion, except in the presence of high-dose steroid use. The presence of a chronic ulcer may result in a prodromal history. Symptoms and signs depend on the size of the defect, degree of soiling, and degree of spontaneous sealing.

Table 13.1.   Ranson criteria for severity of acute pancreatitis.

On Admission	Age >55 years
	White cell count >16,000
	Fasting blood sugar >11.2 mmol/litre
	Serum LDH >350 IU/litre
	Serum AST >250 units %
Within 48 h	Haemocrit decrease >10%
of admission	Blood urea nitrogen increase >1.8 mmol/litre
	Serum calcium <2 mmol/litre
	Arterial PO$_2$ <7.98 kPa
	Base deficit >4 mmol/litre
	Estimated fluid requestration >6 litre

LHD, lactate dehydrogenase; AST, aspartate transaminase; PO$_2$, partial pressure of oxygen.

The **diagnosis** is based on suspicion and confirmed by an erect chest X-ray or a lateral decubitus abdominal film in a debilitated patient. If a pneumoperitoneum is not seen, serum amylase estimation is mandatory. If doubt still exists, a water-soluble contrast study or diagnostic peritoneal tap should be considered.

Initial **management** is supportive (see peritonitis). Thereafter, an operative approach is recommended, particularly if there is a pneumoperitoneum. Surgery should consist of an oversew with omental patch for duodenal ulcers, and excision with primary closure for gastric ulcers. Meticulous peritoneal toilet is required. Although many patients can be successfully managed conservatively initially, the incidence of residual sepsis, requiring intervention, is high and this regimen should be confined to those with severe pre-existing disease.

Diverticular disease (perforation) of the colon

Diverticular disease of the colon remains asymptomatic in 90% of patients. One per cent of patients may suffer from generalized or localized peritonitis secondary to perforation (12). The initial leak may become sealed, resulting in a tender inflammatory mass. Ultrasound or CT examination will confirm abscess formation and, rarely, a water-soluble enema may be required to confirm the leak (13).

Local disease may be treated with intensive supportive measures, broad-spectrum antibiotics, and regular review. Patients with generalized peritonitis require urgent resuscitation and laparotomy. At laparotomy, the length of the involved segment is variable, and the peritonitis may be faecal or purulent. Where local inflammation only is found, any associated sepsis should be eliminated and peritoneal lavage undertaken. Where the peritonitis is faecal, local resection of the affected segment should be performed as either a Hartmann's or a Paul–Mickulicz procedure. Primary anastomosis is not recommended, because of the high risk of subsequent dehiscence.

Approximately 20% of patients with colorectal cancer present with obstruction, and a proportion of these may have localized perforation. The principles of management are as outlined above, but it is important to note that the operation should be as radical in the emergency setting as in the elective. In elective cases, there may be an advantage in performing a proximal diversion alone, with a staged definitive procedure 7–10 days later.

Toxic megacolon occurs in 2–10% of patients with ulcerative colitis. The incidence is influenced by extent of disease and severity of presentation. The transverse colon is the most common site of involvement. Onset is heralded by a deterioration in the patient's general condition and abdominal signs. Initial management is intense medical therapy, with high-dose systemic steroids. In view of the risk of perforation (50–60%), with an associated mortality of 50%, emergency subtotal colectomy with formation of end ileostomy is required if there is no response within 72 h. Spontaneous colonic perforation may also occur in the absence of toxic megacolon and, in the presence of systemic steroid therapy, a high index of suspicion is required.

STOMAS

The stomas most commonly constructed in the emergency setting are the ileostomy and the colostomy. Both may be performed in a loop, split, or end form. The loop and split are variants on a theme. In the latter, the distal bowel is closed or isolated from the proximal limb to ensure complete diversion. Both types may be used to protect an anastomosis or defunction an inflammatory mass or perforation. Construction of an end stoma implies that the distal bowel has been resected. Common examples include an end ileostomy after subtotal colectomy, and an end-colostomy (Hartmann's procedure) after resection of the sigmoid colon. Any remaining distal bowel may be closed and placed in the peritoneal cavity, or brought to the surface as a mucus fistula. In selected patients, after colonic resection, both ends of the colon may be brought out through the same stoma site (Paul–Mickulicz procedure). As in the case of a loop stoma, this allows subsequent closure without re-opening the peritoneal cavity.

When a stoma is being sited, bony landmarks such as the thorax and pelvis should be avoided, with consideration also given to the contact point of clothes and the position of any scars.

The principles of stoma formation are based on accurate mucocutaneous apposition. Eversion is essential for stomas that may leak liquid — such as an ileostomy — to avoid leakage and excoriation. Attachment of the bowel to the parietal peritoneum may reduce the incidence of prolapse, parastomal herniation, and internal herniation. Generally, an ileostomy is considered the procedure of choice, in the absence of a loaded distal colon, because it is associated with greater patient satisfaction and a reduced complication rate (14).

The **complications associated with stoma formation and closure** include:

- skin problems
- incomplete diversion
- prolapse
- retraction
- stenosis
- Parastomal hernia
- internal hernia
- fistulation

References
1. Golledge J, Toms AP, Franklin IJ *et al.* Assessment of peritonism in appendicitis. *Ann R Coll Surg Engl* 1996; **78**: 11–14.
2. Schein M, Assalia A, Bachus H. Minimal antibiotic therapy after emergency abdominal surgery: a prospective study. *Br J Surg* 1994; **81**: 989–991.
3. Suanes C, Salvessen H, Stangeland L. Perforated peptic ulcer over 56 yrs. Time trends in patients and disease characteristics. *Gut* 1993; **34**: 1666–1667.
4. Kronborg, O. Treatment of perforated surgical diverticulitis: a prospective randomised trial. *Br J Surg* 1993; **80**: 505–507.
5. Tudor R, Farmakis N, Keighley MRB. National audit of complicated diverticular disease. Analysis of index cases. *Br J Surg* 1994; **81**: 730–732.
6. Elliott TB, Yego S, Irvin TT. Five year audit of the acute complications of diverticular disease. *Br J Surg* 1997; **84**: 535–538.
7. De Beaux AC, Palmer KR, Carter DC. Factors influencing morbidity and mortality in acute pancreatitis. *Gut* 1995; **37**: 121–126.
8. Neoptolemos JP, Raraty M, Finch M, Stutton R. Acute pancreatitis. The substantial human and financial costs. *Gut* 1998; **42**: 886–891.
9. Glazer G, Mann DV. UK guidelines for the management of acute pancreatitis. *Gut* 1998; **42 (suppl 2)**: 51–13.
10. Windsor ACI, Kanwar S, Li AGK *et al.* Compared with parenteral nutrition, enteral feeding attenuates the acute phase response and unproven disease severity in acute pancreatitis. *Gut* 1998; **42**: 431–435.
11. Powell JJ, Miles R, Siriwardena AK. Antibiotic prophylaxis in the clinical management of severe acute pancreatitis. *Br J Surg* 1998; **85**: 582–587.
12. Senapati A, Marks CG. Management of perforated diverticular disease. *Ann R Coll Surg Engl* 1995; **77**: 161–162.
13. McKee RF, Deigran RW, Krukowski ZH. Radiological investigation in acute diverticulitis. *Br J Surg* 1993; **80**: 560–565.
14. Leong APK, Landono-Schimmer EE, Phillips RK. Life table analysis of stomal complications following ileostomy. *Br J Surg* 1994; **81**: 727–729.

14. Oesophageal Problems

ANTHONY WATSON

Many patients with oesophageal disorders can be managed as outpatients, with the exception of those who present as an emergency, those requiring inpatient assessment, and those undergoing intervention or surgical treatment for their disorder.

Oesophageal disorders that may present as an emergency include acute oesophageal obstruction, oesophageal perforation, oesophageal bleeding, acute inflammatory conditions, and less commonly in the UK, caustic ingestion. Oesophageal bleeding is considered in detail in Chapter 11.2; the remaining conditions will be discussed here. In the category of non-urgent conditions that may require inpatient management, Barrett's oesophagus, oesophageal motility disorders, and carcinoma of the oesophagus will be referred to here, although they are also discussed elsewhere in this volume.

ACUTE OESOPHAGEAL OBSTRUCTION

The many causes of dysphagia are discussed in the next section. Those that may present as acute oesophageal obstruction, include swallowed foreign bodies, acute bolus obstruction and intramural rupture of the oesophagus.

Swallowed foreign bodies

Swallowed foreign bodies occur most commonly in children, the mentally handicapped, or the elderly. Apart from food boluses, swallowed objects are usually solid, such as tablets, coins, marbles, batteries, safety pins, and even dentures in the elderly. The cardinal symptom is dysphagia, often associated with odynophagia (pain on swallowing). If obstruction is complete, the patient may have difficulty even in swallowing saliva. Occasionally, small objects may pass through the oesophagus, particularly after drinking.

Treatment

If the foreign body is small, spontaneous passage through the oesophagus may have occurred by the time the patient reaches hospital, or it may be induced by taking a carbonated drink. If not, endoscopy should be performed, although when a sharp foreign body has been swallowed, it is wise to precede this with a chest X-ray to exclude perforation. Fibreoptic endoscopy is preferable, as it affords a better view and is associated with a lower risk of perforation, although instruments for the retrieval of foreign bodies that will pass through the biopsy channel of a fibreoptic endoscope are smaller than those that can be passed at rigid endoscopy. If the swallowed object is sharp or pointed, an endoscope overtube may be passed to avoid damage to the oesophageal wall during extraction. Foreign bodies may be grasped and recovered by using grasping forceps, snares, or baskets; specially designed accessories for removing coins are available. In children, it may be preferable to perform endoscopy under general anaesthesia.

Acute bolus obstruction

In addition to ingested foreign bodies, food boluses may produce acute oesophageal obstruction. Although this may occur in an entirely normal oesophagus, as a consequence of swallowing an inadequately chewed large food bolus, it occurs most frequently in the presence of oesophageal pathology. Any of the conditions that cause dysphagia (see Chapter 29) may increase the likelihood of a relatively normal-sized food bolus causing obstruction. In practice, this is most common in patients with carcinoma of the oesophagus, an oesophageal stricture, or a motility disorder. It may also occur in patients who have an oesophageal endoprosthesis, particularly with the Atkinson or Celestin types — rather than the more recently introduced self-expanding metallic stents — on account of their relatively small internal diameter.

Clinical features

In addition to dysphagia, complete oesophageal obstruction by a swallowed food bolus can result in severe oesophageal pain. This is usually felt retrosternally, but may radiate to the back, jaws and even to the left arm, and may be so severe as to mimic an acute myocardial infarction. However, the close temporal relationship to eating, together with the associated dysphagia, usually helps distinguish between the two. If the oesophageal obstruction is complete, the patient may be unable to swallow their own saliva, which is particularly distressing.

Treatment

Once the diagnosis is established, if the oesophageal obstruction does not appear to be complete, it is worth the patient trying to ingest a carbonated drink. This may occasionally result in passage of the bolus into the stomach; more usually, endoscopic dissimpaction is necessary. The impacted food bolus may occasionally be withdrawn using a basket or balloon but, if not, it may be pushed onwards into the stomach using a balloon or plastic dilator. If a diagnosis has not been previously made, biopsy examination of any narrowing or suspicious area should be performed, and the opportunity may be taken to perform an endoscopic dilatation, should an organic stricture be present. If a bolus obstruction has occurred in the presence of an oesophageal endoprosthesis, it is important to establish that tumour overgrowth or tube displacement has not contributed to the problem.

Intramural haematoma of the oesophagus

Rapid increases in intraoesophageal pressure — such as during vomiting, particularly against a closed glottis, during violent coughing and, occasionally, during epileptic seizures or status asthmaticus — may result in a variety of traumatic lesions to the oesophagus. The most common is the Mallory–Weiss syndrome, which results in a distal mucosal tear, presenting as haematemesis. Diagnosis is by endoscopy, and conservative treatment, in terms of fluid replacement and a "nil-by-mouth" regimen, is usually all that is required. In a small proportion of patients, bleeding may continue, in which case local injection with noradrenaline, embolization, or even surgical under-running of the bleeding vessel may be required.

Less commonly, sudden increases in intraoesophageal pressure may result in an intramural, as opposed to a mucosal, tear and, particularly in patients with a coagulopathy, this may result in a large intramural haematoma (1). If this is extensive, it may result in an intramural dissection of the oesophagus, which may result in a mucosal breach in relation to the proximal or distal ends of the dissection, and occasionally both. In these circumstances, the condition is known as intramural rupture of the oesophagus, but is distinguished from a Boerhaave's syndrome (see below) in that there is no perforation through the oesophageal wall and into the mediastinum.

Clinical features

Intramural haematoma and intramural rupture of the oesophagus usually present with severe retrosternal pain — and occasionally, epigastric pain — associated with dysphagia and odynophagia. The pain may be very severe, radiating to the back, jaws, and left arm, and may mimic myocardial infarction or aortic dissection. The intramural bulging as a result of the haematoma results in significant dysphagia, which may be complete. Diagnosis may be made by barium swallow, endoscopy, or computed tomography (CT) scanning. If the mucosa is breached, barium swallow will reveal the characteristic double-barrelled appearance because of the false passage. Endoscopy will reveal the intramural bulging into the lumen and the haematoma may be visible, as may associated breaches of the mucosa. CT scan best demonstrates the grossly thickened oesophageal wall with intraluminal narrowing, caused by the haematoma.

Treatment

Despite the often dramatic presentation of this condition, it invariably resolves on conservative treatment. This comprises analgesia, fluid replacement, and a "nil-by-mouth" regimen until the swelling resolves, which may take 10–14 days. Parenteral nutrition may be considered in these circumstances. Progress of the haematoma may be monitored by any of the diagnostic modalities referred to above.

OESOPHAGEAL PERFORATION AND RUPTURE

Perforation of the oesophagus may occur either spontaneously (Boerhaave's syndrome) or as a result of iatrogenic perforation during diagnostic or therapeutic endoscopy. Although both are potentially serious events, there are significant differences in outcome and management, because a spontaneous perforation usually occurs with the stomach full and diagnosis is frequently delayed, whereas instrumental perforation invariably occurs in a fasting patient and diagnosis is often made rapidly, as the patient is under medical supervision at the time of the occurrence. It is therefore appropriate to discuss these two conditions separately.

Spontaneous rupture of the oesophagus (Boerhaave's syndrome)

This condition is relatively uncommon, but serious and potentially fatal (2). Because of its relative infrequency, an accurate and early diagnosis — which is essential to ensure any prospect of survival — depends on awareness of the existence of the condition and of its classical and dramatic clinical presentation. It is usually caused by vomiting against a closed glottis, and is particularly common after excessive alcohol ingestion. During vomiting, the oesophagus develops very high intraluminal pressures, such that its diameter may increase up to fourfold, but release of this normally occurs rapidly

as the cricopharyngeus relaxes. In Boerhaave's syndrome, cricopharyngeal relaxation does not occur, and the oesophagus usually ruptures at its weakest point, which is the extreme lower end on the left side. Occasionally, perforation occurs in the middle one-third of the oesophagus, in which case it is usually on the right side, and more rarely at the site of a Barrett's ulcer or carcinoma. The perforation is usually long, between 1 and 4 cm. As the stomach is invariably full, gastric contents rupture the overlying pleura and rapidly contaminate the pleural cavity.

Clinical features

At the time of rupture, which typically follows an episode of vomiting, excruciating pain is felt retrosternally, frequently in the upper abdomen and usually with interscapula radiation. The pain is so severe that often pethidine and even opiates fail to relieve it, and a diagnosis of myocardial infarction or dissecting aneurysm is frequently made. Physical examination shows the patient to be dyspnoeic, shocked, and cyanosed. Marked epigastric tenderness and rigidity are usually present and, subsequently, surgical emphysema in the neck is evident. Signs of a hydropneumothorax may take several hours to develop.

Diagnosis

Early diagnosis is crucial to the outcome of treatment. Delay in diagnosis may occur if management is instituted inappropriately for myocardial infarction, dissecting aneurysm, or gastroduodenal perforation. Chest X-ray may show only minimal changes immediately after perforation, but within a few hours the presence of air and fluid in the pleural cavity becomes evident. On suspicion of the diagnosis, an emergency gastrografin swallow should be performed both to confirm the diagnosis and to identify the site and size of the perforation, together with any coexisting oesophageal pathology.

Treatment

Early operation after appropriate resuscitation offers the best chance of survival. Ideally, the diagnosis should be made and confirmed, the patient resuscitated, and surgery commenced within 6 h. After this time, the metabolic effects on the patient and the increasing fragility of the oesophageal wall (compromising its ability to heal) make survival progressively less likely.

Lower oesophageal perforations are best approached through a left thoracotomy, and middle-third perforations through a right thoracotomy. If the perforation is relatively early and the margins of the tear appear viable, then closure of the perforation, which may be augmented by adjacent pleura, pericardium, or diaphragm, is appropriate, together with intrapleural drainage, antibiotics, and enteral or parenteral nutrition until a contrast swallow 7–10 days later has demonstrated healing. In late cases in which the extent of contamination is severe and the margins of the perforation may not be viable, the alternatives are drainage, with a cervical oesophagostomy and a gastrostomy, or transhiatal oesophagectomy. The mortality for cases diagnosed and treated within 6–12 h is 10–15%, but this increases to more than 50% for those diagnosed and treated after this time.

Instrumental perforation of the oesophagus

Perforation during diagnostic fibre-optic endoscopy is relatively uncommon, reported rates being between 0.1 and 0.5%. The rate is greater with the use of the rigid oesophagoscope, which is still used by some ear, nose, and throat, and thoracic surgeons. The most common site of perforation is in the proximal oesophagus, associated either with an osteoarthritic cervical spine, resulting in compression of the cervical oesophagus by osteophytes, or with the presence of a pharyngeal pouch, in which case it is common for the endoscope to enter the pouch preferentially. Perforation at other sites is uncommon.

The increasing range of therapeutic endoscopic procedures of the oesophagus has resulted in an increased risk of perforation. Dilatation of benign strictures is associated with a perforation risk of 1–2%, either as a result of direct rupture at the site of the stricture, or caused by passage of the guide-wire distally without the benefit of direct vision, if this form of dilatation is used. In balloon dilatation for achalasia, because of the high pressures used, the risk of perforation increases to around 5%. Dilatation and intubation of carcinomatous strictures carry the greatest perforation risk, which is of the order of 10% for intubation using a semi-rigid system such as the Nottingham introducer, although the risk is proving to be considerably less with the use of self-expanding metal stents, because of the very fine, soft delivery systems.

Clinical features

The clinical features of endoscopic perforation of the oesophagus are less dramatic than those of spontaneous rupture. Contamination is often minimal, as the perforation is usually small, the patient is fasted, and sterilized equipment is used. Furthermore, sedation administered before or during endoscopy often masks the appearance of symptoms. Perforation may be apparent to the endoscopist at the time of endoscopy or therapeutic procedure, or it may become apparent by the appearance of surgical emphysema in the neck. The patient rarely complains of pain at the time, because of the sedation, although tachycardia or cyanosis during the procedure may arouse suspicion. If the diagnosis is not made at the time of endoscopy, pain may be a feature, particularly after swallowing, which may be felt retrosternally or in the back as the patient recovers from the sedation.

Diagnosis

The diagnosis should be suspected in the presence of any of the above clinical features, particularly if a therapeutic procedure has been performed. If perforation is suspected, a contrast swallow is recommended, both to confirm or refute the suspected diagnosis, and to indicate the size and site of the perforation.

Treatment

The relatively small size and limited contamination associated with endoscopic perforations means that conservative treatment is more likely to be successful than in the case of Boerhaave's syndrome (2). If the patient's general condition is good and the perforation less than 1 cm in length on gastrografin swallow, it is worth an initial trial of conservative treatment, which should include a "nil-by-mouth" regimen, broad-spectrum antibiotics, and parenteral feeding. Oral feeding should be withheld until a contrast swallow, usually on the 5th day, has confirmed healing of the perforation. If the patient's condition appears to deteriorate, either as a result of sustaining a perforation or during conservative treatment, or if the initial perforation is greater than 1 cm in size, surgical repair should be performed by a cervical or transthoracic approach, depending on the level. As such lesions are usually diagnosed early and contamination is minimal, simple closure is usually all that is required, together with postoperative antibiotics, withholding of oral fluids, and parenteral nutrition, until a contrast swallow has demonstrated healing.

In the absence of oesophageal carcinoma, the mortality from instrumental perforation is relatively low, at 5% or less. In the presence of carcinoma, mortality is invariably greater, and approaches 50%, partly because of the indication for intubation, either poor general condition or an extensive tumour, and because simple closure is less likely to be successful. In these circumstances, management options include the insertion of an occlusive prosthesis, such as a Cook tube to close over the site of the perforation, or, preferably, the insertion of a covered self-expanding metallic stent.

CORROSIVE INJURY OF THE OESOPHAGUS

Corrosive injuries of the oesophagus are relatively uncommon in Britain compared with rates in many other countries (3). They are usually caused by ingestion of caustic alkaline substances, but occasionally by a strong acid; caustic alkaline agents are most commonly present in bleach and other household cleaning agents. Ingestion is accidental in the case of children but, in adults, such substances are usually ingested in attempted suicide. Caustic substances result in coagulative necrosis of the oesophageal mucosa, with penetration into the muscular layers if the agent is particularly strong or contact time is prolonged. Healing gradually ensues by granulation tissue with a varying degree of epithelialization, but there is inevitably considerable scarring.

Clinical features

The clinical features are quite dramatic, with pain in the chest, mouth, and pharynx. Odynophagia and dysphagia rapidly supervene, and there may be epigastric pain and vomiting as the stomach becomes affected. On examination, the patient is distressed and shocked, with excessive salivation; mucosal damage to the mouth and lips is frequently present at an early stage.

Treatment

Immediate management should be directed towards exclusion of perforation, and the ingestion of a buffer agent in an attempt to neutralize the toxic agent. Analgesics should be given parenterally and fluid replacement commenced. As soon as is feasible, the extent of injury to the pharynx, oesophagus, and stomach should be assessed by gentle fibreoptic endoscopy.

In the rare instances of perforation or gastric necrosis, surgical intervention is mandatory, in the form of oesophagectomy together with cervical oesophagotomy and gastrotomy if the stomach is intact, or gastrectomy and jejunotomy if the stomach is necrotic. The initial aim is to save life and then to plan colonic replacement once full recovery has ensued. Fortunately, the majority of cases can be managed conservatively, with a "nil-by-mouth" regimen and parenteral nutritional support. Both corticosteroids and antibiotics are frequently given, although their value is not proven. Mild cases may recover fully after such measures, but more commonly, a varying degree of stricture formation is present and repeated dilatations are often needed. Unfortunately, many strictures are long and resistant to dilatation, in which case elective oesophageal resection with colon interposition becomes necessary.

BARRETT'S OESOPHAGUS

Barrett's oesophagus is characterized by **replacement of the squamous lining of the distal oesophagus for a variable length by a columnar-lined epithelium**. It occurs as a complication of gastro-oesophageal reflux disease in approximately 12% of patients, in whom, as a result of destruction of the squamous lining in the distal oesophagus, a columnar metaplasia occurs by differentiation of totipotential stem cells into an acid-resistant mucosa, which may resemble gastric mucosa or intestinal mucosa, with goblet cells present; this is known as intestinal metaplasia. The importance of Barrett's oesophagus is that it is a pre-malignant lesion, resulting in adenocarcinoma of the oesophagus or cardia in approximately 10% of cases overall. Over the past two decades, adenocarcinoma of the oesophagus and cardia has increased dramatically in incidence, and whereas adenocarcinoma used to account for fewer than 10% of oesophageal tumours, it now accounts for around 50% in most specialist units, the incidence of this tumour increasing more rapidly than that of any other malignancy in the Western world.

Barrett's oesophagus is visible endoscopically as a salmon-pink mucosa — in contrast to the pale pink squamous lining — which is usually circumferential, although in the early stages it may occur as distinct tongues extending for 1 or 2 cm into the lower oesophagus. **Accurate diagnosis requires careful endoscopic documentation of the location of the gastrooesophageal junction, the squamocolumnar junction, and the diaphragmatic crura.** The length of the columnarized segment may vary from 1 to 2 cm — in the so-called short-segment Barrett's oesophagus — to 10 cm or more. Until relatively recently, the diagnosis of Barrett's oesophagus has been restricted to the presence of at least 3 cm of circumferential columnarization, above the normal squamocolumnar junction, or "Z-line", to allow for the normal variation in the position of the Z-line, the presence of junctional epithelium, and the difficulty in precise location of the oesophagogastric junction. Recent studies have shown, however, that patients with short tongues of columarization or short-segment Barrett's, are at risk of malignant transformation, although the risk is substantially less than that of the traditionally defined "long-segment" Barrett's oesophagus (3). Recent histological studies of biopsy specimens from the apparently normal squamocolumnar junction of patients undergoing upper gastrointestinal endoscopy have shown that 18% show intestinal metaplasia, this proportion increasing to 36% if alcian blue staining is used. Confusion has arisen as a result of this finding also being referred to as "short-segment Barrett's", because macroscopically there is no columnarization, no malignant risk has been established, and the aetiology is controversial, age and *Helicobacter pylori* infection being supported more strongly than a reflux aetiology. Until more is known about this condition, it is wisest to refer to it descriptively as "microscopic intestinal metaplasia of the cardia". The differing characteristics of long- and short-segment Barrett's oesophagus and microscopic intestinal metaplasia at the cardia are shown in Figure 14.1 and Table 14.1.

Pathophysiology of Barrett's oesophagus and malignant transformation

Comparative studies of patients with Barrett's oesophagus and those with erosive oesophagitis show that the former have a greater incidence of lower oesophageal sphincter failure (90% or more) and of oesophageal body peristaltic failure (70% or more), and greater levels of oesophageal exposure to acid and to alkali, as measured by Bilitec monitoring. There is also a significant impairment of mucosal sensitivity to perfusion with acid in Barrett's patients compared with that in patients with erosive oesophagitis. It is apparent, therefore, that patients with Barrett's oesophagus are at the extreme end of the spectrum of patients with gastrooesophageal reflux disease. In these circumstances, one might expect that patients with Barrett's oesophagus have a long history of significant reflux symptoms, before developing their columnar metaplasia. However, this is the case in only a minority of patients, because of the impairment of mucosal sensitivity. Many patients with Barrett's oesophagus, therefore, have very little in the way of symptoms and, occasionally, Barrett's oesophagus is diagnosed during endoscopy for other indications, without any previous history suggestive of reflux. A small proportion of patients have reflux symptoms for some time and suddenly experience spontaneous resolution of their symptoms as a result of columnar metaplasia of the lower oesophagus. It is believed to take at least 10 years from the onset of gastrooesophageal reflux disease to the development of Barrett's oesophagus, although this progression is by no means an inevitability, because of the differing natural history of gastrooesophageal reflux disease. A study from the Mayo Clinic many years ago (4) showed that, in patients with endoscopic oesophagitis, the condition resolved in 35% of patients, decreased in severity in a further 17%, persisted in 20%, and progressed in 28%. It is this last group of patients, who are most at risk of progression and have the more severe pathophysiological profile, who are at greatest risk of developing Barrett's oesophagus. Interestingly, studies of patients with short-segment Barrett's oesophagus have shown that the pathophysiological profile is intermediate between that associated with uncomplicated gastrooesophageal reflux disease and Barrett's oesophagus.

As regards **malignant transformation**, this process also takes up to 10 years in susceptible individuals. Surveillance programmes suggest that the mean individual risk of development of adenocarcinoma is around 1:72 patient years of follow-up, or

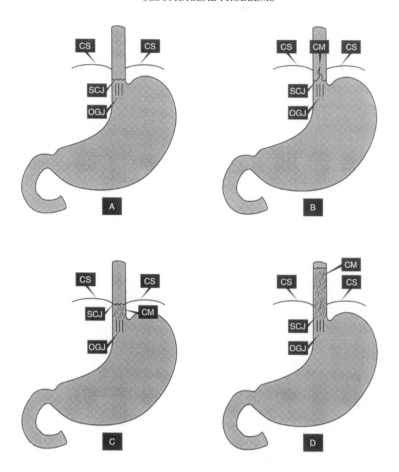

Figure 14.1. The relative relationships between the oesophagogastric junction (OGJ: the upper limit of gastric rugal folds), the squamocolumnar junction (SCJ) and the diaphragmatic crural sling (CS) in the normal situation, and the area of columnarization of the mucosa (CM) in the varying types of Barrett's oesophagus.

(A) **The normal situation**. The oesophagogastric junction is regarded as the point at which the tubular oesophagus flares open to join the stomach, which normally coincides with the proximal limit of the gastric rugal folds. The squamocolumnar junction is normally a few millimetres proximal to this and the crural sling 2–3 cm proximal, unless there is a hiatus hernia. These macroscopic appearances will pertain in patients who have microscopic intestinal metaplasia at the cardia. (B) A "tongue" of **columnarization**, which is confluent but not circumferential. (C) **Short-segment Barrett's oesophagus**, in which the columnarization is confluent and circumferential, although the length of the columnarized segment is less than 3 cm. (D) **Traditional long-segment Barrett's oesophagus**, in which the circumferential columnarization exceeds 3 cm in length.

Table 14.1. The differing characteristics of traditionally defined long-segment Barrett's oesophagus, short-segment Barrett's and microscopic intestinal metaplasia at the cardia.

	Traditional (>3 cm)	Short-segment (<3 cm)	Intestinal metaplasia at cardia
Prevalence (%)	1–3	8–17	18–36
Gastrooesophageal reflux disease	++	+	?
Malignant potential	++	+	?

+, present; ++, present with a higher incidence; ?, unknown

approximately 1.5% per annum overall. However, risk factors have been identified, including the presence of intestinal metaplasia, the length of the columnarized segment — and particularly a length greater than 7 cm — in White men, in smokers, in those with a mixed acid and alkaline refluxate, and in those who develop Barrett's oesophagus at a relatively young age. The process of malignant transformation is a multistep one whereby normal epithelium, possibly in a genetically susceptible individual, passes through the stages of a hyperproliferative epithelium as a result of the action of environmental agents such as acid, bile and tobacco, through columnar metaplasia and, as a result of a series of heterogeneous genetic events progresses to low-grade and then high-grade dysplasia. As the final transition to invasive adenocarcinoma occurs, there is an interaction between mitogens (epidermal growth factor family) and cell adhesion molecules (cadherin and catenin). Whereas low-grade dysplasia may regress, high-grade dysplasia almost inevitably results in invasive adenocarcinoma, and, indeed, by the time high-grade dysplasia has been detected by endoscopic biopsy, a focus of invasive adenocarcinoma is already present in some 40% of patients.

Clinical features

As discussed previously, Barrett's oesophagus is frequently not associated with a significant antecedent reflux history, although it may be diagnosed in some patients with a long history of reflux disease, and particularly the short-segment variety. Sometimes, the occurrence of complications of Barrett's oesophagus — namely stricture, ulcer, or adenocarcinoma — may be the first indication of the precursor lesion. Indeed, the vast majority of oesophageal strictures resulting from reflux disease occurring in the mid or upper oesophagus are associated with Barrett's oesophagus, as reflux-induced strictures tend to occur at the squamocolumnar junction, wherever that may be.

Diagnosis is by fibreoptic endoscopy. In patients with circumferential columnar metaplasia, the transition between the salmon-pink columnar lining and the pale pink squamous lining is apparent, usually with a regular line of demarcation. Diagnostic doubt may arise in the case of short-segment Barrett's oesophagus or tongues of columnarization, and it may be difficult to distinguish the former from a normal squamocolumnar junction or Z-line. The normal oesophagogastric junction is visible endoscopically at the point at which the tubular oesophagus flares to form the oesophagogastric junction, and is marked by the upper limit of the gastric rugal folds. A presumed diagnosis should always be confirmed histologically, and it is the identification of intestinal metaplasia with goblet cells that, par excellence, identifies Barrett's oesophagus and, particularly, the form of columnar metaplasia that has malignant potential.

Treatment

The management of patients with Barrett's oesophagus is a complex issue, which encompasses the primary management of uncomplicated Barrett's oesophagus, surveillance to detect early malignant transformation, and treatment of complications of Barrett's, such as ulcer, stricture and high-grade dysplasia.

Treatment of uncomplicated Barrett's oesophagus
There is no consensus on the most appropriate management of uncomplicated Barrett's oesophagus. Treatment options that are practised include no treatment in the absence of symptoms (despite the fact that there are good pathophysiological reasons why many Barrett's patients do not have symptoms), acid suppression therapy, endoscopic ablation and anti-reflux surgery. Although there is some knowledge about the influence of these modalities on the natural history of the columnarized segment, the influence on the risk of development of adenocarcinoma is currently unknown.

Acid suppression therapy with proton pump inhibitors may produce symptomatic improvement in those patients who have symptoms, although studies have shown that symptomatic improvement does not correlate with normalization of acid exposure in patients with Barrett's oesophagus. Indeed, several studies have reported the difficulty of normalizing acid exposure in Barrett's patients, using doses of omeprazole up to even 80 mg daily (5). This is likely to relate to the previously mentioned pathophysiology of this group of patients, with high levels of acid exposure in association with both lower oesophageal sphincter and peristaltic failure in the majority of patients. Furthermore, acid suppression therapy does not normalize alkaline exposure, as measured by Bilitec monitoring, although it does reduce the degree of exposure to abnormal bilirubin, presumably by a volume-reducing effect. Seven investigative series have examined the reduction in length of the columnarized segment by proton pump inhibitors, and only one of these series reported a small reduction, the others showing no change. It remains to be seen whether titrating the dose of proton pump inhibitor until acid exposure has been normalized will result in different findings.

Endoscopic ablation of the columnarized segment with laser, photodynamic therapy, thermocoagulation, or using an argon-beam plasma coagulator have been deployed in combination with acid suppression therapy or anti-reflux surgery in recent years. Each of these modalities has been shown to result in squamous regrowth, although there is a risk of complications, principally stricture and haemorrhage after photodynamic therapy, and perforation with laser therapy or argon-beam plasma coagulation. Several series have, however, shown residual areas of intestinal metaplasia deep to the neo-squamous lining in up to 60% of patients (6). Clearly, they still retain malignant potential and, indeed, high-grade dysplasia and malignancy have been reported. Furthermore, these areas are relatively inaccessible to biopsy and there is the theoretical risk that neoplasia may be detected at a later stage. For these reasons, the place of endoscopic ablation in the management of Barrett's oesophagus remains controversial.

Anti-reflux surgery has been associated with partial or complete regression of Barrett's oesophagus in a large number of series, the proportion of patients in whom this occurs ranging from 10–40%. Two separate studies have shown that anti-reflux surgery appears to have a more beneficial influence on the natural history of the columnarized segment than has acid suppression therapy, with a greater rate of healing of existing strictures, a lower rate of development of new strictures, a lower incidence of progression, and a greater incidence of regression of the columnarized segment (7). These factors are likely to relate to ability of anti-reflux surgery to correct lower oesophageal sphincter failure, to enable total and continuous normalization of acid exposure and of alkaline exposure. Despite this, however, the development of adenocarcinoma has been reported after successful anti-reflux surgery. It seems likely that, in order to have a beneficial influence on the incidence of adenocarcinoma, anti-reflux surgery must be performed sufficiently early within the multistep process of genomic instability. A more recent study from the Mayo Clinic (8) reported 113 patients with Barrett's oesophagus who were followed for up to 18 years after anti-reflux surgery, on a surveillance programme. Although three patients developed adenocarcinoma, the malignancies all occurred within the first 3 years, after which no carcinomas developed. The incidence in this series was 1:274 patient years of follow-up, which is some four times lower than the mean incidence reported from surveillance programmes of patients treated by acid suppression therapy.

At present, acid suppression therapy, endoscopic ablation, and anti-reflux surgery are utilized depending on personal preference, with no knowledge as to which is the most effective in reducing the incidence of adenocarcinoma. In order to answer this question, an international prospective randomized study of proton pump inhibition and anti-reflux surgery, with or without endoscopic ablation, is being launched as a joint initiative between the Oesophageal Section of the British Society of Gastroenterology and the UK Medical Research Council.

Surveillance
The rationale for surveillance of patients with Barrett's oesophagus is that the condition is undoubtedly a pre-malignant lesion, the detection of high-grade dysplasia identifies tumours at an early stage, and the survival after resection of such lesions is much more favourable than that in patients in whom the condition is detected clinically. Of those tumours detected in surveillance programmes, some 75% are early, node-negative lesions; 5 year survival after resection of such tumours is about 80%, compared with 20% after resection of clinically detected tumours. Notwithstanding these factors, the role of surveillance remains controversial in the UK, because of the cost and labour-intensive nature of surveillance programmes, and the fact that only approximately 3% of patients with Barrett's oesophagus actually die from adenocarcinoma, the majority dying from other causes. However, investigators in several series have concluded that the cost of detecting adenocarcinoma by surveillance programmes is not dissimilar to that in other screening programmes, such as for breast or colorectal cancers.

The current recommendations for surveillance programmes include surveillance endoscopy every 2 years in general, but annually in high-risk patients and in the presence of low-grade dysplasia (9). Biopsies should be taken from four quadrants of the oesophageal wall at 2-cm intervals, together with any raised or suspicious lesion. As there is a certain degree of subjectivity in the diagnosis of high-grade dysplasia, it is recommended that this should be confirmed by two independent pathologists. If there is still doubt, biopsies should be repeated after a 1-month course of high-dose proton pump inhibitor, to exclude the effect of inflammatory change. Other potential markers of malignant potential, such as aneuplody, sulphamucin staining, ornithine de-carboxylase, and expression of *p53* and *APC* genes have not proved as reliable as high-grade dysplasia, which does have the disadvantages of subjectivity, dependence on the site of biopsy, and the fact that, by the time high-grade dysplasia is present, a focus of invasive adenocarcinoma exists in some 40% of patients. Attempts to overcome these problems include the use of optical techniques such as laser-induced fluorescence spectroscopy to facilitate the precise identification of areas of high-grade dysplasia at an early stage. It is anticipated that, ultimately, accurate molecular markers will be identified.

Management of high-grade dysplasia
Currently, majority opinion favours prophylactic oesophagectomy once a diagnosis of high-grade dysplasia has been convincingly made by two independent pathologists, assuming that the patient is fit to undergo surgery. As indicated previously, 5-year survival in this group of patients is excellent and, because these patients are normally relatively healthy and well-nourished, morbidity and mortality after oesophagectomy are considerably less than those associated with resection of clinically detected tumours, operative mortality being 2% or less. If the patient is unfit for surgery, then endoscopic ablation of the area or areas of high-grade dysplasia should be performed by either laser photocoagulation or photodynamic therapy. The results are generally less good than after oesophagectomy, as some 20% of surveillance-detected tumours have nodal metastases, and it is for this reason that these modalities should not be used a primary treatment in otherwise healthy patients.

Management of ulcer and stricture
Barrett's ulcer may cause pain or bleeding, and should be managed by high-dose proton pump inhibitors after biopsy has excluded neoplasia. In the event of failure to respond, which occurs in a greater proportion of these patients than in uncomplicated gastrooesophageal reflux, anti-reflux surgery is indicated.

Reflux stricture should be managed initially by proton pump inhibitors and endoscopic dilatation, which should be repeated as necessary, assuming malignancy has been excluded by biopsy and brush cytology. Anti-reflux surgery has been shown to reduce dilatation requirements in several series, and if frequent dilatations are required, and for reflux stricture in young patients, anti-reflux surgery is indicated. The vast majority of reflux strictures can be managed by these means, and nowadays resection is rarely necessary.

ACHALASIA AND OTHER OESOPHAGEAL MOTILITY DISORDERS

Oesophageal motility disorders may be classified into those that occur as a primary phenomenon, and those that are secondary to other conditions, such as scleroderma, other collagen disorders, diabetes mellitus, myasthenia gravis, cerebrovascular disorders, Chagas' disease, and gastrooesophageal reflux. They may be further classified according to the part of the oesophagus predominantly involved — for example, cricopharyngeal spasm and Zenker's diverticulum, affecting primarily the upper oesophageal sphincter; hypertensive and hypotensive lower oesophageal sphincter; and "nutcracker" oesophagus and diffuse oesophageal spasm, predominantly involving the oesophageal body. This is not entirely satisfactory, as conditions such as achalasia and non-specific motility disorder may involve both the oesophageal body and the lower oesophageal sphincter, and there is frequently transition with time from one type of disorder to another.

Achalasia

Achalasia is a disorder of unknown aetiology, characterized by aperistalsis of the body of the oesophagus, impairment of relaxation of the lower oesophageal sphincter, and frequently, a high resting lower oesophageal sphincter pressure. The combined effect of these factors is to produce a functional obstruction at the lower end of the oesophagus, causing stasis of food and progressive dilation of the oesophagus.

Aetiology and pathophysiology

Infection with a neuropathic virus and an auto-immune process have been postulated as being involved in the aetiology of achalasia, although the exact cause is unknown. Pathological studies have shown that there is degeneration of and a reduction in the numbers of ganglion cells in the Auerbach's plexus of the lower oesophageal sphincter and in the oesophageal body. Abnormalities have also been seen in the vagal dorsal motor nucleus and in vagal nerve fibres. It appears to be the non-adrenergic, non-cholinergic inhibitory intrinsic innervation that is impaired, which is believed to mediate sphincter relaxation. Cholinergic neurones seems to be preserved, which may be responsible for the high resting lower oesophageal sphincter pressure in achalasia. In early cases, it is predominantly the lower oesophageal sphincter that is principally affected, although there may be mild changes affecting the oesophageal body in the lower one-third, with low-amplitude, simultaneous contractions. In severe cases, aperistalsis may occur in the lower two-thirds of the oesophagus, although relatively normal primary peristalsis may be present in the upper one-third. The chronic stagnation of food within the dilated, atonic oesophagus is believed to be a contributory factor to the increased incidence of malignancy in achalasia, which is approximately 5%.

Clinical features

Achalasia can occur at any age, ranging from childhood to old age, although its greatest incidence is in individuals between the ages of 30 and 50 years. It affects both sexes equally. The predominant symptom is dysphagia, which in the early stages may be intermittent. However, it gradually becomes progressive, although it is usually more marked for solids than liquids. The intermittent nature of the dysphagia and the long history are in distinction to those associated with carcinoma of the oesophagus, which is relentlessly progressive over a relatively short period. Regurgitation of food and, occasionally, frank vomiting occur because of hold-up in the dilated oesophagus.

Diagnosis

The diagnosis is made on the basis of the history, together with radiological, endoscopic, and manometric findings. **Chest X-ray** may show a mediastinal shadow caused by the dilated oesophagus, which often contains an air/fluid level. The normal gas bubble in the stomach may be absent, and in some patients pulmonary changes are evident because of recurrent aspiration. Barium swallow is the mainstay of radiological diagnosis; it shows a dilated, atonic oesophagus with poor or absent peristalsis — best seen on cine-radiography. The lower end of the oesophagus shows a charac-

teristic smooth, tapered narrowing exhibiting a typical "rat tail" appearance. This smooth, distal narrowing without evidence of hiatal hernia or reflux usually enables achalasia to be distinguished from carcinomatous or reflux-induced stricture, but doubt may occasionally be expressed by radiologists, making further investigation mandatory.

Endoscopy is necessary in any patient in whom narrowing is demonstrated radiologically. The classical endoscopic feature of achalasia is the ability to pass the endoscope easily through the lower oesophageal sphincter into the stomach in a patient in whom a barium swallow has suggested complete or virtually complete obstruction. The oesophagus may be seen to be dilated and aperistaltic at endoscopy, and if it has attained a sigmoid configuration, entry into the stomach may be somewhat difficult because of the convoluted shape, rather than any organic narrowing. Any suspicious area should undergo biopsy examiniation because, rarely a stenosing adenocarcinoma can present in a manner similar to achalasia — the so-called pseudoachalasia.

Manometry is the most accurate way of making a firm positive diagnosis. The resting lower oesophageal sphincter pressure is usually increased above the upper limit of normality of 20 mmHg and frequently is in excess of 30 mmHg. Sphincter relaxation after swallowing is incomplete or absent. The oesophageal body, particularly in the lower two-thirds, shows weak amplitude contractions that are usually simultaneous and non-propagated. Once the oesophagus becomes dilated, these contractions are of extremely low amplitude and may become undetectable, although relatively normal peristalsis may be present in the upper oesophagus.

Treatment

The **aim of treatment** is to relieve the functional obstruction at the lower oesophageal sphincter sufficiently to allow the feeble oesophageal contractions to propel food into the stomach, but insufficiently to allow gastrooesophageal reflux to occur. The principal treatment modalities are pharmacological, dilatation, or surgical cardiomyotomy.

Pharmacological treatment comprises the use of drugs that reduce the lower oesophageal sphincter pressure. These include anti-cholinergics agents such as dicyclomine hydrochloride, long-acting nitrates such as isosorbide dinitrate, and calcium-channel blocking drugs such nifedipine or verapamil. In general, pharmacological treatment is unsatisfactory, as the effect is short-lived and all the drugs, when used in doses sufficient to have a sustained effect, result in side effects, principally headache.

Botulinum toxin injection has been used in recent years, as it blocks the presynaptic release of acetylcholine at the neuromuscular junction. Studies have shown that intrasphincteric administration of botulinum toxin decreases lower oesophageal sphincter pressure in patients with achalasia, which results in significant symptomatic improvement in more than 60% of them. Unfortunately, the effect is relatively short-lived. Repeated injections are necessary at 6–12 month intervals (10).

Dilatation for achalasia has taken many forms over the years, but is currently most frequently performed using a Rigiflex balloon which is available in 30, 35 and 40 mm diameters. It is generally recommended that treatment be commenced with the smallest balloon, as the risk of perforation is smaller, progressing to the larger balloon in the event of a poor or short-lived response to dilatation. The ballons are passed over an endoscopically placed guide-wire, ideally under fluoroscopic control, and connected to a manometer. Inflation is performed to a pressure of approximately 69 kPa (10 p.s.i.) and is maintained for 1–2 min. A good symptomatic response is achieved in 60–70% of patients, although the duration of this response is variable between several weeks and 1 or 2 years. Complications of pneumatic dilatation include perforation, with an incidence of 1–5%, and gastrooesophageal reflux, with an incidence of about 8% (11).

Surgical treatment is the most effective form of management, and consists of cardiomyotomy, involving division of the circular and longitudinal muscle in the region of the lower oesophageal sphincter down to the submucosa. It is effective in more than 90% of patients, with documented decreasing of the resting lower oesophageal sphincter pressure, restoration of normal lower oesophageal sphincter relaxation, and improvement in oesophageal body motility in approximately 30% of patients (11). Gastrooesophageal reflux may occur in up to 10% of patients, particularly if the procedure is performed transabdominally, and many surgeons perform a prophylactic anti-reflux procedure because of this. Cardiomyotomy can now be performed by a minimally invasive approach, either laparoscopically or thoracoscopically, with results similar to those achieved by open surgery, but with a more rapid convalescence. In many centres, minimally invasive cardiomyotomy is becoming the treatment of choice.

A **practical approach** to the management of patients with achalasia is to try pneumatic dilatation initially, as the response is variable and there are no good predictors of success. If the response to a single dilatation is good, or dilatation intervals are extremely infrequent, this may be considered appropriate treatment. However, if there is rapid recurrence after dilatation, a minimally invasive cardiomyotomy should be offered as a permanent cure. The place of botulinum toxin injection is limited, as its results are generally no better than those of dilatation, and repeated injection makes subsequent cardiomyotomy considerably more difficult.

Diffuse oesophageal spasm

This condition is characterized by disordered and incoordinate oesophageal peristalsis. Instead of the peristaltic wave progressing sequentially down the oesophagus, with relaxation of the segments immediately distal to the peristaltic wave such that contents are propelled down the oesophagus, numerous contractions may occur simultaneously at many levels. High pressures are often reached in an attempt to propel the bolus, which may be trapped between two actively peristalsing segments.

Clinical features

Diffuse oesophageal spasm characteristically occurs in middle age. The cardinal symptoms are dysphagia as a result of ineffective propulsion, and chest pain as a result either of bolus impaction or of high amplitude contractions. Chest pain is often severe and similar to anginal pain, being crushing in character and often radiating to the back, jaws, and arms. Attacks are usually precipitated by eating, but also by anxiety and some workers have demonstrated an abnormal psychological profile in a high proportion of patients suffering from diffuse oesophageal spasm. The dysphagia is frequently paradoxical — that is, worse for liquids than for solids.

Diagnosis

Barium studies frequently demonstrate the presence of spasm, which may be diffuse and constant or segmental and transitory, affecting principally the lower two-thirds of the oesophagus. In extreme cases of segmental contractions, the appearances are very striking, producing the so-called corkscrew oesophagus. **Cine-radiography** is particularly helpful in milder cases and may be augmented by the swallowing of a solid bolus, such a bread or marshmallow, during the study. **Oesophageal manometry** forms the mainstay of diagnosis, particularly in less dramatic cases. The principal findings are of simultaneous, non-propagated contractions and incoordinate peristalsis. Other manometric features include high-amplitude contractions, of prolonged duration. In some cases there may be associated lower oesophageal sphincter abnormalities, predominantly high resting pressure or incomplete relaxation. In milder cases, the manometric features may be intermittent, in which case the diagnostic accuracy may be increased by performing prolonged ambulatory oesophageal manometry over a 24-h period or by performing one of the provocation tests, such as balloon distension or the administration of edrophonium during conventional manometry.

Treatment

In mild cases, reassurance of the absence of a cardiac cause for the symptoms is often all that is required. In more severe cases, treatment is often disappointing. Nitrate compounds such as glyceryl trinitrate may help in curing acute episodes of chest pain. Calcium-channel blocking drugs such as nifedipine or verapamil are helpful as long-term treatment in a proportion of patients. In more resistant cases, oesophageal dilatation and, particularly, balloon dilatation of the lower oesophageal sphincter are occasionally of value; in severe cases, a long oesophageal myotomy is occasionally performed transthoracically or thoracoscopically. However, there is no form of treatment that helps all suffers; this may reflect the high incidence of associated psychiatric disease, which may itself require treatment.

Nutcracker oesophagus

This is a relatively unusual but dramatic variant of diffuse oesophageal spasm, in which extremely high peristaltic pressures are recorded, often as great as 250 mmHg, the contractions often being prolonged. These high-pressure or prolonged contractions most frequently give rise to chest pain, which again may

mimic that of myocardial ischaemia. Dysphagia may also occur. Abnormalities on barium studies are less dramatic than those in diffuse oesophageal spasm, and other manometric criteria — apart from the high-amplitude contractions — are frequently normal. Treatment follows the sequence described for diffuse oesophageal spasm.

Non-specific oesophageal motility disorder

A proportion of patients with symptoms of chest pain or dysphagia demonstrate manometric abnormalities that are not easily categorized, including intermittently absent peristalsis, very-low-amplitude contractions, intermittent repetitive contractions, or incomplete lower oesophageal sphincter relaxation. Treatment is even more disappointing than that of diffuse oesophageal spasm, unless it is secondary to gastro-oesophageal reflux disease.

CARCINOMA OF THE OESOPHAGUS

Carcinoma of the oesophagus is an unpleasant malignancy in that it tends to be relatively advanced at the time of presentation, in the majority of patients. In those who are operable, a major thoracoabdominal procedure is usually required, which results in 5-year survival figures of only around 20%. The incidence of carcinoma of the oesophagus is increasing, because of the increasing incidence of adenocarcinoma consequent upon Barrett's oesophagus, such that adenocarcinoma, which previously comprised fewer than 10% of all oesophageal tumours, now comprises approximately 50%. The principal aetiological factors in the Western world are alcohol and tobacco for squamous lesions, and Barrett's columnar-lined oesophagus for adenocarcinoma. Other pre-malignant lesions include the Plummer–Vinson (Patterson–Kelly) syndrome, achalasia, Zenker's diverticulm, and lye stricture.

Clinical features

Symptoms are usually delayed until the disease is well advanced, because dysphagia, which is the predominant symptom, is not usually experienced until the tumour has encircled some two-thirds of the circumference of the oesophagus. To compound the problem, the average time from the first symptom of dysphagia to presentation to hospital is approximately 4 months.

Dysphagia is the presenting complaint in more than 90% of patients. The first indication is often an undue awareness of the passage of solid food, before actual difficulty in swallowing arises. The patient then usually notices progressive hold-up of solid food, which initially needs to be washed down with liberal amounts of fluid and, subsequently, can not be swallowed at all. The patient can often localize with reasonable accuracy the site of hold-up, although in approximately 30% of lesions in the lower oesophagus, the sensation of hold-up is at the upper end, and *vice versa*. Surprisingly, many patients do not seek medical advice at this stage, but gradually change to a softer diet, and it is only when difficulty in swallowing semi-solids arises that medical advice is sought. A characteristic feature of dysphagia associated with oesophageal carcinoma is that it is relentlessly progressive and, if untreated, difficulty will eventually occur in swallowing liquids, and then in swallowing saliva.

Acute bolus obstruction occasionally occurs if a piece of solid food, usually meat, impacts at the level of the tumour. Such an event may not necessarily have been preceded by a history of dysphagia. Typical oesophageal pain, commencing retrosternally and radiating to the back, jaws and left arm may occur if food impacts, but otherwise pain is an unusual presenting symptom in oesophageal cancer.

As a consequence of dysphagia, there is often considerable **weight loss and nutritional deficiency**, frequently associated with hypoproteinaemia and iron-deficiency anaemia.

Other less common modes of presentation of oesophageal cancer are **bleeding** and **respiratory symptoms**. Bleeding is relatively uncommon, and usually presents as haematemesis, although occasionally melaena or occult gastrointestinal bleeding may occur. Rather surprisingly, this presentation is usually associated with relatively early tumours. Conversely, respiratory symptoms, when they occur, are usually associated with advanced tumours. Unexplained cough may be caused either by overspill of regurgitated oesophageal contents into the respiratory tree, or by the presence of a tracheo–oesophageal fistula associated with erosion of the tumour directly into the bronchial tree. In these circumstances, spasmodic coughing occurs immediately after eating or drinking.

Diagnosis

Barium swallow

Many advocate this as the first investigation in patients with dysphagia. The characteristic radiological appearances of oesophageal carcinoma are those of an irregular stricture, with shouldered margins. The area of narrowing is frequently long and tortuous. These features usually enable the condition to be distinguished from a benign stricture or achalasia. Barium swallow may demonstrate a tracheo–oesophageal fistula, and enable a better assessment of tumour length and gastric involvement than is possible with endoscopy, if the neoplastic stricture is tight and undilatable.

Endoscopy

It is essential to perform endoscopy in all cases of suspected oesophageal carcinoma. First, it enables a tissue diagnosis to be made; second, it allows a more accurate assessment of length and gastric involvement than can be achieved with barium swallow, if the endoscope can be passed through the tumour; third, endoscopic dilatation can be performed to improve swallowing, and hence nutrition, before definitive treatment. If the endoscope can not be passed through the lesion and into the stomach, it is advisable to dilate the neoplastic stricture, to enable a complete assessment to be made and to ensure that representative biopsy specimens are taken from the body of the lesion. Diagnostic accuracy of biopsy is increased by performing brush cytology in addition to taking punch biopsies. With very tight strictures, it may be possible only to biopsy the upper margin of the lesion, which can yield false-negative results. In these circumstances, it is usually possible to pass a brush through the biopsy channel to obtain brushings from the length of the lesion.

Staging

CT scanning is the most widely used modality in staging of oesophageal cancer, and is very accurate in the detection of visceral metastases and gross involvement of contiguous structures. It is somewhat less accurate in defining accurate T (tumour) and N (node) staging, which in this context is approximately 60% and 50% respectively. **Magnetic resonance imaging** has not, as yet, conferred any improvement on these figures, and even positron emission tomography, which is rather more accurate than CT scanning in the detection of distant metastases, is no more accurate in the assessment of locoregional disease. **Endoluminal ultrasound** (EUS) currently affords the most accurate modality for locoregional staging, with rates for T and N staging approaching 90% and 80% respectively. EUS has the disadvantages of being invasive, expensive, and unsuitable for severely stenotic tumours, although the increasing ability of microprobes is reducing this problem. However, the results of EUS can have a significant impact on treatment, particularly in the demonstration of extensive coeliac node involvement, which is uniformly associated with poor prognosis after resection of, in particular, adenocarcinomas, and in the detection of advanced locoregional disease that may indicate preoperative chemoradiation. **Laparoscopy** has proved significantly more accurate than CT scanning in the detection of peritoneal metastases, and slightly more accurate in the diagnosis of liver metastases. **Thoracoscopy** is being used in some centres for assessment of locoregional disease, although there are few data to compare its accuracy with other modalities. **Bronchoscopy** is best reserved for those patients in whom there is suspicion of airway involvement on clinical or radiological grounds, as an oesophago–respiratory fistula is extremely rare in the absence of such features.

Patient selection for treatment

Once a diagnosis of oesophageal carcinoma has been confirmed, it is important to consider the tumour staging and the age and general condition of the patient, in order to consider the therapeutic options available. As resectional surgery, either with or without adjuvant therapy, is the only modality that has been consistently associated with cure in 20–30% of those resected, this should be the objective in relatively fit patients with a relatively favourable tumour. In patient selection, age is a significant factor in the ability to withstand a major thoracoabominal resection, although biological age is more important than chronological age; with improved surgical and anaesthetic techniques, patients in their late 70s and early 80s who are otherwise fit can tolerate resection extremely well. Severe intercurrent disease, and in particular cardiac and respiratory insufficiency, has a significant impact on morbidity and mortality after resection, and these problems are relatively common in the age group in which oesophageal cancer most frequently presents — often against a background of tobacco and alcohol abuse. If resectional surgery is being considered, it is advisable to perform pulmonary function tests on all patients, and a full cardiological assessment in those in whom cardiac disease is suspected.

On the basis of these assessments of tumour staging and patient fitness, most clinical situations will resolve themselves into two groups of patients: those in whom an aggressive and potentially curative surgical approach is justified, and those in whom palliation should be the prime objective. In terms of tumour staging, only unequivocal evidence of distant metastases, contiguous organ involvement, and extensive coeliac nodal involvement are contraindications to an attempt at curative resection. In this context, it should be appreciated that apparent involvement of the aorta on CT scanning is a relatively frequent finding, because of loss of fat planes in malnourished patients and, in practice, adherence to the aorta is much more commonly associated with inflammatory adhesion, rather than infiltration. Also, apparently locally advanced disease should not, in itself, be a contraindication to resection, as 5-year survival in node-positive squamous lesions is 10% if an adequate lymphadenectomy is performed, and the use of neoadjuvant therapy may down-stage tumours in a proportion of patients, resulting in even better survival data. Analysis of a consecutive series of 396 patients with oesophageal cancer, referred to my unit in an area of high incidence, showed that approximately 40% of these patients were deemed suitable for an attempt at curative resection using the selection criteria described. In the remaining 60%, palliation was deemed the principal objective by virtue of advanced tumour staging or contraindications to surgery because of advanced age or severe intercurrent disease (13). Such a selection process has been shown to result in a resectability rate of 97%, and current hospital mortality rate of 4.8%. Attempts to be less selective and more aggressive usually result in a reduction in the resectability rate, or an increase in the operative mortality.

Treatment

As discussed above, the principal treatment modalities are surgical resection, adjuvant therapy, and a variety of palliative modalities.

Resectional surgery

For oesophageal cancer, resectional surgery should be performed in specialist units, where expertise is strong and there is a sufficient throughput of cases to enable teams to become familiar with each stage of management and to anticipate or detect problems early, to enable prompt treatment. The most widely used surgical approach is the Lewis–Tanner oesophagogastrectomy, performed by a laparotomy and right thoracotomy, to which a cervical phase can be added, especially for proximally situated tumours. Trans-hiatal oesophagectomy without thoracotomy has the theoretical advantage of avoiding the complications of thoracotomy. However, the advent of thoracic epidural analgesia has significantly reduced the incidence of ventilatory complications after thoracotomy, and comparative studies have failed to show any advantage of trans-hiatal oesophagectomy over the Lewis–Tanner technique. Furthermore, there is concern, in an era of increasing degrees of lymphadenectomy, that trans-hiatal oesophagectomy is an oncologically inadequate procedure, and there are survival data to support this view. The advent of minimally invasive surgery has led to the application of thoracoscopic and mediastinoscopic mobilization of the oesophagus, with claims that an adequate lymphadenectomy can be performed. However, evidence to date suggests that morbidity and mortality are somewhat greater than after a conventional thoracoabdominal approach.

The outcome after surgical resection remains depressing for the majority of patients with oesophageal tumours. Although technical advances have resulted in a reduction in the incidence of fatal anastomotic leakage and respiratory complications, resulting in a 30-day mortality of 5% in specialist units, overall 5-year survival is only 20–30%, with better results for squamous lesions than for adenocarcinomas. This reflects the fact that the majority of tumours are locally advanced by the time they are diagnosed (T_3N_{1-2}). However, when survival data are stratified for tumour staging, the small proportion of node-negative tumours are associated with a 5-year survival approaching 50% and an even smaller proportion of $T_{1-2}N_0$ lesions have a rate better than 70%, irrespective of cell type (14). Such data highlight the potential rewards of early diagnosis, which is rarely feasible outside surveillance programmes. In the West, the majority of adenocarcinomas diagnosed at the T_1 stage are part of Barrett's surveillance programmes, and 5-year survival approaches 90% (14).

Adjuvant therapy (see also chapter 18.1)

There have been many studies comparing the use of chemotherapy or radiotherapy used alone, either before or after resectional surgery, and none has shown a significant survival advantage. However, the preoperative use of combined chemotherapy and radiotherapy as neo-adjuvant therapy has been much more promising, and is believed to relate to the potentiating effect of chemotherapy on radiosensitivity. Several series have reported improved survival using neo-adjuvant combination chemotherapy and radiotherapy compared with that in historical controls who underwent resection alone, with 5-year survival rates up to 40%. Most series report tumour down-staging in the majority of patients treated by neo-adjuvant therapy; indeed, in 20–40% of patients there is a complete histopathological response, and in this group of patients, 5-year survival is as good as 67%. These encouraging results have been more recently confirmed in a prospective randomized trial of neo-adjuvant therapy before surgery compared with surgery alone for oesophageal adenocarcinoma, with a statistically significant improvement in 3-year survival, to 30% in the neo-adjuvant group. The 3-year survival of the group receiving treatment by surgery alone was only 6%, which is considerably less than that in many published series (15). Nonetheless, there is considerable enthusiasm for the use of neo-adjuvant therapy, particularly in patients with locally advanced tumours.

Palliative treatment

As discussed above, a palliative approach is appropriate in some 60% of patients with oesophageal cancer. In recent years, there have been several major advances in the ability to improve the quality of the relatively short life span of these patients, the average survival being only 6–8 months. For this reason, the less invasive **endoscopic methods** of palliation are preferable to surgical options, except where surgery has been performed with curative intent and complete removal proves unfeasible, in which case palliative resection will restore normal swallowing in 90% of patients — a rate that is greater than that for any other modality. There is now such a good range of endoscopic modalities that surgery is no longer justified as a primary palliative therapy. **Rigid oesophageal prostheses** of the Atkinson or Celestin variety have been used for some 20 years now. They restore the ability of the majority of patients to take a semi-solid diet and a few to achieve a near-normal diet, but have the disadvantage of a perforation risk of around 10%, approximately half of these proving fatal. Tumour overgrowth and tube migration necessitate a subsequent procedure in a minority of patients. The principal advantage of these prostheses is that they enable most patients to tolerate a reasonable diet with only one interventional procedure, which is important when life expectancy is limited.

The recent introduction of **self-expanding metallic stents** has been welcomed, as they have several potential advantages over conventional plastic stents. They have a relatively small unexpanded diameter (8–12 mm), which means that smaller and more flexible delivery systems can be used, thus obviating the need for preliminary dilatation in many patients and virtually abolishing the risk of perforation. Also, the greater diameter when the stent is fully extended (16–22 mm) has enabled a considerably greater proportion of patients to tolerate a substantially normal diet. There are some disadvantages, however, including the high cost of the stent and introducer (£600–800), the risk of tumour ingrowth, which is more common with uncovered stents and stent migration, particularly when the stent traverses the cardia and when a covered stent is used (16). Furthermore, once these stents have expanded, it is very difficult to remove them or change their position should the need arise. One prospective randomized study has compared uncovered Wallstents and conventional plastic prostheses (17). Rather surprisingly, 30-day mortality and relief of dysphagia were similar between the two groups, but the overall cost of palliation was less with the Wallstents because of shorter hospital stay — 5.4 days, compared with 12.4 days with plastic prostheses. However, the latter stay is much longer than that seen in many experienced units, and may relate to the use of general anaesthesia to insert plastic stents in this series. At the present time, therefore, both systems have advantages and disadvantages, although improvements in the design of self-expanding metallic stents are likely to reduce the rate of complications and hence reintervention.

The other principal group of palliative modalities comprises those that achieve tumour debulking, including laser photocoagulation, the Bicap heater probe, photodynamic therapy, radiotherapy, and direct injection of sclerosants. Tumour debulking using the Nd-YAG (neodymium-yttrium-argon-garnet) **laser** results in good quality palliation, superior to that obtained by conventional intubation, but with the principal disadvantages of high capital costs and the necessity for repeat treatments at 6–8-week intervals (18). However, when laser treatment was compared with use of self-expanding metallic stents in a prospective randomized study, the patients treated using stents obtained greater relief of dysphagia (19). **Laser photocoagulation** is a safe technique, with perioperative mortality of 1% and is particularly valuable in the treatment of exophytic tumours and those situated close to the cricopharyngeus, where intubation is less suitable. **Thermocoagulation** using the Bicap heater probe has been reported to achieve palliation similar to that obtained by laser photocoagulation at a considerably lower capital cost, but is only suitable for circumferential stenotic lesions, as mucosal damage occurs in non-circumferential lesions. **Photodynamic therapy**, involving the application of light energies to the tumour after administration of a photosensitizer, has been used more for early lesions than advanced ones, but can be very effective. It does have complications, however, including occasional stricture formation and haemorrhage. The recent development of an orally administered photosensitizer has alleviated the principal disadvantage of avoidance of exposure to sunlight.

External beam radiotherapy has a limited role in palliation; advanced bulky tumours not amenable to surgery require such a large field that the dose per unit tumour volume is so small as to be relatively ineffective. Furthermore, as such lesions are commonly obstructing, the dysphagia often worsens as a consequence of radiotherapy, necessitating intubation. Finally, the duration of the treatment course and the systemic effects of radiotherapy militate against its suitability in patients with limited life expectancy. More useful, however, is **intracavity irradiation (brachytherapy)**, in which a tube containing caesium or cobalt pellets or an iridium wire is placed through the tumour under general anaesthesia, and can deliver an effective dose of 15 Gy in just over 1 h. Relief of dysphagia is, therefore, much more rapid than after external beam radiotherapy and is much more effective, with more than 50% of patients having restoration of normal swallowing. Tumour necrosis by **endoscopic injection of a chemical agent** has been shown to be a remarkably simple and effective means of achieving palliation. The use of ethanol has been shown to produce palliation comparable to that of laser recanalization, and in a prospective, randomized trial comparing laser therapy and injection of the sclerosant, polidocanol, they were equally effective and 80% of patients were relieved of dysphagia after the first treatment course. Multiple treatments were required with both modalities, with the cost of sclerosant injections clearly much less than laser therapy.

Different palliative modalities will be appropriate to different situations and individual patients, depending on such factors as the position of the tumour and its pathological characteristics — that is, whether it is exophytic, circumferential, or stenotic. Indeed, different palliative treatments may be appropriate at different times in the patient's illness; for example, laser photocoagulation may be appropriate for tumour ingrowth or overgrowth after stenting. Furthermore, evidence is emerging to suggest that the use of combined palliative modalities may result in superior palliation and even in increased survival. The combination of laser photocoagulation with radiotherapy — both external beam and brachytherapy — appears to reduce the necessity for repeated laser photocoagulation. Similar results have been obtained by combining laser, chemotherapy, and radiotherapy, with an apparent increase in survival, although the study was non-randomized and undoubtedly some early cases were included. In view of the increasing complexity of palliative regimens and the necessity to tailor and perhaps combine modalities for individual patients, palliative treatment, as with resectional surgery, should be performed in specialist centres with facilities for a choice of the available palliative options.

References

1. Cope C, Watson A. Intramural haematoma of the oesophagus: report of 3 cases and review of the literature. *Aust NZ J Surg* 1994; **64**: 190–193.
   A report of three cases of this unusual condition from the same institution, illustrating the frequent diagnostic difficulty, the classical diagnostic features on investigation, and the excellent clinical course on conservative treatment if the correct diagnosis is made.
2. Jones WG, Ginsberg RJ. Oesophageal perforation: a continuing challenge. *Ann Thorac Surg* 1992; **53**: 534–543.
   A good review article that covers the various types of oesophageal perforation. The importance of early diagnosis and surgical treatment in Boerhaave's syndrome and the good results obtained by conservative treatment in instrumental perforations are discussed.
3. Spechler SJ, Goyal RK. The columnar-lined esophagus, intestinal metaplasia and Norman Barrett. *Gastroenterology* 1996; **110**: 614–621.
   An excellent review that depicts the various stages in our understanding of the condition and its associated malignant risk, together with the confusion in terminology that the recent discovery of short-segment Barrett's and interstinal metaplasia at the cardia have produced.
4. Palmer ED. The hiatus hernia-esophagitis-esophageal stricture complex. Twenty year prospective study. *Am J Med* 1968; **44**: 566–579.
5. Sharma P, Sampliner RE, Camargo E. Normalisation of esophageal pH with high dose proton pump inhibitor therapy does not result in regression of Barrett's esophagus. *Am J Gastroenterol* 1997; **92**: 582–585.
   This study builds on data from recent studies that have shown that elimination of symptoms in Barrett's oesophagus by proton pump inhibitor therapy does not correlate with normalization of acid exposure and, indeed, the latter can be very difficult to achieve in Barrett's patients. The authors demonstrate that, even when acid exposure is normalized, by 60 mg daily of lansoprazole, no regression of the columnar lining occurs.
6. Berenson MM. Ablation therapy of Barrett's esophagus: measures of success and failure. *Am J Gastroenterol* 1998; **93**: 1794–1795.
   An editorial that highlights the fact that results of squamous re-epithelialization after endoscopic ablation of Barrett's oesophagus have to be interpreted with caution, in that up to 60% of patients so treated have residual or recurrent metaplastic epithelium underlying the squamous regeneration.
7. Ortiz A, Martinez de Haro LF, Parilla P. Conservative treatment versus anti-reflux surgery in Barrett's oesophagus: long term results of a prospective study. *Br J Surg* 1991; **78**: 274–278.
   A prospective, randomized study comparing acid suppression with high-dose H_2-receptor antagonists and proton pump inhibitors or with anti-reflux surgery, which showed that patients in the surgical arm had greater symptomatic relief, greater resolution of strictures, and a lesser incidence of new strictures. However, there was no difference in the incidence of adenocarcinoma.
8. McDonald ML, Trastek VF, Allen MS *et al.* Barrett's esophagus: does an anti-reflux procedure reduce the need for endoscopic surveillance? *J Thorac Cardiovasc Surg* 1996; **111**: 1135–1140.
   A longitudinal study from the Mayo Clinic of 113 patients followed for up to 18 years after anti-reflux surgery. Three patients developed adenocarcinoma within the first 3 years of follow-up, suggesting that surgery had been performed after the sequence of genomic instability had commenced in these patients. However, there was no incidence of adenocarcinoma in the subsequent 15 years, giving an overall incidence of 1:274 patient years of follow-up.
9. Sampliner RE. Practice guidelines on the diagnosis, surveillance and therapy of Barrett's esophagus. *Am J Gastroenterol* 1998; **93**: 1028–1031.
   Recommends that patients with Barrett's oesophagus should

undergo surveillance endoscopy and biopsy at an interval of 1–3 years determined by the presence and grade of dysplasia. Also recommends that patients with long-standing reflux symptoms, particularly those older than 50 years, should undergo endoscopy to detect or exclude Barrett's oesophagus.

10. Pasricha PJ, Rai R, Ravich WJ *et al.* Botulinum toxin for achalasia: long-term outcome and predictors of response. *Gastroenterology* 1996; **110**: 1410–1415.
    A study that demonstrates the efficacy of botulinum toxin in producing symptomatic improvement and decreased lower oesophageal sphincter pressure in more than 60% of patients, although the duration of response was relatively short, necessitating repeat injections. Higher success rates were seen in patients older than 50 years and those with vigorous achalasia.

11. Tack J, Janssens J, Vantrappen G. Non-surgical treatment of achalasia. *Hepatogastroenterology* 1991; **38**: 493–497.
    Results of a long experience of conservative management of achalasia, predominantly balloon dilatation, giving good to excellent results in 77% of patients in expert hands, with a perforation risk of 2.6% and gastrooesophageal reflux in approximately 8%.

12. Csendes A, Bighetto I, Henriquez A. Late results of a prospective randomized study comparing forceful dilatation and oesophagomyotomy in patients with achalasia. *Gut* 1989; **30**: 299–304.
    The only prospective randomized trial in the management of achalasia showing a greater incidence of good and excellent results after myotomy than after balloon dilatation.

13. Watson A. Squamous oesophageal cancer: current results in the West. *World J Surg* 1994; **18**: 361–366.
    A large series that demonstrates that some 40% of patients with squamous oesophageal cancer underwent resection, with a hospital mortality less than 7% and overall 5-year survival of 23%. However, stratification for tumour staging showed that, for node-negative patients, 5-year survival was 47%, and for tumours confined within the adventitia it was 71%, emphasizing the potential benefits of early detection and treatment.

14. Peters JH, Clark GWB, Ireland AP *et al.* Outcome of adenocarcinoma arising in Barrett's esophagus in endoscopically surveyed and non-surveyed patients. *J Thoroac Cardiovasc Surg* 1994; **108**: 813–822.
    An interesting study comparing the outcome of resection in 13 patients whose adenocarcinoma was detected as part of a surveillance programme compared with 35 patients with a clinically diagnosed Barrett's adenocarcinoma. Ninety-two per cent of the former were early lesions, compared with 28% of the latter; the respective 5-year survival rates after resection were 88% and 20%.

15. Walsh TN, Noonan N, Hollywood D *et al.* A comparison of multi-modal therapy and surgery alone for esophageal adenocarcinoma. *N Engl J Med* 1996; **335**: 462–467.
    The first prospective randomized study to show a survival advantage for adding chemoradiation as neo-adjuvant therapy before surgery in oesophageal adenocarcinoma. However, the study has been criticized because survival after surgery alone is significantly less than in any other published series.

16. Watson A. Self-expanding metal oesophageal endo-prostheses: which is best? *Eur J Gastroenterol Hepatol* 1998; **10**: 363–365.
    A leading article that reviews the published series relating to self-expanding metallic stents. In general, they are associated with excellent palliation but, surprisingly, a relatively high procedure-related mortality up to 27%. Disadvantages include the high cost, tumour ingrowth with uncovered stents and stent migration, particularly with covered stents that traverse the oesophagogastric junction.

17. Knyrim K, Wagner HJ, Bethge N. A controlled trial of an expansile metal stent for palliation of esophageal obstruction due to inoperable cancer. *N Engl J Med* 1993; **329**: 1302–1307.
    A randomized study comparing self-expanding metallic stents and conventional plastic prostheses, the latter being introduced under general anaesthesia. Somewhat surprisingly, results were identical, apart from a greater treatment cost with plastic prostheses, associated with a rather long mean hospital stay of 12.5 days.

18. Carter K, Smith JS, Anderson JR. Laser recannalisation versus endoscopic intubation in the palliation of malignant dysphagia: a randomised prospective study. *Br J Surg* 1992; **79**: 1167–1170.
    Randomized study showing superior palliation by Nd-YAG laser therapy compared with intubation, but repeat treatments were necessary to maintain this quality of palliation.

19. Adam A, Ellul J, Watkinson AF. Palliation of inoperable esophageal carcinoma: a prospective randomised trial of laser therapy and stent placement. *Radiology* 1997; **202**: 334–348.
    A randomized study comparing self-expanding metallic stents and laser therapy, showing better palliation with the stents and a lower requirement for repeat treatment.

15. Intestinal Obstruction

MARC WINSLET

INTRODUCTION AND CLASSIFICATION

The diagnosis of intestinal obstruction is based on the classic quartet of:

- abdominal pain
- distension
- vomiting
- absolute constipation

Intestinal obstruction may be classified **functionally** into two types:

1. *Dynamic*: Peristalsis is resisted by mechanical obstruction. The obstructing lesion may be intraluminal (e.g. impacted faeces or bezoar), intramural (e.g. malignant or inflammatory strictures), or extramural (e.g. adhesions and hernias).
2. *Adynamic*: May occur when peristalsis is absent (e.g. parlytic ileus), or it is non-propulsive (e.g. pseudo-obstruction). A mechanical element is absent.

In addition, obstruction may be classified **clinically** into

1. *Small bowel (high or low)*: In **high small-bowel** obstruction, vomiting occurs early, and distension is minimal with little radiographic evidence of fluid levels. **Low small-bowel** obstruction is associated with pain and central distension, and vomiting and dehydration are delayed. Radiography reveals classic central fluid levels.

2. *Large bowel*: Distension occurs early. Pain is mild, and vomiting and dehydration are late. Radiography reveals a dilated proximal colon.

The nature of presentation will also be influenced by:

- Whether the obstruction is **acute or chronic**. The former is usually seen in the small bowel, whereas the latter occurs in the large bowel.
- Whether the obstruction is
  - **simple** (i.e. the blood supply is intact) or
  - **strangulating** (there is direct interference to blood flow).

Strangulation may occur secondary to external compression (e.g. hernial orifices, adhesions and bands), interruption of mesenteric flow (e.g. volvulus or intussusception), increasing intraluminal pressure (closed loop obstruction) or primary obstruction of the intestinal circulation (mesenteric infarction). The significance of strangulating obstruction is its associated morbidity and, mortality which are dependent on age, and extent of involvement. Closed-loop obstruction is a special type of strangulating mechanical obstruction, in which the bowel is obstructed at both a proximal and a distal point. The classic form of closed-loop obstruction is seen in the presence of a malignant stricture of the colon with a competent ileocaecal valve.

The most common causes of intestinal obstruction in the western world are:

- adhesions (40%)
- inflammatory strictures (15%)
- carcinoma (15%)
- obstructed herniae (12%)
- faecal impaction (8%)
- miscellaneous causes, including pseudo-obstruction (10%)

ACUTE INTESTINAL OBSTRUCTION

The four cardinal features — **pain**, **vomiting**, **distension**, and **constipation** — vary according to location, age, underlying pathology, and presence or absence of intestinal ischaemia.

Pain is usually the initial symptom, is colicky in nature, and is usually centred around the umbilicus (small bowel) or lower abdomen (large bowel). The development of severe pain is indicative of strangulation.

The time interval between the onset of symptoms and the development of **vomiting** is dependent on the site of obstruction. As obstruction progresses, the character of the vomitus alters from digested food to faecal fluid.

The degree of **distension** is dependent on the site of obstruction and is greater the more distal the lesion. It is delayed in colonic obstruction and may be minimal in the presence of mesenteric vascular occlusion.

Constipation may be relative or absolute, the latter indicating complete obstruction.

Other manifestations may include:

- Dehydration
- Pyrexia
  - may indicate ischaemia, perforation, or inflammation associated with the obstructing lesion, and abdominal tenderness
- Localized tenderness indicates impending ischaemia
- Peritonitis indicates overt infarction or perforation

Radiological diagnosis

This is usually based on a **supine abdominal film** (Figure 15.1).

1. *Obstructed small bowel*: Characterized by central segments that lie transversely. Dilated jejunum is characterized by a concertina or ladder effect, because of the presence of the valvulae conniventes. In contrast, distended ileum is rather featureless.

2. *Obstructed large bowel*: Apart from the caecum, this shows haustral folds which, unlike valvulae conniventes, are spaced irregularly and the indentations are not located opposite one another.

3. *Intestinal obstruction*: Fluid levels appear later than gas shadows. In infants, a few fluid levels in the small bowel may be physiological; whereas in the adult two are not uncommonly seen — one at the duodenal cap and the one in the terminal ileum. The presence of conspicuous, numerous fluid levels indicates the presence of advanced obstruction of the small bowel. Chronic obstruction is usually associated with a large amount of gas in the caecum.

4. *Gas-filled loops and fluid levels*: May also be seen in established paralytic ileus and pseudo-obstruction. These can however, normally be distinguished, on clinical grounds. Fluid levels may also be seen in non-obstructing conditions, such as acute intra-abdominal sepsis.

Other radiological investigations

A limited water-soluble enema may be undertaken to differentiate large-bowel obstruction from pseudo-obstruction. A barium follow-through examination, however, is contraindicated in the presence of acute obstruction and may, indeed, be life threatening.

Treatment

The mainstay of treatment consists of:

- gastrointestinal drainage
- fluid and electrolyte placement
- relief of obstruction (1)

The first two steps are mandatory.

Surgical intervention is necessary for most cases of intestinal obstruction, but should be delayed until resuscitation is complete, provided there is no evidence of strangulation or closed-loop obstruction.

The timing of surgical intervention is dependent on the clinical picture, with early surgery indicated for obstructive or strangulated external herniae, internal intestinal strangulation, and acute obstruction. Indications for delay of surgical intervention

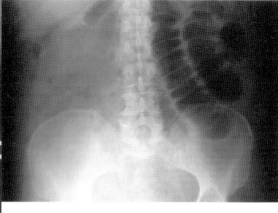

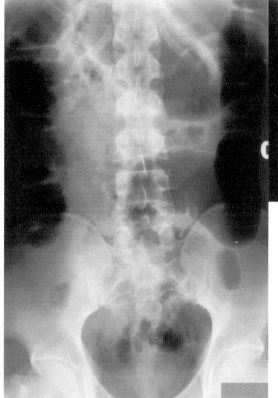

Figure 15.1. Supine abdominal radiographs. (left) Large-bowel obstruction. (top) small-bowel obstruction. See text for details.

include obstruction secondary to adhesions when there is no pain or tenderness. In such circumstances, conservative management may be continued for up to 72 h, in the hope of spontaneous resolution (2,3).

Surgical intervention is focused on the site of obstruction, the nature of the obstruction, and the viability of the gut. The type of procedure will depend on the underlying cause and may include excision, bypass, proximal decompression, or enterolysis.

Large bowel obstruction is usually due to underlying carcinoma (4) or, occasionally, diverticular disease. The presence of pseudo-obstruction should always be excluded by limited contrast study or contrast computed tomography.

The operative procedure of choice is dependent on underlying pathology, but when the removable lesion is found in the caecum, ascending colon, hepatic flexure, or proximal transverse colon, a right hemicolectomy should be performed. If the lesion is not removable, a proximal stoma or an ileo-transverse bypass should be considered. Obstructing lesions at the splenic flexure should be treated by extended right hemicolectomy. Obstructive lesions of the left colon or rectosigmoid region should be treated by resection unless there are clear contraindications, such as a moribund patient or advanced disease (5–7). In such cases, it is safest to raise a proximal stoma, with subsequent further staged procedures (8).

INTRA-ABDOMINAL ADHESIONS

The aetiology of intra-abdominal adhesions is multifactorial and includes areas of ischaemia (anastomosis and raw areas), foreign material (talc and starch), infection (peritonitis, tuberculosis), inflammatory conditions (e.g. Crohn's disease), and radiation.

Numerous agents have been advocated as prophylaxis against adhesion formation. Currently, no single agent has been shown to be safe and effective. The major factor to limit adhesion formation is good surgical technique. Postoperative adhesions giving rise to intestinal obstruction usually involve the lower small bowel. Operations for appendicitis and gynaecological procedures are the most common precursors.

Initial management of intra-abdominal adhesions and bands is based on intravenous rehydration and nasogastric decompression. Occasionally, it may be curative. If an initial conservative regimen is embarked upon, regular reassessment is required, and conservative management should not extend beyond 72 h (9–11).

The treatment of recurrent intestinal obstruction as a result of adhesions is problematic. Surgical management may consist of repeat enterolysis (adhesiolysis) alone, or the use of plication or intubation procedures.

SPECIAL TYPES OF MECHANICAL OBSTRUCTION

Internal hernia

Internal hernias may occur when a portion of the mobile small intestine becomes trapped in a retroperitoneal fossa around the duodenum or caecal area, or in a congenital defect of one of the mesenteries. They are uncommon, and preoperative diagnosis is unusual.

Enteric strictures

Small-bowel strictures usually occur secondary to tuberculosis or Crohn's disease. Malignant strictures may be associated with lymphoma; adenocarcinoma and sarcoma are rare.

Bolus obstruction

Bolus obstruction of the small bowel may be caused by food, gallstones, tricho- and phytobezoars, stercoliths, and worms.

Gallstone obstruction classically occurs in the elderly, and the patient usually presents with recurrent and complete obstruction. Plain radiography will show small-bowel obstruction and an air/fluid level in the biliary tree. At operation, the stone is disimpacted, milked back, and removed. The gallbladder region should not be explored.

Food boluses can normally be managed by intraluminal crushing.

Phytobezoars may be predisposed to by high fibre intake, inadequate chewing, previous gastric surgery, hypochlorhydria, and the loss of the gastric pump.

Stercoliths are usually found in association with jejunal diverticula or ileal strictures.

Ascaris lumbricoides is the most common **worm** to cause small-bowel obstruction. An attack may be initiated by antihelminthics. If worms are not visible, the diagnosis may be indicated by eosinophilia.

Postoperative intestinal obstruction

Differentiation between persistent paralytic ileus and mechanical obstruction in the postoperative period may be difficult. In the early post operative period — in practice, days 1–5 — distinguishing between the two is rarely important. Obstruction beyond 7 days is usually significant, and timely surgical intervention is required.

Acute intussusception

Acute intussusception occurs where a segment of bowel invaginates into an adjacent segment. It is most commonly encountered in children, in an idiopathic form, with a peak incidence of 3–9 months. Hyperplasia of Peyer's patches may be the initiating event. This, in turn, may be related to weaning or to upper respiratory tract infections. Intussusception is an example of strangulating obstruction, as the blood supply is usually impaired. It may be ileoileal, ileocaecal or ileocolic, depending on the size and extent of invagination.

The presentation in the child is classical, with sudden onset of screaming, associated with drawing up of the legs, vomiting and the passage of blood and mucus per rectum. On examination, a mass is felt in 50% of affected patients. Radiography reveals evidence of small- or large-bowel obstruction. Barium enema may be diagnostic, except in the presence of an ileoileal variant. Barium enema may also be used therapeutically in selective cases, to allow hydrostatic reduction. It is successful in 50% of patients, with a recurrence rate of 5%. The differential diagnosis includes acute entercolitis, Henoch–Schönlein purpura, and rectal prolapse.

Operative management is required when hydrostatic reduction has failed or is contraindicated. Reduction is achieved by squeezing the most distal part of the intussusception cephalad. In the presence of an irreducible mass or gangrene, resection is required.

Volvulus

A volvulus is a twisting or axial rotation of a portion of the bowel around its mesentery. When complete, it forms a closed-loop obstruction. Volvuli may be primary (congenital mild rotation of the gut, abnormal vascular attachments, or bands) or secondary (to an acquired adhesion or stoma).

Specific types include neonatal volvulus, which occurs secondary to arrested gut rotation. Volvulus of the small intestine may occur spontaneously, secondary to adhesions to the parietes or female pelvic organs. Caecal volvulus may occur *de novo*.

A barium enema may be used to confirm the diagnosis, with an absence of the caecum and a bird's-beak deformity. Sigmoid volvulus is common in Eastern Europe and Africa. Plain radiograph is usually diagnostic, showing massive colonic distension, with a dilated loop of bowel running diagonally across the abdomen from right to left and two fluid levels, one within each loop of bowel.

The initial management should include endoscopic decompression, with a subsequent stage procedure or early laparotomy with fixation or resection if this fails.

Paediatric intestinal obstruction

Neonatal intestinal obstruction has an incidence of 1 in 2000 live births. The most common causes include congenital atresia or stenosis, neonatal volvulus, meconium ileus, and Hirschsprung's disease.

In **congenital atresia**, the duodenum and ileum are most commonly affected. Multiple sites may be involved. Treatment consists of bypass as soon as resuscitation is complete. Atresia/stenosis of the jejunum/ileum requires early diagnosis, because of the risk of vascular insufficiency, with gangrene and perforation. Arrested rotation may present with repeated vomiting, resulting from the presence of the transduodenal bands of Ladd. Treatment consists of early laparotomy and division of congenital bands.

Meconium ileus presents as a neonatal manifestation of cystic fibrosis, with progressive ileal inspissation *in utero*, resulting in neonatal obstruction. Diagnosis may be confirmed by the absence of trypsin in stool/bile and the concentration of sodium in sweat. This may respond to conservative management with either gastrograffin or Hypaque enema, allowing dispersion. If conservative management fails, laparotomy with resection of the dilated bowel and a Bishop–Koop reconstruction is required.

Necrotizing enterocolitis is a common phenomenon in sick, premature neonates, who may be predisposed to the condition by hypoxia, hypothermia, hypotension, and umbilical artery cannulation. The ileum, caecum, and colon are predominantly affected, with a spectrum from mucosal to transmural necrosis. Initial treatment consists of aggressive resuscitation, with delayed laparotomy.

CHRONIC INTESTINAL OBSTRUCTION

The symptoms of chronic intestinal obstruction may rise from two sources — the cause and the subsequent obstruction. The cause may be organic and intramural, mural, or extramural, as previously intimated. The most common functional courses are Hirschsprung's disease, idiopathic megacolon, or pseudo-obstruction.

The symptoms of chronic obstruction differ from the acute form in their predominance and timing. Constipation occurs early, but the other symptoms may appear late. A plain abdominal film may confirm the diagnosis. In the presence of radiological large-bowel obstruction, a single-contrast enema should be undertaken to exclude functional disease.

Hirschsprung's disease

Hirschsprung's disease is the result of failure of complete migration of the ganglion cells of the large bowel to the anus, resulting in physiological obstruction. Eighty per cent of cases present in the neonatal period with acute large-bowel obstruction; 20% present with failure to thrive or severe constipation. Barium enema reveals a characteristic narrow segment, whereas full-thickness rectal biopsy will show aganglionosis.

Treatment consists of initial decompression, followed by a definitive pull-through procedure.

Paralytic ileus

In paralytic ileus, there is failure of transmission of peristaltic waves secondary to neuromuscular failure. It may occur in the postoperative period or in association with infection, in a reflex form after fractures or retroperitoneal haemorrhage, and in the presence of metabolic abnormalities such as uraemia or hypokalaemia.

Paralytic ileus is characterized by abdominal distension, absolute constipation, and vomiting, but no pain. The essence of treatment is directed towards prevention. Specific treatment is directed towards removal of the primary cause and gastrointestinal decompression.

Pseudo-obstruction

Pseudo-obstruction is an obstruction, usually of the colon, in the absence of a mechanical cause or acute intra-abdominal disease (12). It may occur in the idiopathic form, or be associated with metabolic abnormalities such as diabetes, myxoedema, and porphyria. It may also occur in association with severe trauma, shock, septicaemia, or retroperitoneal irritation. Drugs, particularly antidepressants and laxatives, may be contributory, and it may also occur in association with scleroderma and Chagas' disease.

After confirmation of the absence of organic obstruction by colonoscopy or single-contrast barium enema, colonic decompression should be undertaken if the patient is symptomatic.

The many **factors associated with paralytic ileus and pseudo-obstruction** may be summarized as:

- Postoperative period
- Metabolic
  - hypokalaemia
  - uraemia
  - porphyria
- Endocrine
  - diabetes
  - myxoedema
- Septicaemia
- Drugs
  - tricyclic antidepressants
  - phenothiazines
  - laxatives
- Retroperitoneal inflammation
  - blood

- urine
- pancreatitis
- Tumour
- Trauma
  - fracture lumber spine/pelvis
- Shock
  - myocardial infarction
  - stroke
  - burns
- Secondary gastrointestinal involvement
  - scleroderma
  - Chagas' disease

Acute mesenteric ischaemia

The superior mesenteric vessels are most commonly affected by embolization or thrombosis. Possible sources include the left atrium in association with fibrillation, a myocardial infarct, an atheromatous plaque from an aneurysm, and mitral valve regurgitations. Venous thrombosis may occur in association with factor V Leiden mutation, portal hypertension, portal pyaemia, sickle-cell disease, and use of the oral contraceptive pill. If the main trunk of the superior mesenteric artery is involved, infarction covers an area from the duodenojejunal flexure to the splenic flexure.

The diagnosis is normally clinical, with sudden onset of severe pain and rapid hypovolaemic shock. Abdominal tenderness may be mild initially. Investigation will reveal a profound neutrophil leucocytosis, with an absence of gas in the small intestine on abdominal radiography.

After resuscitation, patients in whom diagnosis was early may be amenable to embolectomy or revascularization. In the majority of those diagnosed late, the situation may be deemed incurable. In those patients undergoing extensive enterectomy, intravenous alimentation may be required.

References
1. Karanjia ND, Walker A, Rees M. Fluids and electrolytes in surgery. *Surgery* 1992; 10(6): 121–128.
2. Bizer LS, Liebling RW, Delaney HM *et al.* Small bowel obstruction: the role of non operative treatment in simple intestinal obstruction and predictive criteria for strangulation obstruction. *Surgery* 1981; **89**: 407–413.
3. Donckier V, Closset J, Van Gansbeke D *et al.* Contribution of computed tomography to decision making in the management of adhesive small bowel obstruction. *Br J Surg* 1998; **85**: 1071–1074.
4. Parker MC, Baines MJ. Intestinal obstruction in patients with advanced malignant disease. *Br J Surg* 1996; **83**: 1–3.

5. Deans GT, Krukowski ZH, Irwin ST. Malignant obstruction of the left colon. *Br J Surg* 1994; **81**: 1270–1276.

6. Carty NJ, Corder AP, Johnson CD. Surgical debate – colostomy is no longer appropriate in the management of uncomplicated large bowel obstruction. *Ann R Coll Surg Engl* 1993; **75**: 46–51.

7. Biondo S, Jaurrieta E, Jorba R *et al.* Intraoperative colonic lavage and primary anastomosis in peritonitis and obstruction. *Br J Surg* 1997; **84**: 222–225.

8. Runkel NS, Hinz V, Lehnert T *et al.* Improved outcome after emergency surgery for cancer of the large intestine. *Br J Surg* 1998: **85**: 1260–1265.

9. Wilson MS, Hawkswell J, McCloy RF. Natural history of adhesional small bowel obstruction: Counting the cost. *Br J Surg* 1998; **85**: 1294–1297.

10. Menzies D. Post operative adhesion: their treatment and relevance in clinical practice. *Ann R Coll Surg Engl* 1993; **75**: 147–153.

11. Thompson JN, Whawell SA. Pathogenesis and prevention of adhesion formation. *Br J Surg* 1995; **82**: 3–5.

12. Mann SD, Debinski MS, Kamm MA. Clinical characteristics of chronic intestinal pseudo-obstruction in adults. *Gut* 1997; **41**: 675–681.

16. Management of Severe Inflammatory Bowel Disease

DAVID RAMPTON

INTRODUCTION

Most patients with inflammatory bowel disease (IBD) are cared for predominantly as outpatients (see Chapter 36). This chapter reviews the management of patients with attacks of ulcerative colitis, Crohn's disease and indeterminate colitis severe enough to require admission to hospital.

If the outcome of severe attacks of IBD is to be optimized, meticulous care must be taken in confirming the diagnosis, establishing disease activity, site, and extent, selecting and giving treatment, and monitoring progress. Such care is best provided by a multidisciplinary team led, unless surgery is necessary, by an experienced medical gastroenterologist. The manifestations, chronicity, and psychosocial impact of IBD mean that, throughout its course, patients must be kept fully informed about the evolution of their illness, and the therapeutic options available.

ACUTE SEVERE ULCERATIVE COLITIS

Who needs admission to hospital?

Immediate admission is required for patients with acute severe attacks of ulcerative colitis defined primarily by clinical features, which include six or more bloody diarrhoeal stools daily, pyrexia and tachycardia (>90 beats/min) (1). Such patients will usually be systemically unwell, may be anaemic, and may have lost weight; in very ill

patients there may be abdominal tenderness, or distension, or both. The decision to admit the patient to hospital is not usually dependent on the results of blood or other tests of disease severity, although these will often be abnormal (see below).

It is also advisable to admit less sick patients who have failed to respond as outpatients to 2 weeks' of treatment with oral prednisolone (see Chapter 36). As the initial attack of ulcerative colitis is more dangerous than subsequent ones, the threshold for admission should be lowered in patients presenting for the first time with bloody diarrhoea.

In-patient management of acute severe ulcerative colitis

The principles involved in managing patients with acute severe ulcerative colitis are summarized in Table 16.1.

General measures

These patients should be admitted immediately to a specialist gastroenterology ward for close joint medical, surgical, and nursing care. Early involvement of the nutrition team, a stoma therapist in patients likely to need surgery, and, if available, a trained IBD nurse, counsellor, or both, is important. A counsellor may be particularly helpful for patients having their first attack of ulcerative colitis: for these, a full and detailed explanation of their

Table 16.1. Principles of inpatient management of acute severe ulcerative colitis.

General measures	
Explanation, psychosocial support	Patient support groups (NACC)
Specialist multidisciplinary care	Physicians, surgeons, nutrition team, nurses, stoma therapist, counsellor
Establishing the diagnosis, extent/site and severity	Clinical evaluation
	FBC, ESR, CRP, albumin, liver function tests, amoebic serology
	Stool microscopy, culture, *Clostridium difficile* toxin
	Sigmoidoscopy and biopsy
	Plain abdominal X-ray
	Consider colonoscopy, air, or instant-contrast enema, leucocyte scan
Monitoring progress	Daily clinical assessment
	Stool chart
	Temperature and pulse 4-hourly
	Daily FBC, ESR, CRP, urea and electrolytes, albumin
	Daily plain abdominal X-ray
Supportive treatment	IV fluids, electrolytes (Na, K), blood transfusion
	Nutritional supplementation
	Subcutaneous heparin
	Haematinics (folate)
	Avoid antidiarrhoeal agents (codeine, loperamide), opiates, NSAIDs
	Rolling manoeuvre (if colon dilating)
Specific treatment Medical	Corticosteroids: IV (hydrocortisone or methylprednisolone) then by mouth (prednisolone)
	Continue 5-aminosalicylic acid by mouth in patients already taking it; otherwise, start it when improvement begins
	Antibiotics for very sick febrile patients, or when infection suspected
	Consider cyclosporin IV then by mouth (with trimethoprim/sulphamethoxazole prophylaxis) for non-responders to steroids at 4–7 days
Surgical (for non-responders at 5–7 days, toxic megacolon, perforation, massive haemorrhage)	Panproctocolectomy with ileoanal pouch or permanent ileostomy
	Subtotal colectomy with ileorectal anastomosis (rarely)

FBC, Full blood count; ESR, erythrocyte sedimentation rate; CRP, C-reactive protein; I.V., intravenous(ly); NSAIDs, non-steroidal anti-inflammatory drugs.

Table 16.2. Differential diagnosis of bloody diarrhoea.

Inflammatory bowel disease	Ulcerative colitis
	Crohn's disease
	Indeterminate colitis
Infective colitis	*Campylobacter, Salmonella, Shigella, Clostridium difficile, Yersinia,* tuberculosis, enterohaemorrhagic *Escherichia coli* (VTEC/O157:H7), amoebiasis, schistosomiasis, herpes*, cytomegalovirus*
Drug-induced colitis	Antibiotics, NSAIDs
Other causes of colitis	Irradiation
	Ischaemia
	Behçet's disease
Other disease	Colorectal cancer
	Diverticulitis

*Mainly in immunocompromised patients (e.g. those with ac-quired immunodeficiency syndrome).

illness, assisted by the written information provided by the National Association for Colitis and Crohn's disease (NACC) (4 Beaumont House, Sutton Road, St Albans, Herts AL1 5HH, UK), is essential. All patients undergoing an acute attack of ulcerative colitis need to be kept fully informed of their treatment and its likely outcome; they must be made aware, from the outset, that they have a 25% chance of needing a colectomy urgently during their admission.

Establishing the diagnosis, extent of disease, and its severity

Investigations are needed to establish the diagnosis in patients presenting for the first time (Table 16.2) and in those with established ulcerative colitis, to

Table 16.3. Confirming the diagnosis, disease extent, and activity in acute severe ulcerative colitis.

Procedure	Diagnosis	Disease extent	Disease activity
History	+		+
Stool microbiology	+		
Sigmoidoscopy	+		+
Rectal biopsy*	+		+
Plain abdominal X-ray		+	+
Colonoscopy, air, or contrast enema*	+	+	+
Radiolabelled leucocyte scan*		+	+
Haemoglobin, platelet count, ESR, CRP, albumin			+

*Sometimes useful (see text).

exclude infection and to assess disease extent (if not already known) and severity (Table 16.3). In most patients, these aims can be achieved by a careful history, sending stool for microbiology, plain abdominal X-ray, sigmoidoscopy and biopsy, and appropriate blood tests. Colonoscopy, air or contrast enemas, and radiolabelled leucocyte scan sometimes merit consideration (Table 16.3).

Clinical evaluation
Abrupt onset of diarrhoea, fever, vomiting, epidemic or contact history, or recent foreign travel suggest infective colitis, even in patients with pre-existing ulcerative colitis. In patients known to be immunosuppressed, cytomegalovirus (CMV), particularly, should be considered. Antibiotic exposure predisposes to *C. difficile* infection, and non-steroidal anti-inflammatory drugs (NSAIDs) may cause either a relapse of established inflammatory bowel disease, or a *de novo* colitis (which usually remits rapidly on withdrawal of NSAID) (2). In patients presenting for the first time, non- or recent cessation of smoking increases the likelihood of ulcerative colitis, whereas previous abdominal or pelvic irradiation make radiation colitis a strong possibility. Ischaemic colitis is usually of sudden onset in older people with other features of vascular disease, and often causes marked abdominal pain in addition to bloody diarrhoea. The very rare Behçet's enterocolitis may be suggested by a history of cyclical oral and genital ulceration, uveitis, erythema nodosum, pathergy, or arthropathy.

Blood tests
Blood tests are better for establishing the activity of ulcerative colitis than for making the diagnosis or identifying its extent. However, an increased platelet count is more common in ulcerative colitis than in infective colitis. In recent travellers to relevant endemic areas, it is worth checking serology, in addition to stool samples, for amoebiasis, strongyloidiasis, and schistosomiasis. No single laboratory variable correlates perfectly with clinical, endoscopic, or histological measures of disease activity (3), but the most useful are haemoglobin, platelet count, erthrocyte sedimentation rate (ESR), C-reactive protein (CRP) (4), and serum albumin.

Sigmoidoscopy and rectal biopsy
Cautious rigid or flexible sigmoidoscopy in the unprepared patient, and without excessive insufflation of air, provides immediate confirmation of active colitis. Sigmoidoscopy also allows biopsy for histology: to minimize the risks of bleeding and perforation, a small superficial biopsy should be taken from the posterior rectal wall, less than 10 cm from the anal margin, using small-cupped forceps. Anecdotally, colonoscopy has a reputation for causing colonic perforation and dilatation in acute severe ulcerative colitis, and although some authorities have reported that it is both safe and useful for decision making (5), most patients can be managed entirely satisfactorily without it.

In patients with established ulcerative colitis, rectal biopsy is not routinely necessary. However, in those presenting for the first time with bloody diarrhoea, infective colitis, as opposed to chronic ulcerative colitis, may be suggested by histology showing an acute, focal, and superficial inflammatory infiltrate with minimal goblet cell depletion and preservation of crypt architecture (6). Although colitis caused by *C. difficile*, CMV, amoebiasis, and Crohn's disease often has characteristic macroscopic appearances, histology may confirm these diagnoses.

Plain abdominal X-ray

A plain film at presentation can be used to assess disease extent, as faecal residue visible on X-ray may indicate sites of uninflamed colonic mucosa. Plain abdominal X-ray is also used to exclude colonic dilatation (diameter >5.5 cm) in very sick patients; note, however, that interpretation of the gas pattern on a plain film may be ambiguous if there has been excessive insufflation of air during a sigmoidoscopy or colonoscopy performed shortly beforehand. Severe active disease is also indicated on plain films by the presence of deep mucosal ulceration and coarse mucosal nodularity, or "mucosal islands". In patients with suspected colonic perforation, diagnosis can be confirmed by an erect chest X-ray or a lateral decubitus abdominal film.

Air and contrast enemas

In some centres, "air enemas", in which air is gently introduced into the unprepared rectum, are performed to enhance the information obtained by plain abdominal radiography, whereas in others, "instant" barium enemas are performed without bowel preparation. Neither technique, however, adds materially to the management in most patients, and both are relatively invasive.

Radiolabelled leucocyte scans

The intensity and extent of colonic uptake 1 h after injection of autologous radiolabelled leucocytes provide, respectively, information about disease activity and (particularly) extent, where doubt exists in patients with ulcerative colitis. Colonic uptake of leucocytes is not, of course, specific for ulcerative colitis and positive results are obtained in other inflammatory colonic diseases. Labelling with technetium-99-hexamethyl propylene amine oxime (^{99}Tc-HMPAO) is preferred to indium-111 because of its superior definition, lower dose of radiation, shorter scanning interval, and lesser cost. For research purposes, faecal excretion of ^{111}In-labelled leucocytes can be used to assess disease activity (3), but this technique is not necessary for routine purposes.

Monitoring progress (Tables 16.1, 16.3)

Progress is monitored by twice-daily clinical assessment (including abdominal examination for gaseous distension, loss of hepatic dullness (which may indicate free gas in the peritoneal cavity) and peritoneal irritation, stool chart (recording frequency, consistency, presence of overt blood, urgency), and 4-hourly measurement of temperature and pulse. Measurement of abdominal girth to predict impending colonic dilatation lacks sufficient reproducibility to be worthwhile. Blood count, ESR, CRP, routine biochemistry, and plain abdominal X-ray should be undertaken daily in sick patients.

Of these variables, the two most useful in predicting the outcome of the acute attack appear to be stool frequency and CRP at 3 days: patients with values greater than 8 stools/day or 45 mg/litre, respectively, have an 85% chance of needing surgery during their admission to hospital (4).

Supportive treatment (Table 16.1)

Intravenous fluids and blood

Most patients require intravenous fluids and electrolytes, particularly potassium, to replace diarrhoeal losses. Serum potassium concentration should be maintained at or greater than 4 mmol/litre, as hypokalaemia predisposes to colonic dilatation. Blood transfusion is recommended if the haemoglobin decreases to less than 10 g/dl.

Nutritional support

Patients can usually eat normally, with liquid supplements if necessary. Very sick patients, many of whom will come to surgery, may need total parenteral nutrition. There is no evidence that bowel rest with total parenteral nutrition in itself influences the course of attacks of severe ulcerative colitis.

Anticoagulation

Because active IBD is associated with a high risk of venous and arterial thromboembolism (7), patients should be given prophylactic subcutaneous heparin (e.g. low molecular weight heparin 3000–5000 units daily). Such treatment does not appear to increase rectal blood loss; indeed, because of anecdotal reports of its efficacy in this setting, controlled trials are under way to assess the primary therapeutic role of intravenous heparin in full anticoagulant (and concomitantly anti-inflammatory) dosage in acute severe ulcerative colitis (8).

Drugs to avoid

Patients should avoid antidiarrhoeal (codeine phosphate, loperamide, Lomotil), opioid analgesic, antispasmodic, and anticholinergic drugs, as they may precipitate toxic megacolon (9).

NSAIDs are also contraindicated, because of their potentially adverse effects on disease activity (2). If relief of mild pain is needed, oral paracetamol appears to be safe; severe pain suggests colonic dilatation or perforation needing urgent intervention.

Because anecdotal reports suggest that iron supplements may exacerbate active inflammation, perhaps by increasing mucosal production of reactive oxygen metabolites, some authorities delay their use until remission has been achieved.

Rolling manoeuvre

In very sick patients, particularly those with clinical or radiological evidence of incipient colonic dilatation, rolling into the prone or knee-elbow position for 15 min every 2 h may aid in the evacuation of gas per rectum, particularly from the transverse colon (which lies superiorly in the abdomen when the patient is supine) (10).

Specific medical treatment (Table 16.1)

The cornerstone of specific medical treatment of acute severe ulcerative colitis remains corticosteroids. Aminosalicylates and antibiotics have minor roles. Cyclosporin is under continuing evaluation, but oral azathioprine and 6-mercaptopurine are too slow to work in patients with acute steroid-refractory attacks. Several new therapeutic approaches are also being assessed (see below).

Corticosteroids

Hydrocortisone 300–400 mg/day or methyl prednisolone 40–60 mg/day are given intravenously. There is no advantage in giving higher doses, although continuous infusion may be more effective than once- or twice-daily boluses (1). Corticosteroid drip enemas (e.g. prednisolone 20 mg or hydrocortisone 100 mg in 100–200 ml water rectally via a soft catheter and intravenous giving-set twice daily with the patient in the left lateral position) are sometimes given in addition to intravenous steroids, but their value is unproven.

With this treatment, about 70% of patients improve substantially in 5–7 days. They are then switched to oral prednisolone 40–60 mg/day, the dose being tapered to zero over 2–3 months. Conventionally, failure to respond to intravenous steroids after 7 days indicates urgent colectomy, but introduction of cyclosporin can now be considered as an alternative (see below).

Aminosalicylates

Aminosalicylates in full dose are continued in those patients already taking them at the time of their admission to hospital and who are well enough to take oral medication, but these drugs do not have a primary therapeutic in acute severe ulcerative colitis. In case patients given aminosalicylates for the first time prove to be allergic to them or intolerant of them, initiation of this treatment is best delayed until the patient shows sufficient improvement on intravenous steroids to switch to oral treatment. Aminosalicylates are contraindicated in patients with a history of sensitivity to aspirin.

Antibiotics

The original Oxford regimen for acute severe ulcerative colitis included intravenous tetracycline in addition to steroids. One study has suggested a role in this setting for adjunctive oral tobramycin (11), but the use of antibiotics is now usually restricted to very sick febrile patients, or to those in whom an infective component to their colitis is strongly suspected. Under such circumstances, a combination of antibiotics — for example ciprofloxacin or a cephalosporin with metronidazole — is often given.

Cyclosporin

The only current evidence-based indication for the use of cyclosporin in IBD is steroid-refractory active severe ulcerative colitis. In a single small controlled trial (12), the results of which have been largely confirmed by subsequent experience elsewhere (13), intravenous (4 mg/kg per day) followed by oral (5–8 mg/kg per day) cyclosporin, given with continued corticosteroids, averted colectomy in the acute phase in 80% of patients failing to respond to 5–7 days of intravenous steroids alone.

Enthusiasm for this approach, however, has to be tempered both by the frequency of relapse necessitating colectomy (up to 50%) that follows withdrawal of cyclosporin, and by its serious adverse effects. These include: opportunistic infections, particularly pneumocystis carinii pneumonia; renal impairment, including a 20% reduction in glomerular filtration rate in most patients, and a sometimes irreversible interstitial nephritis in up to 25% of patients; hypertension (15% of patients); hepatotoxicity (fewer than 20% of patients); epileptic fits (3%), as a result of penetration of the blood-brain barrier by a cremaphor in cyclosporin and confined to patients with low serum concentrations of cholesterol, magnesium, or both; hyperkalaemia; hyperuricaemia; hypertrichosis; gingival hypertrophy; and paraesthesiae. Grapefruit juice and drugs that inhibit the metabolism of cyclosporin (e.g. erythromycin, oral contraceptives, fluconazole, calcium-channel blockers), increase its blood concentration and toxicity. In contrast, phenytoin, carbamazepine, barbiturates, and rifampicin, by inducing hepatic cytochrome P450, decrease blood concentrations of cyclosporin. Long-term oral use of cyclosporin may predispose to lymphoma. Its side effects demand frequent monitoring of its blood concentrations and serum biochemistry in treated patients.

Further studies are needed to define those patients who should be given the drug intravenously, whether a low dose (2 mg/kg per day) will be efficacious and safer, and what oral therapy — for example, cyclosporin, azathioprine, or 6-mercaptopurine — they should be prescribed thereafter. It is already clear, however, that intravenous cyclosporin, perhaps given with trimethoprim/sulphamethoxazole as prophylaxis against *Pneumocystis carinii* infection, is very useful, in the minority of patients with steroid-refractory acute severe ulcerative colitis, for buying time for improving their nutrition before, or preparing them psychologically for, surgery.

Azathioprine and 6-mercaptopurine

Oral azathioprine and its active metabolite, 6-mercaptopurine are very effective in inducing and maintaining remission in patients with steroid-refractory or -dependent IBD. Unfortunately, however, they take 3–4 months to exert their effect and are thus inappropriate for acute severe ulcerative colitis.

Possible new treatments

A report of an uncontrolled trial suggested that anti-tumour necrosis factor (TNF) antibody may be beneficial in active ulcerative colitis (14), as it is in steroid-refractory Crohn's disease (see below) (15,16). The potential benefits of this agent in acute severe ulcerative colitis, in common with those of intravenous heparin (see above) (8), require evaluation in controlled clinical trials. Other new agents targeted at specific points in the inflammatory process are also undergoing initial assessment in ulcerative colitis: these include other cytokines, such as human recombinant interleukin-11, and antibodies and antisense oligonucleotides to leucocyte/endothelial cellular adhesion molecules (17).

Specific surgical treatment (Table 16.1)

A colorectal surgeon should be involved in the care of patients with acute severe ulcerative colitis throughout their stay in hospital. Indications for **urgent colectomy**, which is required in about 20% of patients with acute severe colitis (and in a higher proportion of patients having their first attack) include:

1. Toxic colonic dilatation (more than 5.5 cm diameter on plain abdominal radiograph) not responding, within 24 h, to intensification of medical treatment (see below).
2. Deterioration or failure to respond to intensive medical treatment in 5–7 days.

Emergency surgery, after appropriate immediate resuscitation, including antibiotics and blood transfusion respectively, is required in patients, fortunately rare, who develop (see below):

- colonic perforation
- massive colonic haemorrhage

Details of the surgical options available (panproctocolectomy with ileoanal pouch or permanent ileostomy, or, rarely, subtotal colectomy with ileorectal anastomosis) and their elective indications, are beyond the scope of this chapter.

Other aspects

Toxic megacolon

As mentioned earlier, in very sick patients, the rolling manoeuvre may help prevent toxic megacolon (9,10). If colonic dilatation becomes established, especially if associated with systemic toxicity, immediate surgery is indicated if the intensive treatment outline in Table 16.1, and including rolling, intravenous antibiotics, and a nasogastric tube to aspirate bowel gas and fluids, has not produced improvement in 24–48 h (9).

Colonic perforation and massive haemorrhage

After appropriate urgent resuscitation, including intravenous antibiotics and blood transfusion respectively, emergency surgery is required for both these rare complications of acute severe ulcerative colitis. Even with immediate surgical intervention, the mortality of colonic perforation — which can occasionally also occur in patients without colonic dilatation — is high (up to 50% in published series) (9).

Outcome of attacks of acute severe ulcerative colitis

As indicated above, more than 80% of patients with severe ulcerative colitis avoid colectomy in the acute phase when treated with intravenous corticosteroids, and cyclosporin in addition if necessary. Of these, however, more than 50% will have had a colectomy for recurrent episodes of active disease before 5 years has elapsed. Mortality of acute severe ulcerative colitis should now be less than 1%, the most common cause of death currently being pulmonary embolus.

CROHN'S DISEASE

Whereas the treatment of active ulcerative colitis depends primarily on its severity (see above) and extent, in Crohn's disease the determinants of medical, nutritional, and surgical management include not only the activity and site of disease, but also the nature of the dominant clinical pathology. The **major presentations of active Crohn's disease** include:

- inflammatory ileocaecal disease
- obstructive small bowel disease
- intra-abdominal abscess
- intestinal fistula
- perianal disease
- Crohn's colitis
- oral and upper gastrointestinal disease

Inflammation, obstruction, abscess and fistula require different therapeutic approaches (Tables 16.4–16.6) and often need to be distinguished by appropriate prompt investigation before specific treatment is begun (18).

Drug treatment in Crohn's disease is generally less effective than in ulcerative colitis, and dietary and surgical treatment are therefore more important. As in ulcerative colitis, patients with Crohn's disease should be encouraged to take an active part in deciding which therapeutic approach is best for them (18).

Who needs admission to hospital?

Its heterogeneous presentation makes assessment of disease activity in Crohn's disease more complicated than that of ulcerative colitis. For clinical trials, a large number of multifactorial clinical or laboratory-based scoring systems, such as the Crohn's Disease Activity Index, have been devised, but none is suitable for ordinary clinical use (3,19). The working definitions of the American College of Gastroenterology (Table 16.7) (19) are more practicable. Patients with moderate to severe and severe to fulminant disease need prompt, and in the latter instance immediate, admission to hospital. In patients with Crohn's colitis, indications for admission resemble those for acute severe ulcerative colitis (see above).

Inpatient management of active Crohn's disease

General measures

As in the case of acute severe ulcerative colitis (see above), patients with Crohn's disease that is sufficiently active to necessitate their admission to hospital should be looked after by a multi-disciplinary team with special expertise in IBD, in a specialist gastroenterology ward (Table 16.4). Options for treatment (medical, nutritional, surgical) are often wider than in ulcerative colitis, and it is essential that the patient is kept fully informed about their illness, and takes a place at the centre of the therapeutic decision-making process.

Establishing the diagnosis, clinicopathological problem and severity

In most patients, the diagnosis of Crohn's disease and identification of its principal site will have been made before their admission to hospital. Investigations, therefore, are directed primarily towards clarifying the clinicopathological process (see bulletted list on p. 209), in order to optimize subsequent treatment. In a minority of individuals presenting acutely for the first time, the diagnosis of Crohn's disease will not yet have been made.

Clinical evaluation

Terminal ileal and ileocaecal Crohn's disease usually present with pain, a tender mass in the right

Table 16.4. Current management of active ileocaecal Crohn's disease.

General measures	
Explanation, psychosocial support	Patient support groups (NACC)
Specialist multidisciplinary care	Physicians, surgeons, nutrition team, nurses, stoma therapist, counsellor
Establishing the diagnosis, extent/site and severity	Clinical evaluation
	FBC, ESR, CRP, ferritin, folate, vitamin B_{12}, albumin, liver function tests, Ca, Mg, Zn
	Stool microscopy, culture, toxins
	Plain abdominal X-ray
	Consider colonoscopy and biopsy, small-bowel barium radiology, ultrasound, CT, MRI, leucocyte scan
Monitoring progress	Daily clinical assessment
	Stool chart
	Temperature and pulse 4-hourly
	Alternate-daily FBC, ESR, CRP, urea and electrolytes, albumin
	Daily plain abdominal X-ray (in patients with obstruction)
Supportive treatment	Intravenous fluids, electrolytes (Na, K), blood transfusion
	Nutritional supplementation; low-residue diet if small-bowel strictures
	Subcutaneous heparin
	Haematinics (vitamin B_{12}, folate)
	Analgesia, antidiarrhoeal agents
	Avoid NSAIDs, delayed release drugs
Specific treatment (separately or in combination)	
Medical	Corticosteroids: IV (hydrocortisone or methylprednisolone) then by mouth (prednisolone or controlled-release budesonide)
	Continue high dose mesalazine in patients already taking it; otherwise, start it when improvement begins
	Consider metronidazole; also broad-spectrum antibiotics for very sick febrile patients, or when infection/collection suspected
	Consider azathioprine/6-mercaptopurine (slow response) or anti-TNF antibodies for non-responders to steroids
Nutritional	Liquid formula diet
Surgical	Resection or stricturoplasty

CT, computed tomography; MRI, magnetic resonance imaging.

Table 16.5. Outline of specific treatment of presentations of active Crohn's disease other than ileocaecal disease (Table 16.4) or Crohn's colitis (Table 16.6).

Presentation	Treatment
Subacute obstruction	Trial of IV corticosteroids
	IV fluids and nasogastric suction (if necessary)
	Surgery for non-responders: local resection or stricturoplasty
Intra-abdominal abscess	Broad-spectrum antibiotics
	Percutaneous or surgical drainage
Intestinal fistula	Enteral or parenteral nutrition
	Oral metronidazole (for up to 3 months)
	Oral azathioprine or 6-mercaptopurine
	Consider IV cyclosporin, anti-TNFα antibodies
	Surgery: local resection
Perianal disease	Oral metronidazole (for up to 3 months), ciprofloxacin
	Oral azathioprine or 6-mercaptopurine
	Consider IV cyclosporin, anti-TNFα antibodies
	Surgery: drain abscesses; seton sutures for chronic fistulae
Oral and upper gastrointestinal disease	Treat as in other sites
	Oral, topical, or intralesional corticosteroids; laser for oral ulceration
	Omeprazole for duodenal disease

Table 16.6. Specific treatment of active Crohn's colitis.

Type of treatment	Details
Drug therapy	Corticosteroids: IV (hydrocortisone or methyl prednisolone) then by mouth (prednisolone)
	5-Aminosalicylic acid by mouth
	Metronidazole by mouth an option for mild cases
	Azathioprine/6-mercaptopurine by mouth if response can be postponed for up to 4 months
	Cyclosporin not of proven benefit
Nutritional therapy	Liquid formula diets of uncertain benefit
Surgery	Total colectomy with ileostomy (ileoanal pouch contraindicated)
	Segmental resection for stricture

Table 16.7. Working definition of disease activity in Crohn's disease (adapted from reference 19).

Activity	Features
Remission	Asymptomatic patients
Mild to moderate	Outpatients able to take oral nutrition; with symptoms, fluid depletion, fever, abdominal tenderness, painful mass, or obstruction
Moderate to severe	Patients who have failed to respond to treatment of mild to moderate disease, or those with more obvious symptoms, including fever, >10% weight loss, abdominal pain or tenderness (without rebound), intermittent nausea or vomiting (without obstructive findings), or anaemia
Severe to fulminant	Patients with persisting symptoms despite outpatient oral steroids, or those with high fever, persistent vomiting, intestinal obstruction, rebound tenderness, cachexia, or an abscess

iliac fossa (Table 16.8), or both with or without diarrhoea. In patients with symptoms predominantly caused by inflammation or abscess, the pain tends to be constant and often with fever, whereas in patients with small-bowel obstruction, the pain is more generalized, intermittent, colicky, and associated with loud borborygmi, abdominal distension, vomiting and eventually, absolute constipation.

In patients in whom the diagnosis of Crohn's disease has not yet been made (Table 16.8), acute appendicitis with a mass may be particularly difficult to differentiate from Crohn's disease, except at laparoscopy or laparotomy. In elderly patients presenting *de novo*, caecal carcinoma and lymphoma need careful consideration, and in some ethnic groups — for example South Asian — ileocaecal tuberculosis is more common than Crohn's disease. In about 30% of cases, a chest X-ray, the Mantoux test, or both, may suggest the diagnosis, but colonoscopy with biopsy and culture, laparoscopy, laparotomy, or a trial of antituberculous therapy (to which, confusingly, a small minority of patients with Crohn's disease may respond (20)) — or a combination of any of these — may be necessary.

In **Crohn's colitis**, diarrhoea, which is not usually bloody, is a more prominent symptom than

pain; lines of investigation in previously undiagnosed patients are outlined in the section on acute severe ulcerative colitis, above.

External abdominal or perianal **fistulae** are usually clinically obvious, but direct questions about pneumaturia and faeculent vaginal discharge may be necessary to identify enterovesical or enterovaginal fistulae.

All patients should be carefully assessed in relation to their **nutritional intake and status**, the latter clinically by measurement of weight, height and then body mass index (weight (kg)/height (m)^2; normal range 20–25 kg/m^2) (see Chapter 21).

Blood tests

As in ulcerative colitis, the main value of blood tests is in assessing and monitoring disease activity,

Table 16.8. Causes of a mass in the right iliac fossa.

Ileocaecal	Appendix mass
	Crohn's disease
	Carcinoma, lymphoma, carcinoid
	Tuberculosis, amoeboma, *Yersinia*, actinomycosis
Other	Tubo-ovarian: cyst, tumour, torsion
	Renal: tumour, polycystic kidney, hydronephrosis
	Psoas abscess

which is related directly to the platelet count, ESR, and CRP, and inversely to serum albumin. However, in very sick patients, particularly those with extensive small-bowel disease and steatorrhoea, there may be laboratory evidence of malnutrition and malabsorption (anaemia, low serum concentrations of iron, folate, vitamin B_{12}, albumin, calcium, magnesium, zinc, essential fatty acids) (see Chapter 31). An increased neutrophil count may suggest intra-abdominal abscess, but corticosteroids also cause a neutrophil leucocytosis.

Endoscopy and biopsy

In patients with right iliac fossa symptoms in whom the diagnosis of Crohn's disease is in doubt, colonoscopy to the terminal ileum, with appropriate biopsies, can be helpful. It can also be used to balloon-dilate short strictures (see below). In established Crohn's colitis, colonoscopy during acute relapse is not routinely necessary and may be unsafe (see below). In previously undiagnosed patients, however, because rectal sparing is common in Crohn's colitis, sigmoidoscopy is often not helpful; sometimes, nevertheless, rectal induration or ulceration, or the presence of perianal disease, point to the diagnosis, and 30% of patients with ileocaecal Crohn's disease will have at least microscopic rectal involvement. Furthermore, in about 5% of patients with macroscopically normal rectal mucosa and Crohn's disease more proximally, histology of rectal biopsies may reveal epithelioid granulomata.

Plain abdominal X-ray

A plain film is essential if intestinal obstruction is suspected. It may also hint at a mass in the right iliac fossa, and is occasionally helpful, as in ulcerative colitis, in estimating disease extent or severity in active Crohn's colitis.

Barium radiology

Because it may exacerbate obstructive symptoms and pre-existing perforation, conventional barium follow-through and small-bowel enema (enter-oclysis) should be avoided in severely ill patients with small-bowel disease. Arguments persist as to which technique is preferable for the delineation of small intestinal structure in less sick patients. Enteroclysis may be more sensitive than barium follow-through for the demonstration of small lesions and short strictures, but many patients find the necessary jejunal intubation extremely uncomfortable. In many

centres, because it allows biopsy and, when necessary, balloon dilatation of strictures, colonoscopy is used in preference to barium enema in patients with suspected large-bowel and terminal ileal disease. Contrast fistulography remains a useful technique for the clarification of anatomical connections in patients with abdominal sinuses or fistulae.

Radiolabelled leucocyte scans

^{99}Tc-HMPAO scanning can be helpful to identify, non-invasively, not only sites of large-bowel inflammation, as in ulcerative colitis (see above), but also in the small intestine. Delayed scanning can also be very helpful in identifying intra-abdominal abscesses. Delayed scans in patients with intestinal inflammation outline more of the distal bowel, as the radiolabelled leucocytes that have migrated into the lumen move distally; in contrast, in patients with an abscess, the site of uptake remains constant, often gradually intensifying.

Ultrasound, computed tomography scan, and magnetic resonance imaging (MRI)

Unhelpful in ulcerative colitis, abdominal ultrasound and CT scan can be very useful in active Crohn's disease, allowing not only the evaluation but also the percutaneous drainage of localized collections; both techniques are also increasingly used for the identification of intrinsic gut wall abnormalities, for example areas of thickening or matting of bowel loops. Endoluminal ultrasound and MRI are invaluable for the anatomical delineation of perianal abscesses and fistulae.

Supportive treatment

Patients with active Crohn's disease, like those with acute severe ulcerative colitis, need meticulous supportive treatment — including, as necessary, intravenous fluids and electrolytes, blood transfusion, and prophylactic subcutaneous heparin (see above) (Table 16.4).

Attention to nutritional requirements is essential. Most patients with active Crohn's disease need nutritional supplements — parenterally if they are seriously ill (see Chapter 21) — and haematinics (iron, folate, or intramuscular vitamin B_{12}); however, it may be sensible to delay oral iron therapy until remission has been achieved (see above).

Patients with stricturing small-bowel disease need a low-residue diet, avoiding, for example, nuts, citrus fruits, and vegetables. The management of short bowel syndrome is described in Chapter 20.

In patients without active Crohn's colitis, opioid antidiarrhoeal agents and analgesia can be prescribed as necessary. Cholestyramine (4-g sachets up to four times daily), by binding luminal bile salts, can be used to ameliorate the watery diarrhoea of patients with extensive ileal Crohn's disease or previous resections; note, however, that cholestyramine also binds many other drugs (which should not therefore be taken simultaneously), and may worsen steatorrhoea.

Drugs to avoid include iron salts (see above) and NSAIDs (2). In patients with stricturing small-bowel disease, delayed-release drugs may precipitate obstruction.

SPECIFIC TREATMENT OF DIFFERENT PRESENTATIONS OF ACTIVE CROHN'S DISEASE

Ileocaecal Crohn's disease
Therapeutic options include drugs, liquid-formula diet, and surgery, as separate alternatives or in combination, depending on the individual patient's age, presentation, and personal preference (Table 16.4).

Drug therapy

Corticosteroids
In active disease, oral steroids provide the quickest and most reliable (60–80% of patients) response. Conventionally, prednisolone 40–60 mg/day is used, the dose being tapered by 5 mg every 7–10 days, once improvement, which usually takes 3–4 weeks, has begun. Very sick patients, or those needing to be fasted because of intestinal obstruction, need intravenous corticosteroids at least initially (e.g. methyl prednisolone 40–60 mg/day, hydrocortisone 300–400 mg/day).

In patients able to take oral treatment and in whom systemic steroid side effects are a major problem, controlled-ileal-release budesonide 9 mg/day can be used, albeit at greater financial cost (21). This drug approaches prednisolone in efficacy, but because of its rapid first-pass hepatic metabolism, causes much less adrenocortical suppression, as assessed by plasma cortisol concentrations (21).

Aminosalicylates
In patients with only moderately active ileocaecal disease, few of whom will need to be managed as inpatients, high-dose oral mesalazine (e.g. Pentasa 2 g twice daily, Asacol 1.2 g three times daily) can be tried (22,23); about 40% of them will go into remission in 2–3 months while receiving such treatment, which may be preferred by individuals reluctant to use corticosteroids.

Immunosuppressive drugs
Patients not responding to corticosteroids and who, because of extensive disease or previous surgery, need to avoid operative treatment if possible, can be treated with adjunctive oral azathioprine 2–2.5 mg/kg per day or 6-mercaptopurine 1–1.5 mg/kg per day, the dose of steroids being reduced or phased out altogether as remission is achieved (24). Such patients need to be well enough to wait for up to 4 months for this to occur: use of IV azathioprine does not accelerate the response (25). The side effects of azathioprine and 6-mercaptopurine make blood count and liver function tests mandatory every 2 weeks for 2 months, and then every 3 months indefinitely (see Chapter 36). Homozygous deficiency of 6-thiopurine methyl transferase (TPMT), the enzyme responsible for the safe metabolic dispersal of purine analogues, occurs in about 0.2% of people and predisposes to their side effects. Its assay in the future may help identify patients at particular risk.

Cyclosporin has not been confirmed as useful in active ileocaecal Crohn's disease, and methotrexate, although effective in about 40% of patients with steroid-refractory Crohn's disease, is probably too toxic for widespread use (26). An unblinded trial suggests that oral **mycophenolate mofetil**, a new immunosuppressant increasingly used in renal transplant patients, may be quicker acting and better tolerated than azathioprine (27), but fully blinded trials of this agent have not yet been performed.

Antibiotics
Although metronidazole alone or in combination with ciprofloxacin (28) is moderately effective in mild to moderately active Crohn's disease, it is insufficiently potent to be used as sole treatment in patients ill enough to require admission to hospital (29). Metronidazole and broad-spectrum antibiotics do, however, have a role in the management

of intra-abdominal abscess and perianal disease (see below), in addition to that of diarrhoea resulting from bacterial overgrowth in patients with small-bowel strictures or fistulae.

Possible new treatments

Controlled trials have shown that intravenous infusions of either mouse/human chimeric (cA2) or 95% humanized (CDP571) **anti-TNFα antibody** induce remission in about 30% of patients with active refractory Crohn's disease (15,16), with complete healing of mucosal lesions in some instances. The cA2 antibody (infliximab) has been routinely available in the USA since late 1998 and was launched in the UK in late 1999; it costs about £1500 per infusion. Side effects include infusion reactions and infections. Reassurance is needed that repeated usage (30) will not lead to adverse effects as a result of host antibody induction, or from immunosuppression with consequent opportunistic infection or malignancy; in the latter context, there are isolated reports of lymphoma in patients given anti-TNF antibody. Definition of those patients with Crohn's disease who are most likely to benefit from this very specialist treatment is also needed; this may relate, not only to their disease phenotype (e.g. fistulating disease), but also to their genotype (e.g. TNF microsatellite subtyping).

Other new approaches under evaluation in this setting, as in refractory ulcerative colitis, include **human recombinant interleukin-11** (17), and **antibodies to adhesion molecules**.

Dietary treatment

In patients with a poor response to, or preference for avoiding, corticosteroids, in those with extensive small-bowel disease, and in children, a liquid-formula diet is an alternative primary treatment. This can be either elemental (based on amino acids), protein hydrolysate (peptide-containing), or polymeric (containing whole protein and not therefore hypoallergenic), and is given for 4–6 weeks as the sole nutritional source (31). This approach is probably as effective as corticosteroid treatment in the short term, about 60% of complying patients achieving remission. Unfortunately, after the resumption of a normal diet, many patients relapse (50% at 6 months); whether this can be prevented by selective and gradual reintroduction of particular foods to which individual patients are not intolerant (32), or by the intermittent use of further enteral feeding for short periods, remains to be proven.

The success of enteral nutrition as a primary treatment for Crohn's disease is also limited by its cost, the unpleasant taste of some of the available preparations (polymeric feeds are less unpalatable than elemental ones), the need often to give the feed by nasogastric tube, and the poor compliance of many patients in adhering to the regimen. Such therapy does, nevertheless, offer a valuable alternative in the well-motivated minority of adults for whom it is appropriate.

Surgical treatment

In the 20–40% of patients whose ileocaecal disease fails to respond to drug or dietary therapy — particularly if they have short-segment (less than 20 cm) rather than extensive disease — surgery (limited right hemicolectomy or strictureplasty) is indicated. Indeed, some patients, at presentation, prefer surgery to the prospect of pharmacological or nutritional treatment of uncertain duration; there are no controlled data to confirm which approach is best. After surgery, there is a 50% chance of recurrent symptoms at 5 years and of further surgery at 10 years; taking an aminosalicylate agent long term and stopping smoking may reduce these risks by about 10% and 30%, respectively (33,34). The place of laparoscopic, as opposed to open, surgery in this setting requires further evaluation.

Obstructive small-bowel Crohn's disease

In patients presenting with obstructive symptoms and signs, with appropriate abnormalities on plain abdominal X-ray, the principal difficulty lies in deciding whether stricturing is the result of active inflammation, fibrosis with scarring, or even adhesions (Table 16.5). Sometimes, laboratory markers (e.g. increased platelet count, ESR, CRP) or radiolabelled leucocyte scan can help to identify individuals with active inflammatory Crohn's disease, but in most instances a short trial of intravenous corticosteroids is given, in addition to intravenous fluids and, if necessary, nasogastric suction. Parenteral nutrition is required if resumption of an oral diet is not likely within 5–7 days. If the stricture is in the upper jejunum, terminal ileum, or colon, enteroscopic or colonoscopic balloon dilatation can be undertaken, but in patients not settling in 48–72 h, surgery is needed, options being local resection or, for short or multiple strictures, stricturoplasty. Patients responding to conservative treatment should be advised to take a low-residue diet (see above), to reduce the chance of recurrent symptoms.

Intra-abdominal abscess in Crohn's disease

Ultrasound, CT scan or radiolabelled leucocyte scan are usually used to confirm the diagnosis of intra-abdominal abscess in patients with Crohn's disease presenting with pain, weight loss, diarrhoea, and fever, with or without a tender mass (Table 16.5). Broad-spectrum antibiotics are given, and the abscess drained, percutaneously under radiological control, surgically, or both. When oral food intake is likely to be restricted for more than 5 days, parenteral nutrition should be started. Subsequent treatment is usually of the underlying pathological process, for example, ileocaecal inflammation (see above).

Intestinal fistula

The relevant anatomical connections are clarified using contrast radiology, CT, endoluminal ultrasound, or MRI (see above) (Table 16.6). Restitution of nutritional well-being is required, using enteral or parenteral nutrition; very occasionally, this results in closure of fistulae. Where there is no obstruction distal to the site of intestinal fistulae, medical therapy with oral, rectal, or intravenous metronidazole or oral azathioprine or 6-mercaptopurine, or combinations thereof, will cause some fistulae to heal. Uncontrolled studies suggest that intravenous cyclosporin may heal fistulous Crohn's disease and a controlled trial has shown that anti-TNFα antibody (infliximab) is a promising option (35). Initial hopes that octreotide might reduce output from, and even heal, high small-bowel fistulae were not confirmed in a controlled trial (35). Most patients with enterocutaneous, -enteric, -vesical, or -vaginal fistulae, however, require surgical resection of the fistula and local resection of involved intestine or other viscuses. (See also Chapter 20).

Perianal disease

Non-suppurative perianal Crohn's disease may respond to oral metronidazole (37) or ciprofloxacin, or both, given for up to 3 months, and to azathioprine or 6-mercaptopurine in the long term (24). The role of intravenous high-dose cyclosporin is not yet clear, whereas recent data suggest anti-TNFα antibody (infliximab) therapy (35) is effective. Patients with suppurating perianal Crohn's disease need surgery, minimized as far as possible; abscesses should be drained, and loose (seton) sutures inserted to facilitate the continued drainage of chronic fistulae. Defunctioning ileostomy or colostomy is of uncertain benefit.

Crohn's colitis

The treatment of active Crohn's colitis closely resembles that of active ulcerative colitis (see above and Table 16.1); the differences are outlined in Table 16.6. Oral metronidazole (400 mg twice daily for up to 3 months), if tolerated, can be used in patients with only moderately active disease who wish to avoid corticosteroids or aminosalicylates; the response rate is up to 50% (29). Liquid-formula diets may be slightly less effective than in small-bowel disease, and there are no data to support the use of cyclosporin. In patients who require total colectomy, permanent ileostomy is usually recommended because of the high incidence of pouch breakdown and sepsis in Crohn's disease. In rare individuals with refractory segmental colitis, local resections of short diseased segments can be performed. Toxic megacolon is even more rare in acute severe Crohn's colitis than it has become in ulcerative colitis.

Oral and upper gastrointestinal Crohn's disease

Treatment of oral and upper gastrointestinal Crohn's disease follows the principles outlined above. Patients with **oral Crohn's disease** are best managed in close conjunction with specialists in oral medicine; particular options include topical and intralesional steroids, and laser to painful ulcers. **Duodenal Crohn's disease** may respond to omeprazole (38); endoscopic balloon dilatation of strictures can be helpful, but surgery may be technically demanding, and complicated by fistulation.

Outcome of attacks of active Crohn's disease

The diversity of acute presentations of Crohn's disease, listed earlier, means that quantification of the overall outcome of attacks necessitating the patient's admission to hospital is not readily available and, indeed, would be of dubious clinical value. Figures have been quoted above for the efficacy of different treatments, including surgery, in particular disease settings, and in relation to subsequent management measures (21–28,29–35). About 10% of patients eventually die of their disease; these are usually individuals who have experienced multiple admissions to hospital because of very extensive Crohn's disease, frequent relapses, or major complications of the illness and its treatment.

INDETERMINATE COLITIS

Acute indeterminate colitis, in which the clinical, endoscopic, and histological features of the disease do not allow its definite classification as either ulcerative colitis or Crohn's colitis, is managed as if it were acute severe ulcerative colitis. However, in patients coming to surgery, it is usually advisable to avoid immediate formation of an ileoanal pouch, in view of the high risk of pouch breakdown if the diagnosis proves to be Crohn's disease (see above).

CONCLUSIONS

Sick inpatients with IBD need meticulous supportive treatment, including intravenous fluids and blood, prophylactic heparin, and nutritional supplementation. In both forms of IBD, corticosteroids are at present the most effective medical treatment for active disease. Liquid-formula diets are efficacious in active Crohn's disease, but not in ulcerative colitis. Intravenous cyclosporin is a valuable alternative in steroid-refractory severe ulcerative colitis. Azathioprine and 6-mercaptopurine are useful options in less sick patients with steroid-refractory IBD, although they are slow to act, and their side effects make careful blood monitoring essential. Surgery provides a cure for ulcerative colitis, but not for Crohn's disease.

Improvements in future medical treatments are likely to take two directions. First, conventional therapies — such as steroids, aminosalicylates, and azathioprine — are likely to be made available in formulations that focus delivery more accurately on the site of disease, and thereby reduce systemic side effects. More excitingly, the increase in our knowledge of the aetiology and pathogenesis of IBD will inevitably lead to the development of more selectively targeted pharmacological agents; of these, anti-TNFα antibodies are the first to reach the bed-

side. Gene therapy may eventually prove an important step forward in ulcerative colitis and Crohn's disease as in other chronic inflammatory diseases.

Whatever therapeutic advances are made in the coming years, the management of sick inpatients with IBD will continue to depend on close collaboration between specialist gastroenterological physicians, surgeons, nurses, dieticians, and counsellors. Most importantly, the patient with IBD must be looked after as a person rather than a case. As management becomes more complex and the options more varied, it is essential that the patient remains at the centre of the decision-making process; the individual with IBD must be the final arbiter of the type of treatment he or she is to be given.

References
*Of interest; **of exceptional interest
1.   Marion JF, Present DH. The modern medical management of acute severe ulcerative colitis. *Eur J Gastroenterol Hepatol* 1997; **9**: 831–835.
     Useful review.
2.   *Bjarnason I, Hayllar J, Macpherson AJ *et al*. Side effects of non steroidal anti-inflammatory drugs in small and large intestine in humans. *Gastroenterology* 1993; **104**: 1832–1847.
     Definitive review of effects of NSAIDs on both previously inflamed and normal lower bowel.
3.   Hodgson HJF. Laboratory markers of inflammatory bowel disease. In: Inflammatory Bowel Diseases. RN Allan, JM Rhodes, SB Hanauer *et al*. New York: Churchill Livingstone, 1997; pp. 329–334.
     Useful review of laboratory methods of assessing disease activity in IBD.
4.   **Travis SPL, Farrant JM, Ricketts C *et al*. Predicting outcome in severe ulcerative colitis. *Gut* 1996; **38**: 905–910.
     Survey of 51 Oxford patients with acute severe ulcerative colitis, showing that at 3 days a CRP concentration greater than 45 mg/l or stool frequency greater than 8 per day gives an 85% chance of needing colectomy.
5.   *Alemayehu G, Järnerot G. Colonoscopy during an attack of severe ulcerative colitis is a safe procedure and of great value in clinical decision making. *Am J Gastroenterol* 1991; **86**: 187–190.
     Provocative study of 34 patients, claiming value and safety of colonoscopy in active ulcerative colitis.
6.   *Surawicz CM, Haggit RC, Husseman M *et al*. Mucosal biopsy diagnosis of colitis: acute self-limited colitis and idiopathic inflammatory bowel disease. *Gastroenterology* 1994; **107**: 755–763.
     "Blinded" examination of colorectal biopsies from more than 130 patients with infective colitis or IBD (acute onset and chronic), showing features allowing differentiation of infection (acute lamina proprial inflammation, normal crypt architecture) from IBD (mixed lamina proprial inflamma-

tion, abnormal crypt architecture, goblet cell depletion, etc.).

7. *Thromboembolism Risk Factors (THRIFT) Consensus Group. Risk of and prophylaxis for venous thromboembolism in hospital patients. *BMJ* 1992; **305**: 567–574.
Authoritive report classifying IBD requiring the patient's admission to hospital as being sufficiently high risk for venous thromboembolism to need specific heparin prophylaxis, in addition to early mobilization.

8. *Evans RC, Shim Wong V, Morris AI *et al*. Treatment of corticosteroid-resistant ulcerative colitis with heparin — a report of 16 cases. *Aliment Pharmacol Ther* 1997; **11**: 1037–1040.
Sixteen patients with steroid–refractory active ulcerative colitis treated with heparin, with a 75% success rate; useful references to earlier anecdotal use of heparin in IBD.

9. *Present DH. Toxic megacolon. *Med Clin North Am* 1993; **77**: 1129–1148.
Excellent review.

10. Present DH, Wolfson D, Gelernt IM *et al*. Medical decompression of toxic megacolon by "rolling". *J Clin Gastroenterol* 1988; **10**: 485–490.
Uncontrolled report of apparent value of rolling manoeuvre in preventing toxic megacolon in each of 19 at-risk patients.

11. *Burke DA, Axon ATR, Clayden SA *et al*. The efficacy of tobramycin in the treatment of ulcerative colitis. *Aliment Pharmacol Ther* 1990; **4**: 123–129.
Controlled trial in 84 patients showing that oral tobramycin (with steroids) gave a remission rate of 74% in active ulcerative colitis, compared with 43% in patients given placebo (with steroids).

12. **Lichtiger S, Present DG, Kornbluth A *et al*. Cyclosporin in severe ulcerative colitis refractory to steroid therapy. *N Engl J Med* 1994; **330**: 1841–1845.
Remarkable paper showing that nine of 11 steroid-refractory patients with acute severe ulcerative colitis achieved remission when given intravenous cyclosporin, compared with none of 9 patients given placebo.

13. Sandborn WJ. A critical review of cyclosporin therapy in inflammatory bowel disease. *Inflammatory Bowel Disease* 1995; **1**: 48–63.
Useful review.

14. *Evans RC, Clarke L, Heath P *et al*. Treatment of ulcerative colitis with an engineered human anti-TNF-alpha antibody CDP571. *Aliment Pharmacol Ther* 1997; **11**: 1031–1035.
Open study of 15 patients with mild to moderately active ulcerative colitis, showing that single infusion of CDP 571 gave improvement in disease activity at 2 weeks in most patients.

15. **Targan SR, Hanauer SB, van Deventer SJH *et al*. A short-term study of chimeric monoclonal antibody cA2 to tumour necrosis factor alpha for Crohn's disease. *N Engl J Med* 1997; **337**: 1029–1035.
Controlled trial showing that single intravenous infusion of cA2 produced remission after 4 weeks in 33% of 83 patients with moderate to severe refractory Cohn's disease, compared with 4% of 24 patients given placebo.

16. *Stack WA, Mann SD, Roy AJ *et al*. Randomised controlled trial of CDP571 antibody to tumour necrosis factor-alpha in Crohn's disease. *Lancet* 1997; **349**: 521–524.
Small study showing that a single intravenous infusion of humanized anti-TNFα antibody produced significant decreases in Crohn's Disease Activity Index and remission in six of 21 patients, compared with no change in the index and no remission in 10 placebo-treated patients.

17. Rask-Madsen J. From basic science to future medical options for treatment of ulcerative colitis. *Eur J Gastroenterol Hepatol* 1997; **9**: 864–871.
Useful review of relation between current knowledge of pathogenesis of ulcerative colitis and the development of new treatments.

18. Rampton DS. Management of Crohn's disease. *BMJ* 1999; **319**: 1480–1485.
An up-to-date review of the management of Crohn's disease.

19. *Hanauer SB, Meyers S. Management of Crohn's disease in adults. *Am J Gastroenterol* 1997; **92**: 559–566.
Useful practical guidelines to the management of Crohn's disease produced by the American College of Gastroenterology.

20. *Swift GL, Srivastava ED, Stone R *et al*. Controlled trial of anti–tuberculous chemotherapy for two years in Crohn's disease. *Gut* 1994; **35**: 363–368.
Placebo-controlled trial showing that patients with Crohn's disease gain no consistent benefit from rifampicin, isoniazid, and ethambutol given for up to 2 years.

21. **Rutgeerts P, Lofberg R, Malchow H *et al*. A comparison of budesonide with prednisolone for active Crohn's disease. *N Engl J Med* 1994; **331**: 842–845.
Controlled trial showing that budesonide (remissions in 53% of 85 patients) was not significantly less effective than prednisolone (remissions in 66% of 88 patients) in ileocaecal Crohn's disease, but that it caused much less adrenocortical suppression.

22. *Singleton JW, Hanauer SB, Gitnick GL *et al*. Mesalamine capsules for the treatment of active Crohn's disease: results of a 16-week trial. *Gastroenterology* 1993; **104**: 1293–1301.
Dose-ranging controlled study showing that mesalazine (Pentasa) 4 g/day for 16 weeks produced remission in 43% of 75 patients with active ileocaecal Crohn's disease, compared with 14–18% of patients given placebo or Pentasa 1–2 g/day.

23. Tremaine WJ, Schroeder KW, Harrison JM *et al*. A randomised, double-blind, placebo-controlled trial of the oral mesalamine (5–ASA) preparation, Asacol, in the treatment of symptomatic Crohn's colitis and ileocolitis. *J Clin Gastroenterol* 1994; **19**: 278–282.
Placebo-controlled study of 38 patients showing that mesalamine (Asacol) 3.2 g/day given for 16 weeks produced partial or complete remission in 60% of patients, compared with 22% of placebo-treated patients; interpretation compromised by 53% drop-out rate, and because 47% of patients were taking concurrent steroids (in stable dosage).

24. *Pearson DC, May GR, Fick GH *et al*. Azathioprine and 6-mercaptopurine in Crohn's disease: a meta-analysis. *Ann Intern Med* 1995; **122**: 132–142.
Excellent meta-analysis and review.

25. Sandborn WJ, Tremaine WJ, Wolf DC *et al*. Lack of effect of intravenous administration on time to response to azathioprine for steroid-treated Crohn's disease. *Gastroenterology* 1999; **117**: 527–535.
Controlled trial showing that intravenous azathioprine does not speed response in comparison to the oral route.

26. *Feagan BG, Rochon JR, Fedorak RN *et al*. Methotrexate for the treatment of Crohn's disease. *N Engl J Med* 1995; **332**: 292–297.
Controlled study showing that weekly intramuscular methotrexate 25 mg for 16 weeks induced remission in 40% of 94 patients with steroid-dependent/resistant Crohn's disease compared with 20% of 47 patients given placebo.

27. Neurath MF, Wanitschke R, Peters M *et al*. Randomised trial of mycophenolate mofetil versus azathioprine for treatment of chronic active Crohn's disease. *Gut* 1999; **44**: 625–628.
In comparison with azathioprine, mycophenolate appeared, in this unblinded study, to produce a greater remission rate, quicker remission, and fewer side effects.

28. Prantera CR, Zannoni F, Scribano ML *et al*. An antibiotic regimen for the treatment of Crohn's disease: a randomised controlled clinical trial of metronidazole plus ciproflaxacin. *Am J Gastroenterol.* 1996; **91**: 328–332.
Ciprofloxacin shown to have a useful effect in mild-moderately active Crohn's disease.

29. Rosen A, Ursing B, Alm T *et al*. A comparative study of metronidazole and sulphasalazine for active Crohn's disease: the Co-operative Crohn's Disease Study in Sweden. II Result. *Gastroenterology* 1982; **83**: 550–562.
Cross-over study suggesting metronidazole and sulphasalazine to be of similar efficacy (approximately 50% of patients responding to each) in Crohn's ileocolitis and colitis, but not in small-bowel disease.

30. *Rutgeerts P, D'Haens G, Targens S *et al*. Efficacy and safety of retreatment with anti-tumour necrosis factor antibody (infliximab) to maintain remission in Crohn's disease. *Gastroenterology* 1999; **117**: 761–769.
Controlled study of efficacy and safety of infliximab for remission maintenance for up to 44 weeks.

31. Fernandez–Benares F, Cabre F, Esteve-Comas M *et al*. How effective is enteral nutrition in inducing clinical remission in active Crohn's disease: a meta-analysis of the randomised clinical trials. *JPEN* 1995; **19**: 356–364.
Useful meta-analysis and review.

32. *Riordan AM, Hunter JO, Cowan RE *et al*. Treatment of active Crohn's disease by exclusion diet: East Anglian Multicentre Controlled Trial. *Lancet* 1993; **342**: 1131–1134.
Provocative study comparing benefit for exclusion diet in maintaining remission in Crohn's disease: relapse rate 62% at 2 years on exclusion diet, compared with 79% on normal diet.

33. **Camma C, Giunta M, Rosselli M *et al*. Mesalazine in the maintenance treatment of Crohn's disease: a meta-analysis adjusted for confounding variables. *Gastroenterology* 1997; **113**: 1465–1473.
Meta-analysis showing mesalazine to be of very limited value in maintaining remission in Crohn's disease — overall risk of symptomatic relapse reduced by only 6% compared with placebo.

34. *Sutherland LR, Ramcharan S, Bryant H *et al*. Effect of cigarette smoking on recurrence of Crohn's disease. *Gastroenterology* 1990; **98**: 1123–1128.
Historical survey of 174 patients showed relapse rate at 10 years of 70% in smokers and 41% in non-smokers; odds ratio for relapse in woman-smokers 4.2 and in men-smokers 1.5.

35. *Present DH, Rutgeerts P, Targens S *et al*. Infliximab for the treatment of fistulas in patients with Crohn's disease. *N Engl J Med* 1998; **340**: 1398–1405.
Very interesting study indicating that cA2 anti-TNFα antibody rapidly closes enterocutaneous (mainly perianal) fistulae in most affected patients.

36. Scott NA, Finnegan S, Irving MH. Octreotide and postoperative enterocutaneous fistulas: a controlled prospective study. *Acta Gastroenterol Belg* 1993; **56**: 266–270.
Octreotide shown to be of no value in healing enterocuta-neous fistulae.

37. Bernstein LH, Frank MS, Brandt LJ *et al*. Healing of perineal Crohn's disease with metronidazole. *Gastroenterology* 1980; **79**: 357–365.
Open study suggesting usefulness of metronidazole in perianal Crohn's disease.

38. Dickinson JB. Is omeprazole helpful in inflammatory bowel disease? *J Clin Gastroenterol* 1994; **18**: 317–319.
Useful review.

17. Biliary Colic and Cholangitis

ADRIAN HATFIELD

INTRODUCTION

Most gallstones originate in the gallbladder, but about 15% of patients with gallbladder stones will also have stones in the common bile duct. This incidence increases with age in patients who still have a gallbladder *in situ*. After cholecystectomy, about 10% of patients will represent with bile duct stones. These stones will either have been in the bile duct at the time of original surgery, or would have migrated out of the gallbladder or cystic duct at the time of surgery.

The presence of a benign biliary stricture in the bile duct — which could be due to previous gall-stone disease, previous surgery, or primary sclerosing cholangitis — may encourage primary gallstone formation in the bile duct above the stricture.

Gallstone obstruction in the bile duct can lead to the clinical features of biliary colic, cholangitis, and jaundice in any combination. The same features can be seen with obstruction caused by benign stricturing alone and, occasionally, with malignant stricturing.

CLINICAL FEATURES

Biliary colic presents as upper abdominal pain, often in the central epigastrium and not necessarily just in the right upper-quadrant (see Chapter 1). This pain often radiates to the back on the right side, and sometimes to the right shoulder. On occasions there is referred pain into the chest severe enough to lead to a mistaken diagnosis of myocardial infarction.

Biliary colic occurs suddenly and is severe; usually, the pain lasts for some hours. Once biliary colic, which is often associated with vomiting, subsides, the patient is usually pain free, whereas pancreatic pain can last for 1–2 days, and, once settled, often leaves the patient sore for 2 or 3 days afterwards.

The classic presentation of a patient with right upper-quadrant pain, jaundice, and fever or rigors is called "Charcot's triad" and, in the past, has been considered to indicate gallstone obstruction to the bile duct. In common practice, there are many patients who present with biliary colic without jaundice, and biliary colic without a fever. There are also some patients who present with jaundice with or without cholangitis without any pain and, for these patients, a clinical diagnosis of malignant obstruction is often considered. Although the pain of biliary colic is usually severe, there are some patients who have mild abdominal pain and tenderness over the liver as a result of cholangitis secondary to bile duct obstruction that may not necessarily be caused by gallstones. Nowadays, if endoscopic stenting has been used to relieve malignant obstructive jaundice, these symptoms are a common method of presentation of a patient with a stent occlusion.

Another classic clinical presentation, described in Courvoisier's Law, is the presence of an enlarged and palpable gallbladder in a patient with obstructive jaundice; this is indicative of malignant obstruction. The most common exceptions to this are patients with gallstone disease in whom there is obstruction to the neck of the gallbladder or to a low insertion cystic duct, by a gallstone that also then produces bile duct obstruction and jaundice (Mirizzi's syndrome). Such patients may have a mucocoele of a gallbladder, which may rapidly develop into an empyema of the gallbladder.

LABORATORY INVESTIGATIONS

In a patient with an isolated attack of biliary colic, the liver function tests may remain unchanged or there may just be a transient increase in alkaline phosphatase, γ-glutamyltransferase, or both. In patients with more prolonged biliary obstruction, the bilirubin will be variably increased and the alkaline phosphatase and γ-glutamyltransferase increased. With severe cholangitis, the concentrations of γ-glutamyltransferase may be much higher, and there may also be an increase in aspartate transaminase. The biliary obstruction may lead to malabsorption of vitamin K and an increased in the international normalized ratio. In patients with cholangitis, there may be a neutrophil leucocytosis. Blood cultures tend to be positive only when taken at the height of a fever or during the rigor.

IMAGING

Transabdominal ultrasound scanning is very useful for detecting stones in the gallbladder, but has been found to be far less accurate for common bile duct stones. In general, bile duct stones are less dense, cast less of an acoustic shadow, and are therefore more difficult to see. The bile duct may not always be dilated, but, even if the stone is large and the bile duct dilated, if the stone is impacted, the absence of fluid around it may make it difficult to see on ultrasound. After cholecystectomy, ultrasound may detect a moderately dilated bile duct, and this is often used as suggestive evidence of gallstone obstruction. Such a finding on ultrasound is common after cholecystectomy, when the bile duct can remain dilated, but this situation often leads to the need for further investigation to seek for a retained stone.

Recently, the advent of magnetic resonance scanning with appropriate software programs has led to the ability to reconstruct a cholangiogram from sequential magnetic resonance sagittal views. Such scans give excellent non-invasive views of the biliary tree, and are exceptionally useful in detecting stones larger than 2–3 mm; small stones or air in the biliary tree will diminish the accuracy of this procedure. Not every hospital will have a modern, "one breath-hold" scanner with appropriate software, in which case there will be a need to proceed to more invasive cholangiography such as endoscopic retrograde (ERCP) or, at times, transhepatic cholangiography.

ENDOSCOPIC RETROGRADE CHOLANGIOPANCREATOGRAPHY

ERCP has now become established as the measurement of choice in patients with bile duct stones, as one not only obtains a very accurate cholangiogram, but is able to perform the non-surgical treatment of bile duct stones at the same time. The technique of ERCP and its contraindications and complications are discussed in Chapter 46. Current opinion is that ERCP should not be performed in a patient with suspected gallstone obstruction unless the endoscopist is skilled enough to perform the necessary endoscopic sphincterotomy and gallstone removal at the same time. If, at the time of ERCP, contrast medium is injected above an obstruction and then the duct left undrained, sepsis is bound to follow. In addition to the normal technical limitations of ERCP, the success of removing gallstones from the bile duct endoscopically depends on the number, size, and position of the stones. Generally, one would expect to succeed in clearing the bile duct of stones in 80–90% of patients. If it is impossible to remove the stones at the initial ERCP, a stent is usually left in place past the stones, draining the bile duct pending further management. Large stones can now be crushed up with a mechanical lithotripter at the time of ERCP, and the fragments removed either at the same time or at a subsequent procedure.

DIFFICULT MANAGEMENT SITUATIONS

Failed endoscopic access

In some patients, the presence of a papilla inside a duodenal diverticulum or a previous Polya's gastrectomy, makes it impossible for the endoscopist to reach the biliary tree. In this case, a transhepatic cholangiogram and drainage procedure can be performed. Either at the same time or at a subsequent procedure, a guide-wire can be passed down into the duodenum, allowing the endoscopist to perform a sphincterotomy over the guide-wire (combined procedure technique) and to then gain access to the bile duct to crush up or remove stones.

Large bile duct stones

As already mentioned above, the majority of large bile duct stones are now able to be crushed in a mechanical lithotripter at the time of ERCP. There will, however, be some patients in whom this is impossible and the use of extracorporeal shock wave lithotripsy (ESWL) will be required. Old-style lithotripters relied on ultrasound localization of stones and were therefore unsuitable for common bile duct work. Newer machines with fluoroscopic localization, can now localize bile duct stones, providing the bile duct is opacified at the time of lithotripsy, using a previously placed transhepatic drainage catheter or an endoscopically placed nasobiliary drainage catheter. Once the patient has undergone one or more sessions of ESWL, ERCP is necessary to remove stone fragments, as spontaneous passage of fragments can not be relied on to ensure complete and successful clearance of the bile duct.

The use of dissolution agents has been thoroughly investigated in the past (see Chapter 39). Oral agents such as chenodeoxycholic acid or ursodeoxycholic acid are not successful in dissolving bile duct stones, although they may have some role in preventing further stone formation above strictures, by virtue of a choleretic effect. Direct bile duct infusion of mono-octanoin or methylterbutyl ether are both relatively inefficient in the presence of a previous endoscopic sphincterotomy, as the chemical leaks out of the bile duct into the duodenum, which can produce unpleasant side-effects and anaesthesia of the patient.

Stones above strictures

The presence of a postoperative benign stricture, inflammatory stricture as a result of previous gallstones, or one or more strictures caused by sclerosing cholangitis can encourage stasis and the formation of primary stone formation. Such stones are notoriously difficult to treat endoscopically. Direct-contact lithotripsy using a pulsed dye laser or an electrohydraulic lithotripter probe passed down a small endoscope into the bile duct at the time of ERCP, or through a transhepatic tract, are both highly complex and specialist methods for dealing with such stones as an alternative to major open surgery.

SURGICAL INTERVENTION

There is no place for unplanned or emergency surgery in a patient with biliary colic, cholangitis, or jaundice, as this is associated with a high complication rate and, especially in the elderly, an increased morbidity. Nowadays, surgery is undertaken only when other non-operative methods have failed to clear the bile duct of calculi.

In patients with gallbladder stones awaiting laparoscopic cholecystectomy, there is a need for preoperative ERCP in those with a history of biliary colic, pancreatitis, jaundice, or abnormal liver function, or a dilated bile duct on ultrasound scanning. All these factors would suggest the possibility of common bile duct calculi, and it is essential to perform ERCP in these patients, to clear the bile duct before laparoscopic cholecystectomy. If this is not done, there is an increased risk of postsurgical biliary leakage, which then requires urgent ERCP in the postoperative period, with sphincterotomy, gallstone removal and, sometimes, endoscopic stenting until the leak seals.

18.1. Gastrointestinal Malignancy: Oncology

PAULINE LEONARD AND JONATHAN LEDERMANN

INTRODUCTION

Gastrointestinal cancers account for 25–30% of all cancer deaths in the UK, and colorectal cancer — the most common gastrointestinal malignancy — causes 17 000 deaths annually. Surgery has been the mainstay of treatment of gastrointestinal tract tumours, but there has been only a small improvement in the results of treatment of common gastrointestinal cancers over the past 15 years. Non-surgical treatments, principally chemotherapy and radiotherapy, have been viewed with scepticism, largely because the treatment that has been available for many years has been only moderately active.

Over the past few years, better use of existing agents and carefully conducted clinical trials have shown that chemotherapy and radiotherapy, used appropriately, can improve survival and the quality of life of patients with many types of gastrointestinal tumours. Treatment given as an adjuvant to surgery with the aim of eradicating microscopic residual disease has increased the number of patients cured of large-bowel cancer. Palliative treatment in advanced disease improves the symptoms, survival, and quality of life of patients. Recently, several new chemotherapeutic agents have been introduced into clinical practice, and these may add to the benefit of existing therapies.

Multidisciplinary care provides the patient with the best treatment available and is likely to contribute to better survival and quality of treatment. Discussion of clinical cases with an oncologist has become an important component of the management of patients with cancer. Table 18.1.1 summarizes the essential information required by oncologists to enable them to decide about treatment, and the indicators used to assess the response of patients to treatment.

Gastroenterologists and gastrointestinal surgeons will see a large number of patients with common malignancies of the gastrointestinal tract (Table 18.1.2). This chapter concentrates on the role of non-surgical management of gastrointestinal tumours, with particular emphasis on chemotherapy and radiation. Reference will be made to the integration of these therapies with surgical and other treatments discussed elsewhere.

OESOPHAGEAL CANCER
(see also chapter 14)

The overall survival of patients with oseophageal cancer after 5 years is approximately 10%. The results of surgery have improved over the past 20 years, probably as a result of better selection of patients; even so, only 20% survive to 5 years (1). Squamous-cell tumours are the most common type, but the proportion of adenocarcinomas arising from the distal oesophagus is increasing. After surgery, patients either suffer local relapse from occult metastases, or develop distant recurrence in the liver and peritoneum and upper thoracic and cervical lymph nodes.

Radiotherapy

Traditionally, radiotherapy has been used either alone or with surgery. Several clinical trials have been

Table 18.1.1. Essential requirements for the oncologist's decision-making process and assessment of treatment.

Diagnosis	Histological confirmation of tumour
Staging	Details of surgical procedures
	Imaging of tumour
	Serological tumour markers
Therapeutic choices	Adjuvant treatment
	Radical therapy
	– chemotherapy
	– radiation
	– chemoradiation
	Palliative therapy
	– chemotherapy
	– radiation
	– symptomatic
Patient factors	Patient status (clinical performance score)
	Co-morbid conditions
	Informed consent
Outcome	Adjuvant
	– survival
	Radical/palliative
	– measurable tumour response
	– progression-free survival
	– overall survival
	– quality of life

performed comparing adjuvant postoperative radiotherapy with surgery, or neoadjuvant radiotherapy in which radiotherapy is given before operating. The rationale of this approach is to down-stage the tumour. None of these approaches has shown any survival benefit for the addition of radiotherapy. These studies have been summarised in the review by Wobst *et al.* (2). However, there is a correlation between patients who responded well to neoadjuvant radiotherapy and survival. The view generally held is that squamous-cell tumours are more radiosensitive than adenocarcinomas involving the lower one-third of the oesophagus. However, in many of the radiotherapy and chemoradiation trials (see below), patients with both tumour subtypes were included.

Chemoradiation

The inadequacy of radiotherapy alone as primary treatment of oesophageal cancer have has clearly demonstrated by the randomized trial performed by Herskovic *et al.* (3), in which patients were treated with radiation alone or chemoradiation. The two chemotherapy drugs used were cisplatin and 5-fluorouracil (5-FU). The latter is a drug commonly used in the treatment of many gastrointestinal tumours. It acts mainly by inhibiting the enzyme, thymidylate synthase, that is responsible for the synthesis of thymidine from uracil. The drug also has some direct action on RNA synthesis. Combination treatments, principally with cisplatin, have been shown to produce greater tumour response rates, particularly in squamous-cell tumours. The two drugs were given during and after radiation therapy of squamous or adenocarcinoma localized to the mediastinum and cervical lymph nodes. Although the combination arm was more toxic, there was a significant survival benefit, with 50% of the group who received chemoradiation being alive at 2 years, compared with 38% in those receiving radiation alone ($P < 0.01$). Some of the benefit was due to the systemic effects of chemotherapy, as the proportion of patients with distant metastases was less. The rate of local recurrence was also reduced. This was probably due to the interaction of chemotherapy and radiation, as the total dose of radiation in the combined therapy group was smaller. Thus the use of radiation alone as radical treatment of oesophageal cancer can no longer be justified.

Table 18.1.2. Incidence of gastrointestinal cancer in the UK.

	New Cases (men and women)	Annual Deaths			
		Men (1985)		Women (1988)	
		Deaths	Cancer deaths (%)	Deaths	Cancer deaths (%)
Colon	16 715	5860	7	7110	9
Rectum	10 528	3570	4	2920	4
Stomach	12 315	6320	7	4290	6
Pancreas	6 415	3280	4	3510	5
Oesophagus	4 832	3360	4	2230	3

Data from Cancer Research Campaign Factsheets (1989, 1990).

Chemotherapy

Chemotherapy can be used to reduce the size of the primary tumour to increase its resectability, to reduce local recurrence by eliminating occult metastases in local lymphnodes, or to diminish the chance of systemic disease by eradicating micrometastases. It may also be used in advanced disease to palliate symptoms.

Most randomized studies comparing chemotherapy and surgery to surgery alone have contained only a few patients. A large study from the USA comparing preoperative cisplatin and 5FU showed no improvement in survival (4). However, preliminary analysis of the Medical Research Council (MRC) study OE02 using 2 cycles of pre-operative cisplatin and 5FU has shown in improvment of 10% in the two-year survival (5).

Multimodality therapy

The results of chemoradiation, using cisplatin or mitomycin C and 5-FU, are comparable to those achieved with surgery, although there has never been a randomized trial directly comparing the two approaches. Walsh *et al.* (6) have published the results of a randomized trial in which patients received either chemoradiation followed by surgery, or surgery alone. In the combination group, 25% of patients who underwent surgery had no histological evidence of disease in the resected tissue and 32% of these patients were alive at 3 years, compared with 6% in the surgery-alone arm ($P = 0.01$). The trial has been criticized because of the poor results in the control group. An inter-group trial being conducted in the USA is a similar study, but accrual is slow.

Palliative therapy

Both radiation and chemotherapy have been used successfully to palliate symptoms of oesophageal cancer. Details of the chemotherapy used in gastrointestinal oncology is beyond the scope of this chapter, but a summary of the most commonly used drugs and their mode of action is given in Table 18.1.3. Cisplatin and 5-FU are most commonly used to treat squamous-cell cancers, and the use of epirubicin, cisplatin, and continuous infusion of 5-FU (ECF) is gaining popularity in the UK, particularly for adenocarcinomas of the oesophagus and stomach. This regimen is also active in squamous-cell tumours. In one study, 57% of patients had a partial response (reduction of tumour size by at least 50%) to ECF and, 91% experienced symptomatic benefit (7). ECF has also been shown to reduce the requirement for repeated laser treatments. Brachytherapy (intraluminal radiotherapy), alone or in combination with laser therapy, chemotherapy, or

Table 18.1.3. Cytotoxic drugs commonly used in gastrointestinal oncology.

Drug	Class	Mode of action
5-Flourouracil	Antimetabolite (flouropyrimidine)	Inhibition of thymidylate synthase (TS) required for DNA synthesis. Often given with folinic acid (Leucovorin), a TS cofactor
Epirubicin/doxorubicin (Adriamycin)	Anthracycline	Intercalator of DNA and inhibitor of topoisomerase II required for DNA replication
Cisplatin/oxaliplatin	Platinum analogues	Inhibition of DNA synthesis
Gemcitabine	Antimetabolite	Nucleoside analogue. Inhibitor of ribonucleotide reductase and interferes with DNA synthesis
Mitomycin C	Natural product	Alkylator. Cross-links DNA
Irinotecan	Synthetic camptothecin analogue	Inhibitor of topoisomerase I required for DNA replication
Methotrexate	Antifolate	Binds to and inhibits dyhydrofolate reductase
Raltitrexed	A quinazoline antifolate	Inhibitor of TS
Vincristine (Oncovin)	Vinca alkaloid	Mitotic spindle poison
Cyclophosphamide	Synthetic nitrogen mustard	Alkylator. Cross-links DNA

external beam radiation, has also been shown to produce significant symptomatic benefit (see Chapter 45), emphasizing the value of the multidisciplinary team approach to patients with oesophageal cancer.

Summary

Chemoradiation is superior to radiation in oesophageal cancer, and may yield results equivalent to those of surgery for all but a few patients with early disease. However, no direct comparisons have been made in randomized trials. Adjuvant strategies with chemoradiation may improve survival, but the results of trials in progress are awaited. As there are many options for treatment, it is best for patients to be managed by a multidisciplinary team. In general, patients with squamous tumours receive chemoradiation and patients with adenocarcinomas initially receive chemotherapy, with radiation being reserved for tumour progression.

GASTRIC CANCER

Although more than 90% of stomach tumours are adenocarcinomas, a histological diagnosis of the tumour is essential, as lymphomas, which account for most of the remaining group, can be cured by chemotherapy. In the UK, most patients present with advanced gastric cancers. For those with more limited disease, surgery offers the only real prospect for cure. However, only a small group of patients have tumours confined to the stomach. Once nodal spread has occurred the outlook is poor. European trials of more radical surgery have not altered outcome. Stomach cancers are the most chemosensitive gastrointestinal tumours, and chemotherapy has been used principally in advanced disease, to palliate symptoms and prolong survival. Studies have also been performed in the adjuvant setting after surgery.

Chemotherapy

Many cytotoxic agents have been shown to be active in gastric cancer. Tumour response rates are the most commonly quoted yardstick to assess the activity of these drugs. This is important for comparisons between individual drug regimens, but provides only limited information as to the benefit to pa-

tients. Non-randomized (phase II) trials may report survival times, but these have to be interpreted with caution, as the patients in these studies are a selected group. Survival in randomized (phase III) trials — particularly if reported with quality of life measurements — offer the most useful information to clinicians and patients.

5-FU has been used for almost 40 years in gastric cancer. Over the past 15 years it has become clear that its activity can be increased by co-administration of folinic acid — which provides reduced folate, a cofactor for the enzyme, thymidylate synthase — or by intermittent high-dose infusion or protracted infusion therapy. Most of these findings are derived from extensive research in colorectal cancer (see below). The results have been extrapolated to gastric cancer, although relatively few direct comparisons between biomodulated 5-FU and standard bolus injection exist. The addition of other agents such as cisplatin, epirubicin or doxorubicin (Adriamycin), methotrexate or etoposide leads to greater response rates in phase II studies and moderately increased activity in phase III studies. The original 5-FU, Adriamycin and mitomycin C regimen (FAM) has been replaced by 5-FU, Adriamycin and methotrexate FAMtx in Europe, or FEMtx (a similar regimen, but with epirubicin). Etoposide, folinic acid (Leucovorin) and 5-FU (ELF) is a similar regimen, but none of these appears to be superior. ECF, a regimen popular in the UK, has recently been compared with FAMtx in a randomized phase III trial. A small but significant survival benefit was seen in the group receiving ECF (8).

There have now been four studies comparing combination chemotherapy with FAMtx or ELF and "best supportive care". These were all small trials but, in each case, survival was prolonged in the chemotherapy group. On average, one can expect a 6–9 month prolongation in the median survival of patients receiving modern combination chemotherapy regimens. Attempts to quantify benefit in health-economic terms have been difficult, but the findings of one study by Glimelius *et al.* (9) suggested that palliative chemotherapy for gastric cancer is "cost-effective".

Several new agents have shown activity in gastric cancer. These include irinotecan, an inhibitor of topoisomerase I, docetaxel, a drug that interferes with microtubule assembly, and oxaliplatin, a platinum analogue that seems more active than cisplatin in gastrointestinal tract cancers. It is too early to know how these agents will be incorporated into the treatment of gastric cancer. None will cure advanced disease, but they might improve the results of palliative chemotherapy.

Adjuvant chemotherapy

Most of the historic trials in gastric cancer have been conducted with small numbers of patients and drug regimens that would now be considered to have low activity. It is therefore not surprising that a meta-analysis of 11 trials with 2069 patients concluded that there was no significant survival benefit after adjuvant chemotherapy (10). The inclusion of more recent studies alters the odds in favour of chemotherapy. Trials with the more modern combination chemotherapy are in progress, and their results are awaited. In the UK, there is little enthusiasm amongst surgeons for adjuvant therapy, as the British Stomach Group's second trial comparing FAM, radiotherapy, and surgery alone showed no benefit in 5-year survival. However, the high response rate seen with ECF, making some advanced tumours operable, has led to a new trial conducted by the MRC in which the use of ECF before and after surgery is being compared with surgery alone. A similar approach is being adopted in the Netherlands, with FEMtx.

Transcoelomic and intrahepatic spread of tumour occurs frequently. Intraperitoneal treatment with chemotherapy or immunotherapy with a protein-bound polysaccharide has been studied by several groups. In Japan, there have been studies with continuous hyperthermic peritoneal infusion of chemotherapy to try and improve distribution and uptake of drug. Two chemotherapy trials from Japan and Spain, which also were not included in the meta-analysis, have used carbon-absorbed mitomycin C; both studies have demonstrated an improvement in survival.

Radiation

The results of radiation therapy by the British Stomach Group and others who gave radiation and chemotherapy are not encouraging. Radiation is sometimes used for palliation of pain or bleeding, but there are few data from studies to assess its benefit.

Summary

There is no firm evidence that adjuvant chemotherapy is beneficial, but patients should be encouraged to enter randomized trials of modern chemotherapy. Combination chemotherapy has a high response rate, and this leads to palliation of symptoms in a large number of patients, but it is difficult to recommend any specific regimen. For patients fit and willing to undergo chemotherapy, one can expect an extension in median survival of 6–9 months.

PANCREATIC CANCER

More than 95% of tumours are adenocarcinomas arising from the exocrine pancreas. Surgery has a relatively small role in the management of cancer of the pancreas as the majority of patients present with locally advanced or metastatic disease. Relief of symptoms associated with jaundice or intestinal obstruction is an important part of the management of patients and is discussed in Chapter 17. The role of chemotherapy, radiation, and relief of pain — a common symptom in this tumour — will be discussed here.

Chemotherapy

Chemotherapeutic agents have only modest activity in advanced pancreatic cancer. A decision to use palliative chemotherapy will depend on the symptoms and physical state of the patient. Assessment of the activity of drugs can be difficult, as measurement of the primary tumour is not always possible. Assessment of the response may be assisted by measurement of the serum concentrations of carbohydrate antigen CA 19.9, a serological marker of pancreatic cancer that is related to the Lewis Le[a] blood group antigen; its concentrations are increased in the serum of most patients with pancreatic cancers. However, it is not useful for diagnosis, as it is also increased in other gastrointestinal cancers, particularly stomach, colorectal, and bilary tract tumours, and some non-malignant conditions. However, increases and decreases in concentrations of the marker during or after treatment can provide valuable information to the clinician. Symptomatic responses are clinically important, but less easily defined. Measurements of quality of life are being used more frequently to help assess benefit objectively. A new measure — termed "clinical benefit response" — that takes note of the more clinically meaningful effects of treatment on disease-related symptoms such as pain control, general activity (e.g. WHO performance score), and weight gain has recently been introduced.

Virtually all chemotherapy drugs have been investigated in pancreatic cancer. 5-FU has been used extensively, but the results have not been encouraging. Combination treatments with cisplatin or FAM and ECF are more active, but there is often a narrow therapeutic margin, as the clinical condition of patients is often worse than in metastatic cancer from other primary tumours of the gastrointestinal tract. Three new drugs — docetaxel, irinotecan, and gemcitabine — are currently being evaluated in pancreas cancer. Toxicity with the first two agents is significant, and investigation is best suited to patients with a good clinical performance score. Gemcitabine, a deoxycytidine analogue, has been more extensively studied. A randomized trial of gemcitabine compared with 5-FU in previously untreated patients showed a modest but statistically significant improvement in response rate and median survival compared with those treated with 5-FU (11). The difference between the two treatments was even greater when the clinical benefit response was compared. Improvements in clinical benefit have also been seen in patients treated with gemcitabine after progression on 5-FU (12). These results suggest that gemcitabine will become the accepted first-line treatment for patients with advanced pancreatic adenocarcinoma. Despite the recent results with gemcitabine, the median survival for patients with metastatic disease continues to be less than 6 months, with very few patients achieving long-term stabilization of their disease. Some of the effects attributed to chemotherapy may not be substantially different from those achieved with aggressive supportive care alone.

Tamoxifen, an antioestrogen, luteinizing hormone-releasing hormone analogues, and antiandrogens have been studied in pancreas cancer, because many tumours have sex-hormone receptors. Randomized trials with tamoxifen have not shown any evidence of benefit, but a recent study with flutamide showed a small but significant survival benefit (13).

The poor response to conventional cytotoxic chemotherapy has led to research of other modalities of treatment such as inhibitors of invasion and metastasis, drugs that interfere with cell-surface growth receptors or intracellular signalling, and gene therapy. Inhibitors of the matrix metalloproteinases are undergoing clinical trials. Strategies to block the epidermal growth factor (EGF) receptor and inhibit tyrosine kinase are also under investigation. The oncogene k-*ras*, appears to have an important function in the growth of pancreatic cancers, and studies are being performed with farnesyl transferase inhibitors to prevent the posttranslational processing required to localize proteins on the cell k-*ras* membrane.

Radiotherapy

Radiotherapy has been used alone, or combined with 5-FU. Small-scale randomized trials from the USA have provided conflicting data. One from the Gastrointestinal Tumour Study Group (GITSG) suggested a modest improvement in survival after chemoradiation, and the other larger one from the Eastern Cooperative Oncology Group showed no benefit. The inclusion of cisplatin does not produce any additional benefit. In Europe, few patients are being treated with chemoradiation for locally advanced disease.

In Europe, a randomized trial was launched by the European Study Group for Pancreatic Cancer in 1994, to compare survival after pancreatectomy in patients assigned randomly to groups to receive no adjuvant therapy, 5-FU-based chemoradiation, 5-FU-based chemoradiation followed by systemic 5-FU and folinic acid, or 5-FU and folinic acid without radiation.

Symptom control

Patients with pancreatic cancer can often have marked constitutional symptoms. Some such as jaundice and intestinal obstruction, are directly tumour-related; their management is discussed in Chapter 46. Pain can be severe, and may require large doses of opiate analgesia; a coeliac axis block may provide relief and reduce the need for such large doses. Steroids are sometimes used to stimulate appetite and improve well-being. As the prognosis is so poor, it is important to involve the expertise of palliative care specialists early in the management of patients with advanced pancreatic cancer.

Summary

The outlook for patients with cancer of the pancreas remains poor: modern therapies have had little impact on survival. Selected patients may benefit from chemotherapy or radiation. New agents need further evaluation and new types of treatment require investigation. Where possible, patients with advanced pancreatic cancer should be enrolled in clinical trials. As with most other tumours, patients require the expertise of a multidisciplinary team. This approach will improve the care of the patient, even though there may be a small or no measurable effect on the duration of survival.

COLORECTAL CANCER

The incidence of colorectal cancer is 48 per 100 000. It increases sharply with age, and the median age at diagnosis is 70 years. Colorectal cancer accounts for 12% of all cancer deaths and the UK has one of the highest death rates from colorectal cancer in the Western world. Colon cancer affects men and women with equal frequency, but more men are affected by rectal cancer. The molecular alterations involved in the multistep development of carcinogenesis are understood more fully in colorectal cancer than any other solid tumour. Fearon and Volgelstein (14) have demonstrated the series of mutations that accompany the phenotypic development of the malignant process. K-ras and c-myc are the proto-oncogenes involved and p53 (chromosome 17), APC (chromosome 5) and deleted in colon cancer (DCC) found on chromosome 18 are the tumour suppressor genes involved. About 5–15% of patients suffer from inherited (germ-line) mutations associated with an exceptionally high risk of colorectal cancer. Most are hereditary non-polyposis colon cancers resulting from inherited defects in a group of DNA repair gene abnormalities. About 1% of the cancers are due to familial adenomatous polyposis coli resulting from mutations in the *APC* gene. In other affected individuals there may be a strong family history, but the genetic abnormality has not been identified. Knowledge of these changes is of paramount importance in developing screening and early detection of colorectal cancer, but may also improve our understanding of the biology of established cancers and their susceptibility or resistance to non-surgical therapy.

Non-surgical management of colorectal cancer

The oncologist usually will see patients who have undergone surgery to remove the primary tumour. In some cases, surgeons will discuss the patient with an oncologist before treatment is begun. This applies particularly to rectal cancer, in which radiotherapy is either offered before surgery because of a preference in that centre (see below), or, because the tumour is not operable, it is required either as palliation or in a radical dose to the shrink the tumour so that it becomes operable. Less commonly, oncologists see referred patients with advanced colon cancer in whom surgery is not planned as an initial procedure.

In the first group of patients who have undergone a radical resection of the primary tumour, a decision must be made as to whether the patient requires additional treatment with chemotherapy, radiotherapy, or a combination of these. This is based principally on the stage of the disease, which gives an estimation of the risk of recurrence and the magnitude of benefit of additional treatment in relation to the individual's risk. A similar approach is needed for the second group, referred for either preoperative radiotherapy or palliative treatment. The Dukes' pathological staging system of tumours, first described in 1932 remains the system most commonly used in the UK; it is discussed in Chapter 3.2. Modifications have been made to this system, and other factors in the surgical pathology — for example those defined by the Association of Pathologists — are also important indicators of prognosis; these include penetration of the serosal surface, lymphovascular invasion, and the presence of tumour at the circumferential resection margins of rectal cancers. There has been an increase in the detail of reporting, which assists the oncologist in making decisions about adjuvant treatments to reduce the risk of recurrence. In addition, it is essential that the tumour is thoroughly staged to exclude the presence of metastatic disease. This applies particularly to the liver as metastases may not be apparent, even at laparotomy. It is recommended that liver imaging is performed before surgery. Pulmonary spread without liver involvement is uncommon, but it may be found in rectal cancer. Serological tumour markers such as carcinoembryonic antigen (CEA) and CA19.9 are useful indicators of recurrent disease, but it is not clear whether preoperative concentrations are of independent prognostic value. Early-stage disease is associated with a high cure rate but, overall, 40–50% of patients who undergo "curative surgery" will die of metastatic or recurrent disease within 5 years because of the presence of residual disease after surgery. The first 30 months is the time of greatest risk, as 30% of patients will have a recurrence of tumour during that period.

Adjuvant treatment

Adjuvant therapy is administered with the intention of eradicating micrometastatic disease. The probability of residual disease after curative surgery is based on the full histological report of the tumour excised.

Chemotherapy, principally with 5-FU, has been used for more than 40 years in colorectal cancer. The activity of 5-FU, given alone by bolus injection, is modest and it has been difficult to demonstrate its benefit in the adjuvant setting. However, in 1990, a large randomized trial for patients with Dukes' stage C colon carcinoma (15) showed that 5-FU and the antihelminth, levamisole, reduced local recurrence rates and improved overall survival. This study led the Food and Drugs Administration in the USA to recommend adjuvant chemotherapy for all patients with stage III colon cancer. Subsequent trials have demonstrated that 5-FU is more active when given with the biomodulating cofactor, folinic acid, and that this combination is as good as 5-FU and levamisole, but less toxic. An International Multicentre pooled analysis (16) demonstrated that 71% of patients treated with 5-FU and folinic acid had no recurrence of tumour within the follow-up period, compared with 62% in the untreated group. Differences in recurrence and survival were only significant in patients with Dukes' stage C disease. Since then, other even larger studies have examined combinations of 5-FU, folinic acid and levamisole in different schedules and doses. In summary, they have shown a clear survival benefit for patients with stage III (Dukes' stage C) cancer, the magnitude of which is comparable to the benefit of chemotherapy in breast cancer. The role of adjuvant chemotherapy in Dukes' stage B tumours remains uncertain. Some physicians may offer adjuvant therapy to patients who have tumours with poor prognostic features

associated with Dukes' stage B tumours — such as lymphovascular permeation or penetration of the bowel wall (stage pT4) — but clearer guidelines should become available when the results of large trials in the UK and USA are known.

Alternative strategies such as brief perioperative chemotherapy via the portal vein have also been explored. Several moderately sized trials have reported conflicting results. The results of a large prospective randomized trial by the AXIS (Adjuvant X-ray and Infusion Study) Group has shown a small but significant survival benefit at five years (2.5% overall and 4% for colonic tumours) (17). Higher response rates in advanced disease are seen when 5-FU is given by infusion, and this approach is now being studied in the adjuvant setting. There are now also several new cytotoxic drugs available for the treatment of colorectal cancer. Their use in advanced disease is discussed below. Future adjuvant studies will incorporate these agents, to attempt to increase the benefit of adjuvant therapy. A novel approach to adjuvant therapy has been proposed by Reithmüller et al. (18) who used a mouse monoclonal antibody — 17-1A (Panorex), which is directed against an antigen on the surface of colon tumours — as adjuvant therapy in Dukes' stage C colon cancer. In a randomized trial, antibody therapy reduced the chance of death by the same degree as chemotherapy compared with observation alone. The mechanism of action of the antibody is unclear, and further trials are in progress comparing antibody therapy, which is less toxic than chemotherapy, with standard 5-FU and folinic acid treatment, and a combination of the two treatments.

Adjuvant radiotherapy is used mainly in rectal cancer, although there is an increasing trend to use it in caecal tumours that have breached the serosa (stage pT4). It has been traditionally believed that its function is to reduce the chance of local recurrence. Trials in combination with chemotherapy (19,20) have shown that survival can also be improved. The risk of recurrence depends on the depth of penetration of the tumour into the bowel wall, surrounding tissues, and lymphatics: the presence of tumour at the circumferential resection margin is a particularly adverse factor associated with recurrence (21). Risks of local recurrence vary greatly in different centres. The extent to which this is a function of the surgical technique or appropriate use of radiotherapy is unclear, and a subject of great debate. Some groups offer preoperative radiotherapy.

This can either be given as a course of treatment over several weeks followed, after a suitable gap, by surgery, or as a short 5-day regimen, followed immediately by surgery. The Malmo group reported a marked decrease in local recurrence rates when a short course of preoperative treatment was given and surgery was undertaken within 1 week; a recent Swedish trial has confirmed these results (22). The disadvantage of this approach is that many patients are treated who would not normally require radiotherapy. Also, short-course radiation may lead to long-term side effects. In the USA and in most centres in the UK, it is more common to offer postoperative radiation to a selected group who are deemed to be at high risk of tumour recurrence. A trial conducted by the MRC showed that postoperative radiotherapy significantly reduced local recurrence (23); a benefit in survival using radiotherapy alone was not seen. Two randomized trials, in the UK and the Netherlands, are in progress to compare the outcome, toxicity, and economics of short-course preoperative radiotherapy and selected postoperative chemo-radiation.

Advanced disease

For patients with metastatic disease, the aim of treatment is to palliate symptoms and, for this reason, therapies in which the toxicity does not outweigh the benefit should be chosen. Benefit should not be measured solely by tumour shrinkage, but by using a combination of survival, symptom control, and quality of life. 5-FU is the mainstay of treatment, and several randomized trials have demonstrated beneficial effects of palliative chemotherapy compared with best supportive care. The Nordic Cancer Group Study, in 1991 (24), demonstrated the value of treating patients with clinical or radiological evidence of relapse, before the onset of symptoms. The group receiving immediate chemotherapy had a longer progression-free and overall survival. Other trials comparing treatment with best supportive care have shown similar results. Overall, one can expect the median survival after chemotherapy to be prolonged by 6–9 months. 5-FU is a schedule-dependent drug with a short half-life, so it can be either given by continuous infusion via a central venous line, or biomodulated as described by De Gramont et al. (25), who devised an intensive 5-FU and folinic acid regimen given over 48 h every 2 weeks. They reported improved response rates, with

lower toxicity, compared with the standard bolus treatment of 5-FU and folinic acid. The MRC recently closed a clinical trial comparing these two regimens with a third new thymidylate synthetase inhibitor called raltitrexed (Tomudex) in metastatic colorectal cancer. The theoretical advantage of raltitrexed was that it could be given via a peripheral vein as a short 15-min infusion every 3 weeks. However, results of a randomized trial have shown that raltitrexed is associated with greater toxicity than infusional 5-FU (26).

Patients with small-volume disease confined to the liver should be referred to a specialist centre with a multidisciplinary team familiar with the different options available for treatment. A partial hepatectomy should be considered if only a few (<5) metastases are present and confined to one lobe. About 25% of patients undergoing resection may be cured. A combined approach using surgery and chemotherapy may be superior (27), and the addition of percutaneous or intraoperative thermal ablation (laser, cryotherapy, or radiofrequency) may further improve the results of treatment.

Systemic treatments are used in patients with bilobar disease, but trials of localized intrahepatic arterial therapy are also being performed. Response rates after intrahepatic arterial therapy are greater, but survival comparisons using the most effective biomodulated infusional 5-FU regimens are not available. An MRC study (CRO5) is comparing infusional 5-FU and folinic acid with a much higher dose of intrahepatic 5-FU, which delivers an equivalent systemic dose as a result of "spill over".

Until recently, there was little evidence that second-line treatment after the failure of 5-FU therapy was beneficial. However, new drugs are now available that may have a role in second-line therapy. A significant prolongation in survival has been shown in two trials comparing the topoisomerase I inhibitor, irinotecan, with either best supportive care, or a more dose-intense 5-FU regimen (28,29). The survival benefit for the patients receiving irinotecan was 2.6 times greater than that for those receiving best supportive care. The survival advantage for the irinotecan group remained highly significant after adjustment for performance status — a recognized prognostic factor.

Oxaliplatin, a platinum analogue, in combination with 5-FU and folinic acid produces significantly greater response rates than 5-FU and folinic acid alone, and the activity of irinotecan is also greater when combined with 5-FU and folinic acid. The latter given first-line with 5-FU and folinic acid has shown a survival superior to that achieved with the same 5-FU regimen given alone in one trial. More studies are needed to establish whether oxaliplatin and irinotecan, both expensive drugs, given with 5-FU improve survival, and whether these drugs are best used as first-line treatment or at relapse. The MRC in the UK is about to launch such a trial.

Treatment of metastatic colorectal cancer is likely to change considerably over the next few years, as oral thymidylate synthase inhibitors and orally active 5-FU prodrugs reach the clinic. Although their activity is no greater than that of intravenous 5-FU, capecitabine and tegafur-uracil (UFT) can be administered more easily and cheaply. However, many unanswered questions remain, such as the optimum duration of treatment, and whether there is any difference in outcome between combination therapy and sequential use of different drugs. Current and planned MRC trials will consider these issues.

ANAL CANCER

Anal cancer is a rare tumour, but one in which there has been a significant change in management over the past few years. Historically, an abdominoperineal resection of the anorectum was performed for all but the most superficial external tumours. It has been known for some time that these tumours respond well to radiotherapy, and the response rate can be increased by the use of chemoradiation.

The United Kingdom Co-ordinating Committee for Cancer Research has recently published a clinical trial comparing radiation with chemoradiation using mitomycin C and 5-FU. The results showed that patients treated with chemoradiation had significantly better local control of disease and a reduced requirement for a colostomy. However, the overall survival was not different in the two groups (30). Surgery is still required for those patients who do not have local control of their disease — 20–50%, depending on the stage. Although there has been no trial comparing surgery with chemoradiation, the outcome of the non-surgical approach is similar, and the requirement for a colostomy is significantly less. Practice in the UK has changed as a result of the availability of this treatment: the treatment of choice is now chemoradiation, not surgery. The success of this trial was partly due

to the high proportion of UK patients who were recruited into the study. The collaborative group that was established during this study will help to ensure that, in future, patients continue to be treated by specialists in the field, and will probably be offered the opportunity of entering new studies that are being planned to increase the local control rate and reduce the incidence of distant metastases, which currently affects 30–40% of patients.

GASTROINTESTINAL LYMPHOMAS

Stomach

The gastrointestinal tract, including the stomach, is the most common site for extranodal lymphomas. Although the incidence is increasing, primary gastric lymphoma remains a relatively rare disease, comprising 1–10% of all gastrointestinal malignancies in the Western world. Over half of these lymphomas are mucosa-associated lymphoid tissue (MALT) lymphomas, which are usually localized, and have a very good outcome. Most of the remaining cases are diffuse large-cell or Burkitt's lymphoma. The diagnosis is usually by endoscopy and biopsy, but full staging with computed tomography scanning of the thorax, abdomen, and pelvis, measurement of serum lactic dehydrogenase, and bone marrow examination need to be undertaken.

Management and prognosis are most closely correlated with histological subtype and stage. Debate continues as to the optimum management of the different groups of stomach cancers. Resection, radiotherapy, chemotherapy, and a combination of these have all been used. Retrospective studies spanning several decades and using different procedures make it difficult to draw conclusions. Surgical resection is now rarely performed; the morbidity in advanced disease is high, although in localized stage IE disease, surgery can be curative and high response rates are found with chemotherapy (31). Even with resected localized disease, adjuvant chemotherapy is usually offered. Chemotherapeutic regimens vary, depending on age, performance status, and whether there is associated human immunodeficiency virus (HIV) infection. Generally, regimens contain a combination of alkylating agents, anthracyclines, antimetabolites, and high-dose steroids. CHOP (cyclophosphamide, vincristine, hydroxydaunorubicin, prednisolone) and VAPEC-

B (vincristine, doxorubicin, prednisolone, etoposide, cyclophosphamide and bleomycin) are two well-used regimens. High-grade gastric lymphoma is often localized, and the 5-year disease-free survival of this group of patients is 75%; the outlook is less good for more advanced disease. There is little evidence that the addition of radiotherapy alters the outcome. MALT-derived gastric lymphomas have a more indolent course, and long-term survival is good. Epidemiological and histopathological studies support the concept that gastritis secondary to *Helicobacter pylori* infection is a prerequisite for MALT acquisition and subsequent malignant transformation (32). Antibiotic eradication of *H. pylori* leads to high regression rates of B-cell gastric MALT lymphoma (33). Two to three months after treatment, endoscopy and biopsy are repeated. If persistent disease is found, a second antibiotic course is given; patients then remain on 6-monthly endoscopic follow-up. The long-term results of this treatment are not known, and a multicentre randomized trial run by the UK lymphoma group (LY03) is in progress to study remission rate, time to progression, and whether chlorambucil should be used to prevent relapse. Molecular markers may provide a more sensitive measure of response. The polymerase chain reaction (PCR) to detect monoclonal B cells is frequently positive several months after histological eradication. The significance of this is not yet fully understood, as monoclonal B cells are also observed in *Helicobacter pylori*-associated gastritis, so questioning the correct interpretation of clonality by PCR. The collection, by the UK Lymphoma Group, of data from patients with rare tumours increases knowledge and helps treatment guidelines to be established.

Small bowel

Lymphoma may involve the small intestine primarily or as a manifestation of extensive disseminated disease. Primary small-bowel lymphoma constitutes up to 4% of all gastrointestinal malignancies and approximately 15% of all small-bowel malignancies. It is more common in the Middle East. The relative amount of lymphatic tissue in the wall of the small bowel increases distally, hence the greater incidence of lymphoma affecting the terminal ileum. The incidence of primary lymphoma is increasing, probably reflecting an increase in immunocompromised individuals with acquired immunodeficiency syndrome

and transplant recipients (after transplant lymphoproliferative disorders). Antecedent conditions reported to be associated with the development of primary small-bowel lymphoma include non-tropical sprue, Crohn's and coeliac diseases and dermatitis herpetiformis. T-cell tumours are found in association with the latter two conditions, but most intestinal lymphomas are intermediate or high-grade B-cell tumours. Symptoms at presentation include abdominal pain, change in bowel habit, an abdominal mass, and weight loss. Perforation is uncommon. Dawson *et al.* (34) suggested the following criteria should be present before a diagnosis of primary small bowel lymphoma is made:

1. There must be no peripheral or mediastinal lymphadenopathy.
2. The peripheral blood smear must display a normal white-cell and differential count.
3. Tumour involvement must be predominantly in the gastrointestinal tract.

Because of their location, intestinal lymphomas are often diagnosed at laparotomy and are resected in more than 50% of affected patients. A staging system has been developed by Blackledge *et al.* (35) (Table 18.1.4). The role of adjuvant treatment remains unclear, as this tumour is rare. At present, adjuvant chemotherapy is usually reserved for high-grade lymphoma and factors such as age, performance status, serum lactate dehydrogenase concentrations, and concurrent HIV infection need to be considered before the exact regimen is determined. Tumour grade remains the best predictor for outcome. Auger & Allan (36) reported that the median survival after resection was improved from 14 to 34 months with postoperative chemotherapy. Most of the larger series report a 5-year survival in excess of 50% with aggressive multimodality treatment (37). Abdominal radiotherapy is rarely used, because of the possibility of long-term

Table 18.1.4. Staging of gastrointestinal lymphomas.

I	Tumour confined to the gastrointestinal tract
II	Tumour with local mesenteric nodal involvement
III	Tumour with perforation
IV	Tumour with distant (para-aortic and beyond) nodal involvement
V	Tumour with visceral or bone marrow involvement

Published with permission (31)

gastrointestinal side effects. Prognostic factors include tumour grade, stage at presentation, complete resectability, histological subtype, and use of multimodality treatments. Patients with B-cell tumours fare better than those with T-cell tumours. Primary Hodgkin's disease of the small bowel is very unusual and may, in fact, represent impingement of mesenteric lymphadenopathy rather than primary visceral involvement. Management consists of surgical resection followed by definitive systemic chemotherapy.

SMALL-BOWEL CANCERS

Tumours of the small bowel are rare. Primary small bowel sarcomas or stromal tumours are extremely rare. Metastases to the small bowel are more common than primary tumours. The most commonly found tumours are adenocarcinomas, carcinoid tumour, and lymphomas (38). Coit (39) lists the malignant tumours of the small intestine as:

- Adenocarcinoma   44%
- Carcinoid   29%
- Lymphoma   15%
- Sarcoma   12%

Adenocarcinoma

Adenocarcinomas constitute about 44% of all malignancies affecting the small bowel. About 45% arise in the duodenum; the remainder are distributed in the jejunum and, less commonly, in the ileum. Dysplasia preceding cancer occurs in these tumours, as it does in colorectal cancer, and may be seen in the resected tumour. Primary small-bowel adenocarcinoma is more common in patients with germ-line defects in the *FAP* gene or DNA mismatch repair genes (*hMLH1* or *hMSH2*), or Gardener's or Peutz–Jegher syndrome. Patients with Crohn's disease or long-standing gluten-sensitive enteropathy have an increased susceptibility to small bowel carcinoma.

Distinction is often made between tumours arising in the duodenum and those in the jejunum or ileum but, overall, the presenting symptoms are similar, as are options for treatment. Tumours tend to present with abdominal pain secondary to obstruction, or occult gastrointestinal bleeding leading to anaemia, or both. Most patients undergo surgical exploration and the extent of resection, ranging from segmental resection with primary anastomosis to pancreatoduodenectomy, will depend on the site and stage of the tumour. There is no defined role for adjuvant chemotherapy after complete resection of adenocarcinoma of the small bowel. Systemic chemotherapy using 5-FU can palliate symptoms such as pain and bleeding, but documented response rates are low. Radiotherapy is sometimes considered for those with proximal tumours who present with chronic bleeding from an advanced inoperable mass. Overall, survival is generally poor: typically, 20–30% at 5 years.

Sarcoma

Small-bowel sarcomas are extremely unusual, accounting for 10% of all small-bowel malignancies. The majority are leiomyosarcoma and leiomyoblastoma originating from smooth muscle. Recently, these tumours have been renamed "gastrointestinal stromal tumours". Surgical management is the treatment of choice, with wide local excision to obtain clear resection margins. Lymphadenectomy is unnecessary, as these tumours involve the lymph nodes in fewer than 15% of cases. The overall 5-year survival rate is only 20% and is affected by tumour size, histological grade, local invasion, and resectability (40). Peritoneal and liver metastases are the most common reason for treatment failure. There is no evidence to suggest that adjuvant chemotherapy after surgery improves long-term survival, or decreases the rate of recurrence. Metastatic disease is treated with doxorubicin-containing regimens alone, or with ifosfamide. Response rates up to 40% have been documented.

Carcinoid

Carcinoid tumours represent approximately one-third of all small-bowel malignancies. After the appendix, the small bowel is the most commonly affected site. Approximately 90% of all small-bowel carcinoids are found in the ileum. Most tumours are indolent and non-secretory, and are discovered coincidentally at laparotomy or at post-mortem examination. Secretory tumours produce serotonin, histamine, kinins, peptides, catecholamines, glucagon, and gastrin. Fewer than 20% of patients with small-bowel carcinoid will present with carcinoid syndrome (41), and carcinoid tumours of the gut rarely produce metabolic symptoms when the tumour drains through an intact liver; the carcinoid syndrome is seen more commonly if liver metastases develop. Up to 67% will develop the features of flushing of the head, neck, or upper chest some time in their clinical course. Such symptoms are induced by alcohol, emotion, and tyramine-containing foods. Some patients may develop right-sided valvular heart lesions and bronchial asthma.

The frequency of metastatic disease to regional lymph nodes or to the liver is related to the size of the tumour: metastases are rare in tumours less than 1 cm. Metastases occur in 33–67% of affected patients in whom the primary tumour measures 1–3 cm, and in up to 90% of these in whom the primary is greater than 3 cm.

Surgical management of the primary tumour includes wide local resection of all visible disease. However, as 30% of all small-bowel carcinoids are multiple, a careful preoperative search of the remainder of the small bowel is imperative. When surgical excision or debulking is not possible, management is aimed at control of symptoms. Prolonged remission of symptoms has been observed with the resection of bulk metastases, even if this was incomplete. The tumour often grows slowly; the duration of survival depends on the extent of the disease at diagnosis (42).

There have been some reports of short-term remission of symptoms with hepatic dearterialization. A long-acting somatostatin analogue, octreotide, has been developed that can help to control flushing attacks and diarrhoea by inhibiting secretion of peptides. Objective responses and a reduction in secretion of urinary 5-hydroxyindolacetic acid occasionally occurs (43). In addition, gamma camera imaging after intravenous injection of the two agents ^{111}In-labelled ocreotide (44) and ^{123}I-labelled metaiodobenzylguanidine (MIBG) has been used to localize tumours and select patients who are more likely to benefit from either of these treatments. To use these agents therapeutically, ^{123}I is replaced with ^{131}I and ^{111}In is replaced with [90]Yt. These treatments remain experimental, but are being increasingly used, as the results of systemic chemotherapy have been disappointing. Objective responses to chemotherapy occur in about 20% of patients and are usually short-lived. Doxorubicin and 5-FU are the most active single agents; combination regimens containing streptozotocin, 5-FU, methotrexate, cyclophosphamide, and doxorubicin have all been examined (45). Alpha interferon has also been reported to have single-agent activity in carcinoid tumours (46).

Complete resection of carcinoid tumours without overt metastases results in a 75–94% 5-year survival. Even in the presence of liver metastases, the 5-year survival rates can be as high as 54%. However, the apparent improvement in survival over the past two decades is more probably attributable to earlier detection of this slowly progressive tumour, rather than better treatment.

Metastatic disease

The small bowel is not uncommonly the site of metastatic deposits. The most frequently seen metastasis is malignant melanoma. Other extra-abdominal tumours known to spread to this site include tumours of the cervix, breast, kidney, and lung. More commonly, ovarian, colorectal, gastric, pancreatic, and transitional-cell carcinomas of the genitourinary tract can involve the small bowel, by direct extension or intraperitoneal spread. If bleeding, perforation, or obstruction are the presenting features, surgery is used to palliate symptoms, provided the overall condition of the patient is good. Systemic chemotherapy may palliate symptoms, and radiotherapy is occasionally used for uncontrolled bleeding.

HEPATOBILARY CANCERS

These cancers can be divided into those arising from the bilary tract and those from the liver; both are uncommon in the UK. Bilary tumours may involve the bile ducts or gallbladder, but presentation is often late and the prognosis is poor. Gallbladder tumours are treated by surgery if they are resectable. Only a small proportion of cholangiocarcinomas are resectable. The results of chemotherapy — usually with 5-FU — have been disappointing. Higher response rates occur when the drug is combined with doxorubicin and mitomycin C (FAM), but the duration of response is short lived. Radiation therapy has been used in the postoperative adjuvant setting and as palliation, but clinical trials have reported conflicting information as to its benefit (47). One small Scandinavian study comparing chemotherapy and best supportive care has shown an improvement in the median survival from 2.5 to 6.5 months, and a better quality of life, in patients receiving a combination of 5-FU, folinic acid, and etoposide (48). The absence of large clinical trials makes judgement on the correct use of drugs difficult, and these tumours are best treated in specialized centres of experimental therapeutics. For example, gemcitabine is undergoing investigation, and may have a more important role to play in the future; in particular, it has been shown to sensitize tissue to radiation, and may add to the effect of radiation treatment of cholangiocarcinomas.

Hepatocellular cancers are a major health problem in Asia and sub-Saharan Africa, but uncommon in Europe and North America. They are discussed in detail in Chapter 18.2.

References

1. Pisani P, Parkin D, Ferlay J. Estimates of the worldwide mortality from eighteen major cancers in 1985. *Int J Cancer* 1993; **55**: 891–903.

2. Wobst A, Audisio RA, Colleoni M *et al*. Oesophageal cancer treatment: studies, strategies and facts. *Ann Oncol* 1998; **9**: 951–962.

3. Herskovic A, Martz K, al-Sarraf M *et al*. Combined chemotherapy and radiotherapy compared with radiotherapy alone in patients with cancer of the esophagus. *N Engl J Med* 1992; **326**: 1593–1598.

4. Kelsen DP, Ginsberg R, Pajak TF *et al*. Chemotherapy followed by surgery compared with surgery alone for localized esophageal cancer. *N Engl J Med* 1998; **339**: 1979–1984.

5. Clark PI on behalf of the Upper GI Tract Group. Medical Research Council (MRC) randomized phase III trial of surgery with or without pre-operative chemotherapy in resectable cancer of the oesophagus. *Br J Cancer* 2000; **83** suppl. 1: 1.

6. Walsh TN, Noonan N, Hollywood D *et al*. A comparison of multimodal therapy and surgery for esophageal adenocarcinoma [see comments]. *N Engl J Med* 1996; **335**: 462–467.

7. Andreyev HJ, Norman AR, Cunningham D *et al*. Squamous oesophageal cancer can be downstaged using protracted venous infusion of 5-fluorouracil with epirubicin and cisplatin (ECF). *Eur J Cancer* 1995; **31A**: 2209–2214.

8. Webb A, Cunningham D, Scarffe JH *et al*. Randomized trial comparing epirubicin, cisplatin, and fluorouracil versus fluorouracil, doxorubicin, and methotrexate in advanced esophagogastric cancer. *J Clin Oncol* 1997; **15(1)**: 261–267.

9. Glimelius B, Ekstrom K, Hoffman K *et al*. Randomized comparison between chemotherapy plus best supportive care with best supportive care in advanced gastric cancer. *Ann Oncol* 1997; **8**: 163–168.

10. Hermans J, Bonenkamp JJ, Boon MC *et al*. Adjuvant therapy after curative resection for gastric cancer: meta-analysis of randomized trials . *J Clin Oncol* 1993; **11**: 1441–1447.

11. Burris HA III, Moore MJ, Andersen J *et al*. Improvements in survival and clinical benefit with gemcitabine as first-line therapy for patients with advanced pancreas cancer: a randomized trial. *J Clin Oncol* 1997; **15**: 2403–2413.

12. Rothenberg ML, Moore MJ, Cripps MC *et al*. A phase II trial of gemcitabine in patients with 5-FU-refractory pancreas cancer. *Ann Oncol* 1996; **7**: 347–353.

13. Greenway BA. Effect of flutamide on survival in patients with pancreatic cancer: results of a prospective, randomised, double blind, placebo controlled trial. *BMJ* 1998; **316**: 1935–1938.

14. Fearon E, Vogelstein B. A genetic model for colorectal tumourigenesis. *Cell* 1990; **61**: 759–767.

15. Moertel CG, Fleming TR, Macdonald JS *et al*. Levamisole and fluorouracil for adjuvant therapy of resected colon carcinoma [see comments]. *N Engl J Med* 1990; **322**: 352–358.

16. International Multicentre Pooled Analysis of Colon Cancer Trials (IMPACT) investigators. Efficacy of adjuvant fluorouracil and folinic acid in colon cancer. *Lancet* 1995; **345**: 939–944.

17. James RD. Intraportal 5FU (PVI) and peri-operative radiotherapy in the adjuvant treatment of colorectal cancer — 3681 patients randomised in the UK Coordinating Committee on Cancer Research (UKCCCR) AXIS trial. *Proc Am Soc Clin Oncol* 1999; **18**: 264 abstr 1013.

18. Riethmuller G, Schneider-Gadicke E, Schlimok G *et al*. Randomised trial of monoclonal antibody for adjuvant therapy of resected Dukes' C colorectal carcinoma. German Cancer Aid 17-1A Study Group. *Lancet* 1994; **343**: 1177–1183.

19. Krook JE, Moertel CG, Gunderson LL *et al*. Effective surgical adjuvant therapy for high-risk rectal carcinoma [see comments]. *N Engl J Med* 1991; **324**: 709–715.

20. O'Connell MJ, Martenson JA, Wieand HS *et al*. Improving adjuvant therapy for rectal cancer by combining protracted-infusion fluorouracil with radiation therapy after curative surgery. *N Engl J Med* 1994; **331**: 502–507.

21. Adam IJ, Mohamdee MO, Martin IG *et al*. Role of circumferential margin involvement in the local recurrence of rectal cancer. *Lancet* 1994; **344**: 707–711.

22. Swedish Rectal Cancer Trial. Improved survival with preoperative radiotherapy in resectable rectal cancer. *N Engl J Med* 1997; **336**: 980–987.

23. Medical Research Council Rectal Cancer Working Party. Randomised trial of surgery alone versus surgery followed by radiotherapy for mobile cancer of the rectum. *Lancet* 1996; **348**: 1610–1614.

24. Nordic Gastrointestinal Tumor Adjuvant Therapy Group. Expectancy or primary chemotherapy in patients with advanced asymptomatic colorectal cancer: a randomized trial. *J Clin Oncol* 1992; **10**: 904–911.

25. de Gramont A, Bosset JF, Milan C *et al*. Randomized trial comparing monthly low-dose leucovorin and fluorouracil bolus with bimonthly high-dose leucovorin and fluorouracil bolus plus continuous infusion for advanced colorectal cancer: a French intergroup study. *J Clin Oncol* 1997; **15**: 808–815.

26. Maughan TS, James RD, Kerr DJ *et al*. Preliminary results of a multicentre randomized trial comparing three chemotherapy regimens (de Gramont, Lokich and Raltitrexed) in metastatic colorectal cancer. *Proc Am Soc Clin Oncol* 1999; **18**: 262 abstr 1007.

27. Bismuth H, Adam R, Levi F *et al*. Resection of nonresectable liver metastases from colorectal cancer after neoadjuvant chemotherapy. *Ann Surg* 1996; **224**: 509–520.

28. Cunningham D, Pyrhonen S, James RD *et al.* Randomised trial of irinotecan plus supportive care versus supportive care alone after fluorouracil failure for patients with metastatic colorectal cancer. *Lancet* 1998; **352**: 1413–1418.

29. Rougier P, Van Cutsem E, Bajetta E *et al.* Randomised trial of irinotecan versus fluorouracil by continuous infusion after fluorouracil failure in patients with metastatic colorectal cancer. *Lancet* 1998; **352**: 1407–1412.

30. UK Co-ordinating Committee on Cancer Research. Anal Cancer Trial Working Party. Epidermoid anal cancer: results from the UKCCCR randomised trial of radiotherapy alone versus radiotherapy, 5-fluorouracil, and mitomycin. *Lancet* 1996; **348**: 1049–1054.

31. Salles G, Herbrecht R, Tilly H *et al.* Aggressive primary gastrointestinal lymphomas: review of 91 patients treated with the LNH-84 regimen: a study of the Groupe d'Etude des Lymphomes Agressifs. *Am J Med* 1991; **90**: 77–84.

32. Wootherspoon A, Ortiz-Hildago C, Falzon M *et al.* Helicobacter pylori associated gastritis and primary B cell lymphoma. *Lancet* 1991; **338**: 1175–1176.

33. Bayerdöffer E, Neubauer A, Rudolf B *et al.* Regression of primary gastric lymphoma of mucosa-associated lymphoid tissue type after cure of helicobacter pylori infection. *Lancet* 1995; **345**: 1591–1592.

34. Dawson I, Cornes J, Morson B. Primary malignant lymphoid tumours of the gastrointestinal tract: Report of 37 cases with a study of factors influencing prognosis. *Br J Surg* 1961; **40**: 80–89.

35. Blackledge G, Bush H, Dodge O *et al.* A study of gastrointestinal lymphoma. *Clin Oncol* 1979; **5**: 209–219.

36. Auger M, Allan N. Primary ileocecal lymphoma. *Cancer* 1990; **65**: 358–361.

37. Shepherd F, Evans W, Kutas G *et al.* Chemotherapy following surgery for stages 1E and 11E non-Hodgkin's lymphoma of the gastrointestinal tract. *J Clin Oncol* 1988; **6**: 253–256.

38. Vaughn D, Furth E, Rubesin S. Cancers of the small bowel. In: *Textbook of Uncommon Cancer.* 2nd. edn. Eds D Rahavan, M Brecher, D Johnson *et al.* New York: J Wiley and Sons Ltd, 1999; pp. 427–437.

39. Coit DG. Cancers of the gastrointestinal tract. In: *Cancer Principles and Practice of Oncology*, 5th edn. Eds VT De Vita, S Hellman, SA Rosenberg, Philadelphia: Lippincott-Raven, 1997; pp. 1128–1143.

40. Conolon K, Casper E, Brennan M. Primary gastrointestinal sarcomas: analysis of prognostic variables. *Ann Surg Oncol* 1995; **2**: 26–31.

41. Moertel C. Treatment of the carcinoid tumour and the malignant carcinoid syndrome. *J Clin Oncol* 1983; **1**: 727–740.

42. Goodwin J. Carcinoid tumors — an analysis of 2837 cases. *Cancer* 1975; **36**: 560–569.

43. Kvols L, Moertel C, O'Connell M *et al.* Treatment of the malignant carcinoid syndrome: evaluation of a long-acting somatostatin analogue. *N Engl J Med* 1991; **315**: 663–666.

44. Crithchley M. Octroetide scanning for carcinoid tumours. *Postgrad Med J* 1997; **73**: 399–402.

45. Engstrom P, Lavin P, Moertel G *et al.* Streptozocin plus fluorouracil versus doxorubicin therapy for metastatic carcinoid tumor. *J Clin Oncol* 1984; **2**: 1255–1259.

46. Moertel C. Therapy of metastatic carcinoid tumor and the malignant carcinoid syndrome with recombinant leukocyte A interferon. *J Clin Oncol* 1989; **7**: 865–868.

47. Lee C, Barrios B, Bjarnason H. Bilary tree malignancies: the University of Minnesota experience. *J Surg Oncol* 1997; **65**: 298–305.

48. Glimelius B, Hoffman K, Sjoden P *et al.* Chemotherapy improves survival and quality of life in advanced pancreatic and bilary cancer. *Ann Oncol* 1996; **7**: 593–600.

18.2. Gastrointestinal Malignancy: Diagnosis and Treatment of Hepatocellular Carcinoma

STEPHEN M. RIORDAN

INTRODUCTION

Hepatocellular carcinoma (HCC) is among the most common cancers world-wide, with particularly high prevalence in Asia and sub-Saharan Africa. Detection rates are increasing in Western countries. Most patients are diagnosed only after the disease has reached an advanced stage, as HCC has generally grown to a large size by the time of development of tumour-related symptoms, such as abdominal pain. Such symptomatic cases of HCC carry a poor prognosis, with untreated median survival in the order of only a few months. Treatment options for such patients are limited, especially when extrahepatic dissemination has occurred. In contrast, a wider range of potentially effective treatment options are available for small HCCs confined to the liver — including, in selected patients, hepatic resection, orthotopic liver transplantation (OLT), percutaneous ethanol injection (PEI), and transcatheter arterial chemoembolization (TACE). These facts emphasize the need for reliable screening and surveillance programmes aimed at detecting small tumours at an asymptomatic stage in groups at increased risk of HCC development.

SCREENING AND SURVEILLANCE FOR HCC

Screening is the one-time application of a test that allows the detection of a disease at a stage when intervention may significantly improve the natural course and outcome, whereas **surveillance** is the repeated application of such a test over time. The aims of screening and surveillance for HCC are to detect small tumours that are amenable to curative treatment and thereby to reduce disease-related mortality, although no randomized controlled trials have yet been performed to assess whether current strategies achieve these ends.

Nonetheless, since 75–90% of patients who develop HCC have underlying **cirrhosis** and the annual incidence of development of HCC in this group is 1–6%, it has become widely accepted clinical practice to enter cirrhotic patients into screening and surveillance programmes. Histological evidence of liver cell dysplasia in patients with cirrhosis of varying causes identifies those at particularly high risk of progression to HCC, with a 3-year cumulative incidence of 72% in one series (1,2). In those patients with hepatitis-C-related cirrhosis, high necroinflammatory activity and a disorganized distribution of hepatic regeneration are important predictive factors, the latter being associated with a sevenfold increased incidence of development of HCC and representing an even more important risk factor than liver-cell dysplasia (3,4).

However, cirrhosis is asymptomatic and unrecognized before presentation with HCC in nearly 67% of patients from areas with a high incidence of this tumour, such as Asia, and in almost 50% of patients from low incidence areas, such as the UK and Northern Europe. Thus screening and surveillance programmes can have only a limited impact on early HCC detection rates if they are limited to patients known to have cirrhosis. Many centres extend such programmes to include **non-cirrhotic patients with chronic hepatitis C** and all those **seropositive for hepatitis B virus** (HBV) — including surface antigen carriers, as HBV has direct oncogenic potential, as a consequence of the integration of viral DNA into the host genome and activation of genes controlling cell proliferation — even in the absence of chronic hepatitis or cirrhosis. Screening and surveillance of such patients would be expected to have a particularly strong impact on overall early HCC detection rates in Asia, which is home to an estimated 75% of the approximately 300 million HBV carriers world-wide.

Most **screening and surveillance programmes** for HCC combine measurement of **serum alpha-fetoprotein** (AFP) concentrations with hepatic ultrasonography. An increased AFP concentration (>20 ng/ml) occurs in up to 90% of patients with large, symptomatic HCCs, especially in Asia, but the sensitivity of this measure is substantially reduced in the case of small HCCs. Increased AFP concentrations are found in only in the order of 50% of patients with HCCs less than 3 cm in diameter (5), and in as few as 36% of those with tumours smaller than 2 cm in size (6). As 50–83% of HCCs detected by screening and surveillance are in this size range it is not surprising that studies performed both in Asia and the West, to investigate the value of AFP as a tool in screening/surveillance programmes, found low sensitivity, ranging from 39 to 64% (7,8). Specificity for HCC in these studies ranged from 76–91%, modest increases in AFP (usually in the order of 20–500 ng/ml) also being occasionally found in patients with cirrhosis or chronic viral hepatitis alone, hepatic regeneration after acute hepatic necrosis, metastatic liver carcinoma, (especially of gastric or pancreatic origin), and germ-cell tumours. Specificity for HCC is improved by increasing the cutoff AFP value, but at the expense of substantial reduction in sensitivity.

An alternative means of improving specificity of AFP for HCC is with the use of **lectin-binding analysis**, which has been shown to be a useful tool for discriminating between AFP produced by HCC and other disorders, at least in the research setting. In particular, a less than 10% fraction of AFP that is not bound to concanavalin A differentiates AFP produced by HCC from that originating from metastatic liver carcinoma and germ-cell tumours, but also occurs in benign liver disorders. Conversely, a lens-culinaris-reactive AFP fraction greater than 20%

and a phytohaemagglutinin-reactive fraction greater than 10% are found only with HCC (9).

Nonetheless, as the sensitivity of AFP is suboptimal and lectin-binding analysis is not performed on a routine clinical basis, most screening and surveillance programmes also include **hepatic ultrasonography**. The sensitivity of ultrasound for small HCCs is comparable to that of other non-invasive modalities such as dynamic **computed tomography** (CT) and **magnetic resonance imaging** (MRI). Sensitivity of ultrasound for nodular HCCs 1.1–3.0 cm in diameter is 95%, although the rate of detection by each of these techniques is substantially reduced when the tumour diameter is 1 cm or less (Table 18.2.1) (10). More than 90% of solid lesions detected by ultrasound in patients with cirrhosis who are enrolled in screening/surveillance programmes are subsequently confirmed to be HCCs (7), the differential diagnosis including haemangiomas, regenerative nodules, focal fatty change, and metastases. There are no firm guidelines established concerning the optimum surveillance interval. Surveillance every 3–6 months is a rational approach, based on data from China in which the median doubling time of HCCs was found to be almost 4 months and the time taken for tumour diameter to increase from 1 to 3 cm was no less than 5 months (11).

HCC arising in an otherwise normal liver tends to occur in younger patients. **Fibrolamellar HCC** is one such variant and tends to carry a better prognosis than other varieties of HCC. Liver function tests are less often abnormal in this group of patients and serum AFP concentrations are not usually increased, even in the presence of large tumours. Furthermore, the lack of association with underlying chronic liver disease or chronic HBV carrier status argues against an effective screening programme for this tumour.

Further imaging is necessary in patients with increased serum AFP concentrations but negative hepatic ultrasonography. Although the sensitivity of ultrasound for small HCCs is, in general, comparable to that of other non-invasive imaging modalities, areas immediately below the diaphragm can be relative blind spots. Furthermore, diffuse HCCs, isoechoic with the non-tumorous hepatic parenchyma, may be difficult to detect. The next imaging investigation of choice is **contrast-enhanced CT** or **MRI**. Relative advantages of the latter modality are that it does not involve the use of ionizing radiation or iodinated contrast. **Hepatic arteriography** is required if no lesion is

Table 18.2.1. Sensitivities of non-invasive imaging modalities for HCC according to size.

	Sensitivity (%)	
	HCC diameter ≤ 1.0 cm	HCC diameter 1.1–3.0 cm
Ultrasound	33	95
Contrast-enhanced CT	20	95
Contrast-enhanced MRI	27	86

Adapted with permission (10).

Table 18.2.2. Sensitivities of angiographic modalities (hepatic arteriography, CT after intra-arterial Lipiodol (Lipiodol-CT), and MESA using carbon dioxide) for hepatocellular carcinomas ≤ 2 cm in diameter.

	Sensitivity (%)
Hepatic arteriography	58
Lipiodol-CT	65
Carbon dioxide MESA	88

Adapted with permission (12).

evident on non-invasive imaging. Sensitivity of hepatic arteriography for small HCCs is improved by modifications such as CT scanning 7–10 days after hepatic arterial injection of Lipiodol — an iodized oil retained in HCC rather than in normal hepatocytes (**Lipiodol-CT**) or, especially, **microbubble-enhanced sonographic angiography** (MESA) (Table 18.2.2) (12). Recent evidence suggests that the use of helium, rather than carbon dioxide, in MESA further increases the applicability and sensitivity of this technique (13). These modifications are rarely required to detect tumours greater than 3 cm in diameter, as the sensitivity of hepatic arteriography alone is more than 98% in this circumstance (6). **CT during arterial portography** (CTAP) may be necessary to detect the relatively small proportion of HCCs that are hypovascular. Patients in whom no lesion is definable by any of these imaging modalities should be followed with hepatic ultrasonography with or without CT or MRI, at 3-monthly intervals. The possibility of an unrelated germ-cell tumour must be excluded.

In patients in whom a solid lesion has been detected on imaging — unless the lesion is clearly benign, such as a haemangioma — subsequent investigation is directed at establishing the diagnosis of HCC, tumour staging, and assessing hepatic functional reserve.

Establishing the diagnosis of HCC

The presence of a solid mass on ultrasound or other imaging in association with a serum AFP concentration greater than 1000 ng/ml in a patient with histologically proven cirrhosis provides strong presumptive evidence of HCC. Depending on the specific clinical circumstance, confirmation of the diagnosis is most appropriately sought by either hepatic arteriography (which may already have been performed in the investigative procedure, as discussed above) or percutaneous liver biopsy.

Hepatic arteriography is a rational first choice in most patients, as diagnostic abnormalities may be apparent and, at the same time, important information concerning tumour staging is obtained, as discussed below. The arteriographic diagnosis of HCC is based on the presence of typical arterial neovascularity, with irregular vascular dilatation, vessel proliferation, tumour stain, venous threads and streaks, pooling of contrast medium, and arteriovenous shunting. High velocity Doppler signals reflecting arteriovenous shunting are evident in more than 80% of patients with large HCCs at least 4 cm in diameter, and are specific for this disorder (14). In the case of small tumours not detectable on routine hepatic arteriography, characteristic abnormalities on MESA and Lipiodol-CT have a positive predictive value for HCC of 100% and more than 90%, respectively (15,16).

The place of **percutaneous biopsy** for early tissue confirmation of HCC is controversial, as this procedure carries a small but definite risk of tumour dissemination along the needle tract, thereby precluding potentially effective local treatment. Thus many centres adopt the policy that percutaneous biopsy should be performed only if angiography is non-diagnostic or the patient is known to have extrahepatic disease. In this latter setting, it is appropriate to proceed directly to histological diagnosis.

Tumour staging

Staging of HCC involves establishing the number, site, and size of tumours within the liver in addition to determining the presence or absence of vascular invasion and extrahepatic metastases. This is best assessed by arteriographic techniques (including hepatic arteriography, Lipiodol-CT, MESA, or CTAP), especially in those patients being considered for surgical or other local treatment with curative intent. Venography (including indirect portography, hepatic venography, or inferior vena cavography) may also be necessary to exclude tumour thrombus within venous structures, although this can reliably be determined by Doppler ultrasound in most instances. Intraoperative ultrasound plays an important role in finally determining the number and location of intrahepatic HCC foci, especially when these are small.

Extrahepatic spread — most commonly to local lymph nodes, the thorax, and bone — tends to occur relatively late in the course of the disease, but must be excluded in any patient in whom potentially curative local treatment is contemplated. Abdominal and thoracic CT or MRI and radionuclide bone scanning have important roles in this aspect of the staging process. Reverse-transcriptase polymerase chain reaction techniques are being developed to detect circulating HCC cells in peripheral blood, and may have a future role in identifying patients with micrometastases that are not detectable by other means, in whom surgical and other local options would be inappropriate.

Assessment of hepatic functional reserve

Determination of whether or not underlying cirrhosis is present is of paramount importance in assessing hepatic functional reserve and, hence, in evaluating the risk of hepatic decompensation after treatments such as partial hepatic resection, as discussed below. To this end, representative liver biopsies should be obtained from non-tumorous areas. Consideration of a number of parameters has been proposed for further risk evaluation in patients shown to be cirrhotic, including the residual hepatic volume after planned resection as measured by CT scanning, the indocyanine green and bromosulphthalein retention rates, the serum lecithin transaminase concentration, the Child's classification of the cirrhosis (17) and its individual components, and the hepatic venous pressure gradient. Of these, an increased preoperative serum bilirubin concentration and the preoperative presence of significant portal hypertension — defined by a hepatic venous pressure gradient greater than 10 mmHg — are especially important predictors of postoperative hepatic decompensation (18,19). Consideration of Child's class alone is inadequate for selecting patients for hepatic resection, as unresolved deterioration in hepatic function subsequently

occurs in more than 50% of Child's class A patients (18).

Technetium-99m-diethylenetriaminepenta-acetic acid–galactosyl human serum albumin (Tc-GSA) is a liver scintigraphy agent that binds to hepatic asialoglycoprotein receptors, and Tc-GSA scintigraphy may also be a useful means of stratifying postresection risk. In particular, extended hepatectomies (di- and tri-segmentectomies) are high-risk procedures in patients with maximal removal rates of Tc-GSA less than 35% (20). The comparative prognostic value of this test in relation to the serum bilirubin concentrations and the hepatic venous gradient remains to be determined.

TREATMENT OPTIONS FOR HCC

Possible treatment options for HCC may be categorised as **local** (for disease confined to the liver) or **systemic** (for disease with extrahepatic spread) (Table 18.2.3). The further indications, contraindications, and efficacies of these treatments are discussed below. Few randomized trials have been performed to compare treatments or even to establish whether an antitumour effect of a particular treatment is associated with improved survival.

Partial hepatic resection

Partial hepatic resection is feasible in patients with cirrhosis who have a solitary HCC less than 5 cm in diameter in an anatomically suitable (not central) location, provided hepatic functional reserve is adequate and disease is confined to the liver, with no macroscopic evidence of vascular invasion. The aim is for segmental or subsegmental resection. More extensive resection, up to 75% of liver volume, is

Table 18.2.3. Proposed treatments for HCC.

HCC localised to the liver	Partial hepatic resection
	Orthotopic liver transplantation
	Percutaneous ethanol injection (PEI)
	Transcatheter arterial chemoembolisation (TACE)
	Combined TACE and PEI
	^{131}I-labelled lipiodol
	Thermal modalities
HCC with extrahepatic dissemination	Systemic chemotherapy
	Tamoxifen

often possible in non-cirrhotic patients, including those with the fibrolamellar variant of HCC. Perioperative mortality rates are in the order of 3–7% in non-cirrhotic patients and 15% in those with cirrhosis. Parenteral nutritional supplementation with branched-chain amino acids, dextrose, and medium-chain triglycerides in the perioperative period is associated with significant reductions in the postoperative rate of septic complications and degree of deterioration in liver function, including requirement for diuretics, although the in-hospital mortality rate is not significantly changed (21).

Overall, only in the order of 20% of patients in Asian countries and fewer than 10% in the West are finally deemed to be suitable candidates for hepatic resection after careful preoperative assessment. When only those patients with HCCs detected in screening/surveillance programmes are considered, 43–81% in Asian countries and 7–50% in the West are ultimately operable. Prior embolization of the portal vein branch supplying the segment to be resected, using a mixture of fibrin, thrombin, and Lipiodol, represents a promising approach to increasing preoperative hepatic functional reserve and, hence, the number of patients in whom hepatic resection may be appropriate (22). This approach is based on the observation, in experimental animals, that ligation of a portal vein branch leads to atrophy of that lobe and hypertrophy of the non-ligated lobe, along with increased polyamine metabolism and DNA synthesis.

Five-year **survival** after hepatic resection for HCC is of the order of 45% in non-cirrhotic patients and 30–60% in patients with underlying cirrhosis. In well-compensated patients, survival is predominantly limited by the high rate of tumour recurrence (33% by 1 year, 50% by 2 years and more than 60% by 3 years). Histological factors including vascular invasion, positive resection margins, or the absence of a pseudocapsule negatively influence outcome. In both Asia and the West, most (68–96%) recurrences are found in the remnant liver, rather than in extrahepatic sites. Genomic studies demonstrating a clonal origin distinct from that of the original tumour indicate that these are predominantly new HCCs, rather than previously unrecognized satellite lesions (23,24). Multivariate analysis has demonstrated that necroinflammatory activity in the remnant liver is inversely related to disease-free survival after resection for HCC (3). In patients with chronic hepatitis C infection, a recent retrospective study suggests that treatment with interferon-α reduces the progression from cirrhosis to HCC by more than sixfold (25). Whether such treatment, when used either before or after operation improves long-term survival after hepatic resection for HCC remains to be assessed. In patients with decompensated cirrhosis, liver failure and its complications are as important as HCC recurrence in limiting survival.

Orthotopic liver transplantation

In patients with HCC complicating cirrhosis, OLT is the only treatment that can possibly both cure the tumour and remove the pre-malignant potential of the cirrhotic liver. However, early studies that included patients with large HCCs yielded disappointing results, with 3-year survival rates of only 20–30%, as a result of a high incidence of tumour recurrence and rapid progression attributable to post-OLT immunosuppression. Subsequent studies have shown that excellent results may be obtained when OLT is restricted to patients with a solitary HCC no greater than 5 cm in diameter or with no more than three tumour nodules each no more than 3 cm in diameter, in the absence of vascular invasion or extrahepatic spread (26–28). Low rates of tumour recurrence and survival comparable to that of patients transplanted without HCC have been recorded in these circumstances (Table 18.2.4).

OLT is the treatment of choice in patients with decompensated cirrhosis and HCC fulfilling these criteria. Nonetheless, the applicability of OLT is limited, not only by these restrictive tumour-related criteria, but also by a shortage of donor organs, with the result that the patient often spends a long time on waiting lists, during which period further tumour growth may occur; the high prevalence of general medical contraindications, especially in older patients, is a further limitation. No randomized studies have compared the efficacies of hepatic resection and OLT for the treatment of small HCC in well-compensated cirrhotic patients. However, a non-randomized study comparing 3-year overall and tumour-free survival rates in patients with one or two HCC nodules less than 3 cm in diameter found significantly better results in the transplanted group (83% compared with 43% for overall survival, and 83% compared with 18% for tumour-free survival) (29). Notwithstanding the long-term implications of immunosuppression, OLT has become the surgical treatment of choice in this group.

Table 18.2.4. Survival rates after OLT in patients with HCC.

Centre (reference)	HCC-related criteria	Survival
Pittsburgh (26)	Unifocal, < 5 cm in diameter	68% at 5 years
King's College (27)	Unifocal, < 4 cm in diameter	57% at 5 years
Milan (28)	Unifocal, ≤ 5 cm in diameter, or	75% at 4 years
	Multifocal, ≤ 3 foci, each ≤ 3 cm in diameter	

Five-year tumour-free survival of over 50% has been reported in patients transplanted for the fibrolamellar variant of HCC — even those with large or multifocal tumours not amenable to resection (27). OLT is the treatment of choice in this group.

Percutaneous ethanol injection

PEI, in which up to 10 ml of absolute alcohol is introduced into the lesion under ultrasound guidance, is appropriate in patients with a single HCC no greater than 5 cm in diameter or with no more than three tumour nodules each no greater than 3 cm in size, especially if the lesion is superficially located. The procedure is usually repeated one to three times weekly for six to 10 sessions, although a single treatment using a large volume of ethanol is also effective, and generally well tolerated. Transient local pain sometimes requiring narcotic analgesia is the most common side effect. The prevalence of other complications such as liver abscess or haemoperitoneum is less than 2%. Imaging evidence of tumour necrosis is based on a lack of lesion enhancement on contrast-enhanced CT or MRI.

Contraindications to PEI include ascites, uncorrectable coagulopathy, and extrahepatic dissemination. PEI is not useful in patients with larger tumours, as the diffusion of ethanol is limited, not only by the texture of the tumour parenchyma, but also by the presence of septa, which isolate portions of the tumour and prevent the homogeneous distribution of ethanol within it.

Three-year survival rates of up to 79% have been reported with PEI, depending on the size and number of HCC foci treated and the underlying Child's classification (Table 18.2.5) (30,31). Although randomized comparisons are lacking, a non-randomized study found significantly better survival in treated patients compared with a non-treated control group (32). Furthermore, a cohort study comparing PEI with hepatic resection in patients with HCCs no more than 4 cm in diameter found similar overall 4-year survival, despite less rigorous patient selection in those treated with PEI (33). Consequently, PEI is becoming increasingly used both in Asia and the West, as an alternative to hepatic resection in patients with small, resectable HCCs for whom OLT is not available or is otherwise contraindicated, especially in view of its lower associated morbidity and cost. However, treatment may not modify the overall prognosis in Child's C class patients, in whom survival is often determined by the underlying advanced cirrhosis, rather than by progression of the complicating tumour. Rates of tumour recurrence similar to those occurring after hepatic resection have been reported. As with percutaneous biopsy, needle-tract seeding is a possible complication of PEI — a find-

Table 18.2.5. Survival rates after PEI for HCC.

Reference	HCC characteristics	Child's class	3-year survival (%)
Ebara et al. (30)	No more than three foci, each ≤ 3 cm diameter	A	72
		B	72
		C	25
Livraghi et al. (31)	Single focus, ≤ 5 cm diameter	A	79
		B	63
		C	0
	Two or three foci, each ≤ 3 cm diameter	A	68
		B	59

ing with important implications if this technique is used with curative intent.

Transcatheter arterial chemoembolization

TACE, which combines targeted chemotherapy and temporary hepatic arterial embolization with particulate matter such as gelfoam, is an alternative treatment for patients with HCCs confined to the liver, including large or centrally located tumours not amenable to other local treatments. Emulsifying the chemotherapeutic agent(s) with Lipiodol prolongs the contact time between anticancer drugs and tumour cells, and is associated with improved efficacy of TACE. The procedure is performed at 6–12 week intervals until tumour ablation is documented. Main portal vein occlusion and sepsis are contraindications to TACE. Many centres also exclude patients with Child's class C cirrhosis, on the premise that prognosis would remain poor even if the HCC were successfully ablated, and because the procedure carries a risk of further hepatic decompensation consequent to transient ischaemia of the non-tumorous liver. Most patients experience transient fever and right upper-quadrant pain after TACE. Other uncommon side effects include liver abscess, renal failure, and neutropenic sepsis.

Tumour ablation rates after repeated sessions of TACE are substantially greater for HCCs less than 4 cm in diameter than for larger tumours, and multivariate analysis has identified tumour size, along with underlying liver function, as an important factor influencing survival after this form of treatment (35,36). However, the role of TACE in patients with small HCCs and well-compensated cirrhosis is ill-defined, as randomized studies comparing survival with that achieved after OLT, resection, and PEI have not been performed in this group. In practice, repeated TACE is predominantly used in patients with large HCCs that are not suitable for any of these other treatments. Uncontrolled studies have demonstrated 3-year survival rates of 13–41% in this setting. A non-randomized study in patients with HCCs greater than 5 cm in diameter demonstrated significantly improved mean survival in the treated group (13 months) compared with that in untreated patients (7 months) (36). However, two randomized controlled studies comparing TACE with no treatment have not confirmed this finding (37,38), at least in part because of instances of treatment-related liver failure masking any possible survival benefit resulting from tumour ablation.

Limited published experience suggests that the use of TACE before surgery, to reduce tumour bulk, may improve the postoperative outcome in patients with HCCs considered borderline for resection. Experience with TACE as a means of reducing tumour size in order to fulfill the criteria of suitability for OLT is also limited. This treatment does limit tumour progression in the majority of patients with small HCCs who are already awaiting OLT, but any possible effect on tumour recurrence rates and post-OLT survival has not been adequately assessed.

Complete necrosis of large HCCs is achieved with TACE in approximately 50% or fewer cases. On the basis that TACE disturbs tumour parenchyma and disrupts septa such that ethanol is distributed more evenly throughout large lesions, combined modality treatment with an initial session of TACE followed, after 2 weeks, by a course of PEI has been proposed. The efficacy of such an approach in patients with HCC larger than 3 cm in diameter has been assessed in two randomized studies (39,40). Each found that tumour ablation rates were substantially greater, and survival was significantly better, after combined TACE and PEI treatment than with repeated (up to five) sessions of TACE alone (Table 18.2.6). On the basis of current evidence, combined TACE and PEI should be considered the treatment of choice for patients with

Table 18.2.6. Tumour ablation and survival rates after treatment with TACE followed by a course of PEI (TACE + PEI) or repeated sessions of TACE alone for HCCs greater than 3 cm in diameter.

Reference	Child's class A (%)	HCC ablation rate (%)		1-year survival (%)	
		TACE	TACE + PEI	TACE	TACE + PEI
Bartolozzi *et al.* (39)	47	52	85*	48	85*
Tanaka *et al.* (40)	76	20	83	68	100*

*$P < 0.05$ compared with TACE alone.

large, inoperable HCCs, especially those with Child's class A or B cirrhosis. This finding contrasts with the lack of improved efficacy of combined TACE and PEI over that of PEI alone in the treatment of patients with smaller HCCs.

Iodine[131]-labelled lipiodol and thermal modalities

Intra-hepatic arterial injection of lipiodol labelled with ^{131}I represents an approach to delivering targeted radiotherapy to HCC without inducing radiation hepatitis to non-tumourous liver. Comparable efficiency to that of a lipiodol-based TACE regimen has been reported in a prospective, randomized analysis (41). An anti-tumour effect has been reported in up to 90% of patients with predominantly small HCCs treated with thermal modalities such as radiofrequency ablation, interstitial laser coagulation or microwave coagulation (42–44). Large-scale studies further addressing the efficacy and safety of these forms of treatment are awaited.

Systemic chemotherapy

Systemic chemotherapy with a variety of agents, including doxorubicin, epirubicin, mitoxantrone, cisplatin, and etoposide, either alone or in combination, is often used in patients with HCC disseminated beyond the liver. However, the response rate is of the order of only 15% and the value of systemic chemotherapy has never been confirmed in controlled trials. Consequently, this form of treatment has only a limited role in the management of HCC.

Tamoxifen

A number of randomized controlled trials have now been performed to investigate whether the antioestrogen drug, tamoxifen, improves survival in patients with HCC. Earlier studies performed in relatively small numbers of patients and using varying doses up to 60 mg daily yielded conflicting results. The findings of a recently reported, large, multicentre study of 496 patients randomly allocated to receive 40 mg of tamoxifen daily or no hormonal treatment indicate that tamoxifen has no overall efficacy in prolonging survival in patients with HCC (45). Whether treatment confers any benefit in that subgroup of HCC patients whose tumours express high levels of normally functioning oestrogen receptors has not been investigated.

References
*Of interest; **of exceptional interest

1. *Borzio M, Bruno S, Roncalli M et al. Liver cell dysplasia is a major risk factor for hepatocellular carcinoma in cirrhosis: a prospective study. Gastroenterology 1995; 108: 812–817.
2. *Ganne-Carie N, Chastang C, Chapel F et al. Predictive score for the development of hepatocellular carcinoma and additional value of liver large cell dysplasia in western patients with cirrhosis. Hepatology 1996; 23: 1112–1118.
3. *Ko S, Nakajima Y, Kanehiro H et al. Significant influence of accompanying chronic hepatitis status on recurrence of hepatocellular carcinoma after hepatectomy. Ann Surg 1996; 224: 591–595.
4. *Shibata M, Morizane T, Uchida T et al. Irregular regeneration of hepatocytes and risk of hepatocellular carcinoma in chronic hepatitis and cirrhosis with hepatitis-c-virus infection. Lancet 1998; 351: 1773–1777.
   References 1–4 describe histological features identifying cirrhotic patients at especially high risk of development of hepatocellular carcinoma.
5. Okuda K, Okuda H. Primary liver cell carcinoma. In: Oxford Textbook of Clinical Hepatology. Eds M McIntyre, J-P Benhamou, J Bircher et al. Oxford: Oxford University Press, 1991; pp 1019–1053.
6. The Liver Cancer Study Group of Japan. Primary liver cancer in Japan: clinicopathologic features and results of surgical tretament. Ann Surg 1990; 211: 277–287.
7. Sherman M, Peltekian KM, Lee C. Screening for hepatocellular carcinoma in chronic carriers of hepatitis B virus: incidence and prevalence of hepatocellular carcinoma in a North American urban population. Hepatology 1995; 22: 432–438.
8. Oka H, Tamori A, Kuroki T et al. Prospective study of alpha-fetoprotein in cirrhotic patients monitored for development of hepatocellular carcinoma. Hepatology 1994; 19: 61–66.
9. Endo Y. Lectin-binding analysis of serum alpha-fetoprotein: predictive importance of the change of AFP sugar chain in the development of hepatocellular carcinoma. In: Primary Liver Cancer in Japan. Eds T Tobe, H Kameda, M Okudaira et al. Tokyo: Springer-Verlag, Tokyo, 1992: pp. 163–173.
10. *Bartolozzi C, Lencioni R, Caramella D et al. Small hepatocellular carcinoma: detection with US, CT, MRI, DSA and Lipiodol-CT. Acta Radiol 1996; 37: 69–74.
    A study directly comparing the sensitivities of various non-invasive and invasive imaging techniques for detecting small hepatocellular carcinomas.
11. Sheu JC, Sung JL, Chen DS et al. Growth rates of asymptomatic hepatocellular carcinoma and its clinical implications. Gastroenterology 1985; 89: 259–266.
12. *Arakawa A, Nishiharu T, Matsukawa T et al. Detection of hepatocellular carcinoma by intraarterially enhanced ultrasonography with CO_2 microbubbles. Acta Radiol 1996; 37: 250–254.
    A study directly comparing the sensitivities of various angiographic techniques for detecting small hepatocellular carcinomas and demonstrating, in particular, the value of microbubble-enhanced sonographic angiography.
13. *Nishiharu T, Yamashita Y, Arakawa A et al. Sonographic comparison of intraarterial CO_2 and helium microbubbles for detection of hepatocellular carcinoma: preliminary observations. Radiology 1998; 206: 767–771.

This study demonstrates that the use of helium in microbubble-enhanced sonographic angiography improves its sensitivity, while also extending its applicability by allowing the test to be performed more than 30 min after angiography, compared with the less than 4 min needed as with the use of carbon dioxide microbubbles.

14. Taylor KJW, Ramos I, Morse SS *et al.* Focal liver masses: differential diagnosis with pulsed Doppler US. *Radiology* 1987; **164**: 643–647.

15. Chen RC, Wang CK, Chiang LC *et al.* Intra-arterial carbon dioxide–enhanced ultrasonogram of hepatocellular carcinoma treated by transcatheter arterial embolization and percutaneous ethanol injection therapy. *J Gastroenterol Hepatol* 1998; **13**: 41–46.

16. Lencioni R, Pinto F, Armillotta N *et al.* Intrahepatic metastatic nodules of hepatocellular carcinoma detected at Lipiodol-CT: imaging-pathologic correlation. *Abdom Imaging* 1997; **22**: 253–258.

17. Pugh RN, Murray-Lyon IM, Dawson JL, *et al.* Transection of the oesophagus for bleeding oesophageal varices. *Br J Surg* 1973; **60**: 646–649.

18. Bruix J, Castells A, Bosch J *et al.* Surgical resection of hepatocellular carcinoma in cirrhotic patients: prognostic value of pre-operative portal pressure. *Gastroenterology* 1996; **111**: 1018–1023.

19. *Sitzmann JV, Greene PS. Perioperative predictors of morbidity following hepatic resection for neoplasm. *Ann Surg* 1994; **219**: 13–17.

   References 17 and 18 document the importance of the serum bilirubin and the hepatic venous pressure gradient as predictors of hepatic function after resection in patients with cirrhosis.

20. Kwon AH, Kawa S, Uetsuji S *et al.* Preoperative determination of the surgical procedure for hepatectomy using technetium-99m–galactosyl human serum albumin (^{99m}Tc-GSA) liver scintigraphy. *Hepatology* 1997; **25**: 426–429.

21. Fan ST, Lo CM, Lai ECS *et al.* Perioperative nutritional support in patients undergoing hepatectomy for hepatocellular carcinoma. *N Engl J Med* 1994; **331**: 1547–1552.

22. Kinoshita H, Hirohashi K, Kubo S. Preoperative portal vein embolisation for hepatocellular carcinoma. In: *Primary Liver Cancer in Japan.* Eds T Tobe, H Kameda, M Okudaira *et al.* Tokyo: Springer-Verlag, 1992: pp. 283–290.

23. *Nagasue N, Kohno H, Chang YC *et al.* DNA ploidy pattern in synchronous and metachronous hepatocellular carcinomas. *J Hepatol* 1992; **16**: 208–214.

24. *Chen PJ, Chen DS, Lai MY *et al.* Clonal origin of recurrent hepatocellular carcinomas. *Gastroenterology* 1989; **96**: 527–529.

   References 23 and 24 demonstrate that most hepatocellular carcinomas detected in the remnant liver after resection are *de novo* tumours, illustrating the pre-malignant potential of the cirrhotic liver.

25. **International Interferon-α Hepatocellular Carcinoma Study Group. Effect of interferon-α on progression of cirrhosis to hepatocellular carcinoma: a retrospective cohort study. *Lancet* 1998; **351**: 1535–1539.

   An important retrospective study suggesting that treatment with interferon-α may reduce the incidence of hepatocellular carcinoma in patients with hepatitis-C-related cirrhosis by more than six-fold.

26. *Yokoyama I, Todo S, Iwabuki S *et al.* Liver transplantation in the treatment of primary liver cancer. *Hepatogastroenterology* 1990; **37**: 188–193.

27. *McPeake JR, O'Grady JG, Zaman S *et al.* Liver transplantation for primary hepatocellular carcinoma: tumour size and number determine outcome. *J Hepatol* 1993; **18**: 226–234.

28. *Mazzaferro V, Regalia E, Doci R *et al.* Liver transplantation for the treatment of small hepatocellular carcinomas in patients with cirrhosis. *N Engl J Med* 1996; **334**: 693–699.

   References 25–27 indicate appropriate selection criteria for liver transplantation in patients with cirrhosis who have complicating hepatocellular carcinoma.

29. Bismuth H, Chiche L, Adam R *et al.* Liver resection versus transplantation for hepatocellular carcinoma in cirrhotic patients. *Ann Surg* 1993; **218**: 145–151.

30. Ebara M, Kita K, Yoshikawa M *et al.* Percutaneous ethanol injection for patients with small hepatocellular carcinoma. In: *Primary Liver Cancer in Japan.* Eds T Tobe, H Kameda, M Okudaira *et al.* Tokyo: Springer-Verlag, 1992: pp. 291–300.

31. Livraghi T, Giorgio A, Marin G *et al.* Hepatocellular carcinoma and cirrhosis in 746 patients: long-term results of percutaneous ethanol injection. *Radiology* 1995; **197**: 101–108.

32. Isobe H, Sakai H, Imari Y *et al.* Intratumor ethanol injection therapy for solitary minute hepatocellular carcinoma. *J Clin Gastroenterol* 1994; **18**: 122–126.

33. Castells A, Bruix J, Bru C *et al.* Treatment of small hepatocellular carcinoma in cirrhotic patients: a cohort study comparing surgical resection and percutaneous ethanol injection. *Hepatology* 1993; **18**: 1121–1126.

34. Sakurai M, Okamura J, Kuroda C. Transcatheter chemoembolisation effective for treating hepatocellular carcinoma: a histopathologic study. *Cancer* 1984; **54**: 387–392.

35. Mondazzi L, Bottelli R, Brambilla G *et al.* Transcatheter oily chemoembolisation for the treatment of hepatocellular carcinoma: a multivariate analysis of prognostic factors. *Hepatology* 1994; **19**: 1115–1123.

36. Bayraktar Y, Balkanci F, Kayhan B *et al.* A comparison of chemoembolisation with conventional chemotherapy and symptomatic treatment in cirrhotic patients with hepatocellular carcinoma. *Hepatogastroenterology* 1996; **43**: 681–687.

37. Pelletier G, Roche A, Ink O *et al.* A randomised trial of hepatic arterial chemoembolization in patients with unresectable hepatocellular carcinoma. *J Hepatol* 1990; **11**: 181–184.

38. Groupe d'Etude et de Traitment du Carcinome Hepatocellulaire. Comparison of Lipiodol chemoembolization and conservative treatment for unresectable hepatocellular carcinoma. *N Engl J Med* 1995; **332**: 1256–1261.

39. Bartolozzi C, Lencioni R, Caramella D *et al.* Treatment of large HCC: transcatheter arterial chemoembolization combined with percutaneous ethanol injection versus repeated transcatheter arterial chemoembolization. *Radiology* 1995; **197**: 812–818.

40. Tanaka K, Nakamura S, Numata K *et al.* Hepatocellular carcinoma: treatment with percutaneous ethanol injection and transcatheter arterial embolization. *Radiology* 1992; **185**: 457–460.

41. Bhattacharya S, Novell JR, Dusheiko GM, *et al.* Epirubicin-Lipiodol chemotherapy versus ^{131}iodine-Lipiodol radiotherapy in the treatment of unresectable hepatocellular carcinoma. *Cancer* 1995; **76**: 2202–2210.

42. Solbiati L. New applications of ultrasonography: interventional ultrasound. *Eur J Radiol* 1998; **27**: S200–206.

43. Bremer C, Allkemper T. Memzel J, *et al.* Preliminary clinical experience with laser-induced interstitial thermotherapy in patients with hepatocellular carcinoma. *J. Magn Reson Imaging* 1998; 8: 235–239.

44. Matsukawa T, Yamashita Y, Arakawa A, *et al.* Percutaneous microwave coagulation therapy in liver tumors. *Acta Radiol* 1997; **38**: 410–415.

45. CLIP Group (Cancer of the Liver Italian Programme). Tamoxifen in treatment of hepatocellular carcinoma: a randomised controlled trial. *Lancet* 1998; **352**: 17–20.

19. Ascites and Spontaneous Bacterial Peritonitis

STEPHEN M. RIORDAN

INTRODUCTION

Ascites is excessive free fluid that has formed in the peritoneal space. It has many possible causes, including disorders associated with portal hypertension, peritoneal inflammation, reduced plasma oncotic pressure, or disruption to the lymphatic drainage (Table 19.1). However, in the Western world, ascites is caused by cirrhosis in approximately 80% of cases; hepatic or peritoneal malignancies, heart failure, and tuberculous peritonitis account for most of the remainder. Although acute portal vein thrombosis commonly results in transient ascites, chronic portal vein obstruction does not usually cause ascites in the absence of underlying liver disease. Depending on the cause of ascites, appropriate management includes such diverse measures as simple dietary sodium restriction and use of diuretics (in patients with otherwise well-compensated cirrhosis), use of systemic or intra-peritoneal cytotoxic agents (in selected patients with chemosensitive hepatic or peritoneal malignancies, respectively), use of antituberculous chemotherapy (in those with tuberculous peritonitis), thyroxine replacement (in those with myxoedema), interventional radiological techniques such as percutaneous transluminal angioplasty with or without stenting or surgical or radiological portosystemic shunting (in selected patients with Budd–Chiari syndrome), cardiac surgery (in those with constrictive pericarditis), or orthotopic liver transplantation (OLT) (in those with decompensated cirrhosis and, as an emergency, those with acute liver failure meeting criteria for poor prognosis).

Spontaneous bacterial peritonitis (SBP) is an infection, typically, of pre-existing ascitic fluid and with a single bacterial species, in the absence of any other primary intra-abdominal source. SBP is considered to be present if an increased number of neutrophils, or any bacteria, or both, are recovered from ascites. This broad definition takes into account the existence of culture-negative neutrocytic ascites (CNNA), in which ascitic culture is negative, despite the presence of a high neutrophil count and bacterascites, in which a positive ascitic culture is unaccompanied by an increased neutrophil count. CNNA is taken to represent SBP in which culture is falsely negative because of the relative insensitivity of culture techniques. Bacterascites probably represents an early variant of SBP without an inflammatory response. Prospective studies suggest that SBP, including culture-negative and non-neutrocytic cases, is present in up to 27% of all patients with cirrhosis and who are admitted to hospital, and is associated with a poor prognosis. This chapter reviews current understanding of the pathogenesis of ascites and SBP as background to a clinically focused discussion of evidence-based approaches to diagnosis and management of these disorders.

ASCITES

Pathogenesis of ascites

In patients with liver disease, portal hypertension in combination with reduced plasma oncotic pressure resulting from hypoalbuminaemia was traditionally

Table 19.1. Causes of ascites.

Portal hypertension with liver damage	**Portal hypertension without liver damage**
Cirrhosis ± portal vein thrombosis/infiltration by	Acute portal vein obstruction
hepatocellular carcinoma	trauma
alcohol	acute pancreatitis
chronic viral hepatitis B and C	intra-abdominal sepsis
haemochromatosis	hypercoagulable state
Wilson's disease	
primary biliary cirrhosis	**Peritoneal inflammation**
primary sclerosing cholangitis	Spontaneous bacterial peritonitis[¶]
secondary biliary cirrhosis	Malignancies
autoimmune hepatitis	secondary carcinomatosis
α_1 antitrypsin deficiency	primary mesothelioma
cryptogenic	Tuberculosis
Alcoholic hepatitis	Pancreatic enzymes
Nodular regenerative hyperplasia	Bile
Schistosomiasis	Pelvic inflammatory disease
Acute liver failure	*Chlamydia trachomatis*
viral	*Neisseria gonorrhoeae*
drug/toxin reactions	Connective tissue disorders
ischaemic	systemic lupus erythematosus
autoimmune	sarcoidosis
Wilson's disease	familial Mediterranean fever
cryptogenic	
Massive liver infiltration[†]	**Reduced plasma oncotic pressure[§]**
metastases	Nephrotic syndrome
lymphoma	Protein-losing enteropathy
leukaemia	Malnutrition
Fatty liver of pregnancy/HELLP syndrome[†]	
Veno-occlusive disease	**Impaired lymphatic drainage**
chemotherapy	Lymphatic obstruction
pyrrolizimide alkaloids	lymphoproliferative disorders
irradiation	tuberculosis
Budd–Chiari syndrome[†]	hepatic congestion
hypercoagulable state	right ventricular failure
tumours	Budd–Chiari syndrome
hepatocellular carcinoma	veno-occlusive disease
renal-cell carcinoma	Lymphatic tear
adrenal carcinoma	trauma
membranous webs	cirrhosis
Right ventricular failure	
ischaemic heart disease	
valvular heart disease	
cardiomyopathy	
constrictive pericarditis	
cor pulmonale	
myxoedema	

HELLP, 'haemolysis, elevated liver enzymes, low platelets'; [†]Clinical spectrum includes acute liver failure; [¶]Usually complicates pre-existing ascites; [§]In the absence of liver disease.

considered to be primarily responsible for the development of ascites, with secondary renal sodium and water retention occurring to compensate for a reduction in circulating plasma volume (the "underfilling" theory) (1). However, it is now established that plasma volume is increased, rather than reduced, in patients with cirrhotic ascites, and that renal sodium retention precedes the onset of ascites, indicating that it is a cause, rather than a consequence, of ascites formation (2,3). Current evidence indicates that renal sodium and water retention in patients with cirrhotic ascites occurs as the consequence of a profound vasodilatation of splanchnic arterioles, such that, even though total plasma volume is increased, effective arterial volume is reduced (the "arterial vasodilatation" theory) (4). The subsequent activation of compensatory mechanisms promoting renal sodium and water retention, such as the sympathetic nervous system, the renin–angiotensin–aldosterone axis and the non-osmotic hypersecretion of antidiuretic hormone, also leads to renal vasoconstriction and dilutional hyponatraemia, accounting for the well-recognized clinical association between cirrhotic ascites and hepatorenal syndrome, especially in hyponatraemic patients. A similar disturbance in the splanchnic circulation has been documented in patients with non-cirrhotic, pre-sinusoidal portal hypertension resulting from hepatic schistosomiasis (5).

The findings of recent studies suggest that increased synthesis of nitric oxide, a potent vasodilator produced in vascular endothelium, may be responsible for this dramatic circulatory disturbance, at least in cirrhosis (6–8). Whereas SBP may exacerbate pre-existing ascites in cirrhotic patients as a consequence of peritoneal inflammation, with leakage of free fluid into the peritoneal space, recent evidence suggests that this disorder also results in increased and long-lasting peritoneal synthesis of nitric oxide (9), which may exacerbate splanchnic arteriolar vasodilatation and, for reasons discussed above, worsen cirrhotic ascites, even after the superimposed peritoneal infection has been eradicated.

The mechanism of ascites formation in nephrotic syndrome and other hypoproteinaemic states unrelated to liver disease probably relates to activation of the renin–angiotensin–aldosterone axis as a consequence of reduced circulating blood volume caused by hypoalbuminaemia. In aetiologies both related and unrelated to portal hypertension, ascites ultimately forms and accumulates when the volume of free peritoneal fluid produced exceeds the capacity of lymphatics to return it to the vascular space. Consequently, impaired lymphatic drainage, as may occur as a consequence of trauma or malignant or inflammatory lymphatic obstruction, promotes and exacerbates ascites. Lymphatic obstruction in association with lymphoproliferative disorders or tuberculosis is the most common mechanism underlying chylous ascites, although this may also be seen in patients with nephrotic syndrome and in those with uncomplicated cirrhosis, presumably as a result of rupture of overloaded lymphatics.

Approaches to determining the cause of ascites

Key initial components in determining the cause of ascites include the history, physical examination, laboratory indices of liver function, abdominal imaging (including ultrasound with Doppler assessment of patency and flow patterns within venous structures, with or without computed tomography), and diagnostic paracentesis. At the minimum, the last of these should include culture of ascites and determination of the ascitic white cell count and albumin concentration. In more than 97% of instances (10), calculation of the serum to ascites albumin gradient (SAAG) complements the clinical assessment in correctly differentiating patients with ascites related to portal hypertension (gradient >11 g/litre) from those in whom the aetiology is not related to portal hypertension (gradient <11 g/litre). The accuracy of this ratio obviates the need to measure the hepatic venous pressure gradient or splenic pulp pressure in order to establish the presence of portal hypertension in most patients, although pressure measurements remain useful to guide treatment in certain specific circumstances, as discussed below. Consideration of the SAAG in combination with the ascitic white cell count further helps to categorize the cause of ascites (Table 19.2). The ascitic white cell count is usually normal (total count less that 500/µl; neutrophil count less than 250/µl) in patients with uncomplicated portal hypertension-related ascites and increased in those with non-portal-hypertensive aetiologies, with the exception of nephrotic syndrome and other hypoalbuminaemic states. Consideration of the differential white cell count is important when the total ascitic white cell count is increased. Diuretic therapy increases the total white cell count in ascites, but the neutrophil count does not change with diuresis and, in the absence of haemoperitoneum or a bloody tap, remains a valid index of peritoneal inflammation in this circumstance (11).

Further investigation, as directed by the clinical findings and results of these initial laboratory and radiological investigations, is mandatory to determine the actual cause of ascites within the two broad categories of relation or non-relation to portal hypertension (Table 19.3). For example, **liver biopsy** is usually indicated in patients with portal hypertension-related ascites, in order to establish diagnoses such as cirrhosis or to determine the nature

Table 19.2.   Usual SAAG and ascitic white cell count patterns in various causes of ascites.

	Increased SAAG	Normal SAAG

Normal white cell count[†]	Cirrhosis
	Alcoholic hepatitis
	Nodular regenerative hyperplasia
	Schistosomiasis
	Acute liver failure (including fatty liver of
	    pregnancy/HELLP syndrome)
	Veno-occlusive disease
	Budd–Chiari syndrome
	Right ventricular failure
	Acute portal vein obstruction
	Chronic portal vein obstruction (in association with
	    liver disease)
		Nephrotic syndrome
		Protein-losing enteropathy
		Malnutrition

Increased neutrophils[†]	Spontaneous bacterial peritonitis
	    (complicating pre-existing ascites from the
	    above causes)
		Spontaneous bacterial peritonitis
		    (complicating pre-existing
		    ascites from the above causes)
		Pancreatic ascites
		Biliary ascites
		Pelvic inflammatory disease

Increased lymphocytes	Dual pathology (e.g. tuberculous peritonitis or
	    peritoneal malignancy in a patient with alcoholic
	    hepatitis or cirrhosis)
		Peritoneal malignancy
		Tuberculous peritonitis
		Connective tissue disorders

[†]Normal SAAG: < 11 g/litre; normal ascitic white cell count < 500/µl with neutrophil count < 250/µl.

of any hepatic infiltrative process. Approximately 25% of patients with portal vein thrombosis have underlying cirrhosis. To minimize the risk of complications, percutaneous liver biopsy should be performed only after ascites has been effectively treated; the transjugular route is an alternative if this is problematic. Although liver biopsy is useful for excluding chronic liver disease in suspected cases of acute liver failure, it is often precluded by the severe coagulopathy in such patients. **Echocardiography**, **cardiac catheterization**, and **lung and thyroid function tests** may be required to establish the presence and cause of right ventricular failure. **Cytological examination** of ascitic fluid is positive in more than 90% of cases of peritoneal carcinomatosis, whereas **laparoscope-guided peritoneal biopsy** is the most reliable test for tuberculous peritonitis. Mycobacteria are identified on culture of ascitic fluid in fewer that 20% of cases. Increased **adenosine deaminase** concentrations in ascitic fluid have a specificity of over 90%, although reported sensitivities are widely variable. More than 70% of patients with tuberculous peritonitis have no evidence of pulmonary disease.

An increased **ascitic amylase** concentration, generally of the order of 2000 IU/litre, is typical of pancreatic ascites, whereas an **ascitic bilirubin** value in excess of that in serum is compatible with a biliary aetiology. Further **imaging** of the pancreas and biliary tree, respectively, should be undertaken in these circumstances.

A high index of clinical suspicion, along with liver biopsy and venography with differential right atrial, inferior vena caval, hepatic venous, and portal venous pressure analyses, are important for diagnosing and planning treatment of veno-occlusive disease, which complicates bone marrow transplantation to varying extents in up to 50% of patients, and Budd–Chiari syndrome. An underlying hypercoagulable state, most commonly related to a myeloproliferative disorder, is present in approximately 75% of patients with Budd–Chiari syndrome, and should be sought even when substantial liver necrosis is present, despite the fact that interpretation of any low levels of inhibitors of coagulation is difficult in this circumstance. The possibility of an underlying malignancy should also be excluded. Associated thromboses in the inferior vena cava, portal vein, or both, are present

Table 19.3. Further investigations in patients with ascites, as directed by findings on history, examination, liver function tests, abdominal imaging, and initial analysis of ascitic fluid.

Suspected aetiology	Further investigation
Cirrhosis ± hepatocellular carcinoma	Liver biopsy[†] (distinguish from nodular regenerative hyperlasia); hepatitis B and C serology; autoantibodies; iron and copper studies; α_1 antitrypsin concn ± phenotype; endoscopic retrograde cholangiography or percutaneous cholangiography; AFP concn.
Alcoholic hepatitis	Liver biopsy
Massive liver infiltration	Liver biopsy
Schistosomiasis	Serology; stool examination; rectal biopsy; liver biopsy
Acute liver failure (including fatty liver of pregnancy/ HELLP syndrome)	Liver biopsy (often precluded by coagulopathy); viral serology (hepatitis A, B ± D, C and E; herpes simplex; adenovirus; Ebstein–Barr virus; paramyxovirus); autoantibodies; copper studies; drug and toxin screen; β-hCG concn.
Veno-occlusive disease	Liver biopsy; venography with differential pressure analysis
Budd–Chiari syndrome	Liver biopsy; venography with differential pressure analysis; screen for hypercoagulable state
Right ventricular failure	Chest X–ray; ECG; cardiac echo ± catheterization; lung and thyroid function tests
Portal vein obstruction	Venography; exclude cirrhosis ± hepatocellular carcinoma; screen for hypercoagulable state
Peritoneal malignancy	Ascitic cytology; laparoscope-guided peritoneal biopsy
Tuberculous peritonitis	Chest X-ray; ascitic culture; ascitic adenosine deaminase concn; laparoscope-guided peritoneal biopsy
Pancreatic ascites	Ascitic and serum amylase concn.
Biliary ascites	Ascitic bilirubin concn
Pelvic inflammatory disease	Cervical swab for culture or bacterial antigen detection techniques
Connective tissue disorders	Autoantibodies; angiotensin converting enzyme concn
Nephrotic syndrome	24-h urinary protein concn
Protein-losing enteropathy	Faecal α_1-antitrypsin clearance

[†]After effective treatment of ascites or via transjugular route.
concn, concentration; AFP, alpha-fetoprotein; hCG, human chorionic gonadotrophin; ECG, electrocardiogram.

in up to 20% of patients. When ascites appears milky, the triglyceride content should be measured in order to differentiate between true chylous and pseudochylous ascites, the latter caused by scattering of light by aggregates of cholesterol, phospholipid, and protein derived from degenerating malignant or inflammatory cells.

Approach to the management of ascites

Cirrhotic ascites

Sodium and fluid restriction and use of diuretics
As discussed above, **sodium retention** is a key feature in the pathogenesis of cirrhotic ascites; the aim of medical treatment is, therefore, to induce a negative sodium balance. This is achieved with dietary sodium restriction and use of diuretics in more than 90% of affected patients (Table 19.4). A sodium-restricted diet hastens the mobilization of ascites in patients treated with diuretics (12), but patients are rarely compliant with restrictions to less than 2 g/day (88 mmol/day). **Fluid loss** in patients with cirrhotic ascites is directly related to a negative sodium balance, with water passively following sodium, and water restriction should be reserved for that subgroup of patients with hyponatraemia attributable to antidiuretic-hormone-mediated reduced renal free-water clearance (13). Such

Table 19.4. Treatment options for cirrhotic ascites.

First-line	Dietary sodium restriction
	Diuretics: spironolactone ± frusemide
	Fluid restriction only if hyponatraemic
Second-line	Therapeutic paracentesis
	Peritoneovenous shunt
	Transjugular intrahepatic portosystemic shunt
	Orthotopic liver transplantation

patients have impending hepatorenal syndrome and a poor prognosis.

Spironolactone is the single diuretic agent of choice in patients with cirrhotic ascites: in non-azotaemic patients, a natriuretic response occurs in 95%, compared with only 52% of those treated with frusemide (14). The poor efficacy of **frusemide** used alone may be related to increased sodium reabsorption in the distal convoluted tubule and collecting duct, resulting from secondary hyperaldosteronism. The plasma aldosterone concentration is also an important factor influencing the dosage of spironolactone required to induce adequate natriuresis, with doses in excess of 150 mg/day often required in those with more marked hyperaldosteronism (14). Spironolactone undergoes extensive tissue metabolism to biologically active compounds with relatively long half-lives (15) and, consequently, it may take up to 2 weeks for the onset of a natriuretic effect (16). An additional problem is the development of hyperkalaemia in a high proportion of patients. As the combination of spironolactone with frusemide potentiates the intrinsic effects of each drug, a practical therapeutic approach, especially in those with tense ascites, is to commence with 100 mg/day of spironolactone and 40 mg/day of frusemide. Doses are increased every 4–5 days, to a maximum of 400 mg/day of spironolactone and 160 mg/day of frusemide, if no response, as determined by body weight or 24-h urinary sodium concentrations, is apparent. In the absence of peripheral oedema, the aim should be to achieve weight loss of up to 0.5 kg/day. Greater degrees of fluid loss are associated with a reduction in circulating plasma volume and renal impairment.

Refractory ascites

Refractory cirrhotic ascites is defined as ascites unresponsive to a sodium-restricted diet and high-dose diuretic treatment. Fewer than 10% of patients with cirrhotic ascites fall in to this category. Most have hepatorenal syndrome. The impaired delivery of frusemide and spironolactone to their sites of action consequent to renal hypoperfusion limits the efficacy of these drugs in this circumstance (17). The effect of spironolactone is further limited by the fact that renal sodium reabsorption occurs predominantly in the proximal convoluted tubule in hepatorenal syndrome, such that distal tubular sodium concentrations are low (17). Non-steroidal anti-inflammatory drugs depress the natriuretic effects of both frusemide and spironolactone (18), and should be avoided. Clinical experience is that treatment to reduce portal hypertension, such as with β-blockade, does not render patients with previously refractory ascites responsive to diuretics. Conversely, simultaneous plasma volume expansion and use of the vasopressin analogues, omnipressin or terlipressin, leads to improvement in systemic haemodynamics, the glomerular filtration rate and the serum creatinine level in patients with hepatorenal syndrome, with increased natriuresis reported on occasion (19–23). Similar effects have been observed with use of midodrine, an alpha-adrenergic agonist, in combination with octreotide (24).

Possible **treatment options** for cirrhotic patients with refractory ascites include therapeutic paracentesis, a peritoneovenous shunt, a surgical portocaval or transjugular intrahepatic portosystemic shunt (TIPSS), and OLT. Such treatments must also be considered in those patients with complications of diuretic treatment that preclude the use of effective doses. Large-volume therapeutic paracentesis (either daily 4–6 litre parcenteses until the disappearance of ascites, or a single total paracentesis) should be considered to be first-line symptomatic treatment for refractory cirrhotic ascites. Although ascitic fluid complement protein 3 concentrations are significantly reduced after large volume paracentesis — in contrast to the significantly increased values that occur with effective diuretic treatment (25) and raising the possibility that large-volume paracentesis may predispose cirrhotic patients to SBP, as discussed below — one study demonstrated no significant difference in the incidence of this complication in those treated with total paracentesis followed by diuretics or diuretic treatment alone (26). Nonetheless, fewer than 50% of the paracentesis-treated group required more than one paracentesis during follow-up, and further studies are required to demonstrate that repeated large-volume paracenteses do not predispose patients with cirrhotic ascites to SBP.

After paracentesis a reduction in circulating blood volume, with secondary activation of the renin–angiotensin–aldosterone and sympathetic nervous systems, may ensue after 12–24 h unless patients receive intravenous albumin (6–10 g per litre of ascites removed) as a plasma expander (27,28). The incidences of renal impairment, hyponatraemia, and hepatic encephalopathy after the procedure are significantly increased in patients receiving large volume paracentesis without albumin infusion (28). Several randomized studies have been undertaken to investigate whether albumin can be substituted with less expensive plasma expanders, such as dextran-70 and polygeline. In a study of 289 cirrhotic patients with tense ascites treated with total paracentesis (29), postprocedure circulatory disturbance, as defined by a more than 50% increase from the pretreatment plasma renin activity to a level in excess of 4 ng/ml per h on the 6th day after paracentesis, occurred significantly more frequently in patients allocated randomly to groups to receive dextran-70 (34%) or polygeline (38%) than in those who received albumin (18%). The type of plasma expander used and the volume of ascites removed were independent predictors of circulatory dysfunction after paracentesis, which persisted during follow-up and, contrary to earlier reports (30), was associated with shorter survival. The reduced efficacy of dextran-70 compared with that of albumin can probably be explained on pharma-cokinetic grounds, as most dextran-70 has disappeared from the plasma by the time at which paracentesis-induced hypovolaemia typically occurs (31). In contrast, no change in mean plasma renin activity or other clinical or laboratory variables followed the use of intravenous isotonic saline infusion in 14 cirrhotic patients with tense ascites treated with total paracentesis (32). Further studies of saline infusion are warranted to confirm the safety and value of this potentially cost-effective alternative to albumin.

Peritoneovenous shunts are usually effective in controlling ascites, at least in the short term, but carry a high complication rate. Disseminated intravascular coagulation occurs in virtually every patient in the period immediately after operation, although this is clinically silent in most. Bacterial infection, including peritonitis, is a serious postoperative complication that occurs in approximately

25% of patients. No overall increased prevalence of variceal haemorrhage in the immediate postoperative period has been documented (33), although reports are conflicting as to whether peritoneovenous shunting increases the risk of variceal haemorrhage in that subgroup with a history of this disorder (34,35). Preoperative total paracentesis would eliminate any potential increased risk. Shunt obstruction, including that caused by central vein thrombosis, is the most common problem during long-term follow-up, and only about 50% of patients treated with peritoneovenous shunting remain free of ascites at 1 year (34). These data suggest that a peritonovenous shunt should be reserved for those cirrhotic patients with refractory ascites in whom repeated therapeutic paracenteses are not feasible, and who are not candidates for liver transplantation, as discussed below.

Surgical portocaval shunts are rarely indicated nowadays for the treatment of refractory cirrhotic ascites because of the high postoperative morbidity and mortality rate and the availability of alternative therapeutic modalities. Several studies assessing the efficacy of **TIPSS** have reported that refractory ascites is controlled in most patients, although shunt occlusion occurs in 30–50% of patients by 1 year (36,37). Consequently, TIPSS has been proposed in particular as a short-term "bridge" to OLT. Reversal of hepatorenal syndrome may ensue (38). A randomized study comparing TIPSS with therapeutic paracentesis in a relatively small number of Child–Pugh class B and C patients found that TIPSS was superior in maintaining control of ascites at four months in class B patients. However, both treatments were ineffective in class C patients. Moreover, survival of class C patients was significantly shorter in those who received TIPSS (39). Further randomized studies are required to clarify the place of TIPSS in the treatment algorithm for refractory cirrhotic ascites.

OLT offers definitive treatment for patients with cirrhotic ascites, especially those with other features of severe hepatic decompensation, with overall 5-year survival rates in excess of 70%. In contrast, the 5-year survival rate after the onset of ascites in cirrhotic patients treated medically is of the order of only 20% (27). Plasma renin activity and urinary sodium excretion are sensitive predictors of survival in patients with cirrhotic ascites, with mean survival in excess of 28 months in those with normal plasma renin activity and urinary sodium excretion greater than 10 mmol/day, compared with only 6 months in those with increased plasma renin activity and avid renal sodium retention (40). Mean arterial pressure, plasma noradrenaline concentrations, and the glomerular filtration rate also correlate with prognosis in this setting and these variables, in addition to traditional measures of hepatic function, should be considered in the process of selection of patients with cirrhotic ascites suitable for OLT. Refractoriness of ascites to medical treatment is an important marker of poor prognosis. Fifty per cent of patients with cirrhotic ascites refractory to medical treatment die within 6 months, and 75% within 12 months (41). Although rapid normalization of systemic haemodynamics and renal function usually follows OLT in patients with cirrhotic ascites and hepatorenal syndrome, the probability of survival is reduced compared with that in patients with normal renal function who undergo transplant (42), and OLT should preferably be performed before this stage.

Ascites in other portal hypertensive states

Sodium restriction and diuretic treatment are also important in the treatment of **ascites related to non-cirrhotic portal hypertension**. However, attention should be focused on the specific underlying cause. For example, consideration for OLT according to prognostic criteria is of paramount importance in patients with acute liver failure. An hepatic infiltrative process such as lymphoma may be responsive to chemotherapy. Patients with heart failure, including those with myxoedema, require appropriate treatment. Management of any underlying hypercoagulable state is required in patients with portal vein thrombosis.

Management of ascites arising in the context of acute **Budd–Chiari syndrome** or veno-occlusive disease is dictated by liver histology and the results of venography and pressure studies. In Budd–Chiari syndrome, thrombolytic treatment may have a role when used early in those without marked hepatocellular necrosis or major risk of bleeding. Invasive radiological procedures, such as percutaneous transluminal angioplasty with or without stent placement or TIPSS, have been used as alternative non-operative measures to relieve hepatic outflow obstruction, especially in patients with limited stenosis of the hepatic veins. Surgical intervention is often required, however, and options include a

portosystemic shunt or OLT. A side-to-side portocaval anastomosis, converting the portal vein into a hepatic outflow tract, is indicated to decompress a congested liver and thereby prevent continuing necrosis and allow hepatocyte regeneration, provided that the liver biopsy does not show marked hepatocellular necrosis or features of irrevocable damage, such as fibrosis. A mesoatrial, rather than portocaval, shunt is required when inferior vena caval thrombosis or compression by an enlarged caudate lobe results in a pressure gradient between inferior vena cava and right atrium, especially if the caval stenosis is not amenable to stenting. Survival in carefully selected patients with acute Budd–Chiari syndrome and good hepatocellular function treated with a surgical portosystemic shunt is 65–90% at 3–5 years (43,44). OLT is indicated in those patients with substantial necrosis or fibrosis on biopsy, especially in the setting of acute liver failure. Survival rates of 76% at 3 years and 58% at 5 years have been reported (45,46). Treatment of any underlying hypercoagulable state should be commenced before operation and continued in the postoperative setting.

At present, there is no standard therapeutic approach to the patient with moderate or severe **veno-occlusive disease**. Limited experience suggests that about 40% of such patients may respond to thrombolytic treatment with recombinant human tissue plasminogen activator when this is used early in the course of the disease, although the risk of severe haemorrhage is considerable and, as for acute Budd–Chiari syndrome, the applicability of this approach is limited to carefully selected patients (47). Successful relief of ascites with TIPSS has been reported (48), although experience with this form of treatment is also limited. Considerations similar to those pertaining to Budd–Chiari syndrome should apply to the relative indications and contraindications for surgical portosystemic shunting and OLT. The prognosis of any underlying haematological malignancy must also be taken in to account, especially when considering OLT. No long-term survivors after OLT have been reported to date, despite technical success of the procedure.

Ascites related to peritoneal inflammation

As with ascites related to non-cirrhotic portal hypertension, the primary focus of treatment in patients with ascites related to peritoneal inflammation is on the underlying cause, such as antituberculous chemotherapy in those with tuberculous peritonitis, or endoscopic or percutaneous stenting of a biliary leak in cases of biliary peritonitis. Diuretics may be required, at least while the underlying cause comes under control, although there is usually no indication for dietary sodium restriction. Ascites caused by peritoneal malignancy is often refractory to diuretic treatment and usually requires repeated therapeutic paracenteses, although colloid replacement is not necessary. The intraperitoneal instillation of cytotoxic agents may provide effective palliation in selected patients with chemotherapy-sensitive tumours.

SPONTANEOUS BACTERIAL PERITONITIS

Pathogenesis and risk factors for SBP

Postulated key components in the pathogenesis of SBP include:

- bacterial translocation of gut flora from the intestinal lumen to mesenteric lymph nodes
- disturbance of Kupffer cell and systemic neutrophil function
- impaired antibacterial defences in ascitic fluid

Together, these mechanisms promote bacteraemia of flora derived, not only from the intestine, but also from other sites, such as the urinary and respiratory tracts and the skin, with the potential for secondary seeding of ascitic fluid. Gram-negative enteric-type bacteria, especially *Escherichia coli* and *Klebsiella spp.*, are isolated in approximately 70% of cases of SBP. Aerobic Gram-positive bacteria belonging to the genera *Streptococcus* and *Staphylococcus* constitute most of the remaining isolates. Pathogens of genera *Aeromonas*, *Plesimonas*, *Listeria*, *Salmonella* and *Neisseria* are occasionally responsible. Obligate anaerobes are isolated from fewer than 5% of patients (49).

Most patients who develop SBP (including its culture-negative and non-neutrocytic variants) have cirrhotic ascites. SBP also frequently complicates ascites occurring in the uncommon entity of acute liver failure and is well recognized in ascites resulting from nephrotic syndrome; conversely, it rarely complicates ascites associated with peritoneal inflammation. Clinical studies have identified several **subgroups of patients with cirrhotic ascites who are at particularly high risk for SBP**:

- Child–Pugh class C
- impaired Kupffer cell function (maximum removal capacity < 56%)
- small intestinal bacterial overgrowth
- gastrointestinal haemorrhage
- ascitic total protein concentration ≤ 10 g/litre

More that 70% of cases occur in those classified as Child–Pugh C (50). An increased prevalence of SBP has been reported in patients with cirrhotic ascites and small intestinal bacterial overgrowth compared with their counterparts without such overgrowth, presumably as a result of the increased propensity for bacterial translocation (51). Gastrointestinal haemorrhage is another important precipitant of SBP in this group, presumably also related to the enhanced potential for bacterial translocation secondary to ischaemia-induced disturbance in intestinal permeability. Bacteraemia, SBP, or both, typically with Gram-negative enteric-type flora, develop within 48 h of gastrointestinal haemorrhage in nearly 50% of Child–Pugh class C patients with ascites (52). The likelihood of SBP is related to the functional activity of Kupffer cells, which is impaired in patients with advanced liver disease (53). However, the most powerful predictive factor identified in several series is an ascitic fluid total protein concentration no greater than 10 g/litre, which reflects a low complement protein 3 concentration and, hence, opsonization capacity. Patients in whom this value is so low are at a six- to 10-fold increased risk of a first episode of SBP, compared with cirrhotic counterparts with ascitic fluid total protein concentrations greater than 10 g/litre (54,55).

Clinical presentation and course of SBP

The spectrum of clinical features of SBP extends from a fulminant presentation with peritonism and shock to an asymptomatic state manifest only by deterioration in laboratory variables. Abdominal pain with fever or hypothermia, often with an increased volume of ascites that may become refractory to diuretic treatment, are characteristic features. However, the majority of patients present with such non-specific symptoms as general malaise, anorexia, nausea, or vomiting. Presentation with deterioration in mental status as a result of the precipitation or exacerbation of hepatic encephalopathy is well recognized. Consequently, a high index of suspicion is mandatory if patients with SBP are to be identified, and this diagnosis should be sought in any patient with ascites whose clinical status deteriorates in any way.

Although resolution of SBP is usually achieved with the use of appropriate antibiotics, and despite improvements in the general medical care of cirrhotic patients, the in-hospital mortality rate remains 20–40% (56,57). This is largely related to underlying hepatic decompensation and a high prevalence of hepatorenal syndrome. The latter occurs in approximately 30% of patients with SBP, predominantly in those with pre-existing renal impairment, and is progressive despite cure of infection in 50% of this group (58). The cause is uncertain, but a recent study showing that peritoneal production of nitric oxide is substantially increased in cirrhotic patients with SBP and persists for more than 2 weeks, despite appropriate antibiotic treatment, raises the possibility of even further splanchnic arteriolar vasodilatation with impairment of renal perfusion consequent upon compensatory vasoconstrictor mechanisms. A deleterious effect of bacterial products or cytokines on the renal circulation has alternatively been proposed (59). Use of nephrotoxic antibiotics adds to the risk of renal failure in this setting. The development of renal failure is the most important predictor of mortality in hospital that is associated with SBP. In one recent series, the mortality rate approximated 50% in those with complicating renal failure, compared with only 6% in those without this complication (58). Poorer outcome also correlates with increased ascitic concentrations of interleukin-6, tumour necrosis factor-α, and neopterin (60).

Most studies have found that the in-hospital mortality rate is similar in culture-negative and culture-positive patients with neutrocytic SBP. Symptomatic bacterascites carries an in-hospital mortality rate that is comparable to that associated with neutrocytic SBP. The short-term outlook is appreciably better — approximating that in uncomplicated cirrhotic ascites — in patients with asymptomatic bacterascites, which resolves spontaneously in a large proportion of them. Most evidence suggests that the type of bacterial isolate does not influence survival, although a trend towards a greater mortality rate when infection is with encapsulated strains of *E. coli* associated with tissue invasiveness was reported in one study (61).

The medium-term prognosis for patients with cirrhosis who have recovered from an episode of SBP is similarly poor, with a mortality rate at 1 year of about 80%. Approximately 20% of patients who die within 1 year of an episode of SBP succumb to a further episode of spontaneous peritoneal infection, the remainder dying of causes such as variceal haemorrhage, hepatorenal syndrome, or hepatocellular carcinoma (62–64). The risk of SBP recurrence within 1 year ranges from 40–70% and, as for an initial episode, is influenced mainly by the degree of underlying liver dysfunction and the ascitic fluid total protein concentration (50,63,64).

Diagnosis of SBP

Ascitic fluid culture and **assessment of the neutrophil count** must both be performed in order to facilitate the diagnosis of SBP, including its culture-negative and non-neutrocytic variants. Gram's stain of ascitic fluid is usually negative, as the concentration of infecting bacteria is generally of the order of only one colony forming unit/ml, or less. The SAAG has no value in identifying patients with SBP. This gradient remains greater than 11 g/litre in patients with underlying portal hypertension-related ascites and less than 11 g/litre in those with SBP complicating ascites of another aetiology.

An ascitic fluid neutrophil count of at least 250 μl is the single most reliable test for SBP, with a sensitivity of 87%. Other causes of neutrocytic ascites (as listed in Table 19.2) must be excluded but, because of the relative frequencies with which these occur in cirrhotic patients, the specificity and diagnostic accuracy of an increased ascitic neutrophil count for SBP are about 95% and 93%, respectively, in this setting (65). In contrast, the sensitivity of traditional ascitic fluid culture techniques is only 33%. This is improved to 73% by the bedside inoculation of ascitic fluid into blood-culture bottles (66). The timing of inoculation of ascitic fluid into these bottles is important, as a 4-h delay results in a 25% reduction in sensitivity (67). Bedside inoculation of ascitic fluid into an automated colorimetric microbial detection system has similar sensitivity, but provides an earlier microbiological diagnosis of SBP than is obtained with the use of conventional blood-culture bottles (mean 13 h, compared with 43 h) (66). As neither the ascitic fluid neutrophil count nor ascitic culture have 100% sensitivity for SBP, even in combination, it is appropriate to make a clinical diagnosis of this disorder in patients with a typical clinical picture, even when these tests are negative, provided that other sources of infection are excluded.

Secondary bacterial peritonitis as a result of perforation of the gut or an intra-abdominal abscess must be considered in any patient with neutrocytic ascites and a polymicrobial ascitic culture. The ascitic glucose concentration is usually reduced in this circumstance. Gram's stain may be positive for multiple organisms, especially in the case of secondary bacterial peritonitis related to gut perforation. A polymicrobial culture in association with a neutrophil count less than 250 μl (polymicrobial bacterascites) suggests needle perforation of the gut during diagnostic or therapeutic paracentesis.

Management of SBP

Empirical antibiotic treatment should be commenced immediately after diagnostic paracentesis in patients in whom SBP is clinically suspected, or after the demonstration of neutrocytic ascites in other patients. It is inappropriate to wait for the result of ascitic culture in view, not only of the suboptimal sensitivity of this test, but also of the risk of rapid clinical deterioration. The antibiotic of choice is generally the third-generation cephalosporin, cefotaxime, which has adequate penetration into ascitic fluid and offers good cover against the bacteria most often responsible for SBP, and low toxicity. Treatment with 2 g intravenously every 8–12 h is as effective as 6-hourly dosing (62), and treatment for 5 days is as effective as a 10-day course (68). Findings of a recent randomized study suggested that oral ofloxacin (400 mg every 12 h) may be as effective as intravenous cefotaxime in patients with uncomplicated SBP (69). The appropriateness of the chosen antibiotic regimen may be reviewed when the result of ascitic fluid culture and sensitivity eventually become available. **Granulocyte-macrophage colony stimulating factor** has been shown *in vitro* to reverse defects in neutrophil phagocytosis and chemotaxis in cirrhotic patients (70), and may have a role in the management of SBP in selected patients, such as those with severe infection and an incomplete initial response to antibiotics, although this remains to be assessed adequately *in vivo*.

Complicating **hepatic encephalopathy** should be managed along conventional lines, with lactulose usually considered to be the first-line treatment. Hypokalaemic alkalosis related to the use of frusemide must be corrected. Renal support may be required in those with associated hepatorenal syndrome. Survivors of an episode of SBP should be evaluated for OLT, in view of the high risk of recurrence and poor overall prognosis.

Prophylaxis

Antibiotic prophylaxis for SBP is of proven benefit in three high-risk groups with cirrhosis:

- Short-term prophylaxis
  - those presenting with gastrointestinal haemorrhage
- Long-term prophylaxis
  - survivors of previous episodes of SBP
  - those with ascitic total protein concentration ≤ 10 g/litre

Most studies have aimed to reduce or eradicate aerobic Gram-negative bacilli from the intestine using norfloxacin, a poorly absorbed quinolone highly active against these flora. A double-blind, placebo-controlled trial evaluating the long-term efficacy of norfloxacin (400 mg daily) in 80 patients with cirrhosis who had **survived a previous episode of SBP** found a significantly reduced rate of SBP recurrence in the treated group (12% compared with 35%) during a mean follow-up period of 6 months (71). The overall probability of SBP recurrence at 1 year of follow-up was 20% in the group receiving norfloxacin prophylaxis and 68% in the placebo group.

The efficacy of both short- and long-term primary prophylaxis with norfloxacin has been assessed in cirrhotic patients with **low ascitic fluid protein concentrations**. A randomized, controlled study in those with an ascitic fluid total protein concentration no greater than 10 g/litre found that prophylactic norfloxacin (400 mg/day) during periods of the patients' admission to hospital was associated with a significantly reduced incidence of SBP during the hospital stay (0% compared with 23%) (72). Current data suggest that long-term primary prophylaxis with norfloxacin may be preferable to prophylaxis only during periods of admission to hospital in this group. In 109 cirrhotic patients with ascitic fluid total protein concentrations no greater than 10 g/litre, or serum bilirubin concentrations greater than 2.5 mg/dl, the prevalence of SBP after a mean 43 weeks of follow-up was significantly lower (2%) in those assigned randomly to receive continuous prophylaxis (both as inpatients and as outpatients) than in those receiving prophylaxis only during their stay in hospital (17%) (73).

Short-term prophylaxis with norfloxacin is indicated in patients with **cirrhosis presenting with gastrointestinal haemorrhage**. Treatment with 400 mg twice daily, either orally or via a nasogastric tube, for 7 days commencing immediately after emergency endoscopy was associated with a significantly reduced in-hospital incidence of bacteraemia or SBP, especially with aerobic Gram-negative flora, compared with that in patients receiving no prophylactic antibiotics (3% compared with 17%) (74). Prophylaxis is not required for elective sclerotherapy or variceal ligation, as it is gastrointestinal haemorrhage, rather than therapeutic endoscopy, that predisposes patients with cirrhotic ascites to SBP.

Most episodes of SBP recurrence in patients receiving prophylactic norfloxacin are caused by Gram-positive bacteria rather than resistant Gram-negative bacterial species. Indeed, most evidence suggests that the development of bacterial resistance to quinolones during the period of exposure to norfloxacin is uncommon. Similarly, the incidence of side effects is low. Most studies report a reduction in overall mortality associated with prophylactic norfloxacin treatment, although a statistically significant survival benefit has yet to be demonstrated. This is not surprising, as the likelihood of the patient dying as a result of progressive liver failure, variceal haemorrhage, hepatocellular carcinoma, or other causes is unaffected by the use of prophylactic antibiotics. Nonetheless, several cost analysis studies have shown that prophylactic treatment with norfloxacin in each of these high-risk groups is cost effective, as a consequence of the reduced incidence of SBP and its associated utilization of resources (74–76).

The efficacy of alternative antibiotic regimens for SBP prophylaxis has been assessed in several studies. A weekly dose of 750 mg of ciprofloxacin for the prevention of primary or recurrent SBP in 28 cirrhotic patients with ascitic fluid protein concentrations less than 15 g/litre was associated with a significantly reduced incidence of SBP at 6 months compared with that in patients who received placebo (4% compared with 22%) (77). There were no instances of acquired resistance to ciprofloxacin or other side effects reported over this time. Similarly, in a study in which the presence of cirrhotic ascites was the sole entry criterion, use of trimethoprim–sulphamethoxazole for 5 days per week was associated with a significantly greater reduction in the incidence of bacteraemia or SBP during a median follow-up of 3 months than occurred in non-treated patients (3% compared with 27%) (78). No adverse effects were reported. As with norfloxacin, prophylaxis with trimethoprim–sulphamethoxazole is cost effective in patients with cirrhotic ascites, especially those at high risk for SBP (76). However, as both ciprofloxacin and trimethoprim–sulphamethoxazole demonstrate a broader spectrum of antibacterial activity and are better absorbed than norfloxacin, the risk of development of bacterial resistance and systemic side effects when these agents are used for longer periods will need to be assessed.

References
*Of interest; **of exceptional interest
1. Witte MH, Witte CL, Dumont AE. Progress in liver disease: physiological factors involved in the causation of cirrhotic ascites. *Gastroenterology* 1971; **61**: 742–750.
2. *Levy M. Sodium retention and ascites formation in dogs with experimental portal cirrhosis. *Am J Physiol* 1977; **233**: F572–585.
3. *Jimenez W, Martinez-Pardo A, Arroyo V *et al.* Temporal relationship between hyperaldosteronism, sodium retention and ascites formation in rats with experimental cirrhosis. *Hepatology* 1985; **5**: 245–250.
4. *Schrier RW, Arroyo V, Bernardi M *et al.* Peripheral arterial vasodilation hypothesis: a proposal for the initiation of renal sodium and water retention in cirrhosis. *Hepatology* 1988; **8**: 1151–1157.
    References 2 to 4 report the important observation that renal sodium and water retention precedes the onset of ascites, leading to the arterial vasodilatation theory for the pathogenesis of cirrhotic ascites.
5. Denie C, Vachiery F, Elman A *et al.* Systemic and splanchnic hemodynamic changes in patients with hepatic schistosomiasis. *Liver* 1996; **16**: 309–312.
6. Sogni P, Garnier P, Gadano A, *et al.* Endogenous pulmonary nitric oxide production measured from exhaled air is increased in patients with severe cirrhosis. *J Hepatol* 1995; **23**: 471–473.
7. Campillo B, Chabrier PE, Pelle G, *et al.* Inhibition of nitric oxide synthesis in the forearm arterial bed of patients with advanced cirrhosis. *Hepatology* 1995; **22**: 1423–1429.

8. Martin PY, Gines P, Schrier RW. Nitric oxide as a mediator of hemodynamic abnormalities and sodium and water retention in cirrhosis. *N Engl J Med* 1998; 339: 533–541.

9. *Bories PN, Campillo B, Azaou L *et al*. Long–lasting NO overproduction in patients with spontaneous bacterial peritonitis. *Hepatology* 1997; **25**: 1328–1333.
    An important study potentially explaining the interactions between spontaneous bacterial peritonitis, exacerbation of ascites, and renal impairment in cirrhotic patients.

10. *Runyon BA, Montano AA, Akriviadis EA *et al*. The serum-ascites albumin gradient in the differential diagnosis of ascites is superior to the exudate/transudate concept. *Ann Intern Med* 1992; **117**: 215–220.
    Demonstrates the efficacy of a simple test for assessing the cause of ascites

11. Hoefs JC. Increase in ascites white blood cell and protein concentrations during diuresis in patients with chronic liver disease. *Hepatology* 1981; **1**: 249–254.

12. Gauthier A, Levy VG, Quinton A *et al*. Salt or no salt in the treatment of cirrhotic acites: a randomised study. *Gut* 1986; **27**: 705–709.

13. Bichet D, Szatalowicz V, Chaimovitz C *et al*. Role of vasopressin in abnormal water excretion in cirrhotic patients. *Ann Intern Med* 1982; **96**: 413–417.

14. Perez-Ayuso RM, Arroyo V, Planas R *et al*. Randomized comparative study of efficacy of furosemide versus spironolactone in nonazotemic cirrhosis with ascites. *Gastroenterology* 1983; **84**: 961–968.

15. Sungaila I, Bartle WR, Walker SE *et al*. Spironolactone pharmacokinetics and pharmacodynamics in patients with cirrhotic ascites. *Gastroenterology* 1992; **102**: 1680–1685.

16. Fogel MR, Sawhney VK, Neal EA *et al*. Diuresis in the ascitic patient: a randomized controlled trial of three regimens. *J Clin Gastroenterol* 1981; **3(Suppl 1)**: 73–80.

17. Bataller R, Arroyo V, Gines P. Management of ascites in cirrhosis. *J Gastroenterol Hepatol* 1997; **12**: 723–733.

18. Planas R, Arroyo V, Rimola A *et al*. Acetylsalicylic acid suppresses the renal hemodynamic effect and reduces the diuretic action of furosemide in cirrhosis with ascites. *Gastroenterology* 1983; **84**: 247–252.

19. Gadano A, Moreau R, Vachieri F *et al*. *J Hepatol* 1997; **26**: 1229–1234.

20. Hadengue A, Gadano A, Moreau R, *et al*. Beneficial effects of the 2-day administration of terlipressin in patients with cirrhosis and hepatorenal syndrome. *J Hepatol* 1998; **29**: 565–570.

21. Le Moine O, el Nawar A, Jagodzinski R, *et al*. Treatment with terlipressin as a bridge to liver transplantation in a patient with hepatorenal syndrome. *Acta Gastroenterologica Belgica* 1998; **61**: 268–270.

22. Guevara M, Gines P, Fernandez-Esparrach G, *et al*. Reversibility of hepatorenal syndrome by prolonged administration of ornipressin and plasma volume expansion. *Hepatology* 1998; **1**: 35–41.

23. Arroyo V, Jimenez W. Complications of cirrhosis. II. Renal and circulatory dysfunction. *J Hepatol* 2000; **32**(suppl 1): 157–170.

24. Angeli P, Volpin R, Gerunda G, *et al*. Reversal of type 1 hepatorenal syndrome with the administration of midrodine and octreotide. *Hepatology* 1999; **29**: 1690–1697.

25. Ljubicic N, Bilic A, Kopjar B. Diuretics vs paracentesis followed by diuretics in cirrhosis: effect on ascites opsonic activity and immunoglobulin and complement concentrations. *Hepatology* 1994; **19**: 346–352.

26. Sola R, Andreu M, Coll S *et al*. Spontaneous bacterial peritonitis in cirrhotic patients treated using paracentesis or diuretics: results of a randomized study. *Hepatology* 1995; **21**: 340–344.

27. Gines P, Arroyo V, Quintero E *et al*. Comparison of paracentesis and diuretics in the treatment of cirrhotics with tense ascites. *Gastroenterology* 1987; **93**: 234–241.

28. Gines P, Tito L, Arroyo V *et al*. Randomized study of therapeutic paracentesis with and without intravenous albumin in cirrhosis. *Gastroenterology* 1988; **94**: 1493–1502.

29. *Gines A, Fernandez-Esparrach G, Monescillo A *et al*. Randomized trial comparing albumin, dextran 70 and polygeline in cirrhotic patients with ascites treated by paracentesis. *Gastroenterology* 1996; **111**: 1002–1010.
    An important study in a large number of patients, comparing the efficacy of albumin and non-albumin plasma expanders for use with therapautic paracentesis.

30. Planas R, Gines P, Arroyo V *et al*. Dextran-70 versus albumin as plasma expanders in cirrhotic patients with tense ascites treated with total paracentesis. *Gastroenterology* 1990; **99**: 1736–1744.

31. Terg R, Miguez CD, Castro L *et al*. Pharmacokinetics of Dextran-70 in patients with cirrhosis and ascites undergoing therapeutic paracentesis. *J Hepatol* 1996; **25**: 329–333.

32. Cabrera J, Inglada L, Quintero E *et al*. Large-volume paracentesis and intravenous saline: effects on the renin-angiotensin system. *Hepatology* 1991; **14**: 1025–1028.

33. Stanley MM, Ochi S, Lee KK. Peritoneovenous shunting as compared with medical treatment in patients with alcoholic cirrhosis and massive ascites. *N Engl J Med* 1989; **321**: 1632–1638.

34. Bernhoft RA, Pellegrini CA, Way LW. Peritoneovenous shunt for refractory ascites. *Arch Surg* 1982; **117**: 631–635.

35. Fulenwider JT, Smith RB, Redd SC *et al*. Peritoneovenous shunts: lessons learned from an eight-year experience with 70 patients. *Arch Surg* 1984; **119**: 1133–1137.

36. Rossle M, Haag K, Ochs A *et al*. The transjugular intrahepatic portosystemic stent-shunt procedure for variceal bleeding. *N Engl J Med* 1994; **330**: 165–171.

37. Lind CD, Malisch TW, Chong WK *et al*. Incidence of shunt occlusion or stenosis following transjugular intrahepatic portosystemic shunt placement. *Gastroenterology* 1994; **106**: 1277–1283.

38. Guevara M, Gines P, Bandi JC, *et al*. Transjugular intrahepatic portosystemic shunt in hepatorenal syndrome. *Hepatology* 1998; **27**: 35–41.

39. Lebrec D, Giuily N, Habengue A *et al*. Transjugular intrahepatic portosystemic shunts: comparison with paracentesis in patients with cirrhosis and refractory ascites. *J Hepatol* 1996; **25**: 135–144.

40. Arroyo V, Bosch J, Gaya-Beltran J *et al*. Plasma renin activity and urinary sodium excretion as prognostic indicators in non-aztoemic cirrhosis and ascites. *Ann Intern Med* 1981; **94**: 198–210.

41. Bories P, Garcia-Compean D, Michel H *et al*. The treatment of refractory ascites by the LeVeen shunt: a multi-center controlled trial (57 patients). *J Hepatol* 1986; **3**: 212–218.

42. Rimola A, Gavaler JS, Schade RR *et al.* Effects of renal impairment on liver transplantation. *Gastroenterology* 1987; **93**: 148–156.

43. Klein AS, Sitzmann JV, Coleman J *et al.* Current management of Budd–Chiari syndrome. *Ann Surg* 1990; **212**: 144–149.

44. McCarthy PM, van Heerden JA, Adson MA *et al.* The Budd-Chiari Syndrome. *Arch Surg* 1985; **120**: 657–662.

45. Shaked A, Goldstein RM, Klintmalm GB. Portosystemic shunt versus orthotopic liver transplantation for the Budd–Chiari syndrome. *Surg Gynecol Obstet* 1992; **174**: 453–459.

46. Halff G, Todo S, Tzakis AG *et al.* Liver transplantation for the Budd–Chiari syndrome. *Ann Surg* 1990; **211**: 43–49.

47. Hagglund H, Ringden O, Ericzon BG *et al.* Treatment of hepatic venoocclusive disease with recombinant human tissue plasminogen activator or orthotopic liver transplantation after allogeneic bone marrow transplantation. *Transplantation* 1996; **62**: 1076–1080.

48. Shen-Gunther J, Walker JL, Johnson GA *et al.* Hepatic venoocclusive disease as a complication of whole abdominopelvic irradiation and treatment with the transjugular intrahepatic portosystemic shunt: case report and literature review. *Gynecol Oncol* 1996; **61**: 282–286.

49. Hoefs JC, Canawatti HN, Sapico FL *et al.* Spontaneous bacterial peritonitis. *Hepatology* 1982; **2**: 399–407.

50. Andreu M, Sola R, Sitges-Serra A *et al.* Risk factors for spontaneous bacterial peritonitis in cirrhotic patients with ascites. *Gastroenterology* 1993; **104**: 1133–1138.

51. Morencos FC, de las Heras-Castano G, Martin-Ramos L *et al.* Small bowel bacterial overgrowth in patients with alcoholic cirrhosis. *Dig Dis Sci* 1995; **40**: 1252–1256.

52. Bleichner G, Boulanger R, Squara P *et al.* Frequency of infections in cirrhotic patients presenting with acute gastrointestinal haemorrhage. *Br J Surg* 1986; **73**: 724–726.

53. Bolognesi M, Merkel C, Bianco S *et al.* Clinical significance of the evaluation of hepatic reticuloendothelial removal capacity in patients with cirrhosis. *Hepatology* 1994; **19**: 628–634.

54. Runyon BA. Low-protein-concentration ascitic fluid is predisposed to spontaneous bacterial peritonitis. *Gastroenterology* 1986; **91**: 1343–1346.

55. Llach J, Rimola A, Navasa M *et al.* Incidence and predictive factors of first episode of spontaneous bacterial peritonitis in cirrhosis with ascites: relevance of ascitic fluid protein concentration. *Hepatology* 1992; **16**: 724–727.

56. Llovet JM, Planas R, Morillas R *et al.* Short-term prognosis of cirrhotic patients with spontaneous bacterial peritonitis: multivariate study. *Am J Gastroenterol* 1993; **88**: 388–392.

57. Toledo C, Salmeron JM, Rimola A *et al.* Spontaneous bacterial peritonitis in cirrhosis: predictive factors of infection resolution and survival in patients treated with cefotaxime. *Hepatology* 1993; **17**: 251–257.

58. Follo A, Llovet JM, Navasa M *et al.* Renal impairment following spontaneous bacterial peritonitis in cirrhosis: incidence, clinical course, predictive factors and prognosis. *Hepatology* 1994; **20**: 1495–1501.

59. Bataller R, Gines P, Guevara M *et al.* Hepatorenal syndrome. *Semin Liv Dis* 1997; **17**: 233–247.

60. Propst T, Propst A, Herold M *et al.* Spontaneous bacterial peritonitis is associated with high levels of interleukin-6 and its secondary mediators in ascitic fluid. *Eur J Clin Invest* 1993; **23**: 832–836.

61. Soriano G, Coll P, Guarner C *et al.* Escherichia coli capsular polysaccharide and spontaneous bacterial peritonitis in cirrhosis. *Hepatology* 1995; **21**: 668–673.

62. Runyon BA, McHutchison JG, Antillon MR *et al.* Short-course versus long-course antibiotic treatment of spontaneous bacterial peritonitis: a randomized controlled study of 100 patients. *Gastroenterology* 1991; **100**: 1737–1742.

63. Tito L, Rimola A, Gines P *et al.* Recurrence of spontaneous bacterial peritonitis in cirrhosis: frequency and predictive factors. *Hepatology* 1988; **8**: 27–31.

64. McHutchison JG, Runyon BA. Spontaneous bacterial peritonitis. In: *Gastrointestinal and Hepatic Infections*. Eds C Surawicz, CS Owen. Philadeplhia: WB Saunders Co, 1995; pp. 455–475.

65. *Reynolds TB. Rapid presumptive diagnosis of spontaneous bacterial peritonitis. *Gastroenterology* 1986; **90**: 1294–1297.

66. *Ortiz J, Soriano G, Coll P *et al.* Early microbiologic diagnosis of spontaneous bacterial peritonitis with BacT/ ALERT. *J Hepatol* 1997; **26**: 839–844.

67. *Runyon BA, Antillon MR, Akriviadis EA, McHutchison JG. Bedside inoculation of blood culture bottles with ascitic fluid is superior to delayed inoculation in the detection of spontaneous bacterial peritonitis. *J Clin Microbiol* 1990; **28**: 2811–2812.

References 56–58 demonstrate that the ascitic neutrophil count is the most sensitive marker of spontaneous bacterial peritonitis, and discuss issues relevant to establishing a microbiological diagnosis.

68. Rimola A, Salmeron JM, Clemente G *et al.* Two different dosages of cefotaxime in the treatment of spontaneous bacterial peritonitis in cirrhosis: results of a prospective, randomized, multicenter study. *Hepatology* 1995; **21**: 674–679.

69. Navasa M, Planas R, Clemente G *et al.* Randomized, comparative study of oral ofloxacin versus intravenous cefotaxime in spontaneous bacterial peritonitis. *Gastroenterology* 1996; **111**: 1011–1017.

70. Garcia-Gonzalez M, Boixeda D, Herrero D *et al.* Effect of granulocyte-macrophage colony-stimulating factor on leukocyte function in cirrhosis. *Gastroenterology* 1993; **105**: 527–531.

71. Gines P, Rimola A, Planas R *et al.* Norfloxacin prevents spontaneous bacterial peritonitis recurrence in cirrhosis: results of a double-blind, placebo-controlled trial. *Hepatology* 1990; **12**: 716–724.

72. Soriano G, Guarner C, Teixido M *et al.* Selective intestinal decontamination prevents spontaneous bacterial peritonitis. *Gastroenterology* 1991; **100**: 477–481.

73. Novella MT, Sola R, Soriano A *et al.* Continuous versus inpatient prophylaxis of the first episode of spontaneous bacterial peritonitis with norfloxacin. *Hepatology* 1997; **25**: 532–536.

74. Soriano G, Guarner C, Tomas A *et al.* Norfloxacin prevents bacterial infection in cirrhotics with gastrointestinal haemorrhage. *Gastroenterology* 1992; **103**: 1267–1272.

75. Younossi ZM, McHutchison JG, Ganiats TG. An economic analysis of norfloxacin prophylaxis against spontaneous bacterial peritonitis. *J Hepatol* 1997; **27**: 295–298.

76. Idanomi J, Sonnenberg A. Cost-analysis of prophylactic antibiotics in spontaneous bacterial peritonitis. *Gastroenterology* 1997; **113**: 1289–1294.

77. Rolachon A, Cordier L, Bacq Y *et al.* Ciprofloxacin and long-term prevention of spontaneous bacterial peritonitis: results of a prospective controlled trial. *Hepatology* 1995; **22**: 1171–1174.

78. Singh N, Gayowski T, Yu VL *et al.* Trimethoprim-sulfamethoxazole for the prevention of spontaneous bacterial peritonitis in cirrhosis: a randomized trial. *Ann Intern Med* 1995; **122**: 595–598.

20. Intestinal Failure and Enterocutaneous Fistulae

JEREMY NIGHTINGALE

INTRODUCTION

Intestinal failure occurs when there is reduced intestinal absorption so that macronutrient or fluid supplements, or both, are needed to maintain health. Macronutrient (carbohydrate, fat, or protein) supplements may be given by the oral, enteral, or parenteral route. The term "fluid supplements" implies water and sodium chloride supplements.

Intestinal failure can be acute or chronic. **Acute intestinal failure** is reversible and may have either medical (e.g. chemotherapy) or surgical (fistula, ileus, or obstruction) causes. **Chronic intestinal failure** most commonly arises after an intestinal resection leaves behind a short length of small bowel. Occasionally, chronic intestinal failure results from gut dysmotility (e.g. scleroderma, visceral myopathy, or neuropathy), or inflammation (e.g. extensive small-bowel Crohn's disease or long-term irradiation damage), or from the gut being bypassed, as in the surgical treatment of obesity.

The first part of this chapter will discuss the management of patients with a short bowel; the second part considers the management of enterocutaneous fistulae.

PROBLEMS AND MANAGEMENT OF A SHORT BOWEL

Normal human small intestinal length, measured from the duodenojejunal flexure at post-mortem examination or during surgery, varies in the range 275–850 cm and tends to be shorter in women.

After an intestinal resection, it is much more important to refer to the remaining length of small intestine, rather than the amount removed: a resection of 200 cm will cause few problems to a patient with a starting length of 850 cm, but will cause serious problems if the starting length is 275 cm.

Two groups of patients with a short bowel are commonly encountered in clinical practice (Figure 20.1): those who have had a jejunoileal resection and a colectomy and thus have a jejunostomy; and those who have had a jejunoileal resection leaving a jejuno–colic anastomosis. Occasionally the ileocaecal valve is preserved, however this is not of proven benefit in adults. The causes leading to the two surgical groups are summarized in Table 20.1, and the problems in Table 20.2. Both groups of patient have had

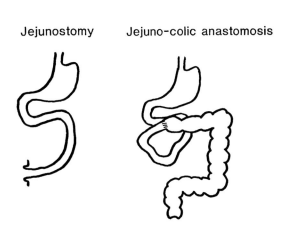

Figure 20.1. The two common types of short bowel in patients who have undergone intestinal resection.

Table 20.1. Causes of a short bowel.

	Jejunostomy	Jejunum–colon*
Number/Sex	15M/31F	12M/26F*
Age (years) (mean and range)	42 (16–68)	46 (7–70)
Cause		
Crohn's disease	33	16
Ischaemia	2	6
Irradiation	3	5
Ulcerative colitis	5	—
Volvulus	—	5
Other	3	6

Data from Nightingale *et al.* (1).
*All had jejuno–colic anastomosis, except seven, in whom the ileocaecal valve was preserved.

Table 20.2. Problems of a short bowel.

	Jejunostomy	Jejunum–colon
Water, sodium, and magnesium depletion	Common	Uncommon
Nutrient malabsorption	Common	Common*
Renal stones	None	25%
Gallstones	45%	45%
Adaptation	No evidence	Gut transit may slow
Social	Large stomal losses, dependant on treatment†	Steatorrhoea

*Bacterial fermentation of carbohydrate salvages some energy, but D(−)-lactic acidosis can occur if the diet is high in mono- and oligosaccharides.
†If a patient with a jejunostomy stops treatment for 1 day, they are likely to become dehydrated.

more than 60 cm terminal ileum removed, so need regular vitamin B_{12} injections. Both groups have a high prevalence of gallstones (45%), which may have resulted from periods of biliary stasis. Fluid and nutritional problems differ in each type of patient (1).

Jejunostomy patients

Patients with a jejunostomy have problems immediately after surgery, with a high volume of stomal output (2–8 litre/24 h) that is greatest after food or drink is consumed, and causes major problems from water, sodium, and magnesium losses (2). There are problems with nutrient absorption, but the consequences of undernutrition are less immediate.

The high volume of stomal output is mainly the result of loss of the normal daily intestinal secretions of about 4 litre (0.5 litre saliva, 2 litre gastric acid, 1.5 litre pancreaticobiliary secretions), which have been added to the 2 litre of food and drink consumed each day. Normally, most of this fluid is reabsorbed in the upper jejunum. If the jejunal length is very short, there is also rapid emptying of liquid from the stomach into the small bowel; this is probably due to loss of the distal ileal and colonic L cells which, on contact with unabsorbed nutrients, would normally release the hormone, peptide YY (3). Peptide YY reduces gastric and pancreatic secretions and slows gastrointestinal transit.

The sodium concentration at the duodenojejunal flexure is about 90 mmol/litre and this gradually increases to about 140 mmol/litre in the terminal ileum. Jejunal mucosa, in contrast to ileal mucosa, is very permeable to water, sodium, and chloride. The absorption of sodium can occur only against a small concentration gradient, and is coupled to the absorption of glucose and some amino acids.

Treatment of a high volume of output from a jejunostomy

The principles of treatment for a high-volume output from a jejunostomy are essentially the same as for a patient with "ileostomy diarrhoea" or a high small-bowel entero–cutaneous fistula:

- Reduce oral hypotonic fluids
- Give glucose/saline solution to sip (sodium concentration at least 90 mmol/litre)
- Give drugs to reduce
  - motility: loperamide or codeine phosphate
  - secretions: proton pump inhibitors, H_2-antagonists or octreotide

Problems of dehydration are likely when the stomal output exceeds 2 litre/24 h. The output may be increased by abdominal sepsis, partial gut obstruction, or recurrent disease.

Treatment strategies for patients with a high volume of output from their jejunostomy include:

1. *Oral intake of hypotonic fluid*: This should be reduced to less than 500 ml/24 h. If oral tea, coffee, orange juice — which all contain little sodium — or, indeed, any solution with a sodium

concentration of less than 90 mmol/litre are given, there is a net secretion of sodium into the lumen and this is then lost through the stoma.

2. *Glucose–saline solution*: A solution with a sodium concentration of 90–120 mmol/litre is sipped or given enterally. As there is coupled absorption of sodium with glucose in the jejunum, glucose and sodium are given together. Most commonly, the World Health Organization (WHO) cholera solution (sodium 90 mmol/litre) without the potassium chloride is given (sodium chloride 3.5 g, sodium bicarbonate 2.5 mg, and glucose 20 g in 1 litre of tap water). This sodium concentration is much greater than that given in the commonly used oral rehydration solutions for diarrhoea.

3. *An antidiarrhoeal drug*: May be given 30 min before food, to slow gut transit. Loperamide 2–8 mg is preferred to codeine phosphate, as it does not cause drowsiness and is not addictive. Loperamide, however, does circulate in the enterohepatic circulation, and as this is disrupted in patients with a short bowel, high doses may be needed. Occasionally, there is an additional benefit if codeine phosphate 30–60 mg is given in addition to loperamide.

4. *Antisecretory drugs*: These may reduce the volume of output if it is greater than that of the food and drink consumed; this occurs if the jejunal length is less than 100 cm. An oral proton pump inhibitor (e.g. omeprazole 40 mg daily) (4), high-dose H_2-antagonists (e.g. ranitidine 300 mg before breakfast and supper), or — if there is insufficient bowel to absorb these (less than about 50 cm of jejunum) — octreotide 50 µg may be given before breakfast and supper (5).

5. *Oral magnesium*: Most patients with a jejunostomy become magnesium depleted, which may cause fatigue, depression, irritability, muscle weakness and, if very severe, convulsions. Treatment is with oral magnesium (usually three magnesium oxide 4 mmol capsules at night), subcutaneous, intramuscular or intravenous magnesium and, sometimes, vitamin D, which may increase magnesium absorption from the gut.

6. *Potassium*: Problems associated with potassium are unusual, and net loss through the stoma occurs only when less than 50 cm of jejunum remains. A low serum potassium concentration is most commonly the result of sodium depletion with secondary hyperaldosteronism, and thus greater than normal urinary losses of potassium, or occasionally it is caused by magnesium depletion.

7. *Nutritional treatment*: If less than 75 cm of jejunum remains, long-term parenteral nutrition is likely to be needed; if 75–200 cm remain, oral or enteral nutrient supplements may be required (1,2). A patient maintained on an oral diet may need to consume twice as much energy as a person with a normally functioning gut. This may be achieved with a nocturnal nasogastric or gastrostomy feed, which must contain additional salt and be relatively iso-osmolar. If an elemental diet that is hyperosmolar and low in sodium is given, it can cause a net secretion of water and sodium, which are then lost through the stoma. Thus a diet of polypeptides, polysaccharides, and triglycerides with added salt is most appropriate.

Adaptation

Patients with an ileostomy experience a reduction in stomal output with time, because the ileal mucosa increases its absorption, partly by the villi becoming longer, the crypts deeper, and the gastrointestinal transit rate slower. There is no evidence for such structural or functional jejunal adaptation occurring in patients with a jejunostomy: the stomal output of water, sodium, and nutrients does not decrease with time.

Jejunum–colon patients

These patients are often well after their resection, except for unpleasant diarrhoea/steatorrhoea, but in the succeeding months they may lose weight and become severely undernourished. If the length of jejunum is less than 50 cm, long-term parenteral nutrition is needed in most of these patients (1). With a length of more than 100 cm, the patient can be expected eventually to maintain their weight on a normal diet with no supplements. As the colon has a large capacity to absorb sodium and water, these patients rarely become dehydrated, and fewer than 50% require magnesium supplements.

Nutritional treatment

Because of malabsorption, the oral diet of patients with a jejunum–colon must contain more energy than that of people with a normal gut. A diet high in **polysaccharides** is recommended, as these are fermented in the colon to produce short-chain fatty acids, which are absorbed and provide a source of energy (6). Such a diet, in additional to being very bulky, can (especially if rich in mono- and oligosaccharides), rarely, cause D(–)-**lactic acidosis**. Lactic acid produced by man is the L(+) isomer, but abnormal bacterial colonization of the colon can result in a metabolic acidosis through formation and absorption of the D(–) isomer, which can not be metabolized. D(–)-lactic acidosis can cause a syndrome of ataxia, blurred vision, ophthalmoplegia, and nystagmus. It is suspected if a patient has a metabolic acidosis with a large anion gap. It is treated with broad-spectrum antibiotics (neomycin or vancomycin), thiamine, and changing the diet to one low in mono- and oligosaccharides and high in polysaccharides.

Unabsorbed free fatty acids in the colon are not beneficial. They reduce water and sodium absorption, increase the colonic transit rate, are toxic to bacteria (so reducing the amount of carbohydrate fermented), and bind to calcium and magnesium, so increasing stool losses. A **low-fat diet** is theoretically ideal and will reduce malodorous steatorrhoea; however, fat does yield twice as much energy as comparable weights of carbohydrate and it makes food palatable, thus it can not be excessively restricted. **Medium-chain triglycerides** can be absorbed in the colon and are an alternative source of energy. Diarrhoea may be treated in the same way as for patients with a jejunostomy, with loperamide and, occasionally, codeine phosphate.

Calcium oxalate renal stones occur in 25% of patients with a retained colon. This is the result of an increased absorption of dietary oxalate by the colon, leading to increased oxalate excretion in the urine, where it may precipitate. The increased colonic absorption of oxalate occurs partly because free fatty acids, which normally bind and thus keep oxalate insoluble, preferentially bind to calcium, thus allowing the oxalate to be soluble, and hence absorbed. Unabsorbed bile salts within the colon also directly increase colonic permeability to oxalate. All patients with a short bowel and retained colon are given advice on a low-oxalate diet (avoid rhubarb, spinach, beetroot, peanuts, and excessive amounts of tea), which should prevent the stones forming. Other preventive measures may include reducing the lipid content of the diet, and giving oral calcium supplements, a calcium-containing organic marine hydrocolloid, or cholestyramine (which binds bile salts).

Adaptation

There is no good evidence in man for structural adaptation in the remaining jejunum when the colon has been retained; however, there is some evidence for functional adaptation with time probably as gut transit time increases (7). The diarrhoea in patients with a jejuno–colic anastomosis does reduce with time.

Medical treatments and intestinal transplantation

Medical treatments have been directed at trying to increase mucosal growth; however, treatment with growth hormone, glutamine, and fibre has not been universally successful.

Small-bowel transplantation has been performed mainly in children, and is becoming a more successful operation. Relatively few patients are suitable for this procedure, and, even when tacrolimus is used for immunosuppression, only 40–47% of patients will be alive 3 years after the transplant, and 29–38% will have a functioning graft. Of those who survive with the transplant, 78% are able to cease receiving parenteral nutrition (8). These figures are not as good as those for survival on long-term parenteral nutrition for non-neoplastic reasons: 70% of these patients will be alive 3 years after starting the nutrition and most will have a relatively good quality of life (9).

ENTEROCUTANEOUS FISTULAE

A fistula is an abnormal communication between two epithelialized surfaces. If a fistula communicates with a hollow viscus (e.g. a colo–vesical fistula), it is termed an "internal fistula"; if it communicates onto the skin, it is "external". A fistula can be single or complicated. Fistulae can occur between many different viscera; however, this chapter will consider only the management of enterocutaneous fistulae from the small bowel.

Aetiology

Enterocutaneous fistulae most commonly arise as a postoperative complication from either partial breakdown of an intestinal anastomosis or injury to the gut during abdominal closure (82%). Other causes include Crohn's disease (6%), neoplasia (4%), iatrogenic (3%), and irradiation damage (1%) (10). One form of enterocutaneous fistula that does not occur postoperatively is commonly from bowel proximal to an obstruction. This is more likely if the proximal bowel is diseased. An abscess develops first, then discharges its contents through the skin. If the distal obstruction persists, the fistula will not close spontaneously or, if it does so temporarily, an intra-abdominal abscess will result.

Death from enterocutaneous fistulae is most commonly as a result of sepsis, although some deaths result from electrolyte imbalance, undernutrition, massive bleeding, or the underlying disease. Spontaneous closure of a fistula may occur within 6 weeks of its first appearance, in up to 60% of patients. **Factors that are associated with spontaneous closure of an enterocutaneous fistula include**:

- no bowel obstruction distal to the fistula
- no diseased bowel at the fistula site (e.g. Crohn's, irradiation or malignancy)
- no mucocutaneous continuity (i.e. no visible bowel mucosa)
- no abscess/sepsis adjacent to the fistula
- single rather than multiple fistulae
- no discontinuity of bowel (i.e. bowel not completely detached)
- jejunum rather than ileum
- well nourished patient
- normal serum transferrin and albumin concentrations
- no other systemic problems (e.g. cardiac, respiratory, renal, or hepatic failure)

Management of enterocutaneous fistulae

1. *Treat sepsis*: As sepsis is the most common cause of death, and as patients can not benefit from nutritional support until sepsis has been treated, the initial management of an enterocutaneous fistula is to treat sepsis. This usually involves detecting an abscess with ultrasound, computed tomography, or magnetic resonance imaging scanning, and subsequently draining it. Occasionally, a laparotomy is required, to drain an abscess or to create a defunctioning stoma proximal to a fistula. An abscess cavity may need to be regularly irri-

gated. Broad-spectrum antibiotics, which usually include metronidazole, are given.

2. *Reduce fistula output*: If the fistula has a high output (more than 500 ml/24 h) then fluid balance becomes important, and it may be helpful to measure the fistula fluid electrolyte content. In general, the management of a high-output fistula is the same as the management of a high-output jejunostomy (see above). This involves restricting oral hypotonic fluids, replacing sodium and water — often with a glucose–saline drink (e.g. the WHO electrolyte solution) — and, giving magnesium and zinc as indicated by plasma concentrations. Drugs either reduce intestinal motility (loperamide or codeine phosphate), or reduce secretions. Gastric acid antisecretory drugs will reduce fistula output, but they have not become as popular as somatostatin or octreotide in treating fistulae. Somatostatin and octreotide both reduce the volume of fistula output by reducing salivary, gastric, and pancreaticobiliary secretions and slowing intestinal transit. They also appear to accelerate the rate of spontaneous closure of a fistula (11). **Immunosuppressive drugs** such as azathioprine and cyclosporin have been reported to heal some fistulae associated with Crohn's disease. Subcutaneous heparin or low-molecular-weight heparin are given when the patient is relatively immobile, to prevent venous thrombosis.

3. *Care of fistula site*: Coupled with managing the output is caring for the skin around the fistula. The more proximal the location of a fistula in the gut, the more likely is its output to damage the skin, as pancreatic enzymes are very corrosive. The two important skin-protective preparations are karaya gum (derived from a tree related to the cocoa tree), made into a paste with glycerine, and compressed, thin (1.3 mm thick) squares made of gelatin, pectin, sodium carboxymethylcellulose, and polyisobutylene (Stomahesive). The paste can be used to fill defects, and the squares cut to cover the skin surrounding a fistula or stoma (12). Stoma bags, which may need to be vented to let gas escape, may need to be connected to a drainage system. Unless undernutrition and zinc deficiency are treated, it can be difficult to get the skin into good condition.

4. *Nutritional support*: Nutritional support is given traditionally by parenteral nutrition, with no oral

intake permitted (13) (this can aptly be called "total parenteral nutrition"). However, enteral nutrition is as effective and certainly safer (14), especially for an ileal fistula. If a fistula output exceeds 2 litre daily, or if there is less than 100 cm of small bowel proximal to the fistula, parenteral support is likely to be needed.

5. *Define anatomy*: Early contrast studies are useful to see if there is distal obstruction or an intra-abdominal leak but, in general, the full anatomy is defined when the patient is free from sepsis, is in fluid balance, and is adequately nourished. This is usually visualized by a fistulogram, in which water-soluble contrast is inserted into the fistula under radiological screening. It aims to determine from which part of the gut the fistula arises, if the bowel at the fistula site is diseased, and if there is a distal obstruction. Using this information, an assessment can be made as to whether a fistula is likely to heal spontaneously or if surgery will be needed.

6. *Elective surgery*: Most uncomplicated enterocutaneous fistulae are given a period of 6 weeks to allow for spontaneous closure. If there is a complex high-output fistula, most advocate waiting for about 6 months before attempting an elective repair (15). At this time, the patient should be in a normal nutritional state, and sepsis should have resolved. The principle of definitive surgery is relatively simple and involves the removal of the fistula tract and diseased bowel, and restoration of intestinal continuity. However, in practice, the surgery can be very difficult. If there is sepsis or hypoalbuminaemia, bowel is defunctioned and the creation of a new anastomosis is avoided.

7. *Psychological support*: The management of a complex enterocutaneous fistula involves a patient being in hospital for a long time, undergoing many procedures, and needing invasive treatments. Thus these patients tend to have large mood swings, with "highs" when treatment seems to be going well and the end is in site, and "lows" when everything seems to be taking too long, with no guaranteed successful outcome. Much psychological support is therefore needed from all carers and, often, specialist psychiatric/psychological workers.

References

1. Nightingale JMD, Lennard-Jones JE, Gertner DJ *et al.* Colonic preservation reduces the need for parenteral therapy, increases the incidence of renal stones, but does not change the high prevalence of gallstones in patients with a short bowel. *Gut* 1992; **33**: 1493–1497.

2. Nightingale JMD, Lennard-Jones JE, Walker ER *et al.* Jejunal efflux in short bowel syndrome. *Lancet* 1990; **336**: 765–768.

3. Nightingale JMD, Kamm MA, van der Sijp JRM, *et al.* Gastrointestinal hormones in the short bowel syndrome. PYY may be the 'colonic brake' to gastric emptying. *Gut* 1996; **39**: 267–272.

4. Nightingale JMD, Walker ER, Farthing MJG *et al.* Effect of omeprazole on intestinal output in the short bowel syndrome. *Aliment Pharmacol Ther* 1991; **5**: 405–412.

5. Nightingale JMD, Walker ER, Burnham WR *et al.* The short bowel syndrome. *Digestion* 1990; **45 (suppl 1)**:77–83.

6. Nordgaard I, Hansen BS, Mortensen PB. Colon as a digestive organ in patients with short bowel. *Lancet* 1994; **343**: 373–376.

7. Dowling RH, Booth CC. Functional compensation after small bowel resection in man: Demonstration by direct measurement. *Lancet* 1966; **ii**: 146–147.

8. Grant D. Current results of intestinal transplantation. *Lancet* 1996; **347**: 1801–1803.

9. Messing B, Leman M, Landais P *et al.* Prognosis of patients with nonmalignant chronic intestinal failure receiving long-term home parenteral nutrition. *Gastroenterology* 1995; **108**: 1005–1010.

10. Kuvshinoff BW, Brodish RJ, McFadden DW *et al..* Serum transferrin as a prognostic indicator of spontaneous closure and mortality in gastrointestinal cutaneous fistulas. *Ann Surg* 1993; **217**: 615–623.

11. Nubiola P, Badia JM, Martinez-Rodenas F *et al.* Treatment of 27 postoperative enterocutaneous fistulas with the long half life somatostatin analogue SMS 201-995. *Ann Surg* 1989; **210** :56–58.

12. Gross E, Irving M. Protection of the skin around intestinal fistulas. *Br J Surg* 1977; **64**: 258–263.

13. MacFadyen BV, Dudrick SJ, Ruberg RL. Management of gastrointestinal fistulas with parenteral hyperalimentation. *Surgery* 1973; **74**: 100–105.

14. Levy E, Frileux P, Cugnenc PH *et al.* High-output external fistulae of the small bowel: management with continuous enteral nutrition. *Br J Surg* 1989; **76**: 676–679.

15. Conte RL, Roof L, Roslyn JJ. Delayed reconstructive surgery for complex enterocutaneous fistulae. *Am Surg* 1988; **54**: 589–593.

21. Nutritional Support

JEREMY POWELL-TUCK

INTRODUCTION

A working knowledge of therapeutic diet, in addition to an ability to diagnose and treat nutritional deficiency, whether of macro- or micronutrients, are essentials to the good practice of gastroenterology. Such care improves the quality of life of outpatients and ensures that critically ill inpatients are supported optimally, particularly if they are at risk of coming to surgery. Undernutrition is associated with malaise, weakness, and prolonged hospital stay (1,2). Although some of the relationship with duration of stay may be the result of an association of weight loss with illness severity, it is clear from randomized controlled studies (see below) that this is not sufficient explanation: many studies show the benefit on outcome of improving nutrition. This chapter concentrates on the practice of nutritional support, with an additional short section on dietary therapy in inflammatory bowel disease.

PRINCIPLES OF NUTRITIONAL ASSESSMENT

"**Subjective global assessment**" (3) is a term coined to express a structured clinical technique for assessing the nutritional status of patients by the bedside. Its components can be summarized as:

- History
  - weight change
  - dietary intake change (relative to normal)
  - gastrointestinal symptoms (that persisted for >2 weeks)
  - functional capacity
  - disease and its relation to nutrition requirements
- Physical
  - loss of subcutaneous fat (triceps, chest)
  - muscle wasting (quadriceps, deltoids)
  - ankle oedema
  - sacral oedema
  - ascites
- Subjective global assessment rating
  - well nourished
  - moderately (or suspected of being) malnourished
  - severely malnourished

It is reasonably effective in separating the clearly undernourished from the normally nourished but is not so good at defining an intermediate group. The term, subjective global assessment, *does not* imply that a rapid visual assessment of the patient is a sufficient means of assessing their nutritional status — indeed, such an approach is the basis of the failure by most clinicians to recognize the high prevalence of undernutrition, present among patients admitted to hospital, which tends to worsen during their stay in hospital. Emphasis has also been placed upon physiological impairment (4) of functions such as grip strength as a supplement to weight-for-height records.

Estimates from the literature of the prevalence of undernutrition at the time of a patient's admission to hospital lie between about 20–40% (5). A simple method of screening all patients is required. For this purpose, body weight, w(kg) and height, h(m) are measured and the **Quetelet (body mass) index** (BMI) calculated as w/h². In the UK the desirable range of values is 20–25 kg/m². For less well-nourished general populations, a lesser value of 18.5 kg/m² may be more appropriate as an indicator of likely physiological impairment. At the Royal London Hospital, among 996 patients entering our acute services, 16% men and 17% of women have a BMI less than 20 kg/m² at the time of their admission. As a routine practice, the weight should also be compared with previous weight records or the patient's stated usual weight, to identify **percentage weight loss**: [(usual weight – weight) × 100/usual weight.

McWhirter & Pennington (6) found the prevalence of undernutrition based on weight loss and BMI to be close to 40% at the time of patients' admission to Ninewells Hospital, Dundee (6). In addition, many of those admitted to hospital without weight loss are *at risk* of undernutrition as a result of their inability to swallow or a catabolic state. A number of assessment scores, such as that of Reilly *et al.* (7) have been developed to document this. Nutritional status tends to worsen during hospital admissions.

Clinicians should be alert to **specific nutrient deficiencies** — most commonly, iron, folate, and vitamin B_{12}, but not forgetting deficiencies of other water-soluble vitamins especially B_1 and B_6, which are common even among non-alcoholic individuals admitted to hospital acutely (8). Steatorrhoea or biliary dysfunction increases the likelihood of fat-soluble vitamin deficiencies presenting as bone pain and proximal weakness (vitamin D), bruising and bleeding tendency (vitamin K), ataxia (vitamin E), and night blindness perhaps with corneal abnormalities (vitamin A). The presence or absence of oedema should be noted, and saline depletion detected by measuring blood pressure with the patient lying and standing, and seeking a postural decrease of more than 15 mmHg.

Serum albumin has (in common with weight loss) been repeatedly shown to be a good predictor of poor surgical outcome, but its status as a *nutritional* indicator is more in doubt. Undoubtedly, undernutrition has an impact upon albumin synthesis, but the dominant determinant of most clinical hypoalbuminaemia is either loss from the intestine or kidney, or redistribution so that a greater propor-

tion of its mass is present in the extravascular space (9). Nonetheless, validated prognostic indices have been derived for surgical practice combining albumin concentration with other nutritional parameters. The most important of these indices is probably the nutrition risk index (NRI) used in the Veterans Administration trial (10) (see below):

$$NRI = \text{serum albumin (g/litre)} \times 1.519 + 0.417 \times (\text{current weight/usual weight}) \times 100$$

This is an index mathematically derived to predict risk of surgical complications. For the trial, a value less than 100 was regarded as indicative of malnourishment, greater than 97.5 borderline, and 83.5–97.5 indicative of mild, and less than 83.5 indicative of severe, undernutrition. Thus, if a serum albumin concentration at the lower end of the normal range is taken — say 35 g/litre — a weight 6% greater than usual would result in an NRI of 97.5; a current weight 72% of usual would result in an NRI of 83.5. Taking a modestly reduced serum albumin concentration of 30 g/litre, a weight loss of 9% results in an NRI of 83.5. The fundamental problem with such scoring systems is whether they predict nutritionally reversible complications, or complications consequent upon the disease process, on which nutritional treatment is likely to have little impact.

Clinical assessment is supplemented with a full blood count, and measurement of urea and electrolytes, calcium, phosphate, magnesium and zinc, the last two being especially relevant in diarrhoeal states and short-bowel syndrome.

INDICATIONS FOR PARENTERAL AND ENTERAL NUTRITION

Nutrition support should always be provided by the simplest, safest, most cost-effective approach acceptable to the patient. Food should be preferred to artificial feeding, and the enteral route used in preference to the parenteral. For the majority of undernourished hospital inpatients, food will be the correct nutritional treatment, but its effectiveness will depend upon catering and nursing practices. Most hospital administrations in the UK have been unhappy to allow patients' relatives to bring cooked food into the hospital since the 1990 Food Safety Act, which made the hospital legally liable if such food is the source of food poisoning. Sip feeds containing complete nutrient mixes and based on whole protein are a convenient and effective means of supplementing inadequate oral intake, but they should seldom replace food. Feeding by artificial means such as enteral tubes or parenteral feeding becomes progressively more indicated the longer the patient is unable to eat and the greater the weight loss; it will be necessary if the swallowing mechanism is unsafe as judged by pharyngeal pooling after a test swallow, a detailed assessment by a speech therapist, or by cine-fluoroscopy. Weight loss greater than 10% or a BMI of less than 20 kg/m^2 favours the need for artificial nutrition, as does an inability to feed that lasts longer than 5 days. In the intensive care setting, particularly in the context of severe catabolism as a result of sepsis, trauma, or burns, delay should not be this long, and artificial feeding is started soon after circulatory stabilization, to *prevent* excess loss of lean tissue mass.

The perception of when sip and enteral feeds are indicated is gradually changing. Endoscopically placed enteral tubes are used, in preference to parenteral feeding, to bypass oesophageal or duodenal partial obstruction. Enteral feeding is increasingly used after operation and in conditions such as acute pancreatitis (see below). Parenteral nutrition most commonly has a place either when nasogastric feeding is intolerable — for example with mucositis complicating chemotherapy — or when there is severe intra-abdominal sepsis resulting in prolonged ileus. High-output enterocutaneous fistula remains an indication for total parenteral nutrition (with no enteral nutrient intake) if restricting enteral intake in this way is shown, *in the individual*, to reduce fistula output. Subacute or partial intestinal obstruction that can not readily be bypassed by an endoscopically placed feeding tube is another indication for parenteral feeding perioperatively. Effective nutritional support, particularly by the enteral route, depends upon the motivation and active participation of the patient, and they should be involved in decisions as to the route of treatment, and their feelings respected.

Long-term and domiciliary enteral feeding are indicated principally to bypass an inadequate swallowing mechanism, in neurological disease especially, and also in oropharyngeal dysfunction. **Home parenteral feeding** (11,12) is primarily used in the UK in **severe short-bowel syndrome** (particularly in those with less than 100 cm of small bowel unattached to the colon, or those with less than 50 cm of small bowel atttached to colon) (13), and in some cases of severe **chronic intestinal pseudo-obstruction**. Improving the nutrition of chronically ill patients tends to improve quality of life (14), but any decision to feed the terminally ill parenterally needs careful weighing of potential benefits, bearing in mind the effects of cancer cachexia, which may not be sufficiently reversible by nutritional means to make intervention worthwhile (15).

The ethical aspects of artificial nutritional support are outside the scope of this chapter, but have been thoughtfully reviewed elsewhere (16).

ORGANIZATION OF NUTRITION SUPPORT — NUTRITIONAL SUPPORT TEAMS

Once the high prevalence of undernutriton in hospitals is appreciated, it becomes clear that the approach to its management has to be organized initially at a strategic level. The British Association of Parenteral and Enteral Nutrition (BAPEN) recommends (17) that there should be a Nutrition Strategic Committee in every hospital in order to coordinate dietetic, catering, nursing, pharmaceutical, and medical input into this problem. A system must be developed whereby patients are routinely nutritionally screened, and effective management for those who are underweight set in motion by nurses and dietitians, using hospital food. Much needs to be done to improve the way in which patients eat in hospital, and doctors and dietitians should be aware of the scientific and economic arguments for optimizing such care. Artificial feeding should be reserved for the minority, and should be supervised by a nutritional support team. On the basis of experience in USA, Canada, and France, the multidisciplinary team approach to artificial nutritional support was advocated in the UK and developed in theory and in practice during the 1970s (18,19) stimulated by the growing awareness of the potential advantages of parenteral feeding, but also of the great risks of using the technique inexpertly. The team approach brought together clinicians, pharmacists, nurses, and dietitians, to bring their individual areas of expertise to overcome difficult clinical problems of undernutrition. By 1992 — when the Kings Fund report, *A Positive Approach to Nutrition as Treatment* was published (20), and at which time BAPEN was founded — the team approach had become widely accepted by experts in the field, and had been demonstrated to be superior to a less organized approach to artificial feeding (20–23). In the context of parenteral feeding, there is evidence that careful attention to procedure reduces complications, with the involvement of a nutrition nurse specialist, in particular, reducing the risk of infective complications.

Day-to-day care is thus either run by, or closely supervised by, a team of a doctor, specialist nurse, dietitian, and pharmacist. After careful overall appraisal of the clinical aspects of the case and a nutritional assessment of the patient, the nutritional requirements are estimated, the route of administration decided, a complete and appropriate feed provided (taking into consideration pharmaceutical aspects of intravenous feed admixtures), the feed delivered safely, efficiently and confidently, and finally, the decision to stop artificial feeding made correctly.

TECHNIQUES FOR DELIVERING ARTIFICIAL FEEDING

Nasogastric tubes for feeding purposes should be fine bore. Polyurethane or silicone rubber tubes of 8F gauge or smaller are used, to minimize nasopharyngeal irritation. Guide-wires are used to stiffen some catheters at the time of insertion, but must never be re-inserted into a partially inserted tube: penetration of the side-wall or through a side-port risks perforation of the viscus. Insertion is performed by trained personnel following a standard-driven procedure; the way in which it is performed sets the tone for the rest of the patient's experience of this approach to feeding. It is vital that this is not a negative inital experience carried out clumsily, insensitively, or too hurriedly. The position of the tube must be checked before infusion commences, using air insufflation or litmus testing of the aspirate. Although it is not desirable to insist on routine radiological checking of the position of the tube, this must be done if doubt remains. Once the tube is in place, it is wise to place an indelible mark on the tube, close to the patient's nose, so that any subsequent accidental withdrawal can easily be assessed. Nasogastric feeds should be delivered by constant infusion with the patient in the head-up position, to reduce risks of pharyngeal aspiration of feed. The use of weighted-tip tubes may carry advantages if transpyloric placement is required.

Fine-bore tubes can also be placed endoscopically. We use lengths of Portex tubing inserted via the biopsy channel, to which hubs are attached after removal of the endoscope and rerouting of the tube from mouth to nose.

Gastrostomies or **enterostomies** can be inserted endoscopically, radiologically, laparoscopically, or surgically. Their place is for enteral feeding in the longer term — months, rather than weeks or days. They may have a place for the patient requiring shorter-term feeding who can not tolerate pernasal tubes, or in the restless or confused patient in whom it can be difficult to keep a nasogastric tube in place, and in whom there may be an increased danger of pulmonary aspiration as a result of infusion after displacement. The endoscopic approach is nearly always preferred, and we use Fresenius size 9 and 15 devices, placed under routine pre-procedural antibiotic cover of cefuroxime 750 mg.

Parenteral feeds may be delivered through peripheral catheters, mid-length fine-bore catheters, peripherally inserted central lines, or dedicated skin-tunnelled central venous catheters.

Standard **peripheral catheters** can be used in the short term; thrombophlebitis, a complication that relates to the time-scale of the infusion and to the osmolarity of the feed, can be minimized by using precise insertion technique, careful asepsis, and glyceryl trinitrate patches. Some advocate the use of heparin, with or without cortisol added to the feeds. Many patients do not need high caloric input, and if the non-protein energy is delivered in large part as lipid, this serves to keep osmolarity, and therefore the risk of thrombophlebitis, low. These principles apply also to the mid-length catheters, which reduce the risk of thrombophlebitis further by being of very fine bore and constructed of non-reactive materials such as polyurethane or silicone rubber. These catheters, such as the Vygon nutriline, inserted from the antecubital fossa, may be suitable for use over periods of weeks.

Peripherally inserted central catheters are introduced via the basilic vein at the antecubital fossa. The radial/lateral cephalic vein is avoided, because it joins the axillary vein at a right angle, which can make advancement beyond this point very difficult. Such catheters must, like any other central line, be screened into a correct position in the superior vena cava (SVC).

Central venous catheters are placed via a sub-cutaneous skin tunnel from a point on the anterior chest wall distant from the point of entry of the catheter into the vein. Insertion is via the infraclavicular or low jugular routes, to facilitate the skin tunnel. In order to minimize the small risk of inducing cardiac arrhythmias, the tip of the line should not be inside the chambers of the heart. In order to avoid the very small risk of cardiac tamponade consequent upon erosion of the catheter through the heart or lower SVC wall, the tip should be placed proximal to the reflection of the pericardium onto the SVC. This is achieved in practice by checking that the tip is placed no lower than 2 cm below a line joining the lower borders of the medial ends of the clavicles on a posteroanterior chest radiograph or placed in the angle formed between the trachea and the right main bronchus on an anteroposterior film. This remains true for any catheter, however fine or soft, because it is not clear whether it is the catheter itself or the jet of fluid coming from the end of the catheter that causes perforation. It should be remembered that long lines placed from the antecubital fossa allow as much as 10 cm of travel of the tip when the arm is abducted. Central venous catheters of this kind are best when parenteral feeding is likely to be more than 1–2 weeks duration, when there is poor peripheral access, and when feeds have an osmolarity of more than 1000 mosmol/litre. **Before infusion of the feed, it is vital to check that the catheter is in the vein by aspirating blood.** Radiographs show the position of the line but, without contrast, can not demonstrate its position in the lumen.

CALCULATING THE REQUIREMENTS AND CHOOSING THE FEED (24)

Calculation of energy requirements

- Calculate basal metabolic rate (25)
- Add 10% for each °C increase in temperature
- Adjust for patient's mobility:
  - on ventilator = –15%
  - unconscious = basal metabolic rate (BMR)
  - bedbound and awake = +10%
  - sitting in chair = +20%
  - mobile in ward = +30%
- Add up to 600 kcal per day if weight gain (lean tissue deposition) is required

For parenteral feeding, it is advisable to keep the glucose infusion to less than 4 mg/kg per min, and a soya-bean emulsion such as Intralipid should not be infused at more than $3.8 + 1.6$ g lipid/kg per 24 h, which in practice translates to 500–1500 ml of the 10% emulsion per 24 h.

Calculation of protein requirements

The "Reference Nutrient Intake" in health — measured as grams of nitrogen (gN) per day — is about 7.5 gN/day and 9 gN/day for adult women and men, respectively. For pregnant women, the figure is 8.5 gN/day.

In disease, increased requirements may need to be estimated. The procedure is as follows: provide about 1 gN/200 kcal in the non-catabolic patient; if patients are septic, burnt, or otherwise catabolic increase the nitrogen relative to the energy intake to a usual maximum of 1 gN/100 kcal, depending on the severity of their condition. Alternatively, use 1–2 g protein/kg per day, depending on the level of catabolism. Check estimates by measuring urinary nitrogen losses or calculating them from the urinary urea excretion and comparing them with the prescribed feed.

Parenteral electrolyte requirements

1. *Sodium*: Provide the patient's weight in kilograms as mmol sodium as a baseline, and add calculated losses (see Table 21.1)
2. *Potassium*: Provide the patient's weight in kilograms as mmol/24 h as a baseline, and add losses. If in doubt, start with less.
3. *Calcium (parenteral)*: 5–10 mmol/day.
4. *Magnesium (parenteral)*: 5–10 mmol/day.
5. *Phosphate (parenteral)*: 10–30 mmol/day.
6. *Vitamins and trace elements (parenteral)*: See Elia (26).

MONITORING OF NUTRITIONAL SUPPORT

Refeeding syndrome

Patients who are severely undernourished may die as a result of overenthusiastic refeeding. Sodium retention, related to insulin elaboration, results in rapid weight gain, oedema, and heart failure. Hypokalaemia and hypophosphataemia may

Table 21.1. Contents of intestinal fluids — a clinical guide.

	Volume (ml/24 h)	Na (mmol/litre or *mmol/day)	K (mmol/litre or *mmol/day)	H (mmol/litre or *mmol/day)	HCO$_3$ (mmol/litre or *mmol/day)
Saliva	500–1500	~20	14	—	14
Gastric juice	2–3000	50–60	8–14	27–40	—
Parietal	—	0	17	149	—
Non-parietal	—	137	6	0	25
Bile	600	146–149	5	—	25–30
Panceatic juice	700–2500	125	8	—	10–45
Intestinal					
Jejunal	~3000	142	5	—	8
Ileal	~1000	140	5	—	30
Faeces	100–150	7*	11*	—	<30/kg*

complicate the situation. Energy intake should be restricted to close to the BMR for the first few days of nutritional support in severely undernourished patients.

Acute vitamin and mineral deficiencies can be precipitated by feeding without appropriate micronutrients. Acute folate deficiency may result in megaloblastosis and thrombocytopenia (27) and acute vitamin B$_1$ deficiency (28,29) with lactic acidosis, Wernicke's encephalopathy may be precipitated by refeeding if these nutrients are inadequately supplied. Acute zinc depletion can be precipitated as protein synthesis responds to an inadequately supplemented feed.

Daily weight

Measurement of weight daily is the best way to monitor fluid balance. Unless dehydration is being corrected, be very cautious if weight gain exceeds 1 kg/week. Remember that, in the presence of ascites or oedema, the clinical goal is likely to be weight *loss* initially, as the expanded extracellular space diminishes.

Blood and urine sugar

Stressed patients are usually insulin resistant. To avoid hyperglycaemia, and therefore a hyperosmolar state, blood or urine glucose must be monitored daily.

Temperature chart

The temperature chart is of especial relevance in parenteral feeding, when a spike of pyrexia, or a

change in an existing pattern of pyrexia, may be the first indication of a catheter infection. Under these circumstances, the nutrition nurse specialist very carefully draws blood for culture from the feeding line and from a peripheral vein. Line infection may be declared by chills or fever occurring soon after the start of a feed given intermittently with "rest" periods, and under these circumstances we advise cessation of the feed until the results of blood cultures are known. Pyrexia in enteral feeding may indicate aspiration pneumionia, or, in the case of a percutaneous endoscopic gastrostomy, infection at the stoma.

Blood tests

Urea and electrolytes should be checked regularly according to the patient's clinical condition, and particularly early on after changes in a regimen; plasma magnesium, calcium, phosphate, and zinc, and liver function tests are checked at least weekly.

Twenty-four-hour urinary nitrogen or urea

As a guide to nitrogen requirements, 24-h urinary nitrogen or urea can be monitored, but interpretation of the measurements requires a sophisticated knowledge of nitrogen balance and its response to feeding and stress. Urinary bacterial contamination may invalidate urinary urea measurements. If plasma urea is not changing across the period of the urine collection urinary urea nitrogen represents approximately 85% of excreted urinary nitrogen — the dominant route of nitrogen excretion.

Energy consumption

In the critically ill, there may be advantages in monitoring energy consumption by indirect calorimetry. The principle is to avoid energy excess, which is more dangerous than slight deficiency under these circumstances. Excess energy provision may cause hyperglycaemia or hyperlipidaemia. Excess glucose (more than 4 mg/kg per min) may cause high outputs of carbon dioxide if lipogenesis is induced, and may result in increased catecholamine production even if it is not. Lipid is usually limited to 3.8 g/kg per 24 h, or 500–1500 ml of 10% Intralipid or 500–750 ml of 20% Intralipid per 24 h. Lipofundin MCT/LCT is limited to 1–2 g lipid/kg per 24 h.

CLINICAL USE AND INDICATIONS

Perioperative Nutritional Support

There is evidence (30,31) of a reduction in postoperative complications and duration of hospital stay if supplementary sip feeding is started as soon after operation as the patient can take fluid. Early oral feeding is clinically safe, but a large trial of this approach failed to show improvements in outcome (32). There is no indication for routine perioperative parenteral feeding in well-nourished or mildly undernourished patients (10,33), in whom parenteral feeding is associated with an excess of infective complications. Similarly, there is no indication for routine intravenous protein-sparing therapy (34) using hypocaloric amino acid mixtures. A large study (10) showed benefits from postoperative parenteral feeding in patients judged to be "severely undernourished" — who had an NRI score (see above) less than 83.5.

Claims based upon the findings of randomized controlled trials have been made for additional benefit from postoperative enteral nutrition delivered by nasoenteral tube compared with routine care, (35,36), and this approach has been well studied in the context of fractured neck of femur, with which the time for undernourished patients to achieve independent mobility is significantly reduced (37). Some studies suggest that this postoperative approach may be better than parenteral feeding (38,39) although the evidence that the enteral approach is intrinsically better than the parenteral has been subject to detailed criticism in a recent review (40).

Routine perioperative nutrition support should be limited to the early use of sip-feed supplements as oral fluids become allowed. Parenteral and enteral nutrition techniques are advised in malnourished patients or in those with an unusually prolonged postoperative course who are at risk of prolonged inadequate oral intake, when the overall rule should be applied and the **simplest, safest, most effective approach acceptable to the patient** should be used.

NUTRITIONAL SUPPORT IN THE CRITICALLY ILL

Short periods of starvation over hours or a day or two may be acceptable for most patients, but the difficulty of maintaining or increasing lean body mass during critical illness is too great to delay instituting artificial feeding longer than this in the intensive care unit (ICU). In patients with weight loss of 10% or more, or who clearly are not going to be able to eat adequately within 2 days, artificial nutrition of one kind or another will be indicated immediately. There should be no delay in initiating nutritional support in those with a BMI less than 20 kg/m^2; even if they are their normal weight, there are insufficient body reserves to allow prolonged unmodified catabolism.

The **route** should be enteral when possible. Enteral feeds tend to be more complete than parenteral feeds, have important economic advantages, and may minimize intestinal mucosal atrophy, bacterial translocation, and endotoxinaemia. Feeds are initiated slowly, through slightly wider than usual tubes, and aspiration is carried out at 3-hourly intervals, to ensure that excess gastric retention does not occur. Lack of bowel sounds alone is not a reason to withhold enteral feeding.

It is important that the nutrition team prescribing the feed, whether parenteral or enteral, work in close cooperation with the ICU staff. Intensive care depends upon the ability to adjust treatment from hour to hour but, once feeds have been provided/compounded, such rapid changes are not practical, apart from changing the rate of infusion or stopping the feed, with major implications for wastage. With expensive parenteral feeds, we commonly exclude from the compounded mixture those nutrients most likely to require hour-to-hour manipulation. Thus we may leave sodium or potassium out of the feed completely, and allow the ICU staff to monitor and replace them separately as required. Similarly, we may use smaller volumes than usual, in the knowledge that our ICU colleagues understand what we are doing and will fine-adjust the volume themselves.

Respiratory failure

Provided energy requirements are calculated correctly, and excess is not provided, special formulations are not normally required for patients in respiratory failure. Lipid produces less carbon dioxide per oxygen consumed than does glucose, and so some advocate the use of fat inputs of up to 60% of non-protein calories in the short term for such patients.

$$C_6H_{12}O_6 \text{ (glucose)} + 6O_2 = 6CO_2 + 6H_2O$$

whereas, taking palmitic acid as a typical fatty acid:

$$CH_3(CH_2)14COOH + 23O_2 = 16CO_2 + 16H_2O$$

Although the synthesis of lipid from dietary carbohydrate probably occurs to only a small extent in normal individuals eating mixed meals, high carbohydrate loads given continuously by artificial feed can give rise to lipogenesis. When one molecule of palmitic acid is made for storage from four molecules of glucose, further carbon dioxide is produced in the process, unlike the process involved in the storage of dietary fat, and the respiratory quotient (carbon dioxide produced/oxygen consumed) increases to greater than 1:

$$4C_6H_{12}O_6 + O_2 = CH_3(CH_2)14COOH + 8CO_2 + 8H_2O$$

This emphasizes the need not to provide excess energy — especially not as glucose — if the patient is retaining carbon dioxide. The excess energy, rather than the choice of energy substrate, is the dominant consideration. Glucose infusion should, in general, be kept less than 4 mg/kg per min, to avoid producing respiratory quotients greater than 1.

Cardiac failure

Sodium and water need to be reduced; potassium and magnesium, particularly in the presence of arrythmias or infarction, may be protective.

Renal failure

The detailed nutritional management of renal failure is beyond the scope of this chapter; the principles are the same whether parenteral, enteral, or oral routes are used. The management of such patients calls for close liaison between intensive care specialists, renal physicians, clinical nutritionists, and specialist dietitians. Optimal dialysis simplifies the nutritionist's role, and calculated requirements for energy and protein can be infused with standard electrolytes, mineral, vitamin, and trace element amounts. Lipid infusion must be carefully monitored, because these patients may develop lipaemia as a result of reduced lipid clearance. A greater problem exists if dialysis is less than optimal, perhaps because of logistical difficulties. Here, feeds can be electrolyte-free, restricted to 7–9 gN or less, and reduced in volume as required in the individual case. A similar approach is used for the patient with renal failure who does not require dialysis. Haemofiltration can be used in inpatients with renal or cardiac failure to "make space" for nutrient infusions in those with overloaded circulating volume. Fat-soluble vitamin supplementation may need to be reduced from routine input quantities, to prevent toxicity.

Liver failure

The cardinal principal in artificial feeding in liver failure is to avoid infusing too much sodium. If ascites is accumulating, sodium may be excluded from the feed altogether. Water overload is also common, and results in a low plasma sodium concentration; its restriction is readily achieved with appropriate prescription of artificial feeds. Protein may need to be restricted in the encephalopathic patient, although if infused over a full 24 h, normal protein intakes are usually tolerated. A minimum 100–125 g glucose is required to be infused to prevent hypoglycaemia in liver failure, because of failure of gluconeogenesis. However, the insulin-resistant, high-insulin state may be worsened by infusion of excess glucose. This will exacerbate reductions in plasma concentrations of branched-chain amino acids, which some believe are involved in the pathogenesis of encephalopathy (41). High-insulin states also tend to increase fluid retention. Lipid is usually cleared satisfactorily in liver failure (42). Some use feeds supplemented with branched-chain amino acids or their ketoanalogues. Standard feeds contain about 20% of their amino acids as branched chains; these can be increased to 40% or more, but will have a bigger impact on plasma concentrations if such infusion is combined with the minimum glucose (100–150 g) necessary to prevent hypoglycaemia.

Adjunctive hormonal therapy

In some catabolic patients, nitrogen balance remains negative despite adequate nutrient input. If the degree of this negative balance and its likely duration demand further protection of the lean body mass, hormones can be tried.

Insulin reduces whole-body protein breakdown and amino acid oxidation in normal individuals under conditions of euglycaemic clamp. This anabolic effect is enhanced if plasma amino acid concentrations, which decrease with insulin, are maintained by feeding (43). Clinical experience has shown the effects of insulin to be small or lost in patients undergoing parenteral feeding — probably because, in the clinical setting, the plasma glucose concentration has been allowed to decrease, albeit within the normal range. Infusion of insulin may be worth trying, therefore, in patients receiving parenteral feeding, if efforts are made to maintain plasma glucose at the patient's pre-insulin, fed value (44).

A number of studies have demonstrated that **recombinant human growth hormone** can increase whole-body protein synthesis and improve nitrogen balance. Hyperglycaemia may be a problem, and optimal dosages are not clear. However, two large-scale multicentre controlled trials (45) have demonstrated an excess mortality when growth hormone is used in acutely ill patients, and it is contraindicated under these circumstances.

Insulin like growth factor-I has also been studied. Its effects on protein metabolism are broadly similar to those of insulin. It has also been used in combination with growth hormone. In view of the results with growth hormone, great caution is needed.

NUTRITIONAL SUPPORT IN INFLAMMATORY BOWEL DISEASE

Active inflammatory bowel disease is characterized nutritionally by a state of increased whole-body protein turnover, modestly increased losses of protein from the intestine, and an energy expenditure which, for practical purposes, can probably be considered as normally predictable when activity and pyrexia are taken into consideration. In **ulcerative colitis**, iron deficiency is common; in **Crohn's disease**, in which the small bowel, especially the terminal ileum, is diseased and bacterial overgrowth is not uncommon, vitamin B_{12}, fat-soluble vitamins, calcium, and folate deficiencies are common, among other deficiencies. As with nearly all other states of undernutrition, it is appropriate to seek and treat these deficiencies actively. The treatment of chronic protein–calorie undernutrition is all too often not given the priority it deserves; it is important in both in- and outpatients, and results in improvement of patient well-being.

Patients with Crohn's disease self-select low-residue, low-fibre diets, and in a large multicentre trial in which an attempt was made to increase fibre intake, there was greater non-compliance and a greater withdrawal rate as a result of increased symptoms among those receiving the high-fibre intake (46). A **polymeric whole-protein liquid nutritional supplement** results in increased nutrient intake, improved nutritional status, and reduced disease activity (47). Interest has been raised in the use of artificial feeding as a primary treatment. **Total parenteral nutrition**, with no enteral intake, has not proved beneficial in acute colitis (48,49), and in one controlled clinical trial in Crohn's disease, bowel rest with parenteral feeding or pure enteral feeding was not superior to enteral support with continued oral intake of food (50). A number of studies have appeared to demonstrate advantages for **enteral feeds** in Crohn's disease. Initial claims centred around small controlled trials (51–54) that compared **elemental diet** with **prednisolone**, in which no difference in outcome was observed, and were based upon the knowledge that prednisolone was an effective treatment; they tended not to discuss the type-two error and to have high remission rates compared with those of the multicentre trials of prednisolone, suggesting some (perhaps unconscious) selection of patients before random assignment to treatment groups. Subsequent studies have shown that prednisolone is the superior treatment, on an intention-to-treat basis (55–57). Nonetheless, there remains a strong consensus that enteral feeding can be of benefit, and this is supported by studies, measuring for example, intestinal permeability (58) and gut albumin loss. Although elemental appeared better than polymeric feeds in an early study (59), the evidence is probably in favour of there being no difference in this respect (57,60–63). Enteral feeding has particular advantages when it is important to avoid the side effects of prednisolone and when the patient is particularly motivated to tolerate a liquid diet, a nasogastric feed, or a temporary gastrostomy. It has a place in patients with severe chronic abdominal pain, and when "something extra" is needed over and above drug treatment with steroids, salicylates, and immunosuppressives, particularly in the presence of undernutrition. There has been interest in the use of **exclusion diet** in Crohn's disease, and a controlled trial has provided some support for its use after induction of disease remission with an elemental diet (64).

Attempts to use specific nutrients to influence mucosal inflammation have centred on the use of **eicosapentanoic** acid (fish oil) to modify patterns of eicosanoid synthesis towards the n-3 series, and thereby reduce the inflammatory response. The rationale for this approach has been well reviewed by Calder (65). This approach has had modest clinical success in rheumatoid arthritis, systemic lupus erythematosus and psoriasis, and in preventing graft rejection. One trial in ulcerative colitis showed a modest reduction in requirements for steroids in active disease, but no effect in reducing the rate of relapse in patients in remission (66); another showed improvements in clinical score, but not in mucosal leukotriene B4 production or mucosal histology (67), and a third showed a slight beneficial effect for evening primrose oil, but not fish oil (68). In Crohn's disease, one trial has shown unequivocable benefit from fish-oil capsules in preventing relapse over 1 year (69). It remains to be seen whether the immunomodulatory enteral feeds prove beneficial in inflammatory bowel disease.

Short-chain fatty acid irrigation appears to be effective in the treatment of distal ulcerative colitis (70–72), as it does in the treatment of diversion colitis and pouchitis (73,74).

ACUTE PANCREATITIS

The nutritional management of maldigestion of chronic pancreatitis and the use of enzyme replacement is outside the remit of this chapter. However, there is current interest in the correct way to feed moderate to severe acute pancreatitis. In the past, it has been assumed that a regimen of nil by mouth was important, to reduce pancreatic enzyme secretion during the acute attack. Under these circumstances it may become necessary to provide parenteral feeding if the period of pryrexia and catabolism is prolonged. This approach carries the disadvantage of increasing intestinal mucosal permeability, with prolongation of the systemic inflammatory response and endotoxinaemia. Infusion of neutral-pH mixed elemental feeds into the jejunum has little effect on pancreatic secretion (75) and, by maintaining gut mucosal barrier function, could reduce endotoxinaemia and the systemic inflammatory response. Two controlled trials support such an approach (76,77).

GLUTAMINE

Of all the amino acids incorporated into protein, glutamine exists in the greatest muscle concentration, at about 25 mmol/litre of intracellular water. Normal plasma concentrations are much lower, at about 650 µmol/litre. Glutamine, a dibasic amino acid, acts as a shuttle for ammonium from peripheral tissues to the liver and the kidney, and its five-carbon skeleton, derived to a large extent from muscle branched-chain amino acids, serves as an important fuel for lymphocytes and gastrointestinal mucosal cells. As judged by glutaminase activity, the oesophagus and stomach are able to use glutamine little, the colon more, and the small intestine most, depending upon it as a primary fuel. After surgical and other stress, muscle and plasma glutamine concentrations decrease, and under these circumstances this normally dispensible amino acid has been considered conditionally indispensible. It represents 6–8% of dietary proteins, so that typical dietary intake is around 5 g/day, but its turnover between and within tissues is much greater, with a net postabsorptive interorgan flux of about 20 g (78) and a total-body daily turnover approaching an order of magnitude greater (79). Protein-based enteral feeds contain 5–8 g/100 g protein, peptide-based feeds 1.3–5.6 g/16 gN (80), and standard parenteral feeds contain none, because of stability problems. Techniques have been developed that allow the addition of free glutamine (81), or its alanine or glycine dipeptides, to parenteral feeds (82). Parenteral glutamine supplementation seems partially to prevent the mucosal atrophy associated with total parenteral nutrition when no nutrients are given by mouth (83), to maintain xylose absorption

(84), and to enhance T-cell DNA synthesis 6 days after operation (85).

Criticized for their statistical methodology which excluded long-stay outliers, early small-scale controlled clinical trials (86,87) have nevertheless produced findings suggestive of benefit from the inclusion of glutamine in parenteral feeds, in the context of haematological malignancy, as judged by reductions in the duration of stay in hospital and in infectious complications. A trial in intensive care patients showed a trend towards an improved rate of mortality in hospital, from 59.5 to 42.9% (88). Oral glutamine supplements have not been beneficial in patients with haematological malignancy or those undergoing cancer chemotherapy (for brief review, see (89)). A trial using an "immune-enhancing" feed that included, among other interventions, glutamine supplementation, showed benefit after operation in trauma patients (90), and a recent study (91) of enteral glutamine supplementation in trauma patients has shown a reduced rate of infective complications. A study in colorectal postoperative surgery appeared to demonstrate a reduced duration of hospital stay for patients allocated to a glutamine-dipeptide-supplemented parenteral feed, but can be criticized on the grounds that overall durations of stay were unusually long, and that there was no clinical indication for routine postoperative parenteral feeding in the well-nourished patients included. Our own study conducted in 168 parenterally fed patients did not show a clear outcome benefit for glutamine, although duration of hospital stay among surgical patients was reduced. There was a trend towards lower overall mortality (92).

References

1. Robinson G, Goldstein M, Levine G. Impact of nutritional status on DRG length of stay. *JPEN* 1987; **11**: 49–51.
2. Reilly JJ, Hull SF, Albert N *et al*. Economic impact of malnutrition: a model system for hospitalized patients. *JPEN* 1988; **12**: 371–376.
3. Detsky AS, McClaughlin JR, Baker JP *et al*. What is subjective global assessment of nutritional status? *JPEN* 1987; **11**: 8–13.
4. Windsor JA, Hill G. Weight loss with physiologic impairment. *Ann Surg* 1988; **207**: 290–296.
5. Powell-Tuck J. Penalties of hospital undernutrition. *J R Soc Med* 1997; **90**: 8–11.
6. McWhirter J, Pennington C. Incidence and recognition of malnutrition in hospital. *BMJ* 1994; **308**: 945–948.
7. Reilly HM, Martineau JK, Moran A *et al*. Nutritional screening — evaluation and implementation of a simple nutrition risk score. *Clin Nutr* 1995; **14**: 269–273.
8. Jamieson CP, Obeid OA, Powell-Tuck J. The thiamine, riboflavin and pyridoxine status of patients on emergency admission to hospital. *Clin Nutr* 1999; **18**: 87–91.
9. Fleck A, Raines G, Hawker F *et al*. Increased vascular permeability: a major cause of hypoalbuminaemia in disease and injury. *Lancet* 1985; **i**: 781–784.
10. Veterans Administration Total Parenteral Nutrition Cooperative Study Group. Perioperative total parenteral nutrition in surgical patients. *N Engl J Med* 1991; **325**: 525–532.
11. Elia M. An internatonal perspective on artificial nutritional support in the community. *Lancet* 1995; **345**: 1345–1349.
12. Powell-Tuck J. Management of gut failure. *Lancet* 1994; **344**: 1061–1064.
13. Powell-Tuck J. Don't expect too much of intestinal adaptation in short bowel syndrome. *Eur J Gastroenterol Hepatol* 1994; **6**: 193–195.
14. Jamieson C, Norton B, Day T *et al*. The quantitative effect of nutrition support on quality of life in outpatients. *Clin Nutr* 1997; **16**: 25–28.
15. Powell-Tuck J. Nutrition support in advanced cancer. *J R Soc of Med* 1997; **90**: 591–592.
16. Lennard-Jones JE. *Ethical and Legal Aspects of Clinical Hydration and Nutritonal Support*. Maidenhead: British Association for Parenteral and Enteral Nutrition, 1998.
17. Silk DBA (Ed.). *Organization of Nutritional Support in Hospitals*. Maidenhead: British Association for Parenteral and Enteral Nutrition, 1994.
18. Ellis BW, Stanbridge R de L, Fielding LP *et al*. A rational approach to parenteral nutrition. *BMJ* 1976; **1**: 1388–1391.
19. Powell-Tuck J, Nielson T, Farwell JA *et al*. A team approach to long-term intravenous feeding in patients with gastrointestinal disorders. *Lancet* 1978; **ii**: 825–828.
20. Lennard-Jones JE. *A Positive Approach to Nutrition as Treatment*. London: Kings Fund, 1992.
21. Nehme AE. Nutritional support of the hospitalised patient: the team concept. *JAMA* 1980; **243**: 1906–1908.
22. Keohane PP, Attrill H, Northover J *et al*. Effect of catheter tunnelling and a nutrition nurse on catheter sepsis during parenteral nutrition. *Lancet* 1983; **ii**: 1388–1390.
23. Faubion WC, Wesley JR, Khalidi N *et al*. Total parenteral nutrition catheter sepsis: impact of the team approach. *JPEN* 1986; **10**: 642–645.
24. Department of Health. *Dietary Reference Values for Food Energy and Nutrients for the United Kingdom*. London: HMSO, 1991.
25. Schofield WN. Predicting basal metabolic rate, new standards and review of previous work. *Hum Nutr Clin Nutr* 1985; **39C (suppl 1)**: 5–41.
26. Elia M. Changing concepts of nutrient requirements in disease: implications for artificial nutritional support. *Lancet* 1995; **345**: 1279–1284.
27. Ibbotson RM, Colvin BT, Colvin MP. Folic acid deficiency during intensive therapy. *BMJ* 1975; **ii**: 145.
28. Nagasaki H, Ohta M, Soeda J *et al*. Clinical and biochemical aspects of thiamine treatment for metabolic acidosis during total parenteral nutrition. *Nutrition* 1997; **13**: 110–117.
29. Anonymous. Lactic acidosis traced to thiamine deficiency related to nationwide shortage of multivitamins for total parenteral nutrition — United States, 1997. *MMWR* 1997; **46**: 523–528.

30. Keele AM, Bray MJ, Emery PW *et al.* Two phase randomised controlled clinical trial of postoperative oral dietary supplements in surgical patients. *Gut* 1997; **40**: 393–399.

31. Rana SK, Bray J, Menzies-Gow N *et al.* Short term benefits of post-operative oral dietary supplements in surgical patients. *Clin Nutr* 1992; **11**: 337–344.

32. Reissman P, Teoh TA, Cohen SM *et al.* Is early oral feeding safe after elective colorectal surgery? A prospective randomized trial. *Ann Surg* 1995; **222**: 73–77.

33. Brennan MF, Pisters PWT, Posner M *et al.* A prospective randomized trial of total parenteral nutrition after major pancreatic resection for malignancy. *Ann Surg* 1994; **220**: 436–444.

34. Doglietto GB, Gallitelli L, Pacelli F *et al.* Protein–sparing therapy after major abdominal surgery: lack of clinical effects. *Ann Surg* 1996; **223**: 357–362.

35. Carr CS, Ling E, Boulos P *et al.* Randomised trial of safety and efficacy of immediate postoperative enteral feeding in patients undergoing gastrointestinal resection. *BMJ* 1996; **312**: 869–871.

36. Sagar S, Harland P, Shields R. Early postoperative feeding with elemental diet. *BMJ* 1979; **1**: 293–295.

37. Bastow MD, Rawlings J, Allison S. Benefits of supplementary tube feeding after fractured neck of femur: a randomized controlled trial. *BMJ* 1983; **287**: 1589–1592.

38. Kudsk KA, Croce MA, Fabian TC *et al.* Enteral versus parenteral feeding. *Ann Surg* 1992; **215**: 503–513.

39. Moore FA, Feliciano DV, Andrassy RJ *et al.* Early enteral feeding, compared with parenteral, reduces postoperative septic complications. *Ann Surg* 1992; **216**: 173–183.

40. Lipman TO. Grains or veins: is enteral nutrition really better than parenteral nutrition? A look at the evidence. *JPEN* 1998; **22**: 167–182.

41. Eriksson LS, Conn HO. Branched chain amino acids in the management of hepatic encephalopathy: an analysis of variants. *Hepatology* 1989; **10**: 228–246.

42. Glynn MJ, Powell-Tuck J, Reavely D *et al.* High lipid parenteral nutrition improves portasystemic encephalopathy. *JPEN* 1988; **12**: 457–461.

43. Castellino P, Luzi L, Simonson DC *et al.* Effect of insulin and plasma amino acid concentration on leucine metabolism: role of substrate availability on estimates of whole body protein synthesis. *J Clin Invest* 1987; **80**: 1784–1793.

44. Powell-Tuck J, Glynn MJ. The effect of insulin infusion on whole-body protein metabolism in patients with gastrointestinal disease fed parenterally. *Hum Nutr: Clin Nutr* 1985; **39C**: 181–191.

45. Takala J, Ruokonen E, Webster NR *et al.* Increased mortality associated with growth hormone treatment in critically ill adults. *N Engl J Med* 1999; **341**: 785–792.

46. Ritchie JK, Wadsworth J, Lennard-Jones JE *et al.* Controlled multicentre therapeutic trial of an unrefined carbohydrate, fibre rich diet in Crohn's disease. *BMJ* 1987; **295**: 517–520.

47. Harries AD, Jones LA, Danis V *et al.* Controlled trial of supplemented oral nutrition in Crohn's disease. *Lancet* 1983; i: 887–890.

48. Dickinson RJ, Ashton MG, Axon ATR *et al.* Controlled trial of intravenous hyperalimentation and total bowel rest as an adjunct to the routine therapy of acute colitis. *Gastroenterology* 1980; **79**: 1199–1204.

49. McIntyre PB, Powell-Tuck J, Wood SR *et al.* Controlled trial of bowel rest in the treatment of severe acute colitis. *Gut* 1986; **27**: 481–485.

50. Greenberg GR, Fleming CR, Jeejeebhoy KN *et al.* Controlled trial of bowel rest and nutritional support in the management of Crohn's disease. *Gut* 1988; **29**: 1309–1315.

51. Gonzalez-Huix F, de Leon R, Fernandez-Banares F *et al.* Polymeric enteral diets as primary treatment of active Crohn's disease: a prospective steroid controlled trial. *Gut* 1993; **34**: 778–782.

52. O'Morain C, Segal AW, Levi AJ. Elemental diet as primary treatment of acute Crohn's disease: a controlled trial. *BMJ* 1984; **288**: 1859–1862.

53. Okada M, Yao T, Yamamoto K *et al.* Controlled trial comparing an elemental diet with prednisolone in the treatment of active Crohn's disease. *Hepatogastroenterology* 1990; **37**: 72–80.

54. Saverymuttu S, Hodgson HJF, Chadwick VS. Controlled trial comparing prednisolone with an elemental diet plus non-absorbable antibiotics in active Crohn's disease. *Gut* 1985; **26**: 994–998.

55. Lochs H, Steinhardt HJ, Klaus-Wentz B *et al.* Comparison of enteral nutrition and drug treatment in active Crohn's disease. *Gastroenterology* 1991; **101**: 881–888.

56. Gorard DA, Hunt JB, Payne-James JJ *et al.* Initial response and subsequent course of Crohn's disease treated with elemental diet or prednisolone,. *Gut* 1993; **34**: 1198–1202.

57. Wright N, Scott BB. Dietary treatment of active Crohn's disease: fewer side effects but poorly tolerated and no more effective than corticosteroids. *BMJ* 1997; **314**: 454–455.

58. Sanderson IR, Udeen S, Davies PSW *et al.* Remission induced by an elemental diet in small bowel Crohn's disease. *Arch Dis Child* 1987; **61**: 123–127.

59. Giaffer MH, North G, Holdsworth CD. Controlled trial of polymeric versus elemental diet in treatment of active Crohn's disease. *Lancet* 1990; **335**: 816–819.

60. Mansfield JC, Giaffer MH, Holdsworth CD. Controlled trial of oligopeptide versus amino acid diet in treatment of active Crohn's disease. *Gut* 1995; **36**: 60–66.

61. Raouf AH, Hildrey V, Daniel J *et al.* Enteral feeding as sole treatment for Crohn's disease: controlled trial of whole protein v amino acid based feed and a case study of dietary challenge. *Gut* 1991; **32**: 702–707.

62. Rigaud D, Cosnes J, le Quintrec Y *et al.* Controlled trial comparing two types of enteral nutrition in treatment of active Crohn's disease: elemental v polymeric diet. *Gut* 1991; **32**: 1492–1497.

63. Royall D, Jeejeebhoy KN, Baker JP *et al.* Comparison of amino acid v peptide based enteral diets in active Crohn's disease: clinical and nutritional outcome. *Gut* 1994; **35**: 783–787.

64. Riordan AM, Hunter JO, Cowan RE *et al.* Treatment of active Crohn's disease by exclusion diet: East Anglian multicentre controlled trial. *Lancet* 1993; **342**: 1131–1134.

65. Calder PC. Immunomodulatory and anti-inflammatory effects of n-3 polyunsaturated fatty acids. *Proc Nutr Soc* 1996; **55**: 737–774.

66. Hawthorne AB, Daneshmend TK, Hawkey CJ *et al.* Treatment of ulcerative colitis with fish oil supplementation: a prospective 12 month randomized controlled trial. *Gut* 1992; **33**: 922–928.

67. Aslan A, Triadafilopoulos G. Fish oil fatty acid supplementation in active ulcerative colitis: a double-blind, placebo-controlled, crossover study. *Am J Gastroenterol* 1992; **87**: 432–437.

68. Greenfield SM, Green AT, Teare JP *et al*. A randomized controlled study of evening primrose oil and fish oil in ulcerative colitis. *Aliment Pharmacol Ther* 1993; **7**: 159–166.

69. Belluzi A, Brignola C, Campieri M *et al*. Effect of an enteric-coated fish-oil preparation on relapses in Crohn's disease. *N Engl J Med* 1996; **334**: 1557–1560.

70. Breuer RI, Soergel KH, Lashner BA *et al*. Short chain fatty acid rectal irrigation for left-sided ulcerative colitis: a randomised, placebo controlled trial. *Gut* 1997; **40**: 485–491.

71. Scheppach W. Treatment of distal ulcerative colitis with short chain fatty acid enemas. A placebo-controlled trial. German–Austrian SCFA study group. *Dig Dis Sci* 1996; **41**: 2254–2259.

72. Kim YI. Short-chain fatty acids in ulcerative colitis. *Nutr Rev* 1998; **56**: 17–24.

73. Scheppach W, Christl SU, Bartram HP *et al*. Effects of short-chain fatty acids on the inflamed colonic mucosa. *Scand J Gastroenterol Suppl* 1997; **222**: 53–57.

74. Sagar PM, Taylor BA, Godwin P *et al*. Acute pouchitis and deficiencis of fuel. *Dis Colon Rectum* 1995; **38**: 488–493.

75. Ragins H, Levenson SM, Signer R *et al*. Intrajejunal administration of an elemental diet at neutral pH avoids pancreatic stimulation. *Am J Surg* 1973; **126**: 606–614.

76. Windsor ACJ, Kanwar S, Li AGK *et al*. Compared with parenteral feeding, enteral feeding attenuates the acute response and improves disease severity in acute pancreatitis. *Gut* 1998; **42**: 431–435.

77. Kalfarentzos F, Kehagias J, Mead N *et al*.. Enteral nutrition is superior to parenteral nutrition in severe acute pancreatitis: results of a randomized prospective trial. *Br J Surg* 1997; **84**: 1665–1669.

78. Elia M, Lunn PG. The use of glutamine in the treatment of gastrointestinal disease in man. *Nutrition* 1997; **13**: 743–747.

79. Darmaun D, Matthews DE, Bier DM. Glutamine and glutamate kinetics in humans. *Am J Physiol* 1986; **251**: E117–E126.

80. Kuhn KS, Stehle P, Furst P. Glutamine content of protein and peptide-based enteral products. *JPEN* 1996; **20**: 292–295.

81. Khan K, Hardy G, McElroy B *et al*. The stability of L-glutamine in total parenteral nutrtion solutions. *Clin Nutr* 1991; **10**: 193–198.

82. Furst P, Pogan K, Stehle P. Glutamine dipeptides in clinical nutrition. *Nutrition* 1997; **13**: 731–737.

83. van der Hulst RWJ, van Kreel BK, von Meyenfeldt MHF *et al*. Glutamine and the preservation of gut integrity. *Lancet* 1993; **341**: 1363–1365.

84. Tremel H, Kienle B, Weilemann LS *et al*. Glutamine dipeptide-supplemented parenteral nutrition maintains intestinal function in the critically ill. *Gastroenterology* 1994; **107**: 1595–1601.

85. O'Riordain MG, Fearon KC, Ross JA *et al*. Glutamine-supplemented total parenteral nutrition enhances T-lymphocyte response in surgical patients undergoing colorectal resection. *Ann Surg* 1994; **220**: 212–221.

86. Ziegler TR, Young LS, Benfell K *et al*. Clinical and metabolic efficacy of glutamine-supplemented parenteral nutrition after bone marrow transplantation. A randomized, double-blind, controlled study. *Ann Int Med* 1992; **116**: 821–828.

87. Schloerb P, Amare M. Total parenteral nutrition with glutamine in bone marrow transplantation and other clinical applications (a randomized, double-blind study). *JPEN* 1993; **17**: 407–413.

88. Griffiths RD, Jones C, Palmer TE. Six-month outcome of critically ill patients given glutamine-supplemented parenteral nutrition. *Nutrition* 1997; **13**: 295–302.

89. Powell-Tuck J. Glutamine supplementation in artificial nutritional support. *Lancet* 1997; **350**: 534.

90. Kudsk KA, Minard G, Croce MA *et al*. A randomized trial of isonitrogenous enteral diets after severe trauma. *Ann Surg* 1996; **224**: 531–543.

91. Houdijk APJ, Rijnsburger ER, Jansen J *et al*. Randomised trial of glutamine-enriched enteral nutrition on infectious mortality in patients with multiple trauma. *Lancet* 1998; **352**: 772–776.

92. Powell-Tuck J, Jamieson CP, Bettany GEA *et al*. A double blind, randomised, controlled trial of glutamine supplementation in parenteral nutrition. *Gut* 1999; **45**: 82–88.

22.1. Liver Failure: Acute Liver Failure

DAVID MUTIMER

DEFINITIONS

Acute liver failure is a syndrome defined by progression to hepatic encephalopathy within 8 weeks of the onset of symptoms, occurring in a patient without antecedent chronic liver disease. The first symptom is usually jaundice. Therefore, if the interval from jaundice to encephalopathy is less than 8 weeks, the patient has acute liver failure — commonly called **fulminant hepatic failure**. Most discussions of acute liver failure include reference to the syndrome of **subacute liver failure**, in which the duration of illness is between 8 weeks and 6 months. Subacute liver failure is also called **subacute hepatic necrosis** and **late onset hepatic failure**. The repertoir of terms is less important than the simple recognition that the syndrome of acute liver failure associated with a short prodromal illness frequently differs from that with a long prodromal illness with respect to aetiology, presenting clinical features, natural history, prognosis, and treatment.

At the **acute** end of the spectrum (for example, severe paracetamol poisoning), a patient may present in deep coma with cerebral oedema and without apparent jaundice (which will develop later if the patient survives). Hypoglycaemia may occur abruptly, serum transaminase concentrations are extremely high, and the prothrombin time is markedly prolonged (international normalized ratio (INR), frequently greater than 10). Recovery may be secured with conservative management, although specific features are suggestive of a poor outcome (see below).

At the **subacute** end of the spectrum (typified by many cases of so-called non-A, non-B, or seronega-tive hepatitis), a patient presents with deepening jaundice before the development of confusion. Hypoglycaemia is not an early feature, transaminase concentrations are modestly increased and the INR is between 2 and 4. Frequently, hepatorenal dysfunction with sodium retention and ascites develops insidiously and before the onset of encephalopathy. When the duration of illness is long, severe protein malnutrition and muscle loss will have been experienced. The prognosis for recovery with conservative management is very poor. In the absence of contraindications, liver transplantation is the best treatment.

Wilson's disease may present with a syndrome resembling acute liver failure. Acute Wilson's disease occurs in the context of chronic liver damage — frequently, undiagnosed cirrhosis. Despite the presence of antecedent liver disease, acute Wilson's disease is usually included in discussions of acute liver failure.

EPIDEMIOLOGY AND AETIOLOGY

Paracetamol poisoning

In the United Kingdom, **paracetamol poisoning** is the most common cause of acute liver failure. The UK has the world's highest incidence of paracetamol poisoning, though the incidence may be diminishing. It seems likely that this high incidence is, to a large extent, due to the methods of sales and marketing of this drug. Large quantities can be purchased by any person at a range of outlets, and without expert advice or scrutiny. The majority of poisoned patients have taken a deliberate overdose, although, occasionally, poisoning is accidental — a so-called "therapeutic misadventure". Most patients present within 12 h of poisoning, and are effectively treated with *N*-acetylcysteine (NAC). Significant hepatic toxicity is rarely observed if NAC is administered early, and most cases of serious toxicity are a consequence of late presentation for treatment. Paracetamol poisoning is the most common indication for admission to the acute liver failure unit. The majority are managed conservatively, but transplantation is indicated for some.

Non-A, non-B hepatitis

Second in incidence to paracetamol poisoning, is the entity called **non-A**, **non-B hepatitis** or **seronegative hepatitis**. Although the nomenclature suggests a viral cause for this disease, the aetiology is unknown (1). Some acute cases clearly resemble severe acute viral hepatitis, and may be complicated by the development of bone marrow aplasia (as may also be observed for hepatitis A and B viruses (HAV, HBV)). Others experience a subacute course, and have some features to suggest an autoimmune aetiology (2). The aetiology of seronegative hepatitis, like the clinical features, is probably quite heterogeneous. Known common viral causes of acute liver failure (HAV and HBV) are easily excluded by serological tests; hepatitis E virus (HEV) is an uncommon cause of the condition in the UK, but it should be considered if there has been recent travel to countries where the incidence is greater. A detailed drug history, including non-prescribed substances, herbal medicines, and recreational drugs, is essential. Wilson's disease should be considered, particularly in a younger patient. Although seronegative hepatitis is much less common than paracetamol poisoning, transplantation is frequently indicated. Therefore, of the causes of acute liver failure, seronegative hepatitis is the most common indication for liver transplantation.

Autoimmune liver disease

Autoimmune liver disease may present as an acute hepatitis, frequently before the development of encephalopathy. Clues to an autoimmune aetiology include a history of autoimmune disease, serum autoantibodies, and notably increased concentrations of serum immunoglobulins. However, autoantibodies — albeit in low titre — are frequently identified in the serum of patients presumed to have seronegative hepatitis. In these circumstances, the potential risks and benefits of corticosteroid treatment should be weighed. In more advanced cases, risks of treatment (including the delay pending possible response to treatment) probably outweigh potential benefit. Early consideration of liver transplantation may be more appropriate.

Viral hepatitis

Acute viral hepatitis (known viruses) is an uncommon cause of acute liver failure in the UK.

1. *Acute liver failure caused by (HBV)*: This is seldom observed in the UK. The Queen Elizabeth Hospital (QEH) Liver Unit sees as few as one or two cases per year. For most cases of acute HBV infection, including those complicated by the development of acute liver failure, a source of infection can be identified. Sexual and parenteral transmission should be considered.

2. *Acute liver failure caused by (HAV)*: Again, this is seldom observed in the UK. The QEH Liver Unit may see as few as one case per year. Frequently, the source of infection is clear. More than 50% of affected patients survive without transplantation. As a consequence of improving hygiene in the Western world, few UK children are exposed to HAV. Exposure at an older age is more likely to be associated with severe hepatitis and acute liver failure. As more non-immune people travel to countries where HAV is endemic, the incidence of HAV-associated acute liver failure may increase.

3. *HEV infection*: In some parts of Asia and central America, HEV infection is endemic. Acute HEV infection may cause acute liver failure, particularly during late pregnancy. HEV should be considered as a cause of liver failure when the patient has recently travelled to affected areas. The Public Health Laboratories are able to examine serum for antibodies to HEV.

Drugs

There are few drugs that have not been associated with acute liver failure, and a complete and thorough drug history is essential. **Isoniazid** remains a common and important cause of acute liver failure, as do **non-steroidal anti-inflammatory drugs** — use of which is ubiquitous.

Wilson's disease

Wilson's disease may present as acute liver failure. Clues to the diagnosis include the patient's age (nearly always younger than 35 years, frequently late teenage), associated clinical features (evidence of haemolysis, renal tubular disorders, or acute renal failure), presence of Kayser–Fleicher rings, and a typical pattern of biochemical derangement (transaminase concentrations in the 100s units/litre range not 1000s, alkaline phosphatase concentration low and decreasing, high bilirubin reflecting liver dysfunction in the context of haemolysis and renal failure). Overt Wilsonian neurological features are seldom present at the time that the patient presents with acute liver failure. Ultrasound examination frequently identifies splenomegaly, which suggests antecedent liver disease with portal hypertension.

Acute fatty liver of pregnancy (AFLP)
(see chapter 9)

AFLP occurs at or near term. Prognosis for mother and baby is good when delivery is expedited. Frequently, the first pregnancy is affected. Liver biochemical dysfunction is modest (transaminase concentrations in the 100s units/litre range, not 1000s). Clinical features may be more apparent or first recognized after delivery, and include asterixis, confusion (often mild), hypoglycaemia (often severe and prolonged), minimal prolongation of INR (often about 2), renal dysfunction (usually self-limiting, rarely requiring dialysis), and haematological derangement (neutrophilia, thrombocytopenia and haemolysis). The combination of <u>h</u>aemolysis, <u>e</u>levated <u>l</u>iver enzymes, and <u>l</u>ow <u>p</u>latelets is sometimes referred to as the HELLP syndrome. It is related to, and simply another perspective of, AFLP.

Other causes of acute liver failure

Malignant infiltration, acute Budd–Chiari syndrome, and ischaemia may lead to acute liver failure.

DIAGNOSIS OF ACUTE LIVER FAILURE

Diagnosis is simple: liver dysfunction is severe, acute, and is responsible for the alteration of mental state. Acute liver failure should be distinguished from conditions that have altered conscious state *associated with* abnormal liver function, but not *caused by* liver failure. Such conditions include:

1. The syndrome observed after major circulatory collapse, including very high serum transaminase concentrations ("ischaemic hepatitis": 1000s units/litre range, not 100s), renal dysfunction, and cerebral dysfunction. Prognosis depends on the cause of the circulatory collapse; if the cause of collapse is remediable, liver dysfunction resolves quickly.
2. Multiple drug overdose, including hepatotoxic and sedative substances.
3. Severe sepsis syndrome is frequently associated with deranged liver biochemistry and altered mental state.

Of the routinely available laboratory blood tests, the prothrombin time (INR) gives the best estimate of the severity of liver dysfunction. It is not possible to substantiate a diagnosis of acute liver failure unless the INR is significantly prolonged. In patients with acute viral hepatitis and drug-induced necrosis, the serum transaminase concentrations may be extremely great, but without prolongation of the INR and without development of acute liver failure. In particular, paracetamol poisoning may be associated with serum transaminases in excess of 10 000 IU/litre, without the associated or subsequent development of acute liver failure.

Acute liver failure should be considered in the differential diagnosis of any patient with altered conscious state, in the presence or absence of jaundice; clinically apparent jaundice may be absent or missed when acute liver failure is very acute.

INVESTIGATIONS

Investigations aim to establish the cause and severity of acute liver damage. When the patient is seen before the development of encephalopathy, appropriate investigation may determine the likelihood of progression to acute liver failure. Paracetamol poisoning, which has a well-defined clinical course and prognostic determinants, will be discussed separately. Most poisoned patients admit to the overdose, but poisoning should be excluded in all cases of acute liver failure of unclear aetiology.

Appropriate investigations include, therefore:

1. *Blood paracetamol concentrations*: Cautious interpretation of blood concentrations of paracetamol is essential. Paracetamol may have been cleared from blood during the first 24 h or so after poisoning, so the drug may be undetectable despite causation. Also, some patients take paracetamol for prodromal symptoms of acute liver failure that is due to other causes. Under that circumstance, paracetamol may be detected in blood, but is not the cause of acute liver failure.
2. *Hepatitis virus serology*: Factors sought should include HAV immunoglobulin M (IgM) antibodies, hepatitis B surface antigen, and hepatitis B core antigen IgM antibodies.
3. *Serum ceruloplasmin*: In patients with acute Wilson's disease, serum ceruloplasmin concentrations are usually low or low/normal. Remember that acute Wilson's disease is frequently associated with haemolysis. Ask for a blood film and reticulocyte count when acute liver failure is associated with anaemia.
4. *Autoantibodies and serum immunoglobulins*: Cautious interpretation of autoantibodies in low titre is necessary, as these may be observed in patients with seronegative hepatitis.
5. *Doppler ultrasound*: This examination may permit recognition of malignant infiltration and acute Budd–Chiari syndrome. Liver size and texture are of interest. Liver size is usually normal or diminished in acute liver failure. Liver enlargement raises the possibility of malignant infiltration, and suggests the need for liver biopsy. Abnormal liver texture, including regenerative nodules, may be observed in acute liver failure. Splenic enlargement may suggest antecedent liver disease. Ascites is common when acute liver failure is subacute.
6. *Liver biopsy*: Biopsy is not indicated unless the liver is enlarged, as the procedure is hazardous. Occasionally, it may be difficult to distinguish subacute liver failure from decompensated cirrhosis. Histology may be helpful, but should only be undertaken if the result will influence management.

CLINICAL FEATURES AND THEIR MANAGEMENT

Acute liver failure is a rare disease. The keys to successful management are early recognition of the syndrome and appropriate triage to specialist units. An important component of care may include liver transplantation; in the UK, therefore, expertise in the management of acute liver failure is now focused in those specialist centres that can offer transplantation to selected patients. Of course, the results of conservative management (i.e. without transplantation) by these units are likely to be superior to those achieved by physicians with little or no experience in the management of this condition.

Immediate management

Hypoglycaemia may be a problem at presentation, and almost invariably develops during the course of acute liver failure. Treatment of hypoglycaemia is ideally achieved by infusion of 50% glucose, rate-adjusted to maintain blood glucose at the upper limit of normal range; the blood glucose concentration should be measured hourly. Frequently, high infusion rates are required, and the rate may provide some index of hepatic deterioration or recovery. Hypertonic glucose solutions require administration via a central venous line. Central lines, either subclavian or via the internal jugular route, may be placed safely by experienced practitioners without the need to correct coagulopathy.

Coagulopathy results from diminished production of clotting factors; an element of consumption may also contribute. Prothrombin time provides an adequate index of the severity of the coagulopathy. Specific clotting factor measurement is interesting, but not essential for management. Severe thrombocytopenia is occasionally observed in patients with serious paracetamol poisoning. Correction of coagulopathy is indicated when there is clinically significant bleeding, but is not required before placement of catheters for vascular access.

Haemodynamic instability is a frequent accompaniment of acute liver failure. Typically, hypotension associated with low vascular resistance and high cardiac output are observed. Furthermore, acute liver failure is often complicated by sepsis, which also causes a hyperdynamic circulation. Most patients, particularly those with paracetamol poisoning, are hypovolaemic at presentation. Hypovolaemia and low vascular resistance can cause profound hypotension. When the neck veins are empty, volume resuscitation can be aggressive and should begin before central lines are placed. Subsequently, measurement of central venous pressures will be an aid to resuscitation. When hypotension is associated with clinical signs of a hyperdynamic circulation, noradrenaline is the pressor agent of choice; it should be infused via the central venous line. Severe acute liver failure is frequently characterized by a rapidly escalating requirement for noradrenaline, associated with progressive metabolic acidosis. These features suggest a poor prognosis.

NAC and **prostacyclin** enhance tissue oxygen uptake and utilization in all patients with acute liver failure (3). The ideal regimen for administration of NAC has not been defined; our practice is to establish a continuous infusion at a rate of 15 mg/kg per 24 h, and to continue the infusion until death or recovery is certain. Severe acute liver failure is nearly always complicated by acute renal failure; continuous venovenous haemofiltration (CVVH) is probably the ideal therapy. Prostacyclin may prevent activation of the platelet in the CVVH circuit, and appears to have added beneficial effects on the patient's microcirculation.

Haemorrhagic gastritis should be prevented by acid-suppression treatment; gastritis is a potentially fatal complication of acute liver failure. It is our practice to administer intravenous ranitidine from the time of the patient's admission to hospital. Blood-stained vomitus is not an indication for endoscopy.

Sepsis, bacterial and fungal, frequently complicates acute liver failure, and their haemodynamic consequences may be difficult to recognize in this context. Patients with severe acute liver failure need broad-spectrum antibacterial prophylaxis from the time of their admission to hospital. Antifungal prophylaxis also appears beneficial. *Candida albicans* is the most frequently identified cause of fungal sepsis in acute liver failure; fluconazole 100 mg/day appears to prevent invasive infection by this organism. When the illness is prolonged, and if transplantation is subsequently required, consideration should be given to the early introduction of antifungal agents with a broader spectrum (such as one of the lipid-associated amphotericin preparations).

The **encephalopathy** that develops during acute liver failure is frequently chracterized by agitation and delerium instead of increasing somnolence, whereas the encephalopathy complicating subacute liver failure more closely resembles that associated with decompensation of chronic liver disease. There is no evidence that lactulose, neomycin or enemas retard the development of encephalopathy in acute liver failure; probably, they should be avoided.

Cerebral oedema is more likely to complicate acute liver failure at the acute end of the spectrum, such as that associated with paracetamol poisoning. Clinical signs of cerebral oedema include sudden haemodynamic change (probably, tachycardia is observed more frequently than bradycardia) and pupillary dilatation, irregularity, or inequality. Under these circumstances, treatment with mannitol (100 ml of a 20% solution) is indicated, and may be repeated as required. Failure to respond to mannitol is an indication for thiopentone. At this juncture, discussion with the specialist unit should have been undertaken. Cerebral oedema probably develops during or after the progression to confusion and agitation has been observed. When agitation develops and when clinical features suggest that progression to more advanced coma is likely, sedation, intubation of the trachea, and mechanical ventilation are indicated. There is no merit in restraining an agitated patient. Sedation, and intubation of the trachea permit safe control of ventilation and essential patient monitoring. When a patient with progressive (or predicted) encephalopathy requires transfer to another hospital, sedation and intubation should be undertaken before the transfer. In the specialist centre, intracranial pressure monitoring and measurement of jugular venous oxygen content permit assessment of cerebral oedema and cerebral oxygenation. The referring physician must depend on clinical signs of cerebral swelling, which are notoriously unreliable in acute liver failure. It is important, therefore, to undertake **measures that will prevent or retard the development of cerebral oedema**, including:

1. Early intervention by sedation of the agitated patient and ventilation of the lungs. Some units recommend paralysis. Certainly, sedation should be profound and should prevent coughing.

2. Maintenance of mean arterial blood pressure with adequate volume resuscitation and pressors.
3. Optimization of partial pressures of arterial blood-gases: oxygen to 10 kPa, and carbon dioxide to 4 kPa (there is no merit in hyperventilation). Of course, an arterial line is required.
4. Avoidance of noxious stimuli. We also infuse narcotics.
5. Slight flexion of the upper body to raise the head — not flexion of the head on the body, as this can impair cerebral venous drainage.

Renal failure is almost invariably observed as a complication of severe paracetamol poisoning. Frequently, oliguria or anuria is established at the time of presentation. Renal failure is a delayed development in acute liver failure from other causes, and reflects the severity of the condition. Intravascular volume depletion aggravates the renal dysfunction and should be corrected. Haemofiltration or haemodialysis may be required. CVVH permits adequate control of chemistry and fluid balance, and avoids the haemodynamic stress that complicates intermittent haemodialysis. Unless fluid overload or electrolyte disturbance dictate an immediate need, CVVH can usually be deferred until the patient's prognosis is clear. At that stage, the majority of patients will be sedated, with the trachea intubated, and dual-lumen dialysis lines are easily placed.

Nutritional support is difficult to provide for the patient with acute liver failure: most critically ill intensive care patients, including those with acute liver failure, have gastroparesis. Consequently, attempts at nasogastric feeding frequently fail. In addition, passage of the nasogastric tube may be complicated by troublesome nasopharyngeal bleeding, and constitutes a noxious experience that may aggravate cerebral oedema. The author does not recommend routine passage of a nasogastric tube.

ASSESSMENT OF PROGNOSIS

An accurate assessment of prognosis determines:

1. **The need for referral to a specialist unit or for management by local experts in the presenting hospital**. For many patients that present before the development of hepatic encephalopathy, a poor prognosis is easily predicted and immediate transfer to a specialist unit should be arranged. This minimizes the risks associated with transfer of the critically ill patient in acute liver failure and with incipient or established cerebral oedema.
2. **The need for liver transplantation or for conservative management**.

Paracetamol poisoning

The majority of poisoned patients present within 12 h of poisoning, are effectively treated with NAC, experience no significant liver damage, and are never seen again. They have no real suicidal intent. Poisoning is usually an impulsive act, undertaken in the late evening or early morning. Acute alcohol excess is frequently associated. Liver damage becomes increasingly likely as the interval from poisoning to administration of NAC increases. NAC should be given to poisoned patients with blood concentrations of paracetamol greater than the cut-off value for treatment more than 4 h after the overdose, to all patients who present more than 12 h after the overdose, to those patients that have taken a staggered overdose, and to unreliable (or unconscious) historians (4).

Those predisposed to paracetamol hepatotoxicity are:

1. people with chronic heavy alcohol ingestion (reduces hepatic glutathione) (5)
2. people with eating disorders (reduces hepatic glutathione)
3. people taking cytochrome-inducing drugs such as anticonvulsants

For these at-risk patients, NAC treatment is indicated at lower blood paracetamol concentrations.

Significant hepatotoxicity should be anticipated when NAC treatment is commenced more than 12 h after poisoning. Under this circumstance, and if liver damage is already apparent at the time of presentation, careful observation of the inpatient is indicated. Serum electrolyte concentrations, liver function tests, blood count, and prothrombin time (INR) should be checked daily until it is clear that clinically significant liver damage has not been experienced. Significant liver damage will not be observed if the INR is normal 48 h after overdose. Significant increases in serum transaminase concentration may be observed, but are of no concern in the context of a normal INR. The magnitude of liver damage is reflected by the INR, which usually peaks on the third day after the overdose. Gross prolongation of the prothrombin time (INR >10) may be observed without the development of liver failure.

Severe liver damage is frequently associated with the development of renal failure. Occasionally, renal failure will be observed despite minimal prolongation of the INR. **Indications for referral to** (or, at least, discussion with) **a specialist unit** include:

1. A prothrombin time (in seconds) greater in magnitude than the interval from overdose to the time of measurement (in hours). For example, a prothrombin time of 60 s measured 48 h after the overdose would be sufficient indication for patient referral.
2. Prothrombin time still increasing on the fourth day after the overdose (usually, criterion number 1 has already been fulfilled).
3. Serum creatinine concentration greater than 150 µmol/litre at presentation.
4. Arterial blood pH less than 7.30 at any time (it is useful to check venous blood pH in all patients at the time of presentation: if venous pH is greater than 7.30, arterial puncture is not required).
5. Encephalopathy or hypoglycaemia (patients have usually fulfilled at least one of the first 4 criteria).

Acute liver failure not caused by paracetamol

Hepatic encephalopathy is an indication for immediate referral to a specialist unit. Sometimes, the progression to acute liver failure can be anticipated and referral can be made before the development of encephalopathy. Aetiology is the principal determinant of prognosis: most cases of acute viral hepatitis A and B are self-limiting. Serum transaminase and bilirubin concentrations can be grossly increased, but INR is usually normal. **Indications for referral to a liver unit** include:

1. hepatic encephalopathy
2. INR >1.5 at any time
3. hepatorenal failure — sometimes observed in patients with subacute liver failure before development of encephalopathy
4. acute Wilson's disease

CONSERVATIVE MANAGEMENT OR LIVER TRANSPLANTATION?

Liver transplantation is the preferred treatment for selected patients with acute liver failure (6). The following clinical and laboratory features predict a poor outcome for conservative management (7).

Paracetamol poisoning

1. Arterial pH less than 7.30, measured on the second day after the overdose. Early acidosis, measured within 24 h of poisoning, is a less reliable predictor of outcome, and frequently resolves with fluid resuscitation.
2. Prothrombin time greater than 100 s and serum creatinine concentration greater than 300 µmol/litre in a patient with grade 3 or 4 encephalopathy (see chapter 22.2 for encephalopathy grading system).

The results of liver transplantation are probably superior to conservative management of patients that fulfil either of these criteria. However, as a result of recent improvements in the management of poisoned patients (in particular, the routine use of NAC), the predictive accuracy of these criteria is now uncertain (8,9). Patients who fulfil these criteria may survive with conservative management. Potential obstacles to successful rehabilitation post-transplantation should be identified before a patient is put forward for transplantation. For instance, it is unlikely that a patient with deep-seated psychiatric problems could cope with the rigours of emergency liver transplantation and post-transplant care; transplantation may have a significant adverse impact on the psychiatric condition and prognosis. Under this circumstance, conservative management may be more appropriate.

Acute liver failure not caused by paracetamol

The following criteria suggest a poor outcome for conservative management:

1. The aetiology of the acute liver failure: seronegative hepatitis and idiosyncratic drug reactions have a poor prognosis. Failure caused by Wilson's disease is nearly always an indication for immediate liver transplantation.
2. Age younger than 10 years or older than 40 years.

3. Long interval (more than 7 days) from appearance of jaundice to development of encephalopathy.
4. Serum bilirubin concentration greater than 300 μmol/litre.
5. Prothrombin time greater than 50 s.

Therefore, **liver transplantation is indicated when**:

- the predicted outcome of conservative management is poor
- there are no physical or psychiatric contraindications
- the predicted outcome of transplantation is acceptable

In the last category, although each case is assessed on its own merits, transplantation of a patient *in extremis* may be inappropriate. Inferior results are predicted for older patients with acute liver failure and pre-transplant renal failure. There is a shortage of donor livers, and waiting-list mortality is increasing. Therefore, the patient with acute liver failure may be competing for resources (in particular, the donor liver) with a patient with chronic liver disease for whom a 90% graft and patient survival is predicted. The allocation of donor organs must reconcile the immediate need of the patient with acute liver failure and the demands of expanding transplant waiting-lists.

Most liver transplantation involves implantation of the entire donor liver into the orthotopic position. Auxiliary partial orthotopic liver transplantation (APOLT) involves partial recipient hepatectomy (usually the left lobe) and then orthotopic implantation of part of the donor liver (usually the left lobe) (10). The theoretical advantage of APOLT is that regeneration of the recipient's own liver may be observed, and immunosuppression might be withdrawn. This avoids some of the long-term morbidity associated with the indefinite need for immunosuppression. However, reflecting the more complex technical aspects of the surgical procedure, results of APOLT may be inferior to those achieved by conventional liver transplantation. Randomized trials have not been undertaken to compare APOLT with conventional transplantation.

EXTRACORPOREAL BIOARTIFICIAL LIVER SUPPORT

There is increasing interest in development of bioartificial livers for the treatment of patients with acute liver failure. Theoretically, the bioartificial liver might sustain life pending availability of a suitable liver for transplantation — a so-called **bridge to transplantation**. It might also sustain life until the patient's own liver recovers spontaneously, obviating the need for transplantation. A single randomized study has been published, but it failed to demonstrate benefit for treated patients (11). However, a greater than expected survival rate was observed for the control group in that study, so it was impossible to show a survival advantage of treatment by means of bioartificial livers. Further controlled studies are required, although concerns as to the biological components of these livers (for example, porcine endogenous retroviruses) will retard clinical development of this type of technology.

References
1. Mutimer DJ, Shaw J, Neuberger JM *et al.*. Failure to incriminate hepatitis B, hepatitis C and hepatitis E viruses in the aetiology of fulminant non-A, non-B hepatitis. *Gut* 1995; **36**: 433–436.
   One of a number of studies that fail to identify a viral aetiology for fulminant non-A, non-B hepatitis.
2. Ellis AJ, Saleh M, Smith H *et al.* Late-onset hepatic failure: clinical features, serology and outcome following transplantation. *J Hepatology* 1995; **23**: 363–372.
   A comprehensive review of the King's College Hospital experience in the management of subacute liver failure.
3. Harrison PM, Wendon JA, Gimson AES *et al.* Improvement by acetylcysteine of haemodynamics and oxygen transport in fulminant hepatic failure. *N Engl J Med* 1991; **324**: 1852–1857.
   Careful physiological studies showed haemodynamic benefits for patients with acute liver failure, regardless of aetiology. This work provides a rationale for routine administration of NAC to all patients with acute liver failure, from the time of their admission to hospital.
4. O'Grady JG. Paracetamol-induced acute liver failure: prevention and management. *J Hepatology* 1997; **26 (suppl 1)**: 41–46.
   A recent and comprehensive review of the subject.
5. Lauterurg BH, Velez ME. Glutathione deficiency in alcoholics: risk factor for paracetamol hepatotoxicity. *Gut* 1988; **29**: 1153–1157.
   Data suggest a mechanism to explain the apparently increased sensitivity to paracetamol toxicity, in patients with chronic alcoholism.

6. Mutimer DJ, Elias E. Liver transplantation for fulminant hepatic failure. *Prog Liver Dis* 1992; **10**: 349–367.
    A comprehensive review of the subject — little has changed since publication.

7. O'Grady JG, Alexander GJM, Hayllar KM *et al.* Early indicators of prognosis in fulminant hepatic failure. *Gastroenterology* 1989; **97**: 439–445.
    An extremely important analysis of prognostic factors in acute liver failure. Provides a basis for selection of patients for liver transplantation.

8. Harrison PM, Keays R, Bray GP *et al.* Improved outcome of paracetamol-induced fulminant hepatic failure by late administration of acetylcysteine. *Lancet* 1990; **335**: 1572–1573.

9. Mutimer DJ, Ayres RCS, Neuberger JM *et al.* Serious paracetamol poisoning and the results of liver transplantation. *Gut* 1994; **35**: 809–814.
    A description of our own experience at the Queen Elizabeth Hospital, Birmingham. Data suggest that transplantation is the appropriate treatment for selected patients with paracetamol-induced acute liver failure.

10. Chenard-Neu M-P, Boudjema K, Bernuau J *et al.* Auxiliary liver transplantation: regeneration of the native liver and outcome in 30 patients with fulminant hepatic failure — a multicentre European Study. *Hepatology* 1996; **23**: 1119–1127.
    This paper describes the outcome in 30 patients with acute liver failure who underwent auxiliary transplantation. Regeneration of the native liver, permitting withdrawal of immunosuppression, was observed for many.

11. Ellis AJ, Hughes RD, Wendon JA *et al.* Pilot controlled trial of the extracorporeal liver assist device in acute liver failure. *Hepatology* 1996; **24**: 1446–1451.
    The only published controlled trial of bioartificial liver support for acute liver failure.

22.2.   Liver Failure: Chronic Liver Disease

DAVID MUTIMER and ANDREW DOUDS

INTRODUCTION

Many of the complications of cirrhosis (bleeding as a result of portal hypertension, ascites and spontaneous bacterial peritonitis, hepatocellular carcinoma) are discussed elsewhere in this volume (see Chapters 11.2, 18.2, and 19). This chapter is mainly concerned with the features of hepatic encephalopathy, and a discussion of some of the causes of chronic liver disease.

HEPATIC ENCEPHALOPATHY

Hepatic encephalopathy is a potentially reversible neuropsychiatric syndrome that is typically observed in the context of severe liver dysfunction (1). It is occasionally observed in patients with large portosystemic shunts without cirrhosis; under this circumstance, the development of clinically evident hepatic encephalopathy requires a major precipitant.

The condition may be subclinical or overt.

Subclinical hepatic encephalopathy

Subclinical hepatic encephalopathy is associated with an abnormal electroencephalogram, and can be diagnosed by psychometric tests (e.g. the Reitan trail test). The impact of the condition on the patient's quality of life is uncertain. Intellectually demanding work might suffer. It has been suggested that ability to control machinery (including motor vehicles) might be impaired; what advice should be given to the driver of heavy goods vehicles who has subclinical encephalopathy? Performance of psychometric tests improves with antiencephalopathy regimens, therefore, treatment might be recommended for selected patients with subclinical hepatic encephalopathy.

Overt hepatic encephalopathy

Overt hepatic encephalopathy is associated with alteration of consciousness and with a generalized movement disorder. The spectrum of the latter is remarkable; it includes pyramidal (spasticity, hyperreflexia, up-going plantar response), and extrapyramidal (Parkinsonian features, bradykinesia, mask-like facies) syndromes. Hepatic encephalopathy should be considered when a patient with cirrhosis develops any neuropsychiatric syndrome.

Overt hepatic encephalopathy is usually graded, and a number of closely related schemes are available. A reasonable consensus is:

1. *Grade 1*: Clear impairment of higher neurological functions such as arithmetic, but no apparent impairment of conscious state. Asterixis is present.
2. *Grade 2*: Disorientation and personality change with inappropriate behaviour.
3. *Grade 3*: Confusion and gross disorientation with increasing somnolence.
4. *Grade 4*: Coma.

When grades 3 and 4 coma have been achieved, some clinicians apply the Glasgow Coma Scale

(15/15 is the best achievable score). This may per-mit a more precise objective measurement of dete-rioration or response to treatment.

Hepatic encephalopathy is a clinical diagnosis. It should be the provisional diagnosis when a patient with liver disease develops any neuropsychiatric symptoms or syndrome. Frequently, a precipitant can be identified. **Common precipitants** include:

1. sepsis (blood and ascitic fluid must be cultured)
2. dehydration/intravascular volume depletion (fre-quently diuretic-induced)
3. hypokalaemia (diuretic-induced)
4. medication (sedatives, analgesics, antiemetics)
5. variceal haemorrhage
6. constipation
7. dietary protein loading.

Investigations are undertaken to identify the precipitants; specific treatment targets the identifi-able precipitants. In addition, the lower bowel should be cleared (by enema) and lactulose should be given (by nasogastric tube if necessary).

Prompt resolution of symptoms is expected, and resolution confirms the provisional diagnosis of hepatic encephalopathy. Resolution is observed during a 24–48 h period. Persistence of symptoms beyond this duration suggests that this provisional diagnosis might not be correct. Other causes of impaired conscious state, including intracranial pa-thology and other forms of intoxication, should then be reconsidered.

TREATMENT OF HEPATIC ENCEPHALOPATHY

Treatment strategies include:

1. management of constipation
2. lactulose
3. neomycin
4. manipulation of dietary protein
5. liver transplantation

Lactulose should be given for treatment and prevention of hepatic encephalopathy. For the pa-tient with advanced stages of the condition (grade 3 or 4), lactulose can be given by nasogastric tube. Treatment aims to establish, and to maintain, at least two semi-solid bowel actions per day. After

resolution of overt hepatic encephalopathy, the pa-tient (or carer) should be encouraged to adjust the dose of lactulose to achieve this bowel frequency. Lactulose prevents constipation and affects bowel flora in a way that reduces the production and absorption of unfavourable nitrogenous substances.

Neomycin has a role in the management of overt hepatic encephalopathy, but it is potentially neph-rotoxic and ototoxic, and its use must be short term (48 h maximum).

For the prevention of hepatic encephalopathy, **dietary protein intake** may be restricted. This may, however, adversely affect the patient's nutritional status. Evidence suggests that vegetable-derived protein may be less harmful than animal-derived protein.

Flumazenil is of little or no clinical benefit for the majority of patients with overt hepatic encepha-lopathy. Use of benzodiazepines, however, is fairly ubiquitous. Flumazenil is more likely to be benefi-cial when the encephalopathy is precipitated by the use of benzodiazepines.

Hepatic encephalopathy is, typically, a late de-velopment in the natural history of chronic liver disease. Frequently, even when a precipitant can be identified, the condition signifies gross impairment of hepatic reserve. Therefore, in the absence of contraindications, the patient who develops the overt form should be considered for liver transplantation.

COMMON CHRONIC LIVER DISEASES

Alcoholic liver disease and viral hepatitis are dis-cussed elsewhere in this volume (see Chapters 23 and 41). In this section, mention will be made of primary biliary cirrhosis, primary sclerosing cholan-gitis, autoimmune chronic active hepatitis, haemo-chromatosis, and Wilson's disease.

Primary biliary cirrhosis

Key points in relation to primary biliary cirrhosis (PBC) can be summarized as:

- anti-mitochondrial antibody (AMA) titre >1:40 is highly suggestive of PBC
- PBC is commonly associated with other autoimmune diseases
- ursodeoxycholic acid (UDCA) is widely used, but the magnitude of treatment benefit is uncertain

- liver transplantation should be considered when the serum bilirubin concentration is greater than 100 μmol/litre.

Epidemiology and genetics

PBC is predominantly a disease of women. The prevalence in the United Kingdom appears to be increasing and the current estimate is about 250 per million. The increasing incidence may, in part, be explained by the more prevalent practice of biochemical and immunological screening. Familial clustering has been described, but there is no consistent human leucocyte antigen (HLA) association.

Clinical features

Frequently, the disease is diagnosed at an asymptomatic stage. Non-specific symptoms may be disabling, and include profound lethargy. **Pruritus** is the most common presenting symptom. **Jaundice** is a late development in the natural history of the disease (2). **Other clinical features** include hepatomegaly, xanthelasma, and osteoporosis. Associated **autoimmune diseases** are common. **Hypothyroidism** is particularly common, and thyroid function should be checked regularly during follow-up. PBC is associated with coeliac disease, which should be excluded when anaemia is present.

Diagnosis

Liver function tests are cholestatic, with increased concentrations of γ-glutamyltransferase and alkaline phosphatase. Serum bilirubin is normal in the early stages. The presence of AMAs (titre >1:40) is highly suggestive of PBC; other diagnoses should be considered when the AMA is negative. Histological features may be characteristic, and include inflammation, then loss, of interlobular bile ducts. The need for liver biopsy of a patient with AMA and cholestatic chemistry is uncertain; probably, it is seldom necessary.

Treatment

Pruritus may be difficult to control. Candidate **drugs** include cholestyramine, antihistamines, UDCA, naloxone, rifampicin, and phenobarbitone. In practice, symptoms are usually controlled by cholestyramine, which should be given with break-

fast. In refractory cases, referral for **liver transplantation** should be considered. Fat-soluble vitamin deficiency is frequently observed, and **supplements of vitamins** A and D should be given (by intramuscular injection).

Randomized controlled trials and meta-analysis have shown that UDCA improves liver function tests and delays disease progression (3). It is well tolerated, with a good side-effect profile. Other drugs — including colchicine, methotrexate, azathioprine, penicillamine, corticosteroids, and cyclosporin — have been used. Most of them improve biochemistry, but clinical benefit is unproven and side effects may be significant. Liver transplantation is the treatment of choice for advanced disease. Five-year survival after transplantation for PBC is of the order of 90%. The timing of transplantation is important. The most useful **prognostic marker** is the serum bilirubin. The median survival of a cohort of PBC patients with serum bilirubin of 150 μmol/litre is 18 months; most will die within 2 years; transplantation should be considered once the bilirubin concentration is 100 μmol/litre. PBC frequently recurs after transplantation, but few patients develop symptoms of recurrence during the 10 years after transplantation.

Primary sclerosing cholangitis

Key features in primary sclerosing cholangitis (PSC) include:

- PSC is commonly (75%) associated with inflammatory bowel disease, particularly ulcerative colitis
- the gold standard for diagnosis is endoscopic retrograde cholangiopancreatography (ERCP); magnetic resonance cholangiopancreatography (MRCP) provides inferior definition, but is safer
- PSC may be complicated by cholangiocarcinoma
- therapeutic options are limited, and UDCA is not clearly beneficial
- liver transplantation is appropriate for selected patients, although results are inferior to those achieved for PBC. Disease recurrence may be observed

Aetiology and epidemiology

The aetiology is unknown. There is an association of PSC with HLA B8 DR3 DRW52A, a haplotype that is commonly associated with autoimmune disease. Sixty-seven per cent of patients with PSC have ulcerative colitis; about 5% of patients with ulcerative colitis develop PSC. PSC is also associated with an increased risk for the development of colonic cancer in patients with ulcerative colitis.

Clinical findings

Men are affected more commonly than women. Symptoms of inflammatory bowel disease may be present, although colitis is frequently asymptomatic and unsuspected. Many cases of PSC are asymptomatic, and are diagnosed during investigation of asymptomatic cholestatic biochemistry. Patients may present with intermittent jaundice, abdominal pain, pruritus, and weight loss. Unlike PBC, in which jaundice (once it appears) is progressive, jaundice tends to fluctuate in PSC.

Diagnosis

The following criteria suggest a diagnosis of PSC:

1. Cholestatic liver function tests.
2. Negative AMA, positive perinuclear pattern of anti-neutrophil cytoplasmic antibodies.
3. No evidence of obstruction on ultrasonography.
4. ERCP or MRCP evidence of intra- and extrahepatic duct stricturing.
5. Histological findings of bile ductopenia, ductular proliferation, periductal fibrosis (onion-skin appearance), and increased copper deposition.
6. Exclusion of other causes of sclerosing cholangitis such as surgical bile-duct injury (secondary sclerosing cholangitis).

Complications

PSC may progress to biliary cirrhosis. As disease progresses, jaundice becomes persistent rather than intermittent. Bacterial cholangitis may supervene, and almost invariably complicates biliary intervention (ERCP or percutaneous transhepatic cholangiography) or biopsy. Cholestasis may be associated with steatorrhea and malabsorption of fat-soluble vitamins. Cholangiocarcinoma is a dreaded complication; sudden onset of jaundice, weight loss, and intrahepatic duct dilatation are suggestive of this condition, but the diagnosis may be difficult to establish with certainty. There is no effective screening procedure that permits early detection of cholangiocarcinoma. Smokers may have an increased risk for its development.

Management

Pruritus is a common symptom. This may be treated with the same agents that are used for the pruritus of PBC, such as cholestyramine, antihistamines, UDCA, or rifampicin. **Bacterial cholangitis** should be treated with broad-spectrum antibiotics. Continuous cyclical antibiotic therapy may be appropriate for the patient with frequent attacks of bacterial cholangitis. If a dominant **extrahepatic stricture** is believed to be responsible for repeated episodes of cholangitis, a stent may be placed endoscopically. Sometimes, however, attempts at endoscopic treatments aggravate, rather than alleviate, the situation. UDCA is of unproven clinical benefit, although further studies of its high-dose usage are required.

Cholangiocarcinoma may be resectable, but frequently extends from the main hepatic ducts into segmental branches; extensive hepatic resection may therefore be required to achieve clearance of the tumour. Hepatic resection is seldom tolerated by patients with **advanced PSC and portal hypertension**. Most units consider cholangiocarcinoma to be a contraindication to liver transplantation. Complete tumour clearance is seldom achieved despite hepatectomy, and 5 year post-transplant survival in most series has been less than 20% (an unacceptable risk in times of donor-organ shortage). Liver transplantation is the treatment of choice for patients with **endstage disease** due to PSC. Indications for transplantation include progressive and persistent jaundice, recurrent and uncontrollable episodes of bacterial cholangitis, and ascites. Portal hypertensive bleeding may be observed at a relatively early stage of disease, and is not, *per se*, an indication for transplantation.

Autoimmune chronic active hepatitis

Key points relating to autoimmune chronic active hepatitis (AICAH) are:

- generally classified into three types on the basis of autoantibody profile
- overlap syndromes may occur with PBC, PSC, or viral hepatitis

- corticosteroids are the mainstay of treatment, and are commonly used with azathioprine
- transplantation is the treatment of choice for decompensated cirrhosis, but disease recurrence may be observed

Epidemiology

Predominantly a disease of young women, AICAH may present in either sex at any age. The incidence in western Europe is 0.69 per 100 000 per annum. The haplotype HLA A1 B8 DR3 is frequently associated with AICAH.

Clinical features

The most common symptom is fatigue, with an insidious onset. Arthralgia occurs frequently. Jaundice may be the presenting symptom and is often episodic. Frequently, the patient is asymptomatic.

Spider naevi are nearly always present. The patient may present with signs or complications of portal hypertension, including ascites and variceal bleeding. All forms of autoimmune hepatitis are commonly associated with other autoimmune diseases.

Diagnosis

The following criteria are necessary to establish a diagnosis of autoimmune hepatitis:

- increased serum transaminase concentrations
- increased immunoglobulins, particularly IgG
- autoantibody positivity for: anti-nuclear antibody (ANA), smooth-muscle antibody (SMA), liver–kidney microsomal antibody (LKM), soluble liver antigen (SLA)
    - ANA+ve, SMA+ve, LKM–ve = **type 1 AICAH** (classical "lupoid" AICAH)
    - ANA–ve, SMA–ve, LKM+ve = **type 2 AICAH**
    - ANA–ve, LKM–ve, SLA+ve = **type 3 AICAH**
- histological finding of piecemeal necrosis, with or without lobular hepatitis or bridging necrosis, and no evidence of biliary features

In addition, there should be absence of hepatitis B virus surface antigen, absence of antibodies to hepatitis C virus, normal serum caeruloplasmin, and no evidence of α_1 antitrypsin liver disease.

Treatment

The need for treatment is determined by the severity of hepatic inflammatory activity; treatment is not indicated for established cirrhosis in the absence of inflammatory activity. **Corticosteroids** are the mainstay of treatment. The initial dose should be 40–60 mg/day, slowly reduced to a maintenance dose of 10 mg/day or less. Most clinicians favour the addition of azathioprine 1–1.5 mg/kg per day as the dose of steroid is reduced. Complete withdrawal of steroids should be attempted after 1 or 2 years of treatment. Azathioprine treatment can be maintained after steroid withdrawal; subsequently, it also may be withdrawn. In more than 50% of patients, withdrawal of treatment may be associated with disease relapse. Under that circumstance, treatment should be reintroduced and continued indefinitely.

Prophylactic therapy to prevent osteoporosis should probably be prescribed for patients receiving corticosteroids. Premenopausal women may be prescribed didronel, and postmenopausal women, hormone replacement therapy.

Cyclosporin can be used for disease that is resistant to steroids.

Liver transplantation should be considered for patients with endstage disease but recurrence may occur in the grafted liver.

Genetic haemochromatosis

Key features include:

- the most common recessive genetic disorder: 1 in 300 of the UK population are homozygous for the principal genetic mutation, C282Y substitution of cysteine by tyrosine at amino acid position 282 of the HFE protein
- most Northern European patients (and descendents of Northern European populations) with clinical expression of the disease are homozygous C282Y
- the family of an index patient must be screened for the condition
- clinical expression of the disease can be prevented by venesection
- patients with cirrhosis are at high risk of developing hepatocellular carcinoma

Epidemiology and genetics

Genetic haemochromatosis is most common in northern Europe, where the prevalence of homozygotes is 1 in 300. It is frequently associated with mutations of the *HFE* gene, which is located on chromosome 6. In northern Europe, and in populations derived from northern Europe, the prevalence of *HFE* mutations in patients with clinical genetic haemochromatosis is nearly 100%, but in southern Europe, the disease is observed in a significant number of patients who express a normal *HFE* gene product; therefore, other gene mutations may lead to this condition. The *HFE* gene product (an HLA class 1-like molecule) combines with β_2 microglobulin, and the complex is then expressed on the cell surface in association with the transferrin receptor, decreasing the affinity of the receptor for transferrin. Therefore, diminished expression of the HFE protein at the cell surface is associated with increased affinity of the transferrin receptor for transferrin.

In northern Europe, most genetic haemochromatosis is associated with homozygosity for C282Y. A second mutation, H63D (aspartate for histidine), is frequently observed. Clinical expression of genetic haemochromatosis may be observed in the compound heterozygote — one allele has C282Y, the other H63D. The clinical significance of homozygous H63D is uncertain.

The degree of iron overload and the associated clinical manifestations are widely variable, and suggest the importance of environmental factors. Important cofactors include sex, alcohol intake, viral hepatitis, and haemoglobinopathies (these may be more relevant in southern Europe). Expression of the disease is the result of excessive deposition of iron in tissues.

Diagnosis

Screening for the *HFE* mutation has not superseded the use of conventional biochemical tests for iron overload. Iron status should be assessed by measurement of serum transferrin saturation and serum ferritin; transferrin saturation is the more sensitive marker, as ferritin concentrations increase at a later stage. Liver biopsy, with histochemical staining and measurement of metallic iron, remains the gold standard for diagnosis. Iron content can be expressed in relation to age — the hepatic iron index — which may be more informative.

Clinical features

Haemochromatosis is underdiagnosed in the population at large; many cases are completely asymptomatic. The diagnosis should be suspected in any male patient with asymptomatic hepatomegaly and mildly abnormal liver function tests. The classical presentation is of a pigmented middle-aged male with hepatomegaly, small testes, loss of body hair, and diabetes.

Management

The key to successful management is **early diagnosis**. Adequate treatment in the precirrhotic phase results in a normal life expectancy. Patients should be venesected weekly until the serum ferritin concentration decreases to the low normal range; this often takes up to 2 years. **Venesection** improves liver function, may reverse cardiac symptoms, and can improve diabetic control. Once sufficient iron has been removed, venesection is usually necessary once every 3 months. Patients with cirrhosis need to be monitored for the development of hepatocellular carcinoma.

First-degree relatives of patients with haemochromatosis must be **screened**. An increase in transferrin saturation is the most sensitive biochemical test. When the proband has C282Y, H63D, or both, genetic testing of first-degree relatives is appropriate.

Wilson's disease

Key points relating to Wilson's disease are:

- the gene is located on chromosome 13. It is an autosomal recessive disorder with a carrier frequency of 1 in 90
- liver disease tends to present at a younger age than neurological disease
- liver disease may present as fulminant liver failure
- a normal serum caeruloplasmin concentration does not exclude Wilson's disease.
- D-penicillamine is the mainstay of treatment.
- liver transplantation may be necessary for patients with fulminant hepatitis or endstage cirrhosis.

Aetiology and pathogenesis

The hepatic, neurological, and other features of Wilson's disease results from excess deposition of copper (4). The genetic defect has been localized to chromosome 13. The *WD* gene encodes a copper-dependent, P-type ATPase that may be responsible for transporting copper into the Golgi apparatus, where it is incorporated into caeruloplasmin. Biliary excretion of copper, the principal route of copper elimination, is impaired in Wilson's disease.

Principal **clinical features** may be hepatic, neuropsychiatric, ophthalmic, haematologic, or renal.

Hepatic manifestations

Early in its course, Wilson's disease may be asymptomatic and liver function tests may be normal. **Chronic hepatitis** may present with jaundice and increased concentrations of serum transaminases, and can be indistinguishable from other forms of chronic hepatitis. At this stage, many patients do not have Kayser–Fleischer rings or neurological symptoms. Patients may present with **acute liver failure**; this frequently occurs in late teenage. It is often associated with intravascular haemolysis, profound jaundice, and renal failure. Clues to the diagnosis of fulminant Wilson's disease include a low and declining serum alkaline phosphatase concentration, increased bilirubin, and Coombs-negative haemolysis. Despite the abrupt presentation of acute Wilson's disease, cirrhosis is usually established at the time of presentation.

Compared with other forms of cirrhosis, in Wilson's disease, hepatocellular carcinoma appears to be an uncommon development.

Diagnosis

Occasionally, the diagnosis is difficult to establish or to exclude with absolute certainty. Diagnostic tests include:

1. *Serum caeruloplasmin*: Concentrations are usually low. They are also low in heterozygotes, and may be normal at the time of presentation with acute liver failure (released by massive hepatic necrosis).

2. *Serum copper*: Concentrations are usually low (but may be increased in fulminant Wilson's disease).

3. *Urinary copper*: Concentrations are increased (and may be massively increased in fulminant Wilson's disease).

4. *Liver histology*: There are no specific diagnostic features associated with liver histology.

5. *Metallic copper content of liver tissue*: This should be measured (remember that copper content is also increased in cholestatic liver diseases).

6. *Genetic screening*: Wilson's disease is associated with a number of mutations in the *WD* gene, therefore genetic screening is not simple, except for family members when the proband's mutation is already known.

Treatment

Copper chelation is the most effective form of treatment. D-Penicillamine is the treatment of choice. The starting dose is 250 mg/day, increasing to 1.5 g/day. Patients should also receive pyridoxine supplements. About 20% of patients develop side effects during the first month. A hypersensitivity-type reaction (malaise, fever, rash) is an indication for reduction in the dose, and then gradual escalation. Serious side effects that require complete withdrawal of the drug include bone-marrow suppression, significant proteinuria, myasthenia, polymyositis, and systemic lupus erythematosus. Trientine is an alternative chelating agent for those patients who exhibit unacceptable reactions to penicillamine.

Zinc may be used when chelation therapy is not tolerated. It induces the formation of copper metallothionein in intestinal cells, preventing copper absorption. The role of zinc in the treatment of established symptomatic Wilson's disease is uncertain.

Liver transplantation is the treatment of choice for fulminant Wilson's disease (no patient survives with conservative management), and for patients with decompensated chronic liver disease. The new liver excretes the body's copper excess.

All siblings of the index case must be screened for Wilson's disease.

References

1.   Jalan R, Hayes PC. Hepatic encephalopathy and ascites. *Lancet* 1997; **350**: 1309–1315.

2.   Neuberger JM. Primary biliary cirrhosis. *Lancet* 1997; **350**: 875–879.

3.   Goulis J, Leandro G, Burroughs AK. Randomised controlled trials of UDCA therapy for PBC: a meta-analysis. *Lancet* 1999; **354**: 1053–1060.
As time goes on, it appears that fewer people are convinced of the benefits of UDCA for treatment of PBC.

4.   Gitlin N. Wilson's disease: the scourge of copper. *J Hepatol* 1998; **28**: 734–739.
A review of the subject, including the molecular aspects.

23. Acute Alcoholic Hepatitis

GEOFFREY HAYDON AND PETER HAYES

The aim of this chapter is to discuss the clinical assessment and management of acute alcoholic hepatitis. Detailed attention is applied to prognostic factors and their role in determining the likely efficacy of second-line treatments such as corticosteroids. Nutritional considerations are discussed in detail.

CLINICAL FEATURES OF ACUTE ALCOHOLIC HEPATITIS

Recognition of alcoholic hepatitis, a potentially reversible injury, is an important aspect of the management of this variant of alcoholic liver injury. It usually occurs during or after a prolonged period of alcohol abuse. Although often a precursor, acute alcoholic hepatitis is not a prerequisite for the development of cirrhosis, and is often more subtle than is generally appreciated. The clinical features are summarized in Table 23.1. Its onset is heralded by anorexia, nausea, vomiting, increasing weakness, and diarrhoea. Patients are usually systemically unwell, malnourished, and pyrexial. About 30% of patients are jaundiced; spider telangiectasiae are common, and other less specific features of chronic liver disease, such as palmar erythema, are also present. Hepatomegaly, usually tender, is detectable in the majority of patients; hepatic bruits are less common, but may be localized over part of the liver. Liver failure characterized by ascites and hepatic encephalopathy (which must be differentiated from Wernicke's encephalopathy, delirium tremens, and hypoglycaemia) often occurs. Gastrointestinal bleeding can occur, but is more often caused by erosions, peptic ulceration, or a bleeding tendency than by portal hypertension. Such patients are very susceptible to infections, which are common both at presentation or later in the course of the illness.

Liver function tests are always abnormal in alcoholic hepatitis. Serum transaminase concentrations are not greatly increased (in contrast to acute

Table 23.1. Clinical features of acute alcoholic hepatitis.

	Features that may be present
Symptoms	Anorexia
	Nausea
	Vomiting
	Malaise
	Lethargy
	Diarrhoea
Signs	Fever
	Poor nutrition
	Jaundice
	Signs of chronic liver disease
	(Tender) hepatomegaly
	Hepatic bruits
	Ascites
	Encephalopathy
	Gastrointestinal haemorrhage
Laboratory indices	Increased serum transaminases
	Poor hepatic synthetic function
	Increased acute-phase proteins
	Peripheral blood macrocytosis
	Leucocytosis (irrespective of infection)
	Thrombocytopenia
	Hypokalaemia
	Hyponatraemia
	Hypocalcaemia
	Hypomagnasaemia

hepatitis A or B infection) and may even be normal. Concentrations of aspartate transaminase (AST) in excess of 500 units/litre are extremely unusual and point to another aetiology. The concentration of AST is usually greater than that of alanine transaminase (ALT), and a ratio of AST to ALT greater than 2 is present in about 70% of patients. This ratio probably reflects both pyridoxal-5-phosphate depletion and the pattern of alcohol-induced damage, which causes release of mitochondrial AST from both the liver and smooth muscle, whereas damage predominantly to hepatocytes causes an increase in ALT. However, the sensitivity and specificity of this particular index have not been tested against a wide range of non-alcoholic liver disease.

Poor synthetic function is reflected by hyperbilirubinaemia, hypoalbuminaemia, or prolongation of the prothrombin time. Concentrations of acute-phase proteins such as ferritin and C-reactive protein are commonly significantly increased, but decrease rapidly as the patient's condition improves. Peripheral blood macrocytosis is characteristic, and 50% of patients have leucocytosis, irrespective of infection. Thrombocytopenia may be a direct effect of alcohol, disappearing quickly when alcohol is withdrawn, or may result from hypersplenism of established portal hypertension. Biochemical screening commonly demonstrates hypokalaemia, hyponatraemia, hypocalcaemia, hypomagnasaemia, and hyperlipidaemia. Imaging may or may not be abnormal, depending on the extent to which cirrhosis and portal hypertension have already developed. Liver biopsy, either percutaneous in those in whom it is not precluded by deficient coagulation, or transjugular in those with prolongation of the prothrombin time, establishes the diagnosis and gives further evidence of the severity of the disease.

HISTOLOPATHOLOGICAL FEATURES OF ALCOHOLIC HEPATITIS

A number of histological changes have been recognized, any combination of which may be superimposed on a background of alcoholic steatosis or cirrhosis. The following features are always associated with alcoholic hepatitis, and are thus **diagnostic**:

1. Hepatocyte ballooning, degeneration and necrosis; these may be associated with cytoskeletal changes such as the formation of Mallory bodies.

2. A neutrophil polymorph infiltrate around dying or necrotic hepatocytes (spotty necrosis).
3. Pericellular and perivenular fibrosis.

Features that sometimes occur, but are **not specific for the diagnosis** of alcoholic liver disease include:

1. Confluent areas of necrosis.
2. Venopathies, including thrombosis and fibrous obliteration of terminal hepatic veins.
3. Ductal metaplasia of hepatocytes and cholangiolitis.
4. Cholestasis.

LABORATORY TESTS IN THE PROGNOSIS OF ALCOHOLIC HEPATITIS

The prognosis for a particular episode of alcoholic hepatitis depends on its severity. Malnutrition, jaundice, fluid retention, and encephalopathy are therefore all associated with a poor outlook. Laboratory investigations can also act as a guide to prognosis; the "**discriminant function**" (DF) was originally developed to identify patients with severe alcoholic hepatitis in whom there was a high short-term mortality and who should be considered for treatment with corticosteroids (1); this is discussed further later in this chapter. The DF is calculated from measurement of the serum bilirubin concentration (μmol/litre) and prothrombin time (s) using the following equation:

$$DF = 4.6 \text{ (prothrombin time} - \text{control time)} + \text{(serum bilirubin/17.1)}$$

Values of 32 or greater denote severe disease, with a 4-week mortality greater than 35%; it has been suggested that this subgroup of patients merits treatment with corticosteroids (2). The value of the DF as a guide to short-term prognosis in acute alcoholic hepatitis has also been confirmed in a series of biopsy-proven cases; values greater than 32 were associated with a 2-month mortality of 50% (3).

Serum creatinine, although not assessed in terms of DF, is also an important laboratory parameter indicative of prognosis in alcoholic hepatitis. One study assessed the management and outcome of 15 patients with severe alcoholic hepatitis complicated by renal failure, who were admitted consecutively to a specialist liver unit. Fourteen of them were managed conservatively; the other one underwent liver transplantation. Among the group of 14, 11 underwent renal dialysis for a mean of 24 days. Three patients, including two requiring dialysis, recovered renal function; however, 12 of the 14 eventually died, the cause of death usually bacterial or fungal sepsis. The authors concluded that most patients with renal failure complicating severe alcoholic hepatitis will die, despite intensive care that includes renal dialysis (4).

The value of **histological examination** in alcoholic hepatitis lies not only in confirming the diagnosis, but also indicating the prognosis. Several prospective trials have evaluated the significance of selected histological features in alcoholic hepatitis, and have provided strong evidence that histology is the single most important indicator of long-term prognosis in the assessment of individual patients. These studies have suggested that the probability of chronic alcoholic hepatitis developing into cirrhosis is about 10–20% per year. In the case of acute alcoholic hepatitis, data suggest that 50–60% of patients with histologically confirmed alcoholic hepatitis are alive after 2 years.

SHORT-TERM TREATMENT OF ACUTE ALCOHOLIC HEPATITIS

General measures for treatment include abstinence from alcohol, nutritional support, correction of vitamin deficiencies, dietary adjustment for ascites and encephalopathy, and management of specific complications such as bleeding and infections. Patients with mild to moderate hepatitis may demonstrate a marked improvement in their condition with these measures, and will not require more specific treatment. In contrast, patients who are severely ill with deep jaundice, hepatic enecephalopathy, and marked increase in prothrombin time have a 30–50% (i.e. 1–3 months) mortality and are candidates for more specific treatment. As the pathogenesis of acute alcoholic hepatitis has not been clarified, specific treatment has been empirical and many agents have been tried for short-term treatment.

Nutrition in acute alcoholic hepatitis

Many patients with alcoholic hepatitis have objective signs of malnutrition and a negative nitrogen balance; there are several findings suggesting that nutritional therapy may be beneficial.

The importance of **protein** in the maintenance of the normal structure and function of the liver outweighs that of fat and carbohydrate. Protein deprivation has profound effects, including marked depletion of liver protein stores, breakdown of hepatocellular protein and RNA, and conversion of polysomes to free ribosomes, especially in the rough endoplasmic reticulum where albumin synthesis occurs. Re-feeding of starved animals with a total amino acid mixture corrects polyribosome disintegration and moves protein synthesis towards normal within hours.

The majority of patients admitted with alcoholic liver disease, whatever its manifestation are moderately or severely **malnourished**. In eight studies reporting 362 patients, 87% had anorexia, 55% had nausea or vomiting, and 60% had weight loss. Protein-energy malnutrition scores have been shown to correlate with the severity of histological disease and prognosis, and multiple vitamin deficiencies have been consistently demonstrated. These observations are the basis of the nutritional hypothesis of alcoholic liver disease: as such patients may consume 250 g of alcohol (29.8 kJ) each day, it is clear that 50% or more of the total energy ingested may come from alcohol, increasing the metabolic requirement for various vitamins and minerals. This hypothesis suggests that malnutrition should be considered a metabolic and exogenous complication of alcoholism that may add to, but is not responsible for alcoholic liver disease. Indeed, there is no good evidence that a good diet will protect against the damage produced by alcohol in the liver.

Conversely, it is unclear whether or not nutritional therapy influences the course of acute alcoholic hepatitis. Certainly, it does not influence the vascular complications of alcoholic hepatitis, but it might aid acutely the recovery of parenchymal function. With the anorexia of the illness and the common occurrence of nausea and vomiting in the disease, patients find it difficult to eat a balanced diet of adequate energy intake. In most studies, the average non-alcoholic energy intake is less than 4.2 kJ — inadequate for either normal bodily function or repair of any disease process. There are several reported studies in which the energy intake in alcoholic patients was supplemented by special formulas either given orally or by enteral intubation. This strategy has successfully improved measures of nutrition, compared with control individuals receiving hospital diets alone, and has not precipitated complications such as salt and water retention or encephalopathy. Data on histological changes within the liver are conflicting, although comparisons are difficult because of different inclusion criteria and methodology.

The first studies reported in the 1970s and 1980s included only small groups and were uncontrolled. In the USA Veterans' Administration cooperative study (5), 23 patients with clinical or biopsy-proven alcoholic hepatitis were assigned randomly to groups to receive supplementary enteral alimentation containing branched-chain amino acids and were compared with 34 patients assigned to a hospital diet alone. The total energy and protein intakes in the diet-supplemented group were 20–30% greater than in the control group, although there was no overall difference in mortality. Encephalopathy and ascites improved in both groups; however, serum albumin and total lymphocytes failed to show a significant improvement in the supplemented patients compared with controls. In a concurrent study that randomly assigned 64 patients to supplements or diet alone, perhaps because of a greater severity of illness, the diet-supplemented patients did not attain a significantly more positive nitrogen balance, and there was no difference in morbidity or mortality between the two groups. Although most studies have demonstrated improvement in conventional liver tests during energy supplementation, a difference between controls and treatment groups at the completion of randomized studies was not apparent.

To summarize the available data, it seems that patients with alcoholic hepatitis are commonly nutritionally deficient, and that this undoubtedly contributes to morbidity and mortality, although it is not responsible for the hepatic histology of the disease. It appears that protein supplements speed recovery of nutritional and liver function tests, although statistically significant results probably require longer periods of study than those used to date. The suggestion that intravenous amino acids may be more effective than oral intake is highly controversial, and not borne out by published data. There are also no convincing data demonstrating that branched-chain amino acids are more effective or safer than cheaper forms of protein. Finally, intravenous treatment carries the associated risk of sepsis, whereas chronic enteral nutrition may have the risk of precipitating variceal haemorrhage.

Vigorous protein supplementation does not appear to precipitate or worsen either encephalopathy or ascites.

It may be concluded that enteral or parenteral nutrition should be reserved for more seriously ill patients. Unlike the use of corticosteroids in alcoholic hepatitis, this treatment strategy can not be guided by determination of the value of DF. Protein may improve function of hepatic subcellular elements, without direct reference to the overall nutritional status of the body.

The role of corticosteroids in the treatment of acute alcoholic hepatitis

More than 50 studies have investigated the beneficial effects of prednisolone in acute alcoholic hepatitis. In general, corticosteroids stimulate the appetite, increase the production of albumin, and inhibit the production of collagen types I and IV. Data suggest that the mechanism of corticosteroid amelioration of the inflammatory response occurs through modulation of the production and release of cytokines, especially interleukin-2 and tumour necrosis factor.

In one of the more widely quoted randomized studies, a step-discriminant analysis of the individual elements believed to be associated with a bad prognosis was performed in 55 selected patients (1). The results of this analysis indicated that only a prolonged prothrombin time, a marked increase in the serum bilirubin concentration, hepatic encephalopathy, and worsening renal function were predictive of a bad prognosis. It is from the analysis of these data that the formula for DF was developed; all deaths occurred in patients with values of DF greater than 93. Six of eight recipients of placebo with values of DF greater than 93 died, compared with one of seven patients treated with prednisolone ($P = 0.03$). Because the results suggested a benefit from corticosteroid treatment for the most severely ill patients, a new multicentre trial was organized that included only patients who had values of DF greater than 32, spontaneous hepatic encephalopathy, or both. In this trial, the 28-day mortality rates were 37% in placebo-treated patients and 6% in patients given prednisolone ($P = 0.006$). In the subgroup of patients who presented with spontaneous hepatic encephalopathy, nine of 19 patients (47%) given placebo died, compared with one of 14 patients (7%) treated with methylprednisolone. However, this study has been criticized because histological assessment was not a component of the trial, and thus background hepatic cirrhosis was not excluded (2).

As a consequence of the differing results obtained from controlled clinical trials of glucocorticoid treatment in acute alcoholic hepatitis, four meta-analyses of this treatment have been published (7–10). In the first three, the results were similar. Corticosteroids significantly improved short-term survival of patients with alcoholic hepatitis, with a 37% reduction in mortality. Mortality was significantly decreased in patients with hepatic encephalopathy, whereas corticosteroids had no effect in patients without this condition. The efficacy of corticosteroids was not demonstrated in trials with lesser quality scores or trials that did not exclude patients with acute gastrointestinal bleeding. In the fourth and most comprehensive meta-analysis (10), weighted logistic regression analysis was applied using the summarized descriptive data (e.g. percentage of patients with encephalopathy; mean bilirubin value) of the treatment and control groups from 12 controlled trials that obtained this information. There was a publication bias favouring glucocorticoid treatment, but its overall effect on mortality was not significant. On subgroup analysis, there was an indication of interaction between glucocorticoid treatment and sex, but not encephalopathy. The authors concluded that the effect of glucocorticoid treatment may be different (beneficial or harmful) in special patient subgroups; also, more significantly, they concluded that the results did not support the routine use of glucocorticoids in patients with acute alcoholic hepatitis. The reasons for the conflicting results in the trials within the meta-analyses were identified as the small size of most of the studies, the wide spectrum of the disease both within and between studies, and the uncertain diagnosis, as liver biopsy was rarely performed. All four multivariate analyses indicated that further randomized trials were required.

In conclusion, there seems to be a subpopulation of patients with alcoholic hepatitis — namely, those with severe disease — who benefit from treatment with corticosteroids; this therapy will not benefit patients with mild or moderate forms of the disease. However, these patients are rarely encountered. For example, in a study form the Liver Unit at King's College Hospital, London, over a 9-month period, only 27% of patients qualified for steroids; indeed, this percentage is probably much greater than is seen in non-tertiary referral centres. The severity of the disease must be assessed by the presence of spontaneous hepatic encephalopathy, or by a value of DF greater than 32, which is the more objective measure. The diagnosis should preferably be confirmed histologically, as study findings suggest that there is only a 20% specificity for confirming the diagnosis on biochemical and clinical parameters alone. Patients with complications of the disease, such as gastrointestinal haemorrhage or sepsis, should have these treated adequately first. Corticosteroids are contraindicated in patients with hepatitis B or C infection, or with infection with the human immunodeficiency virus.

Anabolic steroids

Anabolic steroids might be expected to benefit patients with alcohol-related disease, because they stimulate nucleic acid and protein synthesis. Studies from the early 1990s have demonstrated a more rapid improvement in patients treated with both oxandrolone and enteral nutrition. In the largest study of its kind (11), 237 men were treated with oxandrolone and enteral food supplements. Stratification for the degree of malnutrition revealed that oxandrolone improved mortality at 1 month (9.4% compared with 20.9% in those receiving placebo) and at 6 months (79.7% survival in treated individuals, compared with 62.5% in the placebo-treated group; $P = 0.037$) in the moderately malnourished, but did not influence survival in those with severe malnutrition.

Criticisms of such studies, even those stratified for the degree of malnutrition, have indicated that it is almost impossible to separate the benefit of improvements in nutritional status from that of anabolic steroids. In addition, the side effects of the steroids compounds are not negligible.

Liver transplantation in acute alcoholic hepatitis

The applicability of liver transplantation for acute alcoholic hepatitis remains limited because of ethical arguments, and also because of the perception of poor outcome after transplantation. The ethical arguments revolve around the background of the competing demands of alcoholic and non-alcoholic patients, a shortage of donor organs, the high cost of liver transplantation and the public's perception of alcoholism. Consequently, the majority of UK transplant units exclude patients from transplant assessment if they are actively abusing alcohol.

There has been at least one study, however, that has suggested that severe acute alcoholic hepatitis may not be an appropriate contraindication for liver transplantation, outwith ethical arguments. Nine patients were studied: all had values of DF greater than 32, and most had hepatic encephalopathy and hepatorenal syndrome; eight of the nine had underlying hepatic cirrhosis, and one had fibrosis. After transplantation, episodes of acute cellular rejection responded quickly to treatment and, despite recidivism in some patients, long-term survival was comparable to that of patients with alcoholic cirrhosis alone and those with a milder degree of alcoholic hepatitis and cirrhosis (12). This area currently remains highly controversial.

Future treatments for acute alcoholic hepatitis

The emphasis in the treatment section of this chapter has been on the failings of previous treatments, and the lack of substantial evidence for the efficacy of current modes of treatment. At the very least, additional multicentre controlled trials are required to establish the role of corticosteroids and nutritional therapy in acute alcoholic hepatitis. However, future modes of treatment may more specifically modulate the immune response in acute alcoholic hepatitis.

The findings of a recent controlled trial, which to date have appeared only in abstract form, indicated that **pentoxifylline** is an effective drug in the treat-

Table 23.2. The management of acute alcoholic hepatitis.

Initial assessment	History
	Alcohol abuse?
	Other causes of acute hepatitis?
	Examination
	Signs of sepsis?
	Signs of liver failure?
	Signs of gastrointestinal haemorrhage?
Laboratory indices	Measures should include:
	FBC; coagulation screen; UEs; creatinine; LFTs; CRP
	Hepatitis A B C serology; autoantibody profile
	Urine and blood cultures; diagnostic ascitic tap
	Calculate DF as guide to prognosis and management
Basic management (all patients)	Insert urinary catheter
	Insert CVP line if patient "shocked", bleeding, or in renal failure
	Correct vitamin deficiencies
	Institute prophylaxis for alcohol withdrawal syndrome
	Provide nutritional support
Treat specific complications	1. Renal failure
	Correct hypovolaemia
	Consider dopamine infusion
	2. Sepsis
	Give broad-spectrum antibiotics (e.g. augmentin; cefotaxime)
	3. Gastrointestinal haemorrhage
	Perform endoscopy with therapeutic intervention
	4. Hepatic encephalopathy
	Make dietry adjustment
	Give lactulose
	Give phosphate enema
	5. Ascites
	Make dietary modifications
	Consider small dose of diuretics (if renal function normal)
Secondary investigations and management	Perform liver biopsy (unless obvious contraindications)
	Institute enteral or parenteral nutrition (DF not a guide)
	Give corticosteroids (if DF >32 *or* spontaneous hepatic encephalopathy present)

FBC, full blood count; UEs, urea and electrolytes; LFTs, liver function tests; CRP, C-reactive protein; CVP, central venous pressure.

ment of alcoholic hepatitis. Pentoxifylline is a haemorrheologic agent that decreases blood viscosity, increases red and white cell deformability, inhibits neutrophil adhesion and activation, and modulates the release of cytokines from macrophages. Ninety-six patients with severe alcoholic hepatitis (DF >32) were included; 50% were treated with pentoxifylline and the remainder received placebo. Forty-two per cent of patients in the placebo group, and 23% in the pentoxifylline group died. Most of the benefit derived from the pentoxifylline appeared to be related to a significantly decreased risk for developing hepatorenal syndrome.

CONCLUSIONS

The management of acute alcoholic hepatitis may be summarized as shown in Table 23.2. Although severe alcoholic hepatitis is uncommon, it has mortality rates of 60–80%; less severe disease has proportionately less mortality acutely, but significant long-term complications, namely cirrhosis. Treatment of the malnutrition that frequently accompanies the disease process corrects the metabolic consequences of poor nutrition, but may not decrease the mortality. In those with moderate nutrition or whose nutritional status can be improved by enteral or parenteral nutritional supplements, oxandrolone seems to be beneficial. Current data support the use of corticosteroids in those with severe disease (DF >32) and hepatic encephalopathy, but without gastrointestinal haemorrhage.

References
*Of special interest; **of outstanding interest.

1. **Maddrey WC, Biotnott JK, Bedine MS, *et al*. Corticosteroid therapy of alcoholic hepatitis. *Gastroenterology* 1978; **75**:193–199.

This is the original study outlining the use of DF in alcoholic hepatitis.

2. *Carithers DM, Herlong HF, Diehl AM *et al*. Methylprednisolone therapy in patients with severe alcoholic hepatitis. *Ann Int Med* 1989; **110**:685–690.

3. *Ramond M-J, Poynard T, Rueff B *et al*. A randomised trial of prednisolone in patients with severe alcoholic hepatitis. *N Eng J Med* 1992; **326**:507–512.

References 2 and 3 are studies assessing corticosteroid treatment according to prognosis determined by DF.

4. Mutimer DJ, Burra P, Neuberger JM *et al*. Managing severe alcoholic hepatitis complicated by renal failure. *Q J Med* 1993; **86**:649–656.

5. *Mendenhall C, Bongiovanni G, Goldberg S *et al*. VA co-operative study on alcoholic hepatitis. III. Changes in protein calorie malnutrition associated with 30 days of hospitalisation with and without enteral nutrition therapy. *JPEN* 1985; **9**: 590–596.

This was the first study assessing the use of nutritional therapy in acute alcoholic hepatitis.

6. Calvey H, Davis M, Williams R. Controlled trial of nutritional supplementation with and without branched chain amino acid enrichment in the treatment of acute alcoholic hepatitis. *J Hepatol* 1985; **1**:141–151.

7. *Reynolds TB, Benhamou JP, Blake J *et al*. Treatment of acute alcoholic hepatitis. *Gastroenterol Int* 1989; **2**:208–216.

8. *Imperiale TF, McCullough AJ. Do corticosteroids reduce mortality from alcoholic hepatitis? A meta-analysis of the randomised trials. *Ann Int Med* 1990; **113**:299–307.

9. *Daures JP, Peray P, Bories P *et al*. The role of corticosteroids in the treatment of acute alcoholic hepatitis. Results of a meta-analysis. *Gastroenterol Clin Biol* 1991; **15**:223–228.

10. *Christensen E, Gluud C. Glucocorticoids are ineffective in alcoholic hepatitis: meta-analysis adjusting for confounding variables. *Gut* 1996; **37**:113–118.

References 7–10 are four meta-analyses of the controlled trials of steroids in acute alcoholic hepatitis.

11. Medenhall CL, Moritz TE, Roselle GA *et al*. A study of oral nutritional support with oxandrolone in malnourished patients with alcoholic hepatitis: results of a Department of Veterans' Affairs Co-operative Study. *Hepatology* 1993; **17**:564–576.

12. Shakil AO, Pinna A, Demetris J, *et al*. Survival and quality of life after liver transplantation for acute alcoholic hepatitis. *Liver Transplant Surg* 1997; **3**:240–244.

Part III: A Problem-Based Approach to Gastroenterology Outpatients

24. Nausea and Vomiting

ROBIN VICARY

Nausea is used by patients to describe a variety of sensations and emotions, from those experienced before vomiting to anorexia, a revulsion of food, abdominal fullness, or satiety. Although **anorexia** — literally, lack of appetite — may accompany nausea, it is not the same thing, and has different clinical connotations. Defining **vomiting** is much easier, as the only difficulty here lies in the differentiation from regurgitation. The clinician must establish which of the two is being discussed by the patient. **Regurgitation** is essentially effortless, as opposed to the violence of vomiting. Regurgitation usually relates to the patient's posture, and is often accompanied with a sour or bitter taste (as it is often resulting from a dysfunctional gastrooesophageal sphincter). Vomiting is accompanied by contraction of abdominal wall musculature (particularly the recti) and usually preceded by hypersalivation.

TIMING OF VOMITING IN RELATION TO EATING

Clinical assessment of possible intestinal obstruction can be difficult. The timing of the vomiting is one important pointer, and the clinician should work hard to ensure that he is quite clear on this point. In general, the longer the delay after eating, the more likely it is that the vomiting is obstructive. Vomiting of food eaten the previous evening is always the result of a failure of food to leave the stomach (whether this "obstruction" is by pyloric narrowing or diabetic gastroparesis). The earlier the

vomiting after eating, the more likely it is that it is psychological in origin.

Case history

Miss AB, a patient aged 14 years, presented with vomiting. Her symptoms had started 3 months previously and the past childhood and adolescence had been unremarkable, both physically and emotionally. She was the younger of two sisters, from a stable home environment. She had initially been referred by her general practitioner to the local paediatric surgeon, who had performed blood tests, endoscopy, and barium follow-through. The barium follow-through had shown a band-like appearance at the junction of the second and third parts of the duodenum, and a diagnosis of superior mesenteric artery syndrome had been postulated. No dilatation of the first and second parts of the duodenum had been clearly demonstrated. On examination, the patient appeared well, but was thin and had lost 6.4 kg in weight in the previous 3 months. Otherwise, there were no abnormalities. There were no features of anorexia nervosa and there was no history of laxative abuse. The patient was admitted to hospital. In hospital, the patient and her family were closely observed by the nursing staff. The family seemed quite normal, and relationships appeared supportive. However, a staff nurse, on observation of eating, reported that the patient commenced vomiting after the first mouthful or two of food. In fact, the food returned only a few seconds after leaving the mouth — a classical feature of non-organic vomiting. No further investigations were made and the patient was discharged from hospital. The patient and family were informed that no serious disease was present. The vomiting continued for 3 weeks after her discharge, and then ceased. No final diagnosis has been made.

Comment

This case illustrates a number of important factors. First, the younger the patient, the less likely there is to be organic pathology present. Second, the history of the timing of the vomiting was not properly taken by myself or the consultant surgeon, and consequently the correct diagnosis was not made. Third, observation of eating is an important part of the assessment of vomiting. Finally, it is not always possible to come to a firm conclusion in cases presenting with these symptoms.

PAIN AND VOMITING

By removing acid from the stomach, vomiting relieves peptic ulcer pain. The vomiting in biliary colic does not lead to relief of pain, although the doctor should not confuse biliary tract pain with acid-related pain.

Pain preceding vomiting may suggest a chronic obstructive lesion. These lesions may well be difficult to diagnose.

Case history

Miss ST, a 24-year-old woman of Greek origin, presented with her mother, who was concerned at her daughter's vomiting, and the fact that her bowel sounds were "embarrassing". The vomiting was intermittent and had persisted over 6 months, with occasional preceding colicky pain. The "gurgly noises" of her stomach had started around the same time, and were often audible across a room. She had lost 3 kg in weight. On examination, there were no abnormalities. All investigations, including full blood screen, endoscopy, and barium follow-through, were normal. In spite of this, the vomiting continued and the patient was admitted via the Accident & Emergency department with dehydration after a severe attack. A surgeon (rather bravely) performed a laparotomy and removed a large, relatively benign, carcinoid tumour from the ileum.

Comment

The preceding pain and audible bowel sounds were important clinical pointers.

PROJECTILE VOMITING

Defining this term causes much difficulty to gastroenterologists — some relate it to the general force with which the contents leave the mouth, others to the timing of the vomiting in relation to the ventilatory cycle. There is little evidence that this feature of vomiting is helpful, diagnostically, in adults.

VOMITING AND GASTROINTESTINAL BLEEDING

Gastroenterologists are often asked to see patients with "coffee-ground vomit". This term is used to describe many appearances, but it has been shown to be meaningless unless the event is witnessed by a health-care professional who has a clear idea what they are looking for. Much vomited particulate matter can give the appearance of coffee grounds, and many patients will be presented to a gastroenterologist as a "gastrointestinal bleed" when the vomiting is in reality a symptom of other disease.

Case history

Mrs RT, aged 68 years, presented in Accident & Emergency with a 2-day history of vomiting "coffee grounds". There had been occasional abdominal pains, poorly localized, but otherwise no other symptoms. There was no significant past history, but she was taking a non-steroidal anti-inflammatory drug (NSAID) for osteoarthritis of the right hip, and was scheduled to undergo surgery in 2 weeks. On examination she was pale, but otherwise there were no abnormalities. Investigations showed a haemoglobin concentration of 8.5 g/dl, with hypochromia, and microcytosis. Endoscopic examination revealed gastritis and oesophagitis, with a positive test for *Helicobacter*. She was transfused and treated with a proton pump inhibitor and two antibiotics. Vomiting continued on the ward and was attributed to the antibiotics, which were stopped. The vomiting persisted, and it was noted that the patient often vomited in the morning, food that had been eaten the previous evening. A barium enema was requested and revealed a large tumour at the caecum.

Comment

In addition to the other points of history previously mentioned (e.g. timing of vomiting), this case illustrates first, the dangers of assuming that all "coffee ground" is blood, and second — of course — that, in an anaemic patient, finding minor pathology in the stomach explains the anaemia.

OTHER CLINICAL FACTORS IN THE PATIENT WITH NAUSEA AND VOMITING

Alcohol ingestion

Taking a detailed alcohol history is important. Accepting the patient's figures is often misleading and in taking the history, I will often not only discuss exactly how many drinks are taken, but also establish the difference between weekday, evening, and weekend consumption; discussion of "business" lunches is also useful. Early-morning vomiting in the young male and non-pregnant female should always arouse the suspicion of vomiting induced by alcohol.

Drug history

In the cat, vomiting can be induced by electrical stimulation of part of the medulla (1). However, these experiments can not be repeated in humans, and a discrete anatomical centre has not been unequivocally located in man. Most workers believe that the vomiting centre is best thought of as a pharmacological state, and that complex interactions within the medulla cause the ventilatory changes and hypersalivation (all of which are known to have medullary connections) that are found as features accompanying nausea and vomiting.

There appears, therefore, to be a **chemoreceptor trigger zone** in the medulla that appears to activate the vomiting centre. This zone is acted on by certain drugs to induce vomiting. These drugs include digoxin, opiates, and dopamine agonists such as L-dopa and bromocriptine. Other drugs, such as aspirin and NSAIDs, damage the gastric mucosa and stimulate the vomiting centre via ascending vagal afferents.

Alcohol acts both directly on the chemoreceptor trigger zone and via gastric mucosal damage (2).

Nausea and vomiting are common in gastroenterological cancer patients, both as a direct result of their cancer and from the drugs taken to cure them. In these patients, nausea and vomiting from drugs are complex in origin and can be directly from the vagal afferents — as with cisplatin — and from direct stimulation of the chemoreceptor trigger zone. They are also more common in patients with a history of motion sickness (3).

Pregnancy

Nausea occurs as a normal phenomenon in pregnancy. Fifty per cent of all pregnant women vomit during the first trimester, and it is often the first sign for a woman that she is pregnant after a missed period. Both symptoms are much more common early in the day, but a proportion of women experience nausea throughout the day. "**Hyperemesis gravidarum**" is a physiologically more intense accentuation of this condition, and is discused further in Chapter 9.

Later in pregnancy, nausea and vomiting may herald the onset of acute fatty liver of pregnancy.

Psychological and social factors

Many text books fail to mention anxiety as being a leading cause of nausea and vomiting. Especially in young patients, a history of emotionally disturbing events should be sought. In school children, in my practice bullying is a common factor. The approach of examinations, often in patients from tense, achievement-orientated families, is another important underlying contributor. Psychotic illness such as depression is much less commonly an underlying factor (4). The taking of laxatives or diuretics is an important accompaniment of the range of disorders of eating known as the anorexic–bulaemic syndrome, usually occuring in women (5). The diagnosis can often be suspected after questions about the patient's habitus reveal a contentment with their present (malnourished) state. Some patients have, however, learnt to conceal their views on this subject, and may go to some lengths to conceal their eating disorder. Although it is clear that there are major psychological abnormalities in these patients, it is not entirely clear that this is an exclusively psychological disease.

Neurological features

In particular, questioning about headache, double vision, and gait is important.

Case history

Miss RC, a 22-year-old, presented with vomiting to my outpatient clinic. She was seen by a Registrar who found no other abnormalities on history or examination. Blood screen and endoscopy were normal. Psychogenic vomiting was suspected, and treatment instigated with metochlopropamide, with no effect. I saw her at her third outpatient visit, and she was my first patient of the morning. A few minutes into the consultation, to my — and my students' — amazement and consternation, she turned rapidly in her seat, in the middle of a sentence, and vomited forcefully into the consulting-room sink. She was immediately quite well after the incident, for which she had clearly had no warning. On questioning, she had had a mild bilateral frontal headache for the last few weeks, and had no other symptoms. The vomiting was often, but not exclusively, early in the day and usually came with no warning. On examination, there were definite bilateral mild cerebellar signs, but no papilloedema or other signs of increased intracranial pressure. Scanning revealed a large posterior fossa tumour, which at surgery proved to be a cerebellar glioma.

Comment

The characteristic features of "neurological" vomiting were all present here — in particular, there was no warning nausea for the patient, and the vomiting was forceful. The vomiting is often early morning in occurrence.

Motion

Although motion sickness usually starts and is most troublesome in childhood, it occasionally starts in young adulthood or late in life. Any kind of motion may cause it, from that of aeroplanes to that of underground trains. There are usually accompanying features such as sweating, hypersalivation, etc. In older patients, it is important to exclude labyrinthitis.

Infections

Most gastroenterologists will see only occasional episodes of viral or bacterial food poisoning, as these are normally dealt with in the community. A careful history will normally reveal a suspect meal eaten a few hours before the onset of symptoms, and the patient may well be feverish.

Superior mesenteric artery syndrome

Although it is true that the superior mesenteric artery crosses the third part of the duodenum shortly after leaving the aorta, it is clear that many of the early cases attributed to this syndrome were in fact cases of diseases that also cause duodenal dilatation — for example, diabetes mellitus, scleroderma, pancreatitis, and chronic idiopathic intestinal pseudo-obstruction. In many patients, surgical therapeutic approaches have been unsuccessful in treating the symptoms. A reasonable account of the diagnostic criteria can be found elsewhere (6).

Helicobacter infection

A variable proportion of patients with helicobacter infection have nausea as a symptom, although vomiting is rare. Results of treatment for *Helicobacter pylori* cause variable resolution of the nausea (see Chapter 40).

CLINICAL APPROACH TO DIFFICULT CASES

Diagnosis

In spite of a good history and examination (and any relevant investigations), the clinician may be left without a clear diagnosis. In the patient who is not severely ill, a framework for management is important. In young patients, enlisting the help of a psychiatrist at an early date is important. As mentioned above, two of the most common problems seen in young persons with nausea or vomiting are eating disorders or anxiety. It is important that these conditions are identified and managed correctly. Patients with eating disorders may be extremely deceptive, and a psychiatrist may well tease out factors not apparent to the gastroenterologist, and instigate appropriate management. The anxious patient will similarly be helped, although referral to a psychologist for a planned therapeutic programme may be as useful. Anxiety is infectious, and a patient's symptoms may be worsened by a gastroenterologist's "uncertainty" over the diagnosis.

A therapeutic approach

Abstaining from alcohol

Alcohol is a common cause of nausea and vomiting; abstinence is advisable, almost regardless of what the patient admits to consuming. The abstinence should be complete, and for a minimum of 6 weeks, to see any clinical improvement.

Lifestyle advice

There is evidence that lack of exercise affects gastrointestinal tract function (7). Exercise is also known to stimulate appetite. This author advises those who take no exercise to exercise briskly at least three times weekly.

Alternative remedies

Some patients are helped considerably by homeopathy. There are no controlled studies.

Correction of metabolic abnormalities

Hypokalaemia is a common problem in severe vomiting, and results from loss both in the vomit and in the urine from secondary hyperaldosteronism. Alkalosis and sodium depletion often occur.

Nutritional depletion

Carbohydrate and protein malnutrition may occur; the clinician should watch for deficiencies of vitamins or minerals with small total body pools (folic acid, vitamin B, etc.)

Drugs

Most of the drugs used to combat vomiting have unpleasant side effects. Although their use is important in chemotherapy-induced vomiting and motion sickness, they should be used with care in other patients.

Prokinetic drugs

Dopamine D2 receptor agonists

Metoclopramide is useful for chemotherapy-induced vomiting and diabetic gastroparesis. It is also widely used for psychogenic — and, indeed, all other — causes of vomiting. The unpleasant side effects of the associated dystonia (usually facial, but occasionally affecting the limbs) are so common in the patients younger than 30 years, and especially females, that I have stopped using this drug in these groups. The dystonia is usually dose related, and its incidence can be reduced by using the lower dose of 5 mg twice daily. **Domperidone**, a similar drug, causes fewer side effects because it does not cross the blood–brain barrier.

Selective 5-hydroxytryptamine receptor antagonists

Ondansitron is an effective and much used drug in patients undergoing chemotherapy.

Anticholinergic drugs

Hyoscine (Scopolamine) is effective for motion sickness, and can either be used as patches, or can be purchased without prescription (in the UK), as "Kwells".

Prochlorperazine (Stemetil) is used both orally and intramuscularly as an antiemetic.

Anxiolytic drugs

Anxiolytic drugs undoubtedly help anxiety-induced nausea, and probably the vomiting also. **Lorazepam** or **chlordiazepoxide** are both useful drugs.

Other agents

Marijuana is a well documented drug for treating nausea in patients undergoing chemotherapy (8). For patients not wishing to inhale the active substance in marijuana, **tetrahydrocannabinol** (THC) is marketed as Dronabinol. Clinicians surveyed in the study cited that nausea and vomiting were reduced in 50% of their patients who smoked marijuana or took it orally as THC. However, it ranked well down the list of drug preferences amongst physicians for treating mild or severe chemotherapy-induced nausea or vomiting; prochlorperazine, metoclopramide, lorazepam and corticosteroids all ranked higher.

References
1. Borison HL, Borison R, McCarthy LE. Role of the area postrema in vomiting and related functions. *Fed Proc* 1984; **43**: 2955–2963.

2. Shen WW. A potential link between hallucination and nau-
    sea and vomiting induced by alcohol? *Psychopathology*
    1985; **18**: 212–217.
3. Morrow GR. The effect of a susceptibility to motion sick-
    ness on the side effects of cancer chemotherapy *N Engl J
    Med* 1985; **307**: 1476–1503.
4. Muraska M, Mine K, Matsumoto K. Psychogenic vomiting:
    the relation between patterns of vomiting and psychiatric
    diagnosis. *Gut* 1990; **31**: 526–533.
5. Killen JD, Taylor CB, Telol MJ. Self induced vomiting and
    laxative and diuretic use among teenagers. Precursers of the
    binge–purge syndrome? *JAMA* 1986; **255**: 1447–1556.
6. Hines JR, Gore RM, Ballantyne GH. Superior messenteric
    artery syndrome. Diagnostic criteria and therapeutic ap-
    proaches. *Am J Surg* 1984; **148**: 630–637.
7. Sandler RS, Jordan MC, Shelton BJ. Demographic and
    dietary determinants of constipation in the US population.
    Am J Public Health 1990; **80**: 185–189.
8. Schwartz RH, Beveridge RA. Marijuana as an antiemetic
    drug. *J Addict Dis* 1994; **13**: 53–61.

25. Anaemia

ATUL B. MEHTA

Diagnosis of anaemia must identify the precise cause (Table 25.1). It is important to remember iron deficiency, thalassaemia, and (rarely) inherited sideroblastic anaemia as causes of hypochromic, microcytic anaemia. Megaloblastic anaemia (deficiency of vitamin B_{12}, folic acid or both), liver disease, hypothyroidism, marrow aplasia, haemolysis, alcoholism, and myelodysplasia causes of macrocytic anaemia.

HAEMATINIC DEFICIENCY

Vitamins and minerals essential for normal erythropoiesis (haematinics) include iron, folic acid, copper, cobalt, vitamins A, B_6, B_{12}, C and E, riboflavin and nicotinic acid. Iron, folic acid and vitamin B_{12} are the most important (Table 25.2) (1). **Iron**, in its ferrous (Fe^{2+}) form, is an essential component of haemoglobin; vitamin B_{12} and folic acid are both essential for DNA synthesis. **Vitamin B_{12}** is required as a cofactor in the methylation of homocysteine to methionine by methyl tetrahydrofolate. Lack of vitamin B_{12} leads to deficiency of the folate coenzymes necessary for DNA synthesis. **Folates** are derived from folic acid by the addition of glutamic acid residues, reduction to dihydro- and tetrahydrofolates, or addition of single carbon units. They are needed for a variety of single-carbon transfer reactions in the body, especially those in purine and pyrimidine synthesis. Folate deficiency in pregnancy is associated with an increased incidence of pregnancy complications (including pre-eclampsia and intra-uterine growth retardation) and foetal malfunctions (neural tube defects). Lack of B12 and or folate is associated with elevation of homocysteine and this predisposes to vascular thrombosis.

Table 25.1. Classification of anaemia.

Decreased red cell production	Haematinic deficiency
	Iron, vitamin B_{12} folic acid, other
	Marrow failure
	Aplastic anaemia, pure red-cell aplasia, marrow replacement (e.g. leukaemia, lymphoma, myelofibrosis, secondary carcinoma)
Abnormal red cell maturation	Myelodysplasia
	Sideroblastic anaemia
Increased red cell destruction	Inherited haemolytic anaemia (e.g. sickle-cell anaemia, thalassaemia)
	Acquired haemolytic anaemia
	Immune
	Non-immune (e.g. microangiopathic haemolytic anaemia, disseminated intravascular coagulation)
Effects of disease in other organs	Anaemia of chronic disease
	Liver, renal, endocrine disease

Table 25.2. Haematinic intake and stores.

Haematinic	Source	Average daily dietary intake (% absorbed)	Daily requirement	Stores
Iron	Meat, fish, vegetables, cereals, pulses	10–20 mg (5–6)	1 mg (males) 2 mg (menstruating females)	2–3 months
Vitamin B_{12}	Meat, fish, dairy products	10–30 mg	1–2 µg	2–3 years
Folic acid	Widely distributed — meat, vegetables, fruits, yeast. Easily destroyed by cooking	500–1000 µg (20–50)	100–300 µg	2–3 months

Deficiency of haematinics can arise through:

- inadequate dietary intake
- malabsorption
- excess requirement or utilization
- loss

Examples of such causes of deficiency of the three major haematinics are given in Table 25.3.

Malabsorption

Iron

Malabsorption or poor dietary intake are rarely sufficient to cause iron deficiency *anaemia*, although either on its own may reduce iron stores, and both together may cause anaemia. A diagnosis of iron deficiency anaemia must lead to a search for a source of blood loss.

Iron absorption occurs mainly in the duodenum and upper jejunum. Absorption is adjusted to body needs (increased in iron deficiency and pregnancy, reduced in iron overload). Absorption is regulated by two proteins, DMT-1 at the villous tip and HFE at the basolateral surface of the enterocyte. The DMT-1 level determines the amount of iron absorbed, and the DMT-1 level is in turn regulated by the degree of HFE expression. In genetic haemochromatosis, a mutation in HFE leads to increased iron absorption. Dietary iron is released from

Table 25.3. Causes of haematinic deficiency in gastrointestinal disease.

	Iron	Vitamin B_{12}	Folate
Nutritional	Rarely sole cause	Vegans	Poor diet – elderly, alcoholism, institutions
Malabsorption			
Stomach	Anacidity Atrophic gastritis Gastrectomy	Pernicious anaemia Food-cobalamin malabsorption Atrophic gastritis	Gastrectomy
Small intestine	Coeliac disease Tropical sprue	Intestinal stagnant loop syndrome Ileal resection Crohn's disease Coeliac disease Tropical sprue Fish tapeworm Selective malabsorption with proteinuria	Gastrectomy Tropical sprue Scleroderma Amyloidosis Giardiasis Diabetic enteropathy Lymphoma Whipple's disease
Other		Severe chronic pancreatitis Liver/biliary disease	Liver/biliary disease Alcoholism
Increased Loss or Utilization	Haemorrhage —	— —	Liver disease Crohn's disease

protein complexes by acid and proteases in the stomach. Solubulizing agents, such as sugars and ascorbic acid, enhance absorption. Phosphates and phytates in cereals form insoluble complexes with iron, which inhibit absorption. Iron of animal origin (haem iron) is more readily absorbed than non-haem iron, and the ferrous (Fe^{2+}) form is more soluble than the ferric (Fe^{3+}). **Iron uptake** occurs by both active transport and passive diffusion, and can be increased by 20–30% in iron deficiency and pregnancy. Decreased gastric acid secretion in atrophic gastritis, gastric surgery, and prolonged antacid therapy can predispose to iron deficiency. Gastric surgery may lead to chronic blood loss and rapid intestinal transit. Partial gastrectomy with gastrojejunotomy (Billroth II) results in iron deficiency more quickly than with gastro-duodenotomy (Billroth I), which tends to preserve duodenal absorption. Malabsorption of iron also occurs in small intestinal disease (coeliac disease, tropical sprue).

Vitamin B$_{12}$

Vitamin B_{12} is released from protein complexes in food by gastric acid and enzymes, and binds to a high-affinity binding protein, R protein. Pancreatic proteases in the duodenum degrade R protein, releasing vitamin B_{12} to bind to intrinsic factor, a glycoprotein produced by parietal cells in the body and fundus of the stomach. The intrinsic factor–vitamin B_{12} (IF–B_{12}) complex passes to the liver by the portal circulation; a small amount of vitamin B_{12} enters the enterohepatic circulation.

Malabosorption of unbound vitamin B_{12} can occur through gastric or intestinal causes. Gastric surgery causes loss of intrinsic factor and gastric-acid-producing cells, and warrants prophylactic vitamin B_{12} replacement. Deficiency of this vitamin occurs in 15–30% of individuals after gastrectomy, and may take up to 4 years to develop.

Food-cobalamin malabsorption (2) is a recently recognized syndrome in which absorption of food-bound vitamin B_{12} is impaired, but unbound (and biliary) vitamin B_{12} are normally absorbed. Possible mechanisms of this malabsorption include gastric dysfunction, impaired acid production, and impaired pepsin secretion with reduced R protein degradation. These mechanisms combine to prevent the release of cobalamin from food–protein complexes. Food-cobalamin malabsorption may occur after gastrectomy,

in association with H_2-antagonist and proton pump inhibitor treatment, and with *Helicobacter pylori* infection.

Pernicious anaemia is an autoimmune condition characterized by gastric atrophy, achlorhydria, and loss of secretion of intrinsic factor (3). It occurs in the setting of a type A (autoimmune) gastritis in which parietal cell autoantibodies are directed against the gastric H^+/K^+-ATPase. It is most common in northern Europe, with an overall incidence of approximately 120 per 100 000 population in the UK. It is nearly twice as common in women as in men, has a peak incidence at about 60 years of age, and is associated with other organ-specific autoimmune conditions such as Grave's disease, myxoedema, and Addison's disease (Figure 25.1). Antibodies to gastric parietal cells are present in the serum of more than 90% of patients with pernicious anaemia, but are not specific for the disease, being found in both normal individuals and patients with

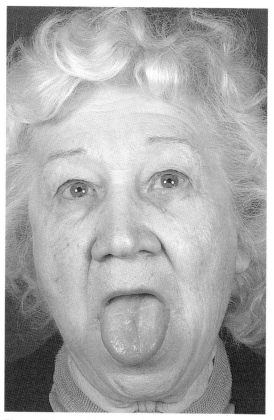

Figure 25.1. Pernicious anaemia in a female aged 65 years. She is wearing a wig to disguise premature greying of the hair. There is a tinge of jaundice in the conjuctivae and skin, blue eyes and an enlarged fleshy sore tongue.

other autoimmune diseases. Antibodies to intrinsic factor are more specific, but are found in only 60% of affected patients. There are two types: type I or blocking antibodies prevent the binding of intrinsic factor to vitamin B_{12}, and type II or precipitating antibodies, present in 35% of patients, inhibit the binding of IF–B_{12} complexes to their ileal receptors. These antibodies are detectable in gastric juice, where they inhibit the function of any remaining intrinsic factor and compound the malabsorption of vitamin B_{12}. The association of pernicious anaemia with gastric cancer is unclear, but it is likely that the risk of gastric carcinoma is increased two- to three-fold, and that of gastric carcinoid tumours perhaps 10-fold.

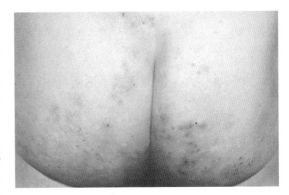

Figure 25.2.   Dermatitis herpetiformis: typical rash over buttocks. This patient also had coeliac disease with iron and folic acid deficiency.

Malabsorption of vitamin B_{12} also occurs in association with colonization of the small intestine by bacteria, such as in **intestinal stagnant loop syndrome** caused by jejunal diverticulosis, Crohn's disease, intestinal fistulae or strictures, postoperative blind loops and resection, or incompetence of the ileocaecal valve resulting, for example, from tuberculosis. Anaerobic organisms metabolize vitamin B_{12} and also deconjugate bile salts, leading to mucosal damage, impaired absorption of IF–B_{12} complexes, and interruption of the enterohepatic recirculation of vitamin B_{12}. The **fish tapeworm** utilizes vitamin B_{12}, and infestation results in vitamin B_{12} deficiency.

Ileal resection, which may be performed for Crohn's disease, bowel obstruction, or lymphoma, often results in vitamin B_{12} malabsorption. In contrast, coeliac disease and tropical sprue are rarely associated with significant vitamin B_{12} deficiency.

Chronic pancreatic insufficiency results in vitamin B_{12} malabsorption as a result of lack of proteases to degrade R proteins and bicarbonate to facilitate binding of vitamin B_{12} to intrinsic factor. However, the deficiency is rarely sufficiently severe to cause megaloblastic anaemia.

Folic acid

Gastric disorders rarely cause significant malabsorption of folate, whereas small-intestinal disease is a common association. **Coeliac disease** is the major cause, although **tropical sprue**, **giardiasis**, and **infiltrations caused by amyloidosis, scleroderma**, or **lymphoma** are also important. Both coeliac disease, and tropical sprue cause villous atrophy and loss of absorptive surface, but coeliac disease affects the proximal intestine preferentially, with less frequent ileal involvement, whereas the lesions of tropical sprue tend to be less severe but more widespread. Coeliac disease may present as dermatitis herpetiformis (Figure 25.2). The most common cause of anaemia in coeliac disease in children is iron deficiency, but folate deficiency, occurs in 10–40% of cases. Megaloblastic anaemia develops in tropical sprue after disease has been present for about 6 months. Significant folate malabsorption with a normal intestinal mucosa characterizes the rare disorder, congenital folate malabsorption. Alcohol may inhibit folate absorption, and several drugs such as sulphasalazine and cholestyramine have been reported to affect folate uptake.

Increased loss or utilization of haematinics

Iron

Blood loss is by far the most important cause of iron deficiency, and the major cause of anaemia, worldwide. Gastrointestinal bleeding frequently betrays occult malignancy and thus thorough investigation and accurate detection and management of the bleeding lesion may be life saving. Assuming a normal Western diet, a steady blood loss of as little as 3–4 ml daily (1.5–2 mg of iron) can result in negative iron balance.

In premenopausal women, iron deficiency is most commonly attributable to menorrhagia but, in men and in postmenopausal women, a search for gastrointestinal blood loss must be initiated.

Table 25.4. Sites of gastrointestinal blood loss leading to iron deficiency.

Site	Lesions
Oesophagus/oropharynx	Oesophaeal varices
	Carcinoma
	Haemangioma, (e.g. hereditary haemorrhagic telangiectasia)
Stomach	Peptic ulceration
	Carcinoma
	Gastritis
	Drugs — NSAIDs, alcohol
	Post-gastrectomy
	Haemangioma (e.g. hereditary haemorrhagic telengiectasia)
Small intestine	Inflammatory bowel disease
	Parasitic infection (e.g. hookworm)
	Ulceration caused by drugs (NSAIDs, potassium chloride)
	Lymphoma
	Meckel's diverticulum
	Whipple's disease
	Radiation enteritis
Large intestine/rectum	Carcinoma
	Inflammatory bowel disease
	Diverticular disease
	Haemorrhoids
	Angiodysplasia
	Radiation colitis
	Haemangioma

NSAIDs, non-steroidal anti-inflammatory drugs.

Table 25.5. Investigations in suspected haematinic deficiency.

Basic	Full blood count
	Haemoglobin concentration
	Red-cell indices (MCV, MCHC, MCH)
	White-cell count and differential
	Platelet count
	Blood film examination
	Reticulocyte count
	Serum iron, total iron-binding capacity, ferritin
	Serum vitamin B_{12} assay
	Serum and red cell folate assay
	Urea and electrolytes
	Liver function tests, including albumin and γGT
Confirmatory (see text for details)	
	Methylmalonic acid – serum/urinary
	Serum homocysteine
	Deoxyuridine suppression test

γGT, γ-glutamyltransferase; MCV, mean copuscular volume; MCHC, mean corpuscular haemoglobin concentration (%); MCH, mean corpuscular haemoglobin (content, μg).

Possible sources are shown in Table 25.4. Most studies in Western populations show that upper gastrointestinal lesions are slightly more common (detectable lesions in 40–60% of cases) than pathology in the lower gut (20–30% of cases). As many as 25% of patients may be harbouring a neoplasm; this increases to 50% of elderly patients with severe iron deficiency. More than one pathology may be present: up to 20% of patients may have lesions in both upper and lower gastrointestinal tract simultaneously. Haematuria, haemoglobinuria, pulmonary haemorrhage, and self-inflicted blood loss are all rare causes of iron deficiency.

Vitamin B_{12} and folic acid

There is no syndrome of vitamin B_{12} deficiency resulting from increased loss or utilization. However, **increased requirement for folate** occurs in the physiological states of pregnancy and lactation, in prematurity, and in pathological conditions with high rates of cell turnover, including inflammatory disorders such as Crohn's disease, rheumatoid arthritis, and exfoliative dermatitis, malignancies such as carcinoma and lymphoma, and haematological disorders, including haemolytic anaemias and myelofibrosis.

Diagnosis of haematinic deficiency

The investigations relevant to diagnosis of haematinic deficiency are summarized in Table 25.5.

Clinical features of iron, vitamin B_{12} and folate deficiency often develop late when tissue haematinic deficiency is severe or well established, and are non-specific. Iron deficiency is associated with epithelial lesions such as glossitis, angular stomatitis, nail dystrophy including koilonychia and, rarely, dysphagia resulting from pharyngeal webs (Paterson–Kelly or Plummer–Vinson syndrome). Atrophic gastritis and reduced gastric acid secretion also occur in a proportion of patients and are corrected with iron replacement. Psychomotor retardation may occur in children. Patients with megaloblastic anaemia may be mildly jaundiced as a result of increased ineffective haemopoiesis and also have painful glossitis, angular stomatitis, and hyperpigmentation. Vitamin B_{12} deficiency may cause an isolated peripheral neuropathy, subacute combined degeneration of the cord, optic atrophy, or psychiatric changes.

Iron

Iron deficiency characteristically leads to a reduction in serum iron and an increase in serum transferrin concentration (reflected as increased total iron-binding capacity, TIBC). However, serum iron may be decreased in the absence of iron deficiency (e.g. in the anaemia of chronic disease) and is increased in inflammatory conditions and liver disease. Infection, inflammation, and liver disease may all decrease transferrin concentrations (and therefore the TIBC). The percentage saturation of transferrin adds useful information: a low value (less than 20% in men, less than 15% in women) occurs in iron deficiency, whereas an increased value may be an early indicator of iron overload, and has been used as a screening test for genetic haemochromatosis. Additional tests are often required. Serum ferritin concentration is an indication of the status of iron stores and a decreased concentration usually indicates deficiency. However, it is an acute-phase protein, and both inflammatory conditions and liver disease may lead to falsely increased (or normal) values even in the presence of iron deficiency. Bone-marrow aspiration and staining by Perl's reaction to demonstrate iron stores remain the reference standards, but two recent methods of diagnosing deficiency are undergoing further evaluation. Some automated red-cell analysers measure percentages of hypochromic or microcytic red cells, and a finding of more than 10% hypochromic cells may be relatively specific for iron deficiency. Serum-soluble transferrin receptor levels reflect the total body mass of the tissue transferrin receptor content, and are increased in iron deficiency, but probably normal in liver disease and anaemia of chronic disorder.

Vitamin B$_{12}$ and folic acid

The effects of vitamin B$_{12}$ and folic acid deficiency on blood count and bone marrow morphology are indistinguishable (see Figure 25.3). Vitamin B$_{12}$ deficiency leads to reduced serum concentrations of the vitamin and increased serum concentrations of methyl-malonic acid and homocysteine. These further tests are not usually required, however. Bone marrow examination will reveal the changes of megaloblastic anaemia, but is rarely required. The deoxyuridine suppression test is a sensitive and specific test for vitamin B$_{12}$ or folate deficiency, but necessitates bone marrow examination, and is rarely required. Serum folate concentrations are markedly affected by recent intake and the red cell folate

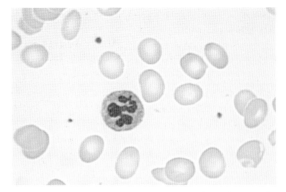

Figure 25.3a. Peripheral blood film in megaloblastic anaemia, showing macrocytic red cells and a hypersegmented neutrophil ($\times$ 40).

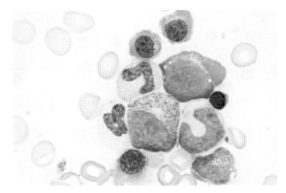

Figure 25.3b. Bone marrow aspirate in megaloblastic anaemia showing a giant metamyelocyte and large nucleated red cells with lacy chromatin (megaloblasts).

content is a better indicator of body stores. Serum concentrations of homocysteine (but not methyl-malonic acid) increase in folate deficiency.

Investigation of the cause of haematinic deficiency

Iron

It is unreliable to use symptoms as a guide to directing investigations, and a significant proportion of patients will have pathology in both upper and lower gastrointestinal tract. Studies have shown that patients with significant colonic pathology may also have upper gastrointestinal lesions; furthermore, iron deficiency should not be attributed to uncomplicated hiatus hernia. Testing for faecal occult blood has low sensitivity, specificity, and predictive value, but coeliac disease may be present in as many as 1 in 20 patients with iron deficiency, and routine small-bowel biopsy is worth undertaking. Thus, in all adult males and non-menstruating females, **investigation of the gastrointestinal tract should include oesophagogastroduodenoscopy, colonoscopy**, and **small-bowel biopsy**. In selected patients, there may also be a role for small-bowel enteroscopy and, occasionally, angiography or labelled-red-cell studies. Prospective studies suggest that the cause of iron deficiency will still not be apparent in 30–40% of patients, but in the majority the anaemia resolves with iron replacement and does not recur (4). Patients who fail to respond or who become transfusion-dependent require further investigation.

Vitamin B$_{12}$

If there is no dietary history of **vegetarianism** in a patient with vitamin B$_{12}$ deficiency, the presence of **serum parietal cell antibodies**, and intrinsic factor antibodies should be sought. The detection of the more specific **intrinsic factor antibodies** obviates the need for an absorption test in nearly all patients. Severe vitamin B$_{12}$ and folate deficiency can affect the bowel mucosa and reduce absorptive capacity, so studies of vitamin B$_{12}$ absorption should, ideally, be performed after 2 months of replacement therapy. Alternatively, if initial absorption studies are abnormal, they can be repeated after treatment. Gastrointestinal absorption of vitamin B$_{12}$ can be assessed using orally administered radioactive cobalt-57-labelled cyanocobalamin and an intramuscular flushing dose of non-radioactive hydroxycobalamin, followed by a 24-h urine collection (Schilling test). The test can be repeated giving radioactive vitamin B$_{12}$ together with a commercial oral preparation of intrinsic factor in order to distinguish between gastric and intestinal causes of vitamin B$_{12}$ deficiency. If intestinal malabsorption is demonstrated and an intestinal stagnant loop is suspected, the test can be repeated after a course of antibiotics. The normal urinary excretion is more than 10% of the test dose within 24 h, although collection for 48 h may be required in patients with renal failure. Food-cobalamin absorption may also be assessed using preparations of B$_{12}$ bound to chick serum or egg yolk. If intrinsic factor antibodies are negative and absorption studies not practicable, response to a trial of treatment with oral vitamin B$_{12}$ suggests food-cobalamin malabsorption. Gastric function studies, including assay of intrinsic factor secretion, are occasionally required, and small-bowel studies are indicated if absorption tests suggest an intestinal problem.

Folate

If the dietary history is unhelpful, the decision as to how far to investigate for malabsorption depends on the clinical status of the individual patient. Coeliac disease can be screened for by non-invasive means. Although anti-gliadin antibodies are non-specific, anti-endomysial antibodies are present in more than 90% of cases (see Chapter 51).

Treatment of haematinic deficiencies

The primary consideration is identification and treatment of the cause. Blood transfusion should be avoided where possible, as replacement of the deficient haematinic alone leads to a rapid increase in haemoglobin of the order of 1 g/dl every week after the commencement of therapy. A reticulocyte response is detectable after 2 or 3 days of treatment and is maximal at 5–7 days.

Iron

Iron is usually given as oral ferrous sulphate (67 mg of elemental iron per 200 mg tablet); gluconate and succinate are equally well absorbed and have a similar frequency of side effects, but are more expensive. Administration of concurrent vitamin C improves absorption. For adults, the optimal response occurs with about 200 mg of elemental iron daily. Optimal iron absorption occurs from an empty stomach but, if side effects occur (e.g. nausea, abdominal pain, constipation), these can be reduced by administration of the iron supplement with food. The use of slow-release preparations is illogical, because most of their iron is released in the lower small intestine, where it cannot be absorbed. Iron therapy should be given for approximately 3–6 months after correction of the anaemia to replenish body iron stores.

Possible reasons for failure of response to oral iron include non-compliance, continuing blood loss, mixed deficiency, malabsorption (rarely), misdiagnosis of thalassaemia trait or sideroblastic anaemia, and coexisting inflammatory or malignant disease. Iron can be given **intramuscularly** or **intravenously**; **parenteral** therapy carries more risks and is more expensive than oral treatment. Iron–sorbitol–citrate can be given intramuscularly, whereas iron–dextran can be given intramuscularly or intravenously. Local reactions to intramuscular injections include pain and discolouration of the soft tissues. Serious **systemic reactions** can occur with both intravenous and intramuscular treatment and may be immediate (anaphylaxis, hypotension, urticaria) or delayed (myalgia, arthalgia, and fever).

Vitamin B_{12}

Vitamin B_{12} is best given as intramuscular **hydroxycobalamin**. A typical regimen for newly-diagnosed **pernicious anaemia** is 1000 µg given at 3–7-day intervals for five injections, followed by 1000 µg every 3 months for life. **Folic acid** should be given simultaneously to allow for the rapid increase in effective haemopoiesis, and potassium supplementation may be required. Intranasal hydroxycobalamin might be an alternative mode of administration. Fortification of the diet with **cobalamin** has been proposed as a means of circumventing some of the complications of the fortification of dietary folate, and this adds to the impetus for research into the prevalence and significance of food-cobalamin malabsorption.

Folate

The form of folate most commonly used for therapy is pteroylmonoglutamic acid or folic acid. Five-milligram tablets are usually given daily, although 100 µg is sufficient for an optimal haematological response. Adequate amounts are absorbed even in coeliac disease. In the USA, flour and other basic foodstuffs are supplemented with folate and this has led to a reduction in the incidence of fetal neural tube defects.

HAEMOLYTIC ANAEMIAS

Haemolytic anaemia arises through failure to compensate for accelerated **red-cell destruction**. Red-cell destruction is predominantly extravascular in the macrophages of the reticuloendothelial system (spleen, bone marrow, and liver). Globin is degraded to amino acids, and haem to protoporphyrin, carbon monoxide, and iron. Protoporphyrin is metabolized to bilirubin, conjugated to a glucuronide in the liver, and excreted in the faeces (as stercobilinogen) and,

after reabsorption, in the urine (as urobilinogen). In addition, the plasma concentrations of haptoglobin are reduced in intravascular haemolysis and by liver disease; haptoglobins are plasma proteins that bind haemoglobin to form a complex, which is removed by the liver.

Unconjugated hyperbilirubinaemia gives rise to jaundice. Deposition of bilirubin in the basal ganglia, to cause kernicterus, may occur if there is rapid haemolysis in the presence of impaired liver function or hepatic immaturity. This is almost unknown in adults, but can occur in neonates and premature babies. Haemolysis in the neonate is conventionally classified as **congenital spherocytic**, or **congenital non-spherocytic anaemia**. The presence of spherocytes indicates hereditary spherocytosis or antibody-mediated red cell destruction. Congenital non-spherocytic anaemia is usually the result of inherited red-cell enzyme defects, the most common of which is deficiency of glucose-6-phosphate dehydrogenase — an important enzyme for generating NADPH in all cells (not only red cells). Deficiency of this enzyme in hepatocytes, together with hepatic immaturity, may contribute to the severe jaundice (with its attendant risk of kernicterus) that occurs in neonates with this condition. Haemolytic anaemias are frequently associated with the presence of **pigment gallstones** which may even be the presenting feature of illness (e.g. in hereditary spherocytosis).

Other haemolytic anaemias

Disseminated carcinoma — with, for example, a gastric primary — can precipitate disseminated intravascular coagulation and the resulting fibrin deposition can lead to a microangiopathic haemolytic anaemia (5). Both mucin-secreting and non-mucin-secreting tumours have been implicated. Intimal proliferation of the pulmonary arterioles (perhaps as a result of micrometastases) has been detected in some patients with microangiopathic haemolytic anaemia associated with carcinoma, and pulmonary hypertension may be a part of the syndrome.

HAEMOGLOBINOPATHIES

The haemoglobinopathies are **autosomal recessive** conditions; they can be divided into the

Table 25.6. Causes of anaemia in liver disease.

Cause	Comments
Dilutional	Increased plasma volume, splenomegaly
Iron deficiency	Bleeding. May be difficult to diagnose
Vitamin B_{12} deficiency	Uncommon
Folate deficiency	Alcoholism. Poor nutrition (e.g. in cirrhosis)
Haemolytic anaemia	Red-cell life span often reduced. Abnormal red cell membrane
	Specific haemolytic syndromes include Zieve's syndrome, spur cell anaemia, Wilsons's disease. Disseminated intravascular coagulation has increased frequency in chronic liver disease
	Autoimmune haemolysis may occur with autoimmune liver disease. Micrangiopathic haemolytic anaemia, [TTP in full], and haemolytic–uraemic syndrome may occur rarely
Aplastic	Associated with viral hepatitis. Impaired hepatic detoxification of organic chemicals may predispose

structural haemoglobin variants (e.g. sickle cell disease) and **disorders of globin-chain synthesis** (the thalassaemia syndromes). The most important affect the β chain (e.g. sickle cell disease, haemoglobin C and β thalassaemia); because the major haemoglobin of late fetal and neonatal life (HbF: α2 γ2) does not contain β chains, these disorders do not present until at least 6–9 months of age. A single amino acid substitution (valine for glutamic acid) in the sixth position of the β chain characterizes haemoglobin HbS and underlies sickle cell disease. HbS tends to polymerize under conditions of low oxygen tension, and this alters the shape of red cells, which in turn leads to thrombosis in small vessels.

Abdominal pain is a frequent presenting feature of sickle cell crisis, and arises through microinfarcts affecting abdominal organs (e.g. liver and spleen) and intestinal mucosa. Mucosal damage predisposes to **bacteraemia** (e.g. caused by *Salmonella*) which may, in turn, cause other recognized complications of sickle cell disease (e.g. gallbladder disease, infection, osteomyelitis). Repeated **infarction of the spleen** during childhood leads to hyposplenism in adults with sickle cell disease, which further predisposes to infection. **Splenic sequestration** crisis in sickle cell disease occurs in children (typically, those younger than 5 years) when red cells sickle within the spleen. Patients present with severe anaemia, splenic pain, and splenomegaly. Splenic sequestration is an acute emergency, and treatment is with blood transfusion; splenectomy is usually performed once the acute event has subsided. **Hepatic sequestration** tends to occur in older children and adults, and presents with severe anaemia and tender hepatomegaly; treatment is by blood tranfusion. Other hepatic complications of sickle cell disease include hepatocellular necrosis, fibrosis, and iron overload.

Blood transfusion is an important modality of **treatment** in the haemoglobinopathies, and is mandatory in thalassaemia major and intermedia. Each unit of packed red cells contains 250 mg of iron, and iron overload occurs frequently, in spite of iron chelation therapy. Intestinal iron absorption is also increased in thalassaemia, probably as an effect of the low mean corpuscular volume on intestinal cells. The major effects of iron overload are similar to those of haemochromatosis (skin pigmentation, diabetes, endocrine disorders, cardiomyopathy, and liver disease).

ANAEMIA IN LIVER DISEASE

A normochromic normocytic anaemia is common in uncomplicated chronic liver disease (Table 25.6) (6). An increased plasma volume as a result of fluid retention and portal venous congestion leads to haemodilution. Splenomegaly also increases plasma volume, causes red cells to pool within the spleen, and can lead to shortened red cell survival. The bone marrow response to anaemia is suboptimal in patients with chronic liver disease, and the precise mechanisms of this remains unclear. Concentrations of erythropoietin are lower in patients with chronic liver disease than in those who are iron deficient but have the same degree of anaemia; however, unlike renal failure, erythropoietin treatment does not lead to a sustained increase in haemoglobin concentration. Increased concentrations of tumour necrosis factor and interleukin-1 may also contribute to the anaemia.

Haematinic metabolism in liver disease

Cirrhosis is a cause of "anaemia of chronic disease" — a common syndrome complicating chronic inflammatory, infective, and neoplastic conditions in which there is defective utilization of iron. The serum concentration of iron is reduced, but (in contrast to iron deficiency) the TIBC is also reduced. The serum ferritin concentration is often increased in cirrhosis, as a result of hepatic inflammation; production of transferrin may decline in chronic liver disease, and the mean corpuscular volume increases. Iron status can therefore be difficult to establish. Iron deficiency, however, commonly occurs as a result of bleeding, and is an easily correctable contributor to the anaemia of chronic liver disease. The liver is an important storage organ for both vitamin B_{12} and folic acid, and their concentrations may increase in conditions in which there is hepatic necrosis. Folic acid deficiency occurs in alcoholism; alcohol also impairs the absorption of folic acid and vitamin B_{12} from the intestine and decreases hepatic stores.

Haemolytic anaemia in liver disease

Red cell life span is frequently reduced in chronic liver disease. This is a consequence of both intracorpuscular and extracorpuscular causes. The major **intracorpuscular cause of haemolysis** is abnormal red cell shape, resulting from alterations in the lipid composition of red cells. Liver disease is frequently associated with an increase in the free cholesterol content of the red cell membrane, which causes an expansion of the membrane. Macrocytosis is the most frequent consequence, but other red cell shape changes in liver disease include those to target cells, echinocytes, and bizarre spiculated cells called acanthocytes; this last severe, haemolytic anaemia is termed "spur cell anaemia". Other intracorpuscular defects include abnormal haem synthesis (e.g. sideroblastic anaemia in association with alcoholism) and reduced activity of red cell enzymes — for example, pyruvate kinase and glucose-6-phophate dehydrogenase deficiencies. An increasingly recognized contributory factor to jaundice in patients with G6PD deficiency is reduced activity of the enzyme in hepatocytes. This is particularly important in neonatal jaundice in G6PD deficient patients (7). The most important

extracorpuscular cause of haemolysis is splenomegaly. The normal spleen plays a central role in "conditioning" the red cell, whereby the spleen progressively erodes the surface of red cells entrapped within its specialized circulation, causing spherocytosis and haemolysis. This effect is enhanced with splenomegaly. Hyperlipidaemia also alters red cell membranes and contributes to haemolysis in Zieve's syndrome; however, this occurs principally in alcoholic individuals, and associated abnormalities (e.g. vitamin E deficiency, folic acid deficiency) may contribute. Haemolysis is often the presenting feature in Wilson's disease, and probably results from a direct toxic effect of copper on erythrocytes.

Aplastic anaemia in liver disease

A transient, mild depression of bone-marrow function leading to mild panyctopenia occurs commonly in viral hepatitis — as, indeed, it does in other viral diseases. However, viral hepatitis is an aetiological factor in up to 10% of patients with aplastic anaemia. Although it is well described in patients with documented hepatitis A and B infection, antibodies to hepatitis viruses A, B, C, and G are usually absent, and the precise cause thus remains unknown (8). The hepatitis is usually mild, the marrow aplasia characteristically severe, and the outcome is often grave. Much of the damage to bone-marrow stem cells (and, indeed, to hepatocytes) us immunologi-cally mediated.

References
1. Pawson R, Mehta A. Diagnosis and treatment of haematinic deficiency in gastrointestinal disease. *Aliment Pharmacol Ther* 1998; **12**: 687–698.
2. Chanarin I, Metz J. Diagnosis of cobalamin deficiency: the old and the new. *Br J Haematol* 1997; **97**: 695–700.
3. Toh BH, Van Dreel IR, Gleeson PA. Pernicious anemia. *N Eng J Med* 1997; **337**: 1441–1448.
4. Rockey DC, Cello JP. Evaluation of the gastrointestinal tract in patients with iron deficiency anaemia. *N Eng J Med* 1993; **329**: 1691–1695.
5. Rytting M, Worth L, Jaffe N. Hemolytic disorders associated with cancer. *Hematol Oncol Clin North Am* 1996; **10**: 276–365.
6. Mehta AB, McIntyre N. Haematological disorders in liver disease. *Forum: Trends Exp Clin Med* 1998; **8**: 8–25.
7. Mehta A, Mason PJ, Vulliamy TJ. Glucose-6-phosphate dehydrogenase deficiency. *Baillieres Clin Haematol* 2000; **13**: 21–38.
8. Brown KE, Tisdale J, Barrat J, *et al.* Hepatitis associated aplastic anemia. *N Eng J Med* 1997; **336**: 1059–1064.

26. Dyspepsia and Gastrooesophageal Reflux

MAGDA NEWTON

DEFINITIONS

Dyspepsia was defined by a panel of experts who met in Rome in 1992 (1) as "pain or discomfort centered in the upper abdomen" and includes symptoms such as early satiety, postprandial discomfort or fullness, nausea, and bloating (2). Heartburn, acid regurgitation, and borborygmi may also be present, but are secondary symptoms in the diagnosis. The classification further subdivides the symptoms into ulcer-like and dysmotility-like dyspepsia, but these definitions are poor predictors of both endoscopic and pathological disease (3). Dyspepsia is caused by peptic ulcer disease in the minority of patients, and a proportion of patients will have gastrooesophageal reflux disease. The majority will have **endoscopy-negative dyspepsia**. This is also known as **functional dyspepsia** or **non-ulcer dyspepsia**. Perhaps a more appropriate term at present is **idiopathic dyspepsia**.

Gastro-oesophageal reflux describes the entry of gastric contents into the oesophagus. This is a physiological event, occurring in healthy asymptomatic individuals, particularly after meals. **Gastro-oesophageal reflux disease** has been defined as "the occurrence of reflux-like symptoms which impair quality of life or the presence of endoscopic erosive oesophagitis" by members of the Genval workshop on reflux disease (4). **Heartburn** is "a burning sensation across the lower chest rising toward or into the neck" often exacerbated by meals or postural change.

EPIDEMIOLOGY

Dyspepsia is very common, with 23–41% of Western populations experiencing dyspepsia and up to 10% experiencing frequent heartburn or acid regurgitation. The incidence of dyspepsia and gastro-oesophageal reflux is, however, believed to be small. Swedish studies have suggested that the incidence of dyspepsia is 0.8% and that of reflux disease 0.5%, over a 3-month period.

A significant health-care resource is applied to the investigation and treatment of dyspepsia. In the UK, more than £4m was spent on ulcer-healing drug prescriptions in 1994. Although 25% of sufferers (5% of the total population) may seek medical help, the majority will self-medicate. Despite this, 4% of general practice consultations are for dyspepsia (5), and it is estimated that 2% of the population undergo either endoscopy or barium meal each year. The hospital gastroenterologist sees only the tip of the iceberg, as only 10% of patients attending their general practitioner with dyspepsia will be referred for hospital consultation. This figure may have changed with the increasing availability of open-access gastroscopy.

Role of *Helicobacter pylori*

Chapter 40 gives a detailed account of the diagnosis and management of *H. pylori* infection.

The role of *H. pylori* infection in dyspepsia is not clear; although it is closely associated with histological gastritis, the correlation between symptoms and endoscopic or histological mucosal abnormality is not good. Currently, there is no convincing evidence to support the importance of *H. pylori* in idiopathic dyspepsia (6). Eradication of this organism in these patients has not been shown to be of benefit (7), although the literature is controversial on this point (8,9).

CLINICAL ASSESSMENT

Symptoms

There are several symptomatic predictors of peptic ulcer disease (10):

- epigastric pain — burning or hunger-like
- relief of pain by food or antacids
- occurrence of pain 1–3 h after meals
- nocturnal pain
- periodic symptoms

Evidence suggests, however, that symptom assessment alone in dyspeptic patients will predict peptic ulceration in fewer than 50% (11). In those in whom heartburn is the predominant symptom and there is good relief with antacids, there is 89% specificity for reflux disease (12), although sensitivity is poor. The relationship between symptoms, oesophageal acid exposure, and oesophageal erosive change in gastrooesophageal reflux disease is not a simple one. Patients may present with atypical symptoms for reflux disease, which include chest pain, dysphagia, asthma, and reflux laryngitis. These patients often require further investigation to establish cause of symptoms.

INVESTIGATION OF DYSPEPSIA

The aims of investigation are to detect significant disease, to direct therapy appropriately, and to reassure the patient. The choice of investigation in patients with dyspepsia may also take into account an aspect of cost–utility, but there is controversy over the most appropriate method of management if this is the only factor. Clinical decisions are therefore important for the individual. **Indications for referral for endoscopy in patients with dyspepsia** include:

- Any patient with dyspepsia and alarm symptoms or signs:
  - unintentional weight loss
  - iron-deficiency anaemia
  - gastrointestinal bleeding
  - dysphagia, odynophagia, or both
  - previous gastric surgery
  - persistent vomiting
  - epigastric mass
  - suspicious results from barium meal
  - previous gastric ulcer
  - use of non-steroidal anti-inflammatory drugs (NSAIDs)
  - epigastric pain severe enough to cause admission to hospital
- Any patient older than 45 years with recent onset of dyspepsia
- Patients younger than 45 years with dyspepsia:
  - who are *H. pylori*-positive who have persistent symptoms despite eradication treatment
  - who are *H. pylori*-negative in whom symptoms persist after reassurance and a course of empirical treatment with antacids or an H_2-blocker
- Patients in whom gastrooesophageal reflux disease is suspected (see later)

Patients with alarm symptoms, regardless of age, should undergo gastroscopy. These symptoms include early satiety, anorexia, vomiting, haematemesis, melaena, dysphagia, weight loss, or anaemia.

In other patients, the need to carry out further investigation depends upon age, other risk factors, and the presence of persisting symptoms (Figure 26.1).

Patients aged 45 years and older who have dyspepsia of recent-onset should be referred for further investigation, as the risk of gastric and other malignancies are significantly increased in this age group.

Patients younger than 45 years with recent-onset dyspepsia and absence of sinister features should be tested for *H. pylori*. This may be done using serological tests or urea breath testing. There is debate as to which patients should then be referred for further investigation. Some, such as the British Society of Gastroenterology (13) advocate endoscopy in *H. pylori*-positive patients (and those taking NSAIDs), as the risk of peptic ulceration in *H. pylori*-negative patients is very low (14,15). Others, including the authors of the Maastricht Con-

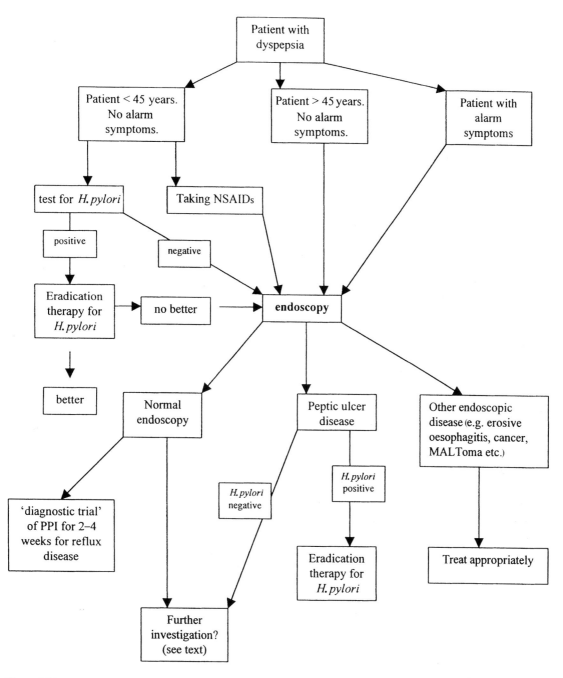

Figure 26.1. Route of investigation for patients with dyspepsia. It takes into account the age of the patient at presentation, the presence or absence of sinister symptoms, and the use of NSAIDs. PPI, proton pump inhibitor; MALToma, mucosa-associated lymphoid tissue lymphoma.

sensus Report (16), suggest that empirical treatment of all patients who are *H. pylori*-positive will ensure that all patients with peptic ulcer disease will be treated, and that this has as good an outcome as the use of endoscopy first in these patients. This approach has been supported by the findings of a randomized study of *H. pylori*-positive patients with 'ulcer-like' dyspepsia who were assigned randomly to receive empirical triple treatment or endoscopy first and treatment of those with mucosal disease only. The outcome in the empirical treatment group was as good or better at 1 year, and only 27% of these patients required subsequent endoscopy for resistant symptoms (17).

Although the majority of patients with gastric cancer are *H. pylori*-positive — which is the argument for endoscopy of *H. pylori*-positive patients in this age group — gastric cancer is rare in patients younger than 45 years; in particular, cancer is rarely found in the absence of sinister symptoms (18).

The **economic arguments** for the benefits of endoscopy over *H. pylori* testing before treatment are weak according to cost—utility or decision analysis based on the American health-care system (19,20). Others have suggested that there is no obvious benefit of one plan of investigation over another (21).

In patients in whom *H. pylori* testing is undertaken and empirical treatment given, it is important to use treatment that will eradicate the organism in 80% of patients. This will vary according to the antibiotic resistance of the local population. These patients require follow-up, ideally to confirm eradication of *H. pylori* by breath testing and to ensure resolution of symptoms.

Use of endoscopy

In patients in whom visualization of the upper gastrointestinal tract is required, endoscopy is the investigation of choice for patients with dyspepsia. The procedure is safe. Mortality associated with diagnostic upper gastrointestinal endoscopy is rare — reportedly varying from 1 in 2000 to 1 in 10 000 endoscopies (22). Among outpatients, this figure is likely to be even lower.

Of the endoscopies undertaken in an open-access endoscopy service, 30% will be normal (personal data). Of those with abnormal findings, 10–17% will have erosive oesophagitis, 10–15% a duodenal ulcer, 5–10% gastric ulcer, 2% gastric cancer, and 30% gastritis, duodenitis, or a hiatus hernia.

Gastric or duodenal mucosal biopsy, have limited roles in the diagnosis of dyspepsia. In all patients with **gastric ulceration**, several biopsies of the lesion should be performed, to exclude malignancy. Gastric antral biopsies should be taken to look for *H. pylori* in patients with gastric and duodenal ulceration. In patients who have been taking proton pump inhibitors (PPIs) before endoscopy, *H. pylori* may migrate proximally within the stomach, and more proximal gastric biopsies may be required to detect the organism. The presence of histological gastritis or duodenitis does not correlate well with endoscopic change or symptoms. Currently, neither specific treatment nor eradication of *H. pylori* is recommended in these patients (16).

A small proportion of patients may not tolerate endoscopy or may not wish to have this investigation. In these patients, a double-contrast barium meal is the investigation of choice.

H. pylori-negative duodenal ulcer disease

The majority of patients with *H. pylori*-negative duodenal ulceration are taking NSAIDs and a careful history of recent use should be taken (23). If patients have not taken NSAIDs and are *H. pylori*-negative, **other causes of duodenal ulceration** should be considered:

- NSAID use
- coeliac disease
- lymphoma
- Crohn's disease
- Zollinger—Ellison syndrome

Patients with *H. pylori*-negative duodenal ulcer who are not taking NSAIDs should be referred to a gastroenterologist for further investigation. At endoscopy these patients should be considered for duodenal biopsy and fasting gastrin studies.

Zollinger–Ellison syndrome

Patients with Zollinger–Ellison syndrome may present with persistent gastric or duodenal ulceration. There is often associated oesophagitis. Presentation may, however, be with diarrhoea and weight loss, or an abdominal mass. The condition is rare, affecting 1 in 1 000 000 of the population. Patients suspected of having Zollinger–Ellison syndrome must undergo a

Table 26.1. Endoscopic classifications of gastrooesophageal reflux disease.

Grade	Description
Los Angeles Classification (27)	
A	One (or more) mucosal break no longer than 5 mm, that does not extend between the tops of two mucosal folds
B	One (or more) mucosal break more than 5 mm long that does not extend between the tops of two mucosal folds
C	One (or more) mucosal break that is continuous between the tops of two or more mucosal folds, but which involves less than 75% of the circumference
D	One (or more) mucosal break that involves at least 75% of the oesophageal circumference
Savary–Monnier Classification (26)	
I	One or more mucosal breaks with or without exudate
II	More than one mucosal break confluent across two or more mucosal folds
III	Mucosal breaks that are confluent and circumferential in the oesophagus
IV	Complications including Barrett's oesophagus, stricture, deep ulcers

fasting gastrin concentration test. This should be taken after the patient has stopped taking PPIs for at least 1 week or H_2-receptor antagonists for at least 3 days. Interpretation of an increased gastrin concentration must be made with caution, as increased values are found in patients with achlorhydria, in addition to those receiving acid-suppressive medication. Diagnosis should be confirmed with gastric secretion studies. In patients found to have Zollinger–Ellison syndrome, a search for the primary tumour is necessary, as these are often malignant.

Further investigation

A few patients are not reassured, despite negative serology and a normal endoscopy. Further investigation may reveal disturbance of gastric motility and delayed gastric emptying, but these findings are not consistent and do not correlate well with symptoms (24). Experimental tools used in the assessment of patients with dyspepsia include radionuclide gastric emptying studies, abdominal ultrasound scanning of gastric antral function, electrogastrography, and assessment of gastric tone using the gastric barostat. The use of the hydrogen breath testing to assess lactose intolerance is controversial (25). These tools are experimental, and as yet have limited clinical value.

INVESTIGATION OF GASTRO-OESOPHAGEAL REFLUX DISEASE

A clinical diagnosis of gastrooesophageal reflux disease can be made in patients presenting with a history of frequent heartburn, often associated with regurgitation, and relieved by antacids. Older patients and those with other symptoms will require further investigation.

Gastroscopy

Gastroscopy is the initial investigation of choice in patients with reflux disease. At endoscopy, a proportion of patients will have erosive oesophagitis. Endoscopic identification of **oesophagitis**, based on the presence of oesophageal erosions, has a high specificity, but poor sensitivity, in the diagnosis of reflux disease. There are many endoscopic classifications of oesophagitis, but the most familiar are those described by Monnier & Savary (26) and the more recent Los Angeles classification (27) (Table 26.1). These classifications of severity correlate well with severity of symptoms and degree of oesophageal acid reflux (28). Minor endoscopic abnormalities such as erythema or friability at the squamocolumnar junction are poor predictors of reflux disease and have a high interobserver variability (28).

Oesophageal mucosal biopsy has little to add in the diagnosis of gastrooesophageal reflux disease, as histological changes are not consistent. Mucosal biopsy, however, is valuable in the diagnosis of oesophageal malignancy, infection, and Barrett's oesophagus.

Endoscopy-negative reflux disease

Absence of endoscopic abnormality does not exclude reflux disease, as a significant number of patients will have "endoscopy-negative" reflux disease. In these patients a diagnostic course of a proton

Table 26.2.   The symptom indices used in the diagnosis and management of gastro-oesophageal reflux disease.

Name of index	Criteria	Reference
Symptom Index	Number of reflux-associated symptom episodes/total number of reflux episodes	32
Symptom Sensitivity Index	Number of reflux-associated symptom episodes/total number of symptom episodes	33
Symptom Association Probability	The probability that a symptom episode has been associated with an episode of gastrooesophageal reflux	34

pump inhibitor is suggested. The good response to such treatment in patients with reflux disease has led to the proposal that higher-dose PPIs — for example omeprazole 40 mg daily for 1 or 2 weeks — given as a "diagnostic trial" will detect patients with endoscopy-negative reflux disease. Evidence for this is scant, but convincing (29–31), and there is controversy over the use of diagnostic trials of these agents in patients who have not undergone endoscopy.

Twenty-four-hour ambulatory oesophageal pH monitoring

Further investigation may be necessary for patients who respond poorly to treatment or who have atypical symptoms such as chest pain. Twenty-four-hour ambulatory pH monitoring has been the "gold standard" in the diagnosis of gastrooesophageal reflux disease, although it is now recognized that up to 25% of patients with reflux disease will have "normal" oesophageal acid exposure times. The acid content of the oesophagus is monitored over a 24-h period with the patient both erect and supine; this is usually an outpatient investigation. After an overnight fast, a nasogastric recording catheter is placed 5 cm above the lower oesophageal sphincter. The position of the sphincter can be determined either by the change in pH as the pH sensor is drawn back from the stomach into the oesophagus, or by a high-pressure zone determined at oesophageal manometry; the latter is the more accurate method of measurement. Patients are usually allowed to eat a normal diet, with some restrictions on alcohol intake and certain acid foods. A diary card is kept of food intake and symptoms during the recording period. A symptom event button on the recording box is used to record symptomatic episodes.

After the 24-h recording, the data recorded are downloaded onto a computer and the results analysed according to a predetermined algorithm. Acid gastrooesophageal reflux is defined as a decrease in the oesophageal pH to less than pH 4. From the data obtained during 24-h oesophageal pH recording, several (**De Meester**) **parameters of oesophageal acid reflux** are usually calculated:

1. Total time of oesophageal pH <4 as a percentage of 24 h
2. Percentage time of pH <4 during erect and supine positions
3. Number of episodes of pH <4
4. Number of episodes of pH <4 for more than 5 min
5. Longest period of pH <4

Various scoring systems have been calculated to define excessive oesophageal acid reflux; most often, it is defined as a total acid reflux time of greater than 4–6% of the total recording period, in association with other abnormal findings.

Correlation of symptoms with episodes of acid gastrooesophageal reflux recorded during 24-h oesophageal pH monitoring has led to the development of a number of "symptom indices" (Table 26.2). Use of the association of symptoms with episodes of acid reflux has increased the sensitivity of oesophageal pH monitoring in the diagnosis of gastrooesophageal reflux disease, particularly for patients whose 24-h oesophageal exposure to acid may be within "normal" limits.

Other investigations

Oesophageal bile reflux

Reflux of bile into the oesophagus can produce the same symptoms as acid reflux. The development of bile sensors that can be used in oesophageal studies has allowed the investigation of bile reflux. Although a proportion of symptomatic patients have excessive oesophageal bile reflux, in the majority of patients symptoms are related more to episodes of acid reflux (35).

Double-contrast barium swallow

As in other dyspeptic patients, a small proportion of patients may not tolerate endoscopy or may not wish to have this investigation. In these patients, a double-contrast barium swallow may be required, to exclude other oesophageal diseases. Excessive reflux of barium during a barium-swallow examination may indicate a tendency to gastrooesophageal reflux, but does not have a good positive predictive value for patients with symptomatic gastrooesophageal reflux disease, and is poorly reproducible in the clinical situation (36).

Provocation tests

Provocation tests such as the Bernstein acid perfusion test, in which the symptomatic response to oesophageal instillation of acid is recorded, are useful in patients who have multiple symptoms or in those with chest pain of non-cardiac origin. These investigations are used in a very small proportion of patients with gastrooesophageal reflux disease.

TREATMENT

Duodenal ulcer

Treatment of *H. Pylori*-positive duodenal ulcer is discussed in detail in Chapter 40. It is likely that management of duodenal ulcers and duodenal erosions should follow the same course.

In **asymptomatic patients with uncomplicated duodenal ulcer disease**, further endoscopic follow-up is unnecessary. In patients with **persistent or recurrent symptoms (after initial response)**, eradication of *H. pylori* should ideally be confirmed by radiocarbon-labelled-urea breath testing more than 1 month after treatment. Use of serology to confirm the eradication of the organism is usually not helpful, as a decrease in antibody titres may not occur for 6 months, if at all. Where breath testing is not available, repeat endoscopy may be required. Recurrence of duodenal ulcer after successful eradi-

cation of *H. pylori* is uncommon (10% over 1 year) and is usually the result of recrudescence of the infection. For those few patients with persistent *H. pylori* infection despite adequate attempts at eradication treatment, long-term treatment with acid suppression may be required.

In **patients with complicated duodenal ulcer disease** (e.g. bleeding or perforation at presentation), *H. pylori* eradication should be confirmed with a radiocarbon-labelled-urea breath test. If this is not possible, repeat endoscopy should be carried out to confirm ulcer healing, and endoscopic biopsies taken to confirm eradication of the organism. Some gastroenterologists would advocate the latter approach in all cases of complicated duodenal ulcer disease.

A **positive repeat breath test** requires further courses of eradication treatment; antibiotic sensitivity and patient compliance may need to be checked.

Patients with *H. pylori*-negative duodenal ulcers require further investigation to exclude other causes listed above. If no other cause is identified, patients may require long-term acid suppression if symptoms recur after treatment. Repeat endoscopy to assess the progress of ulcer healing may be required.

Gastric ulcer

Seventy per cent of gastric ulcers are associated with *H. pylori*. Most *H. pylori*-negative gastric ulcers are associated with use of NSAIDs. In all cases of gastric ulcer, adequate biopsies should be sent for histology to exclude malignant disease. The presence of *H. pylori* should be sought. There is some evidence that additional cytology of gastric ulcers increases the detection of gastric malignancy.

Patients with *H. pylori*-positive gastric ulcers should receive *H. pylori* eradication treatment. In these patients, antisecretory therapy is recommended for up to 2 months, although there is some evidence to suggest that gastric ulcers heal as quickly after *H. pylori* eradication alone.

H. pylori-negative gastric ulcer should be treated with antisecretory therapy for 2 months, with either H_2-receptor antagonists or PPIs. NSAIDs should be discontinued if possible. In patients continuing to take NSAIDs, omeprazole is recommended as the antisecretory agent of choice, as this is more effective than H_2-receptor antagonists (37).

The management of **NSAID-associated gastric ulcer** is currently under review. There is evidence that co-treatment with misoprostol may be beneficial if the NSAID is to be continued, although misoprostol may be poorly tolerated and omeprazole may be as effective (38). The introduction of cyclo-oxygenase-II-selective antagonists for the treatment of arthritis may reduce the prevalence of NSAID-associated peptic ulceration.

Follow-up of gastric ulcers

All patients with gastric ulcer should have follow-up endoscopy after 6–8 weeks, to confirm gastric ulcer healing. If the ulcer is not healed, repeat biopsies should be taken until complete healing occurs. Failure of gastric ulceration to heal despite adequate treatment may be an indication for gastric surgery. The timing of such surgery is not clear, although many endoscopists suggest referral after 6 months of treatment. Patients who are found to have high-grade dysplasia must have early repeat endoscopy with biopsy, as carcinoma *in situ* is common in these patients.

Gastrooesophageal reflux disease

Evidence suggests that *H. pylori* infection is not associated with gastrooesophageal reflux disease (39,40), and that eradication of *H. pylori* in patients with reflux may exacerbate symptoms (41). Management depends upon **adequate gastric acid suppression**.

Patients with mild to moderate erosive oesophagitis and patients with endoscopy-negative reflux disease should be managed in a similar way, as response to treatment and maintenance treatment are similar in the two conditions. It has been suggested that patients with severe (Los Angeles classification C + D; Table 26.1) erosive oesophagitis should be managed more aggressively.

The aims of treatment are symptom relief and prevention of complication. It is preferable to achieve mucosal healing, although evidence for long-term outcome when this is not fully realized is unavailable.

Medical treatments

Although advice to **modify lifestyle** is usually advocated as first-line medical therapy, evidence for short- or long-term benefit is poor (4). Patients with minimal gastrooesophageal reflux symptoms may benefit from advice about weight reduction, avoidance of fatty foods, alcohol, and caffeine, and avoidance of late evening meals and tight-fitting clothes. Elevating the head of the bed at night may help in those patients who have nocturnal symptoms. There is no clear evidence that cessation of smoking is beneficial in these patients.

Antacid therapy may relieve symptoms transiently, but has not been shown to have a significant effect on healing rates in oesophagitis. However, combination of an antacid with an alginate does have symptomatic benefit.

Histamine receptor antagonists

Use of H_2-blockers relieves symptoms and heals oesophageal erosions. The evidence that using larger doses achieves greater acid suppression and improves healing rates is poor, although there may be some value to patients who can not tolerate PPIs. Recent evidence suggests that the addition of a histamine receptor antagonist to PPI therapy at night is beneficial (42).

Motility agents

Cisapride relieves symptoms in patients with mild to moderate disease. Its efficacy appears to be equal to that of H_2-blockers. When it is used in combination with H_2-blockers, healing rates are improved and rates of relapse reduced.

Proton pump inhibitors

PPIs are extremely effective in the treatment of gastrooesophageal reflux disease. Oesophageal mucosal healing occurs in up to 95% of patients with erosive disease. Symptom relief is evident in 85% of patients after 4–8 weeks of treatment maintenance therapy with a PPI is effective at preventing relapse of mucosal and symptomatic disease. PPIs are also more effective than placebo and H_2-blockers in the management of endoscopy-negative reflux disease (43).

Choice of treatment

Management of gastrooesophageal reflux disease can broadly be separated into "step-up" or "step-down" approaches. There is some suggestion that a "step-down" approach to treatment (Figure 26.2) reduces consultation and re-investigation rates. Cost-effectiveness analyses are weak, but favour this approach.

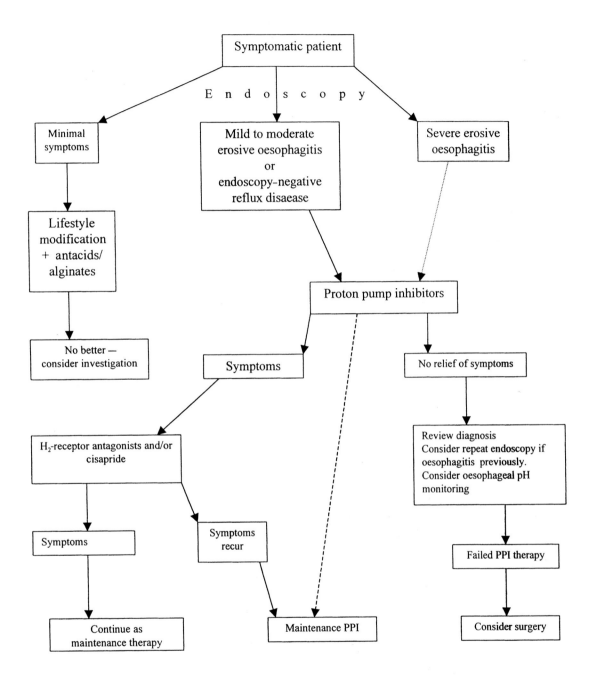

Figure 26.2. The step-down approach to the treatment of gastrooesophageal reflux disease. It results in rapid relief of symptoms for the majority of patients.

For the patient, it is important that symptoms are adequately controlled. There is some evidence that, in the majority of patients, absence of symptoms reflects mucosal healing. Repeated endoscopy is not necessary in patients with mild to moderate disease, but there may be some value in repeating endoscopy in patients with more severe disease, to assess their response to treatment.

Maintenance of symptom-free disease

Relapse rates for gastrooesophageal reflux disease are reported as being between 50 and 90% on cessation of treatment. Prevention of relapse depends largely on long-term acid suppression. PPIs are the most effective form of maintenance therapy, and patients with severe disease should be maintained on one of these drugs (4). Stepping down from this treatment in patients with mild to moderate disease may be largely cost driven. Combination therapy with an H_2-receptor antagonist and cisapride is more effective than treatment with the former alone.

Follow-up

In the absence of oesophageal ulcers, oesophageal strictures, or Barrett's oesophagus, further endoscopy is not necessary after treatment. Patients should be treated with the aim of controlling their symptoms. At present there is no evidence to suggest that, in symptomatic patients who respond to treatment, the incidence of long-term complications is greater than in those who have regular endoscopic follow-up.

Surgery in gastrooesophageal reflux disease

Surgical treatment of oesophageal disease is indicated when there is failure of medical therapy to heal oesophagitis, when symptoms persist despite maximal treatment, or when complications of oesophagitis develop. In infants and children with persisting reflux, surgical procedures may be necessary to reduce the risk of long-term complications. Economically, it appears that the costs of surgery, when compared with those of long-term treatment with PPIs, may be recouped after 10 years of continuous treatment (44), although prospective trials are required to confirm this.

Current recommendations for the management of non-ulcer dyspepsia

1. Stop NSAIDs if possible.

2. Give reassurance.

3. Give a trial of acid suppression with an adequate dose of PPI for at least 2 weeks. If the initial response is good, consider titration of acid suppression for a further 4–6 weeks.

4. Consider use of other symptomatic treatments — for example motility agents (domperidone) with or without further investigation of gastrointestinal motility; however, evidence for the effectiveness of these agents is anecdotal.

5. *H. pylori* eradication is not currently recommended in this group of patients.

6. Consider investigation of the biliary tree as a cause of symptoms.

7. If serious symptoms develop, repeat the investigations.

8. New developments in the management of patients with idiopathic dyspepsia include the use of 5-hydroxytryptamine antagonists and peripheral kappa-receptor antagonists (45), which may have some value in these patients.

References

1. Drossman DA. The functional gastrointestinal disorders and the Rome II process. *Gut* 1999; **45(suppl 2)**: ii1–ii5.
2. Talley NJ, Colin-Jones D, Koch KL *et al*. Functional dyspepsia: a classification with guidelines for diagnosis and management. *Gastroenterol Int* 1990; **4**: 145–160.
3. Talley NJ, Weaver AL, Tesmer DL *et al*. Lack of discriminant value of dyspepsia subgroups in patients referred for upper endoscopy. *Gastroenterology* 1993; **105**: 1378–1386.
4. Dent J, Brun J, Fendrick AM, Fennerty MB *et al*. On behalf of the Genval Workshop Group. An evidence-based appraisal of reflux disease management – the Genval Workshop Report. *Gut* 1999; **44(suppl 2)**: S1–S16.
5. Jones RH, Lydeard SE, Hobbs FSR *et al*. Dyspepsia in England and Scotland. *Gut* 1990; **31**: 40–45.
6. Talley NJ, Hunt RH. What role does Helicobacter pylori play in dyspepsia and non-ulcer dyspepsia? Arguments for and against H. pylori being associated with dyspeptic symptoms. *Gastroenterology* 1997; **113**: S67–S77.
7. Talley NJ. A critique of therapeutic trials in H. pylori-positive functional dyspepsia. *Gastroenterology* 1994; **106**: 1174–1183.
8. Talley NJ, Janssens J, Lauritsen K *et al*. Long-term follow-up of patients with non-ulcer dyspepsia after Helicobacter eradication. A randomized double-blind placebo-controlled trial [abstract]. *Gastroenterology* 1998; **114**: A305.
9. McColl KEL, Murray LS, El-Omar E *et al*. U.K. MRC trial of H. pylori eradication therapy for non-ulcer dyspepsia [abstract]. *Gut* 1998; **42**: A3.
10. Rune SJ. Heartburn and dyspepsia: the utility of symptom analysis. *Aliment Pharmacol Ther* 1997; **11(suppl 2)**: 9–12.
11. Bytzer P, Schaffalitzky de Muckadell OB. Prediction of major pathologic conditions in dyspeptic patients referred for endoscopy. A prospective evaluation of a scoring system. *Scand J Gastroenterol* 1992; **27**: 987–992.

12. Klauser AG, Schindlebeck NE, Muller-Lissner SA. Symptoms in gastro-oesophageal reflux disease. *Lancet* 1990; **1**: 205–208.

13. Axon ATR, Bell GD, Jones RH *et al*. Guidelines on appropriate indications for upper gastrointestinal endoscopy. *BMJ* 1995; **310**: 853–856.

14. Collins JAS, Bamford KB, Sloan JM *et al*. Screening for Helicobacter pylori antibody could reduce endoscopy workload in young dyspeptic patients. *Eur J Gastroenterol Hepatol* 1992; **4**: 991–993.

15. Mendall MA, Goggin PM, Marrero JM *et al*. Role of Helicobacter pylori serology in screening prior to endoscopy. *Eur J Gastroenterol Heptol* 1992; **4**: 713–717.

16. The European Helicobacter pylori Study Group (EHPSG). Current European concepts in the management of Helicobacter pylori infection. The Maastricht Consensus Report. *Gut* 1997; **41**: 8–13.

17. Heaney A, Collins JSA, Watson RGP *et al*. A prospective randomised trial of a 'test and treat' policy versus endoscopy-based management in young Helicobacter pylori positive patients with ulcer-like dyspepsia. *Gut* 1999; **45**: 186–190.

18. Christie J, Shepherd NA, Coding WB *et al*. Gastric cancer below the age of 55: implications for screening patients with uncomplicated dyspepsia. *Gut* 1997; **41**: 513–517.

19. Silverstein MD, Petterson T, Talley NJ. Initial endoscopy or empirical therapy with or without testing for Helicobacter pylori for dyspepsia: a decision analysis. *Gastroenterology* 1996; **110**: 72–83.

20. Ebell MH, Warbasse L, Brenner C. Evaluation of the dyspeptic patient: a cost-utility study. *J Fam Prac* 1997; **44**: 545–555.

21. Briggs AH, Sculpher MJ, Logan RP *et al*. Cost effectiveness of screening for and eradication of Helicobacter pylori in management of patients under 45 years of age. *BMJ* 1996; **312**: 1321–1325.

22. Quine MA, Bell GD, McCloy RF *et al*. Prospective audit of upper gastrointestinal endoscopy in two regions of England: safety, staffing and sedation methods. *Gut* 1995; **36**: 462–467.

23. McColl KEL, El-Nujumi AM, Chittajallu RS *et al*. A study of the pathogenesis of Helicobacter pylori negative duodenal ulceration. *Gut* 1993; **34**: 762–768.

24. Mearin F, Malagdelada JR. Upper gut motility and perception in functional dyspepsia. *Eur J Gastroenterol Hepatol* 1992; **4**: 615–621.

25. Mishkin D, Sablauskas L, Yavolvsky M *et al*. Frustose and sorbitol malabsorption in ambulatory patients with functional dyspepsia: comparison with lactose maldigestion/malabsorption. *Dig Dis Sci* 1997; **42**: 2591–2598.

26. Monnier P, Savary M. Contribution of endoscopy to gastrooesophageal reflux disease. *Scand J Gastroenterol* 1984; **19**: 26–45.

27. Armstrong D, Bennett JR, Blum AL *et al*. The endoscopic assessment of oesophagitis: a progress report on observer agreement. *Gastroenterology* 1996; **111**: 85–92.

28. Lundell LR, Dent J, Bennett JR *et al*. Endoscopic assessment of oesophagitis: clinical and functional correlates and further validation of the Los Angeles Classification. *Gut* 1999; **45**: 172–180.

29. Lind T, Havelund T, Carlsson R *et al*. Heartburn without oesophagitis: efficacy of omeprazole and features determining therapeutic response. *Scand J Gastroenterol* 1997; **32**: 974–979.

30. Schindlebeck NE, Klauser AG, Voderholzer WA *et al*. Empiric therapy for gastroesophageal reflux disease. *Arch Int Med* 1995; **155**: 1808–1812.

31. Johnsson F, Weywadt L, Solhaug JH *et al*. One week omeprazole treatment in the diagnosis of gastro-oesophageal reflux disease. *Scand J Gastroenterol* 1998; **33**: 15–20.

32. Weiner GJ, Richter JE, Copper JB *et al*. The symptom index: a clinically important parameter of ambulatory 24-hour esophageal pH monitoring. *Am J Gastroenterol* 1988; **83**: 358–361.

33. Breumelhof R, Smouth AJPM. The symptom sensitivity index: a valuable additional parameter in 24-hour esophageal pH recording. *Am J Gastroenterol* 1991; **86**: 160–164.

34. Weusten BLAM, Roelofs JMM, Akkermans LMA *et al*. The symptom-association probability: an improved method for symptom analysis of 24-hour esophageal pH data. *Gastroenterology* 1994; **107**: 1741–1745.

35. Marshall RE, Anggiansah A, Owen WA *et al*. The relationship between acid and bile relief and symptoms in gastrooesophageal reflux disease. *Gut* 1997; **40**: 182–187.

36. Johnston BT, Troshinsky MB, Castell JA *et al*. Comparison of barium radiology with esophageal pH monitoring in the diagnosis of gastroesophageal reflux disease. *Am J Gastroenterol* 1996; **91**: 1181–1185.

37. Yeomans ND, Tulassay Z, Juhasz L *et al*. A comparison of omeprazole with ranitidine for ulcers associated with non-steroidal anti-inflammatory drugs. Acid Suppression Trial: Ranitidine versus Omeprazole for NSAID-associated Ulcer Treatment (ASTRONAUT) Study Group. *New Engl J Med* 1998; **338**: 719–726.

38. Hawkey CJ, Karrasch JA, Szezepanski L *et al*. Omeprazole compared with misoprostol for ulcers associated with non-steroidal anti-inflammatory drugs. Omeprazole versus Misoprostol for NSAID-induced Ulcer Management (OMNIUM) Study Group. *N Engl J Med* 1998; **338**: 727–734.

39. Werdmuller BFM, Loffeld RJLF. Helicobacter pylori infection has no role in the pathogenesis of reflux esophagitis. *Dig Dis Sci* 1997; **42**: 103–105.

40. Csendes A, Smok G, Cerda G *et al*. Prevalence of Helicobacter pylori infection in 190 control subjects and 236 patients with gastroesophageal reflux, erosive esophagitis or Barrett's esophagus. *Diseases of the Esophagus* 1997; **10**: 38–42.

41. Labenz J, Blum AL, Bayerdorffer E *et al*. Curing Helicobacter infection in patients with duodenal ulcer may provoke reflux esophagitis. *Gastroenterology* 1997; **112**: 1442–1447.

42. Peghini PL, Katz PO, Castell DO. Ranitidine controls nocturnal gastric acid breakthrough on omeprazole; a controlled study in normal subjects. *Gastroenterology* 1998; **115**: 1335–1339.

43. Lauritsen K. Management of endoscopy-negative reflux disease: progress with short-term treatment. *Alimeny Pharmacol Ther* 1997; **11**: 87–92.

44. Heudebert GR, Marks R, Wilcox CM *et al*. Choice of long-term strategy for the management of patients with severe esophagitis: a cost–utility analysis. *Gastroenterology* 1997; **112**: 1078–1086.

45. Read NW, Abitbol JL, Bardhan KD, *et al*. Efficacy and safety of the peripheral kappa antagonist Fedotozine versus placebo in the treatment of functional dyspepsia. *Gut* 1997; **41**: 664–668.

27. The Irritable Bowel Syndrome

DAVID GERTNER

A panel of experts meeting in Rome in 1992 established what have become known as the "Rome criteria" regarding the description and definition of functional gastrointestinal disorders, including irritable bowel syndrome (IBS) (1). That document may be considered the key reference for this chapter.

The term "irritable bowel syndrome" covers a range of functional gastrointestinal disorders, characterized by the association of abdominal pain with an altered bowel habit. Studies in various parts of the world suggest that up to 25% of the population have symptoms consistent with IBS; in the UK the prevalence of the condition is usually quoted as 14%–22% (2,3). In the developed world, there tends to be a preponderance of females among patients presenting for medical care (4). IBS is more common in cities than rural areas (5). Most patients develop symptoms before the age of 50 years, and many have a history of recurrent abdominal pain starting in childhood (6).

Although IBS is the most common condition diagnosed in most specialist gastroenterology clinics, this represents only the tip of a very large iceberg. About 75% of all the patients with IBS symptoms never consult a doctor about them, and only 10% of the remainder are referred to hospital; the large majority of patients presenting with irritable bowel problems are managed purely in primary care.

Often regarded as a trivial disorder, IBS has a considerable economic impact and a marked effect on the utilization of health-care resources. For example, in the UK, IBS is second only to the common cold as a cause of absence from work, and in the USA it accounts for an estimated 3.5 million visits to physicians per annum.

AETIOPATHOGENESIS

The cause of IBS remains unresolved; a range of mechanisms may be involved in the production of irritable-bowel-type symptoms, and the contribution of these separate factors probably varies from patient to patient. **Possible mechanisms in the pathogenesis of IBS** include:

- Altered motility
  - oesophagus and stomach
  - small bowel
  - colon
- Altered sensation
  - heightened perception of normal motility
  - reduced threshold for noxious sensations
- Central factors
  - altered central processing of stimuli
  - psychological influences
- Food intolerance
- Post infectious

In the absence of specific disease of the viscera, the disorder is commonly classified as functional, and epidemiological evidence suggests that 40–60% of patients have symptoms of depression, anxiety, or both.

Role of motility in IBS

Most studies of intestinal motility suggest that disturbances in gut motor function in IBS are an exaggeration of the patterns present in health, but experiments designed to show motor dysfunction objectively have revealed few clear-cut differences between patients with the syndrome and normal control individuals.

Motor activity in the gastrointestinal tract is based on the **electrophysiological properties of intestinal smooth muscle cells** and the integrative action of the **enteric nervous system** (7). The study of action potentials or electrical spike activity (the electrical equivalent of contractile activity) in the colon is, therefore, a reflection of colonic motility, but recordings of myoelectrical and motor events from the colon are less well defined than those from the upper gastrointestinal tract.

Attempts to record **intraluminal pressures** from the colon rely on the insertion of balloons, water-filled open tubes, and, most recently, solid-state pressure transducers into the colorectal lumen (5). After stimulation of the colon by balloon distension, eating, or cholecystokinin, patients with IBS show a greater response than controls during manometry. Also, the occurrence of frequent sigmoid contractions of greater than normal amplitude in association with the patient's typical pain has been observed.

Some studies have shown that patients with predominant constipation have greater responses than those with predominant diarrhoea, who appear to be hypermotile. Several studies have shown that increased sensitivity to balloon distension of the rectum exists in patients with IBS (8). More recently, the development of systems for the performance of 24-h recordings has allowed some investigators to reproduce typical abdominal pain with balloon distension in the large bowel (7). This indicates that heightened visceral sensation may be a component of IBS, although the balance of evidence speaks against the presence of specific abnormalities in rectosigmoid and colonic spike activity or motility in IBS.

As studies of colonic motor activity failed to provide a pathophysiological marker, investigators looked for motility disturbances in the small intestine. In patients with IBS, prolonged manometry of the upper small intestine shows short bursts of intensive activity (clustered contractions), separated by long intervals of rest more often than in healthy volunteers, but the potentially important abnormality also occurs in individuals free of symptoms. Some clustered contractions seem to coincide with episodes of cramping abdominal pain and discomfort (9). Increased small-bowel motility in response to stress has also been demonstrated in some studies.

Finally, the transit time of a meal, which may be considered the clinical correlate of intestinal motility, has been studied (10). In IBS patients with predominant diarrhoea, both orocaecal and whole-gut transit time appear to be reduced — but again, results are conflicting (11). At least some of the inconsistencies between findings of different studies may be explained by differences in methodology and selection of patients.

Role of nervous regulation

The available evidence suggests that the pathophysiology of IBS is mediated by the nervous system. Although a defect could be confined to the enteric nervous system, with or without an abnormality of smooth muscles, it appears most likely that dysfunction of the extrinsic innervation of the gut also contributes to the condition.

Nociception could be altered at the level of the sensory receptor or the neural pathways transmitting and processing information, as it ascends to the brain. Alternatively, dysfunction could originate in the brainstem, in vagal motor pathways, or within the ears. Such patients with IBS may have evidence of pulmonary (bronchial hyperreactivity) and urogenital (nocturia, urgency, incomplete emptying) dysfunction, in addition to upper gastrointestinal symptoms (nausea, vomiting, early satiety, and gastrooesophageal reflux) (11,12). Disruption of central control, rather than primary organ hyperreactivity, may therefore be responsible for the symptoms in IBS.

Emotional factors can also alter the function of the gut and any acute stress can produce bowel movements, nausea, vomiting, or early satiety, in addition to an increased motility index in the colon and abnormalities of motility in the small intestine of patients with IBS (5). Psychological studies have shown that **anxiety and depression** are more common in patients with IBS than in those with organic gastrointestinal diseases, that patients with IBS are more neurotic and less extroverted, and that traumatic life events frequently precede the onset of symptoms of IBS (13). Patients with IBS score particularly highly on scales measuring anxiety, disease phobia, and hypochondriasis (5). IBS patients also have significantly increased lifetime prevalence rates of major depression, manic disorders, and somatization (14–16).

Other factors

5-Hydroxytryptamine

Postprandial plasma concentrations of 5-hydroxytryptamine (5-HT) are increased in some patients with diarrhoea-predominant IBS (17), but central 5-HT-mediated neural pathways seem to function normally (18).

Food intolerance

Food intolerance, without evidence of true food allergy, may be involved in the production of IBS symptoms in up to 50% of patients (19,20). Findings of a recent study suggested that increased production of colonic gas occurs in patients with IBS compared with controls, and that this may be reduced by dietary manipulation, and may reflect abnormal colonic fermentation by the gut flora (21).

Postinfectious IBS

After severe infectious gastroenteritis, 25–30% of patients develop symptoms suggestive of IBS, and these symptoms frequently persist for months after the acute illness (22,23). Postinfectious IBS is particularly likely to occur in individuals with premorbid anxiety, depression, or a tendency to neuroses and somatization (24).

SYMPTOM PATTERNS AND DIAGNOSTIC STRATEGY

IBS covers a **spectrum of symptom patterns** from "functional diarrhoea" at one extreme to "spastic constipation" at the other. Patients with diarrhoea-predominant IBS tend to have bowel frequency and urgency, particularly in the mornings and after eating. Stool consistency may be normal at first, but become looser with recurrent defecation; total daily stool weight is not usually increased. Nocturnal bowel disturbance is unusual, and abdominal discomfort may not be very marked. Constipation-predominant IBS is relatively more common in

women. Abdominal pain tends to be relieved by defecation; distension, tenesmus, and the passage of mucous per rectum are other frequent symptoms.

A confident presumptive diagnosis of IBS can often be made on the patient's symptoms alone, if these are entirely typical. A reasonably good positive predictive value for the diagnosis of IBS, is provided by the so-called **Manning criteria** (25):

- Abdominal pain
  - with looser stools
  - with more frequent bowel motions
  - relieved by defecation
- Abdominal distension
- Passage of mucous
- Sensation of incomplete evacuation of stool

Use of these Manning criteria, however, tends to under-diagnose IBS in men, and may label as having IBS a relatively high number of patients who prove to have organic bowel disease. Because of these problems with the original definition, a more accurate and restrictive group of criteria (the **Rome criteria**) was produced by a panel of experts in Rome in 1992, and is now accepted as the standard description of IBS (Table 27.1) (26).

In patients with IBS, there is a large overlap with other functional problems, such as:

- functional dyspepsia
- hyperventilation
- atypical chest pain
- chronic pelvic pain
- chronic fatigue syndrome
- "fibromyalgia"
- urinary frequency and urgency

Table 27.1. The Rome criteria for IBS.

1. At least 3 months of continuous or recurrent abdominal pain or discomfort:
   (i)   relieved by defecation, or
   (ii) associated with a change in stool frequency, or
   (iii) associated with a change in stool consistency

2. With two or more of the following at least 25% of the time:
   (i)   altered stool frequency (more than 3/day or fewer than 3/week)
   (ii) altered stool form
   (iii) straining, urgency, or tenesmus
   (iv) passage of mucous
   (v)   bloating or distension

- chronic back pain
- migraine
- sexual dysfunction

Dyspepsia (27) and problems with the genitourinary system (28) are particularly common in patients with IBS and about 67% of claimed sufferers from chronic fatigue also have typical irritable bowel symptomatology (29).

Diagnosis and differential diagnosis

A positive diagnosis of IBS relies on symptom patterns, rather than an exhaustive exclusion of other disorders. Several studies have examined the value of symptomatology in differentiating between organic and functional disease. By increasing the number of symptoms in questionnaires or by using a scale based on a combination of history, physical examination, and routine diagnostic tests, the predicted probability of IBS may be increased — at the expense of practicability. Relatively reliable features are described by the Manning and Rome criteria. Correlation of onset of symptoms with periods of stress or emotional vulnerability is further supportive of the diagnosis of IBS. In contrast, onset of symptoms in old age, progressive course from time of onset, nocturnal symptoms, fever, significant weight loss (not attributable to depression), rectal bleeding, or steatorrhoea are not compatible with the diagnosis of IBS.

Commonly prescribed **drugs may affect gastrointestinal function**. These include:

- antibiotics
- non-steroidal anti-inflammatory drugs
- antidepressants
- β-blockers
- opiate analgesics

Antibiotics may precipitate diarrhoea as a result of altered bacterial flora or, more specifically, pseudomembranous colitis. β-Blockers may cause constipation, and antidepressants often cause chronic constipation.

Investigations

In patients younger than 40 years who have entirely typical symptoms according to the Rome crieria and no "alarm" features, further investigation is not needed, and a confident clinical diagnosis of IBS may positively aid management (30). Patients are frequently referred to specialist gastroenterology clinics from primary care with the comment that they "may be reassured by normal investigations", but this is not necessarily the case. On the contrary, hospital referral may reinforce the patient's belief in a physical cause for their illness, even if an extensive range of tests subsequently proves negative (31). Although most cases of IBS are diagnosed and managed in general practice, about 14% are eventually referred for specialist advice. In 50% of these, the prime reason for onward referral is the dissatisfied patient; in about 30% there is genuine uncertainty as to the precise diagnosis (32).

Not surprisingly, patients seen in hospital clinics tend to complain of more severe symptoms, that occur more frequently, and are more disruptive to activities of daily living, including the loss of more time from work. Outpatient attenders are more likely to attribute their problems to a physical cause, whereas patients managed in primary care tend to relate these symptoms to stress of their way of life.

When the clinical picture is not entirely typical, further investigation may be appropriate. At the minimum, a **sigmoidoscopy** and some **simple blood tests**, including haemoglobin concentration, erythrocyte sedimentation rate, or C-reactive protein concentration should be performed. More detailed investigation is mandatory if alarm symptoms are present, such as first presentation after the age of 50 years, or features such as anaemia, rectal bleeding, or significant weight loss. IBS has a wide differential diagnosis (Table 27.2) (13), and further tests will be influenced by the suspected alternative diagnosis and presenting symptomatology. Common investigations may include stool microscopy and culture, barium radiology, upper or lower gastrointestinal endoscopy, small-bowel biopsy, and breath tests.

The overacceptance of a diagnosis of functional bowel disease in patients with noncharacteristic clinical features is a common cause of delayed diagnosis of physical illness, and hence of medico–legal problems (33).

MANAGEMENT

Seventy-five per cent of all people with IBS-type symptoms do not seek medical advice and, presumably, manage their problem by simple modifications

Table 27.2. Common differential diagnosis in IBS.

Inflammatory bowel disease	Especially Crohn's
Malabsorption states	e.g. Coeliac disease
Infective conditions	e.g. Giardiasis
Diverticular disease	
Colonic neoplasia	Adenocarcinoma, villous adenoma
Lactose intolerance	Lactose deficiency
Vascular insufficiency	Abdominal angina, ischaemic colitis
Gynaecological disorders	Endometriosis
Drug-induced diarrhoea or constipation	e.g. Antidepressants (β-blockers)
Psychiatric disorders	Depression
Thyroid dysfunction	Hypo- or hyperthyroidism

of life style or over-the-counter remedies. The assessment of treatment response in patients seeking consultations is complicated by the observation that 40–70% of such patients improve with placebo therapy alone (34).

The importance of avoiding overdiagnosis and of making a confident, positive diagnosis — taking time to reassure the patient of the absence of serious organic disease, to explain the nature of IBS and the possible mechanisms of symptom production, and to explore aggravating social and psychological factors — cannot be exaggerated.

A step-wise approach to the management of IBS may be summarized as:

1. exclusion of organic disease — where necessary
2. strong reassurance as to normal findings
3. avoidance of dietary precipitants
4. treatment of dominant symptoms
5. modification of central mechanisms

Because luminal factors (carbohydrates, bile acids, food allergens) may have a role in the symptomatology of some patients with predominant diarrhoea, withdrawal of these can be beneficial. A diary of diet and symptoms may be helpful for this purpose. Particular attention should be paid to lactose, fructose, sorbitol, and caffeine intake (35).

Diarrhoea-predominant IBS

In patients in whom diarrhoea is the major problem,

dietary modification may be useful if a genuine food intolerance can be identified. Lactose maldigestion does not seem to be of particular relevance unless a true disaccharidase deficiency is present (36). Control of symptoms with antimotility drugs such as loperamide can be a simple, safe, and effective approach. In more resistant cases, tricyclic antidepressants may be beneficial in low doses, possibly because of their anticholinergic effects (37). Serotonin-5-hydroxytryptamine receptor subtype 3 ($5HT_3$) antagonists such as ondansetron slow colonic transit and are being evaluated for use in the treatment of IBS (38).

Constipation-predominant IBS

Patients with a predominance of constipation benefit from an intensive fibre regimen and bulk-forming laxatives such as ispaghula and stool-softening agents. A modicum of caution needs to be displayed if the patient complains of gas and bloating, as an increased fibre intake may worsen these symptoms. Topical treatment with enemas or suppositories may be helpful. Prokinetic agents, such metoclopramide and domperidone do not slow distal gut activity: cisapride (now withdrawn from the market), acting through release of acetylcholine at the myenteric plexus level and agonism of $5\text{-}HT_4$ receptors, increases small-bowel and colonic transit, but produces little, if any, benefit in clinical practice (39).

Pain-predominant IBS

Patients with a predominance of abdominal pain, distension, and gas may benefit from a range of antispasmodic agents such as peppermint, mebeverine, or hyoscine (37). These smooth-muscle relaxants improve the symptoms of 40–90% of patients, but there is a large placebo response in most studies, and common experience is that individual drugs rarely produce long-term improvement.

Other treatments

If treatment aimed primarily at the supposed source of symptoms proves ineffective, then therapy directed at **central mechanisms** may be tried. Antidepressant agents may be helpful through their central analgesic effects or anticholinergic activity, or by relief of coexisting depression (40).

Non-pharmacological approaches have been investigated, and may be particularly useful in patients with identifiable psychological problems.

Interventions, such as **behavioural therapy**, **stress management**, and **acupuncture** have all been claimed to be beneficial in some cases. **Hypnotherapy** has been investigated in some detail, and has been shown to be useful (41). However, it is time-consuming and expensive treatment and its availability is clearly dependent on local expertise and resources.

PROGNOSIS

IBS is a benign condition but, in terms of continued symptoms, the prognosis is bad. Most patients have fluctuating or recurrent symptoms, but tolerate these with the help of reassurance and the use of simple drug treatment. About 30% eventually become symptom-free and this course is especially likely in cases apparently first triggered by an attack of infective gastroenteritis. The prognosis for continuing and troublesome IBS features is poor in patients who perceive themselves as subject to chronic or recurrent life stress (42). However, observed survival in IBS is not different from that expected in the general population (43).

References

1. Rome II: A Multinational Consensus Document on Functional Gastrointestinal Disorders. *Gut* 1999; **45(suppl 11)**.
2. Thompson WG, Heaton KW. Functional bowel disorders in apparently healthy people. *Gastroenterology* 1980; **79**: 283–288.
3. Jones R, Lydeard S. Irritable bowel syndrome in the general population. *BMJ* 1992; **304**: 87–90.
4. Everhart JE, Renault PF. Irritable bowel syndrome in office-based practice in the United States. *Gastroenterology* 1991; **100**: 998–1005.
5. Farthing MJG. Irritable bowel, irritable body or irritable brain? *BMJ* 1995; **310**: 171–175.
6. Walker LS, Guite JW, Duke M *et al.* Recurrent abdominal pain: a potential precursor of irritable bowel syndrome in adolescents and young adults. *J Pediatrics* 1998; **132**: 1010–1015.
7. Mckee DP, Quigley EMM. Intestinal motility in irritable bowel syndrome: is IBS a motility disorder? Part I. Definition of IBS and colonic motility. *Dig Dis Sci* 1993; **38**: 1761–1772.
8. Spiller RC. Irritable bowel or irritable mind? Medical treatment works for those with clear diagnosis. *BMJ* 1994; **309**: 1646–1647.
9. Kellow JE, Gill RC, Wingate DL. Prolonged ambulant recordings of small bowel motility demonstrate abnormalities in the irritable bowel syndrome. *Gastroenterology* 1990; **98**: 1208–1218.
10. Gorard DA, Farthing MJG. Intestinal motor function in irritable bowel syndrome. *Dig Dis Sci* 1994; **12**: 72–84.
11. Whorwell PJ, Mccallum M, Creed FH *et al.* Non-colonic features of irritable bowel syndrome. *Gut* 1986; **27**: 37–40.
12. Talley NJ, Phillips SF, Bruce B *et al.* Multi-system complaints in patients with irritable bowel syndrome and functional dyspepsia. *Eur J Gastroenterol Hepatol* 1991; **3**: 71–77.
13. Lynn RB, Friedman LS. Irritable bowel syndrome. *N Engl J Med* 1993; **329**: 1940–1945.
14. Masand PS, Kaplan DS, Gupta S *et al.* Major depression and irritable bowel syndrome: is there a relationship? *J Clin Psychiatry* 1995; **56**: 363–367.
15. Walker EA, Gelfand AN, Gelfand MD *et al.* Psychiatric diagnoses, sexual and physical victimisation and disability in patients with irritable bowel syndrome or inflammatory bowel disease. *Psychol Med* 1995; **25**: 1259–1267.
16. Talley NJ, Boyce P, Owen BK. Psychological distress and seasonal symptom changes in irritable bowel syndrome. *Am J Gastroenterol* 1995; **90**: 2115–2119.
17. Bearcroft CP, Perrett D, Farthing MJ. Postprandial plasma 5-hydroxytryptamine in diarrhoea predominant irritable bowel syndrome: a pilot study. *Gut* 1998; **42**: 42–46.
18. Gorard DA, Dewsnap PA, Medbak SH *et al.* Central 5-hydroxytryptaminergic function in irritable bowel syndrome. *Scand J Gastroenterol* 1995; **30**: 994–999.
19. Nanda R, James R, Smith H *et al.* Food intolerance and the irritable bowel syndrome. *Gut* 1989; **30**: 1099–1104.
20. Parker TJ, Naylor SJ, Riordan AM *et al.* Management of patients with food intolerance in irritable bowel syndrome: the development and use of an exclusion diet. *J Hum Nutr Diet* 1995; **8**: 159–166.
21. King TS, Elia M, Hunter JO. Abnormal colonic fermentation in irritable bowel syndrome. *Lancet* 1998; **352**: 1187–1189.
22. Mckendrick W, Read NW. Irritable bowel syndrome – post salmonella infection. *J Infect* 1994; **29**: 1–3.
23. Neal KR, Hebden J, Spiller R. Prevalence of gastrointestinal symptoms six months after bacterial gastroenteritis and risk factors for development of the irritable bowel syndrome: a postal survey of patients. *BMJ* 1997; **314**: 779–782.
24. Gwee KA, Graham JC, Mckendrick MW *et al.* Psychometric scores and persistence of irritable bowel after infectious diarrhoea. *Lancet* 1996; **347**: 150–153.
25. Manning AP, Thompson WG, Heaton KW *et al.* Towards positive diagnosis of the irritable bowel. *BMJ* 1978; **2**: 653–654.
26. Thompson WG, Creed F, Drossman DA *et al.* Functional bowel disease and functional abdominal pain. *Gastroenterol Int* 1992; **5**: 75–91.
27. Agreus L, Svardsudd K, Nyren O *et al.* Irritable bowel syndrome and dyspepsia in the general population: overlap and levels of stability over time. *Gastroenterol* 1995; **109**: 671–680.
28. Francis CY, Duffy JN, Whorwell PJ *et al.* High prevalence of irritable bowel syndrome in patients attending urological outpatient departments. *Dig Dis Sci* 1997; **42**: 404–407.
29. Gomborone JE, Gorard DA, Dewsnap PA *et al.* Prevalence of irritable bowel syndrome in chronic fatigue. *J R Coll Phys* 1996; **30**: 512–513.

30. Spiller R. Investigation and management of gastrointestinal motility disease. *J R Coll Phys* 1997; **31**: 607–613.

31. Van Dulmen AM, Fennis JF, Mokkink HG *et al.* The relationship between complaint-related cognitions in referred patients with irritable bowel syndrome and subsequent health care seeking behaviour in primary care. *Fam Prac* 1996; **13**: 12–17.

32. Thompson WG, Heaton KW, Smyth GJ *et al.* Irritable bowel syndrome: the view from general practice. *Eur J Gastroenterol Hepatol* 1997; **9**: 689–692.

33. Neale G. Reducing risks in gastroenterological practice. *Gut* 1998; **42**: 139–142.

34. Maxwell PR, Mendall MA, Kumar D. Irritable bowel syndrome. *Lancet* 1997; **350**: 1691–1695.

35. Weber FH, McCollum RW. Clinical approaches to irritable bowel syndrome. *Lancet* 1992; **340**: 1447–1452.

36. Tolliver BA, Jackson MS, Jackson KL *et al.* Does lactose maldigestion really play a role in the irritable bowel? *J Clin Gastroenterol* 1996; **23**: 15–17.

37. Camilleri M, Choi MG. Review article: irritable bowel syndrome. *Aliment Pharmacol Ther* 1997; **11**: 3–15

38. Wilde MI, Markham A. Ondansetron. A review of its pharmacology and preliminary clinical findings in novel applications. *Drugs* 1996; **52**: 773–794.

39. Farup PE, Hovdenak N, Wetterhus S *et al.* The symptomatic effect of cisapride in patients with irritable bowel syndrome and constipation. *Scand J Gastroenterol* 1998; **33**: 128–131.

40. Gorrard DA, Libby GW, Farthing MJ. Effect of a tricyclic antidepressant on small intestinal motility in health and diarrhoea predominant irritable bowel syndrome. *Dig Dis Sci* 1995; **40**: 86–95.

41. Houghton LA, Heyman DJ, Whorwell PJ. Symptomatology, quality of life and economic features of irritable bowel syndrome – the effect of hypnotherapy. *Aliment Pharmacol Ther* 1996; **10**: 91–95.

42. Bennett EJ, Tennant CC, Piesse C *et al.* Level of chronic life stress predicts clinical outcome in irritable bowel syndrome. *Gut* 1998; **43**: 256–261.

43. Owens DM, Nelson DK, Talley NJ. The irritable bowel syndrome: long-term prognosis and the physician-patient interaction. *Ann Intern Med* 1995; **122**: 107–112.

28. Diarrhoea

STUART BLOOM

INTRODUCTION AND DEFINITIONS

Increase in frequency of defecation (more than three stools per day) and increase in stool weight (to more than 200–250 g/day) have traditionally been incorporated into definitions of diarrhoea, but patients do not consider increased frequency of defecation alone as diarrhoea, and recent reviews suggest both of these measures should be abandoned, leaving decrease in consistency or increase in liquidity of stool as a single defining criterion (1). Diarrhoea is usually classified as acute (mostly self-limiting infections) and chronic (mostly non-infectious aetiologies) with a somewhat arbitrary cutoff of 4 weeks between the two. One scheme of classification is shown in Table 28.1 (2). The reader is referred to Chapter 35 for a discussion of acute diarrhoea; the present Chapter is concerned mainly with the diagnosis and management of chronic diarrhoea.

Table 28.1. Classification of diarrhoea.

Osmotic diarrhoea
Carbohydrate malabsorption
- Disaccharidase deficiency (congenital or acquired)
- Lactase deficiency
- Sucrase–isomaltase deficiency
- Trehalase deficiency
- Congenital glucose–galactose malabsorption
- Congenital fructose malabsorption

Magnesium-induced diarrhoea

Sodium-containing or anion-containing laxatives

Small intestinal mucosal disease
- Viral gastroenteritis
- Giardiasis

- Coeliac disease
- Lymphoma
- Tropical sprue
- Whipple's disease
- Amyloidosis
- Intestinal ischaemia

Reduced intestinal surface area
- Small intestinal resection
- Enteric fistulas
- Jejuno-ileal bypass

Bile salt malabsorption
- Bacterial overgrowth
- Crohn's disease
- Ileal resection

Pancreatic exocrine insufficiency
- Chronic pancreatitis
- Pancreatic carcinoma
- Cystic fibrosis

Secretory diarrhoea
Bacterial enterotoxins
- *Vibrio cholerae*
- Enterotoxigenic *Escherichia coli*
- *Clostridium perfringens*

Stimulant laxatives
- Aloe
- Bisacodyl
- Cascara
- Danthron
- Dioctyl sodium sulphosuccinate
- Phenolphthalein
- Ricinoleic acid
- Senna

Hormones
- Calcitonin
- Gastrin
- Glucagon
- Prostaglandins

- Serotonin
- Substance P
- Vasoactive intestinal polypeptide

Bile salt diarrhoea
- Bacterial overgrowth
- Crohn's disease
- Ileal resection
- Post-cholecystectomy syndrome

Fatty acid diarrhoea
- Bacterial overgrowth

Mucosal inflammation
- Microsopic colitis
    Collagenous colitis
    Lymphocytic colitis

Diabetic neuropathy

Villous adenoma of the rectum

Inflammatory/exudative diarrhoea
Specific colitides/enterocolitides
- Infections
    Viruses (e.g. rotavirus, adenovirus, Norwalk virus)
    Bacteria (e.g. *Campylobacter* spp., *Salmonella* spp.,
    Shigella spp., *Escherichia coli*, *Yersinia enterocolitica*,
    Clostridum difficile)
    Parasites (e.g. *Giardia lamblia*, *Cryptosporidium*,
    Entamoeba histolytica)
- Ischaemia

Nonspecific colitides
- Ulcerative colitis
- Crohn's disease
- Gut vasculitis

Dysmotility diarrhoea
Functional bowel disorder

Faecal impaction

Endocrine disorders
- Hyperthyroidism
- Phaeochromocytoma

Autonomic neuropathy
- Diabetes melitus
- Multiple sclerosis

Proctitis
- Ulcerative colitis
- Infection
- Radiation/chemical injury

Anal sphincter disturbance
- Surgical and/or obstetric trauma
- Perianal disease

PATHOPHYSIOLOGICAL MECHANISMS

There are four principal mechanisms of disordered water and electrolyte transport in the gastrointestinal tract, one or more of which may have a significant role in causing a particular diarrhoeal state.

Osmotic diarrhoea

Water transport is secondary to electrolyte transport. Unabsorbed or poorly absorbed osmotically active solutes in the lumen of the gut inhibit water absorption, leading to net secretion of water and osmotic diarrhoea. Such solutes (osmolytes) are usually ingested or derived from malabsorption of dietary carbohydrate. The **major clinical hallmarks of osmotic diarrhoea** are:

- the diarrhoea stops when the patient fasts (or stops ingesting the poorly absorbed solute)
- analysis of stool sodium and potassium concentrations reveal an osmotic gap, which represents the osmotically active solutes in the stool. The osmotic gap is calculated as $290 - 2(Na^+ + K^+)$ mosmol/kg. In pure osmotic diarrhoea, the osmotic gap will be greater than 125 mosmol/kg because non-electrolytes account for most of the osmolality of stool water

Secretory diarrhoea

Diarrhoea can arise from a net secretory state as a result of reduced absorption or increased secretion of ions and water. The **processes that cause this state** can be divided into:

- abnormal mediators (e.g. bacterial enterotoxins, neurohumoral agents, immune/inflammatory mediators)
- diffuse mucosal disease (which reduces epithelial cell numbers or impairs their function)
- intestinal resection
- congenital defects in ion transport (e.g. defective sodium bicarbonate transport in the small intestine, which causes congenital chloridorrhoea)

The **clinical hallmarks** of secretory diarrhoea are:

- it persists during fasting, although sometimes at a reduced rate
- the osmotic gap is within normal limits

Inflammatory/exudative diarrhoea

Inflammation, ulceration, or necrosis can disrupt the integrity of the intestinal mucosa and cause pus, mucus, serum, and blood to be discharge into the gut lumen. The stool often contains leucocytes, and there may be obvious blood staining. The main cause of diarrhoea is impaired absorption of water by the inflamed intestine but there may be a component of secretory diarrhoea because of the release of inflammatory mediators.

Dysmotility diarrhoea

Although disordered gastrointestinal motility is an obvious theoretical mechanism for diarrhoea, and there is good evidence for disturbance of gut motility in diarrhoeal disease, it remains unproven whether diarrhoea can be caused specifically and solely by deranged motility. Reduced motility may allow diarrhoea to develop by predisposing to bacterial overgrowth. Motility disorders affecting the anorectum and reflexes involved in defecation may cause increased stool fluidity and frequency of defecation, without increasing stool weight.

CLINICAL APPROACH TO THE PATIENT WITH DIARRHOEA

History

A detailed history is the cornerstone of diagnosis. The following points are relevant; in addition, it should be noted that indicators of functional aetiology are a long history (more than 1 year), lack of significant weight loss (less than 5 kg), absence of nocturnal diarrhoea, and straining with defecation. Taken together, these indicators remain only about 70% specific for functional problems (3).

1. The characteristics of onset should be noted — that is, whether it was congenital, abrupt, or gradual.
2. Exactly what the patient means by diarrhoea and the pattern of diarrhoea should be recorded — are the loose stools continuous or intermittent?
3. Duration of symptoms.
4. Epidemiological factors such as travel or exposure to contaminated water, and illness in other family members. Patients in rural locations may be exposed to farm animals harboring bacterial pathogens (salmonella, brucella).
5. Stool characteristics — is the stool watery, bloody, or fatty? Significant malabsorption can occur with-

out major abnormalities of stool consistency or appearance. Mild or moderate malabsorption may become apparent only when complications supervene after vitamin or metabolite malabsorption, giving clues such as anaemia, osteomalacia, and clotting disorders.
6. Specific enquiry about faecal incontinence is mandatory, because patients seldom report it spontaneously.
7. Pain or other associated symptoms such as cramps, flatulence, bloating, fever, tenesmus, and weight loss must be evaluated. Heat intolerance, palpitations, and weight loss suggest hyperthyroidism; flushing suggests carcinoid.
8. Aggravating factors such as diet and stress should be recorded.
9. Previous evaluations, including biopsy examinations and X-rays should be reviewed. The previous medical history may be very important. Seronegative sponylarthropathy may precede inflammatory bowel disease. A history of diabetes, thyroid disease, or autoimmune phenomena may be important. Previous surgery to the gastrointestinal tract or biliary tract may be the cause of diarrhoea, as may previous radiotherapy.
10. All current medications must be noted, including over-the-counter medications, alcohol, caffeine, and non-absorbable carbohydrates such as sorbitol. Specific enquiries should be made about magnesium-containing products and antibiotics taken over the preceding 6–8-week period.
11. Factitious diarrhoea caused by surreptitious ingestion of laxatives should be considered in all cases of chronic diarrhoea.
12. Discrete but direct enquiry about sexual history should be made. Anal intercourse is a risk factor for proctitis caused by gonorrhoea, herpes simplex, *Chlamydia*, syphillis, and amoebiasis.
13. The family history may disclose congenital absorptive defects, inflammatory bowel disease, coeliac disease, and multiple endocrine neoplasia.

Examination

The most important clues from the physical examination are the extent of fluid and nutritional depletion. Other significant signs include mouth ulcers, flushing, rashes on the skin, thyroid masses, wheezing, arthritis, abdominal masses, ascites, and oedema. The anorectal examination is important, with respect to anal sphincter tone and the presence of perianal fistula or abscesses. Certain physical signs can provide clues to an underlying disorder:

- skin examination may reveal dermatitis herpetiformis (coeliac disease), pyoderma gangrenosum (ulcerative colitis), sclerodactyly (scleroderma), or cutaneous signs of Addison's disease, systemic mastocytosis, glucagonoma, amyloidosis, or carcinoid
- peripheral or lumbosacral arthritis can complicate inflammatory bowel disease and Whipple's disease
- thyroid examination may reveal a goitre or nodule that may be associated with hyperthyroidism
- hepatosplenomegaly, carpal tunnel syndrome, and postural hypotension may occur in amyloidosis
- hepatomegaly and pulmonary stenosis may occur in carcinoid
- signs of peripheral vascular disease raise the possibility of intestinal ischaemia

Investigations

Most patients with chronic diarrhoea need investigation after the history and physical examination. Diagnostic tests can be considered under the headings of spot stool examination, quantitative stool collection and examination, blood and urine tests, endoscopic examination and mucosal biopsy, radiography, and physiological tests.

Spot stool analysis

Randomly collected stool specimens can be tested for the presence of blood, pus, fat, microbes, pH, electrolyte concentrations, and laxatives.

Overt blood
The **overt presence of blood** suggests an inflammatory or ulcerative cause. Approximately 50% of patients with coeliac disease will have stools positive for **occult blood** (4).

White blood cells
The presence of leucocytes in stool is a useful marker of inflammation (5), although the accuracy of the result depends on the skill of the observer.

Sudan staining for fat
The number of stained fat droplets counted in a haemocytometer correlates well with fat output

measured chemically (6). Again, high levels of observer skill are necessary for correct interpretation.

Faecal cultures
At least one culture should be obtained, even in cases of chronic diarrhoea. Poorly sensitive tests for *Giardia* are being replaced by faecal enzyme-linked immunoabsorbent assay for giardia-specific antigen (7). Special techniques are needed to diagnose *Cryptosporidia* and *Microsporidia* in stool. Chronic viral infections (usually in immunocompromised hosts) are usually diagnosed from gastrointestinal mucosal biopsy specimens, rather than from stool samples.

pH, electrolytes, minerals, and laxatives
These are discussed with regard to quantitatively collected specimens, below.

Quantitative stool collection and examination

Usually, if this test is necessary, a 48-h sample is sufficient, especially if the daily stool weight is high. Full analysis includes weight, fat content, electrolyte concentration, pH, occult blood, faecal elastase activity, and screening for laxatives. The patients is usually encouraged to eat a diet containing 80–100 g fat per day.

Electrolytes and calculation of an osmotic gap
This calculation has been described above. The osmolality of stool within the distal intestine (estimated at 290 mosmol/kg because it equilibrates with plasma osmolality) should be used for this calculation, rather than the osmolality measured in the faecal fluid, because measured faecal osmolality begins to increase almost immediately as carbohydrates are bacterially fermented to osmotically active organic acids.

Faecal pH
A low faecal pH is characteristic of diarrhoea caused by carbohydrate malabsorption.

Faecal fat concentration
The upper limit of normal in most laboratories is about 7 g fat/day, or 9% of daily fat intake. However, diarrhoea itself can cause increased excretion of fat ("secondary steatorrhoea" (8)) and therefore a faecal fat content less than 14 g/day has low specificity for the diagnosis of primary defects of fat digestion.

Analysis for laxatives
The simplest test is alkalinization of 3 ml of stool supernatant or urine with one drop of concentrated sodium hydroxide; this mixture will turn pink if phenolphthalein is present. A high faecal sodium concentration in the presence of a low faecal chloride concentration should raise the possibility of ingestion of sodium sulphate or sodium phosphate. A soluble faecal magnesium concentration greater than 45 mmol/litre suggests magnesium-induced diarrhoea.

Tests for protein-losing enteropathy
Hypoalbuminaemia without nephrotic syndrome or significant hepatic dysfunction raises the possibility of loss of protein from the gut. Confirmation of enteric protein loss can come from measuring the faecal clearance of faecal α_1-antitrypsin, measured by a method similar to that for renal clearance of inulin (9).

Blood and urine tests

Urine tests
Urine collection can be helpful for identifying laxatives and measuring 5-hydroxyindole acetic acid as an indicator for carcinoid, vanillylmandelic acid as an indicator for phaeochromocytoma, and histamine as an indicator for mastocytosis.

Vasoactive intestinal peptide and other peptide hormones
Excess secretion of vasoactive intestinal peptide causes a secretory diarrhoea of more than 1 litre/day, which may be associated with hypokalaemia. Measurement of calcitonin (to indicate medullary carcinoma of the thyroid), gastrin for suspected Zollinger–Ellison syndrome, and glucagon can also be useful.

Serological tests
These include anti-nuclear antibodies, perinuclear anti-neutrophil cytoplasmic antibodies, and coeliac antibodies (see Chapter 51).

Endoscopic examination and mucosal biopsy

Sigmoidoscopy and colonoscopy
In most cases of diarrhoea in which histology is helpful in providing a diagnosis, flexible sigmoidoscopy is adequate, rather than full colonoscopy.

Exceptions occur when ileal histology is required, or in the case of patchy change throughout the colon. Microscopic or collagenous colitis are usually diffuse processes, but inflammatory changes or subepithelial collagen-band thickening may occur only in the proximal colon in approximately 10% of patients (10). When there is significant weight loss, bleeding to suggest malignancy, or when imaging has suggested ileal pathology, full colonoscopy is desirable.

Upper gastrointestinal endoscopy
Duodenal biopsies — together, if necessary, with an aspirate of small-bowel contents for aerobic and anaerobic culture — can provide diagnostic information in Crohn's disease, giardiasis, coeliac disease, lymphoma, hypogammaglobulinaemia, amyloidosis, Whipples disease, and various fungal, protozoal, and parasitic infestations.

Radiology

Barium radiography
Although it has not been tested specifically in patients with chronic diarrhoea, the diagnostic yield of small-bowel radiography is about the same whether the barium is given orally (barium follow-through) or via an enteroclysis tube, provided that the study is performed by a radiologist who watches the column of barium and uses fluoroscopy as required (11).

Other techniques
Mesenteric angiography may occasionally help in the diagnosis of mesenteric ischaemia, a rare cause of chronic diarrhoea. The usefulness of magnetic resonance angiography in this setting is not clear. Computed tomography may be useful, to look for pancreatic cancer or evidence of chronic pancreatitis. Inflammatory bowel disease, lymphoma, carcinoid, and other neuroendocrine tumours, may also be revealed by this technique.

Physiological tests

Mucosal absorption
The D-xylose absorption test was used for many years to differentiate small-intestinal mucosal absorptive defects from pancreatic digestive defects. With the modern use of endoscopic biopsies, the role of this test has become less clear.

Tests of ileal absorptive function

The terminal ileum has three unique absorptive functions: absorption of vitamin B_{12}, absorption of sodium chloride against steep electrochemical gradients, and absorption of bile acids. The Schilling test is still used for measuring absorptive capacity for vitamin B_{12}, whereas absorption of bile acids can be measured by the SeHCAT test, which measures the retained fraction of an orally administered synthetic radiolabelled bile acid, selenohomocholic acid, conjugated with taurine. Many clinicians will use a therapeutic trial of cholestyramine as an indirect test for bile-salt malabsorption.

Breath tests for physiological testing

In the main, the breath tests comprise tests for breath hydrogen, to diagnose lactose malabsorption and bacterial overgrowth. The **lactose breath test** exploits the fact that lactose malabsorped by the small intestine in lactase-deficient individuals is fermented rapidly in the colon, to produce organic acids and gases, including hydrogen that is excreted into the breath, where it is measured. The most common procedure uses a 25-g load of lactose, and an increase in breath hydrogen concentration of 20 ppm above baseline within 4 h is taken as the cutoff for a positive test result. As many as 10% of people do not possess an intestinal flora capable of producing hydrogen (12); in such individuals, a negative result will represent a false-negative.

Tests for bacterial overgrowth

A quantitative culture of an aspirate of jejunal fluid can be helpful; more than 10^6 organisms/ml is considered diagnostic. A number of breath tests have been proposed as being useful diagnostically. One widely available test uses non-radioactive glucose and measures breath hydrogen excretion as the signal: 50–100 g glucose is given orally, followed by measurement of breath hydrogen at 15–30 min intervals; an increase of breath hydrogen of 12–20 ppm above baseline is considered positive. Sensitivity and specificity of this test vary from 62–93% and from 78–100%, respectively (13,14). Another breath test using lactulose has been reported to give 100% specificity (15).

Tests of pancreatic exocrine function

These are described in Chapter 51.

EMPIRICAL TREATMENT FOR CHRONIC DIARRHOEA

Symptomatic treatment for undiagnosed or poorly responsive chronic diarrhoea can involve several agents. Opioids such as diphenoxylate and loperamide are satisfactory for most cases. Octreotide is useful in carcinoid tumours and chemotherapy-induced diarrhoea.

References

1. Fine K, Schiller L. AGA technical review on the evaluation and management of chronic diarrhoea. *Gastroenterology* 1999; **116**: 1464–1486.
2. Thillanayagam A. Diarrhoea. *Medicine International* 1998; **26**: 57–64.
3. Bertomeu A, Ros E, Barragan V *et al.* Chronic diarrhoea with normal stool and colonic examinations: organic or functional? *J Clin Gastroenterol* 1991; **13**: 531–536.
4. Fine K. The prevalence of occult gastrointestinal bleeding in coeliac sprue. *N Engl J Med* 1996; **334**: 1163–1167.
5. Harris J, DuPont H, Hornick RB. Faecal leucocytes in diarrhoeal illness. *Ann Intern Med* 1972; **76**: 697–703.
6. Simko V. Faecal fat microscopy. Acceptable predictive value in screening for steatorrhoea. *Am J Gastroenterol* 1981; **75**: 204–208.
7. Rosenblatt J, Sloan L, Schneider S. Evaluation of and enzyme-linked immunoabsorbent assay for the detection of giardia lamblia in stool specimens. *Diagn Microbiol Infect Dis* 1993; **16**: 337–341.
8. Fine K, Fordtran J. The effect of diarrhoea on faecal fat excretion. *Gastroenterology* 1992; **102**: 1936–1939.
9. Strygler B, Nicar M, Santangelo W *et al.* Alpha 1-antitrypsin excretion in stool in normal subjects and in patients with gastrointestinal disorders. *Gastroenterology* 1990; **99**: 1380–1387.
10. Tanaka M, Mazzoleni G, Riddell R. Distribution of collagenous colitis: utility of flexible sigmoidoscopy. *Gut* 1992; **33**: 65–70.
11. Ott D, Chen Y, Gelfand D *et al.* Detailed per-oral small bowel investigation vs. enteroclysis. *Radiology* 1985; **155**: 29–31.
12. Gilat T, Ben Hur H, Gelman-Malachi E *et al.* Alterations of colonic flora and their effect of the hydrogen breath test. *Gut* 1978; **19**: 602–605.
13. Metz G, Gassull M, Drasar B *et al.* Breath hydrogen test for small intestinal bacterial colonisation. *Lancet* 1976; **1**: 668–669.
14. Corazza G, Menozzi M, Strocchi A *et al.* The diagnosis of small bowel bacterial overgrowth. Reliability of jejunal culture and inadequacy of breath hydrogen testing. *Gastroenterology* 1990; **98**: 302–309.
15. Rhodes J, Middleton P, Jewell D. The lactulose hydrogen breath test as a diagnostic test for small-bowel bacterial overgrowth. *Scand J Gastroenterol* 1979; **14**: 333–336.

29. Problems with Swallowing

STEPHEN KANE

INTRODUCTION

Some patients find it easy to provide the doctor with a clear-cut account of their symptoms; for others, it is difficult to get beyond vague and ambiguous terms such as "indigestion" or "I can't swallow" without the encouragement of a carefully taken history. This is vital if one is to untangle whether, for example, the patient is describing exertional angina rather than oesophageal reflux, or anorexia and a lack of desire to initiate swallowing rather than a sensation of a food bolus impacting within the chest, seconds after the voluntary swallow.

Communication problems arising from lack of a shared language between the patient and the physician, dysarthria, or cognitive impairment in the patient, may render history-taking far from ideal, tempting the doctor to fall back onto radiological and endoscopic investigations. However, a detailed assessment of symptoms will go a long way towards a diagnosis and the organization of appropriate investigations, and this chapter will focus mainly on these aspects, particularly as the oesophagus is relatively inaccessible to routine physical examination.

Symptoms of disordered oesophageal function include:

- heartburn (pyrosis)
- oesophageal colic and other pains suggestive of dysmotility
- odynophagia or pain on swallowing
- dysphagia, literally "disturbed eating", but refer-

ring mainly to a symptom complex within which a sensation of food or fluid sticking in transit from mouth to stomach predominates.

In addition, impaired pharyngeal or oesophageal function can result in **regurgitation** into the mouth, either of acid or alkaline gastric contents, happening as part of the gastrooesophageal reflux syndrome, or of undigested food, occurring particularly as an accompaniment to the dysphagia of achalasia.

The oesophagus can, of course, also be a source for **bleeding**, be it from severe oesophagitis or from varices; this symptom is the subject of Chapters 14 and 11.2, and will not be discussed further here.

HEARTBURN

Heartburn is experienced by most of the population on an occasional basis, and with greater frequency by a sizeable minority. It is caused by the reflux of gastric acid and pepsin into the lower, and at times the upper, oesophagus — although alkaline reflux will produce identical symptoms. It is characterized by a burning sensation spreading upwards from the epigastrium, retrosternally, towards the throat. It may radiate to the upper back, and is also sometimes felt in the left or right upper abdomen. It may be preceded by or associated with hypersalivation (waterbrash) or nausea. It is not always distinguishable from the epigastric pain of peptic ulcer disease. Typically, heartburn occurs an hour or so after eating, on stooping forward, or on lying supine or on the right side at night, disturbing sleep. The late evening consumption of a large, spicy, fatty meal with alcohol and coffee is especially likely to precipitate nocturnal symptoms, which are relieved to some extent by sitting up. Heartburn may also occur on an empty stomach, and be relieved temporarily by eating.

Patients may relate their symptoms to the ingestion of particular foods such as cucumbers, citrus fruits, spring onions, and white bread, and to more established inhibitors of lower oesophageal sphincter (LOS) function, such as alcohol and fats. Other precipitants of heartburn are cigarette smoking, xanthine-containing beverages and drugs, and obesity. Calcium-channel blocking drugs such as nifedipine that are used to treat hypertension and ischaemic heart disease lower the pressure in the LOS and may contribute to heartburn, as may tricyclic antidepressants.

Heartburn is an extremely common accompaniment of late pregnancy, as a result either of changes in intra-abdominal pressure or hormonal influences on the LOS.

Patients with heartburn should always be asked whether they notice increased sensitivity to the swallowing of hot or very cold liquids, or neat spirits such as whisky. Retrosternal pain occurring in these circumstances *as* they swallow suggests erosive reflux oesophagitis, although up to 40% of patients subjected to endoscopy for reflux symptoms have no macroscopic changes in the lower oesophagus, and likewise thermal hypersensitivity is not always indicative of visible oesophagitis.

Heartburn may occur as an isolated symptom, or it may accompany the upper abdominal bloating, nausea, fullness, and discomfort of non-ulcer dyspepsia. These symptoms may again be part of a more widespread disorder of gastrointestinal motility that constitutes the irritable bowel syndrome. It may also occur as a consequence of impaired gastric emptying, due either to benign pyloric or duodenal ulceration, or to antral malignancy.

Patients with continuing and severe reflux symptoms, persisting despite treatment with proton pump inhibitors or relapsing frequently when stopping such treatment, should be investigated, particularly if advice on life-style modifications has been adhered to, but has not brought about much improvement. The range of available investigations and their relative values are discussed at the end of this chapter.

OESOPHAGEAL COLIC AND OTHER DYSMOTILITY PAINS

Apart from heartburn, in which the stimulus to pain sensation is largely mucosal, the oesophagus can also be the source of chest pain that is not burning, and which is caused, at least in part, by abnormal patterns of smooth-muscle activity. Such pain may be colicky, but may be described as dull or heavy. Its radiation to the back, throat, and arms adds to its ability to mimic the pain of myocardial ischaemia. It is not necessarily related in its timing to swallowing or eating, may wake sufferers at night, but should not be provoked by exertion. It may be triggered by exposure of the oesophagus to acid, as demonstrated by the observation that patients undergoing a Bernstein test of oesophageal sensitivity to hydrochloric acid will at times experience both typical heartburn and atypical chest pains. Indeed, patients with endoscopically proven reflux oesophagitis frequently have disturbed oesophageal motility, demonstrable on both ambulatory manometry and solid-bolus scintigraphy, which does not disappear when the oesophagitis heals (1). These findings explain why such patients experience both atypical chest pains, and sometimes dysphagia, even in the absence of stricturing.

This type of oesophageal pain also occurs in patients with a variety of oesophageal motility disorders, including achalasia and diffuse oesophageal spasm, in which the other main symptom will be dysphagia. Unlike in those with gastrooesophageal reflux disease, in whom there is a reasonable correlation between physiological disturbance and symptoms, those with disorders of oesophageal motility may manifest disturbed peristalsis within the oesophagus, yet have no concurrent symptoms, and conversely may experience pain in the absence of a simultaneous manometric abnormality. Perhaps for this reason, many patients with atypical chest pain have already undergone negative coronary angiography by the time they are assessed from an oesophageal standpoint. Whereas coronary angiography can almost always exclude coronary heart disease, standard manometry and pH measurement can not always exclude a motility defect. Nonetheless, oesophageal peristaltic abnormalities are common in patients with atypical chest pain who have had normal coronary angiograms (2).

ODYNOPHAGIA

Odynophagia, or pain associated with swallowing, may present as an isolated symptom, or it may accompany either retrosternal pain not provoked by swallowing, or dysphagia.

Typically, patients with a significant degree of reflux oesophagitis will notice heightened burning on swallowing very hot drinks or undiluted alcoholic spirits, as already discussed, and will learn to avoid these.

Acute ulceration of the oesophagus as a result of viral infections, either herpes simplex or cytomegalovirus, causes retrosternal pain, often radiating to the back, but made much worse as each solid or liquid bolus passes down. Severe oesophageal candidiasis can cause similar pain, sometimes with synchronous dysphagia. Endoscopy and biopsies should establish the diagnosis in all these cases, with brushings for cytology if candidiasis is suspected. Evidence of underlying immunodeficiency should be sought.

The same kind of pain results from chemical damage by ingested tablet and capsule medications that, often taken without much water and just before the individual retires to bed, stick in the oesophagus. This syndrome was first described with slow-release potassium tablets, tetracyclines, and the anticholinergic agent, emopronium bromide, but has more recently been associated with a variety of other drugs (3). Alendronate, widely used in the treatment of osteoporosis, has lately been added to the list, and is now dispensed with careful instructions about swallowing the tablets while standing, and with plenty of water. Urgent endoscopy of patients with tablet-related odynophagia reveals irregular mid-oesophageal ulceration. This will usually heal within a few days if the patient stops swallowing the offending drug, but stricturing results in a few.

More uncommon, but probably under-recognized, is the syndrome of spontaneous dissecting intramural haematoma of the oesophagus (4). This is discussed further in Chapter 14.

Odynophagia or impact pain may precede dysphagia in patients with oesophageal carcinoma, well before there is circumferential involvement of the wall, and before the tumour encroaches sufficiently on the lumen to delay the onward passage of a food bolus. It is not a symptom to be taken lightly!

DYSPHAGIA

An important point in the history (5) is whether the patient is describing **true dysphagia** (that is, a sensation of food or fluids sticking either during the voluntary swallow or in the few seconds immediately following it) or **pseudodysphagia**. This can occur in several forms, which are also important features of the history:

1. The complainant says that he or she "can not swallow", but the problem is one of repeated chewing of food, which is then spat out, before swallowing is even attempted. This phenomenon is seen in depression, dementia, and the anorexia of malignant disease.

2. Another form of pseudodysphagia is the complaint that "my food sticks after eating". Here, the sensation is one of fullness or discomfort in the epigastrium shortly after completing a meal, but not within seconds of voluntary deglutition. This symptom may reflect gastric dysmotility (non-ulcer dyspepsia) or, if associated with weight loss, impaired gastric emptying secondary to benign or malignant gastric outflow obstruction.

3. A third form of pseudodysphagia is the sensation of "something stuck", particularly located to the pharynx, but not immediately after swallowing, and if anything made better by a voluntary swallow. This has been described as the "boiled sweet" syndrome — a term that strikes a chord with patients and, unlike "globus hystericus", is not pejorative. It is now appreciated that this abnormal sensation is frequently caused by acid reflux into the pharynx. Its relationship to malfunction of the upper oesophageal sphincter is less clear.

True dysphagia has a variety of causes. It may result from:

-   Neuromuscular incoordination of the voluntary musculature of the pharynx or the involuntary smooth muscle of the oesophagus
-   Mechanical problems of the pharynx and oesophagus, including
    -   pouches and diverticula, webs and rings
    -   benign strictures
    -   malignant strictures

Neuromuscular disorders causing dysphagia (see also chapter 8)

The voluntary swallow

Impairment of the voluntary swallow, with incoordination of muscular activity of the tongue and pharynx, may have its origins in the cerebral cortex, internal capsule, basal ganglia, or brainstem, in the anterior horn cells of the cranial nerves controlling the muscles of deglutition, at the neuromuscular junctions, or in the muscles themselves. Examples of some of the more common conditions encountered are detailed in Table 29.1, and the subject is also discussed in Chapter 8. The causes and management of oropharyngeal dysphagia have recently been comprehensively reviewed elsewhere (6).

Typically, patients with neuromuscular disorders resulting in pharyngeal dysphagia will describe **difficulty** or **delay** in initiating the swallowing process, **immediate hold-up** of the bolus in the neck, and **choking** when they attempt to swallow solids or liquids, together with **nasal regurgitation** of liquids. The last two features are the result of loss of the normal coordinated closure of the nasopharynx and larynx that should accompany the voluntary swallow. Pooling of food and fluid in the pharynx provoke repeated swallowing, and a noticeable "wet voice".

In addition to their swallowing difficulties, such patients are frequently dysarthric, and may also be cognitively impaired, so that a detailed history is not easily obtainable, except perhaps from carers who will have observed choking, and recurrent respiratory infections as a result of aspiration. The prevalence of oropharyngeal dysphagia in elderly, institutionalized patients, particularly those with cerebrovascular disease, is high, but is easily underestimated because of the communication difficulties of the sufferers.

The involuntary swallow

A variety of disorders result from impaired function and coordination of the oesophageal smooth musculature. These include achalasia, diffuse oesophageal spasm, nutcracker oesophagus, Chagas' disease, and oesophageal involvement in systemic sclerosis.

Oesophageal manometry has contributed considerably to a better understanding of the pathophysiology of these disorders (7,8), although radiological investigation prompted by an accurately taken history will often provide the major clues pointing to a diagnosis.

Table 29.1. Neuromuscular causes of oropharyngeal dysphagia.

Anatomical localization	Clinical syndrome
Cerebral cortex and internal capsule	Cerebrovascular accident Head injury
Basal ganglia	Parkinson's disease
Brainstem	Motorneurone disease Multiple sclerosis Cerebrovascular accident
Anterior horn cells	Motorneurone disease Guillain–Barré polyneuritis
Neuromuscular junction	Myasthenia gravis
Striated muscle	Polymyositis Dermatomyositis Thyrotoxic myopathy Dystrophia myotonica

Achalasia (see also Chapter 14) is the best characterized of the oesophageal motility disorders. It occurs in both sexes and at any age from the teens to the 80s, with an annual incidence of 1 in 100 000, the implication being that an average district hospital serving a population of 300 000 will see approximately three new cases per year. The primary abnormality is degeneration of neurones in the myenteric plexus coordinating oesophageal smooth muscle. The cause is unknown, although in **Chagas' disease**, familiar in South America, a similar malfunction results from neuronal degeneration resulting from infection by *Trypanosoma cruzi*. The consequence of neuronal degeneration in achalasia is impairment of normal propulsive peristalsis down the oesophagus, and failure of appropriate relaxation of the LOS when a solid or liquid bolus reaches it. Basal sphincter pressure may be normal or increased. High-amplitude muscle contractions are recorded in the body of the oesophagus in a minority of patients, leading to the term, "vigorous achalasia".

Patients with achalasia often have a history of intermittent symptoms going back for some years. They complain typically of **dysphagia** that is as bad for liquids as for solids, in contrast to patients with a stricturing lesion, who notice difficulty in swallowing solids well before a similar problem develops with liquids. Often, achalasia sufferers will attempt to wash down their solids with copious amounts of fluid. They also complain of **regurgitation** of food and fluids, during or soon after eating. Because the oesophagus empties inadequately, they may suffer nocturnal regurgitation and aspiration, leading to recurrent respiratory infections. **Chest pain**, either with swallowing or unrelated to eating, is a frequent symptom, and one not relieved by endoscopic or surgical interventions that improve dysphagia. **Weight loss** occurs as swallowing difficulties get progressively worse.

Spastic disorders of the oesophagus include **diffuse oesophageal spasm** and **nutcracker oesophagus**. Unlike achalasia, these conditions have no associated pathological abnormalities that have been described to explain the disturbed function. The symptoms that point towards these disorders are similar to those of achalasia: intermittent dysphagia for solids and liquids, regurgitation, and, particularly, non-cardiac chest pain. Classification of these spastic conditions has long been confusing, as they have a number of overlapping clinical, radiological, and manometric features. A scheme of classification has been proposed that is based on four key manometric features: peristaltic performance, contraction abnormalities, LOS basal pressure, and LOS relaxation (7).

In **diffuse oesophageal spasm** there are, in addition to some normal peristaltic waves, intermittent non-peristaltic oesophageal contractions, especially in the lower oesophagus — earlier recognized as tertiary contractions on barium-swallow examinations — with corkscrew oesophagus being the most extreme radiographic example. This contrasts with achalasia, in which there is a complete absence of normal peristaltic contractions. Paradoxically, severe radiographic and manometric abnormalities are frequently associated with a complete absence of symptoms. Contraction waves may be normal, or increased both in amplitude and duration. The term **nutcracker oesophagus** is applied to those patients in whom such high amplitude contractions (>190 mmHg) occur in the absence of non-peristaltic contractions. LOS pressure is increased in a 30% or more of patients with diffuse oesophageal spasm.

Systemic sclerosis often affects the oesophageal smooth muscle, which becomes atrophic, and is replaced by fibrous tissue, with resultant peristaltic impairment. Indeed, in the rather more benign variant of systemic sclerosis, calcinosis, Raynaud's phenomenon, oesophageal dysmotility, sclerodactyly, telangiectasia (CREST) syndrome — oesophageal involvement is an essential criterion for diagnosis. In these disorders, dysphagia resulting from impaired motility alone is usually mild. However,

severe oesophagitis consequent upon failure of the oesophagus to clear refluxed acid, particularly when the patient is supine, frequently results in the formation of a peptic stricture, and this is more likely to be responsible for troublesome dysphagia.

Mechanical causes of dysphagia

Mechanical problems causing dysphagia can be distinguished as pouches or strictures, the latter in turn being benign or malignant.

Pouches

Pouches or **diverticula** may be pharyngeal, mid-oesophageal, or lower oesophageal (epiphrenic). Small lateral pharyngeal diverticula are considered to be embryonic remnants of little importance. The posterior pharyngeal pouch (Zenker's diverticulum) is believed to be secondary to a motility disturbance of the cricopharyngeus muscle, and originates along its upper border. Dysphagia probably results from the full pouch compressing the adjacent normal oesophagus. Undigested food may be regurgitated from the pouch, typically at night. A large pouch may be palpable in the neck. An unsuspected pharyngeal pouch, or even one already diagnosed, can present considerable problems to the endoscopist who is attempting to intubate the true oesophageal lumen, and is one reason for requesting a barium swallow before endoscopy in patients with dysphagia.

Mid-oesophageal diverticula are often small, asymptomatic, and found by chance on radiological or endoscopic investigation. Larger ones occasionally cause dysphagia, either by distorting the main oesophageal lumen, or because food impacts in the diverticular ostium.

Large lower oesophageal diverticula are sometimes noted radiologically in association with gross motility disorders of the "corkscrew oesophagus" type. In contrast, multiple small pseudodiverticula of the lower oesophagus may be observed on barium swallow, or endoscopically, accompanying severe reflux oesophagitis, usually with peptic stricturing.

Strictures

In routine clinical practice, the most common problems presenting to the gastroenterologist as dysphagia are **stricturing lesions** of the oesophagus, principally **Schatzki rings**, benign **peptic strictures**, and

oesophageal carcinomas. Typically, strictures cause dysphagia that is initially experienced only when swallowing solids such as bread and meat, whereas liquids pass freely. As the oesophageal lumen becomes narrower, smaller solids will stick, and eventually dysphagia will be noted with liquids also. This progression happens quickly with cancerous strictures, and slowly with peptic strictures.

A detailed analysis of the symptom patterns of more than 800 patients presenting with dysphagia caused by benign and malignant strictures showed that the **site** at which patients experience their food as sticking is misleading, although it is almost always in the midline, and between the hyoid and the epigastrium. More important is the **time** between the voluntary swallow and the sensation of food impacting, varying from 1 s for lesions in the upper oesophagus to 10 s or more for strictures at the lower end (5).

Schatzki rings

Schatzki rings, usually single, are located at the oesophagogastric mucosal junction, generally above a small hiatus hernia. They consist of squamous mucosa on the superior aspect and columnar mucosa on the underside, with connective tissue and sometimes a little fibrous tissue between the mucosal layers — although, compared with a fibrotic peptic stricture, they are relatively soft and pliable, and easily ruptured with a balloon or bougie. They encroach symmetrically upon the lumen of the lower end of the oesophagus to a variable extent, and may be more evident on a carefully performed barium-swallow examination than on endoscopy.

Typically, this common condition, known in the USA as "steak-house syndrome", presents with intermittent dysphagia for solids, particularly large pieces of meat, which impact on the ring. Relief is obtained by drinking fluids, by regurgitation, or by self-induced vomiting. Long periods may elapse between episodes of dysphagia, although when they occur they may be very distressing, lasting for minutes or hours, and occasionally urgent disimpaction is required.

Emergency or elective endoscopy and dilatation ruptures the ring, but over months or years it will slowly re-develop, requiring occasional further dilatations when symptoms again become troublesome.

Webs

Upper oesophageal mucosal **webs** cause a dysphagia for solids that immediately follows the voluntary swallow. Again, they are better demonstrated radiologically rather than endoscopically, the endoscopist often rupturing the web during intubation, before it can be visualized. The supposed association between such webs and chronic iron-deficiency anaemia, the Plummer–Vinson syndrome, is now in doubt.

Peptic strictures

Benign **peptic strictures** of the oesophagus are a sequel to long-standing gastrooesophageal reflux of hydrochloric acid and pepsin, or occasionally of alkaline bile. Predisposing factors include chronic use of non-steroidal anti-inflammatory drugs, and an edentulous state. Reflux will usually have caused prolonged symptoms, although on occasion the patient will give no prior history of heartburn. Dysphagia for solids is initially intermittent, slowly progressing over months or years, to become persistent. The patient adapts by adopting a softer, more liquid diet, and does not generally lose weight until even this diet becomes difficult to swallow. Dysphagia for liquids is rare, but may occur if the patient does not present until the oesophageal lumen is reduced to a diameter of 3–4 mm. Barium-swallow radiography will show a short, concentrically placed narrowing, without shouldering, located at the lower end of the oesophagus, generally above a sliding hiatus hernia. Peptic strictures may be higher in the oesophagus if the patient has a long segment of Barrett's columnar mucosa, the stricture forming at the squamocolumnar junction.

Upper gastrointestinal endoscopy should follow the radiographic examination. On inspection, the stricture is centrally placed, and the mucosa above it ulcerated circumferentially, but not lumpy. This contrasts with a Schatzki ring, above which there is at most a minor degree of inflammation. A biopsy specimen of the stricture should be examined to exclude malignancy, and brushings for cytological examination may be taken through the stricture also.

Techniques of dilatation vary. Graduated, water-filled "through-the-scope" balloons are particularly useful when the stricture is very tight. Once it has been sufficiently dilated that the endoscope can be passed through it into the stomach, a guide-wire can be placed in the antrum and the stricture further dilated with a tapered bougie such as the Celestin. Dilatation should be repeated on a number of occasions over subsequent weeks if the stricture has proved especially tight and initial dilatation has been felt to be incomplete. Otherwise, further endoscopy and dilatation can be carried out on demand.

Postsurgical strictures

Other forms of benign oesophageal stricture follow operative intervention or chemical damage. **Postsurgical strictures** occur at anastomoses between the oesophagus and the distal stomach or a jejunal loop, generally after resections for lower oesophageal or upper gastric cancer. They are usually short and easy to dilate — although, again, this may need to be repeated. Tumour persistence or recurrence at the anastomosis should be considered, and biopsies taken if the appearances are suspicious.

Chemical strictures

Chemical strictures often follow the accidental or deliberate swallowing of caustic liquids such as lysol, although if the patient presents years after the event, they may deny such ingestion. Such strictures tend to be long and, in contrast to the ulceration of peptic strictures, the mucosa over them is intact. They are best demonstrated initially on a barium-swallow examination. Endoscopic intubation and subsequent dilatation may prove very difficult, particularly if the pharynx has been chemically damaged and is rigid and fibrotic.

Oesophageal carcinoma

Cancer is what the patient most fears when they present with dysphagia, and no patient should be "reassured" that they do not have a malignancy of the upper digestive tract until they have been appropriately investigated. **Carcinomas** of the pharynx, oesophagus, and gastric cardia typically present with a dysphagia for solids that, from its outset, is persistent rather than intermittent. Impact pain may predate dysphagia by many weeks. Once it has started, dysphagia worsens in severity over a few weeks, and difficulty with swallowing liquids is much more likely to be a symptom at presentation than is the case with peptic stricturing.

Ideally, radiographic imaging of the oesophagus should precede endoscopy in any patient presenting with a history suggestive of oesophageal malignancy. A plain chest radiograph is useful at the same time, to look for bronchial carcinoma that is invading the oesophagus or has nodal secondaries that are constricting it from without. A barium swallow

forewarns the endoscopist of the location within the oesophagus where tumour is likely to be encountered, the length of the malignant stricture, and the degree of narrowing of the lumen. Typically, malignant strictures are shouldered, eccentric, irregular, and considerably longer than peptic strictures (>4 cm) by the time they present. Subsequent endoscopy is mandatory in order to confirm the diagnosis, visually and by biopsy and brush cytology. Tumours in the pharynx may preclude standard upper gastrointestinal endoscopy, but should be accessible to nasendoscopy performed by an otolaryngologist.

At endoscopy, oesophageal cancers are usually easily distinguishable from benign strictures. Tumour is encountered bulging into the lumen, often with a leading edge that is 1–2 cm higher on one side than the other. The strictured tumour lumen beyond this is, as noted radiologically, eccentrically placed, and almost invariably ulcerated. The exception to this description is tumour at the oesophagogastric junction that infiltrates submucosally. Its radiographic appearance mimics that of achalasia, with a dilated oesophagus, and beaking at the junction with the stomach. The endoscopist encounters considerable resistance to onward passage of the instrument at this point; indeed, gastric intubation may be impossible. Such resistance is not usually encountered in true achalasia. The mucosa may, however, look normal, and cancer will only be diagnosed if multiple biopsies are taken from the oesophagogastric junction. If the stomach can be entered, the cardia should be viewed on retroflexion and further biopsies taken of normal or malignant-looking mucosa.

The value of balloon dilatation of a malignant stricture, at least to allow inspection of the length of the stricture, is controversial, unless it immediately precedes the placement of a stent. Dilatation carries a much greater risk of perforation than it does for benign strictures, and affords the patient but brief symptomatic relief.

Malignancies of the gastric cardia that impede the onward passage of food reaching this area from the gullet will produce symptoms identical to those associated with squamous or adenocarcimomas of the oesophagus, and should be investigated in the same way. Cancers that involve the body of the stomach, or impede gastric outflow, will lead to a sensation of rapid fullness while the patient is eating or shortly afterwards, rather than true dysphagia, even though the patient's presenting complaint may be "difficulty in swallowing".

APPROPRIATE INVESTIGATION OF OESOPHAGEAL SYMPTOMS

The main **modalities** of investigation are barium-swallow radiography, fibreoptic endoscopy, oesophageal manometry (which until recently has been static, but is moving towards being ambulatory), and 24-h ambulatory pH monitoring. Oesophageal scintigraphy (see Chapter 52) has failed to become a mainstream investigation, in part because of the patchy availability of isotope imaging services. Although non-invasive, it has proved to be less specific and less sensitive than pH monitoring for reflux and manometry for motility disturbances (9).

The **choice** of appropriate investigations relies heavily on a detailed history and a careful physical examination, although it is unusual for the latter to provide valuable clues except in some cases of dysphagia. The presence of enlarged lymph nodes in the neck, or irregular hepatomegaly, raises the suspicion of malignancy. A neurological examination may point towards a diagnosis of pseudobulbar palsy, Parkinson's disease, or motor neurone disease. There may be peripheral stigmata of systemic sclerosis or CREST syndrome.

For mild and uncomplicated reflux, a **barium-swallow examination** will rarely do more than confirming that reflux of barium can be induced in some patients when supine. Indeed, it will fail to demonstrate such reflux in up to 60% of patients. A small sliding hiatus hernia is not a prerequisite for the diagnosis of reflux, and in many instances is of little importance.

When symptoms are persistent, recurrent, severe, or resistant to acid suppression, **endoscopy** is now customary, although its main purpose is to assess the extent of visible oesophageal damage resulting from reflux. Even a minor degree of oesophagitis confirms that reflux is taking place, but macroscopic oesophageal inflammation is absent in 30% or more of reflux sufferers. The diagnostic yield for reflux-induced damage is increased by some 10% if biopsies are taken from the lower oesophageal mucosa. Endoscopy allows for the detection of the two main complications of reflux — Barrett's columnar-lined oesophagus, and stricturing. Paradoxically, patients with Barrett's oesophagus may have little in the way of symptoms, although they almost certainly have had long-standing and marked reflux. In view of the pre-malignant potential of Barrett's mucosa, there is an argument for all patients with reflux, even if it appears to be mild, to undergoing endoscopy. Certainly those with frequent symptoms should be investigated, for they have a considerably increased long-term risk of oesophageal adenocarcinoma (10).

In patients with chest pains that are suggestive of reflux but not typical, or in those with more atypical chest pains which perhaps are caused by reflux, the **Bernstein test** is sometimes used. Here, the pain of reflux is reproduced when dilute hydrochloric acid is perfused into the lower oesophagus, but it is not reproduced when saline is similarly perfused. This test provides only qualitative information. If quantitation of acid reflux is being sought, and particularly if it is to be correlated with typical heartburn or less typical chest pain, then 24-h **ambulatory pH monitoring** is now the "gold standard". This investigation also has considerable value in assessing patients before and after anti-reflux operations. A **scoring system for oesophageal exposure to acid** has been devised that is based on:

- the percentages of total monitored time, of time while the patient is upright, and of time while they are supine, during which oesophageal pH is less than 4
- the number of reflux episodes per 24 h
- the duration of reflux episodes, both the number exceeding 5 min and the duration (in minutes) of the longest episode (11)

Patients who experience atypical chest pains without dysphagia or reflux, and in whom a barium swallow and endoscopy have provided no positive clue, may well have had negative cardiac investigations before an oesophageal motility problem is considered. In such patients, stationary **oesophageal manometry** will frequently demonstrate motility disorders such as diffuse oesophageal spasm, although, unless the patient experiences symptoms concurrently with manometric abnormalities, it remains difficult to attribute symptoms to dysmotility. The intravenous injection of edrophonium, or the inflation of an oesophageal balloon, have been used as **stress tests** to provoke both chest pain and simultaneous changes on oesophageal pressure monitoring. Prolonged ambulatory manometric monitoring is increasingly being combined with pH monitoring, and should be a more satisfactory method of documenting the relationship between atypical chest pain, non-obstructive dysphagia, and disorders of oesophageal motility. In particular, it has shown that there is an increased frequency of high-amplitude, long-duration contractions just before and during episodes of pain (12).

The **sequence of investigations** in patients presenting with dysphagia should be determined by the **history** elicited, and the presence or absence of **physical findings**. If these point to an oropharyngeal problem (6), **nasendoscopy** allows direct inspection of the upper airways and pharynx, permitting identification and biopsy of tumours, and enabling note to be made of residues of ingested foods and fluid in the pharynx suggestive of impaired voluntary deglutition. Function is further assessed with **videofluoroscopy**, a structured radiological examination designed to detect and analyse abnormalities of oropharyngeal swallowing function. This technique should detect delays in the initiation of the pharyngeal phase of swallowing, aspiration, nasal regurgitation, and pharyngeal pooling. It will also demonstrate pharyngeal pouches and webs. Other anatomical abnormalities that are often shown in this area, but are of less certain significance in relation to their contribution to dysphagia, include cricopharyngeal bars, and indentation of the pharynx and upper oesophagus by osteophytes on the cervical spine. **Pharyngeal manometry** is technically more problematic, and the results more difficult to interpret, than is the case with oesophageal manometry. However, when the technique is performed synchronously with videofluoroscopy as **manofluorography**, it enables malfunctioning of the pharyngeal muscles and upper oesophageal sphincter to be more fully assessed.

Those patients who prove to have neuromuscular disorders of oropharyngeal swallowing are ideally **managed by a team** that includes an interested radiologist, a neurologist, an otolaryngologist, and especially a speech and language therapist, all of whom provide vital input in assessing the safety of swallowing, in advising on the consistency of diets, and in contributing to decisions regarding gastrostomy feeding.

A **barium-swallow examination** will be normal in many patients with dysphagia who ultimately prove, on manometry, to have an oesophageal motility disorder, including in some with early achalasia.

However, in most of those with achalasia, there are characteristic radiographic abnormalities, including an absence of peristalsis, together with hold-up of the barium column and smooth-tapered beaking at the oesophagogastric junction. In more advanced cases, copious food debris is visible in a greatly dilated "mega-oesophagus" and a plain chest radiograph will show a much widened mediastinum.

Patients with a history suggestive of a stricturing lesion in the oesophagus often proceed directly to **upper gastrointestinal fibre-endoscopy**. Nonetheless, a prior barium-swallow examination does have certain benefits. It allows for the detection of a pharyngeal pouch — an occasional cause of problems to even the most experienced endoscopist. It may show a Schatzki ring not observed on endoscopy, and may pick up features of motility disorders such as achalasia or diffuse oesophageal spasm in what appears to be an endoscopically normal oesophagus. In particular, radiographic evaluation of strictures provides a longitudinal dimension not available to endoscopists, alerting them to the likelihood of tumour, and to the advisability or otherwise of attempting stricture dilatation.

References

*Of interest; **of exceptional interest

1. McDougall NI, Mooney RB, Ferguson WR *et al*. The effect of healing oesophagitis on oesophageal motor function as determined by oesophageal scintigraphy and ambulatory oesophageal motility/pH monitoring. *Aliment Pharmacol Ther* 1998; **12**: 899–907.

2. Cooke RA, Anggiansah A, Chambers JB *et al*. A prospective study of oesophageal function in patients with normal coronary angiograms and controls with angina. *Gut* 1998; **42**: 323–329.

3. Kikendall JW. Pill-induced esophageal injury. *Gastroenterol Clin North Am* 1991; **20**: 835–846.

4. Shay SS. Benign structural lesions of the esophagus. *Gastroenterol Clin North Am* 1991; **20**: 673–690.
   A useful descriptive review of a number of oesophageal conditions, including webs, rings, and diverticula.

5. *Edwards DAW. Discriminatory value of symptoms in the differential diagnosis of dysphagia. *Clin Gastroenterol* 1976; **5**: 49–57.
   A classic personal paper distilling a lifetime of careful clinical observation.

6. **Cook IJ, Kahrilas PJ. AGA technical review on management of oropharyngeal dysphagia. *Gastroenterology* 1999; **116**: 455–478.
   Detailed and very readable review, which crosses the boundaries of gastroenterology, neurology, and otolaryngology.

7. *McCord GS, Staiano A, Clouse RE. Achalasia, diffuse spasm and non-specific motor disorders. *Baillière's Clin Gastroenterol* 1991; **5**: 307–335.

Comprehensive review of disorders of oesophageal motility and their investigation with stationary manometry.

8. Heading RC, Tebaldi M. Oesophageal symptoms and motility disorders. *Medicine (Gastroenterology)* 1998; **26**: 1–6. An "up-date" style of article, giving a clear exposition on the role of different investigations.

9. Blackwell JN. Oesophageal scintigraphy. In: *Gastrointestinal Motility: Which Test?* Ed. NW Read Petersfield: Wrightson Biomedical Publishing Ltd, 1989; pp. 53–61.

10. Lagergren J, Bergström R, Lindgren A *et al.* Symptomatic gastroesophageal reflux as a risk factor for oesophageal adenocarcinoma. *N Engl J Med* 1999; **340**: 825–831.

11. DeMeester TR. Prolonged esophageal pH monitoring. In: *Gastrointestinal Motility: Which Test?* Ed. NW Read. Petersfield: Wrightson Biomedical Publishing Ltd, 1989; pp. 41–52.

12. Stein HJ, DeMeester TR. Indications, technique, and clinical use of ambulatory 24-hour esophageal motility monitoring in a surgical practice. *Ann Surg* 1993; **217**: 128–137.

30. Postgastrectomy Disorders

MARC WINSLET

A large proportion of patients may suffer from minor postprandial symptoms after gastrectomy, but approximately 10% will develop severe persistent symptoms with physical sequelae. The incidence of postgastrectomy syndrome is influenced by the extent of resection, but not the type of reconstruction. **The most common postgastrectomy disorders** include:

- Nutritional
    - loss of weight
    - anaemia
    - bone disease
- Bile reflux and vomiting
- Small stomach syndrome
- Dumping symptoms
- Reactive hypoglycaemia
- Diarrhoea
- Disease recurrence
- Mechanical
    - afferent loop obstruction
    - efferent loop obstruction
    - intussusception

NUTRITIONAL DISORDERS

Weight loss

This is partly a mechanical phenomenon dependent on the degree of resection (1), but it is also related to the anorexia associated with the presence of severe postcibal symptoms. In a small proportion of patients, an increase in small-bowel transit time may be contributory. A degree of nitrogen and fat malabsorption may also occur, but frank steatorrhoea is unusual.

Anaemia

Iron deficiency anaemia is common after gastric resection and the prevalence increases with time, such that a need for iron supplementation is commonplace. The aetiology is multifactorial and includes bypass of the duodenum — a major site of iron absorption — increased trivalent iron in an alkaline medium, which is less absorbable, and increased levels of iron–protein complexes.

Macrocytic anaemia may occur after high subtotal resection, and is universal after total gastrectomy as a result of the loss of intrinsic factor. Affected patients will require 3-monthly injections of cyanocobalamin for life. **Megaloblastic anaemia** may also occur after partial gastrectomy, in a subclinical form, as the relative hypochlorhydria reduces the release of vitamin B_{12} bound to food. These patients may benefit from the oral administration of crystalline vitamin B_{12}.

Reduced vitamin B_{12} absorption may also occur as a consequence of bacterial overgrowth in the afferent loop (see below) or steatorrhoea. Folate deficiency is rare.

Bone disease

Calcium loss is a late complication that may occur after duodenal exclusion subsequent upon a Polya reconstruction or in association with persistent diarrhoea. This may result in both osteomalacia and osteoporosis. **Symptoms** include bone pain, weakness and stress fractures. Investigation reveals increased serum concentrations of calcium and alkaline phosphatase, with general bony rarefaction on X-ray. **Treatment** includes oral calcium and vitamin D supplements.

BILE REFLUX AND VOMITING

Postcibal gastrooesophageal reflux or bilious vomiting is common after gastric resection, particularly proximal gastrectomy and distal gastrectomy with a Polya reconstruction. The former is the result of the production of cardiooesophageal incompetence after mobilization of the lower oesophagus. The latter is caused by enterogastric reflux of bile and pancreatic juice and, occasionally, intermittent obstruction of the afferent/efferent jejunal loop.

Symptoms include heartburn, epigastric pain, nausea, and vomiting, aggravated by food and unrelieved by antiacid treatment. Long-term enterogastric reflux may produce iron deficiency anaemia and possibly contribute to stomach carcinoma. Endoscopy reveals diffuse oesophagitis and gastritis with pooling of bile in the stomach remnant. A hydroxy iminodiacetic acid (HIDA) scan may confirm the diagnosis.

Symptoms may be **alleviated** by the use of prokinetic agents or oral bile-salt binding agents such as cholestyramine; however, the latter is unpalatable. In severe cases, surgical reconstruction is required with a Roux-en-Y diversion or, less commonly, use of an isoperistaltic interposition (2).

SMALL-STOMACH SYNDROME

Small-stomach syndrome may occur after extensive gastric resection, with severe early satiety and consequent malnutrition. Some patients may be managed by elemental supplementation, but severe cases may require construction of a gastric reservoir and restoration of duodenal continuity.

DUMPING SYNDROME

Up to 50% of patients have some degree of postprandial systemic or gastrointestinal symptoms af-

ter gastric resection or pyloroplasty. True dumping is often referred to as "early" dumping to distinguish it from "late" dumping — which is, in fact, reactive hypoglycaemia (see below).

True dumping is associated with rapid gastric emptying and resultant hypovolaemia, secondary to the large-volume, hyperosmolar enteric load. Enterogastric reflux may also be contributory and several vasoactive peptides (such as vasoactive intestinal peptide, neurotensin, and possibly motilin) have been implicated. The **vasomotor symptoms** occur 15–30 min after meals and may be exacerbated by a carbohydrate load. They include tiredness, fainting, headache, peripheral vasodilatation, sweating, and palpitations. **Gastrointestinal symptoms** occur later and may be absent. They include fullness, distention, nausea/vomiting, borborygmi, and diarrhoea.

Dumping is common in the early postoperative period and tends to improve with time. In resistant cases, dietary manipulation is the mainstay of **treatment**, giving small, dry, high-protein/fat and low-carbohydrate meals. Substances that inhibit gastric emptying may be helpful, and there is some evidence to support the use of octreotide (3). Severe and debilitating cases may warrant formation of an isoperistaltic jejunal interpostion, with or without vagotomy (4).

Reactive hypoglycaemia

This complication is relatively uncommon, but may coexist with other postgastrectomy syndromes. **Symptoms** include sweating, dizziness, and extreme hunger. The condition occurs 2–4 h after a meal, and is caused by the reactive hypoglycaemia that is secondary to the increased insulin concentrations initially needed to cope with the carbohydrate load. The diagnosis may be confirmed by an extended glucose tolerance test, which reveals hyperglycaemia, increased plasma insulin concentrations and subsequent hypoglycaemia — the "steeple curve". The mainstay of treatment is dietary manipulation, with high-protein/low-carbohydrate meals. The addition of acarbose to the diet can delay carbohydrate absorption and can be tried after appropriate dietary changes.

DIARRHOEA

Postgastrectomy diarrhoea has a variable incidence and severity, ranging from mild frequency to episodic or persistent explosive diarrhoea. The aetiology is multifactorial with bile salt/fat malabsorption and increased small-bowel transit time being contributory. Gastric colonization should be excluded. Medical **management** consists of reduced intake of animal fats, and the use of constipating agents, and bile-salt binders. Severe cases may warrant consideration of a reversed jejunal segment or a distal non-propulsive onlay graft.

DISEASE RECURRENCE

Gastric surgery for duodenal ulcer disease is now uncommon and recurrence is a not a practical problem. Resection for gastric ulceration is associated with a 3% recurrence rate and such cases, if intractable, may require re-resection. The most common problem is stomal ulceration after Polya reconstruction for distal gastrectomy. This is uncommon if an adequate antrectomy has been performed. If it occurs, it normally responds to medical treatment and vagotomy is rarely required.

MECHANICAL PROBLEMS

Extrinsic-loop obstruction usually affects the afferent loop of a gastrojejunostomy reconstruction and is predisposed to by a long segment and antecolic anastomosis. Efferent-limb obstruction is normally caused by kinking, adhesions, or stenosis; it is rarely associated with herniation, volvulus, intussusception, or development of a stump carcinoma. The **symptoms** are usually chronic and intermittent, but may be acute. Afferent obstruction presents with early postcibal pain and nausea, relieved by vomiting. Acute unrelieved episodes may be associated with pancreatitis, jaundice, and perforation. Efferent obstruction is clinically associated with pain, absolute constipation, vomiting, and distension, the onset of the last two being influenced by the site of obstruction. **Treatment** is initially conservative, but surgical intervention may be required.

MISCELLANEOUS

There is evidence that previous gastric surgery may predispose to the development of carcinoma in the gastric remnant (**stump carcinoma**). There is a long latent period of 15 or more years (5,6). The aetiology is unclear, but may include enterogastric-reflux-induced intestinal metaplasia, and bacterial overgrowth associated with hypochlorhydria.

Bezoar formation is predisposed to by hypochlorhydria, reduced proteolysis, and loss of the antral pump. This may present acutely with obstructional ulceration, but usually manifests with chronic symptoms of satiety, pain, nausea, and vomiting. The bezoar may respond to enzymatic dissolution or require surgical removal.

There is anecdotal evidence that gastric resection may predispose to cholelithiasis; this may result from vagotomy-induced gallbladder dilation and stasis.

References
1. Keda MI, Ueda T, Shiba T. Reconstruction after total gastrectomy by the interposition of a double jejunal pouch. *Br J Surg* 1998; **85**: 399–402.
2. Kennedy T, Green R. Roux diversion for bile reflux following gastric surgery. *Br J Surg* 1978; **65**: 323–325.
3. Geer RJ, Richards WO, O'Dorisio T, *et al.* Efficacy of octreotide acetate in treatment of severe postgastrectomy dumping syndrome. *Ann Surg* 1990; **212**: 678–687.
4. Miranda R, Steffes B, O'Leary JP *et al.* Surgical treatment of post gastrectomy dumping syndrome. *Am J Surg* 1980; **139**: 40–43.
5. Lundegardh G, Adami HO, Helwick C *et al.* Risk of cancer following partial gastrectomy for benign ulcer disease. *Br J Surg* 1994; **81**: 1164–1167.
6. Kaneko K, Kondo H, Saito D *et al.* Early gastric stump cancer following distal gastrectomy. *Gut* 1998; **43**: 342–344.

31. Malabsorption and Weight Loss

PARVEEN J. KUMAR and MICHAEL L. CLARK

INTRODUCTION

Malabsorption is seen in:

- gastric disease
- small-bowel disease
- pancreatic disease
- liver and biliary tract disease

It may occur:

- as a minor component of a clinical problem — for example, malabsorption of vitamin K in a jaundiced patient
- as failure to absorb a specific substance — for example, the malabsorption of vitamin B_{12} in pernicious anaemia as a result of lack of intrinsic factor

The term **malabsorption syndrome** is used when there is generalized malabsorption. Most cases originally diagnosed as "malabsorption syndrome" have coeliac disease and the term malabsorption syndrome is now rarely used.

Weight loss is invariably the result of anorexia — "insufficient calories being taken in". The only exceptions are hyperthyroidism (increased appetite in addition to increased metabolism) and diabetic ketoacidosis.

Weight loss is seen frequently in association with inflammatory bowel disease (IBD). The potential causes of weight loss in IBD include malabsorption of nutrients from the inflamed gut, steroid treat-

ment, increased energy expenditure, or a reduced energy intake secondary to a loss of appetite (anorexia) (1,2). Of these, **reduced energy intake** has been identified as the single most important factor leading to weight loss; the intake has been documented to be only 42–82% of expected values. Experimental studies have implicated the proinflammatory cytokines — tumour necrosis factor-α, interleukin (IL)-1β and IL-6 — released from inflammatory cells, in causation of anorexia in IBD and other diseased states. In an animal model for human Crohn's disease, administration of an IL-1 antagonist into the brain partially reversed the anorexia and weight loss that occurred with the development of colitis. This would suggest that IL-1 is responsible, at least in part, for the reduction in food intake in this model and, furthermore, that it might be acting by an interaction with the central feeding pathways.

Malabsorption plays only a small role in weight loss, as the malabsorption of any small amount of nutrient can be overcome by increasing the amount of that nutrient in the diet:

1. *Example 1*: A patient with malabsorption and weight loss will have a maximum of about 756 kJ (20 g) of fat in the stool. If the fat intake is 3780 kJ (100 g), then 3024 kJ (80 g) must have been absorbed — therefore the patient can not have lost weight on this diet. Patients who lose weight **must** have a decreased intake.

2. *Example 2*: A morbid obese patient excretes 420 kJ (approximately) in the stool per day. If

a jejuno–ileal bypass is performed with 18 cm of jejunum anastomosed to 18 cm of ileum, the patient malabsorbs and the stool contains 1680 kJ per day. After this operation, patients dramatically lose an enormous amount of weight, which cannot be accounted for by the 1260 kJ malabsorption above. In other words, they lose their appetite and do not eat.

Physiology

Carbohydrate absorption

Dietary carbohydrate consists mainly of starch, with some sucrose and a small amount of lactose. Starch is a polysaccharide made up of numerous glucose units. Its hydrolysis begins in the mouth, by salivary amylase, but the majority of hydrolysis takes place in the upper intestinal lumen, by pancreatic amylase. This hydrolysis is limited by the fact that amylases have no specificity for some glucose/glucose-branching links.

The breakdown products of this carbohydrate hydrolysis, together with sucrose and lactose, are hydrolysed on the brush-border membrane of the enterocytes by their appropriate oligo- and disaccharidases, to form the monosaccharides glucose, galactose, and fructose. These monosaccharides are transported into the cell — galactose and glucose by sodium-linked transport. Fructose is transported across the apical and basolateral membrane down its concentration gradient (Figure 31.1).

Protein absorption

Dietary and endogenous protein (desquamated cells, intestinal secretions) are mainly digested by pancreatic enzymes before absorption. These proteolytic enzymes are secreted as proenzymes and transformed to active enzymes in the lumen of the gut. The presence of protein in the lumen stimulates the release of enterokinase, which activates trypsinogen to trypsin; this, in turn, activates the other proenzymes, chymotrypsin and elastase. These enzymes break down proteins into oligopeptides. Some di- and tripeptides are absorbed intact by a carrier-mediated process, whereas the remainder are broken down into free amino acids by peptidases on the brush-border membranes of the cell. The amino acids released are transported into the cell by a number of carrier mechanisms.

Fat absorption

Figure 31.2 summarizes the normal processes of fat absorption and relates the various stages to the pathologies associated with malabsorption. Dietary fats consist mainly of triglycerides, with some cholesterol and fat-soluble vitamins. The emulsification of fat occurs in the stomach and is followed by hydrolysis of triglycerides by pancreatic lipase in the duodenum, to yield fatty acids and monoglycerides. Bile enters the duodenum after the contraction of the gallbladder. It contains phospholipids and bile salts, both of which are partially water soluble and act as detergents. They aggregate together to form micelles with their hydrophilic ends on the outside. Trapped in the hydrophobic centre of this micelle are the monoglycerides, fatty acids, and cholesterol; these are then transported to the intesti-

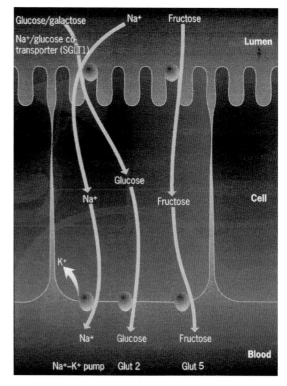

Figure 31.1. Transport of solutes (glucose, galactose, fructose) across the apical membrane, showing glucose/galactose sodium-linked transport. Galactose is transported by the same mechanism as glucose. Fructose is transported across the apical and basolateral membrane down the concentration gradient. The sodium/potassium-ATPase pump is located in the basolateral membrane. SGLT1, sodium/glucose co-transporter; GLUT-2, glucose transporter-2. Reprinted from *Clinical Medicine* 4th Ed, Kumar & Clark, pp. 247, 1998 by permission of the publisher WB Saunders.

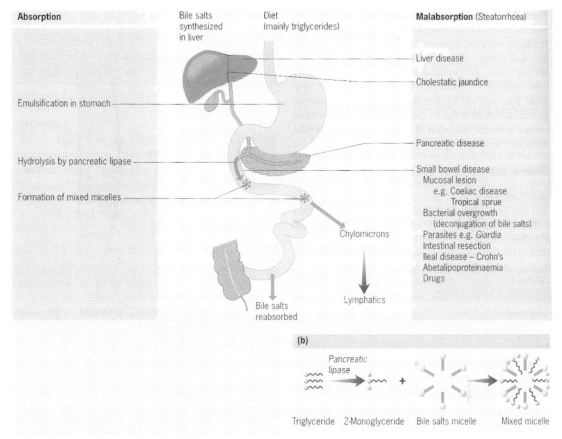

Figure 31.2. A: The pathophysiology of fat malabsorption. B: Diagram showing the formation of mixed micelles. Reprinted from *Clinical Medicine* 4th Ed, Kumar & Clark, pp. 248, 1998 by permission of the publisher WB Saunders.

nal cell membrane. At the cell membrane, the lipid contents of the micelle are absorbed and the bile salts remain in the lumen. Inside the cell, the monoglycerides and fatty acids are re-esterified to triglycerides. The triglycerides and other fat-soluble molecules (e.g. cholesterol phospholipid) are then incorporated into chylomicrons to be transported into the lymph.

Medium-chain triglycerides (which contain fatty acids of chain length 6–12) and a small amount of long-chain fatty acids are transported by the portal vein.

Bile salts are not absorbed in the jejunum, so that their intraluminal concentration in the upper gut is high. They pass down the intestine to be absorbed in the terminal ileum, and are transported back to the liver. This **enterohepatic circulation** prevents excess loss of bile salts into the colon and faeces.

Any interference with the absorptive mechanism produces steatorrhoea (Figure 31.2).

Water and electrolyte absorption

A large amount of water and electrolytes — partially dietary but mainly from intestinal secretion — are absorbed, coupled with solutes such as monosaccharides and amino acids, in the upper jejunum. Some water and electrolytes are absorbed in the ileum and the right side of the colon via an active sodium transport system that is not coupled to solute absorption.

Water-soluble vitamins

These are all absorbed throughout the length of the small intestine. The exception to this is vitamin B_{12} which, like the bile salts, is specifically absorbed in the terminal ileum alone. Malabsorption of these two substances consequently takes place after ileal resection. A small amount of vitamin B_{12} is absorbed by non-specific transport.

GASTRIC DISEASE

Pernicious anaemia (see also chapter 25)

In pernicious anaemia there is an autoimmune gastritis that leads to failure of the secretion of hydrogen ions and intrinsic factor. In the UK, 1 in 800 of the population older than 60 years of age are affected; the condition is more common in females. There is an association with other autoimmune diseases — for example, thyroid disease (50% of patients with pernicious anaemia have thyroid antibodies), Addison's disease, and vitiligo — and an increased incidence of gastric carcinoma in males. Parietal cell antibodies are present in the serum of 90% of affected individuals, but this is not specific. Intrinsic factor antibodies are found in only 50% of patients, but are specific. Intrinsic factor antibodies are either **blocking** (they inhibit binding of intrinsic factor to vitamin B_{12}) or **precipitating** (they inhibit the binding of vitamin B_{12}-intrinsic factor complex to the receptor site in the ileum), but their role in pathogenesis is unknown.

Clinical features

Patients present with an insidious onset, with symptoms of anaemia. There may be mild jaundice as a result of ineffective erythropoiesis. Glossitis and angular stomatitis are present. Neurological symptoms are rare, irreversible, and occur with greatly decreased serum concentration of vitamin B_{12} (<50 pmol/litre). A polyneuropathy involving peripheral nerves and the posterior and lateral columns of the spinal cord (subacute combined degeneration) is seen.

Investigations

A full blood count shows a macrocytic anaemia (see Chapter 25). A bone marrow aspiration will reveal megaloblastic erythropoiesis. The serum concentration of vitamin B_{12} is less than the normal value of 160 pmol/litre. Diagnosis can be confirmed by vitamin B_{12} absorption tests if necessary (see Chapter 25).

Treatment

Pernicious anaemia is treated with intramuscular hydroxocobalamin 1000 µg every 3 months for the remainder of the patient's life, or 5 µg of oral vitamin B_{12} daily — a small amount is absorbed without intrinsic factor and is enough for daily requirements.

Postgastrectomy malabsorption

Anaemia is most commonly due to iron deficiency resulting from poor absorption. Megaloblastic anaemia is uncommon, and can be caused either by folate deficiency (poor intake) or vitamin B_{12} deficiency (long-term gastritis with atrophy resulting in intrinsic factor deficiency). Osteomalacia is an uncommon late complication. Anorexia after gastric surgery may lead to failure to gain weight and, rarely, to severe protein-energy malnutrition.

Diarrhoea is seen usually after vagotomy and is a major problem in 1% of patients. Treatment is with antidiarrhoeal agents. Cholestyramine (a resin that binds bile salts) helps in some patients. Rarely, diarrhoea/steatorrhoea can be the result of bacterial overgrowth in a blind loop of a Polya's gastrectomy.

SMALL-BOWEL DISEASE

The causes of small-bowel disease are shown in Table 31.1.

Presenting features of small-bowel disease

1. *Diarrhoea*: Eighty per cent of patients with small-bowel disease have diarrhoea, some with steatorrhoea. Some patients, however, present with no gastrointestinal symptoms.

Table 31.1. Disorders of the small bowel causing malabsorption.

Reduced absorptive surface	Coeliac disease
	Dermatitis herpetiformis
	Tropical sprue
	Inflammatory bowel disease
	Intestinal resection
	Whipple's disease
	Radiation enteritis
	Parasite infestations (e.g. *Giardia intestinalis*)
	Lymphoma
Interference with bile salts	Bacterial overgrowth

2. *Abdominal pain and discomfort*: Severe pain is unusual, but non-specific abdominal discomfort is not uncommon in all small-bowel disease. Abdominal distension can also cause discomfort and flatulence.
3. *Weight loss*: The anorexia that accompanies small-bowel disease invariably results in weight loss.
4. *Nutritional deficiency*: Deficiencies of iron, vitamin B_{12} and folate — or all of these — leading to anaemia are the only common deficiencies. Occasionally malabsorption of other vitamins or minerals occurs, causing bruising (vitamin K deficiency), tetany (calcium deficiency), oesteomalacia (vitamin D deficiency) or oral ulceration. Ankle oedema may be seen; this is usually nutritional, but may be accompanied by intestinal loss of albumin.

Physical signs of small-bowel disease

Abdominal examination is often normal, but sometimes distension and, very occasionally, hepatomegaly or an abdominal mass is found. In a severely ill patient, gross malnutrition with muscle wasting is seen. There may be evidence of anaemia.

Investigation of small-bowel disease

This will be highlighted in the description of individual diseases given below.

Coeliac disease (gluten-sensitive enteropathy)

In this condition there is an abnormality of the jejunal mucosa, which improves morphologically when the patient is treated with a gluten-free diet. Coeliac disease is common in Europe: the incidence in the UK is approximately 1 in 1000 and in Ireland approximately 1 in 300. The exact mode of inheritance is unknown, but 10–15% of first-degree relatives will have the condition. The haplotype HLA-A1, B8, DR3, DR7, DQ2 (DQA°, 0501, DQB1° 0201) is seen, and is present in more than 90% of patients, compared with 20–30% of the general population. However, 30% of identical twins are discordant for coeliac disease.

Aetiology

Gluten, contained in the cereals, wheat, rye, and barley, has a high molecular weight and can be fractionated to produce α, β, γ and ω gliadin peptides. α-Gliadin is toxic, but there is evidence to suggest that the others have some toxicity also. The exact mechanism of the damage produced is unknown, but it is believed to be T-cell-mediated. There are many immunological abnormalities, but these revert to normal on treatment. The enzyme, tissue transglutaminase (4), has been identified as one of the autoantigens of endomysial antibodies — but its exact role in the pathogenesis is unknown. An environmental factor such as a virus has been suggested. Adenovirus EB12 and gliadin share a sequence homology in their amino acid structure, but this virus has not be substantiated as being an aetiological factor. The aetiological mechanism may well be multifactorial with, for example, a genetically susceptible person being exposed to an environmental antigen that is a molecular mimic of gliadin and stimulates the production of antibodies.

Pathology

The normal small-bowel mucosal structure was described in Chapter 3.2. In coeliac disease there is an absence of villi and a flattened mucosal surface. T cells activated by gluten induce an inflammatory response with an increase in intraepithelial lymphocytes that show an increased expression of the γ/δ T-cell receptor. Crypt hypertrophy occurs, with oedema and infiltration of the lamina propria by chronic inflammatory cells followed by flattening of the mucosa. This sequence of events, described by Marsh (5), is depicted in Figure 31.3. The mucosal damage is predominantly proximal, decreasing in severity towards the ileum.

The term "latent" coeliac disease is used for patients with normal mucosa that becomes abnormal on the introduction of extra gluten into the diet. "Potential" coeliac disease (6) describes patients with normal jejunal histology who have high intraepithelial lymphocyte counts associated with an increased expression of γ/δ T-cell receptors, increased immunoglobulin M and G anti-gliadin antibodies in gut secretions, and increased intestinal permeability (called the coeliac-like intestinal antibody pattern).

Clinical features

Coeliac disease can present at any age. In infants, it appears after weaning onto gluten-containing

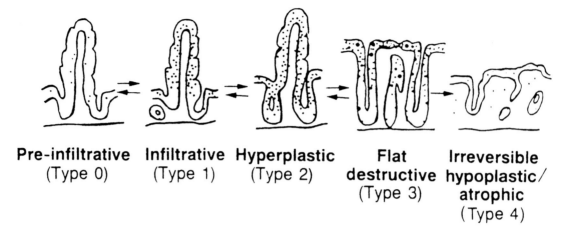

Pre-infiltrative	Infiltrative	Hyperplastic	Flat	Irreversible
(Type 0)	(Type 1)	(Type 2)	destructive	hypoplastic/
			(Type 3)	atrophic
				(Type 4)

Figure 31.3. Various patterns of gluten-induced enteropathy

Type 0 (pre-infiltrative lesion): The mucosa is normal, but patients have the coeliac-like antibody pattern (see text).

Type 1 (infiltrative lesion): There is an increase in intraepithelial lymphocytes.

Type 2 (hyperplastic lesion): Includes pathology of Type 1, with crypt hyperplasia in addition.

Type 3 (destructive lesion): Corresponds to classic flattened mucosa of patients with coeliac disease.

Type 4 (hyperplastic/atrophic lesion): Seen in patients who do not respond to dietary gluten withdrawal (resistant) or patients with lymphoma. EATL, enteropathy-associated T-cell lymphoma. Adapted with permission from Marsh M, 1992 (5).

foods. The peak incidence in adults is in the 3rd and 4th decades. It predominantly affects females. The symptoms are very variable and often non-specific. Gastrointestinal symptoms include diarrhoea or steatorrhoea, abdominal discomfort or pain, and weight loss. Mouth ulcers and angular stomatitis are frequent. Rare complications include tetany, osteomalacia, and gross malnutrition with peripheral oedema. Neurological symptoms such as paraesthesia, muscle weakness, ataxia, epilepsy or polyneuropathy can occasionally occur. There is an increased incidence of atopy and autoimmune disorders such as thyroid disease and, insulin-dependent diabetes mellitus. Other associated diseases include inflammatory bowel disease, chronic liver disease, and fibrosing allergic alveolitis. Physical signs are few and non-specific.

Investigations

Chapter 51 considers in detail the various tests for malabsorption, some of which are relevant to coeliac disease.

Endomysial and transglutaminase antibodies

These are highly sensitive and specific for the diagnosis (see Chapter 51). Antireticulin antibodies are also sensitive (see Chapter 51).

Small-bowel biopsy

This remains the "gold standard" for diagnosis. Under the microscope, the biopsy is flat, with an absence of villi (subtotal villus atrophy); occasionally, very stunted villi are seen (partial villous atrophy). The intraepithelial lymphocytes are increased (more than 30 per 100 epithelial cells), with crypt hypertrophy and an increase of chronic inflammatory cells in the lamina propria.

Other blood tests

There may be a mild to moderate anaemia, and folate deficiency is invariable. Iron deficiency is also common, but vitamin B_{12} deficiency is rare. A blood film may show macrocytosis, microcytosis, in addition to hypersegmented polymorphonuclear leukocytes and Howell–Jolly bodies (resulting from splenic atrophy). In very severely ill patients, other abnormalities such as hypoalbuminaemia are seen.

Absorption tests

These are often abnormal, but are seldom performed (see Chapter 51).

Imaging

A small-bowel follow-through may show dilatation of the small-bowel, with a change in fold pattern.

The folds become thicker and, in severe forms, total effacement is seen. This investigation is only performed if complications are suspected.

Treatment

A gluten-free diet produces a rapid clinical response, with morphological improvement of the jejunal mucosa. Replacement of haematinic agents may be required initially. The major cause of a poor response is poor dietary compliance. A gluten challenge (reintroduction of gluten with evidence of jejunal morphological damage) can confirm the diagnosis; it is performed only if the diagnosis is equivocal and in children whose diagnosis is made before they are aged 2 years, when subtotal villous atrophy can be caused by other disorders, for example an intolerance of cow's milk protein.

Osteoporosis is seen, even in treated cases.

In unresponsive patients, the following **complications** should be considered:

- intestinal lymphoma
- ulcerative jejunoileitis
- carcinoma

T-cell lymphoma is increased in coeliac disease. Ulcerative jejunitis can present with weight loss, hypoalbuminaemia, bleeding, and abdominal pain. Carcinoma of the small bowel and oesophagus, in addition to other gastrointestinal cancers, are seen. The incidence of malignancy compared with that associated with other gastrointestinal disorders is shown in Table 31.2.

Dermatitis herpetiformis

Dermatitis herpetiformis is an uncommon, blistering, subepidermal eruption of the skin associated with a gluten-sensitive enteropathy. The skin condition responds to dapsone, but both the gastrointestinal and dermatological problems improve on a gluten-free diet.

Tropical sprue

Tropical sprue presents with malabsorption and occurs in residents of or visitors to a tropical area where the condition is endemic. It is defined as the malabsorption of two or more substances, usually accompanied by diarrhoea and malnutrition. The condition is endemic in most of Asia, some Caribbean islands, Puerto Rico, and parts of South America. Epidemics, often lasting up to 2 years, occur in some areas, with repeated epidemics at varying intervals.

The **aetiology** is unknown, but it is believed to be an infective agent, as patients improve on antibiotics and removal from the sprue area.

The **presentation** is variable and consists of diarrhoea, anorexia, abdominal distension, and weight loss. The onset can be acute but may be more insidious, occasionally occurring several years after the initial visit to the tropics.

Diagnosis

Diagnosis is usually based on the demonstration of malabsorption — for example of fat or vitamin B_{12}. Infective causes of diarrhoea should be excluded. The jejunal mucosal abnormality is less severe than that in coeliac disease, and consists of a partial villous atrophy.

Treatment

Patients improve on leaving the sprue area and taking folic acid (5 mg) daily. Most patients also require an antibiotic, for example tetracycline 1 g daily. It may be necessary to give this for up to 6 months. Severely ill patients require resuscitation with fluids and electrolytes, and the correction of nutritional deficiencies such as vitamin B_{12}.

The **prognosis** is excellent. Mortality is usually associated with water and electrolyte depletion, particularly in epidemics.

Inflammatory bowel disease

Weight loss is usually related to anorexia. Malabsorption, *per se*, plays a limited part in this disease.

Table 31.2. Incidence of malignancy associated with various gastrointestinal disorders.

Disorder	Incidence %
Familial adenomatous polyposis	100
Barrett's oesophagus	15
Chronic ulcerative colitis	13
Coeliac disease	13
Pernicious anaemia	<5
Postgastrectomy stomach	<5

However, severe extensive Crohn's disease may result in malabsorption of vitamins — for example of niacin, causing pellagra, or of vitamin D, causing osteomalacia. Malabsorption of vitamin B_{12} as a result of ileal disease or bacterial overgrowth is uncommon, but if an intestinal resection has been performed, vitamin B_{12} deficiency becomes likely, and the patient should be monitored, and treated prophylactically if necessary.

See Chapters 16 and 36 for details regarding the **management** of IBD.

Bacterial overgrowth

Bacterial overgrowth is normally found associated with structural abnormalities of the small intestine, but can also occur with motility disorders. Normally, the upper part of the small intestine is almost sterile, containing only a few organisms derived from the mouth. Gastric acid kills most organisms and intestinal motility keeps the jejunum empty. The terminal ileum contains faecal-type organisms such as *Escherichia coli* and anaerobes.

Bacteria such as *E. coli* and *Bacteriodes* are capable of deconjugating and dehydroxylating bile salts. Thus, unconjugated and dehydroxylated bile salts can be detected in aspirates from the upper jejunum, by chromatography. Steatorrhoea occurs as a result of conjugated-bile-salt deficiency. Bacteria are also able to metabolize vitamin B_{12} and interfere with its binding to intrinsic factor, leading to vitamin B_{12} deficiency.

The clinical **presentation** is chiefly with diarrhoea and steatorrhoea.

Investigation is with the hydrogen breath test (see Chapter 51), and with direct aspiration of the jejunal juice followed by culture or chromatography if the diagnosis is in doubt. Vitamin B_{12} deficiency can be demonstrated by the Schilling test (see Chapters 25 and 52). Some bacteria can produce folic acid, therefore this is not usually deficient.

Treatment is usually of the underlying lesion, but with multiple diverticula, grossly dilated bowel, or in Crohn's disease, it may be necessary to use rotating courses of antibiotics — for example metronidazole, tetracycline, or ciprofloxacin.

Intestinal resection

The effects of resection depend on the extent and the area resected. A 30–50% resection can usually be tolerated without severe problems. Massive resection is followed by the short-gut syndrome.

Ileal resection

There are specific receptors for the absorption of bile salts and vitamin B_{12} in the ileum; resection of this area will lead to malabsorption of these substances (Figure 31.4). Ileal resection can therefore lead to the following:

- diarrhoea as a result of bile salts and unabsorbed fatty acids entering the colon and interfering with water and electrolyte absorption
- steatorrhoea resulting from decreased micellar formation caused by excess loss of bile salts in the faeces. Increased bile-salt synthesis can compensate for approximately 30% of the bile salts lost in the faeces
- lithogenic bile and gallstone formation
- renal oxalate stones — caused by increased oxalate absorption as a result of the presence of bile salts in the colon
- low serum vitamin B_{12} concentrations, and macrocytosis

Investigations include a small-bowel follow-through, measurement of serum vitamin B_{12}, and a selenium75 homotaurocholic acid (SeHCAT) absorption study for bile salt loss (see Chapter 52). **Treatment** is with vitamin B_{12} replacements and a low-fat diet if there is steatorrhoea. Diarrhoea may be helped with cholestyramine or aluminium hydroxide mixture, which bind bile salts.

Jejunal resection

As there are no specific sites for the absorption of any substance solely in the jejunum, the ileum can take over the jejunal absorptive function. Gastric hypersecretion, with high gastrin concentrations, can occur with jejunal resection, but the exact mechanism for this is unclear.

Massive resection (short-gut syndrome)

This can occur after resection (in Crohn's disease), mesenteric occlusion, or trauma. Severe symptoms occur when there is less than 90–100 cm of small bowel *in situ*. Symptoms include diarrhoea with severe loss of water and electrolytes, and malnutrition. Parenteral nutrition may be necessary. Intes-

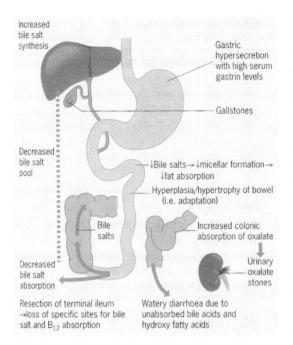

Figure 31.4. The effects of resection of the distal small bowel. Reprinted from *Clinical Medicine* 4th Ed, Kumar & Clark, pp. 257, 1998 by permission of the publisher WB Saunders.

tinal adaptation can lead to an increase in absorption per unit length of bowel with time (see Chapter 20).

Whipple's disease

This rare disease **presents** with steatorrhoea, abdominal pain, and systemic symptoms of fever and weight loss. Peripheral lymphadenopathy, arthritis, and involvement of the heart, lung, and brain may occur.

Diagnosis is based on the clinical picture together with a jejunal mucosa showing stunted villi and diagnostic periodic acid Schiff-positive macrophages. On electron microscopy, bacilli (*Tropheryma whippelii*) (7) are seen within the macrophages. **Treatment** is with antibiotics, which should include an antibiotic that crosses the blood—brain barrier — for example chloramphenicol or cotrimoxazole.

Radiation enteritis

Damage to the intestine can be caused by radiation of more than 50 Gy. As the pelvis is the abdominal area most commonly irradiated, the ileum and rectum are often involved. Clinically, patients **present** with diarrhoea and abdominal pain at the time of radiation. These symptoms improve within 6 weeks after completion of therapy. If symptoms persist for 3 months or more, chronic radiation enteritis is diagnosed. The prevalence is more than 15%.

Patients often present with symptoms of obstruction — partial or complete. Malabsorption can be caused by mucosal damage and by bacterial overgrowth in dilated segments. This occurs because radiation produces muscle fibre atrophy, ulcerative changes (as a result of ischaemia), and obstruction (by strictures) by the radiation-induced fibrosis.

Treatment is symptomatic. Surgery should be avoided. Radiation damage to the rectum produces a radiation proctitis with diarrhoea, which is, again, treated symptomatically or with local steroids.

Parasitic infestation

Giardia intestinalis can produce diarrhoea or malabsorption with steatorrhoea. Minor changes are seen in the jejunal mucosa. The organism can be found in jejunal fluid or histologically, lying on the mucosa. *Cryptosporidium spp.* can also produce malabsorption.

Patients with human immunodeficiency virus infection are also particularly prone to parasite infestations.

Further details of these conditions may be found in Chapter 7.

Miscellaneous causes of malabsorption

Drugs

Drugs that bind bile salts (e.g. cholestyramine) and some antibiotics (e.g. neomycin) can produce steatorrhoea.

Endocrine factors

Thyrotoxicosis can produce diarrhoea and, rarely, steatorrhoea as a result of increased gastric emptying and increased motility.

Diabetes mellitus can cause diarrhoea, malabsorption, and steatorrhoea, sometimes as a result of bacterial overgrowth from stasis. Stasis results from abnormal motility caused by an autonomic neuropathy.

Gastrinoma (Zollinger–Ellison syndrome)

This tumour arises from the G cells in the pancreas and secretes large amounts of gastrin. Gastrin stimulates maximal secretion of gastric acid, which causes peptic ulceration in the stomach and duodenum, but also in the jejunum. Haemorrhage and perforation can occur. The low pH in the upper intestine interferes with lipolysis and this, together with abnormalities of the jejunal mucosa, causes diarrhoea and, rarely, steatorrhoea.

Lymphoma

Lymphoma can be primary or secondary to coeliac disease. When it infiltrates the small bowel mucosa, it causes malabsorption.

Intestinal lymphangiectasia

Diarrhoea and, rarely, steatorrhoea may be produced in intestinal lymphangiectasia.

Hypogammaglobulinaemia

Hypogammaglobulinaemia is seen in a number of conditions, including lymphoid nodular hyperplasia. Steatorrhoea results either from abnormal jejunal mucosa due to malabsorption or from secondary infestation with, for example, *Giardia intestinalis*.

PANCREATIC DISEASE

The pancreas produces enzymes that are released into the intestinal lumen to help in the absorption of fat, carbohydrate, and protein (it also has a small role in vitamin B_{12} absorption, but this is not clinically important).

Severe pancreatic damage (>90%) must occur before the exocrine function is reduced sufficiently to produce malabsorption. This occurs in:

- chronic pancreatitis
- cystic fibrosis
- carcinoma of the body and tail of the pancreas (rarely)

In patients with carcinoma of the head of the pancreas, jaundice occurs as a result of obstruction of the common bile duct; malabsorption of vitamin K can also occur (see below).

Chronic pancreatitis

Steatorrhoea occurs when the secretion of pancreatic lipase is reduced by 90%. Failure of triglyceride hydrolysis because of the lack of lipase can produce severe steatorrhoea, with fat globules being apparent in the stools. Steatorrhoea is often accompanied by diabetes mellitus. Diagnosis of the cause of steatorrhoea is by:

1. *Clinical presentation*: Accompanying severe pain radiating to the back, or a history of high alcohol consumption. Ultrasound is usually the first investigation, but has a sensitivity of only 50%.
2. *Imaging* (see Chapter 49): Computed tomography (CT) is highly sensitive (up to 90%) in the diagnosis of chronic pancreatitis. Magnetic resonance imaging (MRI) requires no ionizing radiation, and is equally sensitive as CT. Endoscopic retrograde cholangiopancreatography is slightly more sensitive in the diagnosis of early pancreatic disease. Magnetic resonance cholangiopancreatography (MRCP) imaging avoids endoscopy and is being used increasingly.
3. *Pancreatic function tests*: (see Chapter 51 for details.)

Treatment is by removal of the precipitating cause (e.g. stop taking alcohol), and use of pain relief. The steatorrhoea is treated with a low-fat diet and pancreatic supplements — for example, pancreatin 2–4 g with each meal, with acid suppression. Diabetes is treated with insulin.

Cystic fibrosis

Many patients with cystic fibrosis have malnutrition resulting mainly from anorexia associated with pulmonary sepsis. About 85% of patients have symptomatic steatorrhoea caused by pancreatic dysfunction.

Diagnosis is by:

- the clinical history in childhood and family history
- high sodium concentration in sweat (more than 16 mmol/litre)
- blood DNA analysis of gene defect
- evidence of bronchiectasis

Tests for malabsorption are not usually necessary.

Treatment of the steatorrhoea is with high-dose pancreatin containing trypsin and lipase, given in microsphere-containing capsules that deliver high doses of enzyme to the duodenum. A rare complication of this, however, is fibrosing colonopathy with stricture formation.

A high-energy diet is required, which must be low in fat.

Carcinoma of body and tail of pancreas

Patients with these pancreatic cancers have non-specific symptoms, but also severe abdominal pain and weight loss. The weight loss is a consequence of anorexia. Malabsorption is not a common feature, as in most patients there is sufficient pancreatic secretion to allow intraluminal hydrolysis to take place.

The **diagnosis** is made with ultrasound, CT, or MRI.

Unfortunately, **treatment** is unsatisfactory, and most patients do not survive longer than 6 months.

LIVER AND BILIARY TRACT DISEASE

Jaundice

Liver and biliary tract disorders that cause malabsorption (all are rare) include:

- Jaundice caused by obstruction
  - carcinoma of the head of pancreas
  - stones in the common bile duct
- Chronic cholestasis
  - primary biliary cirrhosis

Persistent jaundice from any cause will produce malabsorption of fat and, consequently, of fat-soluble vitamins. The steatorrhoea that occurs is not usually a major problem and the jaundice is usually reversible — for example by removal of stones from the common bile duct or insertion of a stent in the case of carcinoma of the pancreas.

Chronic cholestasis in conditions such as **primary biliary cirrhosis** can give rise to occasional troublesome steatorrhoea and a low-fat diet is therefore instituted. However, this is becoming uncommon, as many patients — particularly those with primary biliary cirrhosis — undergo liver transplantation before reaching this stage.

In the short term, the only **fat-soluble vitamin malabsorption** that is clinically important in cases of jaundice is that of vitamin K. This leads to coagulation problems. Water-soluble vitamin K is given by mouth or by intramuscular vitamin K injection.

With persistent cholestasis, malabsorption of vitamins A, D, and possibly E, can become a clinical problem.

References
1. Kelts DG, Grand RJ, Shen G *et al*. Nutritional basis of growth failure in children and adolescents with Crohn's disease. *Gastroenterology* 1979; **76**: 720–727.
2. Kirschner BS, Klich JR, Kalman SS *et al*. Reversal of growth retardation in Crohn's disease with therapy emphasising oral nutritional restitution. *Gastroenterology* 1981; **80**: 10–15.
3. Kumar PJ, Clark ML. *Clinical Medicine*, 4th edn. Edinburgh: WB Saunders, 1998; pp. 247, 248, 257.
4. Dieterich W, Ehnis T, Bauer M *et al*. Identification of tissue transglutaminase as the autoantigen of coeliac disease. *Nature* 1997; **7**: 797–801.
   The first identification of the autoantigen for the endomysial antibody.
5. Marsh M. Mucosal pathology is gluten sensitivity. In: *Coeliac Disease*. Ed. M Marsh. Oxford: Blackwell Scientific Publications, 1992; pp. 136–191.
   An excellent chapter describing the patterns of gluten-induced mucosal change and remodelling in a comprehensive book on coeliac disease.
6. Arranz E, Bode J, Kingstone K, *et al*. Intestinal antibody pattern of Coeliac disease: association wiith α/δ T cell receptor expression by intra-epithelial lymphocytes and other indices of potential Coeliac disease. *Gut* 1994; **35**: 476–482.
7. Relman DA, Schmedt TM, MacDermott RP *et al*. Identification of the uncultured bacillus of Whipple's disease. *N Engl J Med* 1993; **328**: 62–63.
   The bacterial 16 S ribosomal RNA sequence was amplified directly from tissue of patients with Whipple's disease. The bacillus was named *Tropheryma whippelii*.

Further reading
Carey MC, Small DC. The characteristics of mixed micellar solution with particular reference to bile. *Am J Med* 1970; **49**: 590.
Alpers DH. Digestion and absorption of carbohydrates and proteins. In: *Physiology of the Gastrointestinal Tract*, 2nd edn. Ed. LR Johnson. New York: Raven Press, 1987; pp. 1469.
Tso P. Intestinal lipid absorption. In: *Physiology of the Gastrointestinal Tract*. 3rd edn. Ed. LR Johnson. New York: Raven Press, 1994; p. 1873.
Shiau YF. Mechanisms of intestinal absorption of fat. *Am J Physiol* 1981; **3**: G1.
Department of Health Report. Dietary Reference Values for Food Energy and Nutrients for the United Kingdom. *Report of Panel on Dietary Reference Values of the Committee on Medical Aspects of Food Policy.* London: HMSO, 1991.

Davidson S, Passmore R, Brock JF *et al.* (Eds). *Human Nutrition and Dietetics*. Churchill Livingstone: Edinburgh, 1979.

Riley SA, Marsh MN. Maldigestion and malabsorption. In: *Sleisenger & Fordtran's Gastrointestinal and Liver Disease*. 6th edn, vol II. Eds. M Feldman, BF Scharschmidt, MM Sleisinger. Philadelphia: WB Saunders, 1998; pp. 1501–1520.

Marsh MN, Riley SA. Digestion and absorption of nutrients and vitamins. In: *Sleisenger & Fordtran's Gastrointestinal and Liver Disease*, 6th edn, vol II. Eds. M Feldman, BF Scharschmidt, MM Sleisinger. Philadelphia: WB Saunders, 1998; pp. 1471–1495.

(Editorial). Surgery to cure Zollinger–Ellison syndrome. *N Engl J Med* 1999; **340**: 635, 689.

32. Constipation

ANTON EMMANUEL

INTRODUCTION

Constipation is a symptom, not a disease, and reflects slowed colonic transit, impairment of rectal emptying, or both (1). Its severity may vary from the slight, causing no disruption of life, to the severe, when the patient's social and personal functioning is grossly disrupted. Patients referred to hospital tend to be those with more severe impairment of quality of life, and who have failed trials of dietary fibre supplementation.

Patients with slow colonic transit tend to report a reduced frequency of the urge to defaecate, and occasionally the total absence of urge if laxatives are not consumed. Patients with incoordination of the rectum, anus, and pelvic floor present with symptoms of straining, incomplete rectal evacuation and need for anal or vaginal digitation in order to empty the rectum. Variables such as stool frequency and consistency are easy to quantify in the history, but there is no generally accepted normal range; furthermore, these variables differ according to race, personality, and gender. Nonetheless, a working definition of "normal" bowel function is of bowel opening between 3 and 21 times a week and needing to strain on fewer than 25% of occasions to achieve emptying (1).

There are many possible **causes of constipation**:

- Endocrine
  - hypothyroidism
  - glucagonoma
  - diabetes mellitus
- Metabolic
  - hypercalcaemia
  - uraemia
  - hypokalaemia
  - porphyria
  - amyloidosis
  - lead poisoning
- Neurological
  - cortical lesions (tumour, infarction)
  - spinal cord lesions (injury, infarction)
  - peripheral lesions (autonomic neuropathy)
- Neuromuscular disorders
  - systemic sclerosis
  - dermatomyositis
  - dystrophia myotonica
- Psychological
  - anorexia nervosa, bulimia nervosa
  - affective disorder
  - dementia
- Physiological
  - pregnancy
  - old age
- Colonic
  - neuromuscular disorder (Hirschsprung's disease, megabowel, chronic intestinal pseudo-obstruction)
  - stricture (tumour, ischaemia, diverticular)
- Anal
  - fissure
  - polyp, tumour

CLINICAL SUBTYPES

1. *Idiopathic constipation*: This form is often mild. It is most common in the elderly, and is often

ascribable to reduced mental and physical function, low-residue diet, or a drug side effect.

2. *Secondary to coexisting systemic illness*: This is much more rare. It may be necessary to exclude a variety of metabolic, endocrine, and neuromuscular disorders, according to the clinical picture.

3. *Secondary to a colonic cause*: Recent onset of symptoms or the presence of suspicious symptoms should indicate the need to exclude tumours or stenotic lesions of the colon by radiology or endoscopy.

4. *Irritable bowel syndrome*: Constipation is often one feature of the irritable bowel syndrome, and should be suspected when it coexists with complaints of abdominal pain and bloating in an otherwise healthy young person.

5. *Severe constipation with gut dilatation*: This may be caused by:
   - idiopathic megarectum or megacolon (see below)
   - Hirschsprung's disease (see below)
   - chronic idiopathic intestinal pseudo-obstruction: extremely rare (suspect in the presence of a dilated upper intestine)

6. *Severe constipation with a normal diameter colon*: This is a chronic disorder, affecting predominantly women of child-bearing age (2).

CLINICAL FEATURES

Patients may describe a clear precipitant to their symptoms (most commonly abdominal or pelvic surgery, childbirth, or emotional trauma), but the development of symptoms is frequently insidious. In addition to the already described symptoms of infrequent and incomplete defecation, patients presenting to hospital with constipation often report abdominal pain, distension, and nausea (2,3). There is often a history of heavy laxative consumption with unpredictable effects and subsequent development of lack of effect. Malaise and lethargy are invariable; headaches, mood swings and poor concentration are frequently reported. There are often non-specific urinary and gynaecological complaints. Faecal soiling and a history of faecal impaction in a young patient should raise the suspicion of a megarectum.

Up to 50% of women who present with functional gastrointestinal disorders are victims of sexual or physical abuse in childhood (4–6). An important aspect of the consultation in a constipated patient is to create the atmosphere that allows the patient to discuss such matters, as it is known that dramatic relief of constipation can be brought about with the release of emotions relating to the abuse (7). Constipated patients, especially those with slow transit, tend to have specific psychological profiles, with exaggerated levels of somatization, anxiety, depression, and paranoid ideation (8–10).

Examination is usually unremarkable, but the presence of gross abdominal bloating and a faecal mass rising out of the pelvis should raise the suspicion of Hirschsprung's disease or megarectum. Rigid sigmoidoscopy may show the changes of melanosis coli, and should be performed if megarectum is suspected.

INVESTIGATION

Colonoscopy or barium enema examination are helpful only in excluding a primary colonic cause for constipation. There is no pathophysiological significance to the frequent observation of a long colon in these patients. Routine thyroid function and checking of serum calcium concentration rarely reveal any abnormality, unless there is a suggestive history.

Special investigations are only indicated for those patients in whom adequate fibre supplementation has failed to help and who have been referred from the primary-care setting. Careful selection of investigations can give helpful information on which to base subsequent management.

Radio-opaque marker study of whole-gut transit

In addition to being the most useful measure of generalized intestinal motor function, this investigation is simple, non-invasive, and easy to interpret. A well-validated technique involves ingestion of three sets of radioopaque markers at 24-h intervals on three consecutive days during which laxatives are not permitted. A single plain abdominal X-ray is obtained 120 h after the ingestion of the first set of markers and compared against a reproducible normal range of images, allowing the patient to be classed as having slow transit if there is retention of more than the normal for any one of the three sets of markers (11). No stool collection is required and a measure of whole-gut transit can be easily obtained. Such a method also has the advantage of identifying patient compliance and accuracy of reporting — for instance, if the patient reports passing only tiny quantities of stool in the 5 days of the study and yet most of the markers have been passed, it is possible to encourage the patient that, in those small quantities, sufficient colonic clearance was being achieved.

A development of this technique has been to identify regions of slow colonic transit using a mathematical formula based on the assumption that the colon handles all the markers identically (12). There is, however, no evidence that identifying regions of slow transit has any clinical or therapeutic significance.

Rectoanal inhibitory reflex

Testing for this reflex is indicated in patients with suspected Hirschsprung's disease, as its presence excludes the condition without the need for surgical biopsy of the distal rectum. A distensible balloon is inserted into the rectum and inflated to 50 ml while simultaneous recording of anal sphincter pressure is undertaken; the normal reflex is for relaxation of the sphincter in response to rectal filling, whereas patients with Hirschsprung's disease demonstrate no change in sphincter pressure, even with large rectal distension volumes.

Evacuation proctography

Evacuation proctography, or defecography, is a technique used to study anorectal morphology and dynamics during defecation. Semi-solid barium paste is inserted into the rectum and the patient seated on a hollow receptacle; the patient is encouraged to void the rectum while videoradiography is performed (13). Evacuation proctography is indicated if the history is suggestive of a defecatory disorder — functional abnormalities of rectal emptying such as intussusception or frank rectal mucosal prolapse, excess pelvic floor descent, or puborectalis dyskinesis (failure of the puborectalis sling to relax on evacuation) can be readily identified by proctography (14). The ability to evacuate the rectum may also be identified by testing the patient's ability to void the rectum of a water-filled balloon attached to a catheter in the rectum. This however is less "physiological" than proctography and does not offer information regarding the structural abnormalities contributing to or complicating constipation, such as a rectocele (protrusion of the anterior rectal wall into the back of the vagina) or solitary rectal ulcer syndrome, which may be identified by proctography.

Anorectal sensory testing

Rectal balloon distension volumes tend to be greater in constipated patients than in healthy controls, although distension testing is not sufficiently sensitive to be diagnostic. Anorectal mucosal electrosensitivity testing, however, is a specific test of the degree of hindgut innervation. Thus constipation complicating neurological diseases (such as multiple sclerosis, spinal cord injury, Parkinson's disease, or diabetic neuropathy) can be differentiated from constipation that is coincident with neurological disease.

Other investigations

Colonic scintigraphy using a radioisotope incorporated into food can give information regarding segmental transit abnormalities, although the clinical significance of such information is uncertain. Electromyographic and colonic pressure studies are technically complex, and relevant only to research practice, as yet.

TREATMENT

The natural history of constipation is uncertain (15). It is not known what proportion of patients stop presenting with intestinal complaints or displace symptoms to another system, and this factor will undoubtedly affect "success rates" of various treatments. Another factor to bear in mind when reviewing the literature on the treatment of constipation is that, as is common with most functional problems, the longer the period of follow-up after treatment, the worse the outcome.

General measures

Any drugs that may be contributing to the patient's symptoms should be considered. **Common drugs**

that induce constipation include:

- tricyclic antidepressants
- monoamine oxide inhibitors
- antipsychotics
- opiates
- anticonvulsants
- antiparkinsonian agents
- antacids (aluminium- and calcium-containing ones)
- β-blockers
- calcium-channel antagonists
- diuretics
- iron

Once imaging has been performed, where appropriate, to exclude a mechanical cause of their symptoms, many patients simply need reassurance as to what the range of "normal" bowel frequency and stool consistency is amongst the general population. Establishing good rapport with the patient is obvious, but essential — many hospital-referred patients have seen a variety of other medical professionals and may have been left with the impression that their problems are trivial or purely psychological; time spent understanding how the symptoms impact on life gives an insight into what is often the main concern of the patients.

There is no evidence that constipated patients drink less fluid or take less exercise than healthy subjects (16) and it is important to stress the need for a balanced and non-obsessive approach to their lifestyle.

A psychogenic component to the patient's symptoms should be borne in mind. Many patients have been the victims of significant childhood physical and sexual abuse, and many find themselves in occupational or domestic circumstances that are a source of considerable anxiety and stress. The association between stress and gastrointestinal motility is well established (17,18), and there is evidence that demonstrating to the patient the relationship between environmental triggers and subsequent development of symptoms can significantly aid management (19).

Diet

Dietary fibre is not usually effective in the management of constipated patients referred to hospital.

Nevertheless, increasing dietary fibre to 30 g (14.4 g of crude fibre) is the simplest and least expensive first-line treatment of chronic constipation (20). To be most effective, it is probably best achieved by giving formal dietary advice and encouraging the patient to keep a bowel diary for a full month of treatment. However, 30 g of fibre per day can prove difficult for some patients to consume — it amounts to four bowls of bran cereal, or 10 slices of wholemeal bread, or 20 apples! Another problem is that dietary fibre only increases stool weight in proportion to the starting weight, and so the more severely constipated the patient the less effective is the fibre (21). Furthermore, other variables — such as personality and vegetarianism — affect stool output as much as fibre, and so the role of dietary fibre remains questionable.

A further limitation of augmenting dietary fibre is that it may provoke abdominal distension and flatulence in patients with slow-transit constipation (2) and incontinence in those with a megacolon (22).

Pharmacological options

There are many "combination compounds" available to treat constipation, but for clarity a brief outline of the main classes of laxative will be given, classified by mode of action.

Bulk forming laxatives

This class — which includes ispaghula, methylcellulose, and sterculia — comprise naturally based compounds that are helpful only for those patients with mild symptoms who can not obtain adequate dietary fibre. Their role is limited, for the same reasons as described in the section on dietary fibre. In general, their place in the management of the patient with chronic constipation is restricted to improvement of bowel frequency, rather than changes in stool consistency or need to strain (23).

Stimulant laxatives

This class of drugs (e.g. bisacodyl, senna, and sodium picosulphate) are more suited to the management of chronic constipation, because their action is more predictable. The drugs enhance colonic motility (24) and improve stool frequency and consistency (25). Although there is no evidence of significant changes in colonic histological (26) or unwanted motility (27) with their chronic usage, it is usual to attempt to minimize usage to alternate days or every third day (28).

Faecal softeners

These compounds include docusate sodium, liquid paraffin, and arachis oil enema. They can be taken either orally or rectally, but — to judge from the results of available clinical trials — are of limited efficacy. Nevertheless, they are widely used, and can cause side effects related to their detergent or organic chemical composition.

Osmotic laxatives

The osmotic laxatives include lactulose, magnesium sulphate, and phosphate enema.

Lactulose is a syrup derived from lactose, and acts as a laxative by decreasing colonic pH through generation of fatty acids and fermentation products. To achieve a clinically significant effect often requires large doses (of what is an expensive agent) and at least two or three days of treatment (29,30). Other frequently reported problems include the sweet taste, abdominal distension, and flatulence.

Magnesium salts are more potent osmotic laxatives, and have the attraction of being able to be taken in a titrated fashion, the intention being to obtain a semi-solid stool without urgency. The salts have an unpleasant taste and it can be hard to achieve the balance between insufficient dose and watery stool. Excessive dosages run the risk of hyper-magnesaemia, especially in children or patients with renal failure.

Prokinetic agents

Cisapride has proven effective in the management of chronic constipation in one study, although its routine use in chronic constipation is unlicensed (31). It may have a role in constipation associated with neurological diseases (Cisapride has now been withdrawn by the manufacturer). Although **erythromycin** is a potent **upper intestinal** prokinetic, the motilin analogue effects are not clinically relevant in enhancing **colonic** motility. Specific prokinetic drugs are in advanced stages of development as novel, specific, and consistent enhancers of colonic motility.

Biofeedback

Biofeedback for constipation is directed towards three aspects:

1. Habit training, and instruction about diet, exercise, and "normal" bowel function.
2. Addressing specific current or past psychological problems.
3. A physical aspect comprising a sensory component to alter rectal distension sensitivity and a motor component to alter abnormal abdominal, pelvic floor, and anal sphincter function during defecation.

The first two aspects have already been discussed; this section will deal with the practicalities of biofeedback. Although there is a considerable volume of literature on biofeedback for defecatory disorders, the papers are marked by very poor descriptions of the actual practical techniques undertaken.

In essence, the sensory aspect of the physical component comprises "teaching" the individual to perceive gradually smaller volumes of rectal distension, which are normally insensible to many chronically constipated patients (32). A different subset of patients need instruction not to attempt defecation at small volumes, and these are taught to increase rectal capacitance gradually. The motor component is performed with a pressure or myoelectric probe in the anal canal, to monitor external anal sphincter pressure. Patients become accustomed to visual (or, rarely, auditory) feedback of sphincter activity on voluntary contraction of the sphincter. They are then asked to expel a water-filled balloon that is placed simultaneously with the probe in the rectum (33). Failure of the sphincter to relax normally is immediately evident to the patient (as it mimics the voluntary contraction trace performed earlier by the patient), who can then be instructed in techniques to correct this. Similarly, failure of the pelvic floor function on attempted defecation is evident to patient and therapist by poor propulsion of the balloon on attempted evacuation. Many patients with evacuation disorders also have incoordination of abdominal muscles on attempted voiding and they can be taught to correct this. Typically, a patient undergoes four or five sessions of biofeedback at approximately fortnightly intervals, and there is an emphasis on practice at home between appointments.

Controlled trials of biofeedback are, by definition, almost impossible to perform. Nevertheless, an impressive 67% of patients, most of whom are specialist referrals and therefore quite severe and intractable cases, report significant improvement with the technique at long-term follow-up (34,35). Successful treatment is often, but not always, accompanied by improvements in the physiological parameters of defaecation (32,35). Interestingly, success occurs even in those patients with slow transit, suggesting that the effect of biofeedback is at more than just the pelvic level. The only two predictors of failure of treatment are psychiatric co-morbidity and poor compliance with home practice (35). A case can be made for biofeedback as first-line treatment of chronic idiopathic constipation in patients who require laxatives.

Surgical management

Constipation, as has already been made clear, is a complex disorder affecting the brain, spinal nerves, upper intestine, colon, enteric nerves, and intestinal smooth muscle — it is unfeasible that a single surgical intervention could significantly improve symptoms in a permanent fashion. Surgery for chronic constipation has traditionally been reserved for the most intractable cases — often with significant psychological distress (9) — which have failed to respond to conventional management, and the poor success rates seen may in part reflect this fact. Case selection is therefore a crucial element in the identification of possible candidates for surgery. Colectomy has always been restricted to those patients with documented slow transit (12) — no other physiological or radiological variable has proved accurate as a prognostic indicator (36).

Perianal procedures

Anorectal myectomy (37) and puborectalis division (38) have a success rate no greater than 25% in long-term follow-up studies. Slightly greater success is seen in selected patients undergoing repair of a rectocele, among whom up to 50% experience some improvement of perineal symptoms.

Colectomy

Segmental resection, based on removal of the regions of the colon with greatest hold-up of radioopaque markers on a transit study, has not proved to be any more effective than the resection of any other "normal" segment (39). The more commonly performed procedure is a subtotal colectomy and ileorectal anastomosis. Results of the long-term follow-up studies indicate a poor success rate of less than 50% (40,41), with persisting constipation, abdominal pain, and bloating. In addition to the high failure rate, there is a high frequency of complications — in particular, diarrhoea, faecal incontinence, recurrent obstructive episodes, and pelvic sepsis. Critical factors for success after colectomy appear to be the presence of slow transit and the absence of psychological morbidity and defecatory incoordination.

Stoma formation

When a stoma is formed as a primary procedure for constipation or in patients with neurological disease, the outcome can be excellent (42). However, if the stoma is constructed as a salvage procedure after failed previous surgery, it is generally unhelpful.

SPECIFIC CONDITIONS

Megacolon

Megacolon is colonic dilatation in the absence of mechanical obstruction. The radiological definition requires quantification of the width of the caecum as greater than 12 cm, ascending colon greater than 8 cm and the descending colon greater than 6.5 cm (43). Megacolon can be classified as either congenital (Hirschsprung's disease) or acquired (**acute** — Ogilvie's syndrome; **neurological** — Chaga's disease, chronic intestinal pseudo-obstruction; **myopathic** — scleroderma, amyloidosis, chronic intestinal pseudo-obstruction). The term "megabowel" implies dilatation of rectum and colon, whereas "megacolon" describes dilatation of only the abdominal colon. The frequent elongation of the colon seen in chronic constipation is **not** megacolon.

Idiopathic megabowel

Idiopathic megabowel is an uncommon but important condition to consider in patients presenting with constipation, because the aim of management is quite distinct. It occurs equally in men and women and presentation is typically either in early childhood or early adult life (44). Both groups present with intractable constipation but, in childhood, symptoms are typically of faecal impaction and soiling, whereas in adulthood abdominal pain and no soiling are the norm. The soiling results from overflow caused by impacted stool in the rectum, and the resulting fluid is able to leak out through a permanently patent anal sphincter. On examination, anal sphincter dilatation may be evident, in addition to the frequently palpable abdominal mass of a faecal bolus rising out of the pelvis. Investigation by enema contrast study may display faecal loading, dilatation of the colon at the pelvic brim (diameter greater than 6.5 cm) (2), or absence of a "narrowed segment" (see below) on lateral view, thereby excluding Hirschsprung's disease. Idiopathic megacolon can present as recurrent episodes of an acute abdomen as a result of a sigmoid volvulus, and an instant contrast enema is invaluable in demonstrating this. Almost all cases of sigmoid volvulus occur in the context of a megabowel, but not all cases of megabowel present as volvulus.

Management of idiopathic megabowel commences with achieving an empty colon (manual disimpaction may be required, but should be avoided if at all possible, in view of the potential damage to what may already be a weakened anal sphincter). Thereafter a combination of osmotic laxatives (titrated to obtain a stool with the consistency of porridge), habit training (to encourage regular attempts at bowel opening, usually after meals), and biofeedback (to ease defecatory incoordination) should be strictly adhered to. Stimulant laxatives should be avoided, and patients should be encouraged to maintain a liquid intake of at least 2.5 litre per day. Occasionally, suppositories or enemas may be needed if biofeedback has failed to correct an associated difficulty with evacuation. The patient needs to understand that the condition is lifelong and that successful management rests in their own hands.

For those patients in whom strict medical management fails, **surgery** remains an option. The goal, once again, is to obtain a "porridgey" stool, and this may be achieved successfully by colectomy and ileorectal or ileoanal anastomosis (45), or ileostomy (46). Other possible surgical procedures depend on the specific anatomy of the patient: with a megarectum and normal colonic diameter, the rectum should be resected; for megacolon with normal rectal diameter, an ileorectotomy is the operation of choice (47). With medical and, when necessary, surgical management, the outcome of megabowel is usually excellent, with more than 90% of patients achieving normal bowel frequency (45).

Hirschsprung's disease

This is a **congenital megacolon** resulting form absence of intramural enteric nerve plexuses, or aganglionosis, affecting the distal colon. This absence of neural relaxation results in a narrow (unrelaxed) segment of the bowel, which is typically in the rectum or sigmoid colon. Rare variants affecting the anal sphincters alone or the entire colon have also been described. Colonic material is unable to cross the narrowed segment, and there is consequent dilatation of the colon proximally.

Hirschsprung's disease is a familial condition affecting 1 in 5000 births, and affecting predominantly males (five times more often than females) (48). There is an association with Down's syndrome and a variety of congenital anomalies. **Presentation** is usually as a neonate (with abdominal distension and absolute constipation), but rarely some do not come to medical attention until adult life. Presentation in childhood may be with malnutrition or anaemia; in the older age group, faecal impaction is the most common symptom. The presence of overflow incontinence in a severely constipated patient should raise the possibility of idiopathic megabowel, as incontinence never occurs in Hirschsprung's disease. Abdominal examination reveals gross distension, and rigid sigmoidoscopy confirms an empty rectum.

Contrast studies are helpful in showing the hallmark narrow segment (best seen on lateral view), although this may not be seen in cases with very short aganglionic segments. Anorectal physiological testing for the presence of the rectoanal inhibitory reflex can obviate the need for full-thickness biopsy of the rectum (49). Inflation of a balloon in the rectum causes a reflex relaxation of the internal anal sphincter; this reflex is absent in patients with Hirschsprung's disease, because of the aganglionosis. If the reflex is equivocal, biopsy of the rectum is required. Suction biopsy may not give sufficient depth of tissue to stain the neural plexuses, in which case full-thickness biopsy under

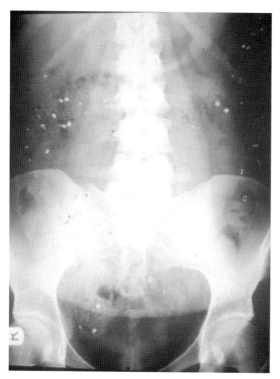

Figure 32.1. Plain abdominal X-ray showing a radioopaque marker transit study. Excessive hold-up of all three kinds of marker indicates slow transit (reference 11: Evans *et al.*, 1992).

anaesthetic is required. Some cases remain uncertain despite these investigations, in which case immunohistochemical techniques and expert pathological input may clarify the situation. Treatment is surgical, the principle being to excise or bypass the narrowed segment, for which there are a variety of techniques. Although the outcome is usually excellent, parents of affected children must be advised that long-term soiling occurs in about 10% of patients (50).

References
*Of interest; **of exceptional interest
1. **Drosmman DA, Sandler RS, McKee DC *et al.* Bowel patterns amongst subjects not seeking health care. Use of a questionnaire to identify a population with bowel dysfunction. *Gastroenterol* 1982; **83**: 529–534.
    The recognised definition "standard" used in studies on constipation.
2. *Preston DM, Lennard-Jones JE. Severe chronic constipation of young women: "idiopathic slow transit constipation". *Gut* 1986; **27**: 41–48.
    A first description of this common clinical entity, and discussion of possible treatments.
3. *Bannister JJ, Timms JM, Barfield LJ *et al.* Physiological studies in young women with chronic constipation. *Int J Colorectal Dis* 1986; **1**: 175–182.
    A descriptive and physiological report of idiopathic constipation.
4. **Drossman DA, Leserman J, Nachman G *et al.* Sexual and physical abuse in women with functional or organic gastrointestinal disorders. *Ann Intern Med* 1990; **113**: 828–833.
    An important early recognition of the prevalence of abuse in idiopathic constipation, although possibly overestimated, given the patterns of patient referral.
5. Leroi AM, Bernier C, Watier A *et al.* Prevalence of sexual abuse among patients with functional disorders of the lower gastrointestinal tract. *Int J Colorectal Dis* 1995; **10**: 200–206.
6. *Preston DM, Pfeffer J, Lennard-Jones JE. Psychiatric assessment of patients with severe constipation. *Gut* 1984; **25**: A582–A583.
    Qualification of psychological traits and overt disorders in idiopathic constipation.
7. Devroede G, Bouchoucha M, Girard G. Constipation, anxiety and personality: what comes first? In: *Stress and Digestive Motility.* Eds. L Bueno, S Collins, JL Junior. London: John Libbey Eurotext, 1989; pp. 55–60.
8. **Wald A, Hinds JP, Camana BJ. Psychological and physiological characteristics of patients with severe constipation. *Gastroenterology* 1989; **97**: 932–937.
    Prospective anal manometry and psychological questionnaire study of patients with slow and normal transit.
9. *Fisher SE, Breckon K, Andrews HA *et al.* Psychiatric screening for patients with faecal incontinence or chronic constipation referred for surgical treatment. *Br J Surg* 1989; **76**: 352–356.
    Recognition of the significant levels of psychiatric morbidity in British patients referred for surgery.
10. Devroede G, Roy T, Bouchoucha M *et al.* Idiopathic constipation by colonic dysfunction: relationship with personality and anxiety. *Dig Dis Sci* 1989; **34**: 1428–1434.
11. *Evans RC, Kamm MA, Hinton JM *et al.* The normal range and a simple diagram for recording whole gut transit time. *Int J Colorect Dis* 1992; **7**: 15–17.
    The production of a simple, single X-ray, transit measurement and a normal range.
12. *Metcalf AM, Phillips SF, Zinsmeister AR *et al.* Simplified assessment of segmental colonic transit. *Gastroenterology* 1987; **92**: 40–47.
    A mathematical assessment of transit times in different segments of the colon.
13. Mathieu P, Pringot J, Bodart P. Defecography: I. Description of a new procedure and results in normal patients. *Gastrointest Radiol* 1984; **9**: 247–251.
14. Mathieu P, Pringot J, Bodart P. Defecography: II. Contribution to the diagnosis of defecation disorders. *Gastrointest Radiol* 1984; **9**: 253–261.
15. *Loening-Baucke VA. Abnormal rectoanal function in children recovered from chronic constipation and encoparesis. *Gastroenterology* 1984; **87**: 1299–1304.
    Description of variable outcome in anorectal physiology variables in children treated for constipation.

16. Klauser AG, Peyerl C, Schinbleck NE *et al*. Nutrition and physical activity in chronic constipation. *Eur J Gastroenterol Hepatol* 1992; **4**: 227–233.

17. **Tache Y, Garrick T, Raybould H. Central nervous system: action of peptides to influence gastrointestinal motor function. *Gastroenterology* 1990; **98**: 517–528.

18. **Bueno L, Gue M. Evidence for the involvement of corticotropin-releasing factor in the gastrointestinal disturbances induced by acoustic and cold stress in mice. *Brain Res* 1988; **441**: 1–4.
    Two definitive studies of intracerebroventricular injection of peptides resulting in altered colonic motility; the importance of corticotrophin-releasing factor as a modulator of the stress response and moderator of colonic motility is established.

19. Creed F, Guthrie E. Psychological treatments of the irritable bowel syndrome: a review. *Gut* 1989; **30**: 1601–1603.

20. *Chaussade S, Khyari A, Roche H *et al*. Determination of total and segmental colonic transit time in constipated patients: results in 91 patients with a new simplified method. *Dig Dis Sci* 1989; **34**: 1168–1174.
    Description of another technique of transit measurement and confirmation of response to dietary modification.

21. *Graham DY, Moser SE, Estes MK. The effect of bran on bowel function in constipation. *Am J Gastroenterol* 1982; **77**: 599–603.
    Recognition that stool output in response to diet varies between subjects, in relation to the original stool output of the patient.

22. Verduron A, Devroede G, Bouchoucha M *et al*. Megarectum. *Dig Dis Sci* 1988; **33**: 1164–1175.

23. Hamilton JW, Wagner J, Burdick BB *et al*. Clinical evaluation of methylcellulose as a bulk laxative. *Dig Dis Sci* 1988; **33**: 993–1000.

24. *Kamm MA, Lennard-Jones JE, Thompson DG *et al*. Dynamic scanning defines a colonic defect in severe idiopathic constipation. *Gut* 1988; **29**: 1085–1090.
    Description of a functional imaging technique, and acceleration of transit with bisacodyl.

25. *Marlett JA, Li BUK, Patrow CJ *et al*. Comparative laxation of psyllium with and without senna in an ambulatory constipated population. *Am J Gastroenterol* 1987; **82**: 333–341.
    A rare comparative study with stimulant laxative, showing significant symptom improvement.

26. Riecken EO, Zeitz M, Emde C *et al*. A prospective study on the effect of anthraquinone-containing laxatives on ultrastructure of colonic nerves. *Gastroenterology* 1987; **92**: 1595–1599.

27. *Fioramtonti J, Dupuy C, Bueno L. *In vivo* motility of rat colon chronically pretreated with sennosides. *Pharmacol* 1993; **41(suppl 1)**: 155–171.
    Important recognition that chronic use of anthraquinones does not lead to slowing of colonic motility.

28. Whitehead WE, Chaussade S, Corazziari E *et al*. Report of an international workshop on management of constipation. *Gastroenterol Int* 1991; **4**: 99–106.

29. Florent C, Flourie B, Rautureau M *et al*. Influence of chronic lactulose ingestion on colonic metabolism of lactulose in man. *J Clin Invest* 1985; **75**: 608–613.

30. Bass P, Dennis S. The laxative effect of lactulose in normal and constipated subjects. *J Clin Gastroenterol* 1981; **3(suppl 1)**: 23–27.

31. *Muller-Lissner SA. Bavarian constipation study group. Treatment of chronic constipation with cisapride and placebo. *Gut* 1987; **28**: 1033–1036.
    Large prospective study showing benefit with cisparide compared with placebo, although it would have been more valid to compare with a laxative.

32. Koutsomanis D, Lennard-Jones JE, Roy AJ *et al*. Controlled randomised trial of visual biofeedback versus muscle training without a visual display for intractable constipation. *Gut* 1995; **36**: 95–99.

33. *Koutsomanis D, Lennard-Jones JE, Kamm MA. Prospective study of biofeedback treatment for patients with slow and normal transit constipation. *Eur J Gastroenterol Hepatol* 1994; **6**: 131–137.
    A description of the technique of biofeedback for constipation.

34. *Enck P. Biofeedback training in disordered defaecation: a critical review. *Dig Dis Sci* 1993; **38**: 1953–1956.
    Recent review of the techniques and outcome of biofeedback.

35. **Chiotakakou-Faliakou E, Kamm MA, Roy AJ *et al*. Biofeedback provides long term benefit for patients with intractable slow and normal transit constipation. *Gut* 1998; **42**: 517–521.
    Important recognition that there is no long-term "dropoff" in outcome of patients who respond initially to biofeedback.

36. Devroede G. Constipation. In: *Gastrointestinal Diseases*, 5th edn. Eds. MH Sleisinger, JS Fordtran. Philadelphia: WB Saunders, 1992.

37. Pinho M, Yoshioka K, Keighley MRB. Long term results of anorectal myectomy for chronic constipation. *Br J Surg* 1989; **76**: 1163–1164.

38. Kamm MA, Hawley PR, Lennard-Jones JE. Lateral division of the puborectalis muscle in the management of severe constipation. *Br J Surg* 1988; **75**: 661–663.

39. Schouten WR. Severe longstanding constipation in adults, indications for surgical treatment. *Scan J Gastroenterol* 1991; **188(suppl)**: 60–68.

40. *Kamm MA, Hawley PR, Lennard-Jones JE. Outcome of colectomy for severe idiopathic constipation. *Gut* 1988; **29**: 969–973.
    Longest follow-up study of outcome, showing disappointing results of colectomy.

41. Coremans GE. Surgical aspects of severe chronic non-Hirschsprung constipation. *Hepatogastroenterology* 1990; **37**: 588–595.

42. *van der Sijp JRM, Kamm MA, Evans RC *et al*. The results of stoma formation in severe idiopathic constipation. *Eur J Gastroenterol Hepatol* 1992; **4**: 137–140.
    Well-described study showing that stoma formation can be a helpful procedure in selected patients.

43. *Preston DM, Lennard-Jones JE, Thomas BM. Towards a radiological definition of idiopathic megacolon. *Gastrointest Radiol* 1985; **10**: 167–170.
    Establishment of validated and reproduced radiological criteria for definition of megacolon and megarectum.

44. Barnes PRH, Lennard-Jones JE, Hawley PR *et al*. Hirschsprung's disease and idiopathic megacolon in adults and adolescents. *Gut* 1986; **27**: 534–538.

45. Hosie KB, Kmiot WA, Keighley MR. Constipation: another indication for restorative proctocolectomy. *Br J Surg* 1990; **77**: 801–803.

46. Stryker SJ, Pemberton JH, Zinsmeister AR. Long term results of ileostomy in older patients. *Dis Colon Rectum* 1985; **28**: 844–848.

47. Stabile G, Kamm MA, Hawley PR *et al.* Colectomy for idiopathic megarectum and megacolon. *Gut* 1991; **33**: 1164–1166.

48. *Passarge E. The genetics of Hirschsprung's disease. Evidence for heterogenous etiology and a study of sixty-three families. *N Engl J Med* 1967; **276**: 138–141.

49. Tobon F, Rein NCRW, Talbert JL *et al.* Nonsurgical test for the diagnosis of Hirschsprung's disease. *N Engl J Med* 1968; **278**: 188–191.
    Two early, but still accurate, descriptive and physiological studies of Hirschsprung's disease.

50. Marty TL, Leo T, Matlak ME *et al.* Gastrointestinal function after surgical correction of Hirschsprung's disease: long-term follow up in 135 patients. *J Paediatr Surg* 1995; **30**: 655–659.

33. Faecal Incontinence

CAROLYNNE VAIZEY

INTRODUCTION

Patients find it very difficult to talk about this most taboo of subjects. Some cannot even talk to their spouses, and go to great lengths to hide the problem from them. Because of this, it may well be necessary to question the patient directly about incontinence. They need to be put immediately more at ease by being told of the relatively high incidence of faecal incontinence, and to be reassured, early on, that there are ways of curing or markedly improving the problem. The specialist's choice of terms and general ease during the discussion are crucial to obtaining a full history.

It has been estimated that 2% of the adult population are faecally incontinent at least once a week (1).

This chapter includes a short section on the background to the mechanisms of continence, followed by a step-by-step approach to the clinical work up of the patient. There is a description of the common conditions causing incontinence, and the final section provides details of the treatments available for faecal incontinence. This last section is intended to give the gastroenterologist information as to when to seek a surgical opinion, and an understanding of the surgeon's choice of treatment.

MECHANISMS OF CONTINENCE

The maintenance of faecal continence is a product of stool consistency, colorectal activity, and the synchronous relationship between the external and the internal anal sphincters. Even the strongest anal canal muscles can not hold back liquid for any length of time. Pressures of up to 500 cm of water have been recorded in the colon, and these far exceed the pressures that can be generated by the sphincter muscles surrounding the anal canal (2). This chapter will concentrate on faecal incontinence that results from weakness of the anal sphincter muscles.

The **external sphincter** is a skeletal muscle that tires easily and, being under voluntary control, it can be exercised, just like the arm and leg muscles. It acts as the "emergency brakes", being used maximally when there is a feeling of impending defecation, thus allowing the individual time to organize a suitable situation for defecation. The **internal sphincter** muscle is a continuation of the circular muscle of the rectum. It is an involuntary smooth muscle, capable of continuous contraction, and maintains a constant tone, preventing stool leakage during everyday activities. Its major activities are therefore relaxation responses. The most common of these is the rectoanal inhibitory reflex. This is a locally mediated response to distension of the rectum, resulting in relaxation of the internal sphincter and a reduction of the resting pressure. The function of this seemingly antisocial reflex is to allow rectal contents to come into contact with the mucosa of the upper anal canal for distinction to be made between solid, liquid, and gas. The external sphincter maintains continence until the rectum relaxes to accommodate the stool and the internal sphincter regains its tone.

CLINICAL EVALUATION OF THE PATIENT

Taking a focused history

Types of faecal incontinence

There may be:

1. *Passive leakage*: The patient looses stool without being aware if it. This usually indicates that there is a weakness or deficiency of the internal sphincter muscle.
2. *Urge incontinence*: The patient can not defer defecation for sufficient time to permit them to reach a toilet. This urgency usually occurs when the external anal sphincter muscle is weak or deficient (3).

Assessing severity of incontinence

Patients may loose solid, liquid, or gas; even the inability to control the passage of gas can be an enormous social disability. The amount of stool lost can vary from a slight stain to the whole stool. Some patients are not, in reality, incontinent, but severely restrict their lifestyles for fear of being so. Frequency of losses is usually recorded as daily or more, weekly, monthly, or less than monthly. The use of pads may give an indication of the severity of incontinence, although there is a variation in the fastidiousness of patients, and there can be an overlap with the need for pads for the presence of urinary leakage.

Determining the cause

In many cases, the cause of the incontinence can be discovered in the history. In women, the most common cause of faecal incontinence is damage to the sphincters during childbirth. Particular risk factors are a forceps-assisted delivery, a large baby, or an occipito-posterior position. The next most common cause of damage to the sphincter muscles is surgical trauma. A history of deliberate or accidental injury or stretching of the anal canal must be sought, including a history of anal intercourse. Abdominal surgery, such as a major bowel resection, may also be significant. Rectal prolapse can cause progressive damage through repeated stretching of the internal sphincter muscle. Confirmation of a rectal prolapse may only be obtained by ask-ing a patient to strain while they are seated on a commode or the toilet. Enquiry should be made as to the presence of systemic illness or neurological disease, and any medication that the patient might be taking. Not only can medication alter the bowel habit and so mask or worsen the incontinence, but some drugs such as indoramin and diltiazem have also been shown to decrease the internal sphincter pressure. Most patients who have a history of a congenital defect affecting faecal continence will be able to provide good details on their particular problem and on any operative procedures that have been performed.

Assessing disruption of the patient's lifestyle

This is essential when planning the appropriate treatments. A woman with ready access to toilets who is planning more vaginal deliveries may not be suitable for an immediate anterior sphincter repair. In contrast, if a woman is the breadwinner for her family, is experiencing major difficulties with working — even with mild incontinence — and is not responding to conservative measures, she may qualify for early surgical intervention.

Use of a scoring system

For the objective comparison of the severity of incontinence before and after treatment, and to compare the efficacy of different treatments, it is necessary to use a scoring system. A well-validated scoring system is the St Marks continence grading scale (4). This is shown in Table 33.1.

Examination of the patient

Routine examination of the abdomen, perianal region, and rectum is essential in all patients. Rigid sigmoidoscopy may, for example, reveal rectal inflammation as a cause of diarrhoea, or a low villous polyp as a source of a mucous leakage. Anal-canal resting tone and squeeze are important to assess, but digital examination of the anal sphincters provides surprisingly poor information as to the presence of sphincter defects. In a study at St Mark's Hospital, UK, the surgeon's clinical assessment of external sphincter defects was correct in only 50% of cases when compared with the subsequent operative and histological findings (5).

Table 33.1.   The St Mark's continence grading scale.

Type of incontinence	Frequency				
	Never	Rarely	Sometimes	Weekly	Daily
Incontinence for solid stool	0	1	2	3	4
Incontinence for liquid stool	0	1	2	3	4
Incontinence for gas	0	1	2	3	4
Alterations in lifestyle	0	1	2	3	4
	No	Yes			
Need to wear a pad or plug	0	2			
Taking constipation medicines	0	2			
Lack of ability to defer defaecation for 15 minutes	0	4			

Never	No episodes in the past 4 weeks	Add one score from each row	
Rarely	1 episode in the past 4 weeks	Minimum score = 0 = perfect continence	
Sometimes	>1 episode in the past 4 weeks but <1 a week	Maximum score = 24 = totally incontinent	
Weekly	1 or more episodes a week but <1 a day	(Adapted from reference 4).	
Daily	1 or more episodes a day		

The investigations

The two essential investigations for defining the status of the anal sphincter muscles are **anorectal physiological testing** and **endoanal ultrasound**. The most important aspect of physiological testing is **anal manometry** to determine the maximum resting and maximum voluntary contraction or squeeze pressures (4): the resting pressure is a reflection of the internal sphincter function and the squeeze pressure a reflection of the external sphincter function. Additional tests can be of importance in selected patients. For example, rectal threshold, urge and maximum tolerated volumes may show a decreased rectal capacity, and an increased rectal electrosensory threshold may reveal an unsuspected neurological deficit.

The introduction of endoanal sonography in the late 1980s radically altered the previously held view that pudendal nerve damage was the underlying cause in most patients with faecal incontinence. Changes in pudendal nerve function were seen to be coexistent with structural damage, the latter corresponding more closely to muscle weakness and incontinence. Ultrasound has not only made it possible to define structural damage to the sphincter complex, but has also allowed for the recognition of degenerative disorders of the sphincter muscles. High-resolution magnetic resonance imaging (MRI), is not an economically practical substitute for the endoanal ultrasound, but can provide improved images of the external sphincter and of fistulous tracks (6). In the investigation of patients who present

equivocal findings on ultrasound, or those who need further definition of possible sepsis related to faecal incontinence, this modality is a major advance.

PATHOGENESIS OF INCONTINENCE

Obstetric damage

Ninety per cent of women with faecal incontinence with obstetric damage as the only risk factor were found to have sphincter damage on endoanal ultrasound. Thirty-five per cent of primiparous women have evidence of damage to the anal sphincters after their first vaginal delivery, and this increases to 80% after a forceps delivery (7).

Surgical damage

With the advent of endoanal ultrasound, surgical damage to the anal sphincter sphincters has been found to be surprisingly common. Perhaps the greatest offender was the anal stretch operation, which has now, hopefully, disappeared from the surgical repertoire. Manual dilatation of the anus under anaesthesia can cause fragmentation of the internal anal sphincter muscle, and sometimes may even damage the external sphincter muscle (8). Sphincter damage may be intentional, as in a lateral sphincterotomy performed to allow healing of a chronic anal fissure. Here, the surgeon aims to perform a controlled cut through only the bottom one-third to one-half of the internal sphincter; however, endoanal ultrasound imaging has shown that full length division of the sphincter sometimes occurs (5). This is more common in the female where there is a relatively short anal canal. The recent introduction of internal sphincter muscle relaxing agents, such as glyceryl trinitrate ointment applied to the anal region, has lessened the need for sphincter-cutting operations for anal fissure (9). In some operations, the damage is totally unexpected — for example, in a haemorrhoidectomy or removal of a low rectal polyp. In cases of anal fistulae, sphincter damage could sometimes be considered less avoidable, as a fistulous tract may pass through, or even above, the sphincter muscles.

Rectal prolapse

Faecal incontinence occurs in 30 to 80% of patients with full-thickness **rectal prolapse**. Endoanal ultrasound can point to this diagnosis, with the demonstration of a thickened submucosa and an abnormal appearance to the internal sphincter. This abnormal appearance can range from a thickened sphincter to a stretched, and even fragmented, muscle ring.

Systemic disease

Diabetes mellitus and systemic sclerosis are of particular interest. Incontinent patients with diabetes mellitus have a combination of somatic neurogenic and autonomic dysfunction. The most consistent anal lesion encountered in patients with faecal incontinence secondary to systemic sclerosis is marked atrophy of the internal sphincter, leading to passive leakage (9). The constipation resulting from disordered colonic motility may mask the sphincter weakness in some patients. Some patients may also have altered rectal compliance, acquired megacolon, or bacterial overgrowth, leading to diarrhoea and greater stress on the sphincter.

Radiation

The use of radiation therapy for malignancies in the region of the anorectum may cause damage to the internal sphincter muscle and this, combined with proctitis and a reduction in rectal capacity, can lead to incontinence.

Spinal injury

Faecal incontinence is present in a high proportion of patients with **spinal injury** (11). This can be a particular problem after the use of laxatives for constipation, as there is no external sphincter activity to oppose bowel contraction. Faecal incontinence also occurs in about 30% of patients with multiple sclerosis. In these disorders, there is often a coexistent problem of constipation, which renders treatment more difficult.

Congenital abnormalities

Faecal incontinence associated with **congenital abnormalities** is common. It may occur as part of the primary abnormality, or after corrective surgery. Fifty-seven per cent of patients have soiling after a posterior sagittal anorectoplasty for anorectal malformations. Fifty-five per cent of patients with spina bifida soil regularly. Thirty-five per cent of children who have had a Duhamel operation for Hirschsprung's disease are incontinent when assessed at age 4 years or older. Twenty-seven per cent of patients operated on for a benign sacral teratoma in infancy have some faecal soiling.

Unknown cause

Finally, there are patients with incontinence of **unknown cause**. Recently, some of these patients have been shown to have degeneration of the internal sphincter, with a fibrotic, thin muscle. Atrophy of the external sphincter muscle may account for further cases previously labeled as idiopathic, but this muscle is harder to characterize on endoanal sonography.

TREATMENT OF FAECAL INCONTINENCE

Treatment will depend as much on the degree of disability experienced by the patient as on the underlying pathology.

Antidiarrhoeal agents

Many patients will improve markedly with the use of an **antidiarrhoeal agent** to firm up the stools. Many of the failures with this treatment come from overdosing, causing the patient such a degree of constipation as to necessitate the use of laxatives, which worsens the incontinence. **Loperamide** is one of the agents of choice and is available in tablet and liquid form, the latter allowing for small dosages to be given and for titration of the dosage according to stool consistency. Another approach is to use suppositories or an **enema** every morning, as this may clear the rectum sufficiently to give the patient the confidence to go out during the day.

Mechanical barriers

Most pads are only effective against minor leakage or staining, and can not contain large amounts of stool. A plug of cotton wool shaped by hand and placed at the anal margin has the added advantage of protecting the perianal skin and preventing subsequent soreness. Commercially available plugs (Convatec, UK) are worn inside the anus and are useful in a minority of patients, but are uncomfortable in most.

Biofeedback

The use of biofeedback to provide focused retraining exercises to strengthen the external sphincter has been successful in patients with a weak but intact external sphincter muscle. Prospective randomized controlled trials are necessary to define accurately the role of such biofeedback programmes in the treatment of incontinence.

Surgical intervention

Some patients with faecal incontinence require **surgical intervention**, although this is not entered into without very careful assessment. The majority of the operations carry a small risk of worsening the condition, have a relatively low success rate, or are extremely complex.

Most patients with a single defect in the **external sphincter muscle** benefit from a simple overlapping repair. The most common cause of a reparable defect in the anal sphincter muscles is obstetric trauma; success rates of up to 80% have been reported (12), although the improvement may not always be sustained (13). In the absence of sepsis, single post-surgical or traumatic injuries to the external sphincter or to both sphincters can usually be treated in the same manner.

The **internal sphincter** is a thin, smooth muscle that is not amenable to surgical repair. Some successes have been reported with the surgical insertion of a flap into the area of a single defect, or with the injection of bulking agents into the defect, the latter also being reported as successful when given as a circumferential injection for a generally weak internal sphincter.

There are, as yet, no surgical treatments with good long-term results reported for weak but intact **anal sphincters** (14). Post-anal repair, which tightens the anal canal posteriorly and improves the anorectal angle, has been shown to have short-term benefit in up to 83% of patients. However, long-term improvement may be present in as few as 28% of patients, and as few as 21% may be fully continent (15). There are preliminary reports on the use of sacral nerve stimulation for patients with weak but intact sphincters. This approach is an alternative to repair of the sphincter muscles, and modifies the neurological supply to the anorectal region, altering reflex activity and appearing to improve squeeze pressures.

In patients with sphincter weakness secondary to **rectal prolapse**, repair of the prolapse by abdominal rectopexy may restore internal sphincter function, and this may be the only intervention necessary to improve continence.

Disruption of the anal sphincters not amenable to simple repair can range from a single defect in the internal sphincter to total disruption of the anal sphincter, with little or no residual muscle tissue. A number of new treatments have been devised for patients with extensive or irreparable sphincter damage or for those who have failed attempted previous repair. Some of these treatments may also have application for patients with profoundly weak but intact sphincters.

Dynamic graciloplasty

The technique of **dynamic graciloplasty** utilizes a chronically stimulated, transposed skeletal muscle to close down the anal canal (16). Chronic stimulation of a skeletal muscle can convert fast-twitch, fatiguable muscle into slow-twitch, less fatiguable muscle. The gracilis muscle is taken from the medial aspect of the thigh and mobilized by cutting its insertion just below the knee. It can then be wrapped around a tunnel outside the anal canal in the manner of a scarf and its distal end anchored to bone or skin. The nerve to gracilis is chronically stimulated with a device based on the design of the cardiac pacemaker. The device is switched off for the patient to pass a stool and on when the patient needs to be continent. This is complex surgery with a high rate of complications and a variable reported success rate; most surgeons reserve it for patients in whom conventional treatments have been tried or have been assessed as inappropriate. Absolute contraindications to dynamic graciloplasty include perianal sepsis, thereby excluding patients with Crohn's disease.

Artificial bowel sphincter

An alternative therapy for these patients is the newly designed artificial bowel sphincter (ABS, American Medical Systems, Minneapolis, USA). This is a silicone device providing an artificial alternative to the sphincter mechanism (17). It was introduced onto the European market on 1 April 1998. It consists of a cuff around the anal canal, a fluid reservoir balloon implanted behind the rectus abdominus muscle in the lower abdomen, and a pump implanted in the scrotum or labia. At rest, the cuff is filled with fluid and closes the anal canal. When the patient wishes to defecate, they squeeze the pump to transfer fluid from the cuff to the balloon reservoir. After a few minutes, fluid passively transfers back to the cuff.

Colostomy

The option of a colostomy for intractable incontinence should be reserved for those not suitable for conventional surgery, and should not be regarded as a treatment failure. For some patients it is the optimum treatment, allowing return to as near normal a lifestyle as possible (18); almost 25% of patients, however, are unable to come to terms with a stoma. Often, those whose quality of life was poor before surgery can regain a normal lifestyle and have a much more positive outlook on life. Further improvement of quality of life can often be achieved by stoma irrigation (19), which is possible in about 80% of patients receiving a colostomy for cancer; it has also been shown to be safe and cost effective. There is no reason why these figures could not be attained by patients with colostomies for faecal incontinence.

An alternative strategy for faecal incontinence involves the creation of a proximal colonic stoma, through which irrigation is performed to keep the distal bowel empty. This is known as the antegrade continence enema or "ACE" procedure, and the stoma is most commonly made from the appendix or from a tubularized caecal flap (20). Long-term problems include stenosis at the mucocutaneous junction, reflux of irrigation fluid into the ileum, and loss of responsiveness to infused fluid.

CONCLUSION

In the past decade, there have been major advancements in both the diagnosis and treatment of faecal incontinence. With increased awareness of the magnitude of the problem by both patients and doctors and the treatment options now available, many patients may now be returned to a more normal lifestyle.

References

1. Kamm MA. Faecal incontinence [review]. *BMJ* 1998; **316**: 528–532..
2. Herbst F, Kamm MA, Morris GP *et al.*. Gastrointestinal transit and prolonged ambulatory motility in health and faecal incontinence. *Gut* 1997; **41**: 381–389.
3. Engel AF, Kamm MA, Bartram CI *et al.* Relationship of symptoms in faecal incontinence to specific sphincter abnormalities. *Int J Colorectal Dis* 1995; **10**: 152–155.
4. Vaizey CJ, Carapeti E, Cahil JA *et al.* Prospective comparison of faecal incontinence grading systems. *Gut* 1999; **44**: 77–80.
5. Sultan AH, Kamm MA, Nicholls RJ *et al.* Prospective study of the extent of internal anal sphincter division during lateral sphincterotomy. *Dis Colon Rectum* 1994; **37**: 1031–1033.
6. deSousa N, Hall A, Puni R *et al.* High resolution magnetic resonance imaging of the anal sphincter using a dedicated endoanal coil. Comparison of magnetic resonance imaging with surgical findings. *Dis Colon Rectum* 1996; **39**: 926–934.
7. Sultan AH, Kamm MA, Hudson CN *et al.* Anal sphincter disruption during vaginal delivery. *N Engl J Med* 1993; **329**: 1905–1911.
8. Speakman CT, Burnett SJ, Kamm MA *et al.* Sphincter injury after anal dilatation demonstrated by anal endosonography. *Brit J Surg* 1991; **78**: 1429–1430.
9. Lund JN, Scholefield JH. A randomised, prospective, double-blind, placebo-controlled trial of glyceryl trinitrate ointment in treatment of anal fissure. *Lancet* 1997; **349**: 11–14.
10. Engel A, Kamm M, Talbot I. Progressive systemic sclerosis of the internal anal sphincter leading to passive faecal incontinence. *Gut* 1994; **35**: 857–859.
11. Glickman S, Kamm MA. Bowel dysfunction in spinal-cord-injury patients. *Lancet* 1996; **347**: 1651–1653.
12. Engel AF, Sultan AH, Kamm MA *et al.* Anterior sphincter repair for patients with obstetric trauma. *Br J Surg* 1994; **81**: 1231–1234.
13. Malouf AJ, Norton CS, Engel AF, *et al.* Long-term results of overlapping anterior anal-sphincter repair for obstetric trauma. *Lancet* 2000; **355**: 260–265.
14. Vaizey C, Kamm MA, Nicholls RJ. Recent advances in the surgical treatment of faecal incontinence [review]. *Brit J Surg* 1998; **85**: 596–603.
15. Setti-Carraro P, Kamm MA, Nicholls RJ. Long term results of postanal repair for neurogenic faecal incontinence. *Brit J Surg* 1994; **81**: 140–144.
16. Baeten C, Geerdes BP, Adang EMM *et al.* Anal dynamic graciloplasty in the treatment of intractable fecal incontinence. *New Engl J Medicine* 1995; **332**: 1600–1605.
17. Lehur P-A, Michot F, Denis P *et al.* Results of artificial sphincter in severe anal incontinence: report of 14 consecutive implantations. *Dis Colon Rectum* 1996; **39**: 1352–1355.
18. Wade B. *A Stoma is for Life*. London: Scutari Press, 1989.
19. Dini D, Venturini M, Forno G *et al.* Irrigation for colostomised cancer patients: a rational approach. *Int J Colorectal Dis* 1991; **6**: 9–11.
20. Malone PS, Ransley PG, Kiely EM. Preliminary report: the antegrade continence enema. *Lancet* 1990; **336**: 1217–1218.

34. Colorectal Cancer Screening and Surveillance

ISIS DOVE-EDWIN and HUW J.W. THOMAS

BACKGROUND AND RATIONALE FOR SCREENING

Colorectal cancer (CRC) is a leading cause of cancer mortality, with 20 000 deaths per year in the UK and approximately 50 000 per year in the USA. Survival is related to the stage at which cancer is detected, and remains poor as the majority of cases are detected at an advanced stage.

Colonic carcinogenesis occurs as a **multistep process of genetic alterations** that result in abnormal growth as colonic mucosa progresses from normal to adenoma and then to carcinoma. This generally occurs over a period of about 10 years, and interrupting this sequence should result in a decrease in the incidence and subsequent mortality from CRC. There is increasing evidence that the incidence and mortality of CRC can be decreased by polypectomy and early detection. As yet, however, there is no systematic population screening programme for CRC in the UK, and the results of the pilot projects of the UK National Screening Group are awaited.

The term **screening** in the context of CRC refers to the process by which asymptomatic individuals who may have colonic adenomas or cancer are identified. The diagnosis is usually presumptive at this stage. **Surveillance** usually refers to monitoring those identified to be at high risk or known to have colorectal disease.

Groups to be screened

The incidence of colorectal carcinoma varies widely. Migration studies show that it is related to environmental factors, the most significant of which is diet. Individuals at greater than average risk include those with a positive family or personal history of colorectal neoplasia (moderately increased risk), and individuals affected by specific genetic syndromes that predispose to CRC, inflammatory bowel disease (IBD), and acromegaly (high risk).

HIGH-RISK INDIVIDUALS

Autosomal dominant syndromes

As many as 2–5% of cases of CRC may arise as a result of highly penetrant autosomal dominant inherited genetic defects. These include familial adenomatous polyposis (FAP), hereditary non-polyposis colorectal cancer syndrome (HNPCC) and the more rare hamartomatous polyposis syndromes, which include Peutz–Jegher's syndrome, juvenile polyposis, and Cowden's disease.

Familial adenomatous polyposis

FAP is a rare autosomal dominant syndrome that accounts for fewer than 1% of cases of CRC. Affected individuals develop hundreds to thousands of colorectal adenomas. The risk of developing CRC is almost 100%, and the median age at diagnosis is 40 years. Individuals from families in which FAP is present should undergo **screening** by flexible sigmoidoscopy at 6-monthly intervals for the presence of polyps (i.e. to see if they express the phenotype) starting from 12–14 years of age. Once polyps are seen, a full colonoscopy should be carried out to assess the severity of the polyposis and to exclude the presence of a cancer. A prophylactic colectomy (either an ileorectal anastomosis or restorative proctocolectomy) should be planned.

FAP is caused by mutations in the *APC* gene on chromosome 5. In families in whom the mutation is known, presymptomatic molecular diagnosis may be feasible, and non-carriers of the gene can be discharged from follow-up.

Hereditary non-polyposis colorectal cancer

HNPCC is another autosomal dominant syndrome characterized by early-onset colorectal cancer. It may account for 1–2% of all cases of CRC. In contrast to FAP, there is no distinct phenotype — in particular, florid polyposis is absent. Gene carriers have a lifetime risk of CRC of approximately 80% (91% in males, 69% in females). In 55–60% of cases of HNPCC, the cancers are right-sided, and affected individuals are also at increased risk of other cancers such as cancer of the endometrium, stomach, small bowel, and genitourinary tract. Mutations responsible for HNPCC are found in DNA mismatch repair genes. In almost all cases, mutations of the DNA mismatch repair genes lead to DNA microsatellite instability (differing lengths of DNA repeat sequences, known as microsatellites, occur throughout the genome), which can be detected in tumour tissue. Individuals at risk are usually identified by their family history, particularly if the International Collaborative Group on HNPCC (ICG-HNPCC) Amsterdam Criteria are fulfilled. These criteria are not a clinical definition of HNPCC, but were established for research purposes at a time when the causative mutation had not been identified. **The Amsterdam Criteria** are as follows:

1. Histologically verified CRC or HNPCC related cancers in three or more relatives, one of whom is a first-degree relative of the other two.
2. CRC affecting at least two generations.
3. One or more cases of cancer diagnosed before the age of 50 years.
4. FAP excluded.

The ICG-HNPCC guidelines suggest that colonoscopic **surveillance** is commenced in gene carriers and at-risk individuals (i.e. family members at risk of inheriting the mutation, in whom gene-

carrier status has not been determined) at 20–25 years of age. Full colonoscopy is imperative, as cancers tend to be proximal. The optimal interval between colonoscopic examinations is not known. There is some evidence that progression from adenoma to carcinoma is accelerated in this syndrome, which is one possible explanation for a relatively high incidence of interval cancers within 3 years of colonoscopy. Thus colonoscopic intervals of 1–3 years are recommended.

The above guidelines are based mainly on retrospective observational studies and the consensus of a panel of experts; a randomized controlled trial to examine the effectiveness of colonoscopic surveillance in these individuals would be unethical. Data from a non-randomized trial are available, and shows a decrease in the incidence and mortality of CRC in a group that accepted colonoscopy and polypectomy, compared with those who declined it. There was also a trend towards a decrease in mortality, although this did not reach statistical significance (1).

Peutz–Jegher's syndrome

In this rare condition (prevalence 1 in 20 000), multiple hamartomatous polyps are found throughout the gastrointestinal tract and melanin spots may be seen on the lips, buccal mucosa, and digits. The majority of hamartomas are found in the small bowel, the most common site for gastrointestinal cancer in affected individuals. Molecular geneticists have identified the causative gene on chromosome 19p, and have also demonstrated that the cancers can arise from hamartomas (2). Current **surveillance** recommendations from St Mark's Hospital Polyposis Registry include biennial upper and lower endoscopy plus barium meal and follow-through, starting when the patient is age 30 years. Polypectomy is recommended for large polyps, to avoid clinical complications such as intussusception. Small-bowel polypectomies may be performed endoscopically via an enterostomy. Affected individuals are also predisposed to gonadal, breast, and cervical cancer, which require annual surveillance.

Familial juvenile polyposis

Juvenile polyposis is characterized by more than 3–5 juvenile polyps in the gastrointestinal tract, although hundreds may be present. They are classified histologically as hamartomas, containing dilated mucin-filled spaces, dilated glands, and an inflamed, abundant stroma. The glands are lined with normal colonic epithelium. In the familial form, there is a 15% incidence of CRC in patients younger than 35 years, and a cumulative risk of 68% by age 60 years. As this condition is so rare, there are no firm management guidelines, but both prophylactic colectomy and colonoscopic surveillance with polypectomy have been suggested. Germline mutations in the gene *SMAD4* (*DPC4*) have been reported in some families in which juvenile polyposis is present (3).

Cowden's disease

Cowden's disease is characterized by multiple hamartomatous polyps in the skin and mucous membranes. It may rarely predispose to the development of CRC. In 40% of cases, hamartomas are found in the gastrointestinal tract, and a mutation in the *PTEN* gene ("phosphatase, tensin-like, deleted on chromosome 10") has been identified in this condition (4). If there is a family history of CRC, 3–5 yearly colonoscopic surveillance is recommended by St Mark's Hospital Imperial Cancer Research Fund (ICRF) Family Cancer Clinic.

Inflammatory bowel disease

Although CRC associated with IBD accounts for less than 1% of the CRC burden in the general population, an individual's risk is related to the extent and duration of the disease. Individuals with extensive disease of more than 10 years duration are at greatly increased risk (10–20 times the population risk). Sclerosing cholangitis associated with **ulcerative colitis** increases the risk of CRC substantially (5). This, too, is related to the duration of disease, with a cumulative risk of approximately 30% after 20 years of illness. Recent evidence (6) suggests that there is also an increased risk of CRC in long-term, extensive Crohn's colitis; patients should be managed as in ulcerative colitis.

IBD-associated cancers tend to occur in individuals at a younger age than the general population, and they tend to be multifocal, infiltrating, and ulcerated. There is evidence that the genetic events involved in the neoplastic process may also be different, in particular, *p53* mutations tend to be an early event, and *ras* mutations may be less common.

Mortality in IBD has decreased considerably as a result of the introduction of and improvements in medical therapy. The aims of CRC **surveillance** in IBD are to define high-risk groups (dysplasia or early cancer) for colectomy. There is no evidence that endoscopic surveillance in colitis improves mortality from CRC, but a prospective randomized controlled study is unlikely to be carried out to answer this question, as it would require a very long period of follow-up, large numbers of patients, and is not likely to be accepted for ethical reasons. Some data do suggest that surveillance and recognition of premalignant changes may both prevent some cancers and identify cancers at an earlier stage, although interval cancers are common, even with surveillance.

Areas of dysplasia in long-standing colitis are frequently not associated with polypoid lesions. It is therefore standard practice to take multiple biopsy specimens from throughout the colon, with up to four biopsies taken every 10 cm. In addition, any gross lesions should be sampled for histopathological examination. Cytological brushings may also improve the diagnostic yield, particularly if samples are being taken from a stricture.

Predictors of malignancy

Dysplasia

The presence of dysplasia is the best predictor of the risk of malignancy in IBD. However, considerable interobserver variation exists when interpreting dysplasia. A standardised classification was introduced in 1983, categorizing dysplasia as low grade or high grade. Colectomy should be advised if high grade dysplasia is present, as there is approximately a 40% chance of finding a cancer at colectomy, and approximately 30% of the patients will develop cancer in the future. The predictive value of low-grade dysplasia is less certain.

Difficulties may also arise in distinguishing between dysplasia associated with a lesion or mass in IBD and that occurring as an incidental finding in an adenomatous polyp. Features that may be helpful in distinguishing the two are that the dysplasia associated with a lesion or mass in IBD is more likely to have dysplastic tissue in the surrounding flat mucosa, be larger than 1 cm in diameter, and occur in younger individuals with a longer disease duration and greater extent of disease. Distinguishing the two lesions is important, because an incidental adenomatous polyp can be managed conservatively, whereas the presence of dysplasia associated with a lesion or mass in IBD may be an indication for surgery.

Alternative markers of precancer
In an effort to increase the predictive value of surveillance, other possible markers of precancer in IBD are being explored:

1. *Aneuploidy*: Aneuploidy results from an abnormal DNA content within cells, with chromosomal instability, and can be detected by flow cytometry. It has been shown to correlate with the degree of dysplasia and presence of cancer, and does provide an objective measurement. At present, it remains largely a research tool.

2. *Abnormal mucins*: Increased concentrations of certain mucins have been demonstrated, in ulcerative colitis, to be associated with dysplasia. In particular, increased concentrations of sialosyl-Tn are seen in the majority of high-grade dysplasia lesions in ulcerative colitis and in sporadic cancers. Use of this marker is limited, as it has a low specificity.

3. *Genetic markers*: Mutations of the gene *p53* have been demonstrated in normal mucosa surrounding dysplastic or malignant tissue, and have also been shown to correlate with the presence of aneuploidy. These mutations may be early events in the neoplastic process, and may therefore have a part to play in surveillance. Microsatellite instability is seen in approximately 20% of IBD-associated neoplasia, and its role as a tool in surveillance has yet to be explored fully.

Colonoscopic surveillance programme

There is still much debate about the value of a structured surveillance programme. There is no evidence to suggest that it is more effective than regular clinical review with early review if symptoms develop. Patients agreeing to enrol in such programmes must be aware of the limitations (i.e. cancers can be missed) and be willing to be compliant. Most importantly, patients must be willing to accept that a colectomy will be recommended if dysplasia is present.

A proportion of patients will be offered colectomy as a means of managing their symptoms and, in practice, this decision may be influenced by the long-term risk of CRC. Otherwise, the extent of disease should be assessed 8–10 years after symptoms/diagnosis. Patients with left-sided or distal disease can be reassured that they are not at significantly increased risk of CRC, and may be managed according to their symptoms. If there is extensive colitis (past or present), colectomy should be considered if symptoms are chronically disabling. If surgery is declined or symptoms are minor, patients may consider colonoscopic surveillance (7). For those who do opt for a surveillance programme, practices vary, but intervals tend to be between 1 and 3 years. This subject remains controversial, and opposing views can be found in the literature (8,9).

Acromegaly

Patients with acromegaly are at increased risk of CRC, and the prevalence of tubulovillous adenomas has also been shown to be increased. The increased risk of CRC does not seem to correlate with concentrations of growth hormone or insulin-like growth factor-I, although the latter has been shown to correlate with epithelial cell turnover. Pending the results of prospective studies examining the issue, the current recommendation is for 3-yearly full colonoscopy in patients older than 40 years. Full colonoscopy is recommended because approximately 25% of adenomas are found in the proximal colon, and the interval of 3 years has been chosen because, in one series, a cancer was detected 3 years after a clear colonoscopy (10).

MODERATE-RISK INDIVIDUALS

Familial CRC risk

Familial clustering of CRC is common and may occur by chance, as a result of shared environmental factors, or because of a hereditary component. In the majority of familial cases, CRC risk is moderately increased (about twofold if one first-degree relative is affected), is proportional to the number of direct relatives affected, and is also greater if a first-degree relative is affected before the age of 45 years. The risk of CRC is also greater if a direct relative has been affected with an adenomatous polyp before the age of 60 years. CRC tends to occur at an earlier age in the group having a familial risk, with the risk of CRC for a

Table 34.1. Familial colorectal cancer: relative risks.

Relatives affected	Risk
None	1 in 35
One first-degree	1 in 17
One first-degree and one second-degree	1 in 12
One first-degree under age 45 years	1 in 10
Both parents	1 in 8.5
Two first-degree	1 in 6
Three first-degree, or three-generation dominant	1 in 2

Reproduced with permission from BMJ Publishing Group: *BMJ* 1990; **301**: 366–368.

40-year-old being equivalent to that of an average-risk 50-year-old.

Currently, screening and subsequent surveillance are offered to individuals according to their empiric lifetime risk of developing CRC, based on their family history (Table 34.1). At St Mark's ICRF Family Cancer Clinic, surveillance is offered to individuals with an empirical lifetime risk of dying from CRC that is greater than 1 in 10 (Table 34.2). Procedures are under regular evaluation.

Many members of the public have a family history of CRC, and increasing demands will be made on the health service for colonoscopic surveillance. In this large group, the actual risk of developing the disease is heterogeneous. At one end of the spectrum, some individuals will have a low to moderate increase in CRC risk: at the other end of the spectrum, carriers of the gene predisposing to HNPCC will have a substantially greater risk. Unlike patients with FAP, individuals with HNPCC can not be distinguished by their phenotype. Identifying high-risk individuals solely by family history is difficult, as details of the family history may be incomplete. Premature deaths from unrelated causes may also confound the picture, as may incomplete gene penetrance. Furthermore, the risk:benefit ratio

of colonoscopy screening will be more favourable in those at truly high risk for CRC.

With increasing knowledge of the molecular genetics involved in inherited predispositions to CRC, molecular testing may have a greater part to play in screening. In the near future, systematic case-finding of gene carriers by mutation analysis may become feasible. Individuals would thus be screened by genetic testing for a high risk of CRC, and would subsequently be offered colonoscopic surveillance or, possibly colectomy. A recent Finnish study has demonstrated the feasibility of molecular screening for HNPCC mutations (12). Consecutive patients with CRC were examined for microsatellite instability and germline DNA mismatch repair mutations. Mutations were found only in those with microsatellite instability, and the likelihood of finding a mutation was greatest in patients with early-onset CRC (before the age of 50 years), a history of multiple CRC or endometrial cancer, and family history of colorectal or endometrial cancer. The efficiency of molecular screening could therefore be increased if testing was limited to these individuals.

Personal history of neoplasia

Previous colorectal cancer

Individuals with a history of colorectal cancer are at increased risk for recurrence of their disease, in addition to the development of a second (metachronous) cancer. After a curative resection, colonoscopy is recommended within 1 year if one was not carried out before surgery, to exclude synchronous polyps or cancer. Otherwise, colonoscopic surveillance at 3-yearly intervals (if adenomatous polyps are seen) or at 5-yearly intervals (if colonoscopy is clear) is recommended, as the rate of adenoma–carcinoma progression is not known to

Table 34.2. St Mark's ICRF Family Cancer Clinic surveillance procedures.

Family members affected	Procedure
At least two relatives affected with CRC, none of whom are under the age of 50 years	Colonoscopy: 5-yearly from age 40–45 years 3-yearly if adenomas are present
One first-degree relative affected under the age of 45 years	Colonoscopy: 5-yearly from age 40–45 years 3-yearly if adenomas are present
Single first-degree relative affected over the age of 45 years	Single flexible sigmoidoscopy at age 50–55 years

be increased in this group. Although there is no evidence from clinical trials that surveillance reduces mortality, the findings of several randomized and non-randomized studies suggest that a more intensive follow-up programme does not influence survival. Six- to 12-monthly colonoscopy with a chest radiograph, and abdominal computed tomography — in addition to a clinical examination and blood tests including carcinoembryonic antigen — results in earlier detection of recurrences, but no change in colorectal cancer mortality (13,14).

Follow-up after colorectal cancer varies widely, with most clinicians encouraging patients to report any new sinister symptoms and to present on a regular basis for history, physical examination, and routine blood tests.

Previous adenomatous polyps

Data from the randomized National Polyp Study (15) show that colonoscopic polypectomy and surveillance decrease the incidence of CRC. Surveillance colonoscopy after 3 years was as effective as at 1 and 3 years. It is therefore recommended that individuals with adenomatous polyps should have a repeat colonoscopy 3 years after colonoscopy and polypectomy, provided the endoscopist is confident that the bowel has been cleared. Surveillance colonoscopy should be carried out 3-yearly if adenomas recur, but 5-yearly intervals should be adequate if the subsequent colonoscopy is clear.

AVERAGE-RISK INDIVIDUALS

In general, the risk of CRC increases with age. In the UK, the cumulative lifetime risk of developing CRC was initially believed to be 1 in 35, but more recent estimates suggest that it is 1 in 25. CRC is rare before the age of 50 years, and, in general, screening could start at this age and finish at about 70 years, as the protective benefits will last an additional 5–10 years.

The ideal method for population screening should be effective, safe, acceptable to the population being screened, and have a favourable cost:benefit ratio. The test itself should be sensitive (low rate of false positives) and specific (low rate of false negatives). Ideally, evidence should be available from randomized controlled trials to test the effectiveness of the screening tool.

Faecal occult blood testing

CRC and large polyps have a tendency to bleed, but in amounts that are not necessarily detectable clinically. There are several test kits available that are able to detect occult blood in the stool. If a test is positive, further investigations are necessary (a full colonoscopy, plus a barium enema if colonoscopy is incomplete) to confirm or exclude the presence of colorectal neoplasia and determine the appropriate treatment.

The **faecal occult blood test** (FOBt) is relatively simple and is usually performed by the patient at home. Individuals are advised to avoid certain foods such as red meat, horseradish, and turnips, which can cause a false-positive result because of their peroxidase activity. Samples are taken from three consecutive bowel motions and the test card is usually sent by post to the screening centre, for interpretation. The reported sensitivity and specificity of the test vary widely and are dependent on many factors. Sensitivity of the non-hydrated test is approximately 70%; with rehydration, this can be increased to 90%, but at the cost of a significant decrease in specificity and the positive predictive value of the test. As a result, although the number of cancers being detected increases, so also does the number of individuals without disease who must undergo colonoscopy as a result of a false-positive result.

Several large, randomized controlled trials have now shown conclusively that mortality from CRC can be decreased (15–33%) by population FOBt screening (16–18). Although mortality was decreased in the group who were screened every 2 years, it was greater if FOBt was carried out annually. Compliance rates for the test are variable; in most clinical studies, they decrease over time, with significant drop-out rates. Knowledge about CRC is one of the factors that improves compliance, and a successful screening programme will require public education. Complications of FOBt screening may arise directly from the diagnostic investigations that follow a positive test.

In the USA, CRC guidelines recommended FOBt screening for the average-risk population, beginning at 50 years of age and with full colonoscopic investigation/treatment if the test is positive. In the UK, the National Screening Committee is establishing a number of screening pilot projects aimed at individuals aged 50–69 years. The primary test

will be FOBt without dietary restriction and without rehydration of the sample. The primary aim of the pilot programmes is to establish whether at a national level, screening will do more good than harm, at a reasonable cost (19).

Sigmoidoscopy

Sigmoidoscopy has the advantage of direct visualization of the colon, and can be used as a screening and diagnostic tool. The fibreoptic flexible sigmoidoscope has replaced the rigid sigmoidoscope as a screening tool as it offers better views of the colon, and has a greater penetration — up to 60 cm, compared with 25 cm. Unlike FOBt, which will mainly pick up cancers (relatively few polyps bleed), sigmoidoscopy has a high sensitivity and specificity for polyps. If polyps are subsequently removed, the use of sigmoidoscopy has the potential to decrease the incidence of CRC.

To date, there are no published randomized controlled trials that test the effectiveness of sigmoidoscopy as a screening tool. Early case–control studies demonstrated that mortality from CRC within the reach of the rigid sigmoidoscope was significantly decreased in those who had the examination, and one would expect that this will also be true of flexible sigmoidoscopy (20–22).

The ideal interval between examinations is not known. A prospective randomized controlled study in Norway (23) demonstrated that flexible sigmoidoscopy with polypectomy performed in an average-risk population showed a significant decrease CRC in the screened group after 10 years. Mortality from CRC was not affected, but this study was limited by its small size. Results from this and a small retrospective case–control study (24) suggest that a 10-year interval is adequate, as polyps are slow growing.

Although the majority of CRCs are left-sided, and potentially within reach of the flexible sigmoidoscope, one of its limitations is that lesions in the unexamined proximal bowel may be missed. There is still some debate as to when a full colonoscopy is required. It seems generally accepted that these high-risk features — multiple adenomas, adenomas larger than 1 cm, and adenomas with tubulovillous histology — are frequently associated with proximal neoplasia and, if seen, mandate a full colonoscopic examination. It is important to note, however, that up to 30% of proximal neoplastic lesions are not associated with distal polyps. Furthermore, small distal polyps may be associated with significant proximal neoplasia, therefore some investigators will proceed to colonoscopy if any adenomas are seen distally.

Many of the uncertainties about flexible sigmoidoscopy screening are currently being investigated in the large multicentre Medical Research Council Flexiscope trial in the UK (25). Average-risk individuals older than 50 years have been assigned at random to receive a "one-off" flexible sigmoidoscopy, with further colonoscopy if high-risk adenomas or cancer are seen. CRC incidence and mortality, in addition to morbidity (including psychological morbidity) are among the various endpoints being assessed.

Colonoscopy

The obvious advantages of colonoscopy are that the entire colon can be visualized, and both diagnostic and therapeutic procedures can be carried out during the test. However, the test necessitates sedation of the patient, requires greater technical expertise than flexible sigmoidoscopy, and is more expensive.

There are no trials that assess the effectiveness of colonoscopy as a population screening tool with respect to CRC mortality and incidence. However, in the USA the National Polyp Study (15) showed that colonoscopic polypectomy reduces the incidence of CRC, and detection of early cancers by colonoscopy decreased the mortality. Furthermore, part of the effectiveness of FOBt screening must be attributed to colonoscopic examination of positive cases, at which time identification of polyps, polypectomy, and identification of cancers take place.

The idea that colonoscopy screening for the population is not feasible has recently been challenged. The Veteran's Affairs Cooperative Study screened asymptomatic average-risk individuals by colonoscopy. The overall serious complication rate was low (0.3%) and the majority of the cancers detected were identified at an early stage (26). The authors believe that population colonoscopy screening may be a feasible reality. Over the long term however, compliance rates are unlikely to be high, and although complication rates are low, they may be unacceptably high in this setting as the great majority of dividuals are disease free. The American consensus group recommends that, if certain

Table 34.3.   CRC screening and surveillance.

Risk Group	Method	Age (years)	Interval (years)	Comments
High risk				
Autosomal Dominant Syndrome				
FAP	Flexible sigmoidoscopy to detect adenomatous polyps	12–14	0.5	Consider genetic diagnosis Colonoscopy to assess phenotype and exclude CRC, then colectomy.
HNPCC	Colonoscopy	20–25	1–3	Consider genetic diagnosis
	Gastroscopy	20–25	1–5	If gastric cancer in pedigree Annual pelvic ultrasound surveillance for endometrial/ ovarian cancer, surveillance for renal cell cancer if in pedigree
Peutz–Jegher's syndrome	Colonoscopy	30	2	Biennial gastroscopy Barium meal & follow-through to screen for upper gastrointestinal cancers
Familial Juvenile Polyposis	Colonoscopy	14		
Cowden's disease (with family history of CRC)	Colonoscopy	20–25	5 if normal 3 if adenomas	
Inflammatory bowel disease				
Ulcerative colitis, extensive disease	Colonoscopy	10 years after onset	1–2	
Crohn's disease, extensive colitis	Colonoscopy	10 years after onset	1–2	
Acromegaly	Colonosopy	40	3	
Moderate risk				
Familial CRC				
Two affected relatives, none <50 years	Colonoscopy	40–45	5 if normal 3 if adenomas	
One first-degree relative, <45 years	Colonoscopy	40–45	5 if normal 3 if adenomas	
One first-degree relative, >45 years	Flexible sigmoidoscopy	50–55	Once only	
Personal history of colorectal neoplasia				
Previous CRC post curative resection	Colonoscopy	3 years after complete perioperative examination	5 if normal 3 if adenomas	Colonoscopy within 1 year of resection if not done before synchronous neoplasia excluded
Previous adenomatous polyps	Colonoscopy	3 years after initial polyps cleared	5 if normal 3 if further polyps	
Average risk				
Individuals at population risk	FOBt	50	1–2	Colonoscopy if FOBt positive
	Flexible sigmoidoscopy	50–55	Once only	Await results of MRC Flexiscope trial

individuals do chose to be screened in this way, 10-yearly intervals are appropriate, on the basis of the indirect evidence that is available.

Barium enema

There is no evidence to support barium enema as a screening tool, and its role is very limited. Incomplete colonoscopy should be followed by a barium study.

Follow up of other gastrointestinal cancers

There is no standardized surveillance regimen for other gastrointestinal cancers, other than clinical review and investigation of new symptoms.

CONCLUSION

CRC is an important public health problem. Clinical trials have shown that mortality from CRC can be decreased by effective screening/surveillance. Individuals should be stratified according to risk, and those at greatest risk offered intensive surveillance. At present, the future of population screening in the UK awaits the results of pilot FOBt studies and a large randomized controlled trial of once-only flexible sigmoidoscopy. Knowledge of the epidemiology and new insights into the molecular biology and genetics of CRC promise to optimize strategies for prevention, screening, and surveillance of this condition. CRC screening and surveillance protocols are summarized in Table 34.3.

References
*Of interest; **of exceptional interest

1. Jarvinen HJ, Aarnio M, Mustonen H, et al. Controlled 15-year trial on screening for colorectal cancer in families with hereditary nonpolyposis colorectal cancer. *Gastroenterology* 2000; **118**: 829–834.
2. Hemminki A, Tomlinson I, Markie D. Localisation of a susceptibility locus for Peutz–Jeghers syndrome to 19p using comparative genomic hybridisation and targeted linkage analysis. *Nature Genetics* 1997; **15**: 87–90.
3. Howe JR, Roth S, Ringold JC et al. Mutations in the *SMAD4/ DPC4* gene in juvenile polyposis. *Science* 1998; **280**: 1086–1088.
4. Nelen MR, Padberg GW, Peeters EAJ et al. Localization of the gene for Cowden disease to chromosome 10q22-23. *Nature Genetics* 1996; **13**: 114–116.
5. Broome U, Lofberg R, Veress B et al. Primary sclerosing cholangitis and ulcerative colitis: evidence for increased neoplastic potential. *Hepatology* 1995; **22**: 1404–1408.
6. Bernstein D, Rogers A. Malignancy in Crohn's disease. *Am J Gastroenterol* 1996; **91**: 434–440.
7. *Lennard-Jones J. Reducing cancer mortality in inflammatory bowel disease. In: *Prevention and Early Detection of Colorectal Cancer*. Eds. GP Young, P Rozen, B Levin. London: WB Saunders, 1996; pp. 217–238.
   Excellent critical review of the literature and practical approach to the prevention of CRC in IBD.
8. Lennard-Jones, JE, Melville DM, Morson BC et al. Precancer and cancer in extensive ulcerative colitis: findings among 401 patients over 22 years. *Gut* 1990; **31**: 800–806.
9. *Lynch DA, Lobo AJ, Sobala GM et al. Failure of colonoscopic surveillance in ulcerative colitis. *Gut* 1993; **34**: 1075–1080. Published results of two IBD CRC colonoscopic surveillance programmes, one for and the other against surveillance programmes.
10. Jenkins PJ, Fairclough PD, Richards T et al. Acromegaly, colonic polyps and carcinoma. *Clin Endocrinol* 1997; **47**: 17–22.
11. Houlston RS, Murday V, Harocopos C et al. Screening and genetic counselling for relatives of patients with colorectal cancer in a family cancer clinic. *BMJ* 1990; **301**: 366–368.
12. Aaltonen LA, Salovaara R, Kristo P et al. Incidence of hereditary nonpolyposis colorectal cancer and the feasibility of molecular screening for the disease. *N Engl J Med* 1998; **338**: 1481–1487.
13. Kjeldsen BJ, Kronborg O, Fenger C et al. A prospective randomised study of follow-up after radical surgery for colorectal cancer. *Br J Surg* 1997; **84**: 666–669.
14. *Schoemaker D, Black R, Giles L et al. Yearly colonoscopy, liver CT and chest radiography do not influence 5-year survival of colorectal cancer patients. *Gastroenterology* 1998; **114**: 7–14.
15. *Winawer SJ, Zauber AG, Ho MN. Prevention of colorectal cancer by colonoscopic polypectomy: The National Polyp Study Workgroup. *N Engl J Med* 1993; **334**: 82–87.
    Large, randomized controlled trial of polypectomy, showing a decrease in CRC incidence. Results showed no significant difference in polyps/CRC at 1 and 3 years after colonoscopy with polypectomy. These results form the basis for many surveillance procedures.
16. *Hardcastle JD, Chamberlain JO, Robinson MHE et al. Randomised controlled trial of faecal-occult-blood screening for colorectal cancer. *Lancet* 1996; **348**: 1472–1477.
17. *Kronborg O, Fenger C, Olsen J et al. Randomised study of screening for colorectal cancer with faecal-occult-blood test. *Lancet* 1996; **348**: 1467–1471.
18. *Mandel J, Bond JH, Church TR et al. Reducing mortality from colorectal cancer by screening for faecal occult blood: Minnesota Colon Cancer Control Study. *N Engl J Med* 1993; **328**: 1365–1371.
    References 13–17 are large, randomised controlled trials showing a decrease in CRC mortality as a result of population-based FOBt screening.
19. *National Screening Committee. First report of the National Screening Committee. Milton Keynes: National Screening Committee, 1998.
    Up-to-date detailed information regarding CRC screening in the UK can be obtained from the National Screening Committee website: http://www.open.gov.uk/doh/nsc/nsch.htm

20. Atkin WS, Morson BC, Cuzick J. Long-term risk of colorectal cancer after excision of rectosigmoid adenomas. *N Engl J Med* 1992; **326**: 658–662.

21. Friedman GD, Collen MF, Fireman BH. Multiphasic health checkup evaluation: a 16-year follow up. *J Chron Dis* 1986; **39**: 453–463.

22. Gilbertson VA, Nelms JM. The prevention of invasive cancer of the rectum. *Cancer* 1978; **41**: 1137–1139.

23. Hoff G, Sauar J, Vatn MH *et al.* Polypectomy of adenomas in the prevention of colorectal cancer: 10 years' follow-up of the Telemark Polyp Study I. *Scand J Gastroenterol* 1996; **31**: 1006–1010.

24. Selby JV, Friedman GD, Quesenberry CPJ *et al.* A case–control study of screening sigmoidoscopy and mortality from colorectal cancer. *N Engl J Med* 1992; **326**: 653–657.

25. *Atkin W, Cuzick J, Northover JMA, *et al.* Prevention of colorectal cancer by once-only sigmoidoscopy. *Lancet* 1993; **341**: 736–740.

    Rationale for the current large, multicentre UK MRC trial of CRC prevention by once-only flexible sigmoidoscopy in patients aged between 50 and 55 years.

26. Lieberman DA, Weiss DG, Bond JH, *et al.* Use of colonoscopy to screen asymptomatic adults for colorectal cancer. Veterans Affairs Cooperative Study Group 380. *N Engl J Med* 2000; **343**: 162–168.

Further reading

Winawer SJ, Fletcher RH, Miller L *et al.* Colorectal cancer screening: clinical guidelines and rationale. *Gastroenterology* 1997; **112**: 594–642.

Burt RW, Colon cancer screening. *Gastroenterology* 2000; **119**: 837–853.

35. Infectious Diarrhoea

MICHAEL FARTHING

INTRODUCTION

Intestinal infection is the most common cause of diarrhoea in both the industrialized and the developing worlds (1). In the latter, microbial enteropathogens are found in great abundance, major reservoirs being water, food, and humans. Intestinal infections continue to have their major impact on those living in the developing world, and are still responsible for the death of up to 4 million pre-school children each year. In some African countries, children may suffer up to seven attacks of acute diarrhoea annually, each of which contributes to the infection–malnutrition cycle that, in many, ultimately results in impaired growth and development.

Despite industrialization, economic wealth, and public health interventions to ensure water quality and sewage disposal, intestinal infections are increasing in the Western world, particularly foodborne (2) (*Salmonella spp.*, *Campylobacter jejuni* and entero-haemorrhagic *Escherichia coli* O157:H7) and waterborne infections (*Giardia intestinalis* and *Cryptosporidium parvum*). Other factors contributing to the increase in acute infectious diarrhoea in the industrialized world include the widespread use of broad-spectrum antibiotics, impaired host immunity caused by human immunodeficiency virus (HIV) infection and anticancer chemotherapy, and the increase in foreign travel from Western countries to the developing world. Figure 35.1 illustrates the continuing increase in reports of *Camp. jejuni*, *Salmonella spp.* and other gastrointestinal infections in the UK.

Chronic gastrointestinal infections, particularly those caused by *Mycobacterium tuberculosis* and the helminths, *Strongyloides stercoralis* and *Schistosoma spp.*, are common in many regions in the tropics, but also appear as imported diseases in the industrialized world.

For the gastroenterologist, the possibility of intestinal infection must always be high on the diagnostic agenda, particularly during the initial investigation of patients with persistent diarrhoea and bloody diarrhoea (Table 35.1). The results of

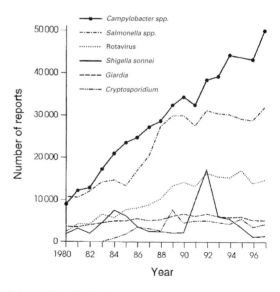

Figure 35.1. Public Health Laboratory Service Communicable Disease Surveillance Centre laboratory reports of selected gastrointestinal infections in England and Wales, 1980–1997.

Table 35.1. Enteropathogens responsible for infectious diarrhoea.

Enteropathogen	Acute watery diarrhoea	Dysentery[*]	Persistent diarrhoea[†]
Viruses			
Rotavirus	+	–	–
Adenovirus (types 40, 41)	+	–	–
Small round structured viruses	+	–	–
Cytomegalovirus	+	+	+
Bacteria			
Vibrio cholerae (rare) and other vibrios	+	–	–
Enterotoxigenic *Escherichia coli*	+	–	–
Enteroinvasive *E. coli*	+	–	–
Shigella spp.	+	+	+
Salmonella spp.	+	+	+
Campylobacter spp.	+	+	+
Yersinia enterocolitica	+	+	+
Clostridium difficile	+	+	+
Mycobacterium tuberculosis	–	+	+
Protozoa			
Giardia intestinalis	+	–	+
Cryptosporidium parvum	+	–	+
Microsporidia	+	–	+
Isospora belli	+	–	+
Cyclospora cayetanensis	+	–	+
Entamoeba histolytica	+	+	+
Helminths			
Strongyloides stercoralis	–	–	+
Schistosoma spp.	–	+	+

[*]Dysentery: diarrhoea with blood.
[†]Persistent diarrhoea: diarrhoea for more than 14–21 days.

the laboratory tests to either confirm or refute a diagnosis of intestinal infection are often not available when management decisions need to be taken. In addition, some organisms are difficult to isolate, and grow slowly in culture (*Campylobacter spp.* and *Yersinia enterocolitica*), and the protozoan parasites — which are generally detected by faecal microscopy, often with the use of special stains — can be missed, as there are relatively few experienced parasitologists in diagnostic laboratories in the developed world. It is vital, however, that intestinal infections are confidently excluded before patients are treated for non-specific inflammatory bowel disease, for example, and before symptoms are attributed to a functional bowel disorder such as the irritable bowel syndrome.

Diagnostic difficulties are also introduced when the severity of the complications of infection are more clinically evident than the diarrhoea. Particular examples include Reiter's syndrome which follows infection with some invasive microorganisms, the haemolytic–uraemic syndrome, which is asso-

ciated with shigellosis and more recently with enterohaemorrhagic *E. coli* infection (EHEC) and the Guillain–Barré syndrome, which has been linked with *Campylobacter jejuni* infection.

Thus the gastroenterologist is increasingly faced with the dilemma as to whether diarrhoea is the result of infection, non-specific inflammatory bowel disease, some other organic gastrointestinal disorder, or a functional bowel disorder. The investigation of diarrhoea, particularly persistent diarrhoea, can consume substantial healthcare resources and it is vital, therefore, that the diagnostic approach should have a carefully thought-through rationale, which should be hierarchical with respect to risk and economic considerations.

DIAGNOSTIC FEATURES AND RISK FACTORS

Acute watery diarrhoea is the most common presentation of acute infectious diarrhoea and is rarely

due to other non-infectious causes. However, many classes of drug, including laxatives, are known to cause diarrhoea, which would usually manifest soon after starting the drug. Another important exclusion is the non-absorbed disaccharide, sorbitol, which is used to sweeten sugar-free confectionery. The **drugs which cause diarrhoea** include:

- Antibiotics
- Anticancer drugs
- Antidepressants
  - lithium
  - paroxetine
- Antihypertensives
  - β-blockers
  - angiotensin-converting enzyme inhibitors
  - hydralazine
- Anticonvulsants
  - valproic acid
- Cholesterol decreasing agents
- Oral hypoglycaemics
  - biguanides
- Gastrointestinal drugs
  - magnesium containing compounds
  - H$_2$-receptor antagonists
  - prostaglandin analogues
  - 5-aminosalicylic acid
- Colchicine
- Diuretics
- Theophylline
- Laxatives

Several groups of individuals are at increased risk of acute intestinal infection, including both watery diarrhoea and bloody diarrhoea (Table 35.2).

Risk factors

Age

Infants and pre-school children and the elderly are particularly susceptible. During the first few months of life, the breast-fed infant is relatively protected from intestinal infection, but exposure to enteropathogens increases during the weaning period and the protective benefits of maternal milk are lost. The elderly appear to have increased susceptibility, partly because of declining immunocompetence, and possibly also to decreased acid secretion, which will be especially evident in those with gastric atrophy as a result of pernicious anaemia and chronic infection with *Helicobacter pylori*.

Immunodeficiency

Primary and secondary impaired immunity are well recognized to be major risk factors for intestinal infection. Common variable immunodeficiency is classically associated with protozoal infections, particularly giardiasis and cryptosporidiosis. HIV/acquired immunodeficiency syndrome (AIDS) has re-emphasized the importance of cellular immunity in host defence against enteric infection, particularly the intracellular protozoa (3). Similarly, anticancer chemotherapy is associated with opportunistic intestinal infection including that caused by cytomegalovirus and *Clostridium difficile*.

Antibiotics

Widespread use of **broad-spectrum antibiotics** in cancer patients and in many other groups of hospi-

Table 35.2. Special risk groups for infectious diarrhoea.

Risk factor	Groups at risk
Age	Infants and young children
	The elderly
Non-immune host defence — gastric acid	The elderly
	Hypo- and achlorhydria
	Recipients of acid-inhibitory drugs
Immunodeficiency	Congential immunodeficiency (common variable immune deficiency)
	HIV/AIDS
	Cancer and cancer chemotherapy
	Undernutrition
Increased exposure to enteropathogens	Travellers
	Food and water-borne disease
Antibiotics	Recipients of antibiotics
	The elderly and cancer patients are at increased risk

AIDS, aquired immunodeficiency syndrome.

tal patients and ambulant individuals has demonstrated the clinical relevance of antibiotic-associated diarrhoea, much of which is attributable to opportunistic infection with *Clostridium difficile*, but other organisms — notably other clostridia — have also been implicated. The importance of gastric acid as a physical barrier to intestinal infection has already been raised with respect to the elderly. However, there is increasing evidence that the use of potent acid-inhibitory drugs such as the H_2-receptor antagonists and the proton pump inhibitors do constitute a small, but nevertheless finite, increased risk of intestinal bacterial infection (4,5). The risk appears to be mainly evident in the elderly.

Travel

Travel from the industrialized world to developing countries continues to be a major risk factor for acute intestinal infection (1). Depending on geographical location, 30–50% of travellers can expect to experience an episode of acute infectious diarrhoea. In general, the infections are of mild or moderate severity and usually self-limiting. However, further investigation and treatment may be necessary for individuals with dysentery, when invasive organisms are involved, or when diarrhoea persists after their return home.

Dietary sources

Food and water continue to be important vehicles for infectious diarrhoea, even in the relatively sanitized industrialized world. Major outbreaks of giardiasis and cryptosporidosis after contamination of domestic water supplies have been well documented in North America and Europe. Food-borne diarrhoeal disease takes two forms: true infection, in which enteropathogens are consumed with food and then colonize and multiply within the intestine producing disease, and the ingestion of preformed toxin in food that has been contaminated by an enterotoxin-producing microorganism (Table 35.3). In the UK, there are major concerns about increasing number of food-related isolations of *Campylobacter jejuni*, *Salmonella spp.*, and EHEC, although major outbreaks have been relatively restricted geographically, particularly to Scotland.

CLINICAL SYNDROMES

Infectious diarrhoea manifests clinically as **three major syndromes**, namely:

1. acute watery diarrhoea
2. diarrhoea with blood (dysentery)
3. persistent diarrhoea

Persistent diarrhoea is sometimes accompanied by overt evidence of intestinal malabsorption. It is usually defined as diarrhoea that has continued for more than 14–21 days. **Intestinal infection may also present in two other ways**:

4. sub-acute intestinal obstruction
5. proctitis

Table 35.3. Microbial pathogens responsible for food-borne diarrhoeal disease.

	Source	Incubation period (h)	Symptoms	Recovery
Bacteria that colonise the gut				
Salmonella spp.	Eggs, poultry	12–48	Diarrhoea, blood, pain, vomiting, fever	2–14 days
Campylobacter jejuni	Milk, poultry	48–168	As above	7–21 days
EHEC	Beef	24–168	As above	7–21 days
Vibrio parahaemolyticus	Seafood	2–48	As above (blood less common)	2–30 days
Yersinia enterocolitica	Milk, pork	2–144	Diarrhoea, fever, pain	1–3 days
Clostridium perfringens	Spores in food, especially meat	8–22	Diarrhoea, pain	1–3 days
Preformed toxins				
Staphylococcus aureus	Transmitted to food by humans	2–6	Nausea, vomiting, pain (diarrhoea)	Few hours
Bacillus cereus	Spores in food, reheated rice	1–2	As above	Few hours
Clostridium botulinum	Spores in home-bottled or home-canned food	18–36	Transient diarrhoea, paralysis	10–14 days

Considering patients in these categories does guide **diagnosis** with respect to both a likely infective aetiologic agent and other possible causes for the symptoms. However, it should be stated clearly that there can be considerable overlap between these infection syndromes, particularly as dysenteric enteropathogens do not always produce bloody diarrhoea. The presence of **macroscopic blood in the stools**, however, almost invariably indicates the presence of an invasive enteropathogen, although the situation can be confused by bleeding from haemorrhoids that has been triggered by acute diarrhoea. Table 35.1 summarizes the enteropathogens commonly responsible for these clinical syndromes, but it also emphasizes the overlap that can occur.

Acute watery diarrhoea

Worldwide, acute watery diarrhoea is the most common presentation of acute infectious diarrhoea. In infants and young children, rotavirus infection is often preceded by a brief prodromal illness with fever and mild respiratory symptoms, after which diarrhoea and vomiting predominate. If fluid and electrolyte losses are not replaced promptly, dehydration and metabolic acidosis soon follow. The degree of dehydration can be assessed clinically by noting skin tone and tissue turgor, intraocular tension and, in young infants, depression of the anterior fontanelle. In addition, there may be dryness of mucous membranes. As the degree of dehydration increases, there is impairment of consciousness ultimately leading to stupor and coma. Typically the illness lasts about 7 days. Adenovirus is a more prolonged illness, with pronounced ventilatory symptoms.

Acute watery diarrhoea in adults is usually bacterial in origin, most commonly caused by enterotoxigenic *E. coli* (ETEC) in travellers, or by one of the food-borne pathogens (Table 35.3) in the indigenous population of industrialized countries. ETEC usually begins after a short incubation period and, on average, lasts 3–5 days. Watery diarrhoea is often accompanied by anorexia, nausea, vomiting, abdominal cramps, bloating, and low-grade fever. In adults, severe dehydration is uncommon, although this may become clinically important in infants and young children and the elderly. Invasive enteropathogens and the intracellular protozoa can all produce acute watery diarrhoea in the initial stages of infection — a clinical presentation that would be indistinguishable from other causes of acute watery diarrhoea. Non-infectious causes of watery diarrhoea include the drugs listed above, bile salt malabsorption, and the neuroendocrine diarrhoeas (vasoactive intestinal peptidoma, carcinoid, medullary carcinoma of the thyroid).

Dysentery

The organisms responsible for acute bloody diarrhoea are the invasive bacterial enteropathogens (*Shigella spp.*, *Salmonella spp.*, *Campylobacter jejuni* and EHEC) and the protozoan, *Entamoeba histolytica*. There is often a prodromal illness of low-grade fever, headache, anorexia, and lassitude. The incubation period is variable, but can range from 1 to 7 days. After an initial period of watery diarrhoea, stool volume may actually decrease, with the appearance of blood in the stools. Moderate or severe cramping lower abdominal pain is an important feature of a dysenteric illness, as are tenesmus and rectal prolapse, particularly in children with shigellosis. Physical examination may confirm the presence of a fever, and there may be mild abdominal distension, with some tenderness over the colon.

Diarrhoea with blood now presents a major diagnostic challenge for the clinician, because of the importance of distinguishing infection from non-specific inflammatory bowel disease and other inflammatory conditions of the colon. The clinical differentiation of infection from these other conditions is usually not easy, although infective colitis generally has a relatively abrupt onset and cramping lower abdominal pain often emerges as the most disruptive symptom, which is usually not the case in ulcerative colitis, for example. The **differential diagnosis of bloody diarrhoea** may be summarized as:

- Invasive infectious diarrhoea (see Table 35.1)
- Non-specific inflammatory bowel disease
  - Crohn's disease
  - ulcerative colitis
  - Behçet's disease
- Ischaemic colitis
- Radiation colitis
- Colorectal cancer (including large polyps, e.g. villous adenoma)
- Diverticular disease
- Intussusception

Persistent diarrhoea

In adults, the most common infective pathogen that produces chronic diarrhoea is the protozoan, *G. intestinalis*; diarrhoea is often associated with anorexia, abdominal bloating, and substantial weight loss. Long-standing infection may be accompanied by overt steatorrhoea. In children, enteropathogenic *E. coli* is an important organism to consider as a cause of persistent diarrhoea. Infection with *Strongyloides stercoralis* may also cause chronic diarrhoea and malabsorption, although this is more common in the hyperinfection syndrome. Amoebic colitis can persist in a relatively indolent manner, without overt blood loss.

Subacute intestinal obstruction

Some chronic infections, such as intestinal tuberculosis and schistosomiasis, cause stricturing in the small and large intestine and give rise to obstructive symptoms. This may or may not be associated with diarrhoea. Other associated features may be fever, malaise, and weight loss; in the case of ileocaecal tuberculosis, there may be an associated tender, right iliac fossa mass (6). Colonic strictures may not produce overt obstructive symptoms with pain, but merely cause irregularity of bowel function. Occasionally, very heavy infections with the round worm, *Ascaris lumbricoides*, can cause small-intestinal obstruction as a result of an entangled mass of worms.

Proctitis and perianal disease

It is now well recognized that *Chlamydia trachomatis*, *Neisseria gonorrhoeae* and herpes simplex virus (HSV) produce inflammatory changes in the rectum. The appearances of *Chlamydia trachomatis* proctitis are indistinguishable from those of non-specific proctitis, but HSV produces typical vesicles in the rectum with periodic proctitic symptoms. The lymphogranuloma venereum strain of *Chlamydia* results in chronic inflammatory changes in the rectum which can progress to stricturing similar to that seen in anorectal Crohn's disease. Rectal tuberculosis may produce discrete ulceration in the rectum with fistulation. In a recent study from India, *M. tuberculosis* was detected in 15% of anal fistulae.

CLINICAL EXAMINATION

Distinguishing infective disorders from non-specific inflammatory bowel disease is of vital importance, particularly in the severely ill patient, for whom a delay in starting appropriate treatment may significantly alter the outcome. Confident exclusion of an infective aetiology is rarely achieved in less than 24–48 h, however, and, in practice, clinical assessment is important for guiding management during the early phase of the illness.

General physical examination in patients with acute watery diarrhoea may reveal signs of **dehydration and acidosis**, but there are no specific signs that would indicate a specific aetiology. However, in adults, severe dehydration and acidosis are likely to occur only in cholera and in diarrhoea caused by related vibrios. Similarly, it is difficult to distinguish the infective causes of dysentery from non-specific inflammatory bowel disease and other forms of colitis. Nevertheless, a careful search should be made for the stigmata of Crohn's disease such as perianal disease, erythema nodosum, oral aphthous ulceration, and pyoderma gangrenosum. Clinical signs of HIV/AIDS — such as Kaposi's sarcoma, hairy leucoplakia, and oral candidiasis — may also guide the final clinical diagnosis. Painful, swollen joints can accompany intestinal infection, particularly that attributable to *Y. enterocolitica* and *Campylobacter jejuni* forming part of Reiter's syndrome, although arthralgia may accompany non-specific inflammatory bowel disease.

Persistent diarrhoea is often accompanied by weight loss and other evidence of **undernutrition**. Again, there are few specific clinical findings that would confirm a specific clinical diagnosis. The most exotic tropical causes of persistent diarrhoea may, however, have clinical stigmata such as larva currens (an erythematous, pruritic, migrating weal) associated with strongyloidiasis and hepatosplenomegaly that may accompany intestinal schistosomiasis.

Endoscopic examination of the rectum with a rigid sigmoidoscope will confirm whether a colitis is present, but it is rarely possible to produce a specific diagnosis with confidence. Discrete ulceration occurs in a variety of conditions (Table 35.4), and although the presence of pseudomembrane strongly suggests infection with *Clostridium difficile*

Table 35.4. Diseases producing "specific" abnormalities in the rectum.

Abnormality	Disease
Deep ulcers	Crohn's disease
	Ameobiasis
	Tuberculosis
	Syphilis
Pseudomembrane	*Clostridium difficile*
	Ischaemic colitis
Vesicles	HSV
Beads of pus	Gonorrhoea

this also occurs in ischaemia. Patchy ulceration and stricturing occur in Crohn's disease, but are also found in tuberculosis and lymphogranuloma venereum. Sexually transmitted diseases of the rectum do have some relatively specific features although chlamydia procitis is clinically indistinguishable from non-specific proctitis. **Microbial enteropathogens that cause proctitis** include:

- *Neisseria gonorrhoeae*
- *Chlamydia trachomatis* (lymphogranuloma venereum)
- *Chlamydia trachomatis* (non-lymphogranuloma venereum)
- *Treponema pallidum*
- HSV

A normal rectum at sigmoidoscopy does not exclude proximal infective or inflammatory bowel disease (Table 35.5).

Table 35.5. Infections and inflammatory conditions of the colon in which the rectum may be spared.

Infections	Ameobiasis
	Pseudomembranous colitis
	Yersiniosis
	Campylobacter jejuni
	Tuberculosis
	Cryptosporidiosis
	Salmonellosis
	Shigellosis
Inflammatory conditions	Crohn's disease (30% of cases of ileocaecal Crohn's have rectal involvement)
	Ulcerative colitis
	Microscopic colitis
	Collagenous colitis
	Behçet's disease

INVESTIGATIONS

The majority of patients with acute infective watery diarrhoea recover without needing to seek medical advice or to undergo any investigations whatsoever. Indeed, routine haematology and blood chemistry are generally not helpful in making a specific diagnosis of acute infectious diarrhoea. If dehydration is present in acute watery diarrhoea, this may be reflected by haemoconcentration, with an increase in haemoglobin and packed cell volume, and possibly an increase in blood urea. If acidosis accompanies the dehydration, there may be a decrease in the serum bicarbonate concentration in venous blood; if the acidosis is severe, a decrease in pH and base excess may be found in arterial blood. In acute bloody diarrhoea, there may be anaemia, an increased neutrophil count, and evidence of an inflammatory process with increased erythrocyte sedimentation rate, C-reactive protein concentration, and platelet count. Anaemia and hypoal-buminaemia may occur in infections that produce persistent diarrhoea; in addition, there may be evidence of intestinal malabsorption, with reduced red-cell folate and serum vitamin B_{12} concentrations. In severe watery diarrhoea, magnesium and potassium losses may become clinically significant. If steatorrhoea is long-standing, biochemical, and sometimes clinical, deficiency of fat-soluble vitamins (A, D, E, and K) occurs. Eosinophilia commonly accompanies helminth infections of the gut (Table 35.6), although only *Strongyloides stercoralis*, *Trichinella spiralis* and *Schistosoma spp.* are associated with diarrhoea.

Microbiology

Microbiological examination of faeces is the usual way to make a specific diagnosis in the majority of

Table 35.6. Eosinophilia and intestinal infection.

Helminths	*Ascaris lumbricoides*
	Hookworm
	Schistosoma spp.[*]
	Strongyloides stercoralis[*]
	Trichinella spiralis[*]
	Trichuris trichura
Protozoa	*Giardia intestinalis*[*] (rare)

[*]Parasites producing diarrhoea that is acute, persistent, or both.

intestinal infections. Light-microscopic examination of three serial faecal specimens is essential to exclude protozoal infection from *G. intestinalis*, *Cryptosporidium parvum*, the microsporidia and *Cyclospora cayetanensis*. Modified acid-fast stains are used to detect *Cryptosporidium parvum* and cyclospora, and calcafluour is used to "highlight" the spores of microsporidia.

Stool culture will isolate the classic invasive enteropathogens, including *Clostridium difficile*, but microscopy is required to detect cysts and trophozoites of *Entamoeba histolytica*. If EHEC is suspected, *E. coli* colonies must be subcultured and serotyped. *Clostridium difficile* toxin A can be detected in faeces by means of an **enzyme-linked immuno-sorbent assay** (ELISA); this investigation should always be requested to confirm the clinical relevance of a *Clostridium difficile*-positive faecal culture.

One of the major disadvantages of faecal culture is the inevitable delay before culture information is available to the clinician. It is unusual for a bacterial enteropathogen to be identified in less than 24–48 h, and for the slower growing organisms, such as *Y. enterocolitica* and *Campylobacter jejuni*, culture information may not be available for 3–5 days. Attempts have therefore been made to develop specific faecal antigen ELISAs, to provide more rapid faecal diagnosis. A faecal antigen ELISA to detect giardia antigens is available in routine diagnostic laboratories. There is also an extremely efficient rotavirus faecal ELISA but, as infection is generally relatively mild and self-limiting, it is difficult to justify clinically, particularly as a positive test does not generally change management.

More recently, attempts have been made to develop **DNA probes** directed towards specific virulence factors of enteropathogens. In principle, this offers the opportunity to make a rapid, highly specific diagnosis (7), but unfortunately, there have been major technical difficulties in developing tests that will work on crude faecal extracts. DNA probes have, however, found a place in the characterization of cultured bacterial isolates — enabling the relatively rapid identification, for example, of the various enterovirulent subtypes of *E. coli*.

Serology

Serology is generally disappointing as a diagnostic aid for acute intestinal infection. However, in persistent diarrhoea it has proved useful to detect invasive colonic disease attributable to *Entamoeba histolytica* (positive in about 80–90% of patients with amoebic colitis), and also for the detection of *Y. enterocolitica* infections, although serology is not usually positive for at least 10–14 days after the onset of the illness. ELISAs are now widely available for the diagnosis of strongyloidiasis and schistosomiasis, and should be regarded as first-line screening tests for these infections. These tests are particularly useful in travellers returning from areas where such infections are endemic.

Abdominal and intestinal imaging

Most patients with acute infectious diarrhoea do not require radiological imaging. However, a **plain abdominal radiograph** can be invaluable in assessing the severity and extent of infectious colitis. A gas-filled colon devoid of faeces indicates a total colitis; loss of haustration and colonic dilatation is indicative of severe ulceration. In acute watery diarrhoea, the plain abdominal radiograph may reveal multiple small-bowel fluid levels and small-bowel dilatation. This does not indicate intestinal obstruction, but probably reflects a partial ileus. The examination is also useful in excluding the presence of free air in the abdominal cavity as a result of bowel perforation.

Barium contrast studies

A double-contrast barium enema is not the examination of choice for colonic infection although, when requested, it can reveal the cone-shaped caecum of amoebic colitis and granulomatous masses in the colon (amoebomata), which may resemble carcinoma. Caecal involvement in tuberculosis may also be demonstrated and can closely resemble Crohn's disease. Colonic strictures occur in tuberculosis, but are radiologically indistinguishable from Crohn's disease. A barium follow-through examination may be useful in revealing ileal abnormalities such as superficial ulceration in yersiniosis and strictures in tuberculosis.

Transabdominal ultrasound

Abdominal ultrasound examination may reveal bowel-wall thickening in invasive ileocolitis, and enlarged lymph nodes in yersiniosis and abdominal tuberculosis. Abdominal ultrasound may also be invaluable in detecting the complications of intestinal infection such as amoebic liver abscess, and in confirming the presence of hepatosplenomegaly and portal hypertension in schistosomiasis.

Ileocolonoscopy

The endoscopic differentiation between acute infectious colitis and other forms of colitis is difficult. The appearances of shigella, salmonella and campylobacter infections are macroscopically indistinguishable from non-specific inflammatory bowel disease. These infections produce a predominantly right-sided colitis that macroscopically resembles ulcerative colitis; this finding should raise the index of suspicion for infection. Ileocaecal and rectal tuberculosis may produce endoscopic appearances identical to those of Crohn's disease. However, the experienced endoscopist may be able to identify the typical amoebic ulcers, which are shallow lesions with undermined edges, often covered with a heaped-up yellow exudate. Intervening mucosa appears normal, which distinguishes it from ulcerative colitis and other invasive bacterial infections of the colon. However, the diagnosis must be confirmed by microscopic examination of ulcer slough for trophozoites.

Ischaemic colitis may be easily identifiable by its regional involvement of the splenic flexure and proximal descending colon (an unusual distribution for other forms of colitis), although both the right colon and the rectum can be involved as isolated segments in an ischaemic process that might be more difficult to distinguish from other forms of colitis. The dark, dusky red appearance of the mucosa may also suggest a diagnosis of ischaemia.

The endoscopic appearances of **radiation colitis** may not be specific, although the presence of telangiectases in an erythematous and spontaneously bleeding mucosa would be highly suggestive. The presence of pseudomembranes in the colon that appear as pale, white/yellow excrescences on the epithelium and which, when removed, leave an area of spontaneous bleeding separated by areas of normal mucosa, are generally indicative of *Clostridium difficile* infection, although pseudomembrane is not specific for this condition and may occur in ischaemia.

Colonic and ileal strictures should be examined endoscopically so that several biopsy specimens can be obtained for histology and microbiology.

Similarly, mass lesions should also be examined endoscopically and by biopsy to exclude neoplasia. The presence of multiple colonic polyps is well recognized in colonic schistosomiasis.

Oesophagogastroduodenoscopy

Endoscopic examination of the upper gastrointestinal tract is indicated only in individuals with persistent diarrhoea, with or without intestinal malabsorption. The macroscopic appearances at endoscopy are usually not helpful, although if there is severe villous atrophy the folds in the second part of the duodenum may be attenuated. *G. intestinalis* and the intracellular protozoa (*Cryptosporidium parvum*, cyclospora and the microsporidia) are all known to be able to produce partial, and in some cases total, villous atrophy — a finding that should be confirmed by endoscopic duodenal biopsy. In addition, duodenal fluid should be aspirated for microscopic examination, particularly for cysts and trophozoites of *G. intestinalis* and for strongyloides larvae.

Histology

The microscopic anatomy of the gastrointestinal tract was considered in detail in Chapter 3.2.

Colon

The histological appearances of colonic mucosa in the later stages of infection with invasive enteropathogens such as *Salmonella spp.*, *Shigella spp.*, and *Campylobacter jejuni* are often indistinguishable from those of non-specific inflammatory bowel disease (8,9). However, if biopsy samples are taken within the first 24–72 h, features that might suggest infectious colitis include mucosal oedema, straightening of the glands, and an acute inflammatory infiltrate including polymorphonuclear leucocytes, which can sometimes be seen penetrating the epithelium. In *Clostridium difficile* infection, an acute inflammatory infiltrate is also apparent, combined with the typical "erupting volcano" lesion that is the histological counterpart of pseudomembrane. Colonic and ileal biopsies in tuberculosis may reveal caseating granulomata and, occasionally, acid-fast bacilli can be detected by light microscopy — although, when tuberculosis is suspected, biopsy specimens should always be sent for microbiological culture. Other organisms that can be identified in mucosal biopsies include the trophozoites of *Entamoeba histolytica* and the "owl's eye" inclusion bodies indicative of cytomegalovirus infection. Ova of *Schistosoma spp.* can also be detected in mucosal biopsy samples, and it is often possible to differentiate one species from another on the basis of egg morphology. *Cryptosporidium parvum* can also be detected by light microscopy of colonic biopsy specimens.

Duodenum

G. intestinalis trophozoites can be visualized entrapped in the adherent mucus layer of the duodenum, whereas *Cryptosporidium parvum* and the microsporidia can be detected in an intracellular location by light microscopy. Transmission electron microscopy is generally required for distinguishing the different species of microsporidia. Adult worms of *Strongyloides stercoralis* may be identified penetrating the small intestinal mucosa. Duodenal biopsies are also necessary to confirm the diagnosis of tropical sprue, in which there is partial villous atrophy and some crypt hyperplasia, although a relative paucity of intraepithelial lymphocytes, which distinguishes it from coeliac disease.

COMPLICATIONS

Worldwide, although the majority of deaths from intestinal infection continue to be the result of dehydration and acidosis, it should always be possible to manage these aspects of the illness by oral or intravenous rehydration. In recent years, it has become increasingly clear that death also occurs as a result of the complications of infection, particularly those caused by the invasive enteropathogens.

Haemolytic–uraemic syndrome

Shigella dysenteriae type 1 infection has been known for several decades to cause haemolytic–uraemic syndrome, and it is now well established that this is also responsible for a substantial proportion of the mortality associated with EHEC infection (2). This syndrome consists of a triad of features:

- acute renal failure
- thrombocytopenia
- microangiopathic haemolytic anaemia

It is also described with *Salmonella typhi*, *Campylobacter jejuni* and *Y. pseudotuberculosis* infections, and occurs in about 6% of patients with EHEC infection. It carries a mortality of 3–5%.

Non-septic arthritis and Reiter's syndrome

These symptoms are commonly associated with several invasive organisms, including *Salmonella spp.*, *Shigella spp.*, *Y. enterocolitica* and *Campylobacter jejuni*. More than 70% of patients who develop non-septic arthritis are positive for the human leucocyte antigen, HLA-B27. Non-septic arthritis may be associated with iritis and conjunctivitis, which may occur in up to 90% of patients with arthritis after shigellosis, and up to 25% of those with salmonella, campylobacter or yersinia infections. The term "Reiter's syndrome" is reserved for the classic triad of symptoms consisting of arthritis, urethritis, and conjunctivitis. Again HLA-B27 positivity strongly predicts the likelihood of developing Reiter's syndrome, and is indicative of its severity.

Guillain–Barré syndrome

A clear link has now been established between *Campylobacter jejuni* infection and the Guillain–Barré syndrome (10). When the syndrome follows campylobacter infection, it appears to be predominantly a motor disorder and has a particularly poor outcome, with an increased risk of the patient's requiring ventilatory support and having severe disability after 1 year of disease.

Septic arthritis

Purulent synovitis during enteric infection is relatively rare, occurring in 0.2–2.5% of individuals with salmonella infection. Infection is usually monoarticular, involving the large joints. Symptoms begin within 2 weeks of the gastrointestinal symptoms, but may occur as late as 7 weeks. There is no association with HLA-B27.

Chronic carrier state

Prolonged carriage is well recognized in salmonella infection particularly in the presence of renal or gallstones. Eradication can be achieved in more than 80% of affected patients by administration of amoxycillin or a quinolone in standard doses for 4–6 weeks.

TREATMENT

The majority of cases of acute infective diarrhoea are self-limiting and resolve without specific treatment, providing attention is paid to restoration of fluid and electrolyte balance. However, there are clear indications for specific anti-microbial chemotherapy in some dysenteric infections such as amoebiasis and dysenteric shigellosis and for infective causes of persistent diarrhoea such as that associated with *G. intestinalis*, the microsporidia, *Cyclospora cayetanensis* and *Strongyloides stercoralis*. Antibiotics may be indicated for other bacterial infections, particularly when symptoms are severe and there is evidence of systemic involvement.

Maintenance of fluid and electrolyte balance

Oral rehydration is the mainstay of management of acute watery diarrhoea (11–13). A glucose–electrolyte solution should be administered early in acute diarrhoea in infants and young children, to prevent the occurrence of dehydration and acidosis. In the developing world, the World Health Organization oral rehydration solution (sodium concentration 90 mmol/litre, osmolality 331 mosmol/kg) is still recommended although there is increasing evidence that solutions with lesser concentrations of sodium (50–60 mmol/litre) and lower osmolality (about 240 mosmol/kg) are as effective in correcting dehydration and acidosis, and have an added advantage in that they appear to be more effective in reducing faecal losses (13,14).

Cereal-based oral rehydration solutions have been shown to reduce stool volume in cholera, but are, commercially, more difficult to prepare than the low-osmolality, glucose-based solutions. In infants and young children with more severe dehydration (>5%), rehydration with intravenous fluids may be required. Food and oral fluids should be commenced as soon as the individual wishes to eat and drink. Breast feeding should be continued throughout the illness in young infants.

In adults, formal oral rehydration therapy is generally not required. It is usually sufficient to recommend increase in oral fluids such as salty soups (sodium), fruit juices (potassium), and a source of carbohydrate (salty crackers, rice, bread, pasta, potatoes) to provide a glucose source for glucose–sodium co-transport.

Antidiarrhoeal agents

Drugs such as loperamide and diphenoxylate/atropine combination reduce bowel frequency and may have a modest effect in reducing faecal losses. These drugs continue to be the first-line self-treatment for travellers, but should not be given to infants and young children. Controversy remains as to whether they should be used in individuals with dysentery; early suggestions that antidiarrhoeal drugs increase faecal carriage of gut enteropathogens or predispose an individual with infective colitis to colonic dilatation are probably unfounded. As yet, there are no true antisecretory agents available for reducing stool volume in acute watery diarrhoea, although the calmodulin antagonist, zaldaride maleate, has been shown to be effective in acute traveller's diarrhoea and may have therapeutic advantages over the traditional antidiarrhoeal agents. Other potential antisecretory drugs include the encephalinase antagonist, acetorphan, the sigma-receptor agonist, igmesine, and certain 5-hydroxytryptamine receptor antagonists.

Antimicrobial chemotherapy

The role of antibiotics in the management of infectious diarrhoea remains controversial (15–18). Although it is clear that antibiotics can reduce the severity and duration of some intestinal infections, particularly those that produce acute watery diarrhoea, the evidence that they alter the natural history in many cases of dysentery is poor, or at best unproven. Antibiotics, however, are clearly indicated for some cases of persistent diarrhoea in which a specific pathogen has been identified.

Acute watery diarrhoea

Antibiotic treatment is not routinely required for acute watery diarrhoea, with the exception of cholera; the severity and duration of *Vibrio cholerae* infection is reduced by tetracycline 250 mg four times daily for 3–5 days and by ciprofloxacin 250 mg daily for three days. *Vibrio cholerae* is also sensitive to doxycycline, ampicillin, chloramphenicol, and co-trimoxazole. The severity and duration of traveller's diarrhoea (predominantly ETEC-related) is also decreased by antimicrobial agents such as doxycycline, trimethoprim, and the fluoroquinolones. Recent evidence indicates that a single dose of ciprofloxacin 500 mg is sufficient (19).

Controversy continues as to the appropriateness of using an antibiotic for a non-fatal, usually mild, self-limiting illness, because of the continuing increase in antibiotic resistance and concerns about an individual developing a life-threatening complication of antibiotic therapy (Stevens–Johnson syndrome, pseudomembranous colitis).

A non-antibiotic approach to treatment has been shown to be moderately effective in the form of bismuth subsalicylate. This reduces the severity of traveller's diarrhoea without exposing the individual to the risks of antibiotic treatment with the associated increasing resistance to antimicrobial drug.

Dysentery

Antibiotic treatment is indicated for dysenteric shigellosis, amoebiasis, and pseudomembranous colitis (Table 35.7) (20,21). However, when these invasive infections are mild and there is no evidence of systemic involvement, the individual will generally recover without specific antimicrobial chemotherapy. In *Campylobacter jejuni* infection, for example, there are doubts that antibiotics significantly influence the natural history, partly because antibiotic treatment is often started once faecal cultures are found to be positive, which is generally several days after the infection has become established. A similar situation may also exist with yersiniosis.

A major controversy exists as to whether antibiotics should be used in EHEC infection. Again, infection is usually well established before the diagnosis is confirmed microbiologically and there is evidence that administration of antibiotics at this stage can promote the development of haemolytic–uraemic syndrome, presumably because of lysis of organisms and release of Shiga-like toxins and endotoxin. Further work is required before firm advice can be given regarding the appropriateness of antimicrobial chemotherapy in EHEC infections, although a recent study indicates that it should not be used in children with suspected or proven EHEC.

Persistent diarrhoea

Some of the organisms responsible for persistent diarrhoea are sensitive to antimicrobial chemotherapeutic agents (Table 35.8) (22). *Cryptosporidium parvum* continues to be resistant to antimicrobial attack, although paromomycin may suppress infection. Recent evidence suggests that high-dose albendazole or the emerging agent, nitazoxanide, may have a role in the treatment of *Cryptosporidium parvum* infection. The micro-

Table 35.7. Antimicrobial chemotherapy for dysentery.

Organism	Drug of choice	Alternative
Bacteria		
Shigella spp.	Ampicillin, 500 mg four times daily, 5 days	Cefixime 400 mg daily, 5–7 days[†]
	TMP–SMX 2, tablets twice daily, 5 days	Nalidixic acid 1 g four times daily, 5–7 days
	Ciprofloxacin 500 mg twice daily, 5 days[‡]	
Salmonella spp.	Ciprofloxacin 500 mg twice daily, 10–14 days[‡**]	
EIEC	? as *Shigella spp.*	
EHEC	?	
Campylobacter jejuni	Erythromycin 250–500 mg four times daily, 7 days	Ciprofloxacin 500 mg twice daily, 5–7 days[‡]
Yersinia enterocolitica	Tetracycline 250 mg four times daily, 7–10 days	
	Ciprofloxacin 500 mg twice daily, 7–10 days[‡]	
	TMP–SMX, 2 tablets twice daily, 7–10 days	
Clostridium difficile	Metronidazole 400 mg three times daily, 7–10 days	Vancomycin 125 mg four times daily, 7–10 days
Protozoa		
Entamoeba histolytica	Metronidazole 400 mg three times daily, 5 days	Paromomycin 25–35 mg/kg three times daily, 10 days
	Diloxanide furoate 500 mg three times daily, 10 days	

[†]And other third-generation cephalosporins; [**]usually only for bacteraemia; [‡]and other fluoroquinolones such as ofloxacin, norfloxacin, fleroxacin and cinoxacin.
TMP–SMX, trimethoprim–sulphamethoxazole; ?, still questioned.

Table 35.8. Antimicrobial chemotherapy for persistent infectious diarrhoea.

Enteropathogen	Drug regimen
Virus	
Cytomegalovirus	Ganciclovir 5 mg/kg every 12 h, 14–21 days
	Foscarnet 60 mg/kg every 8 h, 14–21 days
	Maintenance therapy may be required
Bacteria	(see Tables 35.1 and 35.6)
Protozoa	
Giardia intestinalis	Metronidazole 400 mg three times daily, 7–10 days, or tinidazole 2 g single dose
Cryptosporidium parvum	? Paromomycin 500 mg four times daily
Encephalitozoon intestinalis	Albendazole 400 mg (?800 mg)
Enterocytozoon bieneusi	twice daily, 14–28 days
Isospora belli	TMP–SMX, 2 tablets four times daily, 10 days
Cyclospora cayetanensis	TMP–SMX, 2 tablets twice daily, 7 days
Entamoeba histolytica	(see Table 35.6)
Helminths	
Strongyloides stercoralis	Albendazole 400 mg daily, 3 days
Schistosoma spp.	Praziquantel 40–60 mg/kg per day[†] in two or three doses on one day

[†]40 mg/kg per day for *Schistosoma mansoni* and *Sch. haematobium*; 60 mg/kg per day for *Sch. japonicum*.
TMP–SMX, trimethoprim–sulphamethoxazol.

sporidia have variable sensitivity to albendazole; there is increasing evidence that some microsporidal infections caused by *Encephalitozoon intestinalis* may be cured by albendazole, although *Enterocytozoon bieneusi* is resistant.

PREVENTION

A variety of approaches are available to avoid or prevent intestinal infection; these include interventions to minimize the entry of enteropathogens into the gastrointestinal tract, antimicrobial chemoprophylaxis, immunoprophylaxis, and the more experimental approaches of pro- and prebiotics (Table 35.9).

Avoidance

In principle, all intestinal infections can be avoided if infective microorganisms are not ingested. The usual advice should be followed with respect to uncooked food, focusing — particularly in the UK — on uncooked eggs (chocolate mousse, mayonnaise) and uncooked or partially cooked beef products (steak tartare, hamburgers). In addition, pre-cooked meats can be contaminated by EHEC when sold alongside uncooked beef products by the same retailer. Swimming-pool water, despite adequate chlorination, has been shown to be a vehicle for certain protozoan parasites (*G. intestinalis*, *Cryptosporidium parvum*) because cysts are relatively resistant to chlorination.

Table 35.9. Approaches to the prevention of infectious diarrhoea.

Approach	Specific measures	Reduction in attack rate (%)
Minimize entry of enteropathogens	Avoid uncooked/unpeeled food, ice cubes, tap water etc.	Unknown
	Avoid reheated food at room temperature	
	Food should be heated to more than 65°C	
	Beware swimming pools, lakes, and sea water	
Chemoprophylaxis	Doxycycline	75
Antibiotic	Co-trimoxazole	60
	4-Fluoroquinolones	>85
	(e.g. ciprofloxacin, norfloxacin, ofloxacin, fleroxacin)	
Non-antibiotic	Bismuth subsalicylate	60
Immunoprophylaxis	Vaccines	Unknown
Probiotics	*Lactobaccillus spp.*	Unknown

Prophylaxis

Antimicrobial chemoprophylaxis

A variety of broad-spectrum antimicrobial chemotherapeutic agents can reduce the attack rate of traveller's diarrhoea (16–18). Drugs shown to be effective in controlled clinical trials include sulphonamides, doxycycline, co-trimoxazole, trimethoprim, erythromycin, mecillinam, bicozamycin, and several 4-fluoroquinolone antibiotics. The prophylactic dose is usually 50% of the usual therapeutic dose that produces clinical efficacies of 70–90%. Thus, although the efficacy of antimicrobial chemoprophylaxis is not in doubt, its use is not widely recommended, because of the small, but nevertheless finite, risk of a potentially fatal complication, and because of concerns about increasing drug resistance. However, there may be situations in which chemoprophylaxis for short visits to highly endemic areas might be appropriate, providing the risks are fully discussed.

Non-antibiotic chemoprophylaxis

Bismuth subsalicylate is an effective, non-antibiotic approach to the prevention of traveller's diarrhoea, with an overall efficacy of about 60% (23). When it was available only in the liquid form, compliance was not easy, as a 3-week supply of the drug would add 5 kg to the traveller's luggage. A tablet formulation is now available, the best results being obtained when two tablets are taken four times daily, at meal times and on retiring. Although there are usually no immediate adverse effects, there are concerns about bismuth toxicity after long-term ingestion.

Immunoprophylaxis

A variety of vaccines for enteric infections have been developed or are under clinical evaluation. A reassortant, recombinant rotavirus vaccine has been shown to be effective in the developed world, and recent studies indicate that the simian reassortant is also effective in the developing world, providing several doses are given. However in 1999, rotavirus vaccination received a major setback following a number of reports of serious intussusception in a clinical trial in the USA. A live oral cholera vaccine is also soon to be available, which is based on the pathogenic *Vibrio cholerae* O1, in which the cholera toxin and other virulence genes have been deleted. A variety of oral vaccines are under development that might be useful for travellers and, ultimately, it might be reasonable to pursue a multivalent vaccine covering ETEC, *Salmonella spp.*, *Shigella spp.*, *Campylobacter jejuni*, and possibly some of the protozoal parasites.

Probiotics and prebiotics

The concept of colonizing the gastrointestinal tract with a harmless, but nevertheless protective, microflora in the form of *Lactobacillus spp.* or bifidobacteria is an attractive "natural" approach to the control of enteric infection. A number of lactobacillus strains have been developed and are able to colonize the human gastrointestinal tract. One isolate, *Lactobacillus* GG has been shown to produce modest protection in traveller's diarrhoea (24,25), but *L. acidophilus* and *L. fermentum* were shown to have no effect in a placebo-controlled study in Central America (26). Further studies are required to determine whether this approach has any future.

There is some evidence that feeding preferred bacterial substrates such as oligofructose can increase the numbers of "protective" microorganisms such as bifidobacteria. Again, further evidence is required to confirm that this approach will have clinical benefits.

References
1. Handszuh H, Waters SR. Travel and tourism patterns. In: *Textbook of Travel Medicine and Health*. Eds. HL DuPont, R Steffen. Hamilton: Decker, 1997.
2. Boyce TG, Swerdlow DL, Griffin PM. Escherichia coli O157:H7 and the hemolytic–uremic syndrome. *N Engl J Med* 1995; **333**: 364–368.
3. Farthing MJG, Kelly MP, Veitch AM. Recently recognised microbial enteropathies and HIV infection. *J Antimicrob Chemother* 1996; **37(suppl B)**: 61–70.
4. Neal KR, Brij SO, Slack RCB *et al*. Recent treatment with H2 antagonists and antibiotics and gastric surgery as risk factors for Salmonella infection. *BMJ* 1994; **308**: 176.
5. Neal KR, Scott HM, Slack RCB *et al*. Omeprazole as a risk factor for Campylobacter gastroenteritis: case-control study. *BMJ* 1996; **312**: 414–415.
6. Farthing MJG, Butcher PD. Mycobacterium tuberculosis and paratuberculosis. In: *Enteric Infection: Mechanisms, Manifestation and Management*. Eds. MJG Farthing, GT Keusch. London: Chapman & Hall, 1989; pp. 3–12.
7. Char S, Farthing MJG. DNA probes for diagnosis of gut infection. *Gut* 1990; **32**: 1–3.
8. Allison MC, Hamilton-Dutoit SJ, Dhillon AP *et al*. The value of rectal biopsy in distinguishing self-limited colitis from early inflammatory bowel disease. *Q J Med* 1987; **65**: 985–995.

9. Nostrant TT, Kumar NB, Appelman HD. Histopathology differentiates acute self-limited colitis from ulcerative colitis. *Gastroenterology* 1987; **92**: 318–328.

10. Rees JH, Soudain SE, Gregson NA *et al.* Campylobacter jejuni infection and Guillain–Barré syndrome. *N Engl J Med* 1995; **333**: 1374–1369.

11. Farthing MJG. History and rationale of oral rehydration and recent development in formulating an optimal solution. *Drugs* 1988; **36(suppl 4)**: 80–90.

12. Farthing MJG. Dehydration and rehydration in children. In: *Hydration Throughout Life*. Ed. MJ Arnaud. John Libbey Eurotext, 1998; pp. 159–173.

13. Thillainayagam AV, Hunt JB, Farthing MJG. Enhancing clinical efficacy of oral rehydration therapy: is low osmolality the key? *Gastroenterology* 1998; **114**: 197–210.

14. European Society for Paediatric Gastroenterology and Nutrition Working Group. Recommendations for composition of oral rehydration solutions for the children of Europe. *J Pediatr Gastroenterol Nutr* 1992; **14**: 113–115.

15. Farthing MJG. Prevention and treatment of travellers' diarrhoea. *Aliment Pharmacol Ther* 1991; **5**: 15–30.

16. Farthing MJG, DuPont HL, Guandalini S *et al.* Treatment and prevention of traveller's diarrhoea. *Gastroenterol Int* 1992; **5**: 162–175.

17. DuPont HL, Ericsson CD. Prevention and treatment of traveller's diarrhoea. *N Engl J Med* 1993; **328**:1821–1827.

18. Caeiro JP, DuPont HL. Management of traveller's diarrhoea. *Drugs* 1998; **56**: 73–81.

19. Salam I, Katelaris P, Leigh-Smith S *et al.* A randomised placebo-controlled trial of single dose ciprofloxacin in treatment of traveller's diarrhoea. *Lancet* 1994; **344**: 1537–1539.

20. Keusch GT. Antimicrobial therapy for enteric infections and typhoid fever: state of the art. *Rev Infect Dis* 1988; **10**: S199–S205.

21. Kelly MP, Farthing MJG. Infections of the gastrointestinal tract. In: *Antibiotic and Chemotherapy*. 7th edn. Eds. F O'Grady, HP Lambert, RG Finch, D Greenwood. London: Churchill Livingstone, 1997; pp. 708–720.

22. Kelly MP, Farthing MJG. Intestinal protozoa. In: *Current Therapy of Infectious Diseaes*. Ed. D Schloosberg. St Louis: Moseby, 1997; pp. 574–577.

23. Steffen R. World-wide efficacy of bismuth subsalicylate in the treatment of traveller's diarrhea. *Rev Infect Dis* 1990; **12(suppl 1)**: 80–86.

24. Oksanen PJ, Salminen S, Saxelin M *et al.* Prevention of traveller's diarrhoea by Lactobacillus. *Ann Med* 1990; **22**: 53–56.

25. Hilton E, Kolakowski P, Singer C *et al.* Efficacy of Lactobacillus GG as a diarrheal preventive in travellers. *J Travel Med* 1997; **4**: 41–43.

26. Katelaris P, Salam I, Farthing MJG. Lactobacilli to prevent traveller's diarrhoea. *N Engl J Med* 1996; **333**: 1360–1361.

Further reading

Farthing MJG, Keusch GT (Eds). *Enteric Infection: Mechanisms, Manifestations and Management*. London: Chapman & Hall Ltd, 1989.

Farthing MJG, Keusch GT, Wakelin D (Eds). *Enteric Infection: Mechanisms, Manifestations and Management, vol II: Intestinal Helminths*. London: Chapman & Hall Ltd, 1995.

Gracey M, Bouchier IAD (Eds). *Infectious Diarrhoea. Baillières Clinical Gastroenterology*, vol 7. London: Bailliere Tindall, 1993.

Farthing MJG. Travellers' diarrhoea. In: *Gastroenterological Problems from the Tropics*. Ed. CG Cook. London: BMJ Publishing Group, 1995; pp. 1–9.

Blaser MJ, Smith PD, Ravdin JI, Greenburg HG, Guerrant RL (Eds). *Infections of the Gastrointestinal Tract*. New York: Raven Press, 1995.

La Mont JT (Ed). *Gastrointestinal Infections: Diagnosis and Management*. New York: Marcel Dekker Inc., 1997.

36. Managing Inflammatory Bowel Disease in Outpatients

SIMON TRAVIS

INTRODUCTION

This chapter considers the management issues and clinical dilemmas associated with the treatment of outpatients with inflammatory bowel disease (IBD). It assumes a working knowledge of ulcerative colitis and Crohn's disease; readers seeking accounts of clinical features, investigation, and pathogenesis of IBD are referred to other texts (1,2).

The first two questions that arise in the clinic before treatment is considered are whether the diagnosis of IBD is correct, and whether symptoms are caused by active disease.

Diagnostic accuracy

The specific **diagnosis of IBD depends on four factors**:

- clinical features
- endoscopic appearance
- histopathology
- radiological imaging

When a patient is seen for the first time as an outpatient, it is good practice to review the records of all four factors, because the specific diagnosis influences the therapeutic approach, should disease become refractory. The **duration, distribution, and pattern of disease** should be established, as they also influence treatment. Apart from anything else, the diagnostic label has fundamental implications for the individual patient as far as job security, employment prospects, or life insurance are concerned.

Placing the clinical history in context

Table 36.1 draws attention to cases with diagnostic inconsistencies. The **history** is fundamental for interpreting investigations; for example, visible blood in the stool is so much the hallmark of ulcerative colitis that, if it is absent during active disease, the diagnosis is much more likely to be another form of colitis. This is most commonly Crohn's colitis (which causes diarrhoea without bleeding in 50% of patients), but may be indeterminate, microscopic, or infective colitis. Conversely, a diagnosis of Crohn's disease should be questioned if the history is very short (less than 3 weeks), or if there has been travel abroad, because the endoscopic and radiological features of yersinia ileitis or amoebic colitis can be identical.

Histopathology

Colonic biopsy examinations frequently fail to distinguish between ulcerative and Crohn's colitis. Adequate details about the history and site of biopsy (normal/abnormal colonic mucosa) are essential for interpretation of the biopsy findings (3). Two recognized features of ulcerative colitis that can trap the inexperienced are ill-defined granulomas in association with ruptured crypts, and an apparent skip lesion or "caecal patch" of inflammation. The rectum may also appear to be spared in ulcerative colitis, especially after local treatment, although microscopic inflammation is invariable.

Table 36.1. Discriminating features between ulcerative colitis and Crohn's disease.

	Ulcerative colitis	Crohn's disease
Clinical features		
Diarrhoea		
bloody	90–100%	Only 50% with colitis
non-bloody	Very rare, except in early stages	Very common
Abdominal pain	Usually mild, before defecation	Often severe, colicky
Weight loss	Only in severe attacks	Common
Pyrexia	Only in severe attacks	Common
Aphthoid mouth ulcers	Uncommon	Common, but oral Crohn's is rare
Abdominal mass	Exceptionally rare	Common
Perianal disease	Uncommon and uncomplex if present	Common and often complex
Endoscopic appearance		
Rectal sparing	Exceptionally rare	Common
Aphthoid/serpiginous ulcers	Never	Characteristic
Diffuse granularity	Characteristic	Uncommon
Histopathology		
Inflammatory infiltrate	Diffuse, mucosal	Discontinuous, transmural
Glandular architecture	Distorted; decreased crypt density	Relatively preserved
Crypt abscesses	Common	Uncommon or focal
Goblet-cell depletion	Common when active	Rare
Granulomata	Absent, except near ruptured crypt	Diagnostic if submucosal
Radiological imaging		
Distribution	Continuous, from rectum	Discontinuous
Symmetry	Symmetrical	Asymmetrical
Mucosa	Shallow ulcers	Deep "rose-thorn" ulcers
Strictures	Exceptional; suspect malignancy	Common
Fistulae	Exceptionally rare	Common
Suspicious features:	**No visible blood in stools**	**History <3 weeks**
question the diagnosis	Severe abdominal pain	Travel in Africa, Asia,
	Normal rectal histology	S. America
	CRP >100 mg/litre	CRP <10 mg/litre in active disease

CRP, C-reactive protein.

Indeterminate cases

Tuberculosis, Behçet's disease, carcinoma, lymphoma (especially in the immunocompromised), carcinoid, or infections can and do present with features similar to those of ileocaecal Crohn's disease. Further investigation — including a small-bowel enema (believed by many to be preferable to a barium follow-through), computed tomography (CT) scan, or magnetic resonance imaging (MRI), if available — is then appropriate, but diagnostic laparoscopy or laparotomy is necessary if imaging remains inconclusive. Sometimes, the best investigation is a period of time to allow the diagnosis to become apparent, rather than repeating or arranging invasive intestinal investigation. This is most appropriate when trying to distinguish infective colitis from ulcerative colitis that has presented with *Campylobacter spp.*, *Clostridium difficile*, or other infection. A subsequent relapse will clearly indicate idiopathic IBD.

In around 10% of patients it is impossible to distinguish ulcerative from Crohn's colitis, because the patient has features of both conditions. This condition is termed **indeterminate colitis** and the implication is that, should surgery become necessary, a subtotal colectomy should first be performed and the specimen examined by an experienced gastrointestinal histopathologist, before ileoanal pouch formation. When a diagnosis of indeterminate colitis is made on both clinical and histological criteria, the outcome of pouch surgery is similar to that seen in patients with a definitive diagnosis of ulcerative colitis.

In the future, serological diagnosis may have a greater role, as ulcerative colitis is strongly associated with perinuclear anti-cytoplasmic antibodies (pANCA), whereas Crohn's disease is associated with anti-*Saccharomyces cerevisiae* mannan antibodies (ASCA). In 201 patients with IBD and 167 control individuals, positive pANCA and negative ASCA serology had a 57% sensitivity and 93% positive predictive value for ulcerative colitis; positive ASCA and negative pANCA serology had a 49% sensitivity and 96% positive predictive value for Crohn's disease (4).

Defining active disease

Differential diagnosis of recurrent symptoms

The history is central to the interpretation of investigative findings, although in ulcerative colitis the presence of active disease is readily confirmed by sigmoidoscopy. Active Crohn's disease usually causes anorexia, malaise, weight loss, and often mouth ulcers or arthralgia, in addition to diarrhoea and abdominal pain. In the absence of these clinical features, other causes of diarrhoea and abdominal pain should be considered:

- bacterial overgrowth in Crohn's disease, for instance, causes explosive malodorous diarrhoea, often in the absence of systemic symptoms or abdominal pain
- bile-salt malabsorption is a relatively common cause of diarrhoea after ileal resection
- hypolactasia affects up to 20% of North Europeans and a greater proportion of Asians or Africans

- motility disorders may affect 20% or more of patients with chronic ulcerative colitis (5). Diagnostic criteria for functional gut disorders are difficult to apply in Crohn's disease, as disease activity is not so readily defined as in ulcerative colitis

Initial investigations

Confirmation of active disease should be routine before the initiation of treatment. In practice, this means performing a **sigmoidoscopy** in ulcerative colitis and checking inflammatory markers (C-reactive protein (CRP), plasma viscosity, or erythrocyte sedimentation rate (ESR)) in Crohn's disease. In ulcerative colitis, if the sigmoidoscopy is unexpectedly normal, a **flexible sigmoidoscopy** or **colonoscopy** should be arranged to investigate further any symptomatic relapse and exclude a carcinoma (Table 36.2). In Crohn's disease, if the clinical features favour a diagnosis of active disease, it is reasonable to initiate treatment with **steroids** pending the results of measurements of inflammatory markers; if these are normal, steroids are best withdrawn and other causes of symptoms investigated (Tables 36.3, 36.4).

Further investigations

Further small-bowel **radiology** is only justified when a surgical decision depends on the outcome, as the radiation exposure is considerable. The use of non-

Table 36.2. Diagnosis of recurrent diarrhoea in ulcerative colitis

	Investigation or action
Bloody	
Active disease	Rigid sigmoidscopy and biopsy
Infection	Stool microbiology and *Cl. difficile* toxin assay
Carcinoma	Flexible sigmoidoscopy/colonoscopy (when rectal sparing noted in clinic)
Drugs	Salicylates rarely exacerbate colitis. NSAIDs can provoke relapse
	Observe clinical pattern and response to withdrawal
Non-bloody	Sigmoidoscopy is essential, whether diarrhoea is bloody or not
Drugs	Many, including olsalazine; other salicylates less commonly
Hypolactasia	Lactose-free diet. Lactose-hydrogen breath test if in doubt
Concomitant disease	Consider coeliac disease, Giardia, pancreatic insufficiency
	Weight loss or anaemia are clues. Endoscopy, biopsy, ultrasound
Carcinoma	Pancolitis of more than 10 years duration, or anaemia are clues. Colonoscopy in refractory distal colitis
Poor rectal compliance	Anorectal manometry
Dysmotility (irritable bowel)	Concomitant bloating, pain. Dietary manipulation, anticholinergics

NSAIDs, non-steroidal anti-inflammatory drugs.

Table 36.3. Diagnosis of recurrent diarrhoea in Crohn's disease.

	Investigation or action
Increased inflammatory markers	
Active disease	Corticosteroids or appropriate alternative
Infection	Stool microbiology and *Cl. difficile* toxin assay
Complication (fistula, sepsis, etc.)	Small-bowel radiology, colonoscopy, CT scan
Normal inflammatory markers	
Hypolactasia	Lactose-free diet. Lactose–hydrogen breath test rarely helpful
Bacterial overgrowth	Metronidazole or ciprofloxacin for 1 week. Lactulose breath test uninterpretable after resection
Bile salt malabsorption	Trial of cholestyramine. SeHCAT test results abnormal after ileal resection
Enteroenteric fistula	Small-bowel radiology
Short bowel syndrome	Review surgical notes and small-bowel radiology
Mildly active disease	Isotope white-cell scan. Limited therapeutic trial of steroids
Concomitant disease	Consider coeliac disease, *Giardia*, pancreatic insufficiency. Weight loss or anaemia are clues. Endoscopy, biopsy, ultrasound
Drugs	Many. Review all medication
Excessive sorbitol	Ask about chewing gum, low-calorie drinks, or sweeteners
Dysmotility (irritable bowel)	Concomitant bloating, constant pain. Dietary manipulation, anticholinergic agents

SeHCAT, selenium homocholic acid–taurine.

Table 36.4. Diagnosis of recurrent abdominal pain in Crohn's disease.

	Investigation or action
Elevated inflammatory markers	
Active disease	Corticosteroids or appropriate alternative
Complication (abscess, etc.)	CT scan. (Suspect when CRP >200 mg/litre, or leucocytosis)
Normal inflammatory markers	
Fibrotic stricture	Small-bowel radiology. (History of intermittent colicky pain)
Gall stones	Ultrasound. (Reduced enterohepatic circulation of bile salts)
Renal calculi	Renal ultrasound/intravenous urography. (Hyperoxaluria if calcium binds to unabsorbed fat)
Pancreatitis	Amylase, ultrasound (?gallstones, azathioprine, salicylates, steroids)
Peptic ulcer	Endoscopy (?steroid-induced)
Dysmotility (irritable bowel)	Dietary manipulation, antispasmodics, anticholinergics

ionizing radiation in the form of **MRI scanning** is already valuable in evaluating perineal Crohn's disease (6) and may have a role in determining disease activity in the future. Some investigations (selenium homocholic acid–taurine (**SeHCAT**) scan for bile-salt malabsorption, or **hydrogen breath test** for bacterial overgrowth) are too cumbersome or difficult to interpret after previous surgery to be of use routinely, and therapeutic trials of cholestyramine or metronidazole are clinically justified. Occasionally, it is not possible to exclude active disease as a cause of persistent symptoms — in spite of clinical features, serological markers, contrast radiology, colonoscopy, and therapeutic trials of treatment. In these difficult cases, in which

a decision about continued treatment with steroids or immunosuppression is often essential, an **isotope scan** (white-cells labelled with technetium-99m, using a hexamethyl propylene amine oxime carrier) can help. This appeals as a relatively non-invasive technique for evaluating small-bowel and colonic inflammation, but many units have difficulty in achieving the diagnostic accuracy attained by specialist centres (7).

Disease activity indices

Indices of disease activity should provide an objective and reproducible measure of the severity of colitis or Crohn's disease in order to determine

Table 36.5. Criteria for disease activity in ulcerative colitis.

Feature	Mild	Moderate	Severe
Bloody motions/day	<4	4–6	>6
Heart rate	Normal	Normal	>37.8 beats/min on 2 days out of 4
Temperature	Apyrexial	Intermediate	>90 beats/min
Haemoglobin	Normal	Normal	<10.5 g/dl
ESR	<30 mm/h	<30 mm/h	>30 mm/h

appropriate treatment. Many have been designed, including Truelove & Witts' criteria, the Powell-Tuck Activity Score, or the Simple Clinical Colitis Index for ulcerative colitis (8), and the Crohn's disease Activity, Harvey Bradshaw, or van Hees indices for Crohn's disease (2). Regrettably, these are not widely used outside clinical trials, owing to their complexity or the subjectivity of their evaluation. The **criteria defined by Truelove & Witts** are an exception (Table 36.5): only a single criterion, in addition to a bloody stool frequency of more than six times daily, defines severe disease (9), although these criteria are open to criticism because there are insufficient gradations to monitor progress. What matters, however, is the initial assessment and treatment, so the Truelove & Witts criteria should be more widely used in daily practice. It is easy to underestimate the severity of ulcerative colitis.

MANAGEMENT OF ACUTE RELAPSE

Effective treatment reduces the risk of complications, so oral steroids are recommended in most circumstances, even for mild relapses. All too often, patients are expected to tolerate symptoms that are poorly controlled by local treatment and salicylates for many weeks or months, which is unnecessary. Primary nutritional therapy has a role in some patients with Crohn's disease; moreover, disease sometimes appears to relapse or remit independently of therapeutic approaches. Although recurrent or protracted relapses often indicate inadequate therapy, placebo-controlled trials indicate spontaneous remission in 11% of exacerbations of ulcerative colitis (with clinical improvement in another 30%) and remission in 30% of episodes of active Crohn's disease (10). The inpatient management of severe disease is discussed in Chapter 16.

Ulcerative colitis

Initial treatment

For proctitis and distal colitis, it is appropriate to use **topical steroid** or **mesalazine enemas** for about 2 weeks, before initiating oral corticosteroids if symptoms have not completely resolved. Mild disease of limited extent often resolves in response to such local treatment, without the need to resort to systemic therapy. **Topical mesalazine** (5-aminosalicylic acid (5-ASA)) is more effective than topical steroids for active distal disease, with 70% of patients responding over 3–6 weeks (11). This is independent of dose and preparation, with equivalent responses observed between 1-, 2-, and 4-g rectal preparations (12,13). The choice of suppository, foam, or liquid mesalazine for active distal disease depends on the patient's preference. However, because of the several-fold difference in cost between mesalazine and steroid foam preparations, many clinicians in the UK initiate treatment with topical steroids. There is little advantage in increasing the dose of oral salicylate during active disease.

Further treatment

If symptoms persist after a couple of weeks of local treatment, or if the patient has more extensive disease, oral steroids are indicated, as they are more rapidly effective. There are no data to provide guidance in determining the dose and duration of steroid treatment, but the regimens shown in Table 36.6 are tailored to the objective assessment of disease activity; 75% of patients following these regimens achieve remission within 2 weeks (14). Shorter courses of steroids may be associated with earlier relapse, and doses of 15 mg/day or less are ineffective. This response must be compared with remission rates of 60% after 4 weeks of olsalazine 1 g daily (15) and only 49% after 6 weeks of mesalazine

Table 36.6.   Treatment of active ulcerative colitis.

Treatment	Mild	Moderate	Severe
Prednisolone	20 mg/day for 1 month, 15 mg/day for 1 week, 10 mg/day for 1 week, 5 mg/day for 1 week,	40 mg/day for 1 week, 30 mg/day for 1 week, then as for mild attacks	Admit directly for intensive treatment
Mesalazine or steroid foam enemas	Twice daily until bleeding stops, then at night for 2 weeks	As for mild attacks	
Salicylate	Continue unchanged	Continue unchanged	

2.4 g daily (16), although the combination of oral and rectal **mesalazine** is more effective (17) than either alone. There are understandable reservations about steroids, especially in the USA, but rapid resolution of symptoms is usually the deciding factor for patients when these data are explained. Potential side-effects should be discussed with the patient, but are usually acceptable for the benefit conferred by control of symptoms. **Immunomodulating drugs** should be considered at an early stage if symptoms recur as the dose of steroid decreases, or within 6 weeks of cessation of treatment (see below).

Crohn's disease

Initial treatment

Active Crohn's disease is initially treated with **steroids** in a manner similar to that adopted for ulcerative colitis (Table 36.6). Patients with extensive small-bowel disease, ileal resection, or an ileostomy usually need soluble or non-enteric coated **prednisolone** (with a proton pump inhibitor if necessary for dyspeptic symptoms), as enteric coating delays absorption. Vomiting, severe pain, tachycardia, or hypoalbuminaemia usually indicate a severe attack necessitating the patient's admission to hospital to receive intravenous steroids.

Further treatment

As steroids are ineffective in maintaining remission, they should be withdrawn once the acute episode has settled. The risks of osteoporosis, or growth suppression in children, are thereby kept to a minimum, although it may well be that disease activity, and therefore the need for steroids, is the main factor in bone toxicity (see below). Neverthe-

less, attention has appropriately been directed at **steroids with low systemic bioavailability**, such as **budesonide**. Only about 10% of budesonide administered reaches the systemic circulation after first-pass metabolism, and this component is highly protein-bound, although adrenal suppression is still detectable. Several controlled trials have demonstrated an efficacy of budesonide similar to that of oral prednisolone in active disease, but there is a non-significant trend in favour of prednisolone. In the European study of budesonide 9 mg daily for 6 weeks compared with prednisolone tapered from an initial dose of 40 mg, the remission rates at 10 weeks were 53% with budesonide and 61% with prednisolone, ($P = 0.056$), in 186 patients (18). Budesonide is an order of magnitude more expensive than prednisolone, so most gastroenterologists in the UK reserve it for patients with ileal or ileo-ascending colonic disease who suffer side effects from prednisolone. A practical concern cautions against changing to budesonide without first tapering the dose of prednisolone, as the patient may present with adrenal insufficiency.

ALTERNATIVES TO CORTICOSTEROIDS FOR ACTIVE DISEASE

It is entirely appropriate to discuss the use of alternatives to corticosteroids before the patient starts treatment, or when disease appears steroid-dependent, or in answer to concerns expressed by patients or their relatives. Although steroids are currently the most effective treatment, their inadequacies must be recognized. Around 30% of patients do not respond to these drugs because of refractory inflammatory disease, difficulty in correlating symptoms with disease activity, or complications.

Nutritional therapy

Further details on this subject are to be found in Chapter 21.

Ulcerative colitis

No diet has been shown to alter the pattern of disease in ulcerative colitis, although a **high-fibre diet** may help avoid proximal constipation in patients with proctitis. A **lactose-free diet** may, however, reduce stool frequency if diarrhoea persists after treatment of active disease (Table 36.2).

Crohn's disease

Good nutrition is an important aspect of the management of Crohn's disease, but is itself usually achieved by controlling active disease. This general principle must be distinguished from primary nutritional therapy with **elemental or polymeric liquid diets**, which have been shown to be effective in active Crohn's disease. Steroids are, however, more effective. In a meta-analysis that included 413 patients from eight trials of steroids in comparison with nutritional therapy, clinical remission occurred in 81% of those receiving steroids, compared with 57% of those given nutritional therapy (19). The key issue is compliance with a liquid diet for 6–12 weeks, whether this is given orally or by overnight nasogastric intubation. Even in centres with a special interest, up to 55% of patients fail to complete maintenance studies. Fortunately, it is now apparent that more palatable polymeric feeds are as effective as elemental feeds, which improves compliance. There is some evidence that the effectiveness of polymeric liquid feeds is inversely related to the content of long-chain triglycerides; a controlled trial to test this hypothesis is under way.

An important issue is whether remission induced by nutritional therapy is better sustained than that induced by steroids. One study demonstrated that it was (20), but the meta-analysis found a relapse rate of 65% and 67% for both treatments (19). Consequently, primary nutritional therapy should be reserved for selected patients: these include children with small-bowel disease (see below), patients with extensive small-bowel disease or multiple resections in whom surgery is best avoided, or patients who can not tolerate or who resolutely decline steroids. A polymeric diet should be administered orally or by nasogastric tube for 6–12 weeks. Clinical experience shows that **percutaneous gastrotomy** in patients with Crohn's disease is safe, although it should be avoided in patients with gastroduodenal disease.

Immunomodulators

Immunosuppressants should be regarded as steroid-sparing agents, to enable the withdrawal of steroids while maintaining remission. Unfortunately, their potential toxicity is greater than that of steroids. Other immunomodulators such as anti-tumour necrosis factor (TNF) antibodies offer less toxic, but highly expensive, treatment in some circumstances (see Chapter 16). Table 36.7 summarizes aspects of immunosuppression in IBD.

Azathioprine

Azathioprine 2 mg/kg (or its metabolite 6-mercaptopurine 1.5 mg/kg) takes 6–12 weeks to exert an effect, but when it is used in refractory Crohn's disease, steroid reduction is possible in twice as many patients as is possible with placebo (21). Azathioprine is effective in maintaining remission: in a randomized trial, the postoperative clinical relapse rate was 53% in patients taking 6-mercaptopurine 50 mg/day for 2 years, which was significantly better than was achieved with mesalazine 3 g/day or placebo (22). It is also effective in ulcerative colitis and, once treatment is established, should be continued for 4 or 5 years; earlier withdrawal leads to a greater relapse rate (23). Attempts to induce a more rapid response by intravenous or topical therapy depend on the ability to measure the rate-limiting enzyme, thiopurine methyltransferase (24); however about 15% of patients can not tolerate purine analogues because of nausea or flu-like symptoms. Serious toxicity (pancreatitis, myelo-suppression) occurs in fewer than 5% of patients given azathioprine (25), except during concomitant allopurinol or co-trimoxazole therapy, which should be avoided. Patients should be warned to stop taking azathioprine if they develop sore throat or fever, and blood counts should be monitored regularly.

Cyclosporin

Cyclosporin 4–5 mg/kg is effective in about 60% of patients with severe ulcerative colitis who fail to respond to intravenous steroids (26). There are no

Table 36.7. Immunosuppression in inflammatory bowel disease.

Drug	Indications	Dose	Monitoring
Azathioprine	Established ulcerative colitis or Crohn's disease Relapse when prednisolone <15 mg/day Relapse <6 weeks after stopping steroids Need for steroids >4 months/year Recurrent postoperative relapse (?)	2 mg/kg per day (oral)	Full blood count after 2 weeks, at every clinic review and at 6–8 weekly intervals Clinic review at 6–8 weeks, then at 2–4 month intervals Dose reduction/stop if white cell count <3.5, $\times 10^9$/litre, or neutrophils <1.5 $\times 10^9$/litre
Cyclosporin	Ulcerative colitis, refractory to IV steroids Cholesterol >3.5 mmol, magnesium >0.8 mmol/litre	5 mg/kg per day (oral, after IV therapy)	Whole blood concentration 100–200 ng/ml Clinic review at 2–4 weeks then at 4–6 week intervals Creatinine, blood pressure at every clinic visit
Methotrexate	Active Crohn's disease (increased CRP, endoscopic or radiological confirmation) in spite of steroids Unable to tolerate or refractory to azathioprine Absence of need for early surgery Explicit advice to avoid pregnancy	15 mg/week, up to 25 mg (oral or IM)	Full blood count after 2 weeks, at every clinic review and with liver function tests at 4 weekly intervals Clinic review at 4–6 weeks, then at 2–3 month intervals
Anti-TNFα antibodies	Active Crohn's disease refractory to steroids and other immunomodulators, patients for whom surgery is inappropriate	5 mg/kg (single infusion)	Only at specialist centres

IV, intravenous; IM, intramuscular.

trials of cyclosporin that have initiated treatment in outpatients, but monitoring patients after a successful response to inpatient treatment is necessary to achieve whole blood concentrations of 100–200 ng/ml. Larger doses, concomitant treatment with azathioprine and duration of treatment beyond 12 weeks are associated with appreciable toxicity. Controlled trials have not shown consistent benefit of cyclosporin in refractory Crohn's disease (27).

Methotrexate

Methotrexate 15–25 mg/week by oral or intramuscular injection is an adjunct to steroid treatment for refractory Crohn's disease, but has no role in ulcerative colitis. In 141 patients whose Crohn's disease remained active in spite of the administration of steroids, remission was achieved in 39% after 16 weeks, compared with 19% given placebo (28).

Anti-TNF antibodies

A single infusion of **anti-TNF antibodies** 5 mg/kg provides a short-term response in refractory Crohn's disease, with remission maintained in 30–40% of patients after 12 weeks, and striking endoscopic improvement (29). At present, the role of anti-TNF antibodies is limited to Crohn's disease, especially

fistulating, that is refractory to other treatment, should surgery need to be avoided. The clinical and endoscopic responses to recombinant interleukin-10 in Crohn's disease, although significant, are disappointing (30). Neither of these cytokine agents has fulfilled their initial promise in ulcerative colitis.

Surgery

Surgery is an important part of a therapeutic strategy in both ulcerative colitis and Crohn's disease. Except in emergencies, the timing should be carefully planned with patients and surgical colleagues. It is a viable and appropriate alternative to steroids when disease is refractory or side effects from medical treatment are unacceptable, but is best performed by a gastrointestinal surgeon with a special interest in IBD.

Ulcerative colitis

Indications are discussed in a later section, but surgery implies a **total colectomy**. Segmental resection of limited disease, ileo–rectal anastomosis, or subtotal colectomy leaving a rectal remnant invariably leads to recurrent symptoms, in addition to a persistent risk of neoplasia (31). This is not surprising, given that the disease always involves the rectal mucosa. Although **pouch surgery** is now the operation of choice for patients who maintain good continence during acute exacerbations, **proctocolectomy with a permanent ileostomy** remains an option for patients with poor continence, or those who do not want to risk pouch dysfunction. Expectations must be realistic, although surgery potentially allows withdrawal of steroids and immunosuppression, removes the risk of cancer and improves the quality of life. The prevalence of stomal complications from a permanent ileostomy for ulcerative colitis was 75% in one study over 20 years (32), with intestinal obstruction in 23% and stomal revision necessary in 28% of patients. Pouch surgery does not lead to normal bowel function, because although a good outcome (in 90% of patients) removes urgency and unpredictability, the frequency of evacuation is three to six times daily. This compares very favourably with a permanent ileostomy or active disease, but around 70% of patients thus treated have a complication necessitating readmission to the hospital in the 5 years after surgery, up to 30% develop pouchitis and excision of the pouch is necessary in about 10% (33).

Crohn's disease

Surgery is more commonly necessary in Crohn's disease, but is not curative: 70% of patients will have an operation within 15 years of diagnosis, and 36% will have required two or more operations (34). Much depends on the site of disease, as ileocaecal disease more commonly causes obstructive symptoms requiring surgery than does colonic disease. The range of procedures is beyond the scope of this text, but a few points need to be made. Resection should be as limited as possible: there is no place for a "cancer-type" right hemicolectomy when an ileocaecal resection will relieve obstruction; nor is there a need to resect all macroscopic disease, because a stricturoplasty to relieve a localized (<5 cm) stricture is as effective as resection. **Bowel preservation** should be the rule and, in refractory Crohn's colitis, placement of a defunctioning ileostomy for 12 months allows resolution of disease and successful re-anastomosis in up to 50% of the patients, thus avoiding colectomy. In those in whom **colonic resection** is necessary, segmental resection is often possible, but an ileo–rectal anastomosis should be considered only if the rectum is spared. Lastly, experienced surgeons

measure the remaining length of small-bowel from the duodenojejunal flexure, and recognize that mucosal strictures can be overlooked unless luminal patency is checked by passing ball-bearings or a Foley catheter 2–2.5 cm in diameter down the length of the small bowel. Both these practices should be encouraged.

Relapse after surgery is common, but care must be taken to define the type of relapse. Clinical relapse (60–70% at 2 years) is of most interest to patients and physicians, whereas endoscopic relapse (almost universal within 2 years) provides an objective measure for postoperative trials, although some refer to relapse requiring further surgery (around 50% at 10 years after resection). These issues should be discussed with the patient when considering the relative merits of surgery and steroids, in addition to discussion of appropriate postoperative maintenance therapy (below).

Salicylates

It is controversial to suggest that oral salicylates have a **limited role** in the treatment of active ulcerative colitis, but nevertheless this is the case. Dose-ranging studies have produced conflicting results (35), with no consistent benefit from higher doses in inducing remission (36). Although there is no doubt that salicylates are better than placebo, the evidence does not support doubling the dose of salicylate at the onset of a relapse. Oral salicylates, with or without steroid enemas, take longer to work and are less effective than salicylate enemas or decisive treatment with steroids for acute ulcerative colitis.

Similarly, in acute Crohn's disease, whereas high doses of salicylates (mesalazine 4 g daily for 16 weeks) are more effective than placebo (37), the benefit is limited compared with that from oral corticosteroids. In contrast, there is some evidence that high doses of mesalazine help maintain postoperative remission in Crohn's disease.

Other steroids with low systemic bioavailability

Apart from **budesonide** (see above) designed for ileal release, a different delayed-release formulation has been developed for **colonic release** in ulcerative colitis, although this is not yet commercially available

(38). **Prednisolone metasulphobenzoate**, currently available as an enema (Predfoam), is also being developed in tablet form for treatment of colonic inflammation, because it is poorly absorbed from the colon.

Antibiotics

Antibiotics have no place in the treatment of ulcerative colitis, whatever its severity. Controlled trials of metronidazole, tobramycin, and ciprofloxacin, amongst others, have not shown consistent significant benefit either in active disease or in maintaining remission. In Crohn's disease, however, in which it can be difficult to distinguish active disease from septic complications, metronidazole is appropriate when there is perineal disease or a fever. Some antibiotics (metronidazole and, possibly, clarithromycin) may have an immunomodulatory role in addition to an antibacterial action (39). Antituberculous chemotherapy has not been shown to benefit Crohn's disease in controlled trials (40).

CHOICE OF MAINTENANCE THERAPY

Ulcerative colitis

Salicylates reduce the annual rate of relapse three- to fourfold (41). The question is not so much *whether* they should be prescribed after a first attack of ulcerative colitis, but *which* salicylate, and for how long. The pharmacokinetics and distribution of disease, efficacy, side-effect profile, and cost need to be considered in order that rational therapeutic decisions be made.

Considerations

Pharmacokinetics
Prodrugs (such as sulphasalazine, olsalazine, and balsalazide) have an azo bond that is split by colonic bacteria to release 5-ASA, the active component. This means that they are not released in the small intestine and have a particular role in distal colitis, as luminal concentrations of 5-ASA, probably reflecting tissue concentrations, are greater than those achieved with slow-release mesalazine (42). Controlled-release preparations release 5-ASA in the ileocaecal region (Asacol, coated with an acrylic-based resin, Eudragit-S,

which rapidly dissolves at pH greater than 7.0) or distal jejunum/ileum (Salofalk (UK)/Claversal (Europe)/Rowasa (USA), coated with Eudragit-L, which dissolves at pH greater than 6.0). Once released, 5-ASA acts on the enterocyte or colonic epithelial cell, where it is acetylated. This process is readily saturated, leading to absorption of intact 5-ASA, so the serum concentrations of 5-ASA at ordinary maintenance doses are three- to sixfold greater with controlled-release than with azo-bonded compounds (43). Whether this matters is debated, but it seems reasonable to favour a salicylate with a low systemic load of 5-ASA. Slow-release mesalazine (Pentasa) is coated with ethylcellulose microgranules, which gradually release 5-ASA, starting in the jejunum. Serum concentrations of 5-ASA are similar to those obtained with azo-bonded preparations.

Efficacy
None of the new salicylates is more effective than **sulphasalazine** in maintaining remission. A meta-analysis of maintenance treatment revealed an odds ratio of 0.85 (95% confidence interval (CI) 0.64 to 1.15) when mesalazine was compared with sulphasalazine (36). There have been, however, very few comparative trials between the new salicylates. One trial found **olsalazine** to be more effective than mesalazine (Asacol) in the patients selected. Care must be taken in interpreting this study of 100 patients with left-sided colitis, because it was ended earlier than planned and had an unexpectedly high relapse rate (46% in those receiving mesalazine at 12 months, and 34% in those taking olsalazine) (44). However, the findings are in keeping with the relatively enhanced delivery to the distal colon that is achieved with olsalazine. A comparison of an azo-bonded compound and mesalazine in active disease led to similar conclusions. **Balsalazide** was more effective than 5-ASA for patients with active (predominantly distal) colitis (45).

It is, consequently, logical to select an azo-bonded compound as maintenance therapy for proctitis, distal, or left-sided colitis. (Why the choice and dose of salicylate does not appear to matter for more extensive colitis is an interesting question, but is likely to have something to do with the pathobiology of events at the leading edge (proximal limit) of inflammation; after all, the reason for the sharp demarcation of inflammation in limited colitis has yet to be explained.) If delivery of 5-ASA to the site of inflammation is important, topical treatment may be better than oral therapy. Topical application of 5-ASA as a liquid, foam, or suppository is undoubtedly effective in maintaining remission (12), but is less popular with patients, which is likely to affect compliance, even when suppositories are used on alternate days (13). Topical treatment to maintain remission is therefore best reserved for patients who suffer relapse frequently in spite of oral maintenance therapy.

Duration of treatment

An early study demonstrated that the relapse rate reverted to the frequency observed before treatment, even after sulphasalazine had been continued for 15 years (46). This has been confirmed by other (but not all) studies (41), and a study comparing ulcerative colitis complicated by carcinoma with matched controls found that salicylates taken for at least 3 months significantly protected against cancer (relative risk 0.38; 95% CI 0.20 to 0.69) (47). This strongly favours **long-term maintenance therapy**, but patients in prolonged remission often ask about stopping salicylates, or simply do so of their own accord. The risk of relapse in the next year is approximately inversely related to the duration of remission. One suggestion is that, when a patient has been in remission for 2 years, the nuisance (and potential hazard) of continued therapy outweighs the benefit (48).

Side-effect profile

Eighty per cent of patients tolerate sulphasalazine at the normal maintenance dose of 2 g daily, but one problem encountered is the very occasional occurrence of severe, sometimes fatal, **reactions** to this drug. All the newer salicylates are better tolerated than sulphasalazine. Conversely, renal failure is recorded more frequently with pH-dependent-release mesalazine, and probably persists even when corrected for relative frequency of prescribing. **Nephrotoxicity** appears to be an idiosyncratic reaction (49), but is sufficiently rare that it should influence prescribing only when other factors (pre-existing renal disease, cardiac failure, concomitant use of non-steroidal anti-inflammatory drugs) are present. In these circumstances, pH-dependent-release compounds are best avoided. Whichever 5-ASA preparation is chosen, it is likely to be used for many years or decades. The clinician must be alert to insidious reactions, including late nephrotoxicity, through long-term follow-up, with monitoring of the creatinine concentration, full blood count, and liver function tests on each visit. Other idiosyncratic reactions include **diarrhoea**, which affects around 10% of patients taking olsalazine. This can be disabling, but it can be used to therapeutic advantage: proximal constipation complicates distal colitis or proctitis.

Cost

Considerations of cost are an inescapable part of current prescribing practice. Any figures will be out of date by the time of publication of this volume, but the UK National Health Service costs of all the new salicylates at standard doses are between three- and fourfold greater than a year's prescription of sulphasalazine 2 g daily. This difference amounts to several hundred pounds sterling per patient per year for drugs that will be continued for many years in a large number of patients (typically 500–600 in a district general hospital). As many patients are prescribed higher than standard doses, costs are very appreciable.

Choice

Taking all these factors into consideration, my personal practice is to institute maintenance therapy for ulcerative colitis with sulphasalazine 2 g daily, except in those with a history of drug sensitivities (any previous sensitivity will increase susceptibility to an adverse reaction), or other consideration (such as oligospermia in potential fathers). Patients are warned about relatively common side effects (nausea, headaches, rash) and the need to have a blood test if a sore throat or flu-like symptoms develop. A review appointment is made for 4–6 weeks ahead, when the full blood count, creatinine concentration, and liver function tests are checked. For the 20% or so who can not tolerate sulphasalazine, olsalazine 1 g daily is an appropriate alternative for distal colitis and slow-release mesalazine (Pentasa 1.5 g or Asacol 1.2 g daily) for more extensive disease. Occasionally, there will be patients who can not tolerate any of the salicylates. A few of these will have extended remission without treatment, but if relapses occur more than twice a year, azathioprine is the drug of choice.

Crohn's disease

Many of the considerations concerning the choice of salicylate apply equally well to Crohn's disease. The main differences are that higher doses are necessary and that salicylates are of greater benefit in preventing postoperative relapse than in maintaining medically induced remission. Stopping smoking is probably as effective as any maintenance therapy.

Preventing postoperative relapse

Smoking

In a retrospective study of Crohn's disease, 43% of 144 smokers suffered relapse within 5 years of their first operation, compared with 26% of 143 non-smokers (relative risk 3.1; 95% CI 1.7 to 5.8) (50). The adverse effects of smoking were more pronounced in women, and multiple operations were required in almost 11 times as many smokers as non-smokers. Other studies have drawn similar conclusions.

Drug prophylaxis

Salicylates may, at best, halve the rate of postoperative relapse, but daily doses less than 2 g are ineffective and as much as 4 g may be necessary (41). In one study, mesalazine (Asacol) 2.4 g daily started within 6 weeks of surgery, led to a 55% reduction in severe endoscopic recurrence at 2 years and a corresponding reduction in clinical relapse (51). In another, the endoscopic recurrence rate at 6 months was 31% in patients taking mesalazine (Salofalk/Rowasa) 3 g daily, compared with 41% in those receiving placebo (52). This benefit, while small, is of both clinical and statistical significance, and patients should be prescribed **mesalazine 2–3 g daily** as maintenance therapy for 12 months after surgery. There is, of course, no point in expecting an azo-bonded compound to prevent relapse in small-intestinal disease or an ileo–rectal anastomosis. **Azathioprine** may prove to be more effective than salicylates (22), and should certainly be considered in patients undergoing a second or subsequent operation within 1 or 2 years. Some centres always advise covering surgical procedures with steroids for 1 month, to reduce the risk of an exacerbation in the postoperative period, although this is supported only by anecdotal reports.

Maintaining medically induced remission

In contrast to their effectiveness against postoperative relapse, salicylates probably confer an advantage of only 10% over placebo for medically induced remission (53); routine maintenance treatment with salicylates for patients with Crohn's disease is therefore difficult to justify. Budesonide may help maintain remission (54), although further studies are awaited. Patients should be encouraged to stop smoking, but the most effective pharmacological treatment for preventing recurrent relapse is azathioprine (see above).

INDICATIONS FOR IMMUNOSUPPRESSION

Immunosuppression (Table 36.7) should be considered when patients with ulcerative colitis or Crohn's disease suffer relapse of their disease as steroids are withdrawn (characteristically, when the dose of prednisolone has been decreased to less than 15 mg/day), or within 6 weeks of completing a course of steroids. In ulcerative colitis, **maintenance salicylates** should be continued. It is reasonable to make one further attempt at controlling active disease with steroids and tapering the dose more gradually (by 5 mg every 2 weeks, for example), but increasing awareness of the benefit of **azathioprine** in maintaining remission and manageable toxicity has lowered the threshold for immunosuppression. Because of the delayed action azathioprine, it is appropriate to give a standard course of **prednisolone** (Table 36.6) when azathioprine is begun. Other drugs have more limited applications, and should not be used outside specialist centres. Careful monitoring is essential, with explicit guidance to the general practitioner.

INDICATIONS FOR SURGERY

Ulcerative colitis

Three main indications are well recognized:

1. severe colitis unresponsive to intensive treatment (see Chapter 16)
2. chronic persistent symptoms in spite of or dependent on steroids

3. complications such as dysplasia or frank malignancy

Approach to elective colectomy

The second indication above accounts for the majority of patients, and it is among this group that the patient's views are most important. **Discussion about surgery** is best undertaken in stages. The severity of symptoms (stool frequency, interference with occupation or domestic life) should be carefully discussed, along with realistic expectations of the results. It is helpful to discuss the place of surgery in the management strategy at a relatively early stage with patients who are having troublesome colitis, then to reintroduce it later should immunosuppression fail. The stomatherapist is then contacted for preliminary discussions, followed by an initial surgical consultation, before a final decision is made with the patient. Patients who are soon to have an ileoanal pouch constructed usually appreciate meeting someone of a similar age and sex who has already had undergone the operation. This staged approach allows the patient time to come to terms with the prospect of surgery, while giving time for further medical treatment to work. If surgery proves unnecessary, patients benefit from a greater understanding of the practicalities, in addition to knowing that there is a management strategy rather than delaying difficult decisions until they become unavoidable.

Crohn's disease

Indications for surgery in Crohn's disease include active disease continuing to cause symptoms in spite of medical therapy, strictures causing mechanical obstruction, fistulae, or other local complications such as abscess or perforation. The **timing of elective surgery** is often more difficult than in ulcerative colitis, but, once again, a staged approach helps to avoid repeated courses of steroids and inadequate responses; obstructive pain is most readily managed in this way. The **management** plan should be discussed with the patient, and should include treatment of active disease and review of symptoms after 4–6 weeks. Further immunosuppression (steroids and azathioprine) is reasonable if symptoms are initially well controlled but recur as steroids are reduced, before repeat imaging (small-

bowel radiology), a low-residue diet, and surgery, if obstructive symptoms persist. Surgical decisions are easier if small-bowel radiology shows pre-stenotic dilatation (indicating long-standing strictures) or fistulae, because medical treatment is then unlikely to be effective. It is more difficult if pain is not explained by findings of the investigations. Imaging should be reviewed and a small-bowel enema performed if the clinical history is consistent with obstruction, despite an unremarkable barium follow-through.

SPECIAL SITUATIONS

A variety of management issues arise sufficiently commonly in outpatients that the principles of management require to be outlined, even though the details are beyond the scope of this text.

Children and adolescents

Paediatric IBD is a specialty in its own right, and referral to a tertiary centre is always appropriate if there is doubt about management. With the exception of considerations concerning growth, however, the management is more notable for its similarities to than differences from that in adult practice.

Diagnosis

Crohn's disease is broadly as prevalent as ulcerative colitis in young patients, but cases of indeterminate colitis more commonly turn out to be Crohn's disease than is true in adult practice. One important differential diagnosis not seen in adults is sensitivity to cow's milk protein, which may cause a florid, haemorrhagic colitis shortly after cow's milk has been introduced to the infant's diet. Investigation is best performed by an experienced endoscopist, with both **upper gastro-intestinal endoscopy**, to take small intestinal and gastric biopsy samples, and **colonoscopy** for terminal ileal and serial colonic biopsy specimens (55). This allows a more specific diagnosis than is achieved by barium enema. **Contrast radiology** should be limited to small-bowel studies. A negative **isotope scan** (above) helps in the avoidance of invasive investigation in children, but a positive scan is inadequate for initial diagnosis.

Growth and management

When Crohn's disease affects the small bowel, extensive and proximal disease appears to be more common in children than in adults. **Growth retardation** is a substantial problem, and 30% of children with IBD will be below the fifth centile for height at some stage (56). For this reason, height and weight should be measured routinely and documented on a centile chart at every clinic visit. Growth-velocity charts are more sensitive measures of growth impairment, and are appropriate for complex paediatric cases. The reason for growth failure is largely nutritional and related to disease activity, rather than to the use of steroids (56). Even so, treatment of children aims to minimize steroid use, with primary nutritional therapy favoured for small-bowel Crohn's disease and a lower threshold for surgical intervention (57,58). Growth retardation should be considered to be an indication for early surgery, unless it is rapidly reversed by medical treatment. Relevant surgical procedures include resection or stricturoplasties in Crohn's disease, and colectomy for ulcerative colitis. Pouch surgery in older children (no younger than 8 years) should be performed only at specific specialist centres, but can be very successful.

Adolescence

Adolescence can bring its own problems in the search for personal autonomy — including, in patients with IBD, the rejection of parental support, poor compliance with treatment, and disregard of diet, rather than appear to succumb to unsociable symptoms. The patient's individuality must be respected, and reassurance given that, although it may be delayed, normal height and maturity are almost always achieved (59). Careful consideration must be given to the timing of investigation or surgery with respect to schooling, as successful completion of scholastic exams affects the individuals's employment prospects, which may be put at a disadvantage by a diagnosis of IBD.

Fertility and pregnancy

Fertility

Female fertility is almost normal, apart from a small group who have tubal obstruction as a result of pelvic sepsis in Crohn's disease. In men, the only recognized adverse affect relates to sulphasalazine, which causes reversible oligospermia. Sulphasalazine should be stopped and an alternative salicylate prescribed to men who are planning a family.

Pregnancy

This important issue is covered in detail elsewhere in this volume (Chapter 9). Pregnancy has no predictable effect on the activity of ulcerative colitis or Crohn's disease. Although about 50% of affected women have a better quality and duration of remission, a notable minority (10–15%) have more severe exacerbations. Careful **sigmoidoscopy** is safe in pregnancy. When Crohn's disease appears to present in pregnancy, non-ionizing imaging techniques such as **MRI scanning** at a specialist centre may be helpful in making a diagnosis. The postpartum period is, however, a peak time for relapse and it is sensible to anticipate this by making a clinic appointment for about 4 weeks after the delivery. The greatest risk to pregnancy is active disease, rather than active treatment (60–62).

Breast feeding

Medication is an appropriate source of anxiety when a mother is breast feeding, but **salicylates** appear to be safe, even though the pharmaceutical literature continues to advise caution. Moderate doses of **steroids** may induce cosmetic or other effects in the infant, but breast feeding is desirable rather than essential, and the option of bottle feeding can be discussed. Perceptions vary and maternal views must be taken into account.

Osteoporosis

Cause

Bone density is reduced in both ulcerative colitis and Crohn's disease. This is as much the result of disease activity as it is a consequence of steroid treatment. In those with newly diagnosed Crohn's disease, bone density is already significantly lower than that in age-matched controls, and there is little individual variation in the year after diagnosis, whether or not steroids are used (63). Some studies have found an association between osteoporosis and cumulative dose of steroid over a decade, although this, too, may reflect disease activity.

Treatment

It is possible to halt, or even reverse, the osteopenia that is associated with IBD. An adequate **calcium** intake is important for all patients, and patients taking a lactose-free diet should have calcium supplements (Calcichew, 2 tablets daily). **Hormone replacement therapy** is appropriate for postmenopausal women suffering recurrent relapses who require systemic steroids for more than 4 months in a year, or in those needing multiple operations. **Biphosphonates** are usually well tolerated, despite cautions from the manufacturers concerning potential gastrointestinal side effects, and are appropriate for men or premenopausal women in similar circumstances. Bone densitometry is helpful when there is doubt, but, logically, it should be used in many patients at an early stage in their disease, to determine who will benefit from treatment. Whether this is appropriate or cost effective is uncertain.

MANAGEMENT DILEMMAS

Refractory distal colitis

Approach

Refractory distal colitis can be defined as symptoms caused by colitis distal to the sigmoid-descending junction that persist despite oral and topical steroids for 6–8 weeks. Others have defined refractoriness as an incomplete response to topical steroids and oral salicylates (64), but this might also be interpreted as inadequate initial treatment (above). The situation will be familiar, because such patients are frequent attenders in outpatient departments and, paradoxically, patients with proctitis appear to be over-represented. A consistent approach is essential to avoid a series of haphazard therapeutic trials that are demoralizing to patients and their doctors. The differential diagnosis should first be considered, followed by a trial of mesalazine enemas, treatment of proximal constipation, colonoscopy to reassess the extent of disease, then admission for intensive treatment of persistent symptoms and, finally, surgery.

Treatment strategy

The differential diagnosis includes mucosal prolapse (solitary rectal ulcer syndrome), which may mimic

proctitis, as may radiation proctitis. Rarely, infections (*Chlamydia spp.*, or opportunistic infections in the immunocompromised) may mimic proctitis, but a co-existent irritable bowel commonly accounts for more symptoms than active disease. **Mesalazine** enemas or suppositories for proctitis are often effective when steroids (oral or topical) fail, although the combination of both may be best (65). Proximal constipation may delay the resolution of distal disease. Although there have been no trials to confirm this, when a patient with refractory distal colitis has faecal loading visible on a plain radiograph, administration of **sodium picosulphate** (a sachet of Picolax or Fleet Phosphosoda) may be followed by rapid clinical improvement. When patients remain symptomatic, **colonoscopy** is appropriate to reassess the diagnosis and the extent of disease, and to exclude malignancy. Persistent inflammation is then best treated by admitting the patient to hospital for **intensive treatment**, which was effective in 90% of a group of 39 patients refractory to outpatient treatment (66). **Azathioprine** may then be introduced to maintain remission (Table 36.7).

Alternative treatments including local anaesthetic gels, arsenic suppositories, bismuth enemas, rectal sucralfate, and nicotine patches, amongst others — are of anecdotal interest. Should active colitis persist in spite of the approach outlined above, **colectomy** is appropriate. Of 498 patients who had distal colitis at presentation, 9% came to colectomy in the first year of diagnosis, followed by 1% in subsequent years; this does, however, reflect an active surgical approach to refractory disease (67).

Colonoscopic surveillance

Chapter 34 considers this subject in detail.

Risk of cancer

The risk of colorectal cancer complicating ulcerative colitis has been overestimated, probably because earlier reports came from specialist centres in which patients with extensive colitis were over-represented. As a result of population-based studies, the lifetime risk has been identified as about 10% for extensive ulcerative colitis (or 0.5% per year after the first decade of symptoms). In Denmark, however, the risk over a 25-year period (3.5%) was the same as that in the general population (3.7%), probably because of their surgical approach to treating refractory disease (68). The incidence of colorectal cancer is not increased in distal colitis, although there may be proximal extension of disease in 15–30% of affected patients. For Crohn's disease, the same applies: the risk has not been found to be increased in population-based studies, but referral centres report that patients with extensive Crohn's colitis have an increased risk, similar to that associated with ulcerative colitis of the same extent and duration (34,69).

The value of surveillance colonoscopy in IBD

This topic remains controversial, because the anticipated benefit of surveillance programmes has been difficult to demonstrate. A further perspective will be found in Chapter 34.

In 12 surveillance programmes of 1916 patients, 92 cancers were identified (70). Of these, 52 cancers were early (Dukes' stages A or B), but only 24 were identified during surveillance colonoscopy, rather than during colonoscopy for the investigation of symptoms. If cancers diagnosed at first surveillance colonoscopy were excluded, only 13 were genuinely detected during surveillance, at a cost of 476 colonoscopies for each cancer detected. This is discouraging; however, this analysis took little account of dysplasia, arguing that its detection and interpretation in colitis were uncertain; there is a substantial (20–50%) risk that high-grade dysplasia will be detected once low-grade dysplasia has developed although, in 25% of colitis-related cancer, no dysplasia can be detected at a site separate from the tumour. In a subsequent study of 332 patients, nine of 21 with dysplasia proved to have cancer (71). Taking into account dysplasia and cancers identified by surveillance, this study predicted that 66 colonoscopies were required for each "useful" result. It has to be pointed out, however, that surveillance (biennial colonoscopy) missed six of 20 cancers, with an interval of 10–23 months from the most recent colonoscopy. Lastly, a case–control study of colorectal cancer in ulcerative colitis showed that those patients who died were less likely to have had the benefits of surveillance than were controls with the same extent and duration of disease (72).

Clinical practice

Given the uncertain benefit and possible failure of colonoscopic surveillance, the issues are best discussed with those patients who have extensive ulcerative colitis, to determine their views. Some will prefer to avoid regular colonoscopy and accept the small risk of cancer; others will wish to have anxieties allayed by surveillance colonoscopy. In view of the risk of proximal extension of distal disease, it is appropriate to undertake colonoscopy in all patients 8–10 years after the onset of their disease, to re-evaluate the extent of the disease. Biennial (2-yearly) colonoscopy can then be offered to those with extensive colitis, for as long as colectomy remains an appropriate therapeutic option. Whatever the choice, it is important that patients (and doctors) understand that surveillance is not fail-safe and that new symptoms or anaemia should be investigated. Any patient who develops low-grade dysplasia on two occasions, high-grade dysplasia, or a dysplasia-associated lesion or mass should be offered colectomy. This means that long-term follow-up for patients with extensive colitis is necessary — a view that is supported by the observation that patients who developed colorectal cancer had often been lost to specialist follow-up (70). There is a need to be able to target patients at higher risk of cancer more effectively than by simply determining the extent and duration of disease.

Prognosis

Mortality

Prospective population-based studies have shown that life expectancy, the risk of cancer, and working capacity are very much better than previously reported and are normal for many patients with ulcerative colitis or Crohn's disease (see (73) for a review). Three population-based studies in ulcerative colitis have shown a mortality similar to or slightly less than that in the general population, except in the first year after diagnosis, when the difference is attributable to a small number who present with severe pancolitis. Two other studies have shown a slightly greater mortality (standardized mortality ratio (SMR) 1.4), except in those with proctitis. In Crohn's disease two studies have also shown a slightly greater mortality, which is similar to that of manual labourers (SMR 1.43) from all causes of death. Another three studies have shown no overall increase in mortality, apart from patients with extensive small-intestinal jejunoileal or gastroduodenal disease (SMR 3.5 and 5.9, respectively). In contrast, those with localized ileocaecal disease had a particularly good life expectancy (SMR 0.53).

Surgery

Operation rates vary between centres, with a colectomy rate for ulcerative colitis over 25 years of between 11 and 38%. Patients have a normal life expectancy after colectomy. Furthermore, a relatively high colectomy rate in Copenhagen has probably been the major factor in reducing the incidence of cancer in ulcerative colitis (69). In the case of Crohn's disease, the majority of patients will need surgery (49% at 5 years, 61% at 10 years, 70% at 15 years after diagnosis), especially those with ileocaecal disease, but only about 30% need more than one operation (35). About 10% of patients with Crohn's colitis require an ileostomy.

Working capacity

After the first year, when work is often disrupted, about 90% of patients with ulcerative colitis are fully capable of work; after 10 years, more than 90% of patients are able to work (67). There are fewer data concerning Crohn's disease, but 75% of patients in one population-based study, were able to work normally; 15% who had had Crohn's disease for more than 5 years were disabled, compared with 4% of the general population. This means that it is possible to be relatively optimistic in advising patients, but the key to maintaining working capacity is to ensure that therapeutic decisions are made in good time. When employment has been lost as a result of refractory symptoms, it is much more difficult for the individual concerned to find new employment.

CLINIC ORGANIZATION AND ANCILLARY SUPPORT

Effective outpatient care is enhanced by an open-access appointment system, timing of the clinic, follow-up arrangements, and other details.

Open access appointments

Patients can make these appointments directly; they complement regular review and provide a large measure of reassurance to patients that they will not have to tolerate miserable symptoms for months. Clear advice is needed in the event of a relapse, to avoid undermining the involvement of the general practitioner. Patients should first see their family doctor, but if symptoms have not resolved completely within a couple of weeks, a clinic appointment is appropriate.

Clinic timing

It helps if medical and surgical gastroenterology clinics run simultaneously, to facilitate joint decisions on the management of refractory colitis, perineal Crohn's disease, or other problems. A dietetic clinic at the same time is an added advantage. If the joint histopathology or radiology meeting follows the clinic, so much the better.

Follow-up

Continuity is important, because this helps to avoid deferring decisions on refractory symptoms. The neurosis often attributed to patients with IBD may be partly the result of a lack of continuity of care, with different doctors trying different treatments without an overall management strategy. One way of achieving continuity is to make patient's medical notes available to the doctor before the clinic, with a Consultant review every third visit. Shared care with the general practitioner is attractive once local guidelines have been agreed. Regular follow-up in a specialist clinic is, however, still appropriate.

Ancillary support

A specialist nurse practitioner is a considerable bonus in supporting outpatient care. Continuity of care is facilitated, because such a person tends to remain in one post for longer than is the case for most junior doctors. A direct point of contact for patients is also provided, rather than their making contact through an overworked medical secretary. Information leaflets and videos are often welcomed by patients, but must always be supported by individual explanation, or confusion will arise. Last, and by no means least, patient support groups such as the National Association for Colitis and Crohn's disease (NACC), in the UK offer excellent practical assistance at a local level.

References

1. Fiocchi C. Inflammatory bowel disease: etiology and pathogenesis. *Gastroenterology* 1998; **115**: 182–205.
   An authoritative review; 273 references.

2. Forbes A. Epidemiology, aetiology and pathogenesis. In: *Inflammatory Bowel Disease*. London: Chapman & Hall, 1997; pp. 5–44.
   Excellent, well-referenced monograph on IBD.

3. Jenkins D, Balsitis M, Gallivan S *et al. Guidelines for the initial biopsy diagnosis of suspected chronic idiopathic inflammatory bowel disease*. British Society for Gastroenterology: 1997.

4. Quinton J-F, Sendid B, Reumax D *et al.* Anti-Saccharomyces cerevisiae mannan antibodies combined with anti-neutrophil cytoplasmic autoantibodies in inflammatory bowel disease: prevalence and diagnostic role. *Gut* 1998; **42**: 788–791.
   A useful study that requires confirmation, because analytical techniques vary between laboratories.

5. Nyam DC, Pemberton JH, Camilleri M *et al.* Irritable bowel syndrome in patients with chronic ulcerative colitis: coexistence creates a clinical conundrum. *Gastroenterology* 1996; **110**: A725.

6. Haggett PJ, Moore NM, Shearman JD *et al.* Pelvic and perineal complications of Crohn's disease: assessment using magnetic resonance imaging. *Gut* 1995; **36**: 407–410.
   A comparative study of examination under anaesthetic and MRI. One false-negative MRI result in 25 patients.

7. Weldon MJ, Lowe C, Joseph AEA *et al.* Review article: quantitative leukocyte scanning in the assessment of inflammatory bowel disease activity and its response to therapy. *Aliment Pharmacol Ther* 1996; **10**: 123–132.
   A good review of isotope scanning, but advocates its widespread use, whereas many clinicians would recommend it as a selective basis.

8. Walmsley RS, Ayres RCS, Pounder RE *et al.* A simple clinical colitis activity index. *Gut* 1998; **43**: 29–32.

9. Travis SPL, Farrant JM, Rickerts C *et al.* Predicting outcome in severe ulcerative colitis. *Gut* 1996; 38: 905–910.
   A prospective study of 51 episodes. Provides a clinically useful index based on stool frequency and CRP for identifying patients likely to come to surgery at that admission.

10. Ilnycyj A, Shanahan F, Anton PA *et al.* Quantification of the placebo response in ulcerative colitis. *Gastroenterology* 1997; **112**: 1854–1858.
    A review of 38 placebo-controlled trials. Clinical remission occurred in 9.1% (95% CI 6.6 to 11.6) and clinical improvement in 26.7% (95% CI 24.1 to 29.2) of those taking placebo.

11. Lee FI, Jewell DP, Mani V *et al.* A randomised trial comparing mesalazine and prednisolone foam enemas in patients with acute distal ulcerative colitis. *Gut* 1996; **38**: 229–233.
    A trial involving 295 patients. There was remission in 52% those treated with mesalazine foam, and 31% of those given steroid foam enema, after 4 weeks.

12. Campieri M, Gionchetti P, Rizello F *et al.* Optimum dosage of 5–aminosalicylic acid as rectal enemas in patients with active ulcerative colitis. *Gut* 1991; **32**: 929–931.
    A study of 113 patients. No significant difference was achieved between 1-, 2-, 4-g enemas in distal colitis, although all were better than placebo.

13. Marteau P, Crand J, Foucault M *et al.* Use of mesalazine slow-release suppositories 1 g three times per week to maintain remission of ulcerative proctitis: a randomised double blind placebo controlled multicentre study. *Gut* 1998; **42**: 195–199.
    The 12-month relapse rate was 48% in the treatment group and 62% in the placebo group (*P* = 0.018), among 95 patients.

14. Truelove SC, Watkinson G, Draper G. Comparison of corticosteroid and sulphasalazine therapy in ulcerative colitis. *BMJ* 1962; **2**: 1708–1711.

15. Feurle GE, Theuer D, Velasco G *et al.* Olsalazine versus placebo in the treatment of mild to moderate ulcerative colitis: a randomised double–blind trial. *Gut* 1989; **30**: 1354–1361.
    A trial involving 105 patients. Improvement was achieved for endoscopic score, rather than in clinical symptoms.

16. Riley SA, Mani V, Goodman MJ *et al.* Comparison of delayed release 5–aminosalicylic acid (mesalazine) and sulphasalazine in the treatment of mild to moderate ulcerative colitis relapse. *Gut* 1988; **29**: 669–674.
    A study of 61 patients, with remission in 43% receiving mesalazine 2.4 g daily after 4 weeks.

17. Safdi M, De Micco M, Sninsky C *et al.* A double-blind comparison of oral versus rectal mesalazine versus combination therapy in the treatment of distal ulcerative colitis. *Am J Gastroenterol* 1997; **92**: 1867–1871.
    A study involving 60 patients. Combination therapy was better than either treatment alone, evaluated by a disease activity index.

18. Rutgeerts P, Lofberg R, Malchow H *et al.* A comparison of budesonide with prednisolone for active Crohn's disease. *N Engl J Med* 1994; **331**: 842–845.

19. Griffiths AM, Ohlsson A, Sherman PM *et al.* Meta-analysis of enteral nutrition as a primary treatment of active Crohn's disease. *Gastroenterology* 1995; **108**: 1056–1067.
    In eight trials (413 patients), enteral nutrition was inferior to steroids (odds ratio (OR) 0.35; 95% CI 0.23 to 0.53). In five trials (134 patients), elemental feed was similar to non–elemental feed (OR 0.87, 95% CI 0.41 to 1.83).

20. Riordan AM, Hunter JO, Cowan RE *et al.* Treatment of active Crohn's disease by exclusion diet: East Anglia multicentre controlled trial. *Lancet* 1993; **342**: 1131–1134.
    A trial in 136 patients treated with elemental feed. The rate of withdrawal was 31%. Responders were then assigned at random to receive an exclusion diet or steroids. Median remission was 3.8 months with steroids and 7.5 months by diet (*P* = 0.048).

21. Pearson DC, May GR, Fick GH *et al.* Azathioprine and 6-mercaptopurine in Crohn's disease: a meta-analysis. *Ann Intern Med* 1995; **122**: 132–142.
    In nine trials, azathioprine or 6-mercaptopurine were better than placebo for active disease (OR 3.09, 95% CI 2.45 to 3.91) and maintaining remission (OR 2.27, 95% CI 1.76 to 2.93).

22. Korelitz B, Hanauer S, Rutgeerts P *et al.* Post-operative prophylaxis with 6-MP, 5-ASA or placebo in Crohn's disease: a 2 year multicenter trial [abstract]. *Gastroenterology* 1998; **114**: A4141.

23. Bouhnik Y, Lemann M, Mary J-Y *et al.* Long term follow up of patients with Crohn's disease treated with azathioprine or 6-mercaptopurine. *Lancet* 1996; **347**: 215–219.

A follow-up study of 157 patients. Cumulative relapse rate was 11% at 1 year and 32% at 5 years on therapy; 42 patients stopped treatment; with relapse rates of 38% and 75% at 1 and 5 years.

24. Van Os EC, Zins BJ, Sandborn WJ *et al.* Azathioprine pharmacokinetics after intravenous, oral, delayed release oral and rectal foam administration. *Gut* 1996; **39**: 63–68.
Study in healthy volunteers. Interesting therapeutic potential.

25. Connell WR, Kamm MA, Ritchie JK, Lennard-Jones JE. Bone marrow toxicity caused by azathioprine in inflammatory bowel disease: 27 years experience. *Gut* 1993; **34**: 1081–1085.

26. Scholmerich J. Immunosuppressive treatment for refractory ulcerative colitis — where do we stand and where are we going? *Eur J Gastroenterol Hepatol* 1997; **9**: 842–849.
A useful review; 96 references.

27. Jewell DP, Lennard-Jones JE and the cyclosporin study group of Great Britain and Ireland. Oral cyclosporin for chronic active Crohn's disease. *Eur J Gastroenterol Hepatol* 1994; **6**: 499–505.

28. Feagan BG, Rochon J, Fedorak RN *et al.* Methotrexate for the treatment of Crohn's disease. *N Engl J Med* 1995; **332**: 292–297.
(See text for details.) Total withdrawals were 17% in the methotrexate group (nausea 6%, abnormal liver function 7%) and 2% in the placebo group.

29. Targan SR, Hanauer SB, Van Deventer SJ *et al.* A short-term study of chimeric monoclonal antibody cA2 to tumor necrosis factor α for Crohn's disease. *N Engl J Med* 1997; **337**: 1029–1035.
The largest of two anti-TNFα antibody trials. The other, using a human (rather than murine) monoclonal antibody, showed similar results (*Lancet* 1997; **349**: 521–524).

30. Van Deventer SJH, Elson CO, Fedorak RN. Multiple doses of intravenous interleukin-10 in steroid-refractory Crohn's disease. *Gastroenterology* 1997; **113**: 383–389.
Remission was achieved in up to 50% after 7 days treatment in 46 patients; a 23% response to placebo in 3 weeks is surprising in a "steroid-refractory" group.

31. Varma JS, Browning GGP, Smith AN *et al.* Mucosal proctectomy and coloanal anastomosis for distal ulcerative proctocolitis. *Br J Surg* 1987; **74**: 381–383.
A report on only four patients, but it supports numerous anecdotes of the limitations of segmental resection.

32. Leong AP, Londono-Schimmer EE, Phillips RK. Life-table analysis of stomal complications following ileostomy. *Br J Surg* 1994; **81**: 727–729.
An actuarial analysis of 150 patients with end-ileostomy. There were stomal complications in 56% of those with Crohn's disease, 75% of those with ulcerative colitis, over 20 years.

33. Melville DM, Ritchie JK, Nicholls RJ *et al.* Surgery for ulcerative colitis in the era of the pouch: the St Mark's Hospital experience. *Gut* 1994; **35**: 1076–1080.
A retrospective study of 422 patients who underwent colectomy, 1976–1990.

34. Munkholm P, Langholz E, Davidsen M *et al.* Intestinal cancer risk and mortality in patients with Crohn's disease. *Gastroenterology* 1993; **105**: 1716–1723.

An excellent population-based study of 363 patients followed for 25 years.

35. Riley SA. What dose of 5-aminosalicylic acid (mesalazine) in ulcerative colitis? *Gut* 1998; **42**: 761–763.
Leading article. Brief for the complexity of the topic, but it covers the major issues well; 42 references.

36. Sutherland LR, May GR, Shaffer EA. Sulfasalazine revisited: a meta-analysis of 5-aminosalicylic acid in the treatment of ulcerative colitis. *Ann Intern Med* 1993; **118**: 540–549.
This study demonstrates little benefit from higher doses of salicylates for acute relapse or maintenance therapy. Newer salicylates are no more effective than sulphasalazine, although side effects are fewer.

37. Singleton JW, Hanauer S, Gitnick G *et al.* Mesalamine capsules for the treatment of active Crohn's disease: results of a 16 week trial. Pentasa Crohn's Disease Study Group. *Gastroenterology* 1993; **104**: 1295–1301.
A trial in 310 patients. Remission occurred in 43% of those receiving 4 g mesalazine daily, and 18% of those given placebo.

38. Lofberg R, Danielsson A, Suhr O *et al.* Oral budesonide versus prednisolone in patients with active extensive and left-sided ulcerative colitis. *Gastroenterology* 1996; **110**: 1713–1718.
A study of 72 patients treated for 9 weeks with 10 mg budesonide or 40 mg prednisolone. Endoscopic scores were similar between the groups, but fewer data are given as to the clinical response.

39. Peppercorn MA. Is there a role for antibiotics as primary therapy in Crohn's ileitis? *J Clin Gastroenterol* 1993; **117**: 235–237.

40. Thomas GAO, Swift GL, Green JT *et al.* Controlled trial of antituberculous chemotherapy in Crohn's disease: a five year follow up study. *Gut* 1998; **42**: 497–500.
A long-term follow-up of 130 patients, showing no influence on number of relapses, surgery, or medical therapy.

41. Travis SPL, Jewell DP. Salicylates for inflammatory bowel disease. *Baillière's Clin Gastroenterol* 1994; **8**: 203–231.
A review of salicylate treatment in ulcerative colitis and Crohn's disease, including mode of action; 159 references.

42. Christensen LA, Fallingborg J, Jacobsen BA *et al.* Comparative bioavailability of 5-aminosalicylic acid from a controlled release preparation and azo-bond preparation. *Aliment Pharmacol Ther* 1994; **8**: 289–294.
Useful study on the pharmacokinetics of salicylates.

43. Laursen LS, Stokholm M, Bukhave K *et al.* Disposition of 5-aminosalicylic acid by olsalazine and three mesalazine preparations in patients with ulcerative colitis: comparison of intraluminal colonic concentrations, serum values and urinary excretion. *Gut* 1990; **31**: 1271–1276.

44. Courtney M, Nunes D, Bergin C *et al.* Randomised comparison of olsalazine and mesalazine in prevention of relapses in ulcerative colitis. *Lancet* 1992; **339**: 1279–1281.

45. Green JR, Lobo AJ, Holdsworth CD *et al.* Balsalazide is more effective and better tolerated than mesalamine in the treatment of acute ulcerative colitis. The Abacus Study Group. *Gastroenterology* 1998; **114**: 15–22.

46. Dissanayake AS, Truelove SC. A controlled therapeutic trial of long-term maintenance treatment of ulcerative colitis with sulphasalazine. *Gut* 1973; **42**: 497–500.

47. Pinczowski D, Ekbom A, Baron J *et al.* Risk factors for colorectal cancer in patients with ulcerative colitis: a case control study. *Gastroenterology* 1994; **14**: 923–926.

48. Ardizzone S, Molteni P, Bollani S *et al.* Guidelines for the treatment of ulcerative colitis in remission. *Eur J Gastroenterol Hepatol* 1997; **9**: 836–841.

49. Thuluvath PJ, Ninkovic M, Calam J *et al.* Mesalazine-induced interstitial nephritis. *Gut* 1994; **35**: 1493–1496.

50. Breuer-Katschinski BD, Hollander N, Goebell H. Effect of smoking on the course of Crohn's disease. *Eur J Gastroenterol Hepatol* 1996; **8**: 225–228.

51. Caprilli R, Andreoli A, Capurso L *et al.* Oral mesalazine (5-aminosalicylic acid, Asacol) for the prevention of postoperative recurrence of Crohn's disease. *Aliment Pharmacol Ther* 1994; **8**: 35–43.

52. McLeod RS, Wolff BG, Steinhart AH *et al.* Prophylactic mesalamine treatment decreases postoperative recurrence of Crohn's disease. *Gastroenterology* 1995; **109**: 404–413.

53. Messori A, Brignola C, Trallori G *et al.* Effectiveness of 5-aminosalicylic acid for maintaining remission in patients with Crohn's disease: a meta-analysis. *Am J Gastroenterol* 1994; **89**: 692–698.
    A study concluding that minimal (10%) benefit is obtained from salicylates for medically induced remission in small-intestinal disease.

54. Lofberg R, Rutgeerts P, Malchow H *et al.* Budesonide prolongs time to relapse in ileal and ileocaecal Crohn's disease. A placebo controlled one year study. *Gut* 1996; **39**: 82–86.
    Budesonide extended the median time to relapse after medically induced remission in 176 patients, but at 12 months there was no significant difference between budesonide (3 mg or 6 mg) and placebo.

55. Cameron DJ. Upper and lower gastrointestinal endoscopy in children and adolescents with Crohn's disease: a prospective study. *J Gastroenterol Hepatol* 1991; **6**: 355–358.

56. Hildebrand H, Karlberg J, Kristiansson B. Longitudinal growth in children and adolescents with inflammatory bowel disease. *J Ped Gastroenterol Nutr* 1994; **18**: 165–173.

57. Beattie RM, Schiffrin EJ, Donnet-Hughes A *et al.* Polymeric nutrition as the primary therapy in children with small bowel Crohn's disease. *Aliment Pharmacol Ther* 1994; **8**: 609–616.
    A small descriptive study of seven children; the findings have been confirmed by subsequent experience.

58. Shand WS. Surgical therapy of chronic inflammatory bowel disease in childhood. *Baillière's Clin Gastroenterol* 1994; **8**: 149–180.

59. Ferguson A, Sedgwick DM. Juvenile onset inflammatory bowel disease: height and body mass index in adult life. *BMJ* 1994; **308**: 1259–1263.
    A follow-up study of 87 children previously (more than 5 years earlier) admitted to hospital with inflammatory bowel disease. All those with ulcerative colitis had normal height and body mass index, and fewer than 10% with Crohn's were of short stature.

60. Connell WJ. Safety of drug therapy for inflammatory bowel disease in pregnant and nursing women. *Inflammatory Bowel Diseases* 1996; **2**: 33–47.

61. Diav-Citrin O, Park YH, Veerasuntharam M, *et al.* The safety of mesalamine in human pregnancy: a prospective controlled cohort study. *Gastroenterology* 1998; **114**: 23–28.

62. Modigliani R. Drug therapy for ulcerative colitis during pregnancy. *Eur J Gastroenterol Hepatol* 1997; **9**: 854–857.

63. Ghosh S, Cowen S, Hannan WJ *et al.* Low bone mineral density in Crohn's disease but not ulcerative colitis at diagnosis. *Gastroenterology* 1994; **107**: 1031–1039.

64. Jarnerot G, Lennard-Jones JE, Bianchi-Porro G *et al.* Management of refractory distal ulcerative colitis. *Gastroenterol Int* 1991; **4**: 94–98.
    An expert review of the dilemmas, although now somewhat dated; little more evidence-based medicine has been published to confuse the issue.

65. Mulder CJJ, Fockens P, Meijer JWR *et al.* Beclomethasone diproprionate (3 mg) versus 5-aminosalicylic acid (2 g) versus the combination of both (3 mg/2 g) as retention enemas in active ulcerative proctitis. *Eur J Gastroenterol Hepatol* 1996; **8**: 549–554.

66. Jarnerot G, Rolny P, Sandberg-Gertzen H. Intensive intravenous treatment of ulcerative colitis. *Gastroenterology* 1985; **89**: 1005–1013.
    A model clinical study of practical value, confirming reported therapy and clinical experience.

67. Langholz E, Munkholm P, Davidsen M *et al.* Course of ulcerative colitis: analysis of changes in disease activity over years. *Gastroenterology* 1994; **107**: 3–11.
    The best population-based epidemiological study.

68. Langholz E, Munkholm P, Davidsen M *et al.* Colorectal cancer risk and mortality in patients with ulcerative colitis. *Gastroenterology* 1992; **103**: 1444–1451.

69. Gillen CD, Walmsley RS, Prior P *et al.* Ulcerative colitis and Crohn's disease: a comparison of the colorectal cancer risk in extensive colitis. *Gut* 1994; **35**: 1590–1594.

70. Axon ATR. Cancer surveillance in ulcerative colitis — a time for reappraisal. *Gut* 1994; **35**: 587–589.
    Leading article. (See text.)

71. Connell WR, Lennard–Jones JE, Williams CB *et al.* Factors influencing the outcome of endoscopic surveillance for cancer in ulcerative colitis. *Gastroenterology* 1994; **107**: 934–944.

72. Karlen P, Kornfeld D, Brostrom O *et al.* Is colonoscopic surveillance reducing colorectal cancer mortality in ulcerative colitis? A population-based case control study. *Gut* 1998; **42**: 711–714.
    Among cancer patients who died 5% had received a surveillance colonoscopy, compared with 18% of controls (relative risk 0.29; 95% CI 0.06 to 1.31).

73. Travis SPL. Insurance risks in patients with ulcerative colitis and Crohn's disease: prognosis and pattern of disease. *Aliment Pharmacol Ther* 1997; **11**: 51–59.

37. Motility Disorders of the Oesophagus and Stomach

OWEN EPSTEIN

INTRODUCTION

Motility and sensory disorders of the gastrointestinal tract are frequently encountered in gastroenterological practice, yet they are usually given low priority and are poorly taught in most training programmes. Indeed, when considering "difficult gastroenterology" it is likely that, on close reflection, many gastroenterologists would mention "non-cardiac chest pain, non-ulcer dyspepsia and the irritable bowel syndrome". These and other sensorimotor disorders of the alimentary tract deserve a high profile in gastrointestinal practices, as up to 50% of patients will present with them. It is likely that these disorders will become increasingly important with the decline in acid–pepsin related disorders of the foregut as a result of the introduction of eradication therapy for peptic ulcer disease, and the widespread use of effective antisecretory medication in gastrooesophageal reflux disease.

This chapter reviews the more common motility disorders of the oesophagus and stomach. Relevant clinical anatomy of the oesophagus and stomach is described in Chapter 3.1, and tests of oesophageal and gastric function, together with investigations of gastrointestinal motility are considered in Chapter 50.

Normal oesophageal motility (peristalsis)

The initiation of **swallowing** is both complex and of great clinical importance. As the food or liquid passes through the pharynx and into the hypopharynx, a series of neuromuscular reflexes ensures that the path into the ventilatory tract is closed. A highly coordinated sequence of muscular contractions then occurs: the circular muscle contracts above the bolus as the longitudinal muscle contracts to shorten the oesophagus. The sequential contraction and relaxation of the oesophagus ensure a smooth wave of contraction, which moves in a caudal direction.

Peristaltic contraction is constant at a rate of 2–4 cm/s. Primary peristalsis is initiated by swallowing, whereas secondary peristalsis is stimulated by distension of the lumen at any level, and clears the oesophagus of retained food or gastric refluxate. Within approximately 2 s of swallowing, and before the bolus reaches the distal oesophagus, the lower oesophageal sphincter relaxes for approximately 6–8 s. This sphincter has a resting pressure of approximately 20 mmHg, which decreases to gastric pressures with relaxation. The tone of the lower sphincter is influenced by gastrin, motilin, cholecystokinin and nitric oxide. The role of gastrin is controversial, but cholecystokinin and nitric oxide have roles in relaxation of the sphincter.

An interesting phenomenon occurring in the peristaltic mechanism is "**deglutition inhibition**". If a second swallow is initiated whilst an earlier peristaltic contraction is in progress through the striated muscle, there is rapid and complete inhibition of the initial swallow. However, if the initial swallow has been transmitted to the smooth muscle of the oesophagus, it may proceed, but its amplitude diminishes rapidly. A further observation is that, when swallowing occurs at a series of short intervals, the oesophagus remains quiescent and the lower oesophageal sphincter remains relaxed throughout.

MOTILITY DISORDERS OF THE OESOPHAGUS

Symptoms

Patients may complain of difficulty swallowing and a sensation of food "sticking" in the gullet (dysphagia). The motility disorders may also present with retrosternal pain or discomfort, with or without associated dysphagia and are often confused with ischaemic myocardial pain. Whereas stricturing disease of the oesophagus is usually accompanied by weight loss, this is not a striking feature of the motility disorders. Other symptoms include heartburn and passive regurgitation of food.

Primary motility disorders

Cricopharyngeal dysfunction

Cricopharyngeal dysfunction may cause dysphagia and regurgitation and may underlie the development of a **pharyngeal pouch**. The pouch usually presents in men in mid-life. The usual site of herniation occurs in the midline between of the oblique fibres of the inferior pharyngeal constrictor and the cricopharyngeal muscle. These pulsion pouches are believed to be caused by impaired compliance of the upper oesophageal sphincter (1).

Achalasia of the cardia (see also chapter 14)

This disorder is caused by **functional failure of the oesophagus**. The condition is unusual, occurring in a approximately 1 patient per 100 000 population per year. The disorder presents in adults and has no particular association with either sex. Achalasia resembles the oesophageal involvement in Chagas' disease caused by *Tryponosoma cruzi* which is an endemic parasite in some areas of South America; however, Chagas' disease causes multisystem disease (including cardiac myopathy and involvement of the remainder of the alimentary tract), achalasia is a condition that localizes to the oesophagus.

Achalasia is characterized by increased pressure in the lower oesophageal sphincter, failure of the sphincter to relax completely with swallowing, and complete loss of smooth-muscle peristalsis. The disorder is believed to be caused by **postganglionic denervation of the smooth-muscle component** of the oesophagus. There is a reduction in the number of myenteric ganglionic cells, and inflammation within the myenteric plexus (2). Impairment of the inhibitory neurones appears to be an early manifestation of the disease. In this early phase of the disorder, before the oesophagus has dilated, there is impaired relaxation in both the body of the oesophagus and the lower oesophageal sphincter. Recently, failure of non-adrenergic–non-cholinergic neurones that utilize nitric oxide and vasoactive intestinal peptide as inhibitory neurotransmitters have been implicated. Nitric oxide synthetase is not present at the gastrooesophageal junction in patients with achalasia, and an animal model of the disease has been produced using nitric oxide inhibitors.

Clinical presentation

Patients may present with dysphagia, non-cardiac chest pain, passive regurgitation of food, and aspiration pneumonia. They often report that they attempt to stimulate the passage of food into the stomach by drinking copious amounts of fluid. As the oesophagus dilates, food and fluid are retained within the atonic organ and may regurgitate passively, especially when the patient lies in the supine position.

Diagnosis

Oesophageal manometry is the "gold standard" for diagnosing achalasia, especially in the early stage of the disease. Only about 67% of patients with manometric achalasia have characteristic radiological features, and fewer than 33% of cases are suspected on endoscopic examination (3).

The hallmark of achalasia is **loss of peristalsis and incomplete relaxation of the lower oesophageal sphincter**. This is shown on manometry in almost all patients with achalasia. In the majority of patients (80%), the lower oesophageal pressure is increased (greater than 30 mmHg), and lower oesophageal sphincter relaxation is absent, incomplete, or of abnormally short duration. Simultaneous low-amplitude non-propagated waves dominate, especially in the distal oesophagus. Increased intraoesophageal baseline pressure supports the diagnosis. However, in early disease there may be normal sphincter pressure and activity, but with characteristic pressure and peristaltic profiles in the body.

The **X-ray appearance** is characterized by dilatation of the oesophagus, with an air–fluid level. The lower oesophageal sphincter narrows sharply, giving the appearance of a bird's "beak"; the spastic sphincter does not open with a swallow. Primary achalasia must be differentiated from secondary achalasia, which may have similar manometric and radiological findings. This results from direct infiltration of the oesophageal sphincter by an adenocarcinoma of the gastric fundus and cardia, and may account for the symptoms of up to 5% of patients who have characteristic manometric features of primary achalasia. Consequently, it is usual practice for patients with achalasia to undergo **diagnostic endoscopy**.

Treatment
A number of therapeutic options are available to treat patients with achalasia. **Drug treatments**, including calcium-channel blockers and nitrates have been tried but in practice, any effect is transient and usually ineffective in patients with more progressive disease. Recently, **injection of botulinum toxin** into the lower oesophageal sphincter has been used as a treatment. This endoscopic technique destroys cholinergic neurones, thus restoring the balance between stimulatory and inhibitory input. This approach does seem to be quite helpful but the disorder appears to relapse and repeated injections are required. Currently, **pneumatic dilatation** (with Witzel or Rigiflex dilators) or **surgical myotomy** are favoured treatments. Forceful pneumatic dilatation provides long-term relief in 70–80% of patients. The response is immediate, but between 20 and 50% of patients may require the procedure a second time, and there is a 2–10% risk of perforation using forceful dilatation. A postdilatation pressure of less than 10 mmHg is associated with excellent long-term remission (4). A laparoscopic approach to surgical myotomy is now possible. Previously, the open Heller myotomy required relatively major surgery, but the laparoscopic myotomy in experienced hands appears to be effective, with little morbidity or mortality. Currently, most patients with achalsia are treated by forceful dilatation.

Motility disorders primarily affecting the body of the oesophagus

Clinical presentation
Spastic disorders of the oesophagus present with **non-progressive dysphagia** for both solids and liquids, and may be accompanied by **chest pain**, which may mimic angina (non-cardiac chest pain). Weight loss is not a dominant symptom.

Diagnosis
Disturbed oesophageal peristalsis in the spastic disorder has quite distinct radiological and manometric profiles when compared with those of achalasia. The oesophagus continues to propagate primary peristaltic waves for at least a proportion of the time studied, and there are no pathognomonic radiological findings. There is also a range of manometric abnormality.

In classical **diffuse oesophageal spasm**, manometry demonstrates frequent simultaneous non-peristaltic contractions separated by periods of normal peristalsis; the abnormality must be present for more than 20–30% of wet swallows. Multipeaked waves occur, contractions may be prolonged, spontaneous contractions occur, and the pressure generated may be greater than 180 mmHg. The lower oesophageal sphincter functions normally. On X-ray, classical diffuse oesophageal spasm may appear as a "corkscrew" oesophagus. It is important to recognize that simultaneous oesophageal contractions may be observed in asymptomatic individuals; however, in healthy controls, simultaneous contractions always account for fewer than 30% of swallows (5). Classical diffuse oesophageal spasm is diagnosed in approximately 1–5% of patients with chest pain.

Nutcracker oesophagus is recognized as the most common motility disorder associated with non-cardiac chest pain. This disorder is recognized on manometry by very-high-amplitude peristaltic contractions (>180 mmHg) which, unlike the contractions of diffuse oesophageal spasm, are propagated. The lower oesophageal sphincter pressure may be increased, although this is not necessary for diagnosis.

Classical diffuse oesophageal spasm and nutcracker oesophagus account for a proportion of patients with non-cardiac chest pain but more commonly, patients investigated for chest pain demonstrate **non-specific motility disorders**, which, although appearing abnormal, do not fulfil the strict criteria for achalasia, classical diffuse oesophageal spasm, or nutcracker (5). The most common manometric pattern of the non-specific motility disorders comprises increased wave amplitude, long-duration peristaltic waves, and twin- or multipeaked waves. Most often, these non-specific motility disorders do not correlate in time with chest pain and, although they are likely to be of significance in patients with dysphagia, their significance is much less certain in patients investigated for non-cardiac chest pain.

Treatment

It is likely that gastrooesophageal reflux is the most frequent oesophageal cause of non-cardiac chest pain, whether or not it is accompanied by manometric evidence of a non-specific motility disorder (6,7). It is therefore quite reasonable to offer a clinical trial of intensive **antisecretory medication** as the initial investigation of choice in non-cardiac chest pain, reserving 24-h pH studies and manometry for non-responders.

Attempts to treat diffuse oesophageal spasm, nutcracker oesophagus, and the non-specific motility disorders have all focused on of the use of **smooth-muscle antispasmodic medication**. Drugs similar to those used to manage angina pectoris are most commonly administered; these include calcium-channel blockers and nitrates. There are few data from controlled trials to support their use. Most commonly, patients are offered a trial of **nifedipine** and **sublingual nitrate** taken immediately before a meal or when chest pain develops.

Secondary disturbances of oesophageal motility

Scleroderma

The oesophageal disease associated with systemic sclerosis predominantly affects the smooth muscle of the lower one-third of the organ; the striated muscle is usually spared. Progressive fibrosis of the lower one-third of the oesophagus results in poor peristalsis and incompetence of the lower oesophageal sphincter; in turn, this results in gastro-oesophageal reflux, oesophagitis, Barrett's oesophagus, and strictures.

Diagnosis

A **barium swallow** may reveal little peristalsis and the lumen of the oesophagus may be dilated as a result of generalized hypotonicity. **Oesophageal scintiscanning** often demonstrates delayed oesophageal emptying. On **oesophageal manometry**, the characteristic finding is normal upper oesophageal peristalsis with reduced or absent peristalsis, in the distal oesophagus. The lower oesophageal sphincter pressure is also reduced.

Treatment

Antisecretory medication with a proton pump inhibitor offers excellent protection against reflux. There is no evidence that prokinetic agents are effective.

MOTILITY DISORDERS OF THE STOMACH

Normal gastric motility

The stomach has two functional motor regions. The **proximal one-third** (fundus and proximal part of the corpus) has little peristaltic activity, functioning as a reservoir by maintaining a low resting intraluminal pressure through **receptive relaxation**. When a large meal is consumed, the upper one-third of the stomach wall relaxes, resulting in little pressure change within the gastric lumen: the luminal volume can increase from approximately 300 ml to as much as 1500 ml with little increase in intragastric pressure. This adaptive mechanism is controlled by the vagus nerve and the local release of nitric oxide acting as a potent smooth-muscle relaxant. This protects against sudden pressure surges, which could result in rapid emptying of gastric contents into the small intestine. In addition, receptive relaxation offers some protection against gastrooesophageal reflux through the lower oesophageal sphincter when it is relaxed or is incompetent. In contrast, the **distal two-thirds** of the stomach generates powerful peristaltic activity, which sweeps through from the mid-stomach to the duodenum at a frequency of between two and four peristaltic waves per minute (mean frequency 3 cycles/min).

The rate of gastric peristalsis is regulated by the **gastric pacemaker**, located on the greater curve of the body of the stomach amongst the longitudinal muscle fibres. The pacing frequency is generated by specialized interstitial cells called "**Cajal**" cells. This physiological pacemaker generates a wave of electrical depolarization, which radiates along the stomach from the pacemaker towards the antrum, pylorus, and duodenum. In this state of relative depolarization, gastric smooth-muscle cells can evoke one or more action (spike) potentials which, in turn, provoke muscle depolarization and coordinated muscle contraction. Consequently, not every slow-wave generated by the pacemaker results in contraction of the distal stomach; this only occurs when the muscle is in the appropriate state to generate a spike potential. Immediately after eating has ceased, gastric peristalsis is initiated. This may be irregular at the outset, as only some slow waves have superimposed spike potentials. However, within a few minutes, a stable pattern develops, with peristalsis occurring at the same rate as the pacemaker (3 cycles/min). The contractions of the stomach and duodenum are usually well coordinated and, when a peristaltic wave reaches the pylorus, the duodenal smooth-muscle contracts. **Duodenal contraction** is also dictated by depolarization, which occurs at four times the frequency of that in the antrum. Consequently, the duodenum may produce contractions of 12 cycles/min in response to gastric contraction (3 cycles/min).

The **enteric nervous system**, and in particular the myenteric plexus, is important in determining whether or not the muscle cell contracts in response to the slow wave arising from the pacemaker. Mechanical and chemoreceptors in the stomach and duodenum also determine the **rate of gastric emptying**. In the small intestine there are receptors sensitive to the energy content, osmolality, and pH of the food ingested. High-energy foods inhibit gastric emptying; this is accomplished by the vagal and enteric nervous system, in addition to hormonal feedback. Cholecystokinin may be a mediator, and there is evidence that liberation of nitric oxide may be responsible for some of the inhibitory effect (8). There is also a diurnal variation in the rate of gastric emptying: the emptying rate in the morning is twice that of the evening meal. The consistency of the meal also determines the rate of gastric emptying: a liquid meal usually leaves the stomach at an exponential rate, depending on the energy content and osmolarity. After a solid or semi-solid meal, food begins to leave the stomach only after a lag phase.

The **pressure gradient** between the distal stomach and duodenum during peristalsis is responsible for the **regulated propulsion** of solids and liquids into the duodenum. The pylorus is usually in a state of partial relaxation. The peristaltic wave of the gastric wall accelerates at a faster rate than the gastric contents and, consequently, the wave reaches the pylorus before the gastric contents, thereby constricting the antrum and pylorus and injecting only a small proportion of contents into the duodenum (1–4 ml of chyme per contraction). Most of the food is returned into the stomach by retropulsion

leading to the grinding action that mixes gastric contents and controls the rate of gastric emptying. An important function of the distal stomach is to retain solid food until the particle size is small enough (less than 1 mm) to permit controlled passage into the duodenum. When the concentration of carbohydrate, fat, or protein in the duodenum is too high, feedback through chemoreceptors causes the pylorus to close, followed by the establishment of rhythmic contractions, either at the frequency of antral contraction (3 cycles/min) or, sometimes, at the rate of duodenal contraction (12 cycles/min). This protects the duodenum from being overwhelmed by energy-rich nutrients. Normal gastric emptying is therefore very dependent on a well coordinated interaction between gastric antrum and the duodenum.

In addition to the pulsatile discharge of the gastric pacemaker, a **migrating motor complex** (MMC) also occurs in the stomach and is responsible for emptying indigestible solids (diameter >5 mm) that can not be propelled with digestible solids. These powerful contraction waves occur in the fasting state and are inhibited by feeding. They occur every 60–120 min during the fasting phase, at a time when plasma concentrations of motilin are increased (9). The **interdigestive MMC** is initiated in the stomach and travels distally through the small bowel, but MMCs may also be initiated anywhere along the small intestine. During fasting, this wave of movement is composed of three phases. In the **first phase**, there is no motor activity, and this is associated with absorption of fluid from the small bowel. During **phase 2**, sporadic contractions occur that increase in amplitude and frequency over a period of 30–45 min. This phase is associated with increased gastric acid secretion. In the **final phase** (phase 3) there is a burst of uninterrupted contraction waves occurring at a maximum rate of 3 cycles/min in the stomach and 10–12 cycles/min in the small intestine. This phase lasts for between 2 and 12 min, is associated with an increase in lower oesophageal sphincter pressure, and is responsible for moving the gastric and intestinal contents distally. The MMC migrates distally from the duodenum at a speed of 5–10 cm/min, reaching the terminal ileum after about 1.5 h; some contractions peter out before reaching the distal small bowel. The enteric nervous system appears to control the generation and propagation of the MMC, and motilin appears to be the hormone responsible for mediating phase 3. The MMC is responsible for preventing stasis and bacterial overgrowth.

After a meal, the pattern of the motor complex changes. After the ingestion of food, **intense irregular contractions** develop in the small intestine and these persist for as long as there are nutrients present (in the fed pattern, these random contractions can last between 2.5 and 8 h, after which the fasting pattern resumes). There are **segmental contractions** that facilitate contact between food and the mucosal surface, and **propulsive contractions** that encourage distal movement of the food bolus. Depending on the consistency of the meal, gastric emptying occurs 1–5 h after the meal was eaten. Subsequent passage from the duodenum to the colon takes approximately 1.5 h.

Assessment of gastric physiology

Although abnormalities of gastric motility comprise a significant proportion of foregut disorders, there is a poor correlation between the severity of clinical symptoms and objective measures of gastric physiology, including gastric emptying. A number of techniques have been developed, but all suffer from one or more disadvantages. In practice, most clinicians use clinical, endoscopic, and radiological tests to exclude organic disease, whereas dysmotility syndromes are usually diagnosed by exclusion. Tests of gastric function are described in more detail in Chapter 50.

Abnormalities of gastric emptying

Gastroparesis

The term "gastroparesis" relates to abnormal delay in emptying of food from the stomach, without evidence of mechanical obstruction. The disorder results from muscular, hormonal, or neurological failure. There may be impaired motility of the fundus, with delayed transit of gastric contents into the distal stomach. Antral hypomotility may delay the passage of gastric contents across the pylorus, and gastric dysrhythmias resulting from abnormal pacemaker activity may cause antro–duodenal incoordination.

Clinical features

Patients usually present with symptoms of the early satiety, bloating, anorexia, heartburn, weight loss, nausea, and vomiting. The nature of the vomiting is quite characteristic: the patient often vomits large quantities of partially digested food, and this usually occurs between 2 and 4 h after the meal.

Causes of gastroparesis

In clinical practice, gastroparesis may be idiopathic, a complication of diabetes mellitus, or caused by drugs. **Drugs that may cause delayed gastric emptying** include:

* anticholinergics
* tricyclic antidepressants
* major tranquillisers
* calcium channel blockers
* β agonists
* nicotine
* aluminium containing antacids
* L-Dopa

Most often, the cause of gastroparesis can not be discovered (**idiopathic gastroparesis**). Studies of patients with dyspeptic symptoms in the absence of any mucosal disorder indicate that approximately 50% of them have delayed gastric emptying, mainly for solid food. This has been demonstrated using scintigraphy, manometry, ultrasound, barostat measurement, and transcutaneous electrogastrography.

Gastroparesis may also complicate long-standing **diabetes mellitus**. In this disease, delayed gastric emptying is believed to be caused by a vagal neuropathy. This is supported by evidence of reduced basal gastric acid secretion and abnormality of the beat-to-beat variation in heart rate associated with ventilation. The cause of diabetic gastroparesis remains controversial, as vagotomy usually results in rapid gastric emptying and post-mortem histology of the stomachs of patients with long-standing diabetes has not revealed evidence of abnormal gastric innervation.

Investigation

After a prolonged fast, mechanical obstruction is excluded either by endoscopy or by barium studies. In the absence of obstruction, criteria for diagnosis include the aspiration of more than 1 litre of fluid from the stomach after a 12-h fast, evidence of gastric dilatation on barium studies, or delay in gastric emptying using special tests such as gastric scintigraphy. In diabetic patients, the lag phase may be prolonged and this is believed to be related to abnormal retention in the proximal stomach, in addition to antral hypomotility.

Treatment
Treatment is largely empirical. Predisposing factors (in particular drugs) should be considered when the treatment programme is being initiated. Reflux oesophagitis may occur as a secondary complication of prolonged gastroparesis and, in this setting, the use of H_2-blockers or proton pump inhibitors might be helpful. Attention to diet might be useful; in particular, patients should eat frequent, small-volume meals. Low-residue diets may also be helpful, as may restricting the fat content of the meal, because fat stimulates the release of cholecystokinin, which is a powerful inhibitor of gastric emptying.

Prokinetic agents
Prokinetic agents may be helpful in the symptomatic control of gastroparesis. **Metoclopramide, domperidone and cisapride** are the agents most commonly used. Their effectiveness can not be predicted, and usually depends on a clinical trial of treatment. It is recommended that these drugs are prescribed for 4–8 weeks before symptoms are reassessed and changes made to either dose or class of drug; they should be administered approximately 30 min before food.

1. *Metoclopramide*: A procainamide derivative that has both antiemetic and prokinetic activity. The prokinetic action results from antagonism of dopamine D_2-receptors and augmented release of acetylcholine from the myenteric plexus. The drug passes the blood–brain barrier and central side effects are not uncommon; these include tardive dyskinesia, drug-induced Parkinson's disease, and hyperprolactinaemia — which can result in gynaecomastia, galactorrhoea, and mastalgia. Metoclopramide improves gastric emptying by increasing the amplitude of gastric contractions, relaxing the pyloric sphincter and increasing antral peristalsis.
2. *Domperidone*: This dopamine antagonist does not cross the blood–brain barrier. Like that of metoclopramide, it action is mediated by blocking the gastric dopamine receptors. This prokinetic agent improves antral peristalsis, duodenal contractility, and and antro–duodenal coordination. It has fewer side effects than metoclopramide.

3. *Cisapride*: Enhances release of 5-hydroxytryptamine (5-HT) by an agonist effect on $5HT_4$ receptors whilst antagonizing $5HT_3$ receptors. The net effect is enhanced release of acetylcholine from postganglionic nerve endings in the myenteric plexus. The drug increases lower oesophageal sphincter pressure and enhances peristalsis throughout the gastrointestinal tract. Cisapride has been shown to improve antro–duodenal coordination and antral and pyloric motility. The drug is well tolerated and the only significant side effects are increased stool frequency, abdominal cramps, and very rarely, prolongation of the Q–T interval of the electrocardiogram and cardiac arrhythmias. The drug should not be administered with antifungal drugs or macrolide antibiotics. Care should also be taken when prescribing to patients with any evidence of underlying heart disease. Cisapride has been shown to improve and even completely correct gastric dysrhythmias, and improvement in the electrocardiogram is associated with improved symptoms (10). [Editor's note: cisapride has now been withdrawn from the market, although it is still available on a named-patient basis.]

The antibiotic **erythromycin**, binds to the motilin receptor and functions as a motilin agonist (9). It stimulates gastric emptying by increasing the strength of antral contractions and by a positive effect on antro–duodenal coordination. The drug is associated with side effects, including nausea and vomiting, and idiosyncratic hepatic toxicity has been noticed with certain preparations of this antibiotic.

Non-ulcer (functional) dyspepsia

Non-ulcer dyspepsia (also known as functional dyspepsia) is described by the **Rome criteria of 1991** (11). The disorder is a syndrome of chronic or recurrent upper abdominal symptoms lasting for a period of at least 1 month, with symptoms present for at least 25% of the time and an absence of clinical, biochemical, endoscopic, and ultrasonographic evidence of organic disease to account for symptoms. Whereas the term "gastroparesis" refers to a clear-cut clinical syndrome with readily demonstrable signs of delayed gastric emptying, the term "non-ulcer dyspepsia" is used to describe a foregut syndrome in which the symptoms are less readily explained. The distinction is, however, less clear than previously believed, as physiological changes of both sensory and motor function of the stomach can be demonstrated in up to 50% of patients with non-ulcer dyspepsia.

Clinical features

Non-ulcer dyspepsia accounts for up to 50% of cases of all dyspepsia (12). It has been suggested that patients with this disorder have symptoms that cluster into different subgroups that relate to distinct underlying aetiologies and serve as a guide to investigation and treatment. The three main subgroups are "ulcer-like" dyspepsia (pain dominant), "dysmotility-like" dyspepsia (bloating, early satiety, nausea) and "reflux-like" dyspepsia. Although this classification is widely used, its clinical relevance is questionable, as there is considerable overlap (13). In addition, the subgroup classification does not predict pathophysiology (14).

The pathophysiology of non-ulcer dyspepsia has not been fully established, although a number of mechanisms have been implicated. These include gastrointestinal motor abnormalities, enterogastric reflux, visceral hypersensitivity, and psychosomatic factors.

The considerable evidence for **gastrointestinal motor abnormalities in non-ulcer dyspepsia** includes delayed gastric emptying, impaired antral motility, and abnormal gastric pacemaker function. However, this spectrum of motility disorders is not universal nor is there a clear relationship between the pattern of motility abnormality and symptoms. Abnormalities of gastric motor physiology occur in up to 25–60% of patients with this syndrome (15,16), and it is likely that the remainder have either sensory disorders (17) or, perhaps, motor disorders that are not detectable with current techniques. In addition, it is possible that the motor disorders are intermittent and that negative, "snapshot" investigations in a patient might be positive if long-term studies over hours or days were possible.

Various techniques have been used to evaluate **gastric emptying** in patients with non-ulcer dyspepsia. Gastric emptying is delayed in a substantial proportion of patients. The reported percentage of abnormality varies, depending on the study and method used to study gastric emptying. Gastric emptying measured by scintigraphy was delayed in 30–82% of patients with the syndrome (18); using the carbon-14-labelled-octanoic acid breath test,

30% of patients with non-ulcer dyspepsia had delayed gastric emptying, and gastric clearance of radioopaque markers has been documented to be delayed in 64–68% of patients with the disorder.

Patients with non-ulcer dyspepsia often have **antral hypomotility**, with either decreased frequency or decreased amplitude of phasic pressure waves after a solid meal. However, these abnormalities are not specific, as they have also been detected in patients with peptic ulcer disease and gastritis. Patients with non-ulcer dyspepsia who have severe symptoms may also have small-intestinal dysmotility, which is not evident in those with mild symptoms.

Some scintigraphic studies have indicated that there is **abnormal intragastric distribution of food** in non-ulcer dyspepsia: after a meal, there is impaired filling of the proximal stomach and an increased volume distributing in the more distal stomach (19). Gastric barostat studies indicate that this maldistribution may be related to impaired receptive relaxation in the fundus. This observation is supported by the finding of an abnormally wide gastric antrum on ultrasound in a proportion of patients with non-ulcer dyspepsia. **Gastric myoelectrical abnormalities** have been demonstrated in up to 30% of patients with the disorder. Using the electrocardiogram to assess slow-wave generation by the gastric pacemaker, it has been possible to show significant postprandial tachygastria in non-ulcer dyspepsia (but not irritable bowel syndrome). There is also evidence for impaired antro–duodenal coordination (20).

Against the background of motor abnormalities it is important to recognize that patients with non-ulcer dyspepsia demonstrate an altered pain threshold — **visceral hypersensitivity**. As a group, these patients exhibit thresholds significantly lower for both first perception and the overall pain during gastric distension compared with those of asymptomatic controls.

Other factors such as acid secretion and *Helicobacter pylori* infection have been implicated at one time or another. However, there is no evidence from secretory or provocative tests to support an acid-related aetiology, nor has there been convincing evidence that treatment of *Helicobacter pylori* in non-ulcer dyspepsia is helpful (see Chapter 40).

Treatment

Whereas the treatment of reflux oesophagitis and peptic ulcer disease is well defined, treatment of non-ulcer dyspepsia remains empirical. Indeed, the most practical approach to treatment is for both the doctor and the patient to recognize that a series of therapeutic trials might be necessary. As with all other foregut disorders, change in life style is always worth discussing. In particular, patients should be encouraged to stop smoking, and excessive ingestion of alcohol should be discouraged. Some patients also benefit from dietary manipulation; options include reducing the fat content of the diet and recommending small, regular meals as an alternative to three large traditional meals. **Drug therapy**, however, remains the mainstay of treatment:

1. *Simple antacid treatment*: Many patients have already tried antacid therapy before consulting the doctor. Controlled trials have not supported a beneficial effect of the simple use of simple antacids in non-ulcer dyspepsia. However, some patients do report symptom relief and, although this might be a placebo effect, it is quite reasonable for this form of therapy to be supported.

2. *Antisecretory agents*: Although there is no compelling evidence to implicate acid secretion in the pathogenesis of non-ulcer dyspepsia, there does appear to be a subgroup of patients who benefit from treatment with H_2-blockers or proton pump inhibitors. This might reflect increased sensitivity to an acid load, rather than increased acid production. Both positive and negative clinical trials of H_2-blockers have been published, but there are sufficient data to support the clinical impression that H_2-blockers are helpful in certain patients with non-ulcer dyspepsia. It is therefore quite reasonable to initiate therapy with the trial of an H_2-blocker or proton pump inhibitor, making a judgement after 3 or 4 weeks of treatment.

3. *Prokinetic agents*: The drugs that have been most intensively studied include **metoclopramide, domperidone and cisapride**, and there is quite compelling evidence from clinical trials that these agents are helpful in a proportion of patients with non-ulcer dyspepsia. The three drugs are probably equally effective and the choice should be made on the basis of cost effectiveness and side effects. As with gastroparesis, **cisapride** is the best studied prokinetic agent with the fewest side effects, but because of its effects in patients with under-

lying heart disease, it has now been withdrawn from the market. If antisecretory treatment has been unsuccessful in managing symptoms, it is quite reasonable to introduce the prokinetic agents for a period of between 4 and 6 weeks, to assess the patient's response.

4. *Other drugs*: It is likely that non-ulcer dyspepsia will become a significant therapeutic challenge in gastropharmacology. There are currently a number of agents in the early stages of development and investigation; these include the 5-HT agonists and antagonists, and the κ opioid agonists.

References

1. Cook IJ, Blumberg P, Cash K *et al*. Structural abnormalities of the cricopharyngeus muscle in patients with pharyngeal (Zenker's) diverticulum. *J Gastroenterol Hepatol* 1992; **7**: 556–562.
2. Goldblum JR, Whyte RI, Orringer MB *et al*. Achalasia: a morphologic study of 42 resected specimens. *Am J Surg Pathol* 1994; **18**: 327–337.
3. Howard PJ, Maher L, Pryde A *et al*. Five year prospective study of the incidence, clinical features and diagnosis of achalasia in Edinburgh. *Gut* 1992; **33**: 1011–1015.
4. Eckardt VF, Aignherr C, Bernhard G. Predictors of outcome in patients with achalasia treated by pneumatic dilatation. *Gastroenterology* 1992; **103**: 1732–1738.
5. Kahrilas PJ, Clouse RE, Hogan WJ. American Gastroenterological Association technical review of the clinical use of oesophageal manometry. *Gastroenterology* 1994; **107**: 1865–1884.
6. Bancewicz J, Osugi H, Marples M. Clinical implications of abnormal oesophageal motility. *Br J Surg* 1987; **74**: 416–419.
7. Achem SR, Kolts BE, Wears R *et al*. Chest pain associated with nutcracker oesophagus: a preliminary study of the role of gastroesophageal reflux. *Am J Gastroenterol* 1993; **88**: 187–192.
8. Allescher HD, Daniel EE. Role of NO in pyloric, antral and duodenal motility and its interaction with other inhibitory mediators. *Dig Dis Sci* 1994; **39**: 7S–75S.
9. Peeters T, Matthijs G, Depoortere I *et al*. Erythromycin is a motilin receptor agonist. *Am J Physiol* 1989; **257**: G470–G474.
10. Besherdas K, Leahy A, Mason I *et al*. The effect of cisapride on dyspepsia symptoms and the electrogastrogram in patients with non ulcer dyspepsia. *Aliment Pharmacol Ther* 1998; **12**: 755–759.
11. Talley NJ, Colin Jones D, Koch KL *et al*. Funtional dyspepsia: a classification with guidelines of diagnosis and management. *Gastroenterol Int* 1991; **4**: 145–160.
12. Richter JE. Dyspepsia: organic causes and differential characterisics from functional dyspepsia. *Scand J Gastroenterol Suppl* 1991; **182**: 11–16.
13. Talley NJ, Zinsmeister AR, Schleck CD *et al*. Dyspepsia and dyspepsia subgroups: a population based study. *Gastroenterology* 1992; **102**: 1259–1268.

14. Malagelada J-R. Functional dyspepsia — insights on mechanisms and management strategies. *Gastroenterol Clin North Am* 1996; **25**: 103–112.

15. Malagelada J-R, Stanghellini V. Manometric evaluation of functional upper gut symptoms. *Gastroenterology* 1985; **88**: 1223–1231.

16. Stanghellini V, Tosetti C, Paternico A *et al.* Risk indicators of delayed gastric emptying of solids in patients with functional dyspepsia. *Gastroenterology* 1996; **110**: 1036–1042.

17. Mayer EA, Raybould HE. Role of visceral afferent mechanisms in functional bowel disorders. *Gastroenterology* 1990; **99**: 1688–1704.

18. Malagelada J-R. Gastrointestinal motor disturbances in functional dyspepsia. *Scand J Gastroenterol Suppl* 1991; **182**: 29–32.

19. Troncon LEA, Bennett RJM, Ahluwalia NK *et al.* Abnormal intragastric distribution of food during gastric emptying in functional dyspepsia patients. *Gut* 1994; **35**: 327–332.

20. Jebbink RJ, vanBerge-Henegouwen GP, Akermans LM *et al.* Antroduodenal manometry: 24-hour ambulatory monitoring versus short-term stationary manometry in patients with functional dyspepsia. *Eur J Gastroenterol Hepatol* 1995; **7**:109–116.

38.   Gastrointestinal Aspects of Excess Alcohol Consumption

PETER HAYES

Excess alcohol consumption is defined as an **intake of more than 28 units of alcohol per week for men or 21 units per week for women** (a unit being approximately 10 g of alcohol, equivalent to half a pint of beer, a glass of wine, or a single measure of spirit). The safe limits of alcohol consumption were derived from data that showed the consumption of this amount of alcohol or less was associated with no risk of the development of alcoholic liver disease. These limits take the liver as a reference point, rather than other organs, such as the brain, which may have lower safety limits. It is the alcohol in drinks that is hepatotoxic; the type of alcoholic beverage is unimportant. The effect of alcohol on the liver is determined by a number of factors, including sex, nutrition, and genetics; however, the main factors appear to be the amount and duration of intake.

The term "excessive alcohol intake" is not synonymous with alcohol abuse. It is possible, for example, to abuse alcohol — say in the form of drunk driving — whilst staying within safe weekly limits of alcohol consumption. Excess alcohol consumption affects around 10% of the adult UK population, and is more common in men than in women. Diagnosis is dependent largely on taking an adequate history. Use of questionnaires such as the CAGE and the Michigan MAST test may be helpful as diagnostic tools for identifying alcohol abuse. The CAGE alcohol abuse questionnaire has the form:

C   Have you ever tried to <u>c</u>ut down your alcohol intake?

A   Does someone mentioning your alcohol intake make you <u>a</u>nnoyed?

G   Have you ever felt <u>g</u>uilty about your alcohol intake?

E   Have you ever had to have an <u>e</u>ye opener drink to get you going in the morning?

The MAST test has a list of 12 questions, which makes it less easy to use than the CAGE test but more accurate.

Alcohol abuse can manifest itself in numerous different ways, but in medical practice it tends to be seen in association with accidents, psychiatric disorders, gastrointestinal upset with diarrhoea or vomiting, alcoholic liver disease, and chronic pancreatitis. These last two categories will be considered in more detail below.

ALCOHOLIC LIVER DISEASE

The term "alcoholic liver disease" is reserved for damage caused to the liver for which other possible aetiological factors such as viruses have been excluded, in individuals in whom there is a history of alcohol abuse. In order to make a firm diagnosis, it is essential that as much corroborative information as possible be obtained about a patient's alcohol intake, especially from their family and general practitioner. To label falsely as having alcoholic liver disease someone who does not abuse alcohol is unjust, whereas failing to identify alcohol abuse in someone with liver disease may result in missed therapeutic opportunities.

Alcoholic liver disease is traditionally divided into three types: **alcoholic fatty liver** or steatosis, **alcoholic hepatitis**, and **alcoholic cirrhosis**. It is important, however, to realize that these are not mutually exclusive and are not clear, separable stages of alcoholic liver disease.

Alcoholic fatty liver

Alcoholic fatty liver is common and probably considerably underdiagnosed. The other common causes of fatty liver include obesity and diabetes mellitus.

Presentation

Alcoholic fatty liver is frequently asymptomatic, although patients may present with other problems related to alcohol abuse. On physical examination hepatomegaly is common, but other stigmata of chronic liver disease are less common than may be seen in patients with alcoholic cirrhosis. Characteristic features of portal hypertension — such as the presence of oesophageal varices — may, uncommonly, be identified (1).

Diagnosis

For the diagnosis of alcoholic fatty liver to be made conclusively, a **liver biopsy examination** is required. In clinical practice, however, it is often presumed to be present in a young patient with a history of alcohol abuse who has abnormal liver function tests (typically an increased γ-glutamyltransferase concentration), hepatomegaly on examination, and an ultrasound report that identifies generalized increased echogenicity.

Treatment

Most patients with alcoholic fatty liver will be treated as outpatients, and the most effective form of treatment is **abstinence from alcohol**. One of the major problems in managing patients who abuse alcohol, including those with alcoholic liver disease, is that compliance with the recommendation of alcohol abstinence is very poor. Although most hospitals provide alcohol counselling facilities and involve the services of specialists such as psychiatrists, psychologists and social workers, this has only limited impact on the natural history of liver disease. The introduction of new **drugs**, such as acamprosate, which reduces the craving for alcohol, might help future patients maintain abstinence from alcohol. Currently, this agent holds some promise, but requires more thorough and longer-term evaluation. The use of disulfiram (Antabuse) in alcoholic liver disease remains unclear.

As mentioned above, a minority of patients with alcoholic fatty liver may develop portal hypertension, but it is not generally considered appropriate for all patients to undergo endoscopy to identify varices for the purpose of primary prophylaxis for variceal haemorrhage.

Prognosis

Because the natural history of advanced alcoholic liver disease takes many years, the short- and medium-term prognosis for patients with alcoholic fatty liver is good. It is apparent, however, that some patients will go on to develop alcoholic cirrhosis without passing through a phase of alcoholic hepatitis, and it is now no longer believed that alcoholic fatty liver can be considered a benign, entirely reversible, condition.

Alcoholic hepatitis

This disorder is considered in greater detail in Chapter 23.

Alcoholic cirrhosis

Presentation

Alcoholic cirrhosis is **common**, with a prevalence of approximately 1%; however, because it is commonly asymptomatic, it is often undiagnosed in life. Presentation is usually with one of the complications of cirrhosis, which may be portal hypertension presenting with variceal haemorrhage, liver failure presenting with ascites or encephalopathy, or hepatocellular carcinoma. Sometimes patients present in the clinic having been referred with abnormal liver function tests.

Examination may reveal a wide range of clinical signs that should be sought specifically. **Clinical features of alcoholic cirrhosis** include:

- General features
  - anxious look
  - sweating
  - unkempt or smelling of alcohol
  - tachycardia
  - fever
  - jaundice
- Face
  - parotid enlargement
  - seborrhoeic dermatitis
  - rhinophyma
  - spider naevi
  - telangiectactic facial blood vessels
- Hands
  - finger clubbing
  - Dupuytren's contracture
  - palmar erythema
  - tremor
- Trunk
  - reduced body hair
  - Gynaecomastia
  - spider naevi
- Abdomen
  - extended veins
  - caput medusae (rare)
  - ascites
  - testicular atrophy

Clinical features tend to be more florid in women. The patient's face may reveal **jaundice**, which is usually mild, fine **telangiectatic blood vessels** on the cheeks and nose, seborrheic dermatitis around the nose and eyebrows, **rhinophyma** and **parotid swelling**, and **spider naevi**. The breath may reveal the characteristic smell of alcohol or, alternatively, the smell of foods taken to disguise the smell — typically, garlic or peppermint. Examination of the trunk may reveal **gynaecomastia**, which may be tender; the breast bud should be palpated for, particularly in obese subjects with breast enlargement. Spider naevi are common on the front of the chest and the back and upper arms, and it is generally stated that the presence of more than three or four (as long as the individual is not pregnant) is suggestive of liver disease. The larger the spider naevus, the more likely this is to be the case. Abdominal examination may reveal **hepatomegaly** and, less often, **splenomegaly**, signs of **ascites**, and **dilatation of superficial veins**. The classical **caput medusae** is extremely rare.

Diagnosis

The **diagnosis of alcoholic cirrhosis** is based on:

1. *History*: A combination of history of excess alcohol intake with no other identified risk factor for cirrhosis.
2. *Supporting factors*: Increased γ-glutamyltransferase, increased mean corpuscular volume, increased carbohydrate-deficient transferrin (moderately increased serum ferritin).
3. *Liver histology*: Cirrhosis with features of associated alcohol abuse (e.g. spotty necrosis, Mallory's hyaline, steatosis).

Even in patients in whom diagnosis of alcoholic cirrhosis seems likely, it is important to **exclude other causes of liver disease**, because alcohol abuse is common both in the community and in those with other causes of liver disease. Checking for hepatitis B and C infections, and testing for autoantibodies, in addition to screening for haemochromatosis and α_1-antitrypsin deficiency are advisable. Routinely checking for caeruloplasmin in patients older than 40 years is unnecessary. Laboratory features that would support an alcoholic aetiology of cirrhosis include: increased mean corpuscular volume, an increased concentration of γ-glutamyltransferase, and a serum aspartate transaminase concentration at least twice that of the serum alanine transaminase concentration. Measurement of carbohydrate-deficient transferrin has recently been advocated as a sensitive marker of alcohol abuse that may remain increased for some weeks into a period of abstinence (2); its accuracy in those with active or established liver disease requires to be confirmed.

Other biochemical and haematological features found in cirrhosis of all causes include: hyperbilirubinaemia, which is often mild, hypoalbuminaema, mild anaemia, and a low platelet count. The alpha-fetoprotein concentration may be mildly increased in those with active liver disease, but if an increased concentration is found — particularly if it increases serially — hepatocellular carcinoma should be looked for by ultrasound and computed tomography (CT) scanning.

For a diagnosis of alcoholic cirrhosis to be confirmed, **liver biopsy examination** should be undertaken. This is helpful in staging the disease, although it will not always confirm alcohol as the aetiology, particularly if there has been a period of abstinence from alcohol before the biopsy sample is taken. Diagnosis of cirrhosis is occasionally missed on biopsy examination, particularly if the sample is small and the cirrhosis is macronodular.

Other investigations

Patients in whom cirrhosis is confirmed or suspected should undergo **upper gastrointestinal endoscopy**, to look for varices. If these are present and are medium or large in size, prophylaxis should be with propranolol (160 mg of the long-acting preparation, or a dose titrated to reduce the resting heart rate by 25%). Prophylactic endoscopic treatment with injection has not been proved to be helpful, and should not be undertaken (3). **Endoscopic band ligation** of varices appears to be a promising prophylactic approach, but requires to be evaluated in clinical trials before it can be used routinely. If the varices are small, the patient should undergo endoscopy annually to detect any increase in their size; if they are absent endoscopy should be undertaken every 2 years. In those in whom cirrhosis is identified, 3–4-monthly measurements of alpha-fetoprotein and liver ultrasound should be introduced as screening for liver-cell cancer.

Treatment

Patients attending for treatment of alcoholic cirrhosis can be categorized as those requiring **treatment of complications**, and those requiring the **surveillance measures** described above — regular endoscopy, along with alpha-fetoprotein and imaging tests. It should be emphasized that the most important component of treatment of patients with alcoholic cirrhosis is **abstinence from alcohol**. The evidence of improved survival in patients who are teetotal is good and, although there are some data that suggest that reduced alcohol intake or episodic drinking carries an improved prognosis compared with that in those who continue drinking heavily, it is not generally considered conclusive, and absolute abstinence from alcohol should be insisted upon. In practice, the majority of patients can not or do not adhere to this; nevertheless, the advice should be given forcefully and repeatedly, and this should be documented. This should circumvent any later controversy concerning patients who, when they present with decompensated liver disease and are being considered for transplantation, say they were not told to stop drinking alcohol.

Table 38.1. Child–Pugh classification of liver failure.

Score	1	2	3
Encephalopathy	None	Mild	Marked
Bilirubin (µmol/litre)	<34	34–50	>50
Albumin (g/litre)	>35	28–35	<28
Prolongation of prothrombin time (sec)	<4	4–6	>6
Ascites	None	Mild	Marked
Bilirubin (in primary biliary cirrhosis and sclerosing cholangitis)	<68	68–170	>170

Add the individual scores: <7 = grade A; 7–9 = grade B; >9 = grade C. The survival for patients graded as C, the group with the worst prognosis, is less than 12 months.

Major complications of alcoholic cirrhosis are the same as those as for other causes of cirrhosis — namely, variceal bleeding, liver failure manifest by the development of ascites, encephalopathy, or hepatorenal failure and hepatocellular carcinoma. These are discussed elsewhere in this book.

Prognosis

The prognosis for patients with cirrhosis of all causes, including alcoholic, can be predicted from the **degree of liver failure**. The classification based on the presence of clinical and laboratory tests of liver failure, the Child–Pugh grading (Table 38.1), remains useful in clinical practice (4) (see also chapter 11.2).

Two recent issues concerning alcoholic cirrhosis have received considerable attention: **coexistent hepatitis C infection** and **liver transplantation**.

Hepatitis C infection
Liver disease progresses more rapidly in patients with hepatitis C infection if they drink heavily. In our experience, the majority of patients with such infection who develop cirrhosis within 20–25 years of their infection have a history of heavy alcohol consumption. It is an important aspect of the management of patients with hepatitis C that they should be advised about alcohol intake. The safe amount of alcohol that can be consumed by these patients remains uncertain, although it would appear that an alcohol consumption considered safe in the general population — less than 28 units per week for men and 21 units per week for women — probably does not significantly influence the rate of progression of

hepatitis C liver disease. This issue, however, requires further study. At present, many clinicians advise patients with hepatitis C that they should be teetotal.

Liver transplantation

Orthotopic liver transplantation was originally not considered appropriate for patients with alcoholic liver disease, but over the past decade it has become clear that liver transplantation may be highly effective for patients with endstage and decompensated alcoholic cirrhosis (5). Most units insist that the patient should no longer be abusing alcohol and should have been abstinent for at least 6 months. This inevitably means that some patients will not be considered as candidates for transplantation and may die of their liver disease before 6 months of abstinence can be achieved; conversely, a significant proportion of patients who remain abstinent, even once they have decompensated liver disease, will slowly improve, and this improvement may take place over a prolonged period of time of up to 2 years. The issue of transplantation for treatment of alcoholic liver disease is clearly not one that is solely in the hands of the medical profession, as the transplant community and the public have important views on the subject. Individuals likely to be considered suitable candidates by most units would be those individuals younger than 65 years who have been abstinent from alcohol for at least 6 months, those who have a psychiatrist's opinion that considers it unlikely that they will return to alcohol abuse, and those who have a supportive family. It is becoming increasingly clear that a significant proportion of patients will return to alcohol consumption, but it would appear to be relatively unusual for the liver graft to be lost as a result of accelerated alcoholic liver disease.

ALCOHOLIC-INDUCED PANCREATIC DISEASE

Alcohol abuse may lead to both acute and chronic pancreatitis; as alcohol abuse has increased so has the incidence of both these conditions.

Acute pancreatitis

Alcohol is believed to be the cause of approximately 30–50% of cases of acute pancreatitis,

although this varies from country to country. In the UK, the most common cause remains gallstone disease, whereas in North America alcohol is the most common cause.

Clinical features

The major clinical feature of pancreatitis is **abdominal pain**, but it is not invariably present. The pain is generally epigastric and constant, and unrelieved by vomiting. Sitting forward may relieve the pain in some patients. **Nausea** and **vomiting** are also common. Abdominal examination may not be helpful, although epigastric tenderness and guarding may be present. Jaundice is unusual, and the classical signs of bruising around the umbilicus (Cullen sign) or around the flanks (Turner's sign) are unusual. In severe acute pancreatitis, the patient may be shocked and confused.

Diagnosis

The single most used and valuable investigation is the measurement of **serum amylase**. Concentration increased to more than 1000 IU/litre are diagnostic of acute pancreatitis, but lesser degrees of increase are common in other causes of acute abdominal pain such as perforated peptic ulcer, mesenteric infarction, and dissecting aortic aneurysm. The diagnostically high amylase concentrations may be missed if the patient presents more than 24 h after the acute attack; measurement of amylase in the urine may be helpful in this setting. Although X-rays of the abdomen and chest may be of some help, the most useful investigations are **ultrasonography** and **CT scanning**. Ultrasound is particularly useful in identifying gallstone disease and the serial monitoring of pancreatic pseudocysts and abscesses.

Treatment

The most important aspect of treating acute pancreatitis, other than providing pain relief, is the **identification and management of complications**. These include shock, electrolyte disturbance, and diabetes in addition to respiratory and renal failure. More specific intervention to inhibit pancreatic inflammation by means of steroids or drugs (such as aprotinin and the protease inhibitor, gabexate mesilate (6)), have unproven benefit, as has the prophylactic use of antibiotics.

Chronic pancreatitis

Alcohol is responsible for the majority of cases of chronic pancreatitis; heavy alcohol consumption of over 15 years is the norm. As with alcoholic liver disease, women may be more susceptible to the effects of alcohol on the pancreas, but men make up the majority of patients. The incidence of chronic pancreatitis is increasing, again, particularly in men.

Clinical features

As in acute pancreatitis, **pain** is the predominant symptom of chronic pancreatitis, and is usually epigastric and may radiate to the back The clinical features include **anorexia, nausea**, and **weight loss**. Steatorrohea may be present, as may diabetes mellitus. Clinical examination is often normal.

Diagnosis

Blood tests are of relatively little value in making a diagnosis of chronic pancreatitis, and **endoscopic retrograde cholangiopancreatography** is the most valuable investigation. Other imaging techniques of **ultrasonography** and **CT scanning** may also be valuable. The roles of endoscopy, ultrasound and magnetic resonance imaging at present remain unclear.

Treatment

As with chronic alcoholic liver disease, **abstinence from alcohol** is the most important aspect of treatment but, unfortunately, compliance with this is poor. **Treatment of the pain** is often the main therapeutic problem and opiates are usually required. Interventions such as coeliac plexus blockade have a limited role. Other aspects of management include treatment of diabetes mellitus and improving nutrition, particularly in those with malabsorption, in whom pancreatic enzyme supplements are important.

References

1. Hislop WS, Bouchier IAD, Allan JG *et al*. Alcoholic liver diease in Scotland and North Eastern England presenting features — 510 patients. *Q J Med* 1983; **52**: 232–243.
2. Stibler H. Carbohydrate deficient transferrin in serum: a new marker of potentially harmful alcohol consumption reviewed. *Clin Chem* 1991; **37**: 2029–2037.
3. Stanley AJ, Hayes PC. Portal hypertension and varicael haemorrhage. *Lancet* 1997; **350**: 1235–1239.
4. Pugh RNH, Murray-Lyon M, Dawson JL *et al*. Transection of the oesophagus for bleeding varices. *Br J Surg* 1973; **60**: 646–649.
5. Douds A, Neuberger J. Liver transpslantation for alcoholic cirrhosis: current situation. *Hosp Med* 1998; **59**: 604–605.
6. Buchle M, Malfertheiner P, Uhl W *et al*. Gabexate mesilate in human acute pancreatitis. *Gastroenterology* 1993; **104**: 1165–1170.

39. Gallstones

STEPHEN P. PEREIRA

The purpose of this chapter is to review selected aspects of the non-surgical management of gallbladder stones, and to discuss the role for these treatments in the era of laparoscopic cholecystectomy.

EPIDEMIOLOGY

Gallstone disease is **common**, although there are marked geographical variations, with a high prevalence in Chile and Scandinavia and among native Americans, and a low prevalence in sub-Saharan Africa and some parts of Asia. It affects between 10 and 20% of the world's population. Gallstones occur more frequently in women than in men by a factor of approximately two; this is attributed to the effects of female sex hormones on biliary cholesterol secretion and gallbladder contractility. Most studies report a prevalence of gallstones in women of 5–25% between the ages of 20 and 50 years, and 20–40% after the age of 50 years.

First-degree relatives of patients with gallstones have a prevalence of the disease that is increased at least twofold compared with that in the general population. Genetic factors implicated in the pathogenesis of gallstone disease remain poorly defined and are multifactorial.

Pregnancy and **parity** are other risk factors for cholelithiasis. In a study of 980 Chilean women who underwent ultrasound immediately after giving birth, the prevalence of gallstones was 12.2%, compared with a figure of 1.3% in 150 nulliparous, age-matched controls. Stones that form during pregnancy are composed mostly of cholesterol, are usually asymptomatic and, in up to 30% of women, disappear spontaneously after delivery.

Obesity also predisposes to gallstone formation. In the Nurses' Health Study of 90 302 women followed from 1980 to 1988, the annual incidence of symptomatic gallstones in women with a body mass index greater than 30 kg/m^2 was more than 1% — four times that seen in non-obese women. Those with the greatest body mass index (>45 kg/m^2) had a sevenfold risk of developing symptomatic gallstones. Obesity is associated with enhanced total body cholesterol synthesis and increased secretion of cholesterol into bile, secondary to increased activity of the rate-limiting enzyme, hydroxymethyl glutaryl coenzyme A reductase. Obese patients consuming very low energy diets or having undergone jejunoileal bypass also have a high incidence of cholesterol gallstone formation, of up to 25% during the first 1–4 months of rapid weight loss.

Crohn's disease and **terminal ileal resection** are associated with upto a fourfold increase in the prevalence of gallstones. Their increased frequency in ileal Crohn's disease has been attributed to reduced active bile acid absorption in the terminal ileum, thereby reducing the bile acid pool within the enterohepatic circulation. As a consequence, the hepatic cholesterol:bile acid secretion ratio is increased, resulting in supersaturation of bile with cholesterol. However, a high biliary cholesterol saturation index has been reported in most, but not all studies of patients with ileal disease/resection and in only a minority of post-colectomy and colitis patients, so that this hypothesis remains controversial. An alternative explanation is that malabsorbed bile acids solubilize unconjugated bilirubin in the colon and increase its enterohepatic cycling, which in turn increases the secretion of bilirubin pigments into the bile and subsequent pigment gallstone formation.

Dietary factors implicated in gallstone formation include a high energy intake, increased consumption of unrefined carbohydrate, and diets low in fibre (1). Other associated conditions include hypertriglyceridaemia, diabetes mellitus, and hepatic cirrhosis. Bacterial infection and parasitic infestation of the biliary tree are important factors in the development of pigment stones in Asia, but less so in the West. Patients with haemolytic anaemia caused by hereditary spherocytosis, sickle-cell disease, and thalassaemia also have an increased prevalence of pigment stones.

GALLSTONE COMPOSITION AND MECHANISM OF FORMATION

Cholesterol gallstones

Stones composed predominantly of cholesterol account for about 75% of all gallstones in Europe and North America. Pure cholesterol stones do occur, but most stones are mixed, and contain at least 70% cholesterol in a matrix of calcium bilirubinate, calcium phosphate, and mucin glycoprotein. Mixed stones are usually multiple, hard, and faceted, and have a layered structure when seen in cross-section.

Cholesterol stones form in the presence of supersaturation of bile with cholesterol secondary to hepatic cholesterol hypersecretion, an abnormally rapid appearance of cholesterol microcrystals (the so-called nucleation defect), or crystals retained within the gallbladder, secondary to mucin glycoprotein hypersecretion and gallbladder hypomotility.

Pigment gallstones

Pigment stones can be brown or black, are formed predominantly of calcium bilirubinate, and contain less than 25% of cholesterol. They are usually small and multiple, and about half are radioopaque.

The soft, friable, brown pigment stones are especially common in populations in the Far East, and are associated with **parasitic infestations** and with *Escherichia coli*, *Bacteroides spp.*, and clostridial colonization of the biliary tract. These bacteria contribute to stone formation by deconjugating bilirubin diglucuronide to form free, unconjugated bilirubin, which combines with calcium to form sparingly soluble calcium bilirubinate. Microscopically, brown stones contain cytoskeletons of bacteria. Brown pigment stones are also associated with duodenal diverticula and are more likely to form *de novo* in bile ducts than are other types of stones.

The incidence of black or pure pigment stones increases with age, and they are found in the gallbladders of patients with cirrhosis or haemolytic disorders. Black pigment stones contain an insoluble black pigment, calcium bilirubinate, together with calcium carbonate and phosphate, calcium salts of fatty acids, and bile acids. All pigment stones also contain a large amount of mucin glycoprotein matrix.

Biliary sludge

Biliary sludge is defined ultrasonographically as echogenic, gravitating material in the gallbladder that does not produce acoustic shadowing. It consists of cholesterol microcrystals, calcium bilirubinate granules, and a high concentration of mucin glycoprotein. Groups at risk of sludge formation include critically ill patients in intensive care units, patients with high spinal-cord injuries, and those receiving total parenteral nutrition (TPN). During TPN, the absence of exogenous luminal nutrients leads to reduced meal-stimulated release of peptide hormone and stagnation of bile acids within the enterohepatic circulation. Gallbladder emptying is also impaired. Increases in both the cholesterol saturation index and the vesicular cholesterol concentration, with shortening of the nucleation time, have been documented within 48 h of the commencement of TPN. Gallbladder sludge, in turn, can occur after as little as 3 weeks, and up to 40% of patients will develop gallstones after 4 months of continued treatment.

In a minority of patients, biliary sludge may cause symptoms and precede gallstone formation. In a study of 96 patients with biliary sludge who were followed prospectively for a mean of 38 months, 8% formed asymptomatic gallstones and 6% developed symptomatic stones requiring cholecystectomy. In 60% of the patients, the sludge disappeared and subsequently reappeared, whereas in 18% it resolved completely. Six patients with biliary sludge underwent cholecystectomy for severe biliary pain, recurrent acute pancreatitis, or both. In another study of 286 patients with biliary sludge followed for 20 months, gallbladder stones or complications such as acute cholecystitis occurred in 20% of patients.

Transabdominal ultrasonography is relatively insensitive in detecting biliary sludge or stones that are less than 2 mm diameter. In an early study of 31 patients with acute pancreatitis that was considered to be idiopathic (no gallstones on ultrasound and no other causes found), microscopical examination of duodenal bile revealed bilirubinate granules or cholesterol crystals in 23 (86%), but sludge was seen by ultrasound in only 48%. In contrast, in a recent prospective study of 45 patients with acute pancreatitis or suspected choledocholithiasis but two consecutive "normal" transabdominal gallbladder ultrasound examinations, the sensitivity of **endoscopic ultrasound** for detecting gallbladder microlithiasis was 96%, compared with a sensitivity of 67% for cholecystokinin-induced duodenal bile (compared with the gold standard of cholecystectomy). Thus, biliary sludge/microlithiasis may be responsible for most cases of "idiopathic" acute pancreatitis and, in experienced hands, endoscopic endosonography is currently the most sensitive non-surgical method for detecting microlithiasis.

NATURAL HISTORY OF GALLSTONES

Asymptomatic gallstones

It has been estimated that primary gallbladder stones grow at a rate of 1–4 mm per year, and usually do not cause symptoms until at least 2–7 years after their formation. Stones remain silent or asymptomatic in 66–80% of gallstone carriers. Thus only a minority of patients will ever develop specific, gallstone-related symptoms such as biliary colic — arbitrarily defined as a steady epigastric or right upper-quadrant pain lasting more than 30 min that is unrelated to bowel movement. An even smaller proportion present with "surgical" complications that are mainly the result of obstruction of the cystic duct (acute cholecystitis with or without empyema formation, or even the rare Mirizzi syndrome) or common bile duct (cholestasis/jaundice, cholangitis, or pancreatitis).

In most long-term studies of patients with asymptomatic gallstones, the annual rates of developing biliary pain or gallstone complications vary from approximately 1% to 4%. Asymptomatic stones usually become symptomatic before they cause

complications, and the longer the stones remain quiescent after an initial attack of biliary colic, the less likely it is that complications will occur (2).

Choledocholithiasis in patients with asymptomatic gallbladder stones

On the basis of the evidence above, prophylactic treatment of gallbladder stones in asymptomatic patients is rarely indicated. One exception is choledocholithiasis in patients with asymptomatic gallbladder stones. In patients who are poor risks for surgery and who do not have acute cholecystitis, **endoscopic retrograde cholangiopancreatography** (ERCP) and **sphincterotomy without cholecystectomy** are often used to treat stones in the common bile duct. In one study published more than a decade ago, only 18 of 186 patients treated in this manner required later cholecystectomy, during an average follow-up of 32 months. However, more recent prospective randomized studies have questioned the rationale of adopting a "wait and see" strategy. In one study (3) of 98 elderly and other high-risk patients (mean age 80 years) assigned randomly to undergo either open cholecystectomy with bile-duct exploration or endoscopic sphincterotomy alone, there were no significant differences in immediate morbidity (23% compared with 16%) or mortality (4% compared with 6%). However, during a mean follow-up of 17 months, biliary symptoms recurred in 10 of the sphincterotomy group (20%), seven of whom required later surgery. In a similar study (4) with more than 5 years follow-up, 13 of 35 patients (37%) in the sphincterotomy group required later surgery, compared with two of 41 in the open-cholecystectomy group. There are fewer data comparing laparoscopic cholecystectomy with sphincterotomy, but the former has been shown to have less morbidity and mortality than open cholecystectomy in high-risk patients. In patients who have had a previous sphincterotomy, oral bile-acid treatment is less effective in dissolving cholesterol-rich gallbladder stones because of reduced concentrations of the prescribed bile acid within the underfilled gallbladder.

Symptomatic gallstones

Patients with symptomatic gallstones have a greater risk of developing recurrent biliary colic or gallstone complications than those with asymptomatic gallstones. The average annual rates of developing severe pain (usually requiring cholecystectomy) ranges from 1–8%, with complications (acute chole-cystitis, choledocholithiasis, pancreatitis) occurring in 1–3% per year. These figures suggest that treatment should be offered to patients only after significant biliary symptoms develop. In those with mild, non-specific symptoms, or who have had a single attack of biliary colic, simple observation alone may be appropriate, because as many as 30–50% of patients who have had one episode of pain will not have a recurrent episode.

INVESTIGATIONS

Ultrasonography

Transabdominal ultrasound has a reported sensitivity of 92–96% and specificity close to 100% if a hyperechoic image with acoustic shadowing is seen in the gallbladder. It can not reliably detect individual particles measuring less than 2 mm in diameter, and small stones located in the infundibulum may also be difficult to visualise. Ultrasound can also detect biliary sludge, but is less reliable for stones in the common bile duct, where the sensitivity of detecting choledocholithiasis or a dilated common bile duct ranges from 50 to 70%, compared with a sensitivity of about 95% for ERCP. Endoscopic ultrasonography has a sensitivity comparable to that of ERCP and a specificity approaching 100% in detecting bile-duct stones, and is likely to play an increasing role in the investigation of patients with a low or intermediate pre-test probability of having ductal stones, with associated reductions in costs and morbidity compared with ERCP.

In patients with symptomatic but uncomplicated cholelithiasis who are eligible for cholecystectomy, transabdominal ultrasound is usually the only imaging study required. However, in patients who are being considered for medical dissolution therapy, localized computed tomography of the gallbladder (to determine stone composition) and oral chole-cystography (to assess patency of the cystic duct), are also indicated, for the reasons given below. Alternatively, a significant reduction of gallbladder volume detected in response to a cholecystokinetic stimulus, such as a fatty meal or intravenous cholecystokinin, during ultrasonography predicts patency of the cystic duct with acceptable accuracy.

Computed tomography (CT)

Although radiolucent stones are usually cholesterol-rich, 14–20% of stones that appear lucent by plain X-ray are non-cholesterol in type, whereas at least 50% of stones that are lucent by conventional radiology appear dense by computed tomography (CT) of the gallbladder. The **maximum gallstone attenuation score**, measured by CT *in vivo*, predicts stone composition and dissolvability, and is cost effective in selecting patients for treatment by oral dissolution of the stones; values greater than 100 Hounsfield Units (HU) predict calcium-containing, non-dissolvable stones. The best results with medical dissolution treatment are obtained with stones that have low CT attenuation scores (less than 50–70 HU), or those that are isodense with bile and not visualized at all by CT.

Cholescintigraphy

Although more commonly used in the evaluation of patients with suspected acute cholecystitis or post-operative biliary leak, **isotope scanning** of the gallbladder has been used in the detection of patients with chronic acalculous biliary pain. A technetium-99m-labelled derivative of iminodiacetic acid (e.g. hydroxy iminodiacetic acid) is administered intravenously and images are then recorded by gamma-camera. Serial scans after injection normally show radioactivity in the gallbladder, common bile duct, and small bowel within 30–60 min. An abnormal, or positive, scan is defined as non-visualization of the gallbladder with preserved excretion into the common bile duct and small bowel. False positive results may occur in patients with chronic liver disease, the critically ill, and those maintained on total parenteral nutrition, in whom the gallbladder is atonic. In patients who fail to have the gallbladder visualized within 60 min, the use of intravenous morphine sulphate (which increases pressure within the sphincter of Oddi and induces flow into the gallbladder unless the cystic duct is obstructed) reduces this false positive rate.

Magnetic resonance imaging

Magnetic resonance cholangiopancreatography (MRCP) has the advantage over both ultrasound and ERCP of being completely non-invasive and is also highly specific in detecting bile-duct stones, but recently reported sensitivities have ranged from less than 60% to over 90% — generally because of failure of MRCP to detect small stones (<3–6 mm) in a non-dilated biliary tree (5). Improvements in image acquisition, together with prospective studies to define in which clinical contexts MRCP may obviate the need for ERCP, are awaited.

NON-SURGICAL TREATMENT OF GALLSTONES

Medical treatment

In patients with symptomatic gallstones in whom there is a blocked cystic duct (30% of patients with gallstones diagnosed on ultrasound have a non-visualizing gallbladder on oral cholecystography), there is generally no role for medical treatment and the decision for the specialist usually lies between laparoscopic or open-abdominal removal of the gallbladder. However, in patients with a patent cystic duct who decline or are unfit for surgery, cholesterol-rich (radio- and CT-lucent) gallstones can be removed or dissolved from the gallbladder and bile ducts in a number of ways. These techniques avoid the discomfort and small risks of general anaesthesia and surgical exploration of the abdomen and bile ducts.

In general, for reasons of both clinical and cost effectiveness, the non-surgical treatments should be reserved for patients with mild, uncomplicated gallstone symptoms who decline surgery or in whom the risk of cholecystectomy is high. In a carefully selected group of patients, these medical approaches work moderately well, but they are relatively expensive, require long-term surveillence, and have a rate of recurrence of gallstones of approximately 50% at 5 years.

Oral bile acid therapy

Oral bile acid therapy is the slowest, safest, and best documented of all the non-surgical or minimally invasive alternatives to cholecystectomy. Although the reported rates of dissolution of gallstones vary widely, up to 80% of patients with radio- and CT-lucent stones and a patent cystic duct will progress to confirmed complete dissolution of their gallstones during oral bile acid therapy — given alone, or together with extracorporeal shock-wave lithotripsy (ESWL). Until recently, the preferred oral bile acid regimen in most centres was combination therapy with chenodeoxycholic acid (5–7 mg/kg per day) and its 7-β-hydroxy epimer, **ursodeoxycholic acid** (UDCA; 5–7 mg/kg per day). These bile acids, normal constituents of bile, act by reducing the hepatic synthesis and biliary excretion of cholesterol, resulting in cholesterol desaturation of bile and the leaching out of cholesterol from gallstones. In the UK, chenodeoxycholic acid is no longer available, and UDCA monotherapy is given at a dose of 10–12 mg/kg per day.

Gallstone dissolution usually requires at least 6 months, and up to 2 years, of oral bile acid therapy — depending on the size, number, and composition of the stones. Ultrasonography should be performed every 3–6 months until the gallbladder is clear of stones, followed by a repeat test 3 months later to confirm complete gallstone dissolution, at which time UDCA treatment is stopped. In most patients, treatment should also be discontinued if there is no evidence of partial gallstone dissolution (a decrease in the number or size of the stones) after 1 year, or incomplete dissolution after 2 years.

Recommended **selection criteria** for oral bile acid therapy are given in Table 39.1. The stones should be small (ideally no larger than 5 mm), so that there is a high surface:volume ratio, and

Table 39.1. Selection criteria for oral bile acid therapy and ESWL with or without adjuvant oral bile acids.

Oral bile acids	ESWL ± oral bile acids
Stones ≤5 mm	Single stone ≤20 mm
(≤15 mm acceptable)	(up to three stones ≤30 mm acceptable)
Cholesterol-rich stones	Cholesterol-rich stones
(CT score <50–75 HU)	(calcified rim acceptable)
Patent cystic duct	Patent cystic duct
(OCG or ultrasound with fatty meal)	(OCG or ultrasound with fatty meal)
Non-obese patient	Non-obese patient
Mild biliary symptoms	Mild biliary symptoms
Patient declines or is unfit for cholecystectomy	Patient declines or is unfit for cholecystectomy

cholesterol-rich as determined by a CT attenuation score less than 100 HU. In addition, the cystic duct should be patent (e.g. emptying of more than 30% after cholecystokinin or fatty-meal stimulation) and the patient should not be morbidly obese, so that enrichment of the bile with the prescribed bile acid and cholesterol desaturation can be accomplished. Unfortunately, these selection criteria account for only about 15% of the population with gallstones, with an estimated rate of 80–90% for complete dissolution of the gallstones at 2 years.

Extracorporeal shock-wave lithotripsy

The best results with ESWL are obtained in patients with a patent cystic duct and solitary, radio- and CT-lucent stones measuring less than 20 mm in diameter, although acceptable fragmentation rates are also achieved in patients with up to three large stones no more than 30 mm in diameter. Such patients represent a highly selected subset — an estimated 15% of all patients with symptomatic gallstones — although, only about 7% will have optimal selection criteria of a solitary radiolucent stone less than 20 mm in diameter in a functioning gallbladder. Given the high capital cost of the equipment and its depreciation and maintenance costs, this treatment remains confined to a few specialized centres — usually where the ESWL machine is also used in the treatment of renal stone disease (6).

Most reports suggest that cholesterol-rich gallstones can be targeted and fragmented to less than 10 mm in maximum diameter in 80–100% of patients. However, it is not always possible to target gallbladder stones in the obese and in those with small contracted or high, intrahepatic gallbladders masked by the costal margin. After fragmentation of the stones, oral bile acids are given until complete dissolution of the gallstones is confirmed by serial ultrasound. In general, cholesterol-rich stone fragments measuring less than 10 mm in diameter dissolve readily, although the best results are obtained in those with even smaller stone fragments (less than 5 mm in diameter). Adverse effects of ESWL are usually minor, but include biliary colic, skin petechiae, and microscopic haematuria.

Giant or impacted common bile duct stones that can not be removed after endoscopic sphincterotomy and mechanical lithotripsy are other appropriate targets for ESWL. If the stones are targeted successfully, the fragments can then be extracted by conventional means. Alternative forms of treatment of difficult bile-duct stones are **electrohydraulic lithotripsy** and **laser lithotripsy**. The latter technique involves passage of a fine fibreoptic bundle capable of transmitting laser energy via a T-tube or by the endoscopic retrograde route into the common bile duct. In three published series using a pulsed-dye laser with an optical stone-detection system designed to improve stone targeting, complete stone clearance was achieved in 103 of 114 patients (90%). In a German randomized study comparing ESWL with intracorporeal laser lithotripsy for difficult bile duct stones, bile duct clearance was achieved in 22 of 30 patients (73%) in the ESWL group and in 29 of 30 (97%) in the laser lithotripsy group, after a maximum of three lithotripsy sessions. Next-generation, less costly, pulsed solid-state laser systems are currently under investigation, and may become available in some units in the UK.

Instillation of contact solvents

In symptomatic patients with a functioning gallbladder, cholesterol-rich stones can be rapidly dissolved by the direct instillation into the gallbladder of **methyl *tert*-butyl ether** (MTBE) or **ethyl proprionate**, via a percutaneous, transhepatic catheter — usually performed under local anaethesia. However, some patients experience considerable pain during the placement of the pig-tail catheter, despite intravenous sedation and analgesia, and the procedure is at the limits of acceptability as a technique suitable in conjunction with local anaesthesia.

Despite the initially rapid dissolution rates achieved with contact solvents over 6–12 h, gallstone dissolution is often incomplete. In an early study from the Mayo Clinic, 51 of 75 patients were left with residual gallstone debris. The residual particles usually disappear completely with oral bile-acid therapy, but the need for weeks or months of adjuvant oral bile acids partly defeats the aim of rapid, complete gallstone dissolution by this relatively invasive technique. MTBE has sedative–anaesthetic properties and it can cause other transient side effects, such as oedema of the gallbladder mucosa and duodenitis. Ethyl proprionate seems to lack many of these disadvantages, but experience with it remains limited. There is probably still a small place for contact solvent dissolution of gallstones in patients at prohibitive risk for general anaesthesia, but only in a few specialized (non-UK) centres where there is a large experience with the technique.

Percutaneous cholecystolithotomy

Percutaneous cholecystolithotomy (PCCL) is usually carried out under general anaesthesia. The gallbladder is punctured percutaneously, usually by the subhepatic route, under ultrasound or fluoroscopic control, or both. A guide-wire is then inserted into the gallbladder, and the track is serially dilated until it is wide enough to admit a 22 Fr Amplatz tube, through which an endoscope is passed; the stones are extracted under direct vision.

Because the stones are removed, rather than dissolved, they can be of any composition. The technique has had a particular role, therefore, in symptomatic patients with radioopaque, non-dissolvable stones (those with attenuation scores greater than 100 HU) who are not suitable for the less invasive non-surgical modalities. However, the total in-patient time and cost compare unfavourably with those associated with laparoscopic cholecystectomy, which has largely displaced PCCL from the list of management options.

Reasons for incomplete dissolution of gallstones

Complete dissolution of gallstones (by life table analysis) at 18 months can be achieved in up to 80% of those selected as suitable for medical dissolution treatment. However, even when the stones are lucent by conventional radiology and have CT scores of less than 100 HU, arrested gallstone dissolution (no ultrasonographic response to the oral bile acids after 1 year or partial, but arrested, dissolution after 2 years of treatment) still occurs in 20–35% of patients.

The reasons for incomplete gallstone dissolution in patients selected for treatment using the optimal criteria of a patent cystic duct and a low gallstone CT attenuation score include:

1. *Blocked cystic duct* or *impaired gallbladder emptying*: These may develop during treatment. In a study of 126 patients treated with UDCA alone, cystic duct obstruction developed in approximately 20% of patients after 4 years of treatment. Oral bile acid therapy itself is unlikely to be responsible for the development of cystic duct obstruction, as the (American) National Cooperative Gallstone Study showed that the incidence of acquired cystic duct obstruction during oral bile acid therapy was not different from that in a matched, untreated group of patients with gallstones.

2. *Acquired stone calcification*: this has been reported in 9–21% of patients with no or arrested dissolution of gallstones during oral bile acid therapy, and is attributed to the bicarbonate-rich choleresis induced by the administration of UDCA, which results in the precipitation of calcium carbonate in bile. Acquired gallstone calcification may also occur spontaneously, and is a function of both stone size (large gallbladder stones are more likely to be calcified than small stones) and stone age.

MANAGEMENT OF RECURRENT GALLSTONES

When oral bile acid treatment is withdrawn after complete dissolution, gallstones recur at a rate of 10–15% per annum, reaching a cumulative actuarial plateau of between 40 and 70% (mean around 50%) after 5–10 years. Gallstone recurrence after successful shock-wave lithotripsy and adjuvant oral bile acids is approximately 7% at 1 year and increases to about 30% at 5 years. The lower recurrence rate after ESWL is probably attributable to the fact that some 90% of patients selected for lithotripsy initially have solitary stones — the recurrence rate in such patients is less than that in patients who, before treatment, had had multiple stones.

After confirmed complete dissolution of primary cholesterol-rich gallstones, patients should normally undergo annual ultrasonography to exclude recurrence of their gallstones — at least for the first few years. As calcification of primary cholesterol-rich gallstones is a function of both stone size and age, early detection of recurrent stones explains why, in most studies, even those patients who originally had calcified gallstones develop small, cholesterol-rich stones on recurrence. In two recent reports, recurrent stones were radiolucent by plain abdominal X-ray in approximately 95% of patients, and CT-lucent (attenuation score less than 100 HU) in almost 90%. Thus recurrent gallstones are usually small and cholesterol-rich, and readily dissolvable with oral bile acid therapy.

PREVENTION OF GALLSTONES

Diet

The related factors of obesity, hypertriglyceridaemia, reduced concentrations of high-density lipoproteins and physical inactivity are all associated with an increased risk of gallstone disease, and measures to improve these should be recommended to patients. However, apart from general advice about eating a diet naturally rich in fibre and low in sugar and fat, as recommended for the prevention of heart disease and cancer, consistent evidence for particular dietary factors in gallstone formation is lacking.

Ursodeoxycholic acid

The cost of UDCA means that full-dose treatment is not a practical long-term management option in the prevention of primary or recurrent gallstone formation. The results of most studies also suggest that low-dose oral bile acid treatment reduces, but does not completely prevent, the risk of gallstone formation or recurrence. In the controlled British–Belgian gallstone dissolution trial, UDCA in one-third the full therapeutic dose (3 mg/kg per day) halved the rate of gallstone recurrence after successful dissolution. Short-term UDCA prophylaxis has been recommended in patients at high risk of gallstone formation, such as obese patients undergoing rapid weight loss as a result of gastroplasty or low (2184 kJ/day) energy dieting. In one study, 23% of the placebo-treated group developed gallstones over the 16-week period of the trial, compared with 6% of those treated with 150 mg UDCA twice daily. Moreover, this prevention of gallstone formation by UDCA was dose-dependent, only 2.8% of those taking 600 mg/day, and 1.6% of those taking 1200 mg/day, developed stones.

Aspirin and non-steroidal anti-inflammatory drugs

When aspirin or other non-steroidal anti-inflammatory drugs (NSAIDs) are given to experimental animals together with a lithogenic diet, they inhibit gallbladder synthesis of mucosal prostaglandin and prevent hypersecretion of mucin glycoprotein (which has been implicated both in nucleation and in the trapping of cholesterol microcrystals), in addition to the formation of microcrystals and gallstones.

Subsequent studies in humans have largely confirmed these results in experimental animals, although the only controlled study of low-dose aspirin in preventing the complications of gallstones lacked sufficient power to detect a difference. In an early study of obese individuals during acute weight reduction, the incidence of developing microcrystals or gallstones was significantly reduced if patients were given high-dose aspirin (1300 mg/day). In a retrospective study of 75 patients who had undergone dissolution of gallstones, none of 12 patients who regularly took NSAIDs developed recurrent stones, whereas 20 recurrences occurred among the 63 who had never, or only occasionally, taken NSAIDs. These data provide insights into the pathogenesis of gallstone disease, but do not yet justify the use of, for example, low-dose aspirin for the prevention of primary or recurrent gallstones in high-risk individuals.

Prokinetic agents

In patients at risk of sludge and stone formation, such as those in intensive care or receiving TPN, prokinetic drugs such as cholecystokinin, cisapride, and erythromycin can prevent the development of gallstones. These drugs stimulate gallbladder emptying, but they are also prokinetic to the intestine and may have an effect through decreased 7α-dehydroxylation (by colonic bacteria) of cholic acid to form deoxycholate. Supportive evidence for this hypothesis comes from early studies of constipated people who were given laxatives, with the result that their bile became depleted of deoxycholic acid and less saturated with cholesterol. Similarly, in acromegalic patients receiving long-term treatment with octreotide, oral cisapride shortens large-bowel transit times and reduces the proportion of serum (and presumably biliary) deoxycholic acid to normal. However, as yet there have been no formal prospective studies of the efficacy of intestinal prokinetic agents in preventing cholesterol formation in high-risk groups, and cisapride has now been withdrawn from the market.

References
1. Attili AF, Scafato E, Marchioli R *et al.* Diet and gallstones in Italy: the cross-sectional MICOL results. *Hepatology* 1998; **27**: 1492–1498.
2. Patino JF, Quintero GA. Asymptomatic cholelithiasis revisited. *World J Surg* 1998; **22**: 1119–1124.

3. Tagarona EM, Ayuso RM, Bordas JM *et al.* Randomised trial of endoscopic sphincterotomy with gallbladder left in situ versus open surgery for common bile duct calculi in high-risk patients. *Lancet* 1996; **347**: 926–929.

4. Hammarstrom L-E, Holmin T, Stridbeck H *et al.* Long term follow-up of a prospective randomised study of endoscopic versus surgical treatment of bile duct calculi in patients with gallbladder in situ. *Br J Surg* 1995; **82**: 1516–1521.

5. Adamek HE, Breer H, Karschkes T, *et al.* Magnetic resonance imaging in gastroenterology: time to say good-bye to all that endoscopy? *Endoscopy* 2000; **32**: 406–410.

6. Strasberg SM, Clavien PA. Cholecystolithiasis: lithotherapy for the 1990s. *Hepatology* 1992; **16**: 820–839.

Further reading

Bilhartz EL, Horton JD. Gallstone disease and its complications. In: *Sleisenger and Fordtran's Gastrointestinal and Liver Disease.* 6th edn. Eds. M Feldman, BF Scharschmidt, MH Sleizenger. Philadelphia: WB Saunders Co. 1998; pp. 948–972.

van Erpecum KJ, van Berge-Henegouwen GP. Gallstones: an intestinal disease? *Gut* 1999; **44**: 435–438.

Ko CW, Sekijima JH, Lee SP. Biliary sludge. *Ann Intern Med* 1999; **130**: 301–311.

Dowling RH. Review: pathogenesis of gallstones. *Aliment Pharmacol Ther* 2000; **14(suppl 2)**: 39–47.

40. *Helicobacter pylori*: Diagnosis and Management

A.E. DUGGAN and R.P.H. LOGAN

INTRODUCTION

Current guidelines for the management of patients with dyspepsia increasingly incorporate testing for *Helicobacter pylori*. The guidelines are currently based on consensus, but will become more evidence-based as the results of well designed studies assessing the role of *H. pylori* testing in the management of patients with dyspepsia become available. In addition, the sequencing of the genome of *H. pylori* and the identification of pathogenic strains more frequently associated with peptic ulcer disease and gastric cancer raise the possibility that screening for pathogenic strains may become part of the management of dyspepsia. Indeed, the development of near-patient diagnostic tests for *H. pylori* has already led to the majority of treatment for the organism being undertaken in primary care.

With general practitioners increasingly prescribing eradication therapy, hospital-based gastroenterologists are more frequently facing the challenge of managing patients with symptoms that are persistent despite successful eradication of *H. pylori*. Hospital gastrointestinal specialists need to disseminate evidence-based guidelines for the indications, diagnostic methods, and treatment of *H. pylori* infection to colleagues in primary care, and be familiar with the management issues surrounding treatment failure and antimicrobial resistance.

This chapter will first review the diagnosis of *H. pylori* infection in a variety of settings and then discuss the indications for testing and treatment of such infection in the management of dyspepsia.

DIAGNOSIS OF *H. PYLORI*

No one method for detecting *H. pylori* is suited to all clinical situations, so the clinician must balance the clinical context, indication, cost, convenience, and patient acceptability when deciding which test to use. Currently available tests can be divided into **invasive** (endoscopic) and **non-invasive** (non-endoscopic); their relative merits are summarized in Table 40.1.

Invasive tests

Invasive tests are easy to perform during endoscopy. However, with the exception of *H. pylori* infection that has persisted as a result of multiple treatment failures, diagnosis of *H. pylori* alone is not an indication for endoscopy, because of the small, but not insignificant, morbidity and mortality associated with the procedure. Processing of the biopsy samples for histology and microbial culture are also labour-intensive and expensive.

The risks of sampling error are reduced by using large biopsy forceps — for 2.8-mm-channel rather than for 2-mm-channel endoscopes — and by taking several biopsy samples. The guidelines for the clinical trials in *H. pylori* proposed by the working party of the European *H. pylori* Study Group recommend taking two biopsy specimens from the antrum before treatment and from both the antrum and the corpus after treatment (1).

One problem of all invasive tests is the risk of **false-negative results**, which arises from the nature

Table 40.1.   Advantages and disadvantages of different tests for use in *H. pylori* diagnosis.

	Advantages	Disadvantages
Endoscopic tests		
All	Useful before and after treatment	Expense of endoscopy
		Sampling-error-dependent sensitivity
Microbial Culture	High specificity	Time consuming
	Allows determination of antibiotic resistance	Preparation dependent
Histology	High specificity	Observer-dependent
	Permanent record	Does not allow determination of antibiotic resistance
Urease test	High specificity	Does not allow determination of antibiotic resistance
	Rapid, inexpensive	
Non-invasive tests		
All	Non-invasive	No diagnostic information on *H. pylori* induced disease
		Do not allow determination of antibiotic resistance
Urea breath test	High sensitivity and specificity	^{13}C-urea and isotope ratio mass spectrometry are expensive
	Can confirm efficacy of eradication	
	Using carbon-13 testing, can be performed at a distance from the center performing the analysis	
Serology	Inexpensive	Need local validation
	Quick	Accuracy dependent on purification of strains and suitability
	Easy to perform	of strain types for group being tested
	Require no specialized equipment	
Rapid serology	Inexpensive	Need local validation
(near-patient tests)	Quick	Operator-dependent
	Easy to perform	
	Require no specialized equipment	

of *H. pylori* infection, sampling error, and recent or concurrent therapy with drugs — particularly antibiotics and proton pump inhibitors, which reduce the extent and density of *H. pylori* infection.

H. pylori prefers a mildy acidic environment and is unable to colonize intestinal-type mucosa. The distribution of *H. pylori* infection on the gastric mucosa is not uniform: most patients infected with the organism have infection in the gastric antrum, where parietal cells are absent or scanty. Disease processes that start in the antrum — including progressive gastric atrophy, intestinal metaplasia, and bile reflux — disrupt the favoured mucus habitat of *H. pylori*, leading to an uneven distribution of *H. pylori*, the migration of the organism more proximally or, eventually, the loss of the infection.

Antral biopsy specimens should be taken from the distal antrum, and corpus biopsy specimens from the greater curve in the upper third of the stomach (Figure 40.1). Sampling at the **angular and supra-angular lesser curves** should be avoided unless intestinal metaplasia is being actively sought, because, in long-standing gastritis, antral-type glands

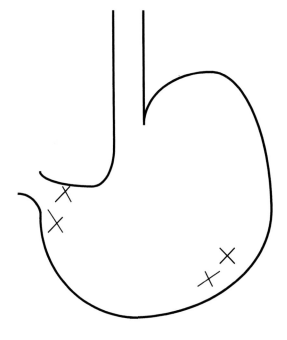

Figure 40.1.   Recommended sites for taking gastric biopsy samples for *H. pylori* testing.

may replace fundal glands and lead to an erroneous diagnosis of corporal atrophic gastritis and failure to detect *H. pylori*. Endoscopists should always be alert to the risk of sampling error, and take additional biopsy samples from elsewhere in the stomach if they are suspicious that infection may be scanty because of the presence of gastric atrophy or intestinal metaplasia.

False positive results rarely occur with endoscopic biopsy samples, provided equipment is properly cleaned, although problems may occur with histology as a result of other gastric bacteria being mistaken for *H. pylori*, especially if special stains are not used (see below).

Effect of concurrent medication on diagnosis

By suppressing gastric acid secretion, **proton pump inhibitors** (PPIs) cause a change in the topography of *H. pylori* infection and a migration of the organism from the antrum to the gastric body. PPIs also cause a diminished bacterial density in both the antrum and body because of their direct antibacterial effect on *H. pylori*. There are no data as to the appropriate period between cessation of PPI treatment and the performance of endoscopic biopsies for *H. pylori*, but data from carbon-13-labelled urea breath testing shows that, in most cases, suppression of infection resolves within 2–4 weeks of the cessation of treatment. Endoscopic studies show that **H$_2$-antagonists** do not affect *H. pylori* density in either the antrum or corpus, and do not need to be stopped before oesophagogastroduodenoscopy (2).

Antibiotics and bismuth also cause diminished bacterial density. Although **bismuth** remains in the gastric body for up to 3 months and may theoretically have a prolonged suppressive effect on *H. pylori*, studies using the ^{13}C-urea breath test have shown recurrence of *H. pylori* within 1 week of the cessation of treatment. Patients should be asked specifically about recent **antibiotic** consumption, as they may not think it important to mention, being neither a reason for their current presentation, or part of their regular medication. Antibiotics should be stopped for 4 weeks before *H. pylori* testing and other drugs known to suppress *H. pylori* infection should be stopped for 2 weeks, both to increase the sensitivity of *H. pylori* diagnosis and to improve the diagnostic yield of oesophagogastroduodenoscopy for detecting peptic ulcer disease and oesophagitis.

Histology

In routine clinical practice, histology is often used as the "gold standard" against which other tests are compared, because of its high sensitivity and specificity, and because it provides a permanent record for future reference. Slides can be reviewed independently and other parameters including intestinal metaplasia and lymphoid aggregates, also assessed.

Although *H. pylori* can usually be detected inexpensively by staining with **haematoxylin and eosin** alone, **special stains** should always be used to distinguish this organism from other bacteria or artefacts in the mucus layer. These stains (modified Giemsa, Steiner silver stain, Genta) are more sensitive than haematoxylin and eosin for detecting the low numbers and abnormal morphologies of *H. pylori* that are likely to occur after ineffective eradication; however, the choice of stain can usually be left to the discretion of the histopathologist.

The accuracy of histology is also dependent on the experience of the observer. The sensitivity and specificity of frequently used stains are similar in the presence of high densities of *H. pylori*, but interobserver variation in the detection of the organism at lower densities of infection can occur. The gastroenterologist is, to a large extent, dependent on the skills of the histopathologist; nevertheless, suspicion should be raised by a report of active gastritis in the absence of *H. pylori* infection: this may be attributable to low levels of infection and should always be an indication for review of slides, the examination of further levels, or assessment of *H. pylori* status by urea breath testing. Biopsy specimens reported as showing extensive intestinal metaplasia should also prompt a more careful assessment of *H. pylori* status by other methods such as urea breath test, because *H. pylori* does not normally colonize this type of epithelium.

Microbiology

Microbiological culture, although highly specific, is the **least sensitive test** for *H. pylori*, because of the fastidious growth requirements of the organism. Specimens need to be transported in physiological saline or semi-solid medium (e.g. Stuart's medium at –4°C) for transportation up to 24 h and then grown on blood or horse serum agar, using both a selective and a non-selective medium in a microaerophilic atmosphere. Culture is time consuming and requires experienced and dedicated personnel for the transport and preparation of specimens. Nevertheless, micro-biology has a major role in determining the antimicrobial sensitivity of clinical isolates either **before treatment** or **after failed treatment**.

Before treatment

Metronidazole resistance was an important predictor of the success of the older bismuth triple-therapy regimens, but may be less important for the PPI-based triple-therapy regimens. Most studies in which these regimens were used have shown that resistance can be overcome in up to 75% of patients, and that clarithromycin is a better choice than amoxicillin as the second antibiotic (see section on treatment). There is, therefore, no current indication for routine culture in non-specialist centres. However, microbial culture may become more important in the future if the prevalence of *H. pylori* resistant to metronidazole or clarithromycin increases.

After failed treatment

Patients failing *H. pylori* eradication treatment as confirmed by urea breath test should have a second course of eradication therapy using **clarithromycin**-based standard triple therapy. However, failure after two courses of eradication therapy is an indication for referral to a specialist centre and follow-up by endoscopy for culture and antimicrobial sensitivity testing.

Currently, there are no standard recommendations for *H. pylori* antimicrobial sensitivity testing, but the E test (AB Biodisk, Soha, Sweden) — which is a quantitative variant of the standard disk diffusion method of assessing antibiotic sensitivity — is a simple and generally reliable method that is commercially available. Confirmation using the reference method for determination of minimum inhibitory concentrations by agar dilution, although recommended by the European *H. pylori* Study Group, is rarely needed in routine clinical practice. Standards for inoculation, incubation, and screening for antibiotic susceptibility are provided in their guidelines for clinical trials in *H. pylori* (1).

Urease tests

Biopsy urease tests are qualitative tests of *H. pylori* infection that are based on the principle that, in the presence of *H. pylori* urease, urea is hydrolysed, leading to an increase in pH and colour change of the pH indicator. Positive results can frequently be interpreted within 1–2 h (especially if kept at 37°C rather than room temperature), but should be reported only as negative after 24 h; false-positive results can occur after 24 h because of other urease-producing organisms in the stomach.

The main **advantages** of biopsy urease tests are that they are simple, quick, and easy tests for detecting *H. pylori*. Several biopsy urease tests are commercially available and direct comparisons of the tests have shown they have similar sensitivities and specificities if performed according to the manufacturers' instructions. The use of two biopsy specimens and incubation of the test at temperatures greater than room temperature gives a quicker result and, unlike other biopsy-based tests, if an adequate biopsy specimen is taken, sensitivity is not affected by the size of the biopsy forceps used. As with all biopsy-based tests, urease tests are prone to sampling error; however, this can be minimized by placing several biopsy specimens from the antrum and body in each test. In financially constrained centres, home-made urease tests can be used, but this is probably not worthwhile, as there is also the option of re-using previously negative tests.

The main **practical problem** of urease tests lies in developing a system to ensure that test results are read and appropriately documented. If the result is not positive by the time the patient leaves the endoscopy suite, it not infrequently arises that the test is left unread at the back of the patient's notes or is taken home in the endoscopist's pocket, with the result not recorded. Few computerized endoscopy reporting systems cater for the late addition of a urease or CLO® result; however, to avoid the need for a further diagnostic test, it is imperative that the result is recorded in the patient's notes. A partial solution for the organized and reliable endoscopist is to enter all the results into the notes at the end of the procedure, so that, subsequently, only those notes relating to late positive results have to be located. If the CLO tests are kept in the endoscopy room, they can be read the next day and the results made available.

Non-invasive tests in secondary care

Serology

Infection with *H. pylori* causes both a local and a systemic immune response. After an initial transient increase in immunoglobulin M (IgM) antibody titres, there is an increase in both IgA and IgG, which are then usually maintained throughout the course of infection. After treatment or spontaneous clearance of infection, titres may take up to 12 months to resolve. Antibodies to *H. pylori* can be detected by **enzyme-linked immunosorbent assay (ELISA)** or latex agglutination, with most assays using serum to detect IgG. Urinary and salivary antibody tests have also been developed, but they have generally been found to be less accurate than serum-based tests.

Serological tests are inexpensive, non-invasive, quick, and easy to perform, and have been independently validated by specialist laboratories. They are commercially available and require no specialized equipment. The accuracy of the numerous commercially available kits varies between populations and between kits, which in part is a reflection of the considerable genetic heterogeneity of *H. pylori* and the even greater antigenic variation; as a consequence, no single *H. pylori* antigen is recognized by sera from all individuals. Pooled preparations from more than one strain avoid non-specific antibody binding, and so have a higher sensitivity, but lower specificity.

Validation studies should always be performed before an *H. pylori* ELISA service is set up, to confirm the sensitivity and specificity of the intended ELISA against endoscopic tests or ideally against the urea breath test, with particular attention paid to the proportion and classification of discrepant results.

Limitations of serology
Serology can not be used to assess the eradication of *H. pylori*, because antibody titres take up to 12 months to decrease below the cutoff value. Children may mount antibody responses that are qualitatively different from those of adults and the elderly, who may have gastric atrophy; lower levels of infection may also stimulate a quantitatively smaller response. Consumption of non-steroidal anti-inflammatory drugs (NSAIDs) has been reported to be associated with reduced accuracy of ELISAs, but there are no data on the duration of this effect, or further studies in progress to confirm this finding.

In the future, the ability to identify pathogenic strains of *H. pylori* associated with peptic ulcer disease or cancer may allow treatment to be targeted at those at risk, without using endoscopy. To date, two bacterial factors have been identified as pathogenic markers associated with peptic ulcer disease: Cag A and Vac A. Cag A seropositivity has also been associated with duodenal ulcer and an increased risk of gastric cancer; however, the clinical significance of Vac A is unclear. Nevertheless, the Vac A genotypes have been shown to be associated with duodenal ulcer, but serological differentiation between the different alleles of Vac A has not yet been possible.

Urea breath testing

Urea breath testing is the most **sensitive** and **specific** method for detecting *H. pylori* infection and assessing its eradication, and is easy to perform. The $^{13/14}$C-urea breath test is based on the principle that a solution of urea isotopically labelled with carbon-13 or -14 will be rapidly hydrolysed by the abundantly expressed urease of *H. pylori*, labelled carbon dioxide being excreted in the exhaled breath.

False-positive results are rare, and are usually the result of poor swallowing technique by the patients; failure to swallow the isotope rapidly allows hydrolysis of the urea by oropharyngeal bacteria. Drugs known to inhibit *H. pylori* infection are the main cause of false-negative or equivocal results and include antibiotics, bismuth, proton pump inhibitors, or high-dose H_2-receptor antagonists. Patients should therefore be advised to cease taking any of the drugs known to cause false-negative results 4 weeks before undergoing their urea breath test. Previous gastric surgery is a less common cause of a false-negative result.

The **^{14}C-urea breath test** is less expensive and more widely available than the ^{13}C-urea version, but uses a radioactive isotope that requires a β scintillation counter for analysis. Scintigraphy although widely available for ^{14}C-carbon dioxide analysis, involves a delay of at least two working days before a result is available; the need to organize an appointment and obtain results from another department is also inconvenient and causes logistic problems for rapid diagnosis. Furthermore, carbon-14 is unsuitable for pregnant women, children, and repeated use. An alternative to the ^{14}C-urea breath test is the **^{13}C-urea breath test**; although more expensive, this has the advantage of using a non-radioactive isotope. Several alternative, cheaper methods for the detection of ^{13}C-carbon dioxide have recently been described, including the use of laser or infra-red spectroscopy. These new technologies are still at an early stage of development and studies of their accuracy are limited, but they promise to enhance considerably the use of the ^{13}C-urea breath test, so that it can be performed in most hospitals or specialist clinics and with results available within 15 min.

Non-invasive tests in primary care

The ^{13}C-urea breath test is commercially available and so can be used by general practitioners in their surgeries. It uses a stable non-radioactive isotope, which means that samples can be sent by post to centres for analysis. However, commercial analysis by mass spectrometry is still relatively expensive (£28 BSIA; Bureau of Stable Isotope Analysis, Chatham, UK). Although improvements in the speed of analysis look promising, there remains a delay in obtaining the result, which does not occur with the near-patient serological tests.

Near-patient testing

Near-patient (or office-based) tests are recent additions to the general practitioner's diagnostic and management armamentarium and allow testing for a wide range of conditions including screening for increased cholesterol, diabetes, and pregnancy. By providing these doctors with easy access to rapid diagnostic methods, they increase the scope of management options available at the time of the patient's consultation.

Rapid serological near-patient tests for detecting *H. pylori* have also been developed, and provide general practitioners with ready access to *H. pylori* diagnosis, which can be used to determine further management. The near-patient tests for *H. pylori* are qualitative tests that are based either on latex agglutination or solid-phase ELISA using serum or whole blood from a venous or capillary sample. Most tests have a test pad that contains immobilized antigen (control zone) and anti-IgG antibody (test zone), to which is added a reconstituting agent and a few drops of the patient's sample. Results are read visually as positive, negative or invalid, after 4–10 min. The tests are therefore easy to perform, require no special-

ized equipment, and provide rapid results. They are also inexpensive (£10–20 per test).

Because near-patient tests are essentially "fancy" ELISAs, it is not too surprising that variable results have been reported (Table 40.2). Other factors also contributing to the wide variation in reported accuracy are commercial competition and lack of independent studies. More importantly, these tests may be prone to observer variation in the interpretation of results. In contrast to the limited numbers of trained staff who perform ELISAs, in primary care a large number of people may be involved with testing, but with insufficient expertise or frequency to become familiar with performing the test and reading the result. In a study undertaken in secondary care of the performance of one type of near-patient tests, 10% of results were considered difficult to read, and in 1% of cases two observers recorded a different result for the same test pad (3).

Other methods

A number of other methods for detecting *H. pylori* infection have been proposed, but are rarely used in clinical practice, because of poor sensitivity and specificity (salivary antibody tests), limited applicability (isotope urine blood tests), limited acceptability (the string test), or lack of refinement of the technique (PCR).

Table 40.2. Accuracy of near-patient tests for *H. pylori*.

Test (reference)	Number of patients	Sensitivity	Specificity
Helisal			
(4)	69	93	88
(3)	100	95	55
(5)	147	78	81
(6)	170	81	73
(7)	256	89	89
(8)	303	85	78
(9)	154	88	91
(10)	110	71	88
FlexSure HP			
(11)	551	94	88
(12)	94	94	79
(13)	64	89	93
Quickvue			
(11)	200	88	83
(14)	99	92	84
(15)	193	82	83

MANAGEMENT OF *H. PYLORI* AND DYSPEPSIA

Dyspeptic symptoms are responsible for 4% of all general practice consultations, in addition to considerable costs from the investigation and treatment of dyspepsia. Expenditure on gastric antisecretory drugs alone accounts for 15% of prescribing costs (£300m per year) in primary care. The increasing demand for oesophagogastroduodenoscopy can not be met; in the UK, annual requirements per head of population for upper gastrointestinal endoscopy have been estimated to have reached 1 in 100. Hence there is great interest in management strategies that might reduce these costs.

Historically, the management of dyspepsia has been mainly **empirical**, with referral to hospital primarily for the management of intractable symptoms, or the need to exclude carcinoma. Recognition of the strong association between *H. pylori* and peptic ulcer disease has changed the management options for dyspepsia, which now include **early endoscopy**, a **trial of empiric therapy**, *H. pylori* **testing and referral of** *H. pylori* **positive patients for oesophagogastroduodenoscopy**, or *H. pylori* **testing and treatment**. However, it needs to be emphasized that testing for the organism has no role in the management of patients with alarm symptoms, which include dysphagia, weight loss, anaemia, jaundice, haematemesis, or melaena. These patients should be referred for urgent endoscopic assessment, as has been recommended for patients older than 45 years with new-onset dyspepsia (although evidence that this measure has improved the early diagnosis of gastrooesophageal cancer in this group is limited).

The most frequent reasons for consultation are concern about serious underlying disease (i.e. cancer) and the severity of symptoms, but psychological distress is also a factor. Widespread publicity about *H. pylori* infection has also contributed to patients' anxiety, leading to consultation with the general practitioner and subsequent requests for testing. In these circumstances hospital-based non-invasive tests provide a very useful alternative to oesophagogastroduodenoscopy and biopsy examinations.

Primary care

The value of *H. pylori* testing and eradication in a dyspeptic patient with a well-established past history of peptic ulcer disease, is widely accepted. However, for the vast majority of patients with dyspepsia, even when the complaint is of reflux or ulcer-like pain, clinical diagnosis is inaccurate and management more complex. With *H. pylori* testing, general practitioners can test for *H. pylori* and refer only *H. pylori*-positive patients for endoscopy, or give eradication treatment to all those who test positive, reserving oesophagogastroduodenoscopy for those with persistent symptoms or whose symptoms fail to respond to empirical therapy. Guidelines have been developed, and randomized controlled trials are under way to determine the place of *H. pylori* testing in the management of dyspepsia in primary care.

Consensus guidelines

Most recent guidelines use *H. pylori* testing to stratify the management of dyspepsia in patients younger than 45 years. For older patients, *H. pylori* testing is not recommended, because of the high proportion of *H. pylori*-negative gastric cancers and the loss of serological responses to *H. pylori* with widespread gastric atrophy, a precursor of gastric cancer. *H. pylori* testing is also appropriate for patients younger than 45 years only if access to accurate diagnostic tests is available. Most guidelines recommend either a **test-and-treat** or **test-and-refer** strategy. The British Society of Gastroenterology guidelines for dyspepsia management recommend referral of *H. pylori*-positive patients to endoscopy, with *H. pylori* eradication reserved for those demonstrated to have gastric ulcer or duodenal ulcer at endoscopy. In contrast, The American Gastroenterology Association guidelines recommend treatment with eradication therapy for positive patients, with referral to endoscopy only if patients continue to be symptomatic. Both guidelines recommend endoscopic investigation of *H. pylori*-negative patients who have continuing symptoms that are unresponsive to antisecretory treatment. A 1–2 month trial of empirical acid-suppression treatment has the benefit of detecting many of the patients with GORD, up to 50% of whom would have no oesophagitis on endoscopy.

Although the majority of dyspepsia management occurs in primary care, most guidelines have been developed in secondary care, and so differences between primary and secondary care need to be considered when these guidelines are used to assess patients presenting with dyspepsia in primary care.

Role of H. pylori testing in primary care

Secondary-care studies confirm that a practice of referring to endoscopy only those patients who are *H. pylori*-positive misses little pathology in the non-referred group. However, the anticipated reduction (23–37%) in the number of endoscopies performed because of the reassurance provided by a negative *H. pylori* test may only be short lived, and has not been substantiated by prospective evaluation in primary care. Treating all *H. pylori*-infected patients younger than 45 years with eradication therapy and performing endoscopy only in *H. pylori*-negative patients has also been proposed; however, this strategy has not been prospectively evaluated and is more labour-intensive.

Clear evidence remains lacking to support a strategy of *H. pylori* testing or eradication treatment in the management of previously uninvestigated dyspepsia. Until randomized trials based in primary care are reported, the best evidence for *H. pylori* testing or eradication treatment in the management of dyspepsia comes from decision-analysis studies that compared *H. pylori*-testing strategies with traditional empirical therapy and with early endoscopy. The findings of studies in the USA suggest that the cost-effectiveness of empiric *H. pylori* eradication strategy, with or without testing, is not greatly different from a strategy of early endoscopy, particularly when endoscopy is as inexpensive as it is in the UK (16).

Although empirical use of *H. pylori* eradication treatment without endoscopic diagnosis of peptic ulcer disease may prove to be the most cost effective for both general practitioners and patients, it is a controversial strategy. There is the risk of increasing antibiotic resistance and of complications such as pseudomembranous colitis. It also assumes that there are no benefits to being infected with *H. pylori*. An increasing incidence of GORD, Barrett's oesophagus, adenocarcinoma of the oesophagus, and gastric cardia has occurred in several Western countries where there has been a decrease in the acquisition of *H. pylori* in childhood. *H. pylori* eradication treatment should be used conservatively until it is established whether these two phenomena are related.

Currently, some general practitioners have access to the near-patient tests that allow testing within primary care. Depending on the test, the cost is £12–20, with eradication treatment costing £20–30. Thus the extra costs involved in testing and successfully eradicating *H. pylori* in a patient with ulcer are relatively modest, and similar to the costs of 3 months of antisecretory treatment. However, the main concerns with test-and-treat strategies are that, among patients seeking primary-care consultations for dyspepsia, only 10–25% of those who are *H. pylori*-positive will have peptic ulcer disease. Cost savings may not materialize if *H. pylori* testing and eradication are also given to the large proportion of patients without peptic ulcer disease whose dyspeptic symptoms are likely to be unaffected by eradicating *H. pylori*, or if poorly effective eradication regimens are used. They are even less likely to materialize in the under-45-years age group, in whom the prevalence of *H. pylori* is much lower, and tests are likely to have a lower positive predictive value than in areas where *H. pylori* infection is endemic.

Secondary care

Role of H. pylori testing in secondary care

Currently, in the UK, abdominal pain is the third most common indication for outpatient referral. The majority of diagnoses will be functional, nevertheless, *H. pylori* testing can be effectively used to stratify the management of patients referred with dyspepsia. The options available to the gastroenterologist are multiple. The traditional approach is to assess all patients in the **outpatient department**. However, this has proved to be time-consuming and costly, and to generate delays in diagnosis without improving the selection of patients for endoscopy. At the other extreme is an unrestricted **open-access service** allowing general practitioners direct access to oesophago-gastroduodeno-scopy referral without any controls to restrict demand.

Many gastroenterology units use selective open-access endoscopy to control the demand for endoscopy. In the absence of *H. pylori* testing in primary care, scrutiny of referral letters to select patients younger than 45 years and with a history of recent-onset dyspepsia for referral for ^{14}C-urea breath testing will identify those who are *H. pylori*-positive and likely to have pathology on endoscopy (provided patients are given sufficient warning to stop acid-suppression therapy before they undergo testing).

Although *H. pylori*-positive patients can then be referred directly to endoscopy, there are no long-term data confirming that *H. pylori*-negative patients are reassured by their negative result and will not require endoscopy at a later date. Thus the benefits of selective endoscopy in terms of reducing work loads may be short-lived. The workloads of gastroenterologists are also likely to increase if general practitioners use near-patient *H. pylori* tests with poor accuracy. This is likely to increase the proportion of inappropriate referral of patients with false-positive results and lead to a failure to identify *H. pylori* in patients with false-negative results. Local validation of *H. pylori* diagnostic tests that are to be used by general practitioners should therefore be the first step in the endorsement of dyspepsia guidelines by the gastroenterologist. Before this, patients should be referred to undergo oesophagogastroduodenoscopy or outpatient department review on the basis of hospital-based and locally validated ELISA testing or by urea breath testing.

Screening

One of the advantages of non-invasive tests for *H. pylori* infection is that they can also be used for screening in either primary or secondary care. However, it is essential to consider the aim and context of screening before deciding which test to use. Selecting a test for screening is often a **trade-off between sensitivity and specificity**. If the aim of screening in secondary care (i.e. patients referred to the outpatient department) is to avoid missing the diagnosis of *H. pylori*-positive duodenal ulcer, tests with a high sensitivity at the expense of specificity are preferable, particularly if the prevalence of *H. pylori* is low in the local population. However, an unacceptably high proportion of patients may be investigated or treated unnecessarily because of false-positive results if the specificity of the test is unacceptably low. In contrast, selecting a test with high specificity will lead to fewer unnecessary oesophagogastro-duodenoscopies from false-positive results, and may provide a useful means of patient reassurance in primary care. However, the prevalence of *H. pylori* and the sensitivity of the test will determine the probability of missing *H. pylori* and peptic ulcer disease. The influence of the prevalence of *H. pylori* on the predictive value of tests is shown in Table 40.3.

TREATMENT

Who to treat

With improvements in the safety, simplicity, and effectiveness of *H. pylori* treatment, eradication therapy is being increasingly prescribed, despite lack of evidence to support its clinical effectiveness in conditions other than peptic ulcer disease and the increasingly rare early MALT lymphoma (Table 40.4).

Duodenal ulcer

H. pylori is present in more than 95% of patients with duodenal ulcer who are not taking aspirin or other NSAIDs, and numerous randomized trials have shown that *H. pylori* eradication, when successful, virtually cures *H. pylori*-positive duodenal ulcer. The **management** of patients with diagnosed duodenal ulcer disease is therefore clear-cut:

- empirical eradication of *H. pylori* without further investigation should be offered to all patients taking intermittent or long-term antisecretory treatment for duodenal ulcer previ-

Table 40.3. Effect of the prevalence of *H. pylori* on predictive value of tests with constant sensitivity and specificity.

Prevalence (%)	Sensitivity (%)	Specificity (%)	PPV	NPV
5	90	90	32	99
15	90	90	64	97
25	90	90	75	96
35	90	90	82	94
50	90	90	90	90

PPV, positive predictive value; NPV, negative predictive value.

Table 40.4. The role of *H. pylori* eradication in the management of gastrointestinal diseases, based on current evidence.

Disease	*H. pylori* eradication
Peptic ulcer disease (non-NSAID)	Indicated
MALT lymphoma	Indicated*
Peptic ulcer disease (NSAID)	Not indicated
GORD	Not indicated
Non-ulcer dyspepsia	Not indicated
Gastric cancer prevention	Not indicated

MALT, mucosa-associated lymphoid tissue; *, insufficient treatment for advanced disease.

ously diagnosed either by endoscopy or by unequivocal barium meal, as there is little value in
confirming the presence of *H. pylori*

- for patients not previously investigated who are
found to have duodenal ulcer at endoscopy, there
is an argument for presumptive eradication treatment without formal testing for *H. pylori*. Alternatively, *H. pylori* can be easily diagnosed by biopsy
urease test (CLO test), which may be positive by
the time the patient is ready to leave the endoscopy
unit and enable eradication treatment to be started
immediately. At endoscopy, biopsy samples can
also be taken for histology, to be sent for processing
only if the urease test remains negative at 24 h. If
both urease and histology are negative the patient
should also undergo a urea breath testing and other
rare causes of gastroduodenal ulceration should be
considered (e.g. Crohn's disease, Zollinger–Ellison
syndrome, and covert use of NSAIDs), particularly
in those patients who have had recurrent duodenal
ulcer

- although the natural history of duodenitis and
duodenal erosions is less well documented, if
seen at oesophagogastroduodenoscopy they
should be treated as part of the spectrum of
duodenal ulcer disease, and *H. pylori* eradicated
if present. Unlike gastritis, macroscopic duodenitis and microscopic duodenal inflammatory
appearances correlate well, and duodenal biopsy
examination is rarely indicated

Gastric ulcer

Gastric ulcers have a much lower prevalence than
duodenal ulcers, except in association with the use of
NSAIDs, but 60–90% of gastric ulcers are associated
with *H. pylori* (17). Several randomized
trials have shown that, in the absence of NSAID use,
H. pylori eradication speeds the healing of ulcers and
prevents their recurrence (18). As the management of
gastric ulceration is dominated by the need to exclude malignancy, testing for *H. pylori* does not
usually pose any problem, provided endoscopic biopsy samples are taken proximal to the ulcer.

Duodenal or gastric ulcer in the presence of H. pylori and NSAIDs

It is not yet known whether eradicating *H. pylori* will
reduce the risk of ulcer disease developing in NSAID
users. The findings of a small randomized study (19)
suggested that eradication of the organism before the

use of NSAIDs is commenced may reduce ulcer
development, but this requires confirmation in a larger
series. For patients already taking NSAIDs, the data
are also unclear and controversial (20,21). A number
of studies have shown no association between long-
term NSAID use and *H. pylori* infection, although
this has not been found consistently. Differences may
exist between type of NSAID or aspirin and ulcer
type. These studies may also be prone to selection
bias if they excluded patients who may have stopped
taking NSAIDs because of dyspeptic or other complications in the past. Randomized trials are needed,
to assess whether an association exists.

In contrast, *H. pylori* eradication may be of no
benefit in patients already taking NSAIDs. Data from
two large randomized trials have shown, compared
with *H. pylori* negative patients, superior rates of
healing and reduced recurrence in *H. pylori* positive
patients taking NSAIDs who are prescribed PPI
prophylaxis, which is consistent with the observation
that *H. pylori* augments the antisecretory effect of
PPIs. As NSAID use accounts for only about 70% of
ulcers developing in NSAID takers (based on a relative risk of 3–4), *H. pylori* colonization is likely to
account for most of the remaining 30% and may
make it prudent, until more data become available,
to eradicate *H. pylori* in those patients taking NSAIDs
who have ulcers and who are also *H. pylori*-positive
— although, in those patients requiring PPI prophylaxis, the benefits may be fewer, if any.

Non-ulcer dyspepsia

A positive definition of non-ulcer dyspepsia remains
elusive but, in operational terms, it can be defined as
**symptoms believed to be arising from the upper
gastrointestinal tract in the absence of endoscopic
ulceration or GORD**. The gastroenterologist or
general practitioner is frequently confronted with the
patient with dyspepsia who is found to be *H. pylori*-
positive, with *H. pylori*-induced gastritis on endoscopy. Given the high prevalence of *H. pylori* infection,
it is not surprising that many patients with non-ulcer
dyspepsia are found to be infected. It is tempting to
think that the infection is responsible for their symptoms; however, there is still no clear evidence that *H.
pylori* eradication is beneficial. Two double-blind
trials of *H. pylori* eradication in patients with non-
ulcer dyspepsia have shown conflicting results, one
study showing benefit in 20% of patients treated,
compared with 7% of those treated with placebo

(22), and the other showing no difference between two such groups (23).

Prescribing *H. pylori* eradication treatment for patients with non-ulcer dyspepsia may generate unnecessary costs, complicate the management of these patients, and cause unnecessary morbidity. As the natural history of the condition is often chronic, prescribing eradication treatment may lead to a proportion of patients representing with un-known *H. pylori* status and unrealized expectations, which, in turn, may generate further consultations or investigations. Prescribing *H. pylori* eradication treatment for patients with non-ulcer dyspepsia also exposes them to a small, but well-recognized, risk of antibiotic side effects, including pseudomembranous colitis.

Gastrooesophageal reflux disease

Symptomatic GORD is a common reason for presentation, both in primary and secondary care. Prevalence data indicate that up to 10% of the adult population experience heartburn on a daily basis. Endoscopic studies of patients referred for investigation of dyspeptic symptoms indicate that erosive oesophagitis accounts for up to 33% of endoscopic diagnosis with pH studies indicating that this is an underdiagnosis of symptomatic gastrooesophageal reflux. Thus the management of GORD is complex, and constitutes a substantial proportion of the gastroenterologist's workload. The three main areas of debate regarding the **role of *H. pylori* in the management of GORD** are:

1. Does *H. pylori* cause GORD?
2. Does *H. pylori* eradication cause, or exacerbate, or cure GORD?
3. Does treatment of GORD with PPIs in the presence of *H. pylori* increase the risk of gastric cancer?

There is no evidence from epidemiological studies that *H. pylori* is implicated in the pathogenesis of GORD. For the clinician, the key question is whether eradicating *H. pylori* exacerbates symptoms or decreases the risk of gastric cancer. Data from *H. pylori* eradication studies in patients with duodenal ulcer have shown that, after *H. pylori* eradication, a proportion of patients have symptomatic reflux. It is unclear whether this is new-onset GORD (because of weight gain after ulcer cure), whether previous GORD symptoms were attributed to duodenal ulcer disease, or whether the symptoms of GORD have now been unmasked as a result of the cessation antisecretory treatment.

***H. pylori* infection augments the antisecretory effect of PPIs and H$_2$-receptor antagonists**, leading to greater acid suppression than in those without infection. Eradication of *H. pylori* decreases the antisecretory effect of both drugs. Theoretically, therefore, *H. pylori*-positive patients whose GORD symptoms are controlled with antisecretory treatment may need higher doses of antisecretory agents to control their symptoms if they have their *H. pylori* infection eradicated. Whether this is clinically relevant needs to be determined.

The main argument to support *H. pylori* eradication in GORD is the hypothesis that, with long-term PPI treatment, *H. pylori* migrates from the antrum to the body of the stomach and thus promotes the development of chronic atrophic pangastritis and intestinal metaplasia. Preliminary data from a randomized trial comparing acid-suppression therapy with antireflux surgery has not confirmed this, although longer follow-up is required. Even if the hypothesis holds true, the increased risk of gastric cancer is likely to be no more than the fivefold increase found in association with pernicious anaemia and, if this proves to be an indication for *H. pylori* eradication, it may be of relevance only to younger patients needing long-term PPI treatment; furthermore, in this group of patients, laparoscopic surgery may be a better management option, given the period of time that would elapse before the development of cancer.

Treatment regimens

In vitro, *H. pylori* is sensitive to a wide range of antimicrobial agents. However, their efficacy *in vivo* is often disappointingly poor because of the unfavourably low pH of the stomach, their failure to penetrate gastric mucus, and the low concentrations obtained in the mucosa of the fundus of the stomach. Although a 2-week bismuth-based triple therapy (bismuth with metronidazole and either tetracycline or amoxycillin) was an effective regimen (efficacy 78–89%), its value was limited by the high rate of side effects and by the complexity of the dosing, both of which led to poor compliance. Efficacy was further compromised in patients with resistant strains of *H. pylori* (24).

First-line treatment is now based on a 1-week regimen of twice-daily PPI and clarithromycin, with either amoxicillin or a nitroimidazole such as tinadazole or metronidazole (efficacy 80–89%). The new triple therapies are less affected by poor compliance, because side effects are less frequent, treatment duration is shorter, and dosing simpler. There is no advantage in using a longer duration of treatment. In addition, the impact of metronidazole resistance on these regimens appears to be less than that of the standard bismuth-based regimens. So far other combinations, including ranitidine-bismuth-citrate triple therapy, appear to be slightly less effective. A recent decision-analysis model has demonstrated that even small differences in the efficacy of eradication regimens can result in big differences in the relative cost effectiveness of different eradication strategies for *H. pylori*. With the availability of the highly effective new triple therapies, regimens with suboptimal or inconsistent efficacy should not be used.

Assessing eradication

If an effective eradication regimen has been used to treat uncomplicated duodenal ulcer, it is more cost effective not to assess eradication, but to treat symptomatic relapse as an eradication failure. Assessing the success of eradication and treating eradication failures with either maintenance acid-suppression therapy or repeat antibiotics generates costs equivalent to many years of symptomatic treatment with acid-suppression therapy. If a decision is made to confirm eradication, it is best done by carrying out a ^{13}C- or ^{14}C-urea breath test, 4 weeks after the discontinuation of treatment.

Second-line treatment for treatment failure

Metronidazole-resistant *H. pylori* is a clinical problem, particularly among patients who have previously been prescribed metronidazole for other indications. The prevalence of metronidazole-resistant *H. pylori* has also increased because of the use of suboptimal *H. pylori* eradication regimens. Fortunately, in both randomized and non-randomized studies, metronidazole resistance can be overcome in up to 75% of cases by combining metronidazole with a **PPI** and either **clarithromycin** or **amoxycillin**. Clarithromycin appears to be a better second antibiotic than amoxycillin.

Quadruple therapies using a combination of standard triple therapies with a PPI have been proposed for patients with metronidazole-resistant strains. **Seven-day treatment** has been shown to have an efficacy of between 90 and 100%, but more data are needed to confirm this finding and to determine whether it is more cost effective than a second course of PPI-based triple therapy for patients in whom eradication of *H. pylori* initially failed.

The prevalence of clarithromycin resistance is much lower, being less than 5% in the UK at present, but up to 10% in parts of Europe. Too few data are available to permit conclusions to be drawn as to the susceptibility of clarithromycin-resistant strains to current antibiotic regimens; however, unlike metronidazole resistance, clarithromycin resistance may be irreversible, which would make it a major problem in the treatment of *H. pylori* in the future.

Recurrence

Patients frequently express concern about transmitting their *H. pylori* infection to a spouse or to children, or re-acquiring it after eradication. There is little place for concern in either case. It is clear from analysis of the whole genome sequence that *H. pylori* can not survive outside its unique gastric habitat and must be transmitted person-to-person either faeco-orally or oro-orally. Infection occurs predominantly in childhood; primary seroconversion in adults from developed countries is uncommon and of the order of less than 0.5% per year. **Rates of re-infection** 1 year after documented *H. pylori* eradication are similar to those for primary infection and are between 0.5 and 1.5%. **Acquisition of *H. pylori*** by handling gastric juice and by giving mouth-to-mouth resuscitation have been reported, therefore clinicians need to be aware of, and avoid transmitting, *H. pylori* inadvertently, via either unclean endoscopes or other material exposed to gastric juice.

FUTURE PRACTICE

In the future, the role of *H. pylori* testing in the management of dyspepsia may change in the light of results of decision-analysis models and community-based trials that are currently being performed in Britain and in Europe. Treatment may become targeted to pathogenic strains, particularly if well-conserved and consistent virulence markers can be found. Although it is difficult to predict to what extent metronidazole resistance will be a problem in the future, because of the poor correlation between minimum inhibitory concentrations and the performance of the triple therapies, the increasing prevalence of clarithromycin-resistant organisms already seen in some countries is a cause for future concern.

It is interesting to speculate on the role of prevention in the future management of *H. pylori*. Vaccination against *H. pylori* infection has been one option that has been seriously investigated. Should a suitable antigen preparation be found, the advantages of vaccination would be its anticipated impact on the incidence of gastric cancer and peptic ulcer in areas where *H. pylori* is endemic. In these areas, vaccination may be an inexpensive public health measure. However, the benefits are likely to be fewer in those areas that are also more likely to be able to afford such treatment. It may be much less justifiable to recommend widespread vaccination in many Western countries where the prevalence of *H. pylori* infection is much lower, there is greater consumer concern about the possibility of vaccination increasing the risk of other diseases, and the survival benefits associated with *H. pylori* infection can not be disregarded.

References

1. Guidelines for clinical trials in *Helicobacter pylori* infection. *Gut* 1997; **41(suppl 2)**: S1–S23.
   Guidelines on the standards for the diagnosis of *H. pylori* infection; particularly for use in trials of *H. pylori* management.

2. Meining A, Kiel G, Stolte M. Changes in *Helicobacter pylori*-induced gastritis in the antrum and corpus during and after 12 months of treatment with ranitidine and lansoprazole in patients with duodenal ulcer disease. *Aliment Pharmacol Ther* 1998; **12**: 735–740.

3. Stone MA, Mayberry JF, Wicks ACB *et al*. Near patient testing for *Helicobacter pylori*: a detailed evaluation of the Cortecs Helisal Rapid Blood Test. *Eur J Gastroenterol Hepatol* 1997; **9**: 257–260.

4. Yapp T, Kapur K, Thomas GAO *et al*. Validation of the Helisal rapid whole blood test for the detection of IgG antibodies to *H. pylori*. *Gut* 1995; **37**: A56 (Abstract).

5. Peitz U, Tillenburg B, Baumann M. Insufficient validity of a new rapid whole blood test for *Helicobacter pylori* (HP) infection. *Gastroenterology* 1996; **110**: A226 (Abstract).

6. Duggan A, Logan R, Knifton A. Accuracy of near-patient blood tests for *Helicobacter pylori*. *Lancet* 1996; **348**: 617.

7. Lahaie RG, Ricard N. Validation of Helisal whole blood test, serum and saliva tests for the non-invasive diagnosis of *H. pylori* infection. *Gastroenterology* 1996; **110**: A167 (Abstract).

8. Reilly TG, Poxon V, Sanders DSA, *et al*. Comparison of serum, salivary and rapid whole blood diagnostic test for *Helicobacter pylori* and their validation against endoscopy based tests. *Gut* 1997; **40**: 454–458.

9. Moayyedi P, Carter AM, Catto A, *et al*. Validation of a rapid whole blood test for diagnosing *Helicobacter pylori* infection. *BMJ* 1997; **314**: 119.

10. Talley NJ, Lambert JR, Howell S, *et al*. An evaluation of whole blood testing for *Helicobacter pylori* in general practice. *Aliment Pharmacol Ther* 1998; **12**: 641–645.

11. Graham DY, Evans DJ, Peacock J, *et al*. Comparison of rapid serological tests (FlexSure HP and QuickVue) with conventional ELISA for detection of *Helicobacter pylori* infection. *Am J Gastroenterol* 1996; **91**: 942–948.

12. Miller S, Sharma TK, Cutler AF. Prospective evaluation of test characteristics of a new method for detection of serum antibodies to *Helicobacter pylori*. *Gastroenterology* 1996; **110**: A197 (Abstract).

13. Kroser J, Faigel DO, Furth EE, *et al*. Comparison of rapid office-based serology with formal laboratory-based ELISA testing for diagnosis of *Helicobacter pylori* gastritis. *Dig Dis Sci* 1998; **43**: 103–108.

14. Williams NR, West JA, Howard AN, *et al*. Validation of a rapid near-patient test for diagnosing *H. pylori* infection. *Gut* 1997; **44**: A81 (Abstract).

15. Duggan AE, Hardy E, Hawkey CJ. Evaluation of a new Near Patient Test for the detection of *Helicobacter pylori*. *Eur J Gastroenterol Hepatol* 1998; **10**: 133–136.

16. Silverstein MD, Petterson T, Talley NJ. Initial endoscopy or empirical therapy with or without testing for *Helicobacter pylori* for dyspepsia: a decision analysis. *Gastroenterology* 1996; **110**: 72–83.
    Decision-analysis model assessing the cost effectiveness of different management strategies for the treatment of patients with dyspeptic symptoms.

17. Penston JG. Clinical aspects of *H. pylori* eradication therapy in peptic ulcer disease. *Aliment Pharmacol Ther* 1996; **10**: 469–486.

18. Labenz J, Borsch G. Evidence for the essential role of *H. pylori* in gastric ulcer disease. *Gut* 1994; **35**: 19–22.

19. Chan FKL, Sung JJY, Chung SCS *et al*. Randomised trial of eradication of *Helicobacter pylori* before non-steroidal anti-inflammatory drug therapy to prevent peptic ulcers. *Lancet* 1997; **350**: 975–979.

20. Wilcox CM. Relationship between nonsteroidal anti-inflammatory drug use, *Helicobacter pylori*, and gastroduodenal mucosal injury. *Gastroenterology* 1997; **113**: S85–S89.

21. Hawkey CJ, Tulassay Z, Szczepanski L, *et al*. Randomised controlled trial of *Helicobacter pylori* eradication in patients on non-steroidal anti-inflammatory drugs: HELP NSAIDs study. *Lancet* 1998; **352**: 1016–1021.

22. McColl K, Murray L, El-Omar E, *et al*. Symptomatic benefit from eradicating *Helicobacter pylori* infection in patients with nonulcer dyspepsia. *N Engl J Med* 1998; **339**: 1869–74.

23. Talley NJ, Janssens J, Lauritsen K, *et al*. Eradication of *Helicobacter pylori* in functional dyspepsia: a randomised double-blind placebo-controlled trial with 12 months' follow up. The Optimal Regimen Cures Helicobacter Induced Dyspepsia (ORCHID) Study Group. *BMJ* 1999; **318**: 833–837.

24. van der Hulst R, Kellar J, Rauws E *et al.* Treatment of *Helicobacter pylori*: a review of the world literature. *Helicobacter* 1996; **1**: 6–19.

A meta-analysis of trials of *H. pylori* eradication regimens.

Recommended reading

Current European concepts in the management of *Helicobacter pylori* infection. The Maastricht Consensus Report. European Helicobacter Pylori Study Group. *Gut* 1997; **41**: 8–13.

Guidelines on the indications for treatment of *H. pylori* infection.

Helicobacter pylori testing kits. *Drug Ther Bull* 1997; **35**: 23–24.

A review of diagnostic tests for *H. pylori* that are suitable for use in primary care.

Penston J, McColl K. Eradication of *Helicobacter pylori*: an objective assessment of current therapies. *Br J Clin Pharmacol* 1997; **43**: 232–243.

A comprehensive review of trials of *H. pylori* eradication regimens.

Blaser MJ. *Helicobacter pylori* and gastric diseases. *BMJ* 1998; **316**: 1507–1510.

A well-presented counter-argument for not eradicating *H. pylori*.

British Society of Gastroenterology. *Dyspepsia Management Guidelines* 1996. London: British Society of Gastroenterology, 1996.

These British guidelines emphasize a *H. pylori* test-and-refer to endoscopy strategy.

American Gastroenterological Association Medical Position Statement. Evaluation of dyspepsia. *Gastroenterology* 1998; **114**: 579–581.

These US guidelines emphasize a *H. pylori* test-and-treat strategy.

American Gastroenterological Association Technical Review. Evaluation of dyspepsia. *Gastroenterology* 1998; **114**: 582–595.

A review of the evidence supporting current concensus guidelines for the management of dyspepsia.

Briggs AH, Sculpher MJ, Logan RPH *et al.* Cost effectiveness of screening for and eradication of *Helicobacter pylori* in management of dyspeptic patients under 45 years of age. *BMJ* 1996; **312**: 1321–1325.

A decision-analysis model assessing the cost effectiveness of *H. pylori* eradication compared with maintenance therapy for diagnosed duodenal ulcer disease, and the cost effectiveness of screening for duodenal ulcer compared with empirical treatment.

Fendrick AM, Chernew ME, Hirth RA *et al.* Alternative management strategies for patients with suspected peptic ulcer disease. *Ann Intern Med* 1995; **123**: 260–268.

Duggan AE, Tolley K, Hawkey CJ *et al.* Varying efficacy of *Helicobacter pylori* eradication regimens: cost effectiveness study using a decision analysis model. *BMJ* 1998; **316**: 1648–1654.

A cost-effectiveness study comparing how small differences in efficacy of *H. pylori* eradication regimens for patients with duodenal ulcer can lead to large differences in their relative cost-effectiveness.

Logan RPH, Walker MM, Misiewicz JJ *et al.* Changes in the intragastric distribution of *Helicobacter pylori* during treatment with omeprazole. *Gut* 1995; **36**: 12–16.

An endoscopic study showing that 4 weeks of treatment with PPIs causes a significant decrease in the histological density of *H. pylori* infection in the antrum and corpus, and an increase in the density of *H. pylori* infection in the fundus.

37. Kuipers EJ, Lundell L, Klinkenberg-Knol EC *et al.* Atrophic gastritis and *Helicobacter pylori* infection in patients with reflux esophagitis treated with omeprazole or fundoplication. *N Engl J Med* 1996; **334**: 1018–1022.

A cohort study (with a number of methodological problems) of two groups of patients with *H. pylori* and oesophagitis treated with PPIs or fundoplication, and their rate of progression of atrophic gastritis over a mean follow-up of 5 years.

38. Lundell L, Havu N, Andersson A *et al.* Gastritis development and acid suppression therapy revisited. Results of a randomised clinical study with long-term follow-up [abstract]. *Gastroenterology* 1997; **112**: A28.

A randomized study not confirming that *H. pylori*-positive patients treated with long-term PPIs have an increased risk of atrophic gastritis.

41. Viral Hepatitis

SIMON WHALLEY, GEORGE WEBSTER, ELLIE BARNES and GEOFFREY DUSHEIKO

INTRODUCTION

This chapter reviews the clinical features of liver disease caused by hepatitis viruses A to E and the hepatitis G virus. Recent trials of treatment against hepatitis B and C have revealed some factors predictive of response. Current management issues include monitoring for complications of the disease or the therapy administered, together with how to prevent disease transmission. Hepatitis A and E are similar; they are both RNA viruses, primarily spread via the faecal–oral route, and do not lead to chronic liver disease. In contrast, both hepatitis B and hepatitis C can lead to acute and chronic liver disease. Hepatitis D coexists with hepatitis B. There is little evidence for a pathological role for hepatitis G in causing liver disease. These viral infections will be discussed and examples of case reports presented, with questions posed to exemplify some of the common management issues.

CLINICAL FEATURES OF ACUTE VIRAL HEPATITIS OF ANY CAUSE

Viral hepatitis may present acutely with clinical features that are common to all hepatotropic infections. However, hepatitis C rarely presents in the acute phase, as symptoms are often minimal, and there is little evidence that hepatitis G causes liver injury. The early clinical phase of acute hepatitis often starts with a variety of non-specific symptoms, such as fatigue, anorexia, malaise, and myalgia. A few days later, anorexia, nausea, vomiting, and right upper-quadrant abdominal pain can appear, followed by passage of dark urine and pale faeces, and the development of jaundice. With the appearance of jaundice, there is usually improvement in symptoms. The jaundice usually deepens during the first few days and persists for 1 or 2 weeks. The faeces then darken and the jaundice diminishes over an additional period of 2 weeks or so. The liver may be palpable in acute severe hepatitis, but the spleen is palpable in only a minority of patients.

Non-specific blood tests

The leucocyte count usually is normal but, often, some atypical lymphocytes are found. Serum C3 and C4 concentrations may be decreased, perhaps reflecting antigen–antibody complex formation. Autoantibodies, including abnormalities in rheumatoid factor, and anti-nuclear and anti-smooth muscle antibodies may also be detectable.

HEPATITIS A

Virology

Hepatitis A virus (HAV) is a small RNA virus of the family *Picornaviridae*. The virus is not cytopathic; liver cell damage is caused by the host immune response.

Epidemiology

HAV occurs **world-wide**, sporadically or in epidemics. Its exact prevalence is difficult to estimate, as infection is frequently asymptomatic and therefore under-reported. In temperate zones HAV infection increases in the autumn, whereas in developing countries the incidence of HAV infection peaks in the rainy season. The group most often affected world-wide are children aged between 5 and 15 years, but infection may occur at any age. In developing countries, 90% of children have immunoglobulin G (IgG) antibodies to HAV by the age of 10 years, confirming previous exposure. However, in areas where there has been an improvement in socioeconomic conditions, the mean age at first exposure has increased, such that only 5–10% of young adults in developed countries have serological evidence of exposure to HAV. Travellers from areas of low prevalence who visit developing countries are at particular risk of acquiring this infection.

Transmission

HAV is transmitted by the faecal–oral route and the infection is therefore common in areas of poor sanitation and overcrowding. Common-source outbreaks usually occur from faecal contamination of food or drinking water. The eating of raw shellfish cultivated in contaminated water is associated with a high risk of HAV infection. Other risk factors include male homosexual practice. Rarely, HAV has been transmitted parenterally after transfusion of blood products from a donor who was in the incubation period of the disease.

Clinical course

The incubation period of HAV infection is 3–5 weeks. Clinical disease is uncommon in young children. In adults, however, severe hepatitis is not uncommon, the illness may be protracted, and the patient may be incapacitated for several weeks. HAV infection does not lead to chronic liver disease. Rarely (in fewer than 1 in 1000 cases), HAV may cause fulminant liver failure. Approximately 5% of patients with clinically apparent HAV infection develop cholestatic hepatitis.

Laboratory diagnosis

Diagnosis is confirmed by specific **serological tests for antibodies to HAV**, including radioimmunoassay and enzyme-linked immunosorbent assay (ELISA); anti-HAV antibody develops during the early phase of the illness and increases rapidly. Hepatitis A IgM is detectable in serum for 45–60 days after the onset of symptoms and is the simplest way to establish the diagnosis of acute disease, whereas titres of anti-HAV IgG increase with convalescence and persist for many years after infection. HAV antigen can be detected in faeces using immune electron microscopy or by the polymerase chain reaction (PCR), but these tests are not routinely performed.

Case history

- a 30-year-old man presents feeling non-specifically unwell with jaundice. He returned 3 weeks ago from Turkey. He has no risk factors for liver disease. He is found to be hepatitis A IgM-positive

Management issues

1. Should the patient be admitted to hospital?
   HAV IgM antibodies imply recent infection and confirm the diagnosis. Patients do not require admission to hospital unless vomiting occurs, the prothrombin time is prolonged, or there are signs of fulminant liver failure. Prognosis is excellent and recovery is usually complete. Hepatitis A infection accounts for fewer than 1 in 1000 cases of fulminant hepatitis.

   Liver biopsy examination is not indicated. The average adult with hepatitis A will feel unwell for 6 weeks. Chronicity does not develop, and the development of anti-HAV IgG antibodies results in long-term immunity to the disease.

2. Six weeks later, the patient is still jaundiced and itching has become intolerable. What are the therapeutic options?

   Prolonged cholestasis lasting 42–100 days affects about 5% of patients with hepatitis A, causing severe pruritis and steatorrhoea. A short course of prednisolone, starting at a dose of 30 mg/day and reducing over 3 weeks usually curtails the cholestasis (1).

3. Should he have been vaccinated for hepatitis A infection before travelling?

   Yes. Before the availability of a vaccine, human immunoglobulin to HAV was recommended for patients without HAV antibody who were travelling to endemic areas. A highly immunogenic vaccine may now be offered to travellers, with the option of a booster 6–12 months later. Vaccination should also be offered to armed forces personnel, staff of children's day-care centres and institutes for intellectually handicapped people, male homosexuals, intravenous drug abusers, sewage workers, and patients with haemophilia or chronic liver disease. If immediate protection is necessary, travellers require HAV-immunoglobulin, followed by vaccination.

4. Should patients and their contacts be isolated? The virus is excreted in faeces for up to 2 weeks before the onset of jaundice. The virus is therefore disseminated before the diagnosis is made, and strict isolation of patients is therefore not useful. Immune serum globulin prophylaxis prevents HAV infection in 80–90% of people if it is given within 6 days of exposure; it may be given to close contacts of the patient. The dosage should be at least 2 IU anti-HAV/kg body weight, but in special cases, such as pregnancy or in patients with liver disease, the dosage may be doubled.

HEPATITIS E

Hepatitis E virus (HEV) infection has been reported in Asia, the Middle East, North Africa, and Central America. Sporadic cases have been observed in developed countries in travellers returning from these areas. As with HAV, **transmission** is via the faecal–oral route. Large epidemics have been reported.

The **incubation period** is 6 weeks and, in common with HAV infection, the illness is self-limiting, with no progression to chronic liver disease. High mortality rates of 20%, as a result of fulminant hepatitis, have been reported in women in the third trimester of pregnancy.

Serological assays are available for HEV infection. IgM is detected infrequently at presentation and disappears by 3 months after jaundice; IgG titres may be high, but disappear over time. The diagnosis may also be confirmed by PCR on faeces from acutely infected patients.

HEV immunoglobulin and vaccine are not yet available for the prevention of infection.

HEPATITIS B

Virology

Hepatitis B virus (HBV) is a partially double-stranded circular DNA virus of the family *Hepadnaviridae*.

Epidemiology

World-wide, hepatitis B infection remains the ninth leading cause of death, with an estimated 350 million people chronically infected. There is a wide variation in prevalence of the carrier rate in the world, ranging from 0.3% in the UK and the USA, to 5% in southern Europe, and to as high as 20% in parts of Africa and South East Asia. The incidence of HBV infection in Western and Northern Europe, and the USA is declining. Infection rates in children have declined in those high-prevalence areas in which the universal immunization of infants has been introduced.

Risk factors

The main routes of **transmission** of HBV are perinatal, horizontal, sexual, and intravenous.

Perinatal transmission
Perinatal transmission of HBV is an important factor in causing the high prevalence of chronic hepatitis B in some regions, particularly in China, where there are 100 million carriers. Transmission occurs because of peripartum haemorrhage and subsequent ingestion or inoculation into the blood circulation of the baby. The risk of perinatal infection is greatest for children born to hepatitis B Espmark antigen (HBeAg)-positive mothers with high levels of serum HBV DNA. For infants born to HBeAg-positive mothers, there is a substantial risk (90%) that chronic hepatitis B will develop.

Horizontal transmission
Perinatal transmission accounts for about 50% of cases of childhood chronic hepatitis B; the remaining 50% are acquired via child-to-child transmission. The prevalence in children is quite low at 1 year of age, but increases rapidly thereafter; in many endemic regions the prevalence reaches a peak in children aged 7–14 years. HBV is endemic in closed institutions, including those for the mentally handicapped and orphanages, and is more prevalent in adults in urban communities with poor socioeconomic conditions.

Intravenous transmission
Blood-bank screening of donor blood for HBV came into effect in the UK in 1972, and since then the risk of transmission by transfusion of blood or blood products has become remote. Transmission of HBV

may result from accidental inoculation of minute amounts of contaminating blood or fluid during: medical, surgical, and dental procedures; intravenous and percutaneous drug abuse; tattooing; body piercing; acupuncture; laboratory accidents; and accidental inoculation with razors and similar objects. In the tropics, other factors may be important, including traditional tattooing and scarification, blood-letting, and ritual circumcision.

Sexual transmission

Transmission of HBV can occur by intimate sexual contact. The sexually promiscuous, particularly male homosexuals, are at a very high risk. Heterosexual transmission accounts for more than 30% of new cases in the USA.

Acute hepatitis B

Clinical manifestations

The incubation period of HBV varies from about 60 to 180 days. The **clinical spectrum of disease** varies considerably, from an asymptomatic or mild anicteric illness to acute disease with jaundice or fulminant hepatitis. Inapparent or subclinical and anicteric infections are common. Jaundice is very uncommon in children younger than 5 years, but it occurs in 50% of older children or adults. In children, the prodromal features may be mild or even absent, although anorexia, when present, tends to be severe. Occasionally, extrahepatic manifestations occur. These relate to immune-complex phenomena and include vasculitis, nephritis, arthritis, and polyarteritis nodosa.

Liver function tests

The serum concentrations of aspartate aminotransferase (AST) and alanine aminotransferase (ALT) are increased; usually, the concentration of ALT is greater than that of AST. Increased concentrations of these enzymes may be the only abnormality to be found in patients with asymptomatic and anicteric infections. Serum bilirubin concentrations increase in proportion to the severity of hepatic damage.

Laboratory diagnosis

The first *marker* to appear in the circulation is hepatitis B surface antigen (HBsAg), which becomes detectable 2–8 weeks before biochemical evidence of liver damage or the onset of jaundice. Measurement of HBsAg is the test most widely used for diagnosis of hepatitis B infection. Current immunoassays are able to detect HBsAg in concentrations of 100–200 pg/ml serum, corresponding to about 3×10^7 particles/ml. After HBsAg, markers of viral replication appear, namely HBV DNA and HBeAg.

Serum HBV DNA can be **quantified** by DNA hybridization, the Chiron bDNA assay (a chemiluminescent signal amplification assay based on oligonucleotide amplification), or the Roche Amplicor Monitor assay (based on PCR). The Chiron assay has a level of sensitivity of 0.7×10^6 genome equivalents/ml, whereas the Roche Amplicor Monitor assay has a greater level of sensitivity — about 1000 copies/ml. HBV DNA usually reaches 10^5–10^8 genome equivalents/ml with the onset of symptoms, after which the concentrations decrease.

By the time the patient consults a physician, HBV DNA and HBeAg are often no longer detectable in serum. Figure 41.1 shows the typical profile of antigen and antibody response in hepatitis B. Antibody to the viral core (anti-HBc) is detectable 2–4 weeks after the appearance of the surface antigen, which persists throughout the infection and after recovery. A positive IgM anti-HBc test typically

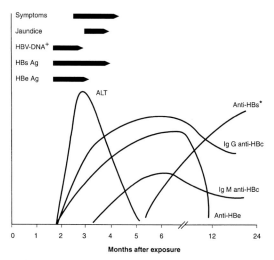

Figure 41.1. Acute icteric hepatitis B infection: serological markers. [†]HBV DNA measured by liquid hybridization assay. [*]Anti-HBs is not detected in 10% of patients.

distinguishes acute from chronic hepatitis B. In acute infections, clearance of the virus is marked by seroconversion, with appearance of anti-HBe antibodies and disappearance of HBeAg. The loss of HBeAg is a sign that the patient will clear HBsAg; usually this occurs later during convalescence, along with the production of antibody to surface antigen (anti-HBs). In fulminant hepatitis, rapid clearance of HBeAg and HBsAg may occur.

Prognosis

Approximately 2–3% of patients with acute hepatitis B develop fulminant hepatic failure: mortality is 0.2%. Convalescence after acute hepatitis may be prolonged, although complete recovery in adults usually takes place within a few months. The vast majority of patients make a **full recovery** without progression to chronic liver disease.

Case history

- a 30-year-old man presents to clinic with a one week history of malaise. His only risk factor for HBV infection is homosexual intercourse three months ago. Examination is unremarkable. Blood tests show ALT 1200 IU/litre and serology positive for HBsAg plus anti-HBc IgM, indicating acute HBV infection

Management issues
1. Is interferon therapy indicated?

Anti-viral treatments

Although non-specific symptoms may be improved, there are no data to indicate anti-viral treatment accelerates healing or clearance of virus, or that early treatment with interferon prevents the development of chronic disease. Interferon-α has not been found to be beneficial in patients with fulminant hepatitis B, in whom only low levels of viral replication are usually found.

Chronic hepatitis B

Definition

Chronic hepatitis B is defined as persistence of HBsAg in the circulation for more than 6 months after clinical infection. The "carrier" state may be lifelong and may be associated with liver damage varying from mild chronic hepatitis to severe active hepatitis, cirrhosis, and primary liver cancer.

Risk factors for chronicity

Risk factors identified as leading to the development of chronic HBV infection include **acquisition in childhood**, **male sex**, and the presence of **congenital or acquired immune deficiencies**. Chronic hepatitis B infection occurs in 90% of neonates or young infants, but in only 1–5% of immune-competent adults. In countries where hepatitis B infection is common, the greatest prevalence of HBsAg is found in young children, with steadily declining rates among older age groups. HBeAg has been reported to be more common in young than in adult carriers of hepatitis B, whereas the prevalence of anti-HBe seems to increase with age.

Diagnosis

Many carriers are diagnosed as a result of screening for HBsAg, or the detection of abnormal liver function tests. Older patients may present for the first time with complications of cirrhosis, or hepatocellular carcinoma.

Natural history and prognosis of chronic hepatitis B

Chronic carriage of hepatitis B may be divided into two phases. In the **first phase**, high levels of viral replication occur and the patient is seropositive for HBeAg with detectable HBV DNA (by molecular hybridization) in serum. The **second phase**, of non-replication, is characterized by disappearance of HBV DNA from serum, followed by loss of HBeAg. Although HBeAg correlates with the presence of the virus, in some cases when virus replication declines to very low levels or when "pre-core mutants" are present (see p 492), seroconversion to anti-HBe may occur without clearance of the virus. Chronic hepatitis B generally lasts for many years, but may not necessarily be lifelong.

The concentrations of **aminotransferases** fluctuate with time; typically they are increased in patients with HBeAg, HBV DNA-positive chronic hepatitis, but some of these patients may have normal values. Spontaneous remission in disease activity may occur in approximately 10–15% of HBeAg-positive carriers per year. This may occur after a sudden, asymptomatic increase in serum

ALT associated with seroconversion to anti-HBe-positive status and clearance of HBeAg. Serum aminotransferase concentrations become normal, although they remain HBsAg-positive. The term "healthy hepatitis B carriers" has been used for these patients, but is somewhat inappropriate, as they are at risk of reactivation of viral replication, and, if cirrhosis has developed, they may ultimately develop hepatocellular carcinoma, in the face of relatively low levels of viraemia. For HBsAg-positive patients with compensated cirrhosis, the cumulative probability of survival is 84% at 5 years and 68% at 10 years. The worst survival is for HBeAg and HBV DNA-positive individuals.

Case history

- a 28-year-old lady of Chinese origin is referred to clinic by the obstetric department. After routine ante-natal screening, they find her to be positive for HBsAg. Further serology reveals she is HBeAg-positive, anti-HBe negative, total anti-HBc-positive, but anti-HBcore IgM-negative, indicating chronic HBV infection with active viral replication. ALT is moderately increased at 160 IU/litre, suggesting current hepatic inflammation

Management issues

1. How may her baby be prevented from acquiring HBV infection?
2. In the long term, what anti-viral treatments should be considered, and what factors are predictive of response?

Prevention and control of hepatitis B

Passive immunization

Hepatitis B immunoglobulin (HBIg) is prepared from pools of plasma with high titres of HBsAg, and may confer temporary passive immunity.

Active immunization

HBV vaccines currently used in the UK and elsewhere in developed countries are prepared from yeast (*Saccharomyces cerevisiae*) using recombinant techniques. They are relatively safe; side effects occur in only a few patients and include inflammation at the site of inoculation and mild pyrexia. A variety of vaccines containing surface protein other than HBsAg that are derived from pre-S sequences are now undergoing clinical trial, and there are some indications that the rate of non-responsiveness may be lower than that with vaccines containing HBsAg alone.

Combined immunoprophylaxis

The development of **acute illness** may be ameliorated and the **carrier state** of HBV may be prevented in many patients by the administration of combined immunoprophylaxis. Whenever immediate protection is required — for example, for babies born to HBsAg-positive mothers or after accidental inoculation — active immunization with vaccine should be combined with simultaneous administration of HBIg at a different site. The Department of Health in the UK recommends that the upper arm be used as the site for hepatitis B vaccination in adults. Many studies have shown that the antibody response rate was significantly greater in centres using deltoid injection than centres using the buttock. Passive immunization with HBIg does not interfere with an active immune response.

HBIg should be administered as early as possible after exposure to HBV — preferably within 48 h — usually 3 ml (containing 200 IU/ml of anti-HBs) in adults; it should not be administered 7 days or more after the exposure. Two doses of HBIg should be given 30 days apart.

The dose of HBIg recommended in the **newborn** at risk of infection with HBV is 200–400 IU of anti-HBs. This should be given within 12 h of birth. With the use of combined passive and active immunization, the chance of the baby developing chronic hepatitis B is reduced to about 10%. Failure to respond to vaccination has been ascribed to mutations in the HBV genome (substitution of arginine for glycine at amino acid 145 appears to be the most common) that lead to altered HBsAg, which escapes neutralization by HBIg (2).

Indications for immunization against hepatitis B

The World Health Organization recommended, a decade ago, that universal immunization should occur in all countries by 1997. This aim has not been achieved, and universal immunization of infants world-wide remains a goal. However, an important success of vaccination has emerged in Taiwan, where the risk of hepatocellular carcinoma has decreased (3).

In 1996, the Department of Health in the UK recommended **active immunization for the following risk groups:**

1. Babies born to mothers who are chronic carriers of HBV or to mothers who have had acute hepatitis B infection during pregnancy. In addition, babies born to mothers who are HBeAg positive or who had acute hepatitis B during pregnancy should receive HBIg. Currently, vaccine without HBIg is recommended for babies born to mothers who are HBsAg-positive but known to be anti-HBe-positive.

2. Sexual contacts of patients with acute hepatitis B, who should also receive HBIg.

3. Parenteral drug misusers.

4. Close family contacts of a patient with hepatitis B infection or carrier, or families adopting children from countries with a high prevalence of hepatitis B.

5. Patients with haemophilia (and others receiving regular blood transfusions or blood products, and carers responsible for the administration of such products).

6. Patients with chronic renal failure. Higher doses of vaccine may be required in those who are immunocompromised.

7. Occupational risk groups, including health-care workers. Staff and students of residential accommodation for those with severe learning disabilities, members of the emergency and prison services, and inmates of custodial institutions.

8. Those travelling to areas of high prevalence.

Antiviral treatment for chronic hepatitis B

Two classes of drug will be discussed: interferon-α, and nucleoside analogues.

Interferon-α

Interferons are naturally occuring glycoproteins that have antiviral and immunomodulatory effects. The **interferon-α** group are produced by leucocytes. Several human recombinant forms of interferon-α, including HuIFN-α-n1 (Wellferon, a mixture of interferon species), HuIFN-α-2b (Intron A), and HiIFN-α-2a (Roferon-A) have been licensed for the treatment of chronic hepatitis B. All are administered parenterally, either intramuscularly or subcutaneously, but can be given intravenously for patients with bleeding disorders. Interferon-α-2a and -2b have similar antiviral activity.

The standard dose of interferon-α in the treatment of hepatitis B infection is 9–10 MIU subcutaneously, three times a week for 4–6 months. Contraindications

to and side effects associated with interferon are discussed in the section on hepatitis C.

Treatment of chronic hepatitis B is aimed at patients with active disease and viral replication, preferably at a stage before cirrhosis has developed. Patients should be selected who have increased ALT, detectable HBV DNA, and HBeAg in their serum. Liver biopsy examination should, ideally, be performed before the institution of treatment, both to assess the grade of necroinflammatory change and to stage the amount of fibrosis; it is not routinely performed after treatment.

Close monitoring is required throughout treatment. Monitoring requires regular clinical examinations, checking vital signs, urinalysis, usually monthly measurement of serum biochemistry, full blood count, and clotting screen, and thyroid function tests. There are no adequate data on the safety of interferon in pregnancy; however, it has been shown to have abortifacient effects in rhesus monkeys and is therefore contraindicated in pregnancy. A pregnancy test may be necessary before treatment is begun. Side-effects of interferon-α are discussed on p. 498.

Response to treatment is defined as loss of serum HBV DNA and HBeAg, with normalization of serum transaminase concentrations. A "flare" of hepatitis with an increase in serum ALT, which is often subclinical, occurs in up to 70% of responders, usually 4–8 weeks into treatment. This is associated with seroconversion to positive anti-HBe, and subsequently, to clearance of HBV DNA and HBeAg, with normalization of aminotransferase concentrations. This response results in improvement of necroinflammatory damage, and reduced infectivity. For patients who tolerate treatment, there is some evidence — although controversial — that interferon may reduce the rate of progression to hepatocellular carcinoma (4).

A large trial in the USA demonstrated that 37% of patients treated with interferon 5×10^6 U/day for 16 weeks lost HBV DNA and HBeAg, compared with 7% of controls (5). Long-term follow-up of responders has shown that up to 65% of those who lose HBeAg also lose HBsAg (6). Relapse of hepatitis with reappearance of HBeAg and increases in transaminase concentrations occurred in 13% of patients, generally within the first 12 months of discontinuing interferon. HBsAg was negative in the serum of 10% of patients at the end of treatment and, notably, 5 years after interferon treatment this clearance of HBsAg was seen in 70% of patients. A dose of 10 MIU on alternate days for 4 months appears to be equally as efficacious (7).

Several **pre-treatment factors** have been identified as being **predictive of achieving a response to interferon in chronic hepatitis B**:

- female
- White
- heterosexual
- acquired HBV after 6 years of age
- disease duration less than 4 years
- history of jaundice
- serum ALT concentration >100 IU/litre
- high-grade hepatic inflammation
- HBV DNA concentration in serum less than 200 pg/litre
- HBeAg-positive
- IgM anti-HBc-positive
- absence of human immunodeficiency virus or immunosuppression

The absence of any of these factors should not necessarily exclude patients from treatment, although they may guide the physician in selecting appropriate patients to receive interferon therapy.

Special considerations should be taken into account when the following patient groups are being considered for interferon therapy:

1. *Children*: Children infected perinatally, and having mild disease activity, respond poorly to interferon treatment. Conversely, children with active disease and notably increased serum transaminase concentrations respond to interferon therapy in a manner similar to adults and usually tolerate treatment reasonably well. The appropriate dose of interferon for children is 3 MU/m^2 three times weekly for 4 months.

2. *ALT <100 IU/litre*: These patients have a poor chance of achieving a response to interferon. Although prednisolone priming before interferon is commenced has been shown to confer no additional benefit, subgroup analysis revealed that it was beneficial for patients with ALT values less than 100 IU/litre (5). Although such priming is uncommon now, for this group there may be some justification in prednisolone priming with 2-weekly decrement-dose scheduling of 60/40/20 mg daily. The rationale for prednisolone priming is that it suppresses the immuno-

logical response and is followed by a rebound flare in the immune response; this hepatitis may be sufficient to cause seroconversion to anti-HBe, and clearance of HBV DNA from serum.

3. *Advanced cirrhosis*: These patients should be treated with interferon only with extreme caution. Compared with that in the non-cirrhotic groups, the response rate in this group is not favourable. Side effects and complications are more likely, and interferon may exacerbate the hepatitis, leading to decompensation and fatal bacterial peritonitis. Low-dose interferon, perhaps just 1 MIU three times a week, may be tried at centres with access to liver transplantation, although nucleoside analogue treatment may be a more appropriate option.

4. *Glomerulonephritis*: Patients with chronic hepatitis B may develop membranous or membrano-proliferative glomerulonephritis as a result of deposition of immune complexes in the kidneys. Interferon can be effective in these patients, with normalization of transaminase concentrations and clearance of HBeAg; furthermore, urine protein excretion also decreases and resolution of the glomerulonephritis may occur.

5. *Pre-core mutants*: Patients with HBV pre-core mutants do not synthesize HBeAg, most commonly because of a stop-codon mutation at nucleotide 1896. In Mediterranean Europe, and elsewhere, disease caused by this variant of HBV is more common than that caused by the "wild type" (HBeAg-positive chronic hepatitis). Typically, the patients have lower concentrations of serum HBV DNA. The natural history is variable: some patients with fulminant hepatitis B have been shown to have pre-core mutants. Response to interferon is not good: approximately 10–25% of patients have a long-term response to treatment doses of 9–10 MIU three times a week for 6–12 months, and relapse rates tend to be high in these patients (8).

Nucleoside analogues

In the light of their success in treating human immunodeficiency virus (HIV) infection, nucleoside analogues are currently undergoing evaluation in the treatment of chronic hepatitis B infection. HBV, although a DNA virus, replicates via a reverse transcriptase activity of the DNA polymerase on an RNA intermediate. Nucleoside analogues act by blocking the production of this enzyme thereby preventing viral replication. Generally, replication resumes when the drug is discontinued. The long-term efficacy and safety of nucleoside analogues are unknown, as is the optimal duration of treatment. Viral resistance to nucleoside analogues may occur; this problem may be overcome by using combination therapies. Several analogues have been developed:

1. *Lamivudine*: The (–) enantiomer of 2',3'-dideoxy-3'-thiacytidine (also known as 3TC or Epivir). This is currently the most widely studied analogue and is established as a potent inhibitor of HBV replication. It acts by inhibiting DNA synthesis through chain termination. The (–) stereoisomer is more active than the (+) form, which is degraded by deoxycytidine deaminase. Lamivudine is rapidly absorbed after oral administration, and is remarkably well tolerated. Serious side effects have been observed in only 5% of patients; these include anaemia, neutropenia, increase in liver enzymes, nausea, and neuropathy. Increased concentrations of lipase may occur. Severe exacerbation of hepatitis accompanied by jaundice has been reported in patients in whom HBV DNA became positive after they discontinued treatment, or after the development of resistance. HBV DNA becomes undetectable (by hybridization assay) by 4 weeks in more than 90% of patients who receive 100 mg–300 mg/day (9). The optimal dose is 100 mg daily, but this should be reduced in patients with renal impairment. Up to 40% of patients treated with lamivudine for 1 year have sustained suppression of HBV DNA, and in a large Asian trial (10), approximately 15% of patients became HBeAg-negative after 12 months of treatment, compared with 4% of placebo recipients; this efficacy is similar to that of interferon. Histological improvement has been noted after 1 year of treatment. Lamivudine resistance is apparent in about 15% of patients after 1 year of treatment. This appears to be related to the appearance of resistant HBV variants (M552I and M552V) with a methionine to valine or isoleucine substitution in the highly conserved Tyr-Met-Asp-Asp (YMDD) motif of the HBV polymerase gene.
2. *Ganciclovir*, a guanine analogue: This drug has been used intravenously to treat recurrence of hepatitis B after liver transplantation. Oral ganciclovir has been used to treat HBeAg and anti-HBe-positive hepatitis B in a preliminary trial.
3. *Famciclovir*: This guanine analogue is readily absorbed, being the oral precursor of penciclovir. A significant reduction in HBV DNA and ALT concentrations within the treatment period was observed in a group receiving 500 mg three times a day, and the HBeAg seroconversion rate was increased compared with that achieved with placebo. However, some patients appear not to be sensitive to famciclovir, and resistant mutations have been reported.
4. *Adefovir dipivoxil*: This new agent is an adenine analogue. Preliminary *in vitro* evidence suggests that M552I and M552V variants of HBV, which are relatively resistant to lamivudine, are susceptible to inhibition by adefovir.
5. *Lobucavir*: This is a new cytidine analogue that is under investigation, pending satisfactory safety in preclinical trials.

Hepatitis B virus and primary liver cancer

HBsAg carriers are 200-fold more likely to develop hepatocellular carcinoma than are members of the non-carrier group. For White patients with compensated cirrhosis, the incidence of hepatocellular carcinoma is approximately 2 per 100 patient-years (11).

Primary liver cancer is more common in males than among females and the incidence of the tumour increases with age, reaching a peak in the 30–50 years age group. There is often a considerable interval between the initial virus infection and the development of carcinoma, although the tumour does occur in younger age groups in high-risk populations. Cirrhosis is not always a prerequisite for the development of hepatocellular carcinoma in chronic HBV infection, as it is in chronic hepatitis C. Frequent (3–6-monthly) measurement of alpha-fetoprotein and ultrasound of the liver are recommended to screen patients with cirrhosis for hepatocellular carcinoma.

HEPATITIS D

Virology

Hepatitis delta virus (HDV) was first identified in 1977, after the detection of delta antigen (HDAg), by immunofluorescent staining, in the nuclei of hepatocytes from patients with hepatitis B infection.

The HDV particle consists of an RNA genome associated with HDAg, coated by an envelope of HBsAg, which is needed for release and entry into hepatocytes.

Epidemiology

The mode of **transmission** of hepatitis D is similar to the parenteral spread of hepatitis B virus. HDV has a world-wide **distribution**, with predominance in Italy, Eastern Europe, parts of Russia, the Middle East, and parts of Africa and South America. About 5% of HBsAg carriers world-wide (approximately 15 million people) are infected with HDV. In areas of low prevalence of HBV, those at risk of hepatitis B — particularly intravenous drug users — are also at risk of HDV infection. Epidemics with high mortality have been described in South America in association with severe hepatitis B. Delta infection is associated with acute and chronic hepatitis, always in the presence of hepatitis B.

Clinical features

HDV causes acute, fulminant, and chronic hepatitis. HDV requires HBV for its transmission. There are **two patterns of hepatitis D infection**:

- **co-infection with HBV and HDV**, often leading to a more severe form of acute hepatitis caused by HBV. Vaccination against HBV prevents such infections
- **superinfection with HDV** in a patient chronically infected with HBV. This may exacerbate the course of the chronic liver disease and cause overt disease in a previously asymptomatic HBsAg carrier. Superinfection with HDV often leads to chronic HDV infection

Laboratory diagnosis

Serological tests are available to detect antibody to HDV: anti-HD IgM and anti-HD IgG. Hepatitis D viraemia is marked by an anti-HD IgM, and then an anti-HD IgG, response. HDV RNA and HDAg can be detected in serum, but tests for these are not routinely available. Co-infection is determined by the presence of anti-HBc IgM with anti-HD IgM. Markers of HBV replication may be suppressed during acute HDV infection. Superinfection of HDV in HBV carriers often leads to chronic HDV infection. The virus reaches greater concentrations in the circulation than does HBV; up to 10^{12} particles/ml have been recorded.

Case history

- a 30-year-old man with a known history of chronic hepatitis B is seen in clinic after his return from a visit to Italy. He feels ill and blood tests reveal a markedly increased ALT concentrations of 800 IU/litre. Serology shows that he remains HBeAg-positive and has not developed anti-HBe antibodies. However, serology has become positive for anti-HDV IgM, indicating superinfection with HDV.

Management issues

What is the efficacy of interferon therapy?

Treatment

Interferon 10 MIU three times a week for a prolonged period of 9–12 months is often required to treat HDV. Unfortunately, relapse when treatment is stopped is a major problem, and sustained response rates of 25% are the best that can be expected (12).

Vaccination

Vaccination against hepatitis B helps prevent HBV infection and therefore HDV infection.

HEPATITIS C

Virology

Hepatitis C virus (HCV) is an RNA virus and a member of the family *Flaviviridae*. The 10 000 nucleotide genome, first identified in 1989, encodes for both structural and non-structural proteins. The non-structural proteins, including protease, helicase, and RNA polymerase, appear important for viral replication, and are the likely targets for antiviral treatments in the future. Nucleotide sequence variations form the basis of the classification of **six major genotypes** (1–6), divided further into **three subtypes** (a–c). Further nucleotide variability in viruses circulating within an individual are referred to as quasispecies. Genotype appears to have an influence on the response to treatment, and perhaps to the rate of disease progression. The predominant genotype varies widely between geographical locations and patient populations.

Epidemiology

The prevalence **world-wide** of hepatitis C is estimated at 150 million people, with a disease spectrum ranging from mild to severe chronic hepatitis, cirrhosis, and hepatocellular carcinoma.

Serological testing has shown that 1–2% of people in developed countries have been exposed to HCV, with an estimated 4 million infected in the USA. Higher rates are found in Asia and Africa, with up to 15% of people in Egypt infected. Genotypes 1, 2, and 3 are most prevalent in the USA and Europe, and type 4 is most prevalent in Egypt and the Middle East. Type 1b appears more frequent in patients older than 50 years, and type 3a in people infected through intravenous drug usage. Approximately 50% of anti-HCV-positive blood donors in South Africa are infected with type 5a. Type 6a was originally found in Hong Kong.

Transmission

HCV is a blood-borne virus, and the majority of patients have been infected through blood or blood-product transfusion, or abuse of injected drugs. More than 60% of cases in the UK are associated with previous **abuse of injected drugs**. Specific groups affected by HCV include patients with **haemophilia** who, before 1985, received unsterilized factor-concentrate; in this group, up to 90% of patients are anti-HCV-positive. Solvent detergent inactivation and heat treatment have eliminated the risk of transmitting hepatitis C infection to this group. The prevalence of hepatitis C is high in those who, in the 1970s and 1980s, received multiple **blood transfusions**, and, in Ireland and Germany, **rhesus-negative mothers** who received anti-HD immunoglobulin that was contaminated with HCV. In the UK, screening of donated blood for anti-HCV antibodies since 1991 has virtually eliminated blood products as a source of transmission. The widespread **use of non-disposable needles** during treatment of schistosomiasis may have contributed to the high prevalence of HCV in Egypt. HCV is poorly transmitted via the **sexual** route, although those with several partners are at greater risk. In the absence of barrier contraception, only 5–10% of regular sexual partners of infected patients are found to be infected. Likewise, transmission from **infected mother to infant** occurs only in about 5% of cases, the risk being greatest in those with high titres of circulating virus. Caesarean section, instead of vaginal delivery, does not appear to reduce the rate of HCV transmission from mother to infant. **Co-infection with HIV** markedly increases the rate of vertical transmission of HCV, up to 18%. Infection of an infant through **breast feeding** has not been reported. In 10–20% of patients, no risk factors for virus transmission can be identified.

Acute hepatitis C

The mean incubation period of hepatitis C is 6–12 weeks, but this may be reduced after infection by a large inoculum. The acute course is generally mild and the peak serum ALT concentration is typically less than that found in hepatitis A or B. Fewer than 15% of patients develop an acute icteric hepatitis after infection. Subclinical disease is common, and many patients may first present decades after the original infection with sequelae such as cirrhosis. Fulminant hepatitis is a relatively rare outcome of HCV infection, but has been reported in patients superinfected with HAV and in patients withdrawn from immunosuppressive treatment.

Chronic hepatitis C

Clinical manifestations and prognosis

Chronic HCV is usually **clinically silent**, with liver damage occurring over many years. A number of outcomes may occur after infection. Up to 85% of infected patients develop chronic HCV, as defined by persistence of HCV RNA in the serum. Approximately 20% of patients with chronic HCV will develop cirrhosis and endstage liver disease after 20 years of infection. The reason for the differing clinical course between patients is uncertain, but **risk factors for disease progression** include long duration of disease, male sex, older age at time of infection, alcohol excess, and co-infection with HIV or HBV. An association of more advanced disease with viral genotype 1 is most probably attributable to the older age group of the patient cohort infected with this genotype. Per year, up to 4% of patients with HCV cirrhosis develop hepatocellular carcinoma, and this may be a more common complication in those infected with genotype 1b. Although many patients are asymptomatic at the time of diagnosis, a range of non-specific complaints, including fatigue, headache, and poor concentration, are common in chronically infected patients. Clinical features may be most clearly linked to HCV infection in association with cirrhosis and endstage liver disease. A number of **extrahepatic manifestations have been associated with chronic HCV**:

- Essential mixed cryoglobulinaemia
  - detectable in 36–54% of patients
  - most patients asymptomatic
  - arthralgia, pruritis, and purpura in 18%
  - neuropathy and glomerulonephritis in 2%
  - more common in patients with chronic HCV
- Sjögren's syndrome/focal lymphocytic sialadenitis
- Lichen planus
- Porphyria cutanea tarda
- Polyarteritis nodosum
- Autoimmune hepatitis
- Thyroiditis
- Polymyositis
- Membranous glomerulonephritis
- Idiopathic pulmonary fibrosis

The pathogenesis of these extrahepatic manifestations remain uncertain; a causative link with HCV is stronger for some conditions than others. Up to 45% of patients with chronic HCV have cryoglobulins in their serum, but fewer than 10% of them develop the vasculitic syndrome of mixed essential cryoglobulinaemia, including a purpuric rash, weakness, arthralgia, and neuropathy. Antibodies to HCV are found in 8–10% of patients with porphyria cutanea tarda, a disease characterized by the appearance of skin fragility and a vesicular rash on sun-exposed areas, especially the back of the hands. The frequency of HCV in patients with membranoproliferative glomerulonephritis appears high, especially in those with associated cryoglobulinaemia.

Liver function tests

Mildly increased **serum aminotransferase concentrations** (ALT/AST) — at approximately 1.5–2.5 times the upper limit of normal — are a characteristic feature of chronic HCV. Serum ALT concentrations can be used as a surrogate marker of hepatic inflammation; fluctuations in ALT are common throughout the course of disease. There is, however, a poor correlation between the concentration of ALT and either the level of viraemia, or the severity of histological disease. Although simple and cheap to perform in patients as part of assessment and follow-up, measurement of serum transaminases provide inexact information about disease activity.

Laboratory diagnosis

Antibody tests

A positive anti-HCV antibody may confirm exposure to HCV, but in itself it provides no information concerning disease activity. The most widely used antibody tests are sensitive ELISAs, which detect a combination of antibodies to HCV proteins. False-positive results are not infrequent, even when third-generation ELISAs are used, and specificity may be confirmed by using a recombinant immunoblot assay (RIBA). In clinical practice, RIBA tests are usually necessary only when there is doubt concerning the diagnosis, or in patients with autoimmune hepatitis, in whom false-positive ELISA test results are particularly common.

HCV RNA analysis

Unlike anti-HCV antibody tests, detection of HCV RNA confirms the presence of **current infection**. Amplification of circulating viral RNA is performed by PCR, which has a level of sensitivity of approximately 100–1000 viral copies/ml. High viral loads are associated with a poor response rate to antiviral treatment.

Other blood tests

Chronic hepatitis C may occur in conjunction with **other liver diseases**. Haemochromatosis, α_1-antitrypsin deficiency, and Wilson's disease should be excluded, if appropriate, during initial assessment. We also test for anti-smooth-muscle and liver kidney microsomal antibodies; although these are frequently seen as an epiphenomenon in patients with chronic HCV, true autoimmune hepatitis is a rare disease association, which can, however, be exacerbated by interferon-α treatment. Similarly, thyroid function tests and anti-thyroid autoantibodies should be measured, as **thyroid dysfunction** may occur with interferon-α treatment, particularly in the presence of pre-existing anti-thyroid antibodies. HBsAg should be tested for, as active HBV infection is associated with more progressive histological disease in those with HCV. **HIV** testing may be appropriate in those with particular risk factors. Knowledge of the HCV genotype is important, as recent studies suggest that a longer course of combination treatment with ribavirin is indicated for genotype 1 than for other genotypes (12 months compared with 6 months, respectively).

Liver biopsy examination

Histological examination of the liver is the only definitive method of assessing the **degree of dam-**

age incurred by HCV. It allows identification of the degree of inflammation (grade) and extent of fibrosis (stage), and may guide a decision concerning the need for treatment. Unless there are specific contraindications, liver biopsy examination should be performed in HCV RNA-positive patients with chronic hepatitis C and increased concentrations of ALT. The procedure is not routinely necessary after treatment, as response is most conveniently assessed by clearance of serum HCV RNA and normalization of transaminase concentrations.

Case history

- a 53-year-old business man is referred to clinic by his general practitioner. He has a 3-year history of fatigue and general malaise. His doctor found no abnormalities on examination, but routine blood tests revealed mildly increased serum transaminase concentrations. On the basis of these findings, a third-generation ELISA anti-HCV antibody test was performed and found to be positive. The patient was very distressed at this finding. He reported very occasional use of intravenous drugs in his 20s, but none since, and he drank only minimal amounts of alcohol. He is married with two children.

Management issues

1. What general advice would you give him?
2. What are the potential side effects of antiviral therapy?
3. How successful are antiviral therapies for hepatitis C and what factors can predict this response?

Management of chronic hepatitis C

General advice

A diagnosis of HCV infection often raises considerable anxieties in the patient, and a crucial aspect of management is for the patient to be fully informed of the natural history of the disease. Many people erroneously believe that progression to endstage liver disease is inevitable, and that treatment is ineffective. The plan of investigations, and reason for these should be discussed, in addition to the efficacy and limitations of available treatments. The factors associated with progressive disease may be discussed. It should be stressed that alcohol and HCV have a synergistic effect upon liver injury.

Regular **alcohol use** should be discouraged, although a safe lower limit has not been defined.

Particular anxiety often surrounds **transmissibility**. Patients should be advised not to donate blood, and the risks for drug users of sharing needles and solutions should be reiterated. Specific advice to avoid sharing razors and toothbrushes should be given. It should be explained that sexual transmission of HCV is unusual, but that condoms should be used during casual sexual contacts, to lower the risk of a range of transmitted infections (e.g. HIV). It is prudent to advise regular sexual partners that the risk of transmission is low, but can not be excluded. Individuals in monogamous sexual relationships should be advised of this low risk, and barrier sexual intercourse thus appears to be unnecessary in this setting.

Antiviral therapy

The only licensed treatment for chronic HCV is **interferon-α**, either as monotherapy or in combination. The USA National Institute of Health consensus statement on HCV (13) and the European Association for the Study of the Liver consensus statement (14) declared that treatment was indicated in a patient with positive anti-HCV antibody, positive HCV-RNA by PCR, increased liver enzymes (AST, ALT), and moderate to severe hepatitis on liver biopsy examination. Studies are in progress to assess the benefit of treating patients who have only mild histological disease. Treatment of HCV should, ideally, be given before the development of cirrhosis, and is contraindicated in patients with decompensated cirrhosis. However, for patients who tolerate the treatment there is some evidence, albeit controversial, that interferon-α may reduce the incidence of hepatocellular carcinoma. Studies in children have investigated interferon monotherapy but not combination therapy; response rates were similar to those seen in adults. For patients with extrahepatic manifestations of HCV, sustained remission is unlikely.

Response to treatment is defined as normalization of serum ALT (**biochemical response**) or the development of negative HCV RNA by PCR (**virological response**). The long-term response is categorized as end-of-treatment response, sustained response, or relapse. Relapse, if it is to occur, generally happens within 6 months of the discontinuation of treatment. The efficacy of treatment is therefore usually judged by the sustained virological response at 6 months after the treatment has been discontinued. Early clearance of virus predicts a sustained response. Therefore, patients who do not show a biochemical and virological response after 3 months of treatment should be considered for discontinuation of treatment.

Patients who achieve a sustained virological response usually have histological improvement, with a reduction in hepatic inflammation. Thus by clearing HCV, or at least halting active viral replication, antiviral therapy appears to be advantageous in preventing the progression of hepatic fibrosis or the development of cirrhosis.

The potential **side effects of interferon-α** include:

- influenza-like symptoms, chills, fever (common; may be relieved by paracetamol)
- nausea
- lethargy
- weight loss
- depression (even suicidal ideation)
- myelosuppression (usually neutropenia and thrombocytopenia)
- hypersensitivity
- autoimmune reactions (especially hyper/hypothyroidism)
- hypotension/arrhythmias
- hair loss (usually mild and diffuse)
- retinopathy

Flu-like symptoms (fever, lethargy, headache, myalgia) can be treated with paracetamol. **Myelosuppression** may be an early feature: full blood-count monitoring is required and the dose of interferon may need to be reduced or the drug withdrawn completely. **Psychological complications** include depression, anxiety, irritability, and pyschosis.

About 67% of patients with chronic hepatitis C are positive for anti-nuclear antibody, smooth-muscle antibody, or both, whereas only 4% are positive for anti-mitochondrial antibody. Anti-liver-kidney microsomal antibody is rare in the USA, but the prevalence is about 4% in European and Japanese patients (15). In these patients, liver histology shows the features typical of chronic hepatitis C and lacks the appearances of autoimmune hepatitis. There is a risk that interferon, because of its immunostimulatory properties, may cause a hepatitis in patients with concomitant autoimmune phenomena. In practice this

is uncommon, but patients must be monitored closely for a flare of their hepatitis while they are receiving interferon (16). Rarely, interferon can cause autoimmune phenomena; during treatment, up to 50% of patients develop anti-nuclear, anti-smooth-muscle, or anti-thyroid antibodies. Thyroid dysfunction occurs in about 5% of patients and requires cessation of therapy. Hypothyroidism usually resolves but, occasionally, long-term replacement is needed.

Interferon is **contraindicated** in the presence of significant psychological disease, neutropenia, thrombocytopenia, symptomatic heart disease, decompensated cirrhosis, uncontrolled epilepsy, pregnancy, and inadequate contraception. Relative contraindications to its use include autoimmune disease and diabetic retinopathy. It is difficult to justify commencing treatment in patients who continue to abuse alcohol and use intravenous drugs. Predictors of long-term response to interferon are shown in Table 41.1.

Initial reports showed that, of patients who receive a 12-month course of interferon-α 3 MIU subcutaneously three times weekly, 50% achieved end-of-treatment response, but, overall, only 25% of patients had a sustained virological response (17). It is not proven that increased dose, daily administration, or high induction dose lead to an increase in sustained virological response. Recent studies have shown that the **combination of ribavirin with interferon** leads to considerable improvement in response rates (18). There is now little justification for using interferon as monotherapy.

Table 41.1. Predictors of long-term response to interferon.

Viral factors	Non-viral genotype 1
	Low level of viraemia (fewer than 1×10^6 copies/ml) before treatment
	Limited quasispecies diversity
	Mutations in the NS5A region (reported mainly in Japan)
	Loss of detectable virus (negative HCV RNA) after 1 month of treatment
Host factors	Younger age
	Female
	Low body mass
	Absence of cirrhosis on biopsy examination
	Low hepatic iron stores
	Absence of iatrogenic or natural immunosuppression
	ALT normalized in first 12 weeks of treatment

Ribavirin is a guanosine nucleoside analogue that, on its own, has minimal virological effect on HCV. The side effects of ribavirin include haemolysis and it is also potentially teratogenic, therefore patients of either sex should be advised to avoid conceiving a child during and for at least 6 months after completing their course of treatment. The drug is contraindicated in endstage renal failure, haemoglobinopathies, severe heart disease, and pregnancy.

For interferon- naïve patients, a 12-month course of interferon–ribavirin achieves a sustained virological response of 40%. For those with genotype 1 and a viral load of greater than 2 million copies/ml, a 12-month duration of treatment appears to be optimal. If the level of viraemia is less than 2 million copies/ml, 6 months of treatment is sufficient. For genotypes 2 and 3, the sustained virological response is improved (69%, compared with 29% in genotype 1) and a 6-month course of combination therapy appears to be equally effective, whatever the viral load.

In the case of interferon monotherapy, failure to clear HCV RNA from serum within 12 weeks predicts a failure of sustained virological response and indicates that interferon can be withdrawn. Combination of ribavirin with interferon leads to considerable improvement in response rates, with late clearance of HCV RNA from serum, and an associated sustained virological response. Approximately 45–50% of patients who have suffered disease relapse after interferon-α monotherapy will have sustained biochemical and virological responses to combined therapy.

Endstage liver disease as a result of chronic HCV is now the most common indication for **orthotopic liver transplantation**. The number of patients requiring liver transplantation will increase further over the next 15 years. Recurrence of HCV in the grafted liver is almost universal, with cirrhosis sometimes occurring at an accelerated rate in these immunosuppressed patients. The 5-year rate of HCV-related cirrhosis of the graft is about 10%.

Future developments

Further studies will allow the **optimal duration and dosing regimen** of interferon–ribavirin to be defined, and will identify the need to tailor these to individual factors, such as genotype. Alternative interferons are under evaluation, including second-generation long-acting pegylated interferon (which can be administered once a week), "natural" interferon and interferon-β. The use of combination therapies, with the addition to interferon-α of ribavirin, amantadine, non-steroidal anti-inflammatory agents, or thymosin, is undergoing evaluation. In response to the recent definition of the molecular structure of HCV, new antiviral agents including potential protease and helicase inhibitors are in the process of development, and an effective vaccine is being sought. Treatments to prevent re-infection of the graft after liver transplantation would be particularly important, in view of the predicted increase in the numbers of transplants that will be performed to treat chronic HCV over the next 20 years.

GBV-C AND HEPATITIS G VIRUS

The identification of this virus originated when serum obtained from a surgeon with acute hepatitis (who had the initials GB) induced experimental hepatitis in tamarins. It is now recognized that the two newly discovered isolates, GBV-C and hepatitis G, are the same virus. However, this awkward nomenclature persists. Two further viruses were given the nomenclature GBV-A and GBV-B, and are now known to be primate viruses.

Virology

GBV-C/hepatitis G virus (HGV) is a single-strand RNA virus of the *Flaviviridae* family.

Transmission and epidemiology

GBV-C/HGV has a **global distribution** and is present in up to 3% of the volunteer blood-donor population in Western countries. Despite the extremely high level of HGV contamination of non-virus-inactivated blood products, their use has not been associated with very high rates of persistent infection, although such infection has been reported.

Clinical significance

Overall, the high prevalence of this virus in the asymptomatic blood-donor population suggests it is not an important cause of chronic hepatitis. The virus is of **unknown pathogenic significance**.

The evidence against the relationship of GBV-C/HGV and chronic liver disease includes the fact that there is currently no clear relationship of GBV-C/HGV infection to liver disease. No definite causal relation between GBV-C/HGV and chronic hepatitis has been established and, although this human virus may be responsible for some cases of non-A–E hepatitis, surveillance studies in the USA do not implicate GBV-C /HGV as a major aetiological agent of non-A–E hepatitis. Persistent infection with HGV is quite common, but infection does not appear to lead to chronic hepatitis, and does not affect the clinical course in patients with hepatitis A, B, or C infection. Most post-transfusion HGV infections have not apparently been associated with classic hepatitis (19).

Fulminant hepatitis

There are reports of GBV-C/HGV RNA in serum detected by PCR in patients with fulminant hepatitis of unknown aetiology. It has been suggested that a specific strain of GBV-C/HGV may occur in serum of German patients with fulminant hepatic failure. It is unknown whether the virus was the cause of this, or whether it was merely a secondary infection acquired by blood or plasma transfusions received by patients with fulminant hepatitis from other causes.

Diagnosis

Reverse transcriptase PCR and serological assays are available for detection of GBV-C/HGV. The presence of antibodies to the envelope (anti-E2 AB) of GBV-C/HGV indicates resolution of infection.

Treatment and prevention

Interferon-α treatment results in clearance of HGV RNA in serum. However, in view of the lack of data confirming the pathogenicity of this virus, antiviral therapy is not indicated. GBV-C/HGV co-infection does not affect the responsiveness to interferon-α treatment of patients with chronic hepatitis C infection. Blood products are not routinely screened for GBV-C/HGV.

References
*Of interest; **of exceptional interest

1. *Gordon S, Reddy R, Schiff L *et al*. Prolonged intrahepatic cholestasis secondary to acute hepatitis A. *Ann Int Med* 1984; **101**: 635–637.
    A short review with six case presentations, emphasizing the fact that an awareness of cholestatic viral hepatitis avoids unnecessary investigation of suspected obstructive jaundice.

2. Oon CJ, Lim GK, Ye Z *et al*. Molecular epidemiology of hepatitis B virus vaccine variants in Singapore. *Vaccine* 1995; **13**: 699–702.

3. *Chang MH, Chen CJ, Lai MS *et al*. Universal hepatitis B vaccination in Taiwan and the incidence of hepatocellular carcinoma in children. *N Engl J Med* 1997; **336**: 1855–1859.
    A large trial reported from Taiwan that vaccination of children against HBV has had an impact in reducing the incidence of hepatocellular carcinoma.

4. International Interferon-alpha Hepatocellular Carcinoma Study Group. Effect of interferon alpha on progression of cirrhosis to hepatocellular carcinoma: a retrospective cohort study. *Lancet* 1998; **351**: 1535–1539.

5. *Perrillo RP, Schiff ER, Davis GL *et al*. Hepatitis Interventional Therapy Group. A randomized, controlled trial of interferon alfa-2b alone and after prednisone withdrawal for the treatment of chronic hepatitis B. *N Engl J Med* 1990; **323**: 295–301.
    The largest US trial of interferon for the treatment of chronic hepatitis B demonstrated its efficacy, and that prednisolone priming before interferon was efficacious for a subgroup of patients with serum ALT concentrations less than 100 IU/litre.

6. Korenman J, Baker B, Waggoner J, *et al*. Long-term remission of chronic hepatitis B after alpha-interferon therapy. *Ann Int Med* 1991; **114**: 629–634.

7. Di Bisceglie AM, Fong TL, Fried MW, *et al*. A randomised controlled trial of recombinant alpha-interferon therapy for chronic hepatitis B. *Am J Gastroenterol* 1993; **88**: 1887–1892.

8. Brunetto MR, Oliveri F, Colombatto P, *et al*. Treatment of chronic anti-HBe-positive hepatitis B with interferon alpha. *J Hepatol* 1995; **22(suppl)**: 2–44.

9. **Dienstag JL, Perrillo MD, Schiff ER *et al*. A preliminary trial of lamivudine for chronic hepatitis B infection. *N Engl J Med* 1995; **333**: 1657–1661.
    An early report that 12 weeks of lamivudine therapy was well tolerated, and daily doses of 100 mg and 300 mg reduced HBV DNA to undetectable levels.

10. **Lai CL, Chien RN, Leung NW, *et al*. A one-year trial of lamivudine for chronic hepatitis B. Asia hepatitis lamivudine study group. *N Engl J Med* 1998; **339**: 61–68.
    This study showed that lamivudine was associated with substantial histological improvement and loss of HBeAg plus undetectable HBV DNA in 16% of patients after 1 year of treatment. Sustained normalization of ALT concentrations was seen in 72% (68 of 95) patients. YMDD mutations were seen in 14% of patients, and were not associated with decreased histological response.

11. Fatovich G. Progression of hepatitis B and C to hepatocellular carcinoma in Western countries. *Hepatogastroenterology* 1998; **45(suppl 3)**: 1206–1213.

12. *Rosina F, Pintus C, Meschievitz C *et al*. Long-term interferon treatment of chronic delta hepatitis: A multicenter Italian study. *Prog Clin Biol Res* 1991; **364**: 385–391.
    This study highlighted that chronic delta hepatitis requires a long duration of interferon therapy and that relapse is a major problem.

13. **NIH Consensus Development Conference Panel. Statement: management of hepatitis C. *Hepatology* 1997; **26**: 2S–10S.

An important and authoritative declaration on the management of hepatitis C.

14. **EASL International Consensus Conference on Hepatitis C. Consensus statement. *J Hepatol* 1999; **30**: 956–961.
This statement takes into careful consideration data from the latest trails, in defining guidelines for management of a spectrum of HCV-related disease.

15. Miyakawa HE, Kitazawa E, Abe K, *et al.* Chronic hepatitis C associated with anti-LKM-1 antibody is not a subgroup of autoimmune hepatitis. *J Gastroenterol* 1997; **32**: 769–776.

16. Todros L, Saracco G, Durazzo M, *et al.* Efficacy and safety of interferon alpha therapy in chronic hepatitis C with autoantibodies to LKM. *Hepatology* 1995; **22**: 1374–1378.

17. **Davis GL, Balart LA, Schiff ER, *et al.* Treatment of chronic hepatitis C with recombinant interferon alpha. A multiceter randomized, controlled trial. *N Engl J Med* 1989; **321**: 1501–1506.

An early study reporting on the efficacy of interferon therapy for hepatitis C.

18. **McHutchison JG, Gordon SC, Schiff ER, *et al.* Interferon alfa-2b alone or in combination with ribavirin as initial treatment for chronic hepatitis C. Hepatitis Interventional Therapy Group. *N Engl J Med* 1998; **339**: 1485–1492.
A large multicentre study reporting on the superior efficacy of interferon plus ribavirin combination therapy over interferon monotherapy, and of the need for a longer course of treatment for HCV genotype 1.

19. *Alter HJ, Nakatsuji S, Melpolder J, *et al.* The incidence of transfusion-associated hepatitis G virus infection and its relation to liver disease. *N Engl J Med* 1997; **336**: 747–754.
This large study reported that there was no clear relationship between GBV-C/HGV infection and liver disease.

42. Abnormal Liver Function Test in an Asymptomatic Patient

LUCY DAGHER and ANDREW K. BURROUGHS

INCREASED SERUM TRANSAMINASES

The incidental discovery of asymptomatic patients with mild to moderate increases in serum transaminase concentrations represents a common clinical problem. Blood donors, "routine check-ups", or preoperative evaluations account for many of these patients. The **history and physical examination** should guide the evaluation of asymptomatic patients with increased serum transaminases. The **history** should focus on:

- use of prescription and over-the-counter medications and alcohol
- occupational exposures to hepatotoxins
- risk factors for hepatitis
- family history of liver disease

Repeat testing is essential in asymptomatic patients who lack risk factors and signs of liver disease. Obtaining medical records is useful in determining the chronicity of the problem. Patients with an isolated increase in ALT should be evaluated for extrahepatic sources of this enzyme, particularly from muscle.

Identifying the cause of the increased transaminase concentrations is possible with assessment of the pattern of the liver enzyme tests and additional testing. **The ratio of aspartate transaminase (AST) to alanine transaminase (ALT)** appears to be a useful index for distinguishing non-alcoholic steatohepatitis from alcoholic liver disease: although values less than 1 suggest the presence of non-alcoholic steatohepatitis or viral hepatitis, a ratio of

2 or more is strongly suggestive of alcoholic liver disease (1,2). An increase in γ-glutamyltransferase strengthens the diagnosis of alcohol abuse. A drug-related effect is possible if there is a correlation between the increase in liver enzyme concentrations and the start of administration of the drug; the most common drugs causing increased transaminases are non-steroidal anti-inflammatory drugs, antibiotics, hydroxymethyl glutaryl coenzyme A reductase inhibitors, antiepileptic drugs, and antituberculous drugs. In addition to prescribed medication, over-the-counter medications, herbal preparations, and illicit drug use may also be the cause. The first step in determining if a medication or alcohol is responsible is for the patient to stop taking these, to see if the tests then return to normal.

If the abnormalities persist, and particularly if transaminase values remain high, **markers of autoimmune disease** should be tested, particularly in young women; serological analyses for hepatitis B and C should be obtained in all patients. Investigation of the patient's iron status should be routinely performed to exclude the possibility of **haemochromatosis**, and measurements of ceruplasmin and copper concentrations are appropriate in patients aged 45 years or younger, to detect **Wilson's disease**. Most patients should be tested for α_1-antitrypsin if the above evaluations fail to explain the aetiology of persistently increased transaminases.

All patients with persistently increased concentrations of transaminases that are of uncertain cause should be advised to discontinue unnecessary medications and abstain from alcohol for several weeks,

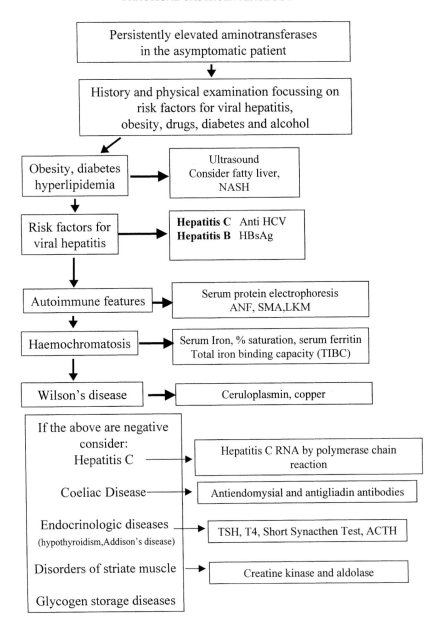

Figure 42.1. Investigation of persistently increased transaminase concentrations in the asymptomatic patient.
NASH, non-alcoholic steatohepatitis; anti-HCV, antibodies to hepatitis C virus; HBsAg, hepatitis B surface antigen; ANF, anti-nuclear factor; SMA, smooth-muscle antibody; LKM, liver–kidney microsomal antibody; TSH, thyroid-stimulating hormone; T_4, thyroxine; ACTH, adrenocorticotrophic hormone.

then tested again. Findings of a recent study also suggested that **expectant clinical follow-up** is the most cost-effective strategy for managing asymptomatic patients with negative viral, metabolic, and autoimmune markers and chronically increased transaminase concentrations (3). If these interventions have little or no effect and the concentrations remain increased over 6–12 months in the absence of discernible causes, then the patient should be counselled, and a liver biopsy examination recommended.

Figure 42.1 summarizes the approach to the investigation of asymptomatic patients with persistently increased transaminase concentrations.

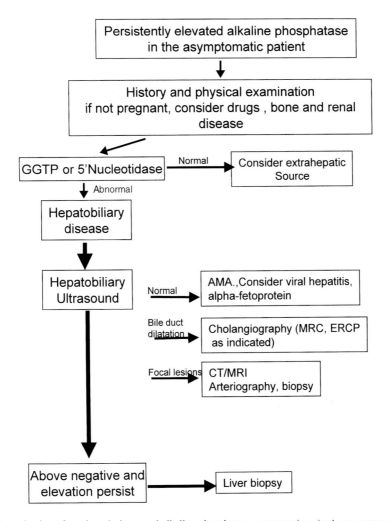

Figure 42.2. Investigation of persistently increased alkaline phosphatase concentrations in the asymptomatic patient. GGT, γ-glutamyltransferase; AMA, anti-mitochondrial antibody; MRCP, ERCP, magnetic resonance and endoscopic retrograde cholangiopancreatography; CT, computed tomography; MRI, magnetic resonance imaging; ALP, alkaline phosphatase.

INCREASED ALKALINE PHOSPHATASE

The patient's history may allow diagnosis or exclusion of increased concentrations of alkaline phosphate as a result of physiological bone growth (children or teenagers), or primary bone disease such as Paget's disease or multiple fractures, and osteoporosis. Women in the third trimester of pregnancy have increased serum alkaline phosphatase concentrations that are attributable to placental alkaline phosphatase.

Before further laboratory tests or imaging procedures are undertaken, in patients in whom increased alkaline phosphatase has been demonstrated, measurements of the enzyme should be repeated, as isolated increases can be caused by laboratory errors. Subsequently, the γ-glutamyl-transferase or 5'-nucleotidase concentration should be determined. If these enzymes are normal, the increased alkaline phosphatase is unlikely to be of hepatic origin and additional investigations relating to bone or kidney should be considered. If the increase in alkaline phosphatase is of liver origin and persists, an **ultrasound scan** should be performed, to exclude biliary obstruction and space-occupying lesions. If the ultrasound is normal, this is suggestive of chronic cholestatic or infiltrative disease. Cholestatic diseases include partial bile-duct obstruction, primary biliary cirrhosis, primary sclerosing cholangitis, and adult paucity of intrahepatic bile ducts. Infiltrative diseases include sarcoidosis and other granulomatous diseases.

A scheme of investigation of asymptomatic patients with persistently increased concentrations of alkaline phosphatase is summarized in Figure 42.2.

INCREASED γ-GLUTAMYLTRANSFERASE

Because of its lack of specificity, γ-glutamyltransferase is not useful as a screening test for liver disease. Occasionally, an increased γ-glutamyltransferase concentration is detected as an isolated finding on routine testing; invasive investigations are probably unjustified in these asymptomatic patients, as significant liver disease other than fatty liver is rare in such cases. Ireland et al. (4) showed that the results of liver biopsy examinations in patients with an increase in γ-glutamyltransferase alone were normal, or showed only reversible changes, on histological examination. In the presence of other enzyme abnormalities, an appreciable proportion of patients had fibrosis or cirrhosis, often with active inflammation. Patients with an isolated increase in γ-glutamyltransferase should be followed up, with clinical evaluation and measurement of other liver functions, at intervals of few months. If symptoms or signs appear, other tests become abnormal, or the γ-glutamyltransferase concentration continues to increase over many months, an ultrasound or computed tomography scan, or both, should be performed, to exclude a space-occupying lesion, and liver biopsy examination should be considered.

References
1. Cohen JAKM. The SGOT/SGPT ratio: an indicator of alcoholic liver disease. *Dig Dis Sci* 1979; **24**: 835.
2. Sorbi D, Lindor KD. The ratio of aspartate aminotransferase to alanine aminotransferase: potential value in differentiating nonalcoholic steatohepatitis from alcoholic liver disease. *Am J Gastroenterol* 1999; **94**: 1018–1022.
3. Das A, Post AB. Should liver biopsy be done in asymptomatic patients with chronically elevated transaminases: a cost–utility analysis [abstract]. *Gastroenterology* 1998; **114**: 3241A.
4. Ireland A, Hartley L, Ryley N *et al.* Raised gamma-glutamyltransferase activity and the need for liver biopsy. *BMJ* 1991; **302**: 388–389.

43. Perianal Problems

CAROLYNNE VAIZEY

SYMPTOMS

The most common symptoms associated with peri-anal disease are bleeding, and discomfort ranging from mild irritation to severe pain (1). It is impor-tant to gain an accurate description of any perianal bleeding. Spots of fresh blood seen only on the toilet paper suggest pathology localized to the peri-anal skin or anal canal. Blood dripping into the pan after the passage of stool is most commonly associated with haemorrhoids. Blood mixed in with the stool or darker blood are more suggestive of pathology higher up the colon. These descriptions serve only as guidelines, however, and there are always exceptions to the rules that can catch the unwary. Always enquire as to whether the patient is taking anticoagulant medication, as this will be a contraindication to most outpatient treatments of piles and to taking any biopsy samples. Severe perianal pain is a truly disabling symptom, and can also be frightening to a patient who does not understand the cause. The most frequently seen cause of severe pain is an anal fissure, but the list of possible pathologies is long. In any patient with anal pain you must always think of, and exclude, perianal sepsis. This, in some cases, and particu-larly in the scarred anus, can be difficult to define in the clinic setting. If there is any doubt, an endoanal ultrasound scan performed by an expert, or referral for an examination under anaesthesia are mandatory.

ANAL LESIONS

Common minor anal disorders

Haemorrhoids

The two most common **presentations** of haemor-rhoids are bleeding and prolapse. The bleeding corresponds to the presence of dilated capillaries just below the surface epithelium. Prolapse occurs with degeneration of the supporting structure of the haemorrhoids. Pain, especially when any more than a dragging sensation, is generally only a feature of thrombosed piles; if these are not present, other pathological processes should be excluded. The **diagnosis** is established on proctoscopy. A rigid sigmoidoscopy is an essential part of the physical examination, to exclude other pathologies.

Symptoms are often intermittent, which makes assessment of the efficacy of **treatments** difficult. The most conservative approach is to increase the fibre in the diet, discourage straining, and prescribe one of the many local agents that claim to decrease vascularity. Treatments possible in the clinic setting include the application of Baron's bands, injection of oily phenol, infra-red photocoagulation, cryo-therapy, and laser treatment. None of these options provides long-term cures, usually giving only tem-porary alleviation of the symptoms (2).

Haemorrhoidectomy has been a notoriously pain-ful operation and, until recently, patients were kept in hospital for a number of days after operation.

Improved patient acceptability can be achieved with a combination of **measures aimed at decreasing the postoperative discomfort**; these may include:

1. Administration of mild laxatives before operation, to avoid passage of a hard stool.
2. Avoidance of an intra-anal dressing at the end of the operation.
3. Use of a local anaesthetic agent, injected into the skin bridges at operation, an anti-inflammatory suppository at the end of the operation, and then patient-administered analgesia after the operation.
4. Administration of metronidazole postoperatively to avoid local infection.
5. Internal sphincter-relaxing agents administered as ointments after operation.

With these measures, combined with improved patient information and access to advice, it has now proved possible to perform day-case haemorrhoidectomies with improved patient satisfaction and acceptable pain control.

Skin tags

Excess skin, forming tags, can be associated with haemorrhoids or may be present on their own. Removal cannot comfortably be performed in most outpatient settings and therefore necessitates a minor operation. Patients may opt to live with the tags once they are reassured of their benign nature; some, however, find that the tags lead to difficulty with hygiene and they therefore request operation.

Fibroepithelial polyps

Fibroepithelial polyps are well-defined, firm, often stalked polyps that arise from the anal canal. They may be asymptomatic or may cause acute discomfort, or they may prolapse through the anus. Removal is by simple surgical excision.

External thrombosed pile

An external thrombosed pile is a well-defined, tender lump that is a blood clot beneath the perianal skin caused by excessive straining. Most cases can be treated by conservative means such as warm baths and analgesics, but occasionally the patient will demand incision and expression of the clot.

Mucosal prolapse

Often mistaken for haemorrhoids, this form of prolapse is of the mucosa only, and is most commonly found anteriorly. Local treatments for haemorrhoids are often applied to the prolapsed mucosa — most commonly sclerotherapy. There is however, no evidence to support the success of these treatments in the long-term.

Full-thickness rectal wall prolapse

This disorder must be included as part of the differential diagnosis of haemorrhoids, and must also be differentiated from anterior mucosal prolapse. The usually elderly or chronically malnourished patient may give a good history of the bowel prolapsing, with straining at stool or even on minor physical effort. If the diagnosis is not obvious, the patient should be transferred from the examination couch to a toilet and asked to strain. The rectal wall will then be found to protrude through the anal canal. In addition to a history of constipation and straining, symptoms of faecal incontinence should be enquired after, the incidence varying from 21 to 83% (3). Discomfort is often a feature of this disorder; surgical referral is appropriate even in the elderly and infirm, as a perineal operation, such as the Delorme's procedure, can be performed with little risk (4). The previously favoured abdominal operations for rectal prolapse have been associated with a high incidence of constipation after operation, and these are now often combined with a sigmoid resection in an attempt to avoid this complication.

Fissure

Fissure, a usually exquisitely painful linear ulceration of the anal canal, can often be diagnosed on history alone. The pain is especially sharp on the passage of a stool, and there can be an incapacitating perianal aching for many hours after. Spots of blood on the toilet paper are less impressive than the blood which can drip into the pan with bleeding haemorrhoids. It may be possible to see the ulcer on gently everting the anal canal. The term "sentinel pile" is used for the tag-like lesion that is a marker for a chronic fissure, being sited on the skin side of the ulceration. In the case of an acute fissure, if the anal canal spasm is extreme, the diagnosis can only be confirmed on examination under anaesthesia, at which time biopsy sampling of the ulcer edge and rectum is worthwhile in cases with a high clinical suspicion of Crohn's disease or an infectious aetiology.

With the recent introduction of **internal sphincter muscle relaxing agents**, most fissures can now be treated without surgery. Most hold with the view that relaxing the internal sphincter allows an increase in the blood supply to the anal margin, which allows for ulcer healing. Glyceryl trinitrate cream is the agent most commonly used at present, but there is a high incidence of headache with this agent (5). Research is currently aimed at alternative medications such as diltiazem or botulinum toxin. In some persistent cases, referral to the surgeon is still required. A **lateral sphincterotomy** is then the operation of choice (6), with the uncontrolled destruction of an anal stretch now thankfully an historical manoeuvre. The patient must still be warned of the small risk of passive faecal leakage after a sphincterotomy. In persistent cases deemed to be at high risk for incontinence, an alternative surgical approach is the insertion of a well-vascularized flap of skin into the fissure site.

Perianal sepsis including anal fistula

Perianal abscess usually occurs after infection of an anal gland. It is most common in patients between the ages of 20 and 50 years. Urgent drainage is essential before the pus breaks through into other areas in the perineum. More rarely, perianal sepsis can occur secondary to accidental or surgical trauma, or after infection of a haematoma, haemorrhoid, or other local pathological process. Only occasionally do patients present to outpatients with acute sepsis; more commonly, they are seen in the casualty department. A **perianal abscess** is usually easy to diagnose, presenting as a visible, red, exquisitely tender swelling next to the anus. An **ischiorectal abscess** may be less obvious, with the loose areolar tissue accommodating the pus without as much discomfort or swelling. Deep sepsis higher up the anal sphincter mechanism may present as rectal pain and an examination under anaesthesia or radiological imaging may be necessary to make the diagnosis. A submucous abscess may only be diagnosed after *per rectal* examination reveals a tender intra-anal lump. A **communication between the abscess cavity and the anorectum** may be obvious at the operation

for abscess drainage or it may present later as a fistulous track. Any discharging area or small area of granulation tissue near the anus should be assumed to communicate with the anorectum until proved otherwise. The path of the track can often be felt on careful palpation of the perianal region. Most colorectal surgeons use operative exploration as their first diagnostic test for a fistula, but magnetic resonance imaging (MRI) may be used to define complex cases. The external and internal openings must be located. The track must be followed and the presence of any unsuspected extensions established. The existence of an underlying disease process such as Crohn's disease, an infection, or the presence of a foreign body must not be missed; biopsy examination and cultures are frequently necessary.

Subcutaneous and submucous fistulae are sited away from the sphincter muscles, and therefore should be readily cured by a laying open of the track. The remaining fistulae are classified according to their relationship to the internal and external anal sphincter muscles. This is a practical approach, as these sphincter muscles are all important in planning the surgical treatment of the fistula. The St Mark's Hospital (Middlesex, UK) classification has **four major categories**: intersphincteric, transphincteric, extrasphincteric, and suprasphincteric (7). Only those tracks passing through the most distal parts of the sphincter tissue can be laid open without fear of incontinence. Preoperative assessment with anorectal physiological testing and an endoanal ultrasound scan to define any pre-existing sphincter defects are wise when any degree of sphincter damage is anticipated. This is particularly so in parous women or those with a previous history of perianal surgery.

For **fistulae not amenable to fistulotomy** (laying open with healing by secondary intention), the surgeon has limited options. The muscle can be cut and repaired, but this does carry a risk of poor healing and incontinence. The fistulous track can be cored out with repair of the opening in the muscle, but again this does not always heal. The insertion of a **seton suture** is a safer option. A seton is a suture, wire, or tubing that is threaded along the track and secured outside the anus, usually with a knot. It can be left loose to allow for drainage and subsidence of the associated inflammation, or tied tightly to cut slowly through the muscle — in theory, maintaining muscle-fibre alignment and allowing healing to occur behind it. Complex or high fistulae require complex surgery, details of which can be found in specialist colorectal surgery text books.

Pruritis ani

The anogenital region is the most common site for intractable itching of the skin. Once an individual has acquired a heightened awareness of an area, only the smallest of stimuli is necessary to initiate further paroxysms of scratching. Scratching, in turn, sensitizes the skin further, and a vicious cycle is established that is very difficult to break. Local lotions applied to the skin can cause further irritation.

The cause may be a **benign anorectal condition** such as haemorrhoids or fissure, or a **neoplastic condition** such as Bowen's disease, Paget's disease, or anal carcinoma. It may also be caused by a **dermatological condition** such as dermatitis or lichen sclerosis, or an **infection or infestation** such as *Candida albicans* or threadworm. Most of these conditions can be excluded with careful examination, with the addition of skin scrapings or biopsy examination where necessary. Those who appear to have **idiopathic pruritis** should be questioned in detail about the presence of faecal leakage. Wiping the anal skin with damp cotton wool before examination of the patient may reveal unsuspected contamination of the area. Where leakage is suspected, anorectal physiological testing and an endoanal ultrasound scan may define a defect or weakness in the internal anal sphincter. It is always useful to have a general advice sheet available for patients with pruritis. The following are the main points to be included when drawing up such an **advice sheet**:

1. Avoid all creams and ointments unless these have been prescribed for you. Some soaps are also irritant. Short-term use of steroid ointments can alleviate symptoms; long-term use may damage the skin and worsen the problem.
2. Wash the skin with water after each stool when possible. Pat dry; do not rub. When you are unable to use running water to clean, have a kit available with a small bottle of water and some soft but strong cotton wool.
3. Wear cotton under clothing and, for women, try to wear stockings instead of tights.
4. Avoid hot and spicy foods and foods that cause flatulence or loose stools.
5. If faecal leakage is suspected, improvement may be made by firming up the stools with an antidiarrhoeal agent such as loperamide (Imodium), but care must be taken to avoid constipation. A cotton-wool plug shaped by hand to fit the anus will absorb any excess mucous coming through the anus.
6. Scratching must be avoided at all costs; nothing encourages irritation more than this. Wearing cotton gloves to bed may be necessary in habitual offenders. Vigorous washing or drying can be just as damaging as a good scratch.

If you fail to make progress with the patient with intractable pruritis, be prepared to seek a dermatological opinion.

Crohn's anus

The incidence of **perianal disease in Crohn's disease** (8,9) is variably quoted as from less than 25% to more than 90%, but is certainly more common in the patient with colonic, as opposed to ileal, disease. Although the patient with perianal Crohn's disease has common pathologies such as skin ulcers, fissures, fistulae, and perianal sepsis, there is often a **specific and diagnostic appearance** to the anus. It is characteristically oedematous and angry, with a purple hue, and symptoms are often less impressive than the signs. When there is significant pain, sepsis should be suspected and examination under anaesthesia is indicated to exclude this complication. Skin erosion, ulceration, and the development of juicy tags are common. Haemorrhoids are rare, but when they do occur, treatment should be conservative. Excision of haemorrhoidal tissue or large skin tags is said to lead to proctectomy in up to 20% of cases. Fissures may be atypical, in that they are often off the midline and may be less painful than the non-Crohn's fissure. An increased resting pressure is not a feature, and treatment that leads to any form of sphincter damage is contraindicated. Fistulae can be complex and medical management may provide the best chance of healing. No data from controlled trials are available, but it has been suggested that up to 30% of fistulae will heal with drug treatment such as a combination of antibiotic therapy and immunosuppression with intravenous azathiaprine or 6-mercaptopurine. Control of any concomitant rectal disease is also essential.

Defunctioning ileostomy for anal disease has a limited place, with 25% of patients showing no improvement and 25% suffering relapse at stoma reversal. Even proctectomy can lead to problems, as this operation is notorious for poor healing in patients with severe anal Crohn's disease.

Sexually transmitted diseases causing anal manifestations

When the specialist is confronted by a patient with anorectal symptoms, a diagnosis of sexually transmitted disease is dependent on a high index of suspicion. The gastroenterologist must also be aware that these patients are commonly found to have more than one disease. Opportunity to discuss sexual preferences and practices is not easy to provide in a busy outpatients department, often taking time and tactful questioning in a private environment. Some patients feel more relaxed and able to discuss topics that cause them embarrassment after the examination has been completed. The most commonly seen problems are outlined here.

Human papilloma virus or condylomata acuminata

Perianal warts or condylomata acuminata are the most common and easy to recognize perianal lesion. Patients may give a direct history of having warts, or they may complain of perianal wetness, irritation, discomfort, or bleeding. Lesions vary from single pinhead-sized outgrowths to confluent, cauliflower-like clusters that cover the perianal region and extend out onto the buttocks. The lesions may also be found on the genitalia and inside the anal canal, so a full examination — including a proctoscop — is essential.

A wide range of treatments has been used for perianal warts: observation, the application of chemicals, and surgical excision are the most widely used. Immunotherapy and laser therapy are more expensive and less accessible forms of treatment in most centres. Awareness of the association of human papilloma virus with the development of **dysplastic change** or **invasive malignancy** is essential for the long-term follow up of these patients.

Herpes simplex virus

The typical lesions are a crop of small vesicles or ulcers (1–2 mm in size) and, later, larger ulcerated areas resulting from coalescence of the lesions. The lesions can be found on the genitalia or the perianal region, and can extend up into the anal canal or, more rarely, into the rectum. The lesions are often painful; typically, they resolve by complete healing over a period of about 2 weeks. There may be associated systemic symptoms of fever and malaise, and some patients will also describe a deep aching pain typical of a lumbosacral radiculopathy. Severity of attacks can vary from an almost unnoticed, fleeting discomfort to exquisite tenderness necessitating admission for control of symptoms or secondary infection. In 40% of affected patients the course is chronic and relapsing, with the new attacks often heralded by buttock and leg pain. In most cases a clinical diagnosis and symptomatic treatment are sufficient; the diagnosis can be confirmed on cytology of ulcer beds. Acyclovir appears to be effective in reducing repeated episodes of infection.

Molluscum contagiosum

Caused by a large virus from the "pox" group, the typical lesions of molluscum contagiosum are small (3 mm), discrete, pearly, rounded nodules with umbilicated centres. The lesions are painless and self-limiting, but local destruction can be used to prevent further spread and to improve the eventual cosmetic result.

Syphilis

The manifestations of syphilis most commonly seen on the perianal skin are the primary sore or chancre, which occurs about 3–5 weeks after the infection has been acquired, and condylomata lata, which are part of the spectrum of secondary syphilis. The primary lesion is a painful erosion, ulcer, or papule up to about 1 cm in diameter; the lesion can be lifted up, like a button in the skin. Painless rubbery enlargement of the regional lymph nodes follows about 1 week after the appearance of the initial lesion, and the lesions resolve after about 1 month. Several weeks later, in addition to the systemic manifestations of secondary syphilis multiple, flat moist plaques and nodules, often purplish in colour, can occur in the perianal region. These are condylomata lata.

Antibiotic treatment is curative for this disease, but the high incidence of other sexually transmitted disease means that a thorough screening is necessary.

RECTAL LESIONS

Rectal discomfort or dissatisfaction, difficulty with defecation, and the passage of blood with the stool are the most common symptoms of rectal disease. Digital examination, rigid sigmoidoscopy with biopsy forceps, and proctoscopy should all be possible in outpatient clinics. Exclusion of a rectal tumour, inflammatory bowel disease, or a solitary rectal ulcer is then always possible. The first two of these pathologies are dealt with in other chapters, solitary ulcer will be detailed here.

In patients with rectal bleeding, the cause should always be defined. If examination in the outpatient department is normal, further investigations — including endoscopy and, sometimes, an examination under anaesthesia — will be necessary. Many patients with rectal discomfort will have a normal outpatient examination and here the progression to further investigations may be less productive. A defecating proctogram may help to define problems such as intrarectal intussusception or a rectocele. Ultrasound scanning or MRI may reveal occult sepsis or a thickened internal anal sphincter, but other investigations should be used selectively.

Solitary rectal ulcer syndrome

The term "solitary rectal ulcer syndrome" is used to describe a spectrum of clinicopathological abnormalities that can affect both adults and children. It is generally agreed that occult or overt rectal prolapse and paradoxical contraction of the pelvic floor muscles are amongst the factors involved in the development of the condition.

The main **clinical features** are:

1. Passage of blood and mucus *per rectum*, associated with straining and a feeling of incomplete emptying, although some cases are asymptomatic.
2. Evidence of rectal prolapse, either internal or external, with or without abnormal perineal descent on evacuation proctography.
3. Sigmoidoscopic appearance varying from erythema to ulceration or polypoid lesions. These lesions are commonly solitary and between 5 and 10 cm from the anal margin, but they can be multiple. Although most commonly on the anterior rectal wall, they can be more extensive, and even circumferential.
4. Histological evidence of fibrous obliteration of the lamina propria, with disorientation of the muscularis mucosa and extension of smooth muscle fibres into the lamina propria.

There is a general lack of awareness of the syndrome, as a direct result of its rarity. Ulcerated solitary rectal ulcer syndrome may be mistaken for inflammatory bowel disease, and some patients have been treated with high-dose oral steroids. Polypoid lesions may be confused with neoplasia. Histological examination therefore plays a key role in **diagnosing solitary rectal ulcer syndrome**, as the proctoscopic appearance can be misleading. Radiological and physiological investigations are of limited diagnostic value, although endoanal ultrasound may show a markedly thickened internal sphincter, and defecating proctography may reveal internal prolapse.

There is **no specific cure** for solitary rectal ulcer syndrome. Symptoms may be improved by treatment, but it is uncommon to achieve endoscopic and histological normality. **Biofeedback behavioural retraining** has become the first line of treatment in those centres in which it is available. Most other non-invasive therapies remain unproven, and long-term surgical results are poor, with the most extensive series reported showing that, overall, 52% of patients who did not have a stoma were improved after surgery (10). For some patients a stoma, either temporary diverting or permanent, is required. Many, however, continue to experience functional symptoms.

Rectocele

Bulging of the rectum anteriorly into the vagina is a common finding in women, especially in those who have delivered their children vaginally. Most remain asymptomatic, but some may present with complaints of difficulty with defecation, which can be both with the initiation of defecation and with the completion of defecation. More specifically, the patient may complain of a bulge into the vagina or of having to press on the posterior vaginal wall to defecate. A large rectocele can be **diagnosed** on examination, and the confirmatory investigation of choice are a defecating proctogram or dynamic MRI. A patient with specific symptoms and the presence of trapping of contrast within the rectocele on proctogram will probably benefit from **surgical repair** of the rectocele. Those without specific symptoms and without trapping of contrast may benefit from **biofeedback training** as the first line of treatment.

Sexually transmitted diseases causing rectal disease

As with sexually transmitted diseases that cause anal manifestations, the diagnosis is dependent on a high index of suspicion. Some of the most commonly encountered pathologies are outlined here.

Herpes simplex

A **diagnosis** of Herpes simplex should be considered in a patient with exquisitely painful proctitis. On proctoscopy, the mucosa is friable and there may be vesicles and pustules. The diagnosis can be made on cytology of ulcer scrapings or culture of the fluid from the vesicles. **Treatment** is mainly symptomatic, but acyclovir may reduce the duration and severity of symptoms.

Cytomegalovirus

Cytomegalovirus is extremely common in the immunosuppressed patient and it can cause ileocolitis with inflammation, haemorrhage, ulceration, or perforation. Significant *per rectal* bleeding can be a memorable feature, especially for the unwary surgeon. **Diagnosis** can be made on viral culture, viral inclusion bodies seen on biopsy examination, antigen assay, or by polymerase chain reaction. **Treatment** with intravenous ganciclovir is usually successful.

Chlamydia

The most common sexually transmitted disease, chlamydia causes systemic symptoms and can involve the rectum with proctitis. Tenesmus, rectal pain, blood and mucus *per rectum*, and a non-specific infective picture on histology are typical features. Late complications can include rectal stricturing. **Diagnosis** is made by tissue culture or microimmunofluorescent antibody titre. Chlamydia is **sensitive to** oral tetracycline or erythromycin.

Gonorrhoea

Up to 50% of rectal infections with gonorrhoea can be asymptomatic. A mucopurulent discharge, a feeling of rectal fullness, or pruritis may be present. **Diagnosis** by Gram stain or culture may be difficult, and **treatment** may have to be instituted on a high index of suspicion. The antibiotic usually used is penicillin, but resistant cases may need a combination-drug regimen.

Syphilis

A painful anal canal ulcer or ulcers, or proctitis with rectal pain, tenesmus, and a mucous discharge may occur in anorectal syphilis. Serological testing confirms the diagnosis and treatment is with penicillin or erythromycin.

Radiation injury to the anorectum

A majority of patients receiving pelvic radiotherapy experience acute anorectal symptoms and up to a fifth suffer from late-phase radiation proctitis.

Patients referred for a gastroenterological outpatient opinion may present with rectal bleeding from mucosal friability or neovascular telangiectasia, anorectal pain, diarrhea, tenesmus, fecal frequency, fecal urgency or frank incontinence. Chronic inflammation can lead to a marked reduction in rectal capacity and symptoms of diarrhea may be worsened by the presence of small intestinal injury to loops of bowel caught in the pelvic field. There is conflicting evidence as to the nature of radiation induced anal canal injuries, based on mainly retrospective works on different groups of patients undergoing varying radiotherapeutic regimens.

Proctitis can be scored on symptoms, endoscopic appearance and histology (Table 43.1) (11). Conservative therapy has been shown to be of limited value, although endoscopic laser therapy may be useful to control rectal bleeding and antidiarrheal agents such as Imodium, used judiciously, can control frequency, urgency and incontinence.

Longer term sequelae of severe proctitis can be disabling and these include rectal stricture and rectovaginal fistula. The risk of rectal cancer is increased. Surgical reconstruction in these cases is associated with a high morbidity and is reserved for those with adequate anal sphincter function and no evidence of recurrent disease. The simplest option for the incapacitated is often a colostomy.

CONCLUSION

The prospect of discussing anorectal symptoms and having an anorectal examination is frightening for most people, and this should be borne in mind

Table 43.1. Scoring system for radiation proctitis based on symptoms, endoscopic findings and histology results (adapted from (12)).

	Score	0	1	2
Symptoms	Urgency	Nil	Mild (5–20 mins)	Moderate/severe (<5 mins)
	PR bleeding/week	0	<4	>4
	PR blood quantity	None	Streaks	Obvious
	Diarrhea (days per week)	0	1	>1
	Number of stools	<1	2–3	>3
	Pain (rectal)	Nil	Pain present	—
Endoscopy (rectum)	Erythema	Nil	Mild	Moderate
	Granularity/edema	Nil	Mild	Moderate
	Telangiectasia	Nil	Few or some	Sparse or florid
	Ulcers	Nil	Few or numerous	—
Histology	Overall grade	Normal	Abnormal	—

PR = per rectum

during any consultation for anorectal conditions. A confident diagnosis, reassurance, and a clear explanation of the problem and the available therapies will go a long way to putting the patient at their ease and making any further visits less of an ordeal. In a busy outpatient departments, it is often very helpful to have available a broad spectrum of explanatory leaflets about the various conditions and the treatments, as many patients are too nervous to remember all that is said to them, or to ask all the necessary questions.

References
1. Metcalf A. Anorectal disorders. Five common causes of pain, itching, and bleeding. *Postgrad Med* 1995; **98**: 81–84, 87–89, 92–94.
2. Loder PB, Kamm MA, Nicholls RJ *et al*. Haemorrhoids: pathology, pathophysiology and aetiology [review]. *Br J Surg* 1994; **81**: 946–954.
3. Wassef R, Rothenberger D, Goldberg S. Rectal prolapse. *Curr Probl Surg* 1986; **23**: 397–451.
4. Monson JR, Jones NA, Vowden P *et al*. Delorme's operation: the first choice in complete rectal prolapse? *Ann R Coll Surg Engl* 1986; **68**: 143–146.
5. Lund JN, Scholefield JH. A randomised, prospective, double-blind, placebo-controlled trial of glyceryl trinitrate ointment in treatment of anal fissure. *Lancet* 1997; **349**: 11–14.
6. Williams N, Scott NA, Irving M. Effect of lateral sphincterotomy on internal sphincter anal function. *Dis Colon Rectum* 1995; **38**: 700–704.
7. Phillips RKS. *A companion to Specialist Surgical Practice: Colorectal Surgery*. London: WB Saunders, 1997.
8. Enriquez-Navascues JM, Leal J, Tobaruela E, *et al*. The value of Hughes–Cardiff classification in the management of perianal Crohn's disease. *Rev Esp Enferm Dig* 1997; **89**: 583–590.
9. Winter AM, Hanauer SB. Medical management in Crohn's disease. *Semin Gastroint Dis* 1998; **9**: 10–14.
10. Sitzler PJ, Kamm MA, Nicholls RJ, *et al*. Long-term clinical outcome of surgery for solitary rectal ulcer syndrome. *Br J Surg* 1998; **85**: 1246–1250.
11. Stockdale AD, Biswas A. Long-term control of radiation proctitis following treatment wth sucralfate enemas. *Br J Surg* 1997; **84**: 379.
12. Talley NA. Chen F, King D, *et al*. Short-chain fatty acids in the treatment of radiation proctitis: a randomized, double-blind, placebo-controlled, cross-over pilot trial. *Dis Colon Rectum* 1997; **40**: 1046–1050.

Part IV: Procedures and Investigations in Gastroenterology

44. The Gastrointestinal Endoscopy Unit: Information for Users

RUSSELL E. COWAN

CLEANING AND DISINFECTION OF ENDOSCOPY EQUIPMENT (for particular aspects of gastrointestinal endoscopy in HIV positive patients, see Chapter 7.)

The most important aspect of this process is manual cleaning of the endoscopes with detergent. If this is not performed thoroughly, organic material may become fixed, and disinfection will not then be possible.

All modern endoscopes are fully immersible (provided the video connection terminals are covered by the cap). Automated endoscope washer/disinfectors have become an essential part of most endoscopy units. They increase instrument throughput and reduce staff contact with disinfectant, but they do not negate the need for manual cleaning of the insertion tube, suction/biopsy channel, instrument tip, and valve recesses. Although they offer several advantages, for example the complete irrigation of all channels, more reliable and reproducible decontamination, and reduction in staff contact with the disinfectant, they are not without some disadvantages. These are listed in the British Society of Gastroenterology Working Party Report on cleaning and disinfection (1).

Some special features or performance characteristics of washer/disinfectors are optional, but all machines should clean, disinfect, and rinse in accordance with local hospital infection control committee procedures or national guidelines. A number of other optional features may be offered, but it is essential to confirm that a machine is compatible with the disinfectant to be used (2); the disinfectant will remain in contact with the machine for much longer periods than with the endoscope.

Selection of disinfectant

The ideal disinfectant should be effective against a wide range of micro-organisms including pathogenic spores, *Mycobacterium tuberculosis* and blood-borne viruses, compatible with instruments and processors, non-irritant, environmentally friendly and affordable.

Glutaraldehyde

A 2% solution of glutaraldehyde is the most widely used agent. It is a very effective disinfectant with good microbicidal activity against non-sporing bacteria, viruses and Mycobacteria, while its action against spore-producing bacteria is only moderate and slow. It is inexpensive, and is non-damaging to endoscopes, accessories, and automated processing equipment; however health and safety issues related to its use are a source of considerable concern (3,4).

The major problem associated with the use of aldehyde disinfectants is that of **adverse reactions** among workers in endoscopy. These problems have been recognized by the Health and Safety Executive (HSE). The Health and Safety at Work Act 1974 requires employers to ensure, as far as is reasonably practicable, the health, safety, and welfare of all employees. The Act also requires employees to comply with the precautions established to ensure safe working. The Control of Substances

Hazardous to Health Regulations 1994 (COSHH) require employers to assess the risks to the health of staff that are posed by exposure to hazardous chemicals, such as glutaraldehyde, to avoid such exposure where this is reasonably practicable, and otherwise to ensure adequate control (5).

It is likely that, within the next few years, the use of aldehydes will be reduced because of these difficulties; safe alternatives are currently under consideration. Such an alternative is **orthophthalaldehyde (OPA)**, which appears to be similarly efficacious to 2% glutaraldehyde, although it is a poor sporicidal agent. It does not require activation, is more stable and produces little or no odour. It is not yet listed as a respiratory sensitizer although it has been identified as a skin irritant. The relatively high cost of OPA may be offset, in part, by its greater stability during storage and reuse.

Glutaraldehyde toxicity

Glutaraldehyde is both an irritant and a sensitizer. It is therefore not only good clinical practice, but also a COSHH requirement, that employees who may be exposed to glutaraldehyde receive regular health surveillance. Pre-employment health assessment should include inquiry regarding asthma, and skin and mucosal symptoms, such as rhinitis and conjunctivitis (3). Simple lung-function testing by spirometry should be carried out (6). Employees should be reassessed annually, by questionnaire, for the development of symptoms; subsequent records should be retained for 30 years.

Any **potential contact** with glutaraldehyde liquid or vapour necessitates the wearing of protective equipment. This should include long-sleeved gloves, impermeable plastic aprons, chemical-grade eye protection or face shields, and respiratory equipment suitable for removing toxic organic vapours (6). Monitoring of atmospheric concentrations of glutaraldehyde vapour can be used to record effectiveness of the control systems, including local exhaust ventilation, but atmospheric monitoring should only be carried out by a person competent in the task; occupational hygienists are trained in the monitoring and analysis of exposure data (3).

Endoscopy staff must be informed of the **risk of exposure** to glutaraldehyde and trained in the safe methods of its control. Only staff who have completed such an education and training programme should be allowed to disinfect endoscopes.

The unsafe use of glutaraldehyde has significant health and legal consequences; the safe use of glutaraldehyde may have revenue consequences that contribute significantly to the cost of gastrointestinal endoscopy. Switching to alternative, supposedly less toxic disinfectants also carries cost implications.

Peracetic acid and chlorine dioxide

Both peracetic acid and chlorine dioxide are highly effective disinfectants. Experience with these agents in the context of endoscopy is gradually increasing; certainly, adequate ventilation and other protective measures will continue to be required. Freshly prepared, both disinfectants are **rapidly active** against vegetative bacteria, including *Mycobacterium tuberculosis*, *M. avium intracellulare* and other atypical mycobacteria, and against a range of viruses, including poliovirus, rotavirus, hepatitis B virus (HBV) and human immunodeficiency virus (HIV). Sporicidal activity has been substantiated in 10 min or less (7,8). There are two commercially available preparations of peracetic acid: 0.2% peracetic acid (Steris) and 0.35% peracetic acid (Nu-Cidex), and now only one preparation of chlorine dioxide (Tristel). There is some concern about the effects of both these disinfectants on disinfection machines, and in the case of chlorine dioxide, on endoscopes, but these effects seem to be mostly cosmetic, with no functional consequences.

Although peracetic acid is not currently listed as an irritant, its principle ingredients are (ie hydrogen peroxide and acetic acid). Chlorine dioxide is listed as an irritant.

The disinfection contact time for these two agents is 5 min, and sporicidal activity is achieved in 10 min. These times are very favourable by comparison with 2% glutaraldehyde, for which the disinfection contact times range from 10 min before a session and between cases, to 60–120 min after use in a patient known to have *M. avium intracellulare* or other highly resistant mycobacteria. Table 44.1 summarizes the recommendations concerning contact times.

Other disinfectants

Peroxygen compounds and **quaternary ammonium derivatives** are less suitable because of unsatisfactory mycobacterial or virucidal activity, or incompatibility with endoscopes and automated washer/disinfectors.

Table 44.1. Recommended contact times for different disinfectants.

	Disinfectant contact time (min)		
	2% Glutaralderhyde	0.35% Peracetic acid	Chlorine dioxide
Before a session	10	5	5
Between cases	10	5	5
End of session	20	5*	5*
High level disinfection	20	5*	5*
Before ERCP			
Before use in immunocompromised patients			
After use in patients with pulmonary tuberculosis			
After a patient with known infection with *M. avium intracellulare* or other highly resistant mycobacteria	60–120	5*	5*

*Sporicidal activity is achieved in 10 min.
ERCP, endoscopic retrograde cholangiopancreatography.
Adapted with permission (from BMJ Publishing Group (1)).

Alcohol is effective but, on prolonged contact, is damaging to lens cements. It is also flammable. It has a useful role in flushing endoscope channels to dry them before storage.

Superoxidised water (Sterilox), an electro-chemical solution containing a mixture of radicals with strong oxidizing properties, is highly microbicidal when freshly generated. Practical experience of its use is, to date, limited, so its safety for users can not yet be determined. Its speed and effectiveness as a disinfectant are appealing, but problems concerning its compatibility with endoscopes somewhat undermine its potential to become a popular alternative to glutaraldehyde. The lacquered polymer sheath of Olympus flexible endoscopes is damaged by Sterilox.

Use of new disinfectants

Alternatives that are safer than the aldehyde disinfectants for endoscopy staff to use may be less effective as disinfectants or may damage endoscopes and processing equipment. If an alternative to glutaraldehyde is to be tried, the following steps should be taken (1):

1. Inform the instrument and processing equipment manufacturers, as the use of an alternative to glutaraldehyde may invalidate guarantees or service contracts.
2. Carefully cost the change, bearing in mind the life of the disinfectant.
3. Ensure that processed items are thoroughly cleaned and that the manufacturers' stated contact times are achieved, unless advice from professional organizations recommends otherwise.
4. Establish what is required in terms of COSHH regulations with respect to ventilation, personal protective clothing, health risk screening, and so on.
5. Keep the British Society of Gastroenterology and other organizations informed of your experience, be it favourable or not.

Cleaning and disinfection of accessories

Endoscopic accessories require the same attention to detail as the endoscopes. An increasing number are single use — for example, cytology brushes, polypectomy snares, injection needles, and most endoscopic retrograde cholangiopancreatography (ERCP) accessories (9). The Medical Devices Agency bulletin DB9501 advises on potential hazards, both clinical and legal, associated with the reprocessing and re-use of medical devices intended for single use only (10).

OBTAINING CONSENT FOR ENDOSCOPIC PROCEDURES

Information and explanation are essential to the success and safety of endoscopic practice. Many patients are fearful of endoscopy, not helped by the frightening experiences of their friends and relatives, and by inappropriate remarks made by endoscopy staff.

Whenever possible, patients should remain responsible for themselves, and clinicians must make every effort to maintain the autonomy and self-determination of their patients. Correctly obtained informed consent also helps to protect against complaints by patients and claims of malpractice against doctors (11). In the UK, there are now Department of Health guidelines produced by the National Health Service Management Executive (12). These list the patient's rights and outline the health professional's role in advising the patient and obtaining their consent to treatment. Although oral consent may be sufficient for the majority of contacts with health professionals, written consent will be required for the vast majority of procedures performed by gastroenterologists, especially those carried out in the endoscopy unit. It has been suggested in the British Society of Gastroenterology guidelines that the patient should be told of adverse events of a minor or temporary nature that have an incidence of more than 10%, and of serious events with an incidence of more than 0.5% (13).

The doctor should answer all questions put to him by the patient fully and truthfully. It is emphasized by the British Society of Gastroenterology Working Party that these instructions are no more than guidelines, and that the law will judge every case on its merits (14). In practice, this translates to patients being provided with **written information** warning them of the risks, particularly in the case of certain procedures (Table 44.2), although it is important not to overlook the fact that **all endoscopic procedures carry a risk**, however small, of producing bleeding or perforation to the lining of that part of the gastrointestinal tract being examined.

Obtaining consent in practice

To ask the patient to sign a consent form **immediately** before the procedure is not ideal. Instead, the patient should be fully informed by the endoscopist at least 24 h before the procedure, and then be asked to sign a consent form. For busy units and endoscopists, these are impossible standards to reach and maintain. Instead, strenuous efforts should be made to approach this ideal, and for most units these measures are already in place:

1. An explanation of why the endoscopic procedure needs to be done and the essential elements of it should be covered by the referring clinician (general practitioners in the case of open-access endoscopy services).
2. An appropriate pamphlet on the endoscopic procedure should be sent to the patient along with the appointment details.
3. A general health assessment should be made and confirmation should be obtained that the pamphlet has been read and the procedure understood.
4. A qualified nurse with endoscopy experience should welcome and interview the patient when they arrive at the endoscopy unit, when further explanation and reassurance can be given, and any residual concerns may be passed on to the endoscopist.
5. The endoscopist should deal with any last minute questions. If the consent form has not been signed previously, the endoscopist should ask for signature.

No protocol can substitute for careful and friendly discussion with the patient both before and after the procedure.

Table 44.2. Gastrointestinal endoscopic procedures and their potential complications.

Procedure	Complication
Dilatation of a stricture	Perforation
ERCP	Acute pancreatitis, cholangitis, perforation, bleeding, gallstone impaction
Percutaneous endoscopic gastrostomy	Perforation, infection, aspiration
Colonoscopy and flexible sigmoidoscopy (especially with polypectomy)	Colonic perforation and bleeding

Special situations relating to obtaining consent

There are a number of situations in which obtaining consent needs particular care and attention.

Obtaining consent from hospital inpatients

Sick patients may require time and extensive explanation before they can give consent. If they do not wish to give consent, their wishes should not be ignored. Ideally, the endoscopist should see and assess the patient on the ward. This is particularly important for ERCP, percutaneous endoscopic gastrostomy (PEG) insertions and other interventional procedures, and also for high-risk patients (e.g. those with severe gastrointestinal bleeding). If the specialist or deputy decides to carry out the procedure despite the increased risks then he or she should explain the procedure and mention the risks to the patient before requesting their consent.

Assessment on the ward is not always possible, so hospital wards should have appropriate information leaflets to give to the patient, and an informed member of the referring team should explain the procedure.

Close contact between the wards and the endoscopy unit can help the exchange of relevant information. A well-designed request card that accompanies the verbal request for the endoscopy should impart important information about the patient's condition, both general and gastroenterological.

Endoscopic procedures involving insertion of long-term prostheses

These endoscopic procedures are:

- insertion of a stent through oesophageal or other strictures
- insertion of biliary stents
- insertion of gastrostomy tubes

The explanation of these procedures should be comprehensive and include details, not only of early complications, but also long-term potential problems.

The patients requiring these procedures are often very ill. It is important, therefore, that the appropriateness of a procedure in the patient's overall management should be agreed with those looking after the patient.

For the mentally incompetent, the doctor makes the decision as to the appropriate procedure after discussion with all concerned in the care of the patient, basing the decision on the patient's best interest.

Obtaining consent for procedures in minors

In this situation, much responsibility falls upon the parents. It is important to be aware of the following rules:

1. Parents or guardians provide consent on behalf of the child up to the age of 16 years. Children younger than 16 years who have sufficient understanding and intelligence to appreciate the issues involved may consent for themselves when there has been parental refusal. Indeed, parents can not override a child's consent, but can override a refusal.
2. Parental consent *must* be obtained when a child does not have sufficient understanding and is younger than 16 years, except in an emergency when there is no time to obtain it.
3. Parents or guardians should consent on behalf of the mentally impaired adolescent to the age of 18 years.
4. If parents were married at the time of the birth of the child, both have parental responsibility. An unmarried mother has sole responsibility (unless the father has acquired responsibility by court order or a Parent Responsibility Agreement).
5. If parents refuse to give consent for an essential procedure or if there is conflict between the parents, it may be necessary for the endoscopist to obtain permission from the Court to proceed, where time permits. This should be considered only as a final option. The hospital authorities should, instead, rely on the judgement of the clinicians — usually the consultant in charge — who should obtain a written supporting opinion from a medical colleague that the patient's life is in danger if the treatment is withheld, and should discuss the need for the endoscopic intervention with the parents or guardians in the presence of a witness. In the UK, the witness can be a directorate manager, senior nurse (not below G grade), a doctor (not below registrar), another consultant or the on-call manager. **In these circumstances the appropriate directorate manager and the customer-care department or the on-call manager must be notified**.

Patients who are incapable of consenting

1. For a mentally impaired adult, the clinician has the responsibility "to do his best for the patient". The issue should be discussed in detail with relatives and carers, but they should *not* be expected to sign a consent form. Moreover, it would be unlawful for them to do so unless the patient is a minor. In difficult cases, especially if parents or carers express misgivings, the support of a clinical colleague should be sought.

2. In an emergency, the endoscopist takes responsibility and no consent is necessary. Instead, the legal principle of "necessity" can be used.

3. No-one can give or withhold consent to treatment on behalf of a mentally impaired patient, except in Scotland where a "tutor-dative" with appropriate authority may make medical decisions on behalf of the patient (15).

Withdrawal of consent during a procedure

Almost always, it is a struggling patient under the influence of drugs who withdraws consent. The endoscopist then has the responsibility of doing what he considers best for the patient.

In the context of the trend for endoscopies to be performed without intravenous sedation, the patient may struggle a lot and, in effect, withdraw consent to continue. If it is likely that the procedure will take more than an extra few minutes, it is prudent to withdraw the endoscope, allow the patient time to recover, then discuss with him or her how best to proceed. An alternative would be to give the patient intravenous sedation during the procedure, using a previously established venous access, having agreed to this option with the patient at the time of obtaining consent.

Legal defence unions and professional bodies

If the clinician is concerned about any aspect of patient consent or refusal, he should contact his legal defence union or professional body. If the clinician has followed the above guidelines and has acted in the best interests of the patient, and with due professional competence and according to his or her own professional conscience, he or she is unlikely to be criticized by a court or a professional body.

STANDARDS OF SEDATION AND PATIENT MONITORING DURING ENDOSCOPY

There are striking national differences in the practice of sedation for gastrointestinal endoscopy. Until recently in the UK, more than 80% of patients undergoing upper gastrointestinal endoscopy received sedation, whereas only a minority do so in Germany. In France, intravenous sedation techniques are almost entirely practised by anaesthetists. In recent years, an increasing number of patients in the UK have been undergoing diagnostic upper gastrointestinal endoscopy and flexible sigmoidoscopy without sedation, in response to the greater demands for endoscopy, in particular in the open-access services.

Endoscopic procedures can be painful and can cause considerable anxiety (16). These problems can be alleviated by giving some form of sedation, analgesia, or both — often termed "conscious sedation" to distinguish it from anaesthesia. As sedation-induced respiratory depression is the most common cause of endoscopy-related deaths, it is clear that strict rules related to sedation should be established. The benefits of intravenous sedation in terms of better patient tolerance and increased ease of examination for the endoscopist must outweigh any cardiorespiratory morbidity (17).

Sedative and analgesic agents

Pharyngeal anaesthesia

This is useful when little or no intravenous sedation is to be used. Spray application is preferred, as it can be directed to the posterior pharyngeal wall to suppress the gag reflex. It is not necessary when heavy sedation is used, as it may increase the risk of pulmonary aspiration. Patients must be asked not to open their pharynx by making a noise at the time of spraying, as this exposes the larynx to the anaesthesia and may suppress the cough reflex.

Benzodiazepines

The benzodiazepines are the only class of drug used for intravenous sedation during gastroenterological procedures. They are remarkably safe, with a wide margin of safety and high therapeutic index.

Midazolam is well established as the drug of choice for endoscopic procedures in the UK (18). The plasma elimination half-life of this water-soluble agent is 1.5–2.5 h in normal individuals, compared with more than 40 h when the lipid-emulsion formulation of diazepam (Diazemuls) is used (19).

Overall, the doses of benzodiazepines used to induce sedation for endoscopy are higher than necessary, and higher than the manufacturers' recommended doses (18). Doses should be kept to the minimum that is compatible with patient comfort and successful performance of the procedure. Midazolam is now recognized as being three to four times more potent than diazepam in terms of sedative effect, not merely twice as potent as reported initially (20). For equipotent sedative doses, there is approximately a twofold increase in achieving amnesia for the procedure with midazolam compared with that achieved with diazepam (20).

A dose of 5 mg midazolam intravenously is usually sufficient for the majority of patients undergoing either diagnostic or therapeutic endoscopy, including ERCP, even in young fit patients. In the elderly and in those with coexisting medical diseases, such as cardiac, renal, and hepatic failure, this dose must be reduced: a dose of 1 or 2 mg midazolam intravenously may be sufficient. It is important that time is allowed for the sedative to work before the procedure is commenced.

Successful sedation for endoscopy should result in anxiolysis and amnesia rather than ptosis and marked muscle relaxation. It is usually entirely appropriate for the patient to be lying on the endoscopy trolley with eyes wide open. If the patient is deeply sedated, then it could be construed that he or she has received a general anesthetic. In medico–legal terms, this situation could give rise to serious problems.

The benzodiazepines do not have analgesic properties. Local anaesthestic spray on the pharynx is commonly used to provide analgesia. It should be noted, however, that lignocaine is itself a respiratory depressant and can cause bradycardia, hypotension and cardiac arrest. Aspiration pneumonia has been reported up to 30 days after upper gastrointestinal endoscopy, and this may relate to the use of an anaesthetic throat spray (18).

In a double-blind placebo-controlled trial, patient tolerance has been shown to be significantly improved by **midazolam and lignocaine throat spray**, compared with midazolam alone (17). It follows therefore that, for the patient experiencing pain during endoscopy, it may not be appropriate simply to administer an additional dose of sedative.

Opiates

If there is a clinical indication for the use of an analgesic, such as ERCP or colonoscopy, then the doses of the opiate and the benzodiazepine must be reduced. The opiate should be given first and the benzodiazepine dose titrated carefully against the response. There is an eightfold synergism between opiates and benzodiazepines (21). For improved safety, therefore, the dose of opiate should be 25–30% of the usual intravenously administered dose (22).

Elderly patients and those with coexisting pulmonary disease are sensitive to **respiratory depression**, which may occur when opiates and benzodiazepines are used in combination. In the two UK surveys of endoscopic practice, adverse events were more common in patients who received a combination of pethidine and benzodiazepine (18,23). Intravenous pethidine is most commonly used in the UK, usually in a dose of 25–50 mg (18). Fentanyl, a potent opioid with a rapid onset of action and a rapid recovery, is an alternative. Nalbuphine, an opiate analogue, is also popular, being about 10 times more potent than pethidine and with the added administrative advantage that it is not a controlled drug.

Miscellaneous agents

Droperidol, a neuroleptic agent, can be useful in sedating agitated patients and appears to be particularly helpful in alcoholism. It is given in increments of 0.5 mg up to 3 mg (occasionally 5 mg) in total, while the blood pressure is monitored regularly for hypotension.

Nitrous oxide gas, self-administered, provides useful analgesia during colonoscopy and recovery from its effects is almost instantaneous. It does tend to encourage relaxation of bowel peristalsis, which can be a disadvantage to the endoscopist.

General anaesthesia

General anaesthesia may be required in special circumstances, such as complex procedures in young children or uncooperative patients. **Propofol** is a popular agent among anaesthetists, providing short-term anaesthesia that is easily reversed.

Intravenous access

Adequate, **reliable intravenous access through-**

out the endoscopic procedure is essential, for the following reasons:

- Drugs given intravenously have rapid and relatively consistent effects
- It offers speed and ease of administration of multiple drugs
  — Sedative drug: initial and top-up doses
  — Opioid analgesics
  — Anticholinergics (and glucagon)
  — Antibiotics
  — Flumazenil (for sedative reversal)
- Resuscitation by means of emergency drugs can be delievered rapidly
- It facilitates volume expansion with crystalloids, colloids, and blood

Despite these considerations, the prospective audit of upper gastrointestinal endoscopy carried out on behalf of the British Society for Gastroenterology recorded the use of continuous intravenous access in only 60% of inpatients and 40% of outpatients undergoing endoscopy (18). It is to be hoped that practice has improved significantly in the 5 years that have elapsed since this audit was reported.

Intravenous access should be provided by a plastic cannula in all patients until recovery is complete. The preferred site of access is the back of the hand or the forearm — ideally on the right arm, as the use of the antecubital fossa carries the risk of accidental placement in the brachial artery. There is a good case for establishing intravenous access in those receiving only pharyngeal anaesthesia, as this allows the administration of sedative drugs easily and promptly if tolerance of the procedure is poor. Anticholinergics may be required also during the endoscopy.

Cardiorespiratory monitoring

Clinical monitoring

The general condition and well-being of the patient should be monitored throughout the procedure and until the recovery is complete. This should be the responsibility of both the endoscopist and a qualified nurse trained in endoscopic techniques, but, as the endoscopist may be preoccupied by the technical complexities of the procedure, the role of the nurse is paramount.

More than 50% of serious adverse reactions during endoscopy are cardiopulmonary (23,24). Decreases in oxygen saturation occur commonly during gastroscopy and colonscopy, but clinical observation of early signs of respiratory depression and hypoxia is unreliable. Moreover, there is no close correlation between the decrease in oxygen saturation and the type or dose of sedative used and the age and sex of the patient (25). The use of pulse oximeters and the prophylactic use of supplementary oxygen are recommended. Pulse oximeters can detect oxygen desaturation that is not apparent clinically, and alarm systems on the oximeter may alert the endoscopist and nurse to a deterioration in the patient's condition.

Preoxygenation and supplementary oxygen

The provision of oxygen-enriched air for the patient to breathe before and during endoscopy has been shown to diminish greatly, or even prevent, hypoxaemia (26–28). The amount used (2–4 litre/min) usually will not compromise respiratory function in patients with chronic obstructive airways disease. Oxygen supplementation has been recommended, therefore, for those "at risk" patients (29), but its routine use in every case is arguably more appropriate and can be achieved with minimal expense.

During upper gastrointestinal endoscopy, the patient may switch from nasal breathing to mouth breathing, prompted by the endoscope touching the soft palate (29). It is therefore best that oxygen is delivered via a special mouthguard with apertures to direct the oxygen up the nose and to the back of the mouth simultaneously, thus filling the deadspace with oxygen (30).

Electrocardiography

In patients with a history of ischaemic heart disease or known arrhythmias, continuous electrocardiographic (ECG) monitoring during and after the procedure should reduce the number of adverse cardiopulmonary events encountered during endoscopy.

Patient recovery

Clinical monitoring must be continued into the recovery period, when pulse oximetry and supplementary oxygen may be needed for some patients. Day-case patients receiving sedation should be accompanied home by a responsible adult, who should

Table 44.3. Risk of endocarditis.

Level of risk		
High risk	Moderate, low or theoretical risk	No increased risk
Prosthetic heart valve	Mitral valve prolapse with insufficiency	Mitral valve prolapse without insufficiency
Previous endocarditis	Rheumatic valvular or congenital cardiac lesion	Uncomplicated secundum atrial septal defect
Surgically constructed systemic–pulmonary shunt or conduit	Ventriculo-peritoneal shunt	Cardiac pacemaker Coronary artery bypass graft
Synthetic vascular graft less than 1 year old	Heart transplant	Implanted defibrillator

be given written discharge instructions in case of complications.

ANTIBIOTIC PROPHYLAXIS

This is recommended for endoscopic procedures if the patient is at high risk of endocarditis or of symptomatic bacteraemia as a consequence of immunosuppression or neutropenia. Antibiotics are also routinely recommended for those patients undergoing ERCP with evidence of biliary stasis, with prior or active cholangitis, and with pancreatic pseudocyst.

Identification of at-risk patients

Endoscopy units should establish a method (such as a checklist) for identifying at-risk patients and drawing them to the attention of the endoscopist.

Endocarditis

The number of patients with cardiac prosthetic implants has increased steadily over the years, during which time many millions of gastrointestinal endoscopic procedures have been performed. It is reassuring, therefore, that there is **no evidence of any increase in the incidence of endocarditis affecting prosthetic valves**. A handful of reports of endocarditis associated with endoscopic procedures have been published (31–34) and it is not certain, for each case reported, whether the association was causal. The widespread use of antibiotic prophylaxis in gastrointestinal endoscopy would, there-

fore, seem to be unnecessary, making it important that the high-risk patients are identified.

The risk of endocarditis varies with the nature of the underlying cardiac condition, and is dependent on the incidence and intensity of bacteraemia and on the organism(s) causing the bacteraemia (endocarditis is most commonly caused by streptococci and enterococci). Table 44.3 lists the conditions associated with the risk of endocarditis or symptomatic bacteraemia, ranking the level of risk. The incidence and intensity of bacteraemia vary with the type of endoscopic procedure (Table 44.4).

It follows from the data presented in these Tables that patients with cardiac lesions associated with a high risk of endocarditis who undergo gastro-

Table 44.4. Incidence of bacteraemia after various gastrointestinal procedures.

Procedure	Incidence of bacteraemia (%)[†]
Tooth brushing	25
Dental extraction	30–60
Diagnostic oesophagogastroduodenoscopy	4
Oesophageal dilatation/prosthesis insertion	34–54
Oesophageal laser therapy	35
Oesophageal sclerotherapy	10–50[*]
Oesophageal band ligation	6
ERCP	
Obstructed ducts	11
No duct obstruction	6
Rectal digital examination	4
Proctoscopy	5
Sigmoidoscopy	6–9
Barium enema	11
Colonoscopy	2–4

[†]Summary of published data.
[*]Greater after emergency than elective management.

Table 44.5. Recommendations for antibiotic prophylaxis in gastrointestinal endoscopy.

Endoscopic procedure	Patient risk group	Antibiotic prophylaxis*
All procedures	Higher risk of endocarditis	Regimen 1a or 1b
	Severe neutropenia	Regimen 3
	Moderate or low risk of endocarditis	Not necessary
ERCP	Higher risk of endocarditis	Regimen 1a or 1b
	Bile stasis	Regimen 2
	Pancreatic pseudocyst	
	Recent cholangitis	

[†]See Table 44.6 for regimens.

Table 44.6. Recommended antibiotic regimens.

1a. High endocarditis risk
Patients not allergic to penicillin and who have not received penicillin more than once in previous month

Adults	**Children (up to 10 years)**
Amoxycillin 1 g IV	Amoxycillin 500 mg IV
+	+
Gentamicin 120 mg IV	Gentamicin 2 mg/kg IV
then 500 mg amoxycillin orally 6 hours later	**then** one oral dose of amoxycillin 6 hours later
	Age 5–9 years 250 mg
	Age 0–4 years 125 mg

1b. Patients allergic to penicillin or who have received penicillin more than once in previous month

Vancomycin 1 g IV slowly	Vancomycin 20 mg/kg IV
+	+
Gentamicin 120 mg IV	Gentamicin 2 mg/kg IV
or	**or**
Teicoplanin 400 mg IV	Teicoplanin 6 mg/kg IV
+	+
Gentamicin 120 mg IV	Gentamicin 2 mg/kg IV

2. Biliary endoscopic patients
Ciprofloxacin 750 mg orally 60–90 minutes before procedure
or
Gentamicin 120 mg IV just before procedure
or
Parenteral quinolone, cephalosporin or ureidopenicillin IV just before procedure

3. Patients with severe neutropenia
(neutrophils $<100 \times 10^9$/litre)
Adults and children:
As for endocarditis risk and for ERCP + Metronidazole 7.5 mg/kg IV

IV, intravenous.

intestinal endoscopic procedures with a known high risk of bacteraemia run a greater risk of endocarditis and should be given antibiotics preventatively. Table 44.5 gives recommendations on the antibiotic prophylaxis to use, and Table 44.6 lists the regimens of recommended antibiotics for different circumstances.

Bacteraemia

Transient bacteraemia during gastrointestinal endoscopy is well recognized, as shown in Table 44.4. As no blood culture is completely sensitive, the reported rates of bacteraemia will inevitably provide underestimates. One study of upper gastrointestinal endoscopy in immunosuppressed patients reported a high rate (9/47; 19%) of clinically significant bacteraemia (35).

Although bacteraemia during **endoscopy** has been studied extensively, the incidence of **symptomatic bacteraemia** is far less well known. In the vast majority of cases, endoscopy-induced bacteraemia is not associated with recognizable symptoms and is probably unimportant. It is of no greater importance than asymptomatic bacteraemia that occurs after tooth brushing.

Neutropenia appears to confer an increased risk of symptomatic bacteraemia after endoscopy, although the size of the increased risk is not known (35). It is recommended that patients with severe neutropenia (<1000/mm^3 ($<10^9$/litre)) should be given prophylactic antibiotics for gastrointestinal endoscopic procedures known to be associated with a high risk of bacteraemia. Gram-negative aerobic and, less frequently, anaerobic bacteria are the most likely pathogens in these circumstances, and the choice of prophylactic antibiotics should reflect this.

No data have been established to show that **immunocompromised patients with normal neutrophil counts** (e.g. those receiving drug treatment for organ transplantation) are at an increased risk of symptomatic bacteraemia after endoscopy. Routine antibiotic prophylaxis is not recommended for this group of patients, and the same advice pertains in patients with HIV infection.

The relevance of **antibiotic prophylaxis** for various groups of **immunocompromised patients** can be summarized as:

1. *Neutropenia*: Increased risk of symptomatic bacteraemia after endoscopy. Give antibiotic

prophylaxis for high-risk gastrointestinal endoscopic procedures.

2. *Normal neutrophil count*: No data to show an increased risk of symptomatic bacteraemia after endoscopy. Antibiotic prophylaxis not required.

3. *Cirrhosis*: No data available to support use of antibiotic prophylaxis unless there is associated severe neutropenia.

Endoscopic retrograde cholangiopancreatography

Bacteraemia during ERCP is well recognized (36–38). Sepsis is the principal cause of death after ERCP (38,39); it occurs almost exclusively in patients with poor drainage of the pancreatic and biliary systems. Patients with **biliary stasis** invariably have infected bile, and cholangitis and septicaemia may occur as a result of dissemination of bacteria already present, if adequate endoscopic drainage is not provided (40).

Administration of prophylactic antibiotics is recommended for patients likely to undergo a therapeutic procedure in the bile duct, or when there is a pancreatic pseudocyst. Data suggest a reduction in clinically significant sepsis when antibiotics are used (41).

Other factors essential for reducing the likelihood of biliary and pancreatic sepsis during diagnostic and therapeutic ERCP are optimal cleaning and disinfection of the endoscope, the use of sterile contrast medium, and the use of sterile, mostly single-use accessories.

Non-cardiac prostheses

Infections of orthopaedic prostheses, urethral prostheses, central nervous system vascular shunts, pacemakers, and even intraocular lenses may result from haematogenous spread of bacteria. Endoscopic procedures may cause bacteraemia, but the fact that simple and frequent activities, such as toothbrushing, are also associated with bacteraemia suggests there is likely to be little benefit from antibiotic prophylaxis in patients with these prostheses. At present therefore, the British Society of Gastroenterology, in agreement with the American Society of Colon and Rectal Surgeons, hold the view that, in the setting of gastrointestinal endoscopy in patients with prostheses, prophylactic antibiotics are not recommended (42).

Percutaneous endoscopic gastrostomy

Wound infection associated with PEG is low. There are no data available at present to support the case for routine antibiotic prophylaxis; however, with increasing experience with this procedure, this advice may need to be revised.

Recommended antibiotics

Ampicillin and amoxycillin

Ampicillin and amoxycillin are preferred to penicillin for prophylaxis against Gram-positive bacteria, especially streptococci and enterococci, which are the most common cause of infective endocarditis. Enterococcal bacteraemia is most likely after endoscopic instrumentation of the lower gastrointestinal tract.

Aminoglycosides

Gentamicin and other aminoglycosides enhance the bactericidal power of ampicillin and amoxycillin against streptococci and enterococci. Gentamicin is also active against most aerobic coliforms and most *Pseudomonas spp.* It is suitable for use in the context of neutropenia, when metronidazole should be added to provide anaerobic cover. The use of one or two doses only of gentamicin causes very little risk of either nephro- or ototoxicity.

Ciprofloxacin

Ciprofloxacin is probably the preventative antibiotic of choice for ERCP. It is generally highly active against Gram-negative bacteria, but is much less active against Gram-positive infections, including enterococci. It is therefore not suitable for prevention of endocarditis. Oral ciprofloxacin about 4 h before the procedure is not only less expensive than the intravenous preparation, but delivers good blood concentrations.

Other antibiotics

Cephalosporins have poor activity against enterococci and therefore are not appropriate for prevention of endocarditis. Otherwise, they have a broad spectrum of activity and they penetrate relatively freely into bowel contents. Their heavy use in some countries has been associated with outbreaks of *Clostridium difficile* enterocolitis. Glycopeptides such as vancomycin and teicoplanin, with a very broad spectrum of activity against Gram-positive bacteria, can be used in patients who are allergic to penicillins or have recently been exposed to them. Although still uncommon in the UK, vancomycin-resistant enterococci are being encountered with increasing frequency in some hospitals. Most enterococci of bowel origin remain sensitive to the traditionally used antibiotics, but trends of antibiotic resistance in the UK must be closely watched.

USE OF ELECTRICAL CURRENT IN ENDOSCOPY

The reasons for using electrosurgical or diathermy currents are to cut or coagulate tissue in the following situations:

* Sphincterotomy during ERCP
* Polypectomy
* "Hot" biopsy
* Haemostasis
    — bleeding ulcer
    — hereditary haemorrhagic telangiectasia
    — angiodysplasia
* Debulking of tumours and hyperplastic tissue

These aims are achieved by the diathermy current causing **heat**, with resultant coagulation of blood vessels, especially the large ones. Coincidentally, the heated tissue becomes easier to transect or cut, but this is of secondary importance. Heat is generated in tissue by the passage of electricity (electrons), the flow of which causes collisions between intracellular ions and release of heat energy in the process. The electrical current used is high frequency or "radio frequency", alternating in direction at up to 1 million times per second. At such frequencies, there is no time for muscle and nerve membrane to depolarize before the current alternates again; heat is produced, but no "shock". Electrosurgical current is not felt by the patient and, similarly, there is no danger to cardiac muscle.

Cardiac pacemakers

The relatively low power used for endoscopic diathermy means that cardiac pacemakers are **unaffected**.

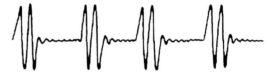

Cutting current - continuous (high power) low-voltage pulses unable to pass through desiccated tissue

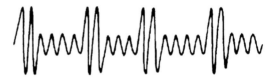

Coagulating current - intermittent high - voltage pulses able to pass through desiccated tissue

Blended current - combines the characteristics of both cutting and coagulating currents

Figure 44.1. Coagulating, cutting and blended currents in diagrammatic form.

Another safety factor is the remote position from the pacemaker of the patient plate, usually on the thigh. This remote position helps to ensure that the return pathway of the electrical current does not involve the pacemaker. This risk applies only to monopolar electrosurgery, as used in endoscopy, whereas bipolar electrosurgery offers a very short return pathway (e.g. between the two tips of the forceps).

Coagulating and cutting currents

Generally, pure **coagulating current** is used for endoscopic electrosurgery and **cutting current** for surgical incisions. Cutting current has an uninterrupted waveform of relatively low-voltage spikes. By contrast, coagulating current has intermittent higher-voltage spikes with alternating "off periods" (Figure 44.1). The higher voltage allows a deeper spread of current across the tissues, thus prompting desiccation, whereas the off periods reduce the tendency to local tissue destruction as produced by the cutting current.

Blended current combines both wave forms (see Figure 44.1), which, in combination with some diathermy units providing a selection of blends, offers a facility for relatively more cutting than coagulation and *vice versa*.

As different diathermy units from different manufacturers have different output characteristics, it is essential to be cautious when changing from one unit to another.

Monopolar and bipolar electrosurgery

These two systems differ in one important way: the position of the return electrode. In monopolar diathermy the return electrode is placed at some distance from the active electrode, usually in the form of a plate on the patient's thigh, whereas in bipolar electrosurgery the return electrode is incorporated into the same instrument as the active electrode, such as the two tips of diathermy forceps. Current flow through the tissues is completely different for these two systems. Bipolar techniques produce extremely localized heating effects, a potential advantage for polypectomy of sessile polyps, in which there is a danger of deep-tissue damage and perforation, whereas monopolar techniques produce deeper heating of the tissues and therefore of local vasculature, reducing the potential for bleeding.

With bipolar diathermy the current never travels through the patient's body, so it can not cause problems. Bipolar current is inherently safer than monopolar. Its applications, therefore, are those situations in which low-power current is used, such as neurosurgery, ophthalmic surgery, and plastic surgery in which cutting tissue is not required. With the exception of bipolar diathermy for haemostasis, gastrointestinal endoscopy utilizes monopolar diathermy. Indeed, as the opposing cusps of the biopsy forceps would be the active and return electrodes, bipolar diathermy for "hot" biopsy during endoscopy would not be suitable, as the tissue within the forceps would be denatured.

Current density

Tissue heats when current is passed through it because of its high electrical resistance. This varies according to the particular tissue, so that fat conducts poorly and heats little, whereas muscle conducts well and heats easily. To coagulate tissue effectively, the flow of current must be restricted to the smallest possible area of tissue — for example, the closed snare loop during polypectomy. This is the principle of current density that is basic to all forms of electrosurgery. It explains why there is no significant generation of heat between the patient plate and the broad areas of skin in contact with that plate. Even a relatively small area of contact between the thigh and the plate is sufficient, and with the low power used in endoscopic diathermy, extra moisture or electrode jelly are not necessary.

Equipment

The electrosurgical generator

The electrosurgical generator produces the diathermy current. There are usually two controls:

1. the selector: cut, coagulation, and blend
2. the intensity: this controls the electrical output

The unit should be switched off until ready to be used. Confirmation of the settings should always be obtained before use.

The active cord

The active cord carries the electrosurgical current from the power unit to the instrument. More than one type of active cord may be needed if all instruments are not made by the same manufacturer. Standardization of equipment in endoscopic electrosurgery is now more the rule than the exception.

The return electrode

The return electrode carries the current out of the patient and back to the power unit. Single-use, disposable adhesive pads are now almost universally used. These general rules of use should be followed:

1. The plate should have a minimum surface area of 25 cm², to avoid burns.
2. The plate should be located as close to the operating area as possible to reduce the length of the return pathway and minimize the risk of alternative pathways developing.
3. The plate should not be placed over joints, as it may become displaced during movement.

4. Hairy, scarred, and wet areas of skin should be avoided, as these diminish conductivity.

There is no known problem with accidental burns when the plate is placed over the site of metal prostheses, such as metal hip replacements and orthopaedic plates.

Foot-pedal control

The foot-pedal control allows the operator to control the electrosurgery with the foot while the hands are deploying the electrosurgical instrument. It should be "shielded" to prevent accidental usage, and it should be waterproof.

The S-cord system

An S-cord system is essential for endoscopic electrosurgery if capacitive coupling between the active electrode and the endoscope itself is to be prevented. Such coupling can cause burns via the metal parts of the endoscopy, and can cause the patient, the endoscopist, or the nurse assisting to receive an electrical shock. The S-cord effectively "earths" the endoscope by transferring any leaked current back to the patient electrode.

Electrosurgical instruments

The main types of electrosurgical instrument used in gastrointestinal endoscopy are:

- polypectomy snares
- "hot" biopsy forceps
- sphincterotomy knives (papillotomes)
- needle knives (needle papillotomes)
- electrosurgical probes

All these instruments require:

- a small area of contact with the patient's tissues, to encourage high current density
- an insulated shaft to prevent current leakage
- an insulated handle and connector, to protect the operator

Dangers of electrosurgery

The main dangers are:

1. Explosion. This danger arises from the explosive combinations of oxygen (from inflated air) and methane (from bacterial fermentation of protein residues) or hydrogen (from bacterial fermentation of carbohydrates). If bowel preparation is poor, carbon dioxide insufflation should be used in place of air to prevent these explosive combinations.
2. Mains current electrocution.
3. Interference with other electromedical devices (e.g. ECG monitoring).
4. Thermoelectric burns — the greatest danger. In Scotland between 1981 and 1991, there were 26 reported cases of accidental patient burning (43). During passage of electrosurgical current, patients must not be in direct contact with any metal part of the trolley that might serve as an alternative path for electrical current return.

HEPATITIS AND HIGH-RISK REGULATIONS

The invasive nature of endoscopic procedures presents a potential risk for occupationally acquired infection in endoscopists and endoscopy assistants. The increasing demand for endoscopic procedures, coupled with the increasing prevalence of viral infection, especially hepatitis C virus, make the risks of acquiring infection even greater.

Two routes of infection are of particular importance: **needle-stick injuries** may cause exposure to blood-borne pathogens, and there is the risk of infection associated with the **endoscopic procedure** itself, including contact with blood in patients with bleeding peptic ulcer disease or varices, and the handling of endoscopic equipment and biopsy specimens.

Parenteral transmission

The three blood-borne pathogens that are most commonly involved are hepatitis B (HBV) and C (HCV) viruses, and HIV. The risk of acquiring infection after needle-stick injury is greatest with HBV (44,45), but the availability of an effective vaccine for HBV substantially reduces the risk. Patients with these infections do present for gastrointestinal endoscopy and the endoscopy staff will not always be aware of their pathology.

HBV infection

More than 33% of the world's population has been infected with HBV (46), and between 5 and 10% of adults and up to 90% of infants infected will become chronic carriers. In Europe, one million people are infected with HBV every year, of whom 90 000 become chronic carriers (46). In this context, it is not surprising that **health-care workers** have prevalence rates of HBV infection three to five times greater than that of the general population (47,48). In the USA it has been calculated that up to 190 health-care workers die annually from HBV causes (49,50).

The **risk of transmission** of HBV to those health workers who are not immune, after needle-stick injury, correlates with the presence or absence of hepatitis B envelope antigen (HBeAg) in the source patient. The presence of HBeAg indicates very high blood titres of HBV and consequently an increased infectivity (40% when HBeAg is present; 2% when HBeAg is absent (45)). The amount of HBV in many body fluids has not been quantified but, reassuringly, the titre in saliva is generally 1000–10 000 times less than the corresponding titre in serum (45). The virus is usually not detectable in faeces. Transmission of the virus from human bites has been reported, but the risk of transmission is low (45).

All **endoscopy staff** should be **immunized** against HBV, but those exposed to HBV who have not been tested for anti-HBs antibody in the previous 2 years should be tested for immunity, as 10–15% will not have protective titres (45). HBV prophylaxis after occupational exposure includes the administration of hyperimmune globulin, whereas susceptible persons are given recombinant HBV vaccine.

HCV infection

The world-wide prevalence of HCV infection is unknown, but is likely to be greater than is currently appreciated. Prevalence among blood donors in north Europe and in the northern parts of the USA and Canada ranges from 0.01 to 0.05% (51); however, HCV antibody testing is performed routinely in donors, but not in patients presenting for gastrointestinal endoscopy.

The parenteral route is the main route of **transmission** and it has been estimated that, after needle-stick injury, the risk is between 3 and 10% (45,50). Transmission via saliva and by human bite has been reported (52), but, as in the case of HBV, faeces are

unlikely to be a source of infection (45). No vaccine for HCV is available, so exposed staff should be tested soon after exposure and at intervals for 6–9 months to detect HCV antibodies or evidence of hepatitis (45).

HIV infection

It is estimated that at least 25 million people have already been infected with HIV and that almost 10 000 new infections occur each day across the world. Inevitably, therefore, some of these people will present for an endoscopy, placing endoscopy staff at increased risk of **occupational infection**. The risk associated with occupational exposure is variable and depends on the titre of the virus in the patient. The mean circulating titre is 100–1000 times greater in patients with AIDS than in asymptomatic HIV-infected patients, so it is likely that the risk of transmission is greater in the former group. Other possible variables include the volume of blood involved, the gauge of the needle and the depth of penetration, but data are not yet available to quantify the effect of these factors on transmission (45). Periodic testing for HIV antibody in exposed endoscopy workers should continue for up to 6–12 months after exposure. Seroconversion is rare beyond this time.

The high prevalence of pulmonary and extrapulmonary **tuberculosis** in HIV-positive patients and the development of multidrug-resistant tuberculosis introduces another potential route of occupation-related infection for endoscopy staff. Data relating specifically to the setting of the endoscopy unit are not available, but the association in other medical departments, between exposure to tuberculosis for periods as short as 2 h, and subsequent positive skin testing or the development of active tuberculosis should serve to heighten the awareness of such a potential problem for endoscopists and assistants alike.

Preventing parenteral transmission

Patients with HBV, HCV, or HIV infections can not always be reliably identified before endoscopy. Universal precautions should thus be recommended. All endoscopy staff should be immunized against HBV and antibody titres checked after immunization. General precautionary measures should also be taken, including the wearing of masks and eye protection, when splashing of blood is likely to occur. Staff with exudative skin disease should not perform or assist with invasive procedures. Cuts and abrasions on both patients and staff should be covered with waterproof dressings (1). Disinfection and sterilization of work surfaces and equipment is also important, especially as HBV remains relatively stable and potentially infective for at least one week after contamination.

Transmission of infection from patient to patient via endoscopic procedures is, thankfully, rare (53). The major reasons identified for transmission of infection are improper cleaning and disinfection procedures, endoscope contamination by automated washer/disinfectors, and the design of some of the endoscopes. The lipid viruses such as HIV and HBV are readily inactivated by high-level disinfection, as long as this is coupled with thorough cleaning before immersion in disinfectant. Vegetative bacteria such as *Pseudomonas* and *Salmonella spp.*, are next most sensitive, and *Mycobacterium tuberculosis* and atypical mycobacteria are the most resistant (53).

Helicobacter pylori infection

Endoscopic transmission of *H. pylori* from patient to patient has been reported (54), but conventional cleaning and disinfection techniques have been shown to be highly effective in eliminating this organism (55,56). A number of studies have investigated whether gastroenterologists are at increased risk of acquiring *H. pylori* infection; the majority of these did associate the performing of endoscopy with an increased likelihood of being infected (57,58), but in one Norwegian hospital no increased risk was reported (59). Endoscopy nurses are also at increased risk of acquiring this infection (58).

Endoscopists and endoscopy nurses maybe at increased risk of acquiring *H. pylori* infection, and patient-to-patient transmission of *H. pylori* has been documented; nevertheless, endoscopy procedures do not contribute greatly to the overall problems associated with *H. pylori*. Until its exact mode of transmission is established, steps to prevent the transmission of *H. pylori* can not be defined.

Conclusion

The risk of occupational infection in endoscopy staff is poorly defined, and has not been extensively investigated. In general, the prevention of transmission of infection between patients and endoscopy staff is based on the execution of adequate cleaning and disinfection of endoscopic equipment. This should be performed for all patients with due care and attention, irrespective of whether they have risk factors for blood-borne infections.

References

1. Cowan RE, Ayliffe GAJ, Babb JR *et al*. Cleaning and disinfection of equipment for gastrointestinal endoscopy. Report of a Working Party of the British Society of Gastroenterology Endoscopy Committee. *Gut* 1998; **42**: 585–593.
   The most recent working party report on behalf of the British Society of Gastroenterology, giving the definitive views of the Society on cleaning and disinfection of endoscopic equipment, including a review of all the available disinfectants and sterilants.

2. Babb JR, Bradley CR. A review of glutaraldehyde alternatives. *Br J Theatre Nurs* 1995; **5**: 22–24.

3. Cowan RE, Manning AP, Ayliffe GAJ *et al*. Aldehyde disinfectants and health in endoscopy units. *Gut* 1993; **34**: 1641–1645.
   A comprehensive review of health problems with aldehyde disinfectants, covering COSHH regulations, methods of dealing with the problem, and health surveillance of endoscopy staff.

4. Taylor EW, Mehtar S, Cowan RE *et al*. Endoscopy: disinfectants and health. *J Hosp Infect* 1994; **28**: 5–14.

5. *Control of Substances Hazardous to Health Regulations 1994*. London: HM Stationery Office, 1994.

6. Department of Health. Glutaraldehyde disinfectants: use and management. *Safety Action Bulletin* 1992; **17**: appendix 4.

7. Baldry MGC. The bactericidal, fungicidal and sporicidal properties of hydrogen peroxide and peracetic acid. *J Appl Bacteriol* 1983; **54**: 417–423.

8. Kline LB, Hull RN. The virucidal properties of peracetic acid. *Am J Clin Pathol* 1960; **33**: 30–33.

9. Wilkinson M, Bramble M, Boys R *et al*. Report of the Working Party of the Endoscopy Committee of the British Society of Gastroenterology on the reuse of endoscopic accessories. *Gut* 1998; **42**: 304–306.
   Useful recommendations on behalf of the British Society of Gastroenterology, listing the re-usable and single-use accessories.

10. Medical Devices Agency. The reuse of medical devices supplied for single use only. *Medical Devices Agency Bulletin* January 1995; MDA DB 9501.

11. Neale G. Reducing risks in gastroenterological practice. *Gut* 1998; **42**: 139–142.

12. NHS Management Executive. Consent to treatment – Summary of Legal Rulings. *EL* 1997; 32.

13. Bell GD, Neale G, Wilkinson M *et al*. Guidelines for informed consent for endoscopic procedures. *BSG Guidelines in Gastroenterology*, January 1999.
    British Society of Gastroenterology guidelines on this difficult subject, complementing the most recently updated Department of Health guidelines (12).

14. Davies N. Medico–legal issues in endoscopy. In: *Quality Control in Endoscopy*. Ed. R McCloy. Berlin, Heidelberg: Springer Verlag, 1991; pp. 93–99.

15. General Medical Council. *Seeking Patients' Consent: the Ethical Considerations*. London: GMC Publications, 1999.

16. Gebbensleben B, Rohde H. Anxiety before gastrointestinal endoscopy — is it a significant problem? *Dtsch Med Wochenschr* 1990; **115**: 1539–1544.

17. Froehlich F, Schwizer W, Thorens J *et al.* Conscious sedation for gastroscopy: patient tolerance and cardiorespiratory parameters. *Gastroenterology* 1995; **108**: 697–704.

18. Quine A, Bell GD, McCloy RF *et al.* A prospective audit of upper gastrointestinal endoscopy in two regions of England: safety, staffing and sedation methods. *Gut* 1995; **36**: 462–467.
    The first large-scale prospective audit undertaken on this subject in the UK on behalf of the British Society of Gastroenterology and both Royal Colleges, producing some surprising results.

19. Greenblatt DJ, Schader RI. Pharmacokinetic understanding of anti-anxiety drug therapy. *South Med J* 1978; **71(suppl 2)**: 2–9.

20. Whitwam JG, Al-Khudhairi D, McCloy RF. Comparision of midazolam and diazepam of comparable potency during gastroscopy. *Br J Anaesth* 1983; **55**: 773–777.

21. Ben-Shlomo I, Abd-El-Khalim H, Ezry J *et al.* Midazolam acts synergistically with fentanyl for induction of anaesthesia. *Br J Anaesth* 1990; **64**: 45–47.

22. Geller E. Report of workshop on drugs for sedation. In: *Quality Control in Endoscopy*. Ed. R McCloy. Berlin, Heidelberg: Springer Verlag, 1991; pp. 22–29.

23. Daneshmend TK, Bell GD, Logan RFA. Sedation for upper gastrointestinal endoscopy: results of a nationwide survey. *Gut* 1991; **32**: 12–15.
    Useful review of sedation practice in the UK for gastroscopy alone, now providing 8–10-year-old data.

24. Hart R, Classen M. Complications of diagnostic gastrointestinal endoscopy. *Endoscopy* 1990; **22**: 229–233.

25. Fleischer D. Monitoring the patient receiving conscious sedation for gastrointestinal endoscopy: issues and guidelines. *Gastrointest Endosc* 1989; **35**: 262–266.

26. Bell GD, Brown NS, Morden A *et al.* Prevention of hypoxaemia during upper gastrointestinal endoscopy by means of oxygen via nasal cannulae. *Lancet* 1987; **i**: 1022–1024.

27. Griffin SM, Chung SCS, Leung JWC *et al.* Effect of intranasal oxygen on hypoxaemia and tachycardia during endoscopic cholangiopancreatography. *BMJ* 1990; **300**: 83–84.

28. Gross JB, Long WB. Nasal oxygen alleviates hypoxaemia in colonscopy patients with midazolam and meperidine. *Gastrointest Endosc* 1990; **36**: 26–29.

29. Bell GD, McCloy RF, Charlton JE *et al.* Recommendations for standards of sedation and patient monitoring during gastrointestinal endoscopy. *Gut* 1991; **32**: 823–827.
    "Gold Standard" working party report on behalf of the British Society of Gastroenterology, making ground-breaking recommendations on safe practice in endoscopy that have since been widely adopted.

30. Bell GD, Quine A, Antrobus JHL *et al.* Upper gastrointestinal endoscopy: a prospective randomised study comparing the efficacy of continuous supplemental oxygen given either via the nasal or oral route. *Gastrointest Endosc* 1992; **38**: 319–325.

31. Logan R, Hastings J. Bacterial endocarditis: a complication of gastroscopy. *BMJ* 1988; **296**: 1107.

32. Watanakurakorn C. Streptococcus bovis endocarditis associated with villous adenoma following colonoscopy. *Am Heart J* 1988; **116**: 1115–1116.

33. Baskin G. Prosthetic endocarditis after endoscopic variceal sclerotherapy: a failure of antibiotic prophylaxis. *Am J Gastroenterol* 1989; **84**: 311–312.

34. Norfleet R. Infectious endocarditis after fiberoptic sigmoidoscopy. *J Clin Gastroenterol* 1991; **13**: 448–451.

35. Bianco JA, Pepe MS, Higano C *et al.* Prevalence of clinically relevant bacteraemia after upper gastrointestinal endoscopy in bone marrow transplant recipients. *Am J Med* 1990; **89**: 134–136.

36. Kullman E, Borsch K, Lindtrom E *et al.* Bacteraemia following diagnostic and therapeutic ERCP. *Gastrointest Endosc* 1992; **38**: 444–449.

37. Sauter G, Grabein B, Huber G *et al.* Antibiotic prophylaxis of infectious complications with endoscopic retrograde cholangiopancreatography: a randomised controlled study. *Endoscopy* 1990; **22**: 164–167.

38. Deviere J, Motte S, Dumonceau JM *et al.* Septicaemia after endoscopic retrograde cholangiopancreatography. *Endoscopy* 1990; **22**: 72–75.
    Detailed review of septicaemia complicating diagnostic and therapeutic ERCP during a 3-year period at the Erasme Hospital in Brussels, a centre of endoscopic excellence.

39. McArdle CS. Oral prophylaxis in biliary tract surgery. *J Antimicrob Chemother* 1994; **33**: 200–202.

40. Motte S, Deviere J, Dumomceau JM *et al.* Risk factors for septicaemia following endoscopic biliary stenting. *Gastroenterology* 1991; **101**: 1374–1381.

41. Alveyn CG, Robertson DAF, Wright R *et al.* Preventation of sepsis following endoscopic retrograde cholangiopancreatography. *J Hosp Infect* 1991; **19(suppl C)**: 65–70.

42. British Society of Gastroenterology. Antibiotic prophylaxis in gastrointestinal endoscopy. *BSG Guidelines in Gastroenterology 2*. September 1996.
    One of a series of guidelines prepared by members of the British Society of Gastroenterology with the assistance of other experts, under the aegis of the Clinical Services and Standards Committee, giving comprehensive advice on antibiotic prophylaxis in a wide range of gastrointestinal endoscopic activities.

43. Wicker CP Electrosurgery. In: *Practical Endoscopy*. Eds. M. Shephard, J Mason. London: Chapman and Hall, 1997; pp. 382–410.

44. Shapiro CN. Prevention of transmission of blood borne pathogens: occupational risk of infection with hepatitis B and hepatitis C virus. *Surg Clin North Am* 1995; **75**: 1047–1056.

45. Gerberding JL. Management of occupational exposures to blood borne pathogens. *N Engl J Med* 1995; **332**: 444–451.

46. Zuckerman AJ. Progress towards the comprehensive control of hepatitis B. *Gut* 1996; **38(suppl 2)**: S1.

47. Denes AE, Smith JL, Maynard JE. Hepatitis B infection in physicians: Results of a nationwide seroepidemiologic survey. *JAMA* 1978; **239**: 210–214.

48. Dienstag JL, Ryan DM. Occupational exposure to hepatitis B virus in hospital personnel: infection or immunization? *Am J Epidemiol* 1982; **115**: 26–27.

49. Sepkowitz KA. Occupationally acquired infections in health care workers. *Ann Intern Med* 1996; **125**: 826–834.

50. Mast EE, Alter MJ. Prevention of hepatitis B virus infection among health-care workers. In: *Hepatitis B Vaccines in Clinical Practice*. Ed. RW Ellis. New York: Marcel Dekker, 1993; pp. 295–307.

51. van der Poel CL, Cuypers HT, Reesink HW. Hepatits C virus 6 years on. *Lancet* 1994; **344**: 1475–1479.

52. Dushieko GM, Smith M, Scheuer PJ. Hepatitis C transmitted by a human bite. *Lancet* 1990; **336**: 503–504.

53. Spach DH, Silverstein FE, Stamm WE. Transmission of infection by gastrointestinal endoscopy and bronchoscopy. *Ann Int Med* 1993; **118**: 117–128.
    Useful article that documents all the published examples, up to that time, of infections apparently transmitted by endoscopy, both gastrointestinal and bronchoscopic.

54. Miyaji H, Kohli Y, Azuma T *et al.* Endoscopic cross-infection with Helicobacter pylori. *Lancet* 1995; **345**: 464.

55. Fantry GT, Zheng QX, James SP. Conventional cleaning and disinfection techniques eliminate the risk of endoscopic transmission of Helicobacter pylori. *Am J Gastroenterol* 1995; **90**: 227–232.

56. Roosendaal R, Kuipers EJ, van den Brule AJC *et al.* Importance of the fiberoptic endoscope cleaning procedure for detection of Helicobacter pylori in gastric biopsy specimens by PCR. *J Clin Microbiol* 1994; **9**: 319–324.

57. Lin SK, Lambert JR, Schembri MA *et al.* Helicobacter pylori prevalence in endoscopy and medical staff. *J Gastroenterol Hepatol* 1994; **9**: 319–324.

58. Goh KL, Parasakthi N, Ong KK. Prevalence of Helicobacter pylori infection in endoscopy and non-endoscopy personnel: results of field survey with serology and ^{14}C-urea breath test. *Am J Gastroenterol* 1996; **91**: 268–270.

59. Berstad K, Hjartholm A-SE, Pederson E *et al.* Helicobacter pylori infection among health employees at the section of gastroenterology, Haukeland Hospital, Norway. *Tidsskr Nor Laegeforen* 1990; **110**: 713–715.

45. Laser Therapy and Photodynamic Therapy

STEPHEN BOWN

For gastroenterologists, lasers are a convenient but sophisticated source of light in the red and infra-red parts of the spectrum. They are easy to control and the light beam can be focused to a small spot. This makes it feasible to transmit most beams via thin, flexible fibres, so treatment can be delivered to any site accessible to such a fibre through a puncture site or in conjunction with a flexible endoscope. The **attractions of laser therapy** may be summarized as:

- precise, localised treatment
- fibreoptic light delivery
- predictable biological response
- suitable for minimally invasive, image guided therapy
- no cumulative toxicity

Early interest centred on the endoscopic control of haemorrhage, particularly from peptic ulcers. Lasers worked well, but simpler and cheaper options later proved to be just as effective. The next major application was for the palliation of advanced cancers of the upper and lower gastrointestinal tract. Lasers still have a role in this indication, although as stent technology improves — particularly for the upper gastrointestinal tract — the percentage of patients in whom a stent is placed at any early stage of their disease is increasing. Nevertheless, fundamentally, lasers and stents remain complementary rather than competitive options. Probably the most important future of lasers in gastroenterology lies in **photodynamic therapy** (PDT), in which laser light is used to activate a previously administered photosensitizing drug. PDT has the potential to ablate the abnormal mucosa in Barrett's oesophagus without damaging the underlying muscle, to destroy small tumours in the wall of the gastrointestinal tract in patients unsuitable for surgery, and even to destroy localized pancreatic cancers by a percutaneous, image-guided procedure, although these techniques are only at the stage of early clinical trials.

INTERACTION OF LASER LIGHT WITH LIVING TISSUE

The most important effects of laser light are thermal and photochemical. The thermal applications are simplest to understand, the effect depending on how much heat is delivered, how fast it is delivered, and the volume of tissue in which it is absorbed. A short laser shot at an appropriate power level can cause **thermal contraction of tissue**, which is of particular value for **haemostasis**. This works either by shrinking the walls of a small vessel, or by closing the lumen of a vessel by contraction of surrounding soft tissue. More energy leads to **tissue necrosis**, the main value of which is in treating **neoplasms**. A lot of heat in a short time (**high laser power**) **vaporizes** the top layer of tissue. Below this, tissue is necrosed and later sloughs, and under this there are inflammatory changes that heal with fibrosis. The depth of each effect can be controlled by the amount of energy delivered. **Low laser powers** delivered via fibres positioned interstitially can be used to **coagulate lesions** in the centre of solid organs such as the liver, without any vaporization.

PDT is the main photochemical application. This involves local or systemic administration of a photosensitizing drug and subsequent activation of the drug by low-power red light, usually from a laser. The **mechanism** is initial photoactivation of the drug, which then converts ground-state triplet oxygen to the active radical, singlet oxygen, which is cytotoxic. Thus PDT requires drug, light, and oxygen; without all three, there is no effect. The real attraction of PDT is the nature of the tissue effect. As there is no increase in tissue temperature during treatment, there is little effect on connective tissue such as collagen, so the mechanical integrity of hollow organs like the gastrointesinal tract is maintained, even if there is local necrosis of all layers of the bowel wall.

Another application used in a small number of centres is to apply **pulsed lasers** endoscopically to break up gallstones in the biliary tree, the pulses of light creating shock waves to break the stone into small fragments that can pass spontaneously or be removed by endoscopic trawling.

These various effects of lasers are summarized in Table 45.1.

All the light transmitted via a fibre is emitted from the distal end of that fibre, and has no effect on the tissues through which the fibre passes. Thus it is possible to produce precise, localized biological effects at sites deep within the body, with little or no trauma to overlying normal tissues. The predictability of both the nature and extent of the biological changes is better than for most other means of producing localized tissue necrosis. Unlike radiotherapy, there is no chronic, cumulative toxicity as the photon energies used are too low to cause ionization, so treatment can be repeated at the same site, if necessary. Thus lasers provide a powerful technique for local coagulation or destruction of diseased tissue; however, the extent of laser effects must be matched to the lesion being treated and one must be sure that all treated areas will heal safely.

HAEMOSTASIS

The first application of lasers in gastroenterology dates back to the 1970s and was for the endoscopic control of **haemorrhage**, particularly from **peptic ulcers**. Early reports were anecdotal and there was considerable controversy over the relative efficacy and safety of the argon ion laser (blue-green beam) and the neodymium yttrium aluminium garnet (**NdYAG**) **laser** (near infra-red beam at 1064 nm). Nevertheless, animal studies showed that, when used appropriately, the NdYAG was both safe and effective. Although other endoscopic techniques such as various forms of electrocoagulation were available at the time, it was largely the novelty of laser technology and the rapid improvements in endoscope technology that stimulated many studies on the potential for endoscopic haemostasis. Perhaps most important was identification of the ulcers most likely to rebleed after an index bleed (those with a bleeding or non-bleeding visible vessel in the ulcer crater). Those in whom the crater was well seen, but which did not have a visible vessel, were at very low-risk of further haemorrhage. Several controlled trials showed that, in the high-risk ulcers, endoscopic treatment with the NdYAG laser significantly reduced the risk of rebleeding and the need for emergency surgery (1). Nevertheless, other simpler and cheaper techniques were developed that worked just as well. Most bleeds from peptic ulcers are now controlled with injection sclerotherapy, often using no more than epinephrine. With subsequent *Helicobacter pylori* eradication and appropriate ulcer-healing medication, this is usually sufficient to produce a good long-term result.

One area in which endoscopic laser therapy still has an important part to play in the treatment of blood loss from benign lesions is with **vascular ectasias** such as telangiectasiae, angiodysplasia, and "water-melon stomach" (gastric antral vascular ectasia or GAVE) (2). With the tip of the laser fibre held

Table 45.1.   Laser effects used in gastroenterology.

High power thermal:	Haemostasis
	Debulking of neoplastic tissue by vaporization and coagulation
Low power thermal (ILP):	Gentle coagulation of lesions within solid organs
Photochemical (PDT):	Non-thermal destruction of tissue by activation of a previously administered photosensitizing drug
Pulsed shock-wave	Fragmentation of gallstones

ILP, interstitial laser photocoagulation; PDT, photodynamic therapy above the target lesion without direct contact, it is easy to define and target the area to be treated and coagulate it rapidly under direct vision. The laser shots may induce some oozing from these lesions, just as may happen with all the other endoscopic modalities — such as sclerotherapy — that are used for these lesions, but this often provides some reassurance that the treated site was indeed a relevant site of blood loss. Laser treatment coagulates the fragile microvessels in these lesions. This leads to superficial erosions that heal with a little local scarring. Whichever modality is used, for larger lesions (more than 5–10 mm in diameter), particularly watermelon stomachs, it is wiser to administer the treatment in several sessions, to minimize the risk of perforation. About 1 month between treatments is adequate time for healing before another adjacent area is treated. This is clinically acceptable, as the blood loss from most of these lesions is chronic rather than acute.

PALLIATION OF ADVANCED CANCERS

Upper gastrointestinal tract cancers

The main role of high-power, thermal lasers such as the NdYAG in current practice is for **palliation of advanced, inoperable cancers** of the upper and lower gastrointestinal tract. Most patients with carcinomas of the oesophagus and gastric cardia have no prospect of cure at the time of presentation, because of the extent of their disease. The dominant symptom is usually dysphagia and the therapeutic challenge is to relieve the dysphagia with the minimum upset to the patient. For those unsuitable for surgery or radical radiotherapy, one is left with the endoscopic options, the most important of which are stent insertion and laser therapy. Further, a patient who can swallow reasonably and is well nourished will tolerate radiotherapy and chemotherapy much better, so the techniques are complementary.

Endoscopic NdYAG laser recanalization of advanced oesophageal cancers was first reported in 1982 (3). The aim of the procedure is to reduce the intraluminal tumour bulk, concentrating on those parts causing the worst obstruction. Prominent nodules can be vaporized. Smaller nodules can be coagulated, and the dead tissue then sloughs over a few days. The deep penetration of the NdYAG laser beam ensures haemostasis in the underlying tissues. Care must be taken to allow for the tissue that will slough in the days after treatment as, if this is not done, there is a risk of delayed perforation; however, for exophytic tumour and an endoscopist with reasonable experience, the **risks are few**. The **incidence of complications is low**, although it often takes several treatments at intervals of a few days to achieve optimum recanalization, as dead tissue must be allowed to slough to see what is underneath. The NdYAG laser beam (up to 70 W) is dangerous if viewed directly, so safety filters must be fitted to fibreoptic endoscopes. There is no risk to operators with videoscopes, as long as the laser is fired only when the fibre is in the endoscope and the endoscope is in the patient. Filters may be required to protect the chips on the camera, although the risk of damage from laser light reflected back up the endoscope is small. Care must be taken to ensure that the laser is not fired with the fibre tip still in the biopsy channel, as this will cause serious damage to the endoscope.

An international inquiry soon after the introduction of this technique in the mid 1980s reported results in 1184 patients in 20 centres (4). After a mean of three laser treatments, 83% of patients could swallow at least some solids. Major complications (perforation and fistulation) were seen in 4.1%, with a 1% treatment-related mortality. The main problem is the need to repeat laser treatment every 4–6 weeks to maintain good palliation, which has led to studies of **adjuvant radiotherapy** to slow down local tumour regrowth. Options include palliative external-beam irradiation and brachytherapy (intraluminal radiotherapy). The simplest, and probably the most effective option, is **brachytherapy**, which can increase the duration of palliation of dysphagia from an average of 5 weeks using laser alone to 19 weeks in those also receiving a single dose of 10 Gy brachytherapy, although it does not change the median survival (32 weeks) (5).

For some years, tumour dilatation and endoscopic insertion of a **silicone-rubber stent** was standard practice in Europe, and enabled most patients to swallow at least semi-solids, but there was about a 10% risk of perforation. These stents were never popular in North America. Over the past few years, several types of **expanding metal stent** have become available. Their insertion is simpler and requires less dilatation (hence less risk of perforation). Many such stents are now placed as an outpatient procedure, and this has become by far the most

Table 45.2.   Laser compared with Stent for palliation of malignant dysphagia.

	Laser	Conventional stent	Expanding metal stent
Endoscopic Technique	Basically safe (risk of perforation if dilatation also needed)	10% risk of perforation	Usually simple and safe
Contraindications	Fistula No endoscopic target	High lesion Tracheal compression Care with angulated lesions	High lesion Tracheal compression
Dysphagia after therapy	Variable, can be close to normal	Semi-solids, some solids	Variable, can be close to normal
Enhancement of dysphagia relief with radiotherapy	Yes	No	No
Follow-up	Therapy can be repeated	Stent can be adjusted	Stents difficult to adjust
Cost	High to set up, low per patient	Low per patient	High per patient

popular technique for palliating advanced malignant dysphagia, although the cost is high (6). The enthusiasm for these has been slightly tempered, as it has become clear that they can have as many long-term problems as the old type of stent and, once in, they are difficult to adjust. Nevertheless, new designs are appearing at regular intervals and these avoid at least some of the problems encountered with the earlier designs.

Lasers are compared with conventional and expanding metal stents in Table 45.2. Common sense dictates that stents and lasers are complementary rather than competitive. An eccentric, exophytic tumour is best debulked with the laser, whereas a circumferential tumour with little exophytic component is best stented. A fistula must be stented, whereas high cervical tumours can seldom be stented. The few available data on comparative costs suggest that the lifetime treatment costs are similar for each of these approaches.

Haemorrhage or obstruction caused by advanced cancers of the distal stomach and duodenum can be treated with endoscopic laser therapy, but the results are often less satisfactory than with lesions of the oesophagus and gastric cardia. Malignant gastric outlet obstruction can now sometimes be relieved by expanding metal stents designed for enteral use.

Lower gastrointestinal tract cancers

Most colorectal cancers are best treated surgically, but 5–10% are unsuitable for resection because of the general condition of the patient or the extent of local or metastatic disease. A defunctioning colostomy palliates obstruction, but does not relieve bleeding or mucus discharge from advanced rectal cancers. A range of non-surgical options has been explored to relieve symptoms from tumour bulk in the rectum, including radiotherapy, cryotherapy, electrocoagulation, and laser sigmoidoscopy. Laser therapy has the advantages of being applied under direct vision (so can be applied safely above the peritoneal reflection), can be carried out as a day-case procedure with little or no sedation, and can be repeated as necessary. Initial **palliation** of obstruction, tenesmus, bleeding, mucus discharge, and diarrhoea can be achieved in up to 90% of patients and maintained for the remainder of the patient's life in up to 80% of those treated this way (7). The effect can be prolonged by the addition of palliative, external-beam radiotherapy, although laser treatment can not help pelvic pain or obstruction caused by extraluminal tumour. Expanding metal stents are now available to relieve some distal colonic strictures, but they are unlikely to have an important role in palliating low rectal cancers.

Some patients with small cancers that have not metastasized and who are unfit for surgery because of their general condition, can justifiably be treated just with laser endoscopy, but PDT, as discussed below, is more appropriate than thermal laser treatment.

INTERSTITIAL LASER PHOTOCOAGULATION

Endoscopic applications of the NdYAG laser use high powers, typically 50–80 W, with short shots of 1 or 2 s. The laser fibre is held a few millimetres above the surface of the target, to vaporize and coagulate tumour tissue under direct vision. An alternative approach is to use a much lower power (3–5 W) to **"cook" the diseased tissue gently**, over a period of several minutes, with the tip of the laser fibre inserted directly into the target area. This is known as **interstitial laser photocoagulation** (ILP). This causes gentle thermal coagulation without vaporization, centred around each fibre tip, with no more damage to the overlying normal tissues than the minimal trauma of inserting the needles. The technique was first described in 1983. Subsequently, a series of *in vivo* experiments showed that it was possible to produce an area of necrosis about 1.5 cm in diameter around each fibre site in normal liver, and that these lesions healed safely, mainly by regeneration of normal liver. This led to the first clinical report of the percutaneous treatment of small hepatic secondary tumours, in 1989 (8). There is no selectivity of effect. Normal or malignant tissue will be necrosed if it is heated to a great enough temperature for a sufficient period of time.

The relevance of ILP in gastroenterology is for the **percutaneous treatment of small hepatic metastases** (particularly from previously resected, primary colorectal cancers) in patients who are unsuitable or unfit for partial hepatectomy. The key to using this technique succesfully is the imaging, to position fibres correctly and to assess the results, both at the time of treatment and during follow-up. It must be possible to define the limits of the target lesion and to match the treatment to these limits, to maximize the prospects of destroying the entire lesion and minimize the risk of unacceptable damage to adjacent normal tissues. Fibres can be inserted through needles positioned percutaneously under ultrasound, computed tomography (CT) or magnetic resonance imaging. Although changes can be seen in real-time, ultrasound is poor at documenting the extent of the tissue response. The simplest way to assess the effect is on contrast-enhanced CT scans taken 24 h after treatment, which show laser-necrosed areas as new zones of non-enhancement. A series using magnetic resonance guidance reported 1048 laser applications in 383 hepatic metastases (mostly from previously resected colorectal primary tumours) in 134 patients. There were no major complications, and the mean survival time was 35 months (9).

It may prove possible to obtain real-time images of the laser-induced thermal changes by undertaking treatments in an interventional magnetic resonance scanner, but this approach is still in the experimental stage. The size of the zone of necrosis depends on the number of laser fibres used, but it is possible to necrose lesions up to about 4–5 cm in diameter. Treated areas heal mainly with regeneration of normal liver. ILP is appropriate only for hepatic metastases in patients with a small number of clearly identifiable lesions and no evidence of extrahepatic disease; for these individuals, it may slow down the progression of their disease, and is likely to be complementary to chemotherapy.

An increasing number of therapeutic options are being considered for the **localized destruction of diseased tissue within solid organs**. In addition to ILP, these include injection of alcohol or chemotherapeutic agents, heating by microwaves, radiofrequency waves or high-intensity focused ultrasound, cryotherapy, brachytherapy, or PDT. ILP and PDT have the advantage that the fibres are thin and can be inserted percutaneously through needles, and so can be positioned relatively easily within firm tissue, such as in secondary tumours. Furthermore, the area of necrosis produced is well defined, roughly ellipsoidal, and does not depend on the physical properties of the tissue to the same extent as is the case with the other techniques. Radiofrequency heating may give comparable results, but the necrosis produced is more dependent on the electrical properties of the target tissue. It is difficult to inject alcohol into hard tissue, although this is a much cheaper option and works reasonably well for softer lesions such as primary hepatomas. Focused ultrasound is completely non-invasive, but is more difficult to use on deeper lesions.

ILP is a technique still in the evolutionary stage, and there are few reported large studies with long-term follow-up, but it does appear safe, effective, and relatively simple.

PHOTODYNAMIC THERAPY

PDT is a method of producing **localized tissue necrosis** by means of light, after prior administration of a photosensitizing agent (10). It attracted considerable interest initially, as many photosensitizing agents are retained slightly more in cancers than in the adjacent normal tissue in which the tumour arose, which raised the possibility of truly selective destruction of cancers. Regrettably, the selectivity of uptake of photosensitizers is rarely sufficient to produce selective necrosis when both tumour and normal tissue are exposed to the same light dose although, under appropriate circumstances, it is possible to produce selectivity of necrosis between different layers of normal tissue.

The real attraction of PDT is the nature of the **biological effects** produced. In contrast to the laser applications discussed above, no heat is involved, and there is only an effect in **oxygenated tissue**. Red light activates the photosensitizer, which then interacts with molecular oxygen to produce singlet oxygen, which is the cytotoxic agent. Different photosensitizers locate at different sites within cells, but the main targets are probably mitochondria and cell membranes. There is also considerable variation as to which cells retain photosensitizer; many photosensitizers localize predominantly in the microvasculature, whereas others go to normal and neoplastic glandular cells. These differences can be exploited to match the biological effect to the disease being treated.

One of the most striking aspects of PDT-induced necrosis is that **connective tissues** like collagen and elastin are **largely unaffected** (11). Thus the mechanical integrity of hollow organs such as the gastrointestinal tract can be maintained, even in the presence of full-thickness necrosis, as long as the tissue contains enough connective tissue. Also, many PDT necrosed tissues heal with more regeneration and less scarring than after other local insults such as heat. Although it is difficult to obtain selective necrosis of tumours compared with the adjacent normal tissue in which the tumour arose, it is possible to obtain selectivity between different normal

tissues, and sometimes between different layers of the same tissue (12). PDT is compared with ILP in Table 45.3.

Like all laser treatments, **PDT is a local treatment**. Even if the photosensitizer is given systemically, there will be a biological effect only in areas that contain sufficient photosensitizer *and* receive an adequate dose of light; neither photosensitizer alone nor light alone will produce any effect. Thus, for there to be any prospect of local control, it must be possible to define the limits of a lesion being treated and deliver an adequate dose of light to all relevant areas. It must also be remembered that ambient light may activate drug in the skin, and care must be taken to avoid this sunburn-like reaction. Using the photosensitizer, porfimer sodium (Photofrin), skin sensitivity to bright sunlight can last for up to 3 months. For meso-tetrahydroxyphenyl chlorin (mTHPC, Foscan), the period is 2–3 weeks and for 5-amino laevulinic acid (ALA, Levulan) it is only 1–2 days. These are the three photosensitizers that have been studied most extensively in the context of the gastrointestinal tract to date.

Tumours of the gastrointestinal tract

Most small, localized cancers of the gastrointestinal tract are best treated with surgery. However, for **unfit patients**, the relatively gentle nature of PDT is an attractive, non-surgical alternative, although no endoscopic option can treat tumour that has spread beyond the wall of the gastrointestinal tract — for example, to local lymph nodes. The preser-

Table 45.3. Comparison of ILP and PDT.

	ILP	PDT
Biological effect	Thermal	Photochemical
Effect on connective tissue	Destroyed	Largely unaffected
Healing	Resorption & scarring, some regeneration	Regeneration, sometimes with scarring
Selectivity of necrosis between tumour and tissue of origin of tumour	None	Minimal
Selectivity of necrosis between tissue of origin of tumour and other adjacent tissues	None	Possible between mucosa and underlying muscle in hollow organs
Cumulative toxicity	None	None
Wavelength of light used	Infra-red (805–1064 nm)	Red (630–675 nm)
Typical laser power per fibre	3–5 W	0.1–0.3 W (higher for illuminating hollow organs)

vation of collagen means that it is safe to produce full-thickness PDT necrosis with little risk of perforation, even if the cancer involves the muscle layer, as histological studies have shown that most early cancers in these organs have as much, if not more, collagen in them as the normal tissue. In a series of 123 patients with early oesophageal cancers treated with PDT using porfimer sodium, the complete response rate at 6 months (no disease detectable on endoscopy and biopsy) was 87%. Although the overall 5-year survival was only 25%, the disease-specific 5-year survival was 74%, so effectively, half the patients died of the underlying cardiorespiratory problems that made them unfit for surgery, without major problems from their cancer (13). Care must be taken not to treat too extensive a lesion, as circumferential scarring in the muscle layer can cause a stricture. Strictures occurred in 35% of the patients in this series, although they did respond to dilatation.

PDT has been proposed as an option for **palliating** advanced cancers of the aerodigestive tract, particularly **obstructing oesophageal cancers**. It is questionable whether PDT can offer more than is achieved with endoscopic thermal laser recanalization or stent insertion, and it has the major disadvantage of making these patients sensitive to bright lights for much of their remaining life (14); nevertheless, using porfimer sodium, this was the first application of PDT to be licensed by the Food and Drug Administration in the USA. It is understandable that the first approval should be for patients with advanced, incurable disease, but a clinically useful role for PDT is far more likely to be established in the treatment of early disease. It seems more logical to licence PDT for treating early oesophageal cancers, as has been done by the Japanese authorities, although the UK is following the American pattern, at least initially. PDT may be of value to treat tumour that has grown over or through an oesophageal stent that can not be adjusted and which can not tolerate the heat from a NdYAG laser.

Pre-malignant lesions of the gastrointesinal tract

The pre-malignant lesion that poses the greatest therapeutic challenge to gastroenterologists is **Barrett's oesophagus**, with or without dysplasia. Endoscopic management of this condition is a difficult problem, but is attracting increasing research

attention. Thermal ablation of the abnormal mucosa with an argon plasma coagulator or KTP (potassium titanyl phosphate) laser involves moving a small therapeutic beam across the area to be treated under direct endoscopic vision. It is easy to under-treat, and leave abnormal mucosa, or overtreat, with the risk of muscle scarring or even perforation, although the technique is very straightforward and, using the argon plasma coagulator, is also inexpensive.

PDT has considerable potential in the management of Barrett's oesophagus, although the best way of applying it has not yet been established. Endoscopically, it is difficult to identify areas of dysplasia or carcinoma *in situ*, so the challenge is to destroy all the Barrett's mucosa without damaging the underlying muscle. As no heat is involved, it is possible to use a balloon light-delivery system to illuminate all the relevant mucosa much more evenly than can be achieved with the thermal techniques, and there is very little risk of perforation because of sparing of collagen. When **porfimer sodium** is used as the photosensitizer, this works well to ablate the mucosa, but unfortunately there is an up to 50% risk of producing an oesophageal stricture (15), as there is no selectivity of effect between the mucosa and underlying layers, and PDT-necrosed muscle heals with scarring and fibrosis. These strictures are difficult to manage, and often require several dilatations over a period of many months.

If **ALA** is used as the photosensitizing agent, the situation is quite different. ALA is a naturally occurring substance that, *in vivo*, is converted, through a series of intermediates to protoporphyrin IX (PPIX) and haem. PPIX is a photosensitizer and, after exogenous administration of ALA, sufficient PPIX accumulates to produce a PDT effect in response to activation with red light. However, in contrast to porfimer sodium (which goes to all layers), PPIX accumulates primarily in the mucosa of the gastrointestinal tract. This makes it possible to destroy mucosa (normal or abnormal) without damaging the underlying muscle layer, which is exactly what is required in the treatment of Barrett's oesophagus (12). ALA can be given by mouth, produces clinically useful concentrations of PPIX in target tissues in 3–6 h, and is cleared from the body in 24–48 h.

In a recent report of ALA PDT, high-grade dysplasia was cleared in 10 of 10 and carcinoma *in situ* was cleared in 17 of 22 patients with Barrett's oesophagus (16). There were no oesophageal strictures, but there were other problems because, with ALA, the depth of necrosis never exceeded 2 mm and this was not always sufficient to cover the full thickness of the mucosa. It is reassuring that the necrosed, neoplastic Barrett's mucosa healed with regeneration of normal squamous mucosa, but follow-up biopsy examinations showed that, in some cases, there remained untreated columnar mucosa under the new squamous mucosa. The clinical significance of such residual columnar mucosa is not clear, but it could retain the potential for malignant change.

PDT with ALA is the only technique at present that seems able to offer a **selective effect**, destroying mucosa but not the underlying muscle; however, more research is required, to find reliable ways of ensuring that the full thickness of the abnormal mucosa is ablated. Various options are being explored, such as fractionating the light dose and adding an iron chelator to increase the tissue concentrations of PPIX. Another possibility is to use a different photosensitizer, such as mTHPC, which localizes in the mucosa and submucosa, but not in the muscle; however, it not yet known whether this can be exploited to give selective mucosal necrosis.

In the current state of knowledge, surgery remains the treatment of choice for patients with high-grade dysplasia or early carcinoma in Barrett's oesophagus. **PDT should be reserved for those who are unfit for surgery**. Endoscopic treatment of Barrett's oesophagus without evidence of dysplasia should be limited to the context of clinical trials. However, if PDT can be developed satisfactorily, particularly using a photosensitizing agent such as ALA, which clears from the body so rapidly, it could become the treatment of choice for many cases of Barrett's oesophagus, with or without dysplasia.

It is possible that a role might develop for ALA PDT in the management of other pre-malignant conditions in the gastrointestinal tract such as chronic ulcerative colitis, but no data on such indications are available.

Tumours of the pancreas and bile duct

Although most work to date on PDT in gastroenterology has concentrated on lesions of the luminal gut, interest has also moved to its potential for treating **localized tumours of the pancreas and bile ducts**. Animal studies have shown that the pancreas and adjacent normal tissues can tolerate PDT, and that necrosis can be produced safely in cancers transplanted into the hamster pancreas. These results justified a **pilot clinical study**. Twelve patients with small, **localized pancreatic cancers**, not involving major blood vessels, were sensitized intravenously with mTHPC. Three days later, up to four needles were inserted into the tumour percutaneously under CT guidance and laser fibres were passed through the needles to activate the drug in the tumour. Most patients had pain for a few days after treatment, but none had clinical or biochemical pancreatitis and most were discharged from hospital within 1 week. A mesenteric haematoma related to needle insertion was found in two patients (one requiring transfusion). Evidence of duodenal wall necrosis was seen endoscopically in five patients, but was asymptomatic in all but one, who developed late duodenal stenosis, successfully treated with an enteral metal stent. Contrast-enhanced CT scans a few days after PDT showed new areas of devascularization in the pancreas consistent with PDT-induced necrosis. The first patient lived for 16 months after PDT and two more were alive more than 1 year after treatment (17). These preliminary results are encouraging, but it is far too early to judge what role may develop for PDT in the management of this unpleasant cancer.

PDT may also have a role in the treatment of **bile-duct cancers**, particularly for relief of obstructive jaundice when biliary stents are ineffective or become occluded (18).

Future applications of PDT

A logical application of PDT is as an adjunct to surgery, to destroy small tumour deposits that are not visible to the naked eye or that involve areas that can not be resected. One randomized trial has been reported in which PDT was examined as an adjunct to resection of rectal cancers, but there was no difference between the groups receiving and not receiving adjunctive PDT with respect to the incidence of local recurrence of tumour (19).

A more speculative application of PDT is for the treatment of *H. pylori*. With the increasing incidence of antibiotic resistance, it would be attractive to have an alternative treatment. All sites colonized by *H. pylori* are easily accessible endoscopically for purposes of light delivery. The organism is certainly sensitive to PDT in culture using methylene blue as the photosensitizer, and preliminary *ex vivo* experiments have also given encouraging results (20); however, it would take considerable technical ingenuity to get adequate drug and light to all relevant sites to make this worth attempting clinically.

The **potential targets for PDT in gastroenterology** can be summarized as:

- endoscopically accessible, small, inoperable tumours
- Barrett's oesophagus
- localised pancreatic cancer
- bile-duct cancer
- as an adjunct to surgery
- palliation of advanced cancers — controversial
- eradication of *H. pylori* — speculative

CONCLUSIONS

The NdYAG laser has a useful and established role to play in the endoscopic palliation of advanced gastrointestinal tract cancers, and is complementary to stent insertion. ILP may help in the management of patients with a small number of isolated hepatic metastases. However, the most important new applications of lasers being developed in gastroenterology are in PDT, particularly for the endoscopic treatment of dysplasia in Barrett's oesophagus and for the treatment of small inoperable tumours in the gastrointestinal tract and in the pancreas. The latter techniques are only at an early stage of clinical trials, but if these studies are successful, PDT could have an important role in gastroenterology practice.

References

1. Swain CP, Kirkham JS, Salmon PR *et al*. Controlled trial of NdYAG laser photocoagulation in bleeding peptic ulcers. *Lancet* 1986; **i**: 1113–1117.
2. Sargeant IR, Loizou LA, Rampton D *et al*. Laser ablation of upper gastrointestinal vascular ectasias: long term results. *Gut* 1993; **34**: 470–479.
3. Fleisher D, Kessler F, Haye O. Endoscopic Nd:YAG laser therapy for carcinoma of the esophagus: a new palliative approach. *Am J Surg* 1982; **143**: 280–283.
4. Ell C, Riemann JF, Lux G *et al*. Palliative laser treament of malignant stenoses in the upper gastrointestinal tract. *Endoscopy* 1986; **18(suppl 1)**: 21–26.
5. Spencer GM, Thorpe S, Sargeant IR *et al*. Laser and brachytherapy in the palliation of adenocarcinoma of the oesophagus and cardia. *Gut* 1996; **39**: 726–731.
6. Gevers AM, Macken E, Hiele M *et al*. A comparison of laser therapy, plastic stents and expandable metal stents for palliation of malignant dysphagia in patients without a fistula. *Gastrointest Endosc* 1998; **48**: 383–388.
7. Brunetaud JM, Manoury V, Ducrotte P *et al*. Palliative treatment of rectosigmoid carcinomas by laser endoscopic photoablation. *Gastroenterology* 1987; **92**: 663–668.
8. Steger AC, Lees WR, Walmesely K *et al*. Interstitial laser hyperthermia: a new approach to local destruction of tumours. *BMJ* 1989; **299**: 362–365.
9. Vogl TJ, Mack MG, Straub R *et al*. Magnetic resonance imaging guided abdominal interventional radiology: laser induced thermotherapy of liver metastases. *Endoscopy* 1997; **29**: 577–583.
10. Dougherty TJ, Gomer CJ, Henderson BW *et al*. Photodynamic therapy. *J Natl Cancer Inst* 1998; **90**: 889–905.
11. Barr H, Tralau CJ, Boulos PB *et al*. The contrasting mechanisms of colonic damage between photodynamic therapy and thermal injury. *Photochem Photobiol* 1987; **46**: 795–800.
12. Loh CS, MacRobert AJ, Buonaccorsi G *et al*. Mucosal ablation using photodynamic therapy for the treatment of dysplasia – an experimental study in the normal rat stomach. *Gut* 1996; **38**: 71–78.
13. Sibille A, Lambert R, Souquet JC *et al*. Long-term survival after photodynamic therapy for esophageal cancer. *Gastroenterology* 1995; **108**: 337–344.
14. Bown SG, Millson CE. Photodynamic therapy in gastroenterology. *Gut* 1997; **41**: 5–7.
15. Overholt BF, Panjehpour M. Photodynamic therapy for Barrett's oesophagus. *Gastrointest Endos Clin N Am* 1997; **7**: 202–220.
16. Gossner L, Stolte M, Sroka R *et al*. Photodynamic ablation of high grade dysplasia in Barrett's esophagus by means of 5-amino levulinic acid. *Gastroenterology* 1998; **114**: 448–455.
17. Rogowska AZ, Whitelaw DE, Lees WR *et al*. Photodynamic therapy for palliation of unresectable pancreatic cancer [abstract]. *Gastroenerology* 1999; **116**: G5026.
18. Ortner MA, Liebetruth J, Schreiber S *et al*. Photodynamic therapy of nonresectable cholangiocarcinoma. *Gastroenterology* 1998; **114**: 536–542.
19. Ansell JK, Abulafi AM, Allardice JT *et al*. Adjuvant intraoperative photodynamic therapy for colorectal cancer (abstract). *Br J Surg* 1996; **83**: 694.
20. Millson C, Wilson M, MacRobert AJ *et al*. Ex vivo treatment of gastric helicobacter infection by photodynamic therapy. *J Photochem Photobiol B* 1996; **32**: 59–65.

46. Endoscopic Retrograde Cholangiopancreatography

ADRIAN HATFIELD

INDICATIONS

With the improvement in ultrasound scanning, computed tomography (CT), magnetic resonance (MR) scanning and, in particular, MR cholangiography and pancreatography, there has been a decreasing need for endoscopic retrograde cholangiopancreatography (ERCP) as a diagnostic modality. However, there will remain a certain number of patients who, after scanning, need further assessment to achieve a diagnosis in both biliary and pancreatic disease. To some extent, the choice of investigations may depend on the local availability of equipment and expertise; the range of therapeutic options is considerable. In the biliary tree, stones can be removed after endoscopic sphincterotomy or, if they are large, crushed or shattered with various forms of lithotripsy. Benign strictures can be dilated or repeatedly stented with plastic endoprostheses (stents). Malignant strictures can be stented with either a plastic or self-expanding metal stent. In pancreatitis, there remains a considerable, but lessening, role in diagnostic pancreatography and there is also a wide range of therapeutic procedures that are applicable to some patients. Pancreatic duct stenoses can be dilated or stented, stones removed, duct leaks stented, and pancreatic pseudocysts drained into the stomach or duodenum internally. **Indications for ERCP** (adapted from (1)) include:

- Suspected biliary-duct disorder
  - jaundice or obstructive cholestasis
  - acute cholangitis
  - gallstone pancreatitis
  - clarification of biliary lesions seen on other imaging
  - biliary fistula
- Suspected pancreatic duct disorder
  - pancreatic cancer
  - mucinous or cystic neoplasm
  - unexplained recurrent pancreatitis
  - clarification of pancreatic lesion seen on other imaging
  - ascites or pleural effusion of suspected pancreatic origin
  - pancreatic pseudocyst
- To direct endoscopic therapy
  - sphincterotomy
  - biliary drainage
  - pancreatic drainage
- To direct endoscopic tissue/fluid sampling
  - biopsy, brush; fine needle aspiration
  - bile/pancreatic juice collection
- Preoperative ductal mapping
  - malignant tumours
  - benign strictures
  - chronic pancreatitis
  - pancreatic pseudocysts
  - mucinous or cystic tumours
- To perform manometry
  - sphincter of Oddi
  - ductal

CONTRAINDICATIONS

There are very few contraindications to performing ERCP as long as it is justified for diagnostic or therapeutic reasons. In therapeutic ERCP, the seriousness of the clinical situation — such as biliary sepsis or pancreatitis — is not a contraindication if the patient is going to undergo a therapeutic procedure to try and improve that condition. There is one particular area in which views have changed in recent years, and that is in the timing of ERCP and sphincterotomy in severe pancreatitis. It is no longer believed to be of great value to perform early ERCP and sphincterotomy, which can be delayed until a time when the patient's condition is stable and an expert team is available. Perhaps the most absolute contraindication to ERCP is in a patient in whom pancreatic or biliary therapy is required and the endoscopist only has the skills to perform a diagnostic manoeuvre. In such a situation, it is better to defer that diagnostic procedure and refer the patient to a centre with appropriate full therapeutic skills.

ENDOSCOPIC TECHNIQUES AVAILABLE

Biliary tract

Endoscopic sphincterotomy is now a standard procedure. It enables division of the sphincter of Oddi and safe removal of bile-duct stones. The sphincterotomy is not a long-term drainage procedure, and should be only as large as is required for removal of the stone. Where access to the biliary tree is difficult or impossible, a small pre-cut can be made in the sphincter with a needle knife and this can then allow a full sphincterotomy to be performed subsequently, whether immediately or at a later date. In the majority of situations, stones can be safely removed through a standard endoscopic sphincterotomy but, with large bile-duct stones, initial extraction may fail and other **more complicated manoeuvres** such as mechanical lithotripsy or extracorporeal shock wave lithotripsy (ESWL) — or even more complex techniques such as mother-and-baby scope intraduct lithotripsy, or percutaneous choledochoscopy and direct contact lithotripsy using either an electrohydraulic lithotripter or a pulsed-dye laser — would be needed. If several attempts at removing gallstones are necessary, pigtail stents must be inserted beside the stones, in order to drain the upper biliary tree to prevent infection.

In the case of **post-laparoscopic cholecystectomy leaks**, if there is a simple leak from the cystic duct, with or without a stone, a sphincterotomy with a stent placed in the common hepatic duct will always seal these leaks satisfactorily within a short period of time. More complex damage to the bile duct itself may need more prolonged stenting and subsequent balloon dilatation of stricturing, if this persists once the stent is removed. If the damage to the bile duct is caused by ischaemia, ascending stricturing may occur; in these circumstances, long-term stenting may not be appropriate in younger patients, in whom reconstructive surgery will ultimately be necessary.

In most cases of benign stricturing, the clinical situation will dictate management. If the patient is elderly or presents a high surgical risk, long-term endoscopic stenting with a change of stent every 6–9 months will usually keep the patient well and free from symptoms. The same rationale would apply in patients with sclerosing cholangitis with dominant extrahepatic stricturing. In a younger patient with a postoperative bile-duct stricture, failure of the stricture to resolve satisfactorily after 1 year will usually indicate the need for a surgical bypass procedure. Long-term stenting itself can lead to an increase in fibrosis and in the length of the bile-duct stricture, making further surgery more difficult if this fibrosing process extends to involve both right and left intrahepatic ducts at the hilum.

Pancreatic disease

In patients with **malignant obstructive jaundice secondary to pancreatic cancer**, the standard endoscopic method of **palliation** is to perform a small sphincterotomy and position a polyethylene prosthesis over a guide-wire and catheter system passed through the bile-duct stricture. Most centres now place 10-French gauge plastic stents, as there is no evidence larger sizes confer any advantage in the short-term, whereas they are more difficult to insert. Far superior palliation can be obtained by placing a self-expanding metal stent into the biliary tree. Such a stent would afford the patient palliation for almost 1 year, whereas plastic stents tend to block after 4–5 months. The cost of self-expanding metal stents, at present between £400 and £500, is vastly greater than that of a standard plastic stent (£10–15). If one were to be able to predict those patients who would survive for longer than 6 months, the use of self-expanding metal stents in such patients would be ideal. Overall, about 67% of patients with malignant obstructive jaundice that is attributable to pancreatic cancer receive successful palliation by means of a simple plastic stent and will die, non-jaundiced, of their original disease. Only the remaining 33% of patients return with jaundice or cholangitis as a result of stent blockage during their life span and will need a change of stent.

The use of ERCP to perform **therapeutic manoeuvres on the pancreas** in patients with chronic pancreatitis — and, to a lesser extent, on the complications of acute pancreatitis — has evolved over the past 10 years. After acute pancreatitis, **peripancreatic fluid collections** or **pseudocysts** can be managed endoscopically if they persist. Pseudocysts can now be drained into the lumen of the stomach or duodenum after a puncture into the cyst cavity and positioning of one or two pigtail stents. Sometimes, a small cut can be made through the stomach or duodenum into the cyst to improve drainage. Other **pancreatic-duct leaks** can be managed by endoscopic stenting, either proximal to the leak or with the stent passed across the site of leakage into the distal pancreatic duct. Pancreatic stents are small, and occlude within a few months; for temporary treatment, a nasopancreatic drain positioned in the pancreatic duct across the site of duct rupture can be an alternative solution. **Pancreatic calculi** obstructing the proximal duct adjacent to the papilla can be removed in some patients after a selective pancreatic sphincterotomy, although in many patients, the presence of a fibrotic stricture between the papilla and pancreatic duct precludes this therapy. In other patients in whom the stones are too large to remove directly, ESWL can be used to fragment the pancreatic calculi, which can then pass spontaneously, or be extracted at a later stage, through a pancreatic sphincterotomy. **Pancreatic-duct stricturing** is common in chronic pancreatitis, and may represent the result of the disease process and not be the cause of further symptoms. Pancreatic duct stenting through such strictures is potentially more harmful than beneficial as it rarely improves the situation and can cause further iatrogenic damage to the duct. Pancreatic endotherapy should be considered as an alternative to pancreatic surgery providing the case is carefully selected and discussed in a multidisciplinary way, and the therapy is performed by experts.

Gastric-outlet obstruction

In many patients with pancreatic or biliary malignancy, a late complication is the development of gastric-outlet obstruction as a result of **neoplastic involvement of the duodenum**, usually at the junction of duodenal cap and second part or in the mid-second part and, more rarely, in the third part of the duodenum. In recent years, the development of longer large-bore self-expanding metal stents, enteral stents, has allowed patients with such late gastric-outlet obstruction to be managed endoscopically, without the need for surgical bypass. At this stage of their disease process, many patients are quite frail and have a very short period of time to live. In this situation, surgery has a high mortality and often poor results. The endoscopic insertion of a large-bore stent into the duodenum is safe and, in most patients, leads to an instant relief of gastric outlet obstruction. The immediate disadvantage is that it will usually preclude further endoscopic access to the papilla for biliary stent placement, and it is prudent to position a self-expanding metal stent in the bile duct before placing an enteral stent in the duodenum.

COMPLICATIONS OF ERCP

Table 46.1 lists the complications of ERCP.

Conventional therapeutic procedures

Complications occur after **ERCP, endoscopic sphincterotomy and gallstone removal**, or **stenting** in about 10% of patients. Such complications are often unpredictable and are not age related, affecting young and old patients alike.

Relative inexperience of the endoscopist, use of the needle-knife for a pre-cut sphincterotomy, a papilla in or on the edge of a duodenal diverticulum, and the presence of a polya gastrectomy are all factors that may increase the complication rate. The use of a needle-knife pre-cut, particularly in inexperienced hands, can increase the complication rate considerably.

There is a small mortality rate related to **therapeutic ERCP**; in most series, this is usually not more than 0.1–0.2%. Deaths have usually followed severe bleeding after sphincterotomy or severe pancreatitis.

Complex endoscopic therapy

More difficult cases of bile-duct obstruction with **large stones** or **segmental hilar stricturing** are accompanied by a greater rate of post-procedure

Table 46.1.   Approximate frequencies of complications from ERCP and sphincterotomy.

	Frequency (%)			
	Average-risk patients		High-risk patients[*]	
Complication	ERCP	Sphincterotomy	ERCP	Sphincterotomy
Pancreatitis	3	5	8	20
Bleeding	0.2	1.5	0.4	3.5
Perforation	0.1	0.8	0.3	1.5
Infection	0.1	0.5	2	2
Sedation reaction or cardiopulmonary	0.5	0.5	2	2
Total (%)[†]	3.9	8.3	12.7	29

[*]Certain patient characteristics and technical aspects of the procedure increase the risk of complications, including suspected sphincter of Oddi dysfunction, recurrent pancreatitis, difficult cannulation, precut sphincterotomy, coagulopathy, renal dialysis, cirrhosis of advanced cardiopulmonary disease.
[†]Some patients have more than one complication.
Adapted from (1).

sepsis, hence it is always important not to fill up the biliary tree beyond benign or malignant obstruction without adequate stent drainage afterwards. The most serious septic complications can occur when diagnostic ERCP is performed in an obstructed bile duct without appropriate endoscopic therapy.

In recent years, the development of **pancreatic endotherapy** has led to a new and quite wide range of manoeuvres in the treatment of acute and chronic pancreatic disease. If pancreatic strictures are stented or drained, there is usually a need for a pancreatic sphincterotomy, which is associated with more complications than biliary sphincterotomy. **Indwelling pancreatic stents** can themselves cause iatro-genic pancreatic duct strictures and should be left in only for short periods of time, about 2–3 months. The **endoscopic drainage of pseudocysts** carries a substantial risk of bleeding, and also perforation or infection. This procedure is best performed in experienced hands, with prior assessment by abdominal CT, and endoscopic assessment by endoluminal ultrasound to select the best site for puncture, where the distance between the stomach wall and pseudocyst is small and there are no intervening vessels.

Reference

1.   Yamada T, Alpers DH, Laine L, *et al.* (Eds.). *Textbooks of Gastroenterology.* Philadelphia: Lippincott Williams and Wilkins, 1999.

47. Liver Biopsy: Indications and Procedure

LUCY DAGHER and ANDREW K. BURROUGHS

INTRODUCTION

The **principal indications for liver biopsy examination**: are:

- evaluation of abnormal liver function tests
- grading and staging of chronic hepatitis
- identification and staging of alcoholic liver disease
- recognition of systemic inflammatory or granulomatous disorders
- evaluation of fever of unknown origin
- evaluation of the extent and type of drug induced liver injury
- identification and diagnosis of space occupying lesions
- diagnosis of multisystem infiltrative disorders
- evaluation of cholestatic liver disease (primary biliary cirrhosis, primary sclerosing cholangitis)
- diagnosis and follow-up of treatment of heritable disorders (haemochromatosis, Wilson's disease)
- after liver transplantation

Prominent among the indications is the evaluation of otherwise unexplained abnormalities of liver function tests, with or without associated hepatomegaly (1–6). In **chronic viral hepatitis**, liver biopsy examination is useful to assess those patients who will benefit from treatment, and to assess the response to the treatment. The use of percutaneous liver biopsy sampling in the diagnosis of **focal liver lesions** depends on the clinical picture. In most patients with **hepatocellular carcinoma**, ultrasound scanning, computed tomography (CT), and measurement of alfa-fetoprotein concentration allow diagnosis to be made; obtaining samples of liver for biopsy examination carries documented risk of seeding tumors down the biopsy track (7,8). Modern imaging techniques can also help to define other types of focal hepatic lesions such as **haemangiomata** and **focal nodular hyperplasia**. The use of fine-needle aspiration to obtain biopsy speciments may be a safer option if material for histological examination is required in case of suspected **angioma** (2).

Liver biopsy examination can be useful in the evaluation of unexplained fever (4); for example, in patients with acquired immunodeficiency syndrome, it is the fastest method by which to diagnose viral and mycobacterial involvement of the liver. Other well-established indications include the diagnosis of drug-induced liver injury (5), granulomatous liver disease, infiltrative processes such amyloidosis, and quantifying iron or copper concentrations in genetic haemochromatosis or Wilson's disease, respectively. In liver transplantation, examination of liver biopsy specimens is essential, to diagnose acute rejection and assess disease recurrence.

Contraindications to liver biopsy examination (9) include:

- the unco-operative patient
- extrahepatic biliary obstruction
- bacterial cholangitis
- abnormal coagulation indexes
- tense ascites
- cystic lesions
- hypervascular tumours

- amyloidosis
- congestive liver

METHODS OF OBTAINING LIVER SPECIMENS FOR BIOPSY EXAMINATION

Liver biopsy sampling may be carried out percutaneously or via a transjugular route, and may be plugged or unplugged. The choice of technique is dictated by the coagulation profile, the presence of ascites, and the results of previous imaging technique.

Percutaneous liver biopsy sampling

Procedure

Someone experienced in the technique should perform liver biopsy sampling in hospital inpatients. According to data obtained from the 1991 British Society of Gastroenterology audit, the frequency of complications was slightly greater if the operator had performed fewer than 20 biopsy samplings; the frequency of complications was 3.2%, compared with 1.1% if the operator had performed more than 100 procedures (3). Outpatient biopsy sampling should be limited to centres where they are performed routinely, and when patients can be observed for at least 6 h. Before the biopsy procedure is commenced, **it is necessary to ensure**:

1. That there are clearly defined indications for the procedure, for which the risk to the patient should not outweigh the potential benefit, and that the patient has had the risks explained to them.
2. That ultrasound examination of the liver has been performed; this applies to every patient. Information provided by ultrasound helps in the choice of procedure for liver biopsy sampling, and it is essential in recognizing two contraindications to blind liver biopsy sampling — namely, dilatation of intrahepatic bile ducts and the presence of hydatid cysts. Moreover, the size of the right lobe of the liver, the absence of vascular tumours (haemangiomas), and the position of the gallbladder can be assessed by ultrasound examination.

Other requirements are that:

- the patient's platelet count and prothrombin time should be checked in the week before the pro-

cedure, providing that patient's liver disease is stable
- the patient's blood group is known
- transfusion facilities are available
- the haemoglobin concentration is more than 10 g/dl
- the platelet count is at least 60 000/mm^3
- the prothrombin time is prolonged by no more that 3 s
- the bleeding time has been checked if drugs affecting platelet function have been taken
- if vitamin K 10 mg IM/day for 2 days, has not improved the prothrombin time sufficiently, fresh frozen plasma may be tried before the procedure. If it is successful, it may be used to cover the procedure; however, there is no evidence that this reduces the risk of bleeding.

Technique

The patient is placed supine with their right side close to the edge of the bed and their right hand behind their head. Intravenous midazolam (10), is useful in anxious patients. Careful explanation and instructions should be given, particularly in holding the breath at full expiration; the patient must be able to perform this satisfactorily.

The point of maximum dullness to percussion at full expiration in the right mid-axillary line in an 8th to 10th intercostal space is marked. After skin antisepsis, 1% lignocaine (without adrenaline) is infiltrated, firstly subcutaneously, then into the intercostal area, and finally down the diaphragm and capsule of the liver, care being taken to infiltrate each layer adequately.

Menghini technique

The Menghini technique is the easiest to teach and perform. A skin incision facilitates penetration of a standard 1.4-mm diameter Menghini needle; the disposable type is preferred, as the bevel is consistently sharp. A 20-ml syringe containing 10 ml isotonic sterile saline is attached to the proximal end of the needle after the 3-cm nail has been inserted, to prevent aspiration of the specimen into the syringe; 1 ml saline is injected to clear any tissue after insertion of the needle down to the parietal pleura. Aspiration is started and maintained with the right thumb, while the left thumb is placed on the proximal end of the needle as a guard. The needle is rapidly introduced, perpendicular to the skin, and immediately removed in a single smooth motion while the patient holds their breath at full expiration; the needle remains in the liver for little more than 1 s. Occasionally, small, fragmented specimens are obtained from cirrhotic livers; a second pass usually yields sufficient tissue, but no further passes should be attempted (11,12).

Tru-Cut needle biopsy

The Tru-Cut needle consists of an inner solid needle (the obdurator) and an outer hollow needle. The obturator has a pointed end for tissue penetration and, immediately behind this, a notch for the biopsy specimen.

The needle is inserted, perpendicular to the skin. When the needle reaches the intercostal space, the patient holds his breath in expiration. The needle, in the closed position, is advanced 4–5 cm into the right lobe. The obturator, with its biopsy slot, is thus advanced further into the liver parenchyma, to its full extent (2 cm). Liver tissue prolapses into the biopsy slot. With the obturator kept firmly in position, the cannula, with its cutting surface, is advanced over the obturator, separating a core of the liver in the slot. The needle is now in the fully closed position and is withdrawn. The total time that the needle is in the liver is 2–8 s. If no specimen is obtained at the first pass, a second attempt can be made, after a careful reappraisal of the point of entry and depth of penetration (13,14). The likelihood of complications increases with the number of punctures made.

After care

The patient should be kept in hospital for at least 6 h after the procedure. Vital signs are monitored every 15 min for the first 2 h, every 30 min for 2 h, and then hourly for the remaining period.

Mild oral analgesics, and occasionally parenteral analgesia, are required for pain at the puncture site or referred to the shoulder.

If discharged from hospital within 24 h, the patient should be advised to remain within easy reach of the hospital overnight, and should be provided with the hospital telephone number and name of the member staff to contact should severe pain, syncope, or other symptoms develop.

Complications

Mortality from the percutaneous liver biopsy sampling is approximately 0.017%. Major complications are puncture of the gallbladder or major bile ducts, and haemorrhage. Bile leakage causes immediate severe abdominal pain, which rapidly progresses to biliary peritonitis unless the leak seals itself. Haemorrhage from capsular tears usually takes a few hours to become apparent. Haemobilia causes biliary colic with melaena and bilirubinuria some days later. Cholangitis may occur, particularly in bile-duct obstruction. Puncture of the kidney or colon usually has no sequelae, but pancreatic puncture may be serious. Intrahepatic haematomas and arteriovenous fistulae are seldom clinically significant and resolve spontaneously (3,6,15,16).

Transvenous jugular liver biopsy sampling

The transjugular route of obtaining specimens of liver for biopsy examination is used if there is impaired haemostasis, if gross ascites is present, or if measurement of hepatic venous pressure is needed. Liver transplant has increased the demand for transjugular liver biopsy sampling, because histological examination is frequently required in these patients, who initially have coagulation disorders. The tranjugular route of biopsy sampling can be part of a combined procedure: in our hospital, a day-case procedure can be performed as a "one-stop liver shop" during which hepatic venography, wedge hepatic venous pressure measurements, and carbon dioxide portography are performed using the same minimal access (17).

Technique

The patient is positioned supine. Intravenous sedation with a benzodiazepine is often useful. The right internal jugular vein is punctured under local anaesthesia. When venous blood is aspirated, a 7- or 10-F Arrow sheath is introduced by a Seldinger technique. A 7-F Cobra catheter is introduced into the hepatic vein and the sheath advanced over it. The catheter is removed and the biopsy needle is inserted via the sheath into the hepatic vein; in our centre, we use a quick-core Tru-Cut type biopsy needle. After each pass, contrast medium is injected. With this technique, mortality ranges from 0 to 0.5% (17), which is notably low, considering that the procedure is performed in high-risk patients. The most common major complication is capsular perforation (1.3%) with bleeding; this occurs particularly in those with small livers, and can be detected and treated during the procedure by injecting gelatin material or coils at the site of leak (17).

Percutaneous plug liver biopsy sampling

When coagulation disorders do not allow conventional percutaneous biopsy sampling, and when the transvenous approach is not available or has been unsuccessful, the injection of 2 ml of gelatin sponge through the cannula of a Tru-Cut needle has been used (18,19).

Ultrasound-guided liver biopsy sampling

Ultrasound-guided percutaneous liver biopsy sampling is used extensively in investigation of focal liver lesion; however, its use in diffuse liver disease is more controversial. Although ultrasound has not been rigorously tested, it is reasonable to use it to try to prevent complications in those patients in whom the landmarks of the liver are difficult to ascertain by physical examination — for example, in obesity. In patients with suspected tumour, use of ultrasound or CT-guided biopsy is the safest technique and has the greatest diagnostic yield. If it is easily available, an ultrasound scan before biopsy sampling can exclude the presence of any anatomical abnormalities. It has been reported (20) that the use of ultrasound led to relocation of the site for biopsy in sampling 12% of patients, by demonstrating intervening structures. Most commonly, gallbladder and lung were the reason for altering the position chosen by percussion. In that study, there were no complications and a 100% first-pass success rate. However, using the criteria of difficult percussion, obesity, and unusual chest shape, the investigators were unable to predict when ultrasound would be useful. There are no data to indicate that ultrasound reduces morbidity, mortality, or costs (21–25).

References

1. Alberti A, Morsica G, Chemello L *et al.* Hepatitis C viraemia and liver disease in symptom-free individuals with anti-HCV. *Lancet* 1992; **340**: 697–698.
2. Caldironi MW, Mazzucco M, Aldinio MT *et al.* Echo-guided fine-needle biopsy for the diagnosis of hepatic angioma. *Minerva Chir* 1998; **53**: 505–509.
3. Gilmore IT, Burroughs AK, Murray-Lyon IM *et al.* Indications, methods, and outcomes of percutaneos liver biopsies in England and Wales: an audit by the British Society of Gastroenterology and The Royal College of Physicians of London. *Gut* 1995; **36**: 431–437.
4. Holtz T, Moseley RH, Scheiman JM. Liver biopsy in fever of unknown origin. A reappraisal. *J Clin Gastroenterol* 1993; **17**: 29–32.
5. Ruijter ThE, Schattenkerk E, Van Leeuwen DJ *et al.* Diagnostic value of liver biopsy in symptomatic HIV-1 infected patients. *Eur J Gastroenterol Hepatol* 1993; **5**: 641–645.
6. Sherlock S, Dick R, Van Leeuwen DJ. Liver biopsy. The Royal Free Experience. *J Hepatol* 1984; **1**: 75–85.
7. Vergara V, Garripoli A, Marucci MM *et al.* Colon cancer seeding after percutaneous fine needle aspiration of liver metastasis. *J Hepatol* 1993; **18**: 276–278.
8. Schotman SN, De Man RA, Stoker J, *et al.* Subcutaneous seeding of hepatocellular carcinoma after percutaneous needle biopsy. *Gut* 1999; **45**: 626–627.
9. Grant A, Neuberger J. Guidelines on the use of liver biopsy in clinical practice. *Gut* 1999; **45(suppl IV)**: IV1–IV11.
10. Brouillette DE, Koo Y-K, Chien M-C *et al.* Use of midazolam for percutaneous liver biopsy. *Dig Dis Sci* 1989; **34**: 1553–1558.
11. Menghini G. One-second needle biopsy of the liver. *Gastroenterology* 1958; **35**: 190–199.
12. Menghini G. One-seconds biopsy of the liver- problems of its clinical applications. *N Engl J Med* 1970; **283**: 582–585.
13. Westaby D, Williams R. Practical procedures: how to biopsy the liver. *Br J Hosp Med* 1980; **23**: 527–529.
14. Maharaj B, Pillay S. "Tru-Cut" needle biopsy of the liver: importance of the correct technique. *Postgrad Med J* 1991; **67**: 170–173.
15. Froehlich F, Lamy O, Fried M *et al.* Practice and complications of liver biopsy. result of a Nationwide Survey in Switzerland. *Dig Dis Sci* 1993; **38**: 1480–1484.
16. McGill DB, Rakela J, Zinsmeister AR *et al.* A 21-year experience with major hemorrhage after percutaneous liver biopsy. *Gastroenterology* 1990; **99**: 1396–1400.
17. Papatheodoridis GV, Patch D, Wathinson A *et al.* Transjugular liver biopsy in the 1990s: a 2-year audit. *Alim Pharmacol Ther* 1999; **13**: 603–608.
18. Riley SA, Ellis WR, Irving HC *et al.* Percutaneous liver biopsy with plugging of needle track: a safe method for use in patients with impaired coagulation. *Lancet* 1984; **ii**: 436.
19. Tobin MV, Gilmore IT. Plugged liver biopsy in patients with impaired coagulation. *Dig Dis Sci* 1989; **34**: 13–15.
20. Riley TR. Can one predict when ultrasound will be useful with percutaneous liver biopsy? [abstract] *Hepatology* 1999; **30**: 479A.
21. Celle G, Savarino V, Picciotto A *et al.* Is hepatic ultrasonography a valid alternative tool to liver biopsy? Report of 507 cases studied with both techniques. *Dig Dis Sci* 1988; **33**: 467–471.
22. Pasha T, Gabriel S, Therneau T *et al.* Cost-effectiveness of ultrasound guided liver biopsy. *Hepatology* 1998; **27**: 1220–1226.
23. Lindor KD, Jorgensen RA, Rakela J *et al.* The role of ultrasonography and automatic needle biopsy in outpatient percutaneous liver biopsy. *Hepatology* 1996; **23**: 1079–1083.
24. Caturelli E, Giacobbe A, Facciorusso D *et al.* Percutaneous Biopsy in diffuse liver disease: increasing diagnostic yield and decreasing complications rate by routine ultrasound assessment of puncture site. *Am J Gastroenterol* 1996; **91**: 1318–1321.
25. Shah S, Mayberry JF, Wicks AC, *et al.* Liver biopsy under ultrasound control: implications for training in the Calman era. *Gut* 1999; **45**: 628–629.

48. Ultrasound for Gastroenterologists

KATE WALMSLEY

INTRODUCTION

Diagnostic ultrasound is accepted as a first-line imaging investigation for many disorders suspected to be gastroenterological in origin, being a low-cost, painless, repeatable procedure requiring little preparation and limited patient cooperation, and with no known harmful effects at diagnostic frequencies. An anatomical rather than a functional tool with which to image solid or fluid structures, its diagnostic efficacy is compromised by air, gas, or bone, and to a lesser extent, scar tissue and fat.

Superficial structures are best imaged with high-frequency ultrasound probes (5–10 mHz); the higher the frequency, the greater the resolution, but the less the depth of penetration. For **general abdominal imaging**, frequencies in the range of 5–2 mHz are in general use, but the choice of probe will, to some extent, depend on the manufacturer's specification. All probes should have an integral Doppler ultrasound facility that includes duplex, colour, and power Doppler.

To optimize diagnostic accuracy, clinical history, findings on clinical examination and the results of basic haematological and biochemical blood tests, including liver function tests, should be available at the time of the scan.

Indications for abdominal ultrasound imaging include:

1. Abdominal pain or fever when origin suspected of being from:
   — liver
   — pancreas
   — kidneys and urinary tract
   — spleen
   — appendix/uterus and ovaries
   — retroperitoneum (computed tomography (CT) better).
2. Palpable abdominal mass.
3. Abdominal distension — fat, fluid or tumour.
4. Jaundice.
5. Unexplained weight loss.
6. Preoperative history and investigation, and staging of malignant disease. CT is the investigation of choice, but ultrasound scan is useful in characterising a mass.
7. Unknown location of primary tumour (e.g. ovary).
8. Need to monitor response to treatment
9. Need for a portable scan to obtain diagnostic imaging of an unconscious patient or a patient who is too sick to move, and who has suspected liver or renal disease, intra-abdominal fluid, or abscess.
10. Need for ultrasound-guided biopsy or drainage.
11. Need to reassure anxious patient with normal scan.

Information obtained about:

- Diaphragm
  — supraphrenic spaces
  — subphrenic spaces
- Liver, gallbladder, biliary tract
- Pancreas
- Spleen
- Aorta, coeliac axis, superior mesenteric artery

- Portal veins, superior mesenteric vein, splenic vein
- Inferior vena cava and hepatic veins
- Retroperitoneum
  — kidneys
  — adrenal masses
  — lymph nodes
  — psoas muscles
- Pelvic organs

TECHNIQUE

The patient should be fasted for 4–6 h before the scan. Clear, non-fizzy fluids are permitted. No preparation is required in an emergency. The examination should not be confined to a single organ (e.g. the gallbladder), unless the single question being asked is "are there gallstones?"

LIVER ULTRASOUND

Ultrasound as a first line imaging modality gives anatomical not functional information and it is mandatory to be able to recognise normal appearances i.e. size, shape and echopattern.

The **normal liver** has smooth, straight, or concave margins, acute inferior and marginal angles, and a homogeneous internal echopattern; it is more echogenic than the right kidney.

Hepatic veins run straight, generally with non-echogenic walls, to reach the confluence with the inferior vena cava just below the diaphragmatic orifice. The **portal vein and its branches** have "bright" echogenic walls. The normal, non-dilated branches of the **intrahepatic bile ducts** can be seen at the porta hepatis and traced accompanying the portal vein branches. The **hepatic artery**, with echogenic walls, can be identified at the porta hepatis, and the **ligamentum teres** can be seen as a bright (echogenic) area casting an acoustic (black) shadow.

Pitfalls in normal anatomy

1. Ultrasound is a poor technique for estimating **liver size**. Dimensions are more accurately delineated on a radioisotope study.
2. A normal **caudate lobe** may appear less echogenic than the surrounding liver and be misinterpreted as a hepatic mass.

3. A **Reidel's lobe** causes the right inferior marginal angle to be convex; if this is not recognized it may be erroneously interpreted as hepatomegaly.
4. In the region of the right dome of the diaphragm, the **muscle slips** may be misinterpreted as a subphrenic collection.
5. An incorrect **time gain curve** can make the back of the right lobe of the liver appear poorly echogenic (black) and the front appear (bright) or *vice versa*.
6. If the right kidney is more echogenic than the liver, the **gain** may be incorrectly set.

Abnormal liver ultrasound appearances

Diffuse homogeneous enlargement of the liver with smooth, round, convex margins

Questions to be asked:

- are the hepatic veins and inferior vena cava (IVC) dilated, and does the calibre of the IVC alter with ventilatory and the cardiac cycle?
- are the hepatic veins patent?
- is there a pleural or a pericardial effusion?
- is there free fluid in the abdominal cavity?
- are the bile ducts of normal calibre, and is the gallbladder seen?

The differential diagnosis is as follows.

Hepatitis — any cause
The **liver** may have a normal echopattern or be less echogenic than normal, making the portal tracts stand out brightly and reversing the liver/right kidney difference in echopattern. If the liver appears less echogenic than the right kidney, the sonographer must decide if the cause is diffuse liver disease (e.g. hepatitis) or diffuse renal disease (Figure 48.1).

The **gallbladder** often has a bizarre appearance, with thick walls and little or no bile within it, associated with the abnormal liver function.

Acute fulminating hepatitis will be associated with ascites and pleural effusions.

Cardiac failure
Characterized by dilated hepatic veins and IVC that fail to change calibre with ventilation, pleural effusions with or without a pericardial effusion and ascites. The liver may be less echogenic than normal.

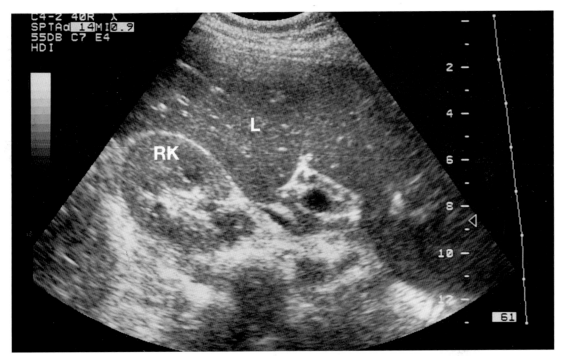

Figure 48.1. Acute hepatitis. Liver (L) less echogenic than the right kidney (RK).

Fatty change

Fatty change is seen as a diffuse increase in internal echogenicity (**bright liver**). It may be a normal variant, with normal liver biopsy findings (1).

It may be **associated with** obesity, diabetes mellitus, and increased alcohol intake.

Micronodular cirrhosis has an identical appearance, and can be differentiated only by histological biopsy examination.

There may be **segmental sparing**, with abrupt transition between affected and non-affected areas; sparing is also common in the region of the porta hepatitis (Figure 48.2).

CT scan will confirm diagnosis of selective fatty infiltration, without the need to perform biopsy studies.

Chronic active hepatitis, primary biliary cirrhosis, haemochromatosis

Diffuse non-specific hepatomegaly with minor changes in internal echopattern with or without prominent portal tracts before the disease progresses to cirrhosis.

Any acute hepatic insult (e.g. toxins, drugs, severe infection or septicaemia, haemolytic anaemia, hepatic disease of pregnancy)

These appear as non-specific diffuse homogeneous hepatomegaly, with normal or minor reduction of echogenicity, with or without splenomegaly.

Budd–Chiari syndrome

Budd–Chiari syndrome is very rare in clinical practice. Diffuse homogeneous hepatomegaly, with caudate lobe enlargement. Disturbed or abnormal blood flow detected using Doppler and colour Doppler scanning.

Diffuse heterogeneous enlargement of the liver

Questions to be asked:

- are the hepatic margins irregular? If so, are the "humps" large or small?
- is the internal echopattern nodular? If yes, are the nodules large or small, and are they of similar sizes?
- are the nodules more or less echogenic than the surrounding liver parenchyma? Do they have a mixed pattern, including very bright areas casting an acoustic shadow that could be calcifications and trans-sonic areas with "bright up" behind that could be fluid?
- can normal liver tissue be distinguished separately?

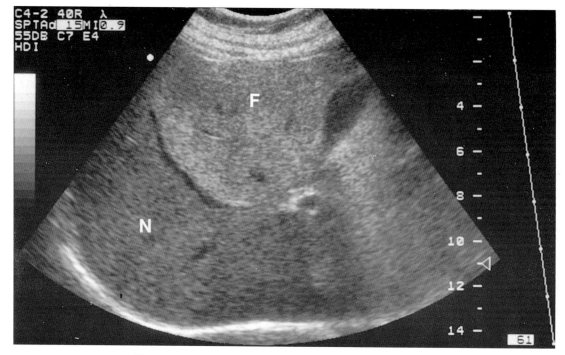

Figure 48.2. Segmental fatty change. N, Normal liver; F, fatty liver.

- are there areas of local dilatation of the intrahepatic bile ducts?
- are the main hepatic ducts, common bile duct, and gallbladder normal?
- is the portal vein patent or dilated?
- is the portal venous flow reversed on pulse wave/colour Doppler examination?
- are there collateral vessels at the porta hepatis, in the gastric or pancreatic bed or subcapsular (2)?
- is there ascites? Look for a triangle of subhepatic fluid between liver and gallbladder if the amount of free fluid suspected is small (Figure 48.3).

The differential diagnosis will be as follows.

Cirrhosis — any cause
Appearances will be determined by the duration of the illness. Look for additional signs for clues to diagnosis: small shrunken liver, large liver with echogenic, less echogenic or mixed nodules, splenomegaly, collateral vessels, blocked or dilated portal vein, ascites, pleural effusions, local dilatation or irregularity of groups of intrahepatic bile

ducts, additional intrahepatic mass (tumour). A biopsy examination will still be required for a definitive diagnosis (3) (Figure 48.4).

Mutiple metastases
Look for:

Irregularity of hepatic margins (these may be very subtle especially in the presence of miliary metastases). Micro- or macro-nodules that may be poorly echogenic, echogenic, of mixed echogenicity, or cystic (Figure 48.5).

Local intrahepatic bile-duct dilatation.

Enlarged, poorly echogenic nodal masses at the porta hepatis.

Ascites.

Lymphoma
Lymphoma may appear as diffuse tiny, poorly echogenic nodules, or large, poorly echogenic nodules, and these may be associated splenomegaly and nodal masses.

Fungal infection
Mutiple small, poorly echogenic nodules (which may be difficult to detect if smaller than 1 cm).

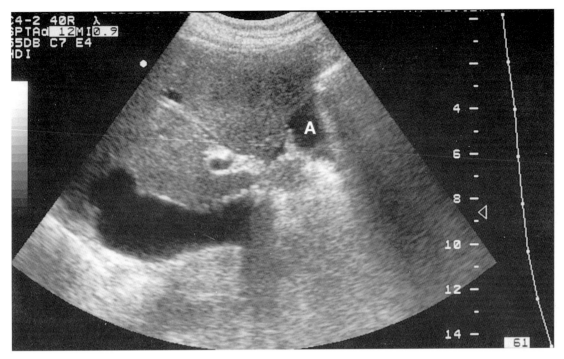

Figure 48.3. Subhepatic triangle of free fluid (arrow).

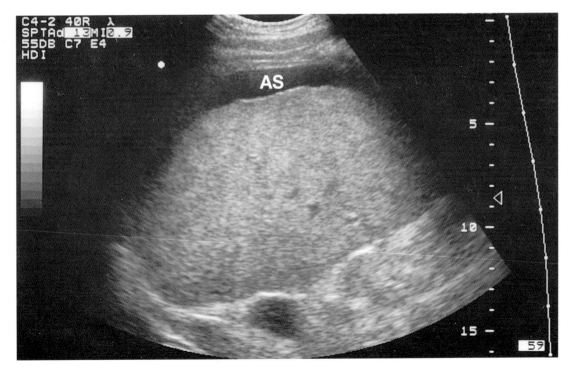

Figure 48.4. Macronodular cirrhosis with ascites (AS).

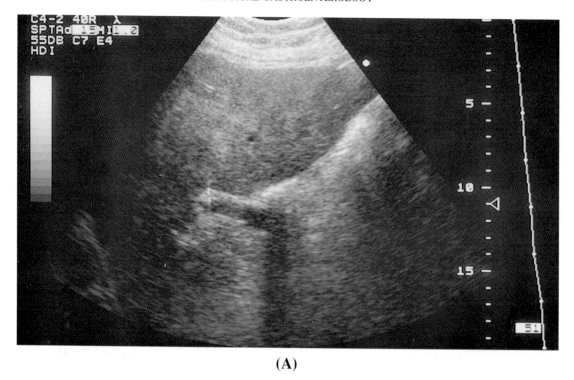

(A)

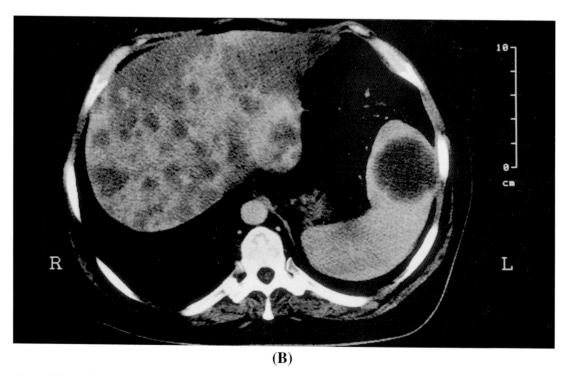

(B)

Figure 48.5. A: Ultrasound image of multiple small hepatic metastases — primary tumour malignant melanoma. B: Corresponding CT image of the same area of the liver.

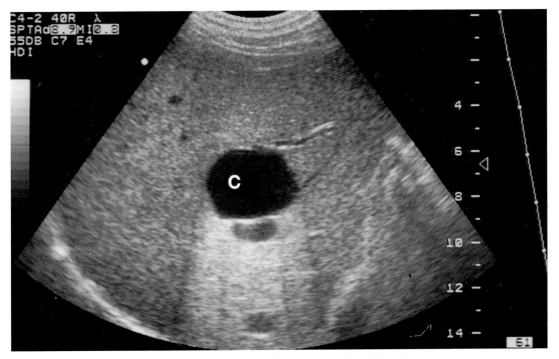

Figure 48.6. Simple hepatic cyst (C) trans-sonic, with "bright-up" behind.

Focal liver defect with or without hepatic enlargement

Questions to be asked:

- single or multiple lesions?
- cystic, solid, or mixed echopattern?
- more or less echogenic than the surrounding liver?
- well or ill defined?
- central or peripheral/subcapsular?
- abnormal blood flow on colour Doppler (e.g. avascular, hypervascular, low-flow tumour blood flow?

The differential diagnosis of focal liver defects is extensive.

Simple cyst
Simple cyst may be single or multiple (Figure 48.6). Large cysts may be multilocular. Ultrasound will detect polycystic kidneys if they are present on the same scan.

Hydatid cyst
Hydatid cyst may be single or multiple, have internal septae and internal echoes, have daughter cysts, or contain calcification in the wall. Ultrasound can not determine if viable parasites remain after treatment, but is a useful technique for follow-up. CT more accurately provides a baseline record of number, size, and site of multiple cysts (Figure 48.7).

Pyogenic abscess
The appearance of pyogenic abscesses depends on their age. They may appear as an ill-defined area of reduced echogenicity, a cystic mass containing low-level echoes, a thin-walled cystic area, or a thick-walled area with a part-cystic mass having multiple internal septa. They may be indistinguishable from, or associated with, primary or secondary necrotic tumour (Figure 48.8).

Amoebic abscess
Seventy-five per cent of amoebic abscesses are single, the remainder multiple. They are sited in right

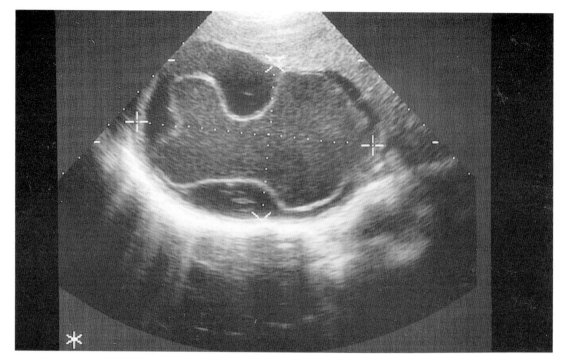

Figure 48.7. Hydatid cyst.

lobe of liver more often than in the left, and always touch a capsular surface. The appearance depends on age. **Young** abscesses have no capsule, are well defined and less echogenic than the surrounding liver, are trans-sonic, often with a posterior "bright-up", and fill with low-level echoes if the gain setting is increased. If the abscess penetrates the diaphragm, this is diagnostic (there may be sympathetic pleural effusion even if the diaphragm is intact). **Older** abscesses have irregular, thick walls with internal projections, and calcification may be present in the wall. If serology is positive and the patient is responding to treatment, aspiration is unnecessary (aspirate if the diagnosis is uncertain or there is suspicion of secondary infection). It can take up to 1 year for abscess to disappear completely. (Figure 48.9).

Fungal disease

Fungal disease presents as multiple small, poorly echogenic nodules; appearances may be confused with those of metastatic disease. Lesions less than 1 cm in diameter may only be detected on CT scan.

Haematoma

Haematoma may be found after blunt abdominal trauma. Appearances depend on the age of the haematoma which may be cystic, multicystic, solid, or of a mixed internal echopattern. CT scan with intravenous contrast, not ultrasound, is the investigation of choice in the acute situation.

Primary benign neoplasms

Adenomas are usually well defined, with a mixed internal echopattern that is slightly more or less echogenic than the surrounding liver parenchyma.

Haemangiomas may be single or multiple, and are usually well defined and more echogenic than the surrounding liver. They may have a lobulated margin and, if large, may show central poorly echogenic areas of necrosis. Often, a prominent adjacent hepatic vein can be identified, especially with colour Doppler (common in the region of the porta hepatis). Haemangiomas can not be differentiated from echogenic liver metastases on ultrasound, but CT with intravenous contrast and delayed scans in which the lesion becomes of the same attenuation as the surrounding liver

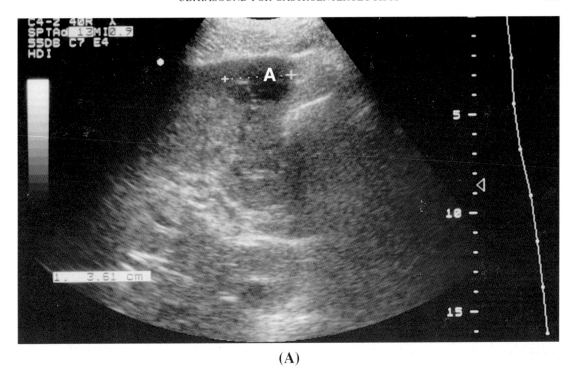

(A)

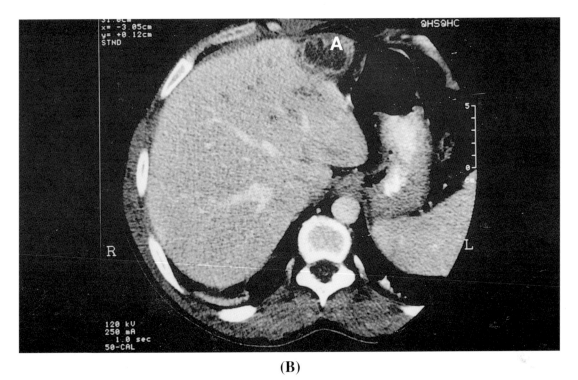

(B)

Figure 48.8. A: Ultrasound image of pyogenic hepatic abscess (A). B: CT image of same abscess.

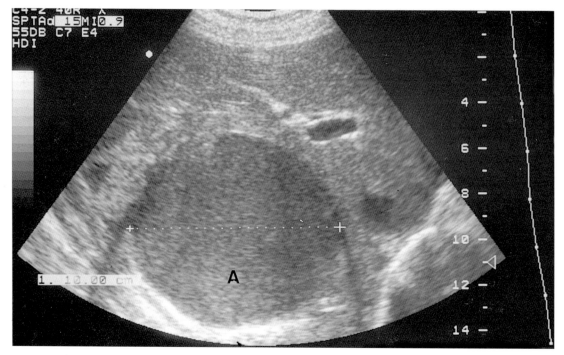

Figure 48.9.   Amoebic abscess (A) abutting capsular surface, with uniform low-level internal echoes.

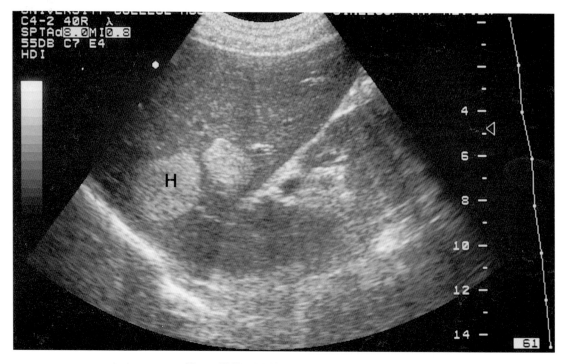

Figure 48.10.   Multiple haemangiomata (H).

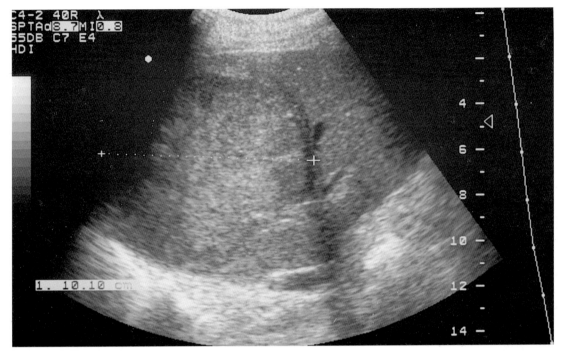

Figure 48.11. Large hepatoma.

will confirm the diagnosis without the need for biopsy examination and its inherent risk of haemorrhage (Figure 48.10).

Schwannomas and **other benign tumours** appear well defined, with a mixed echopattern. CT and biopsy examination are needed for their diagnosis.

The well-defined "tumour" nodules of **focal nodular hyperplasia** may be more or less echogenic than surrounding liver parenchyma. They may concentrate radio-colloids on isotope study. A diagnosis may be made on CT scan or magnetic resonance imaging, but often the diagnosis is one of exclusion after biopsy examination.

Primary malignant neoplasms

Hepatomas (hepatocellular carcinomas) can be single (Figure 48.11) or multiple. They are usually of mixed internal echopattern, but are predominantly poorly echogenic, with ill-defined margins. They are easy to miss in cirrhotic liver, with its heterogenous nodular internal echopattern. A tumour blood flow or obstructed portal vein may be found on colour Doppler.

Angiosarcomas appear highly vascular on colour Doppler.

Diagnostic pitfalls in liver ultrasound

1. Detecting lesions less than 1 cm in size.
2. Detecting capsular/subcapsular lesions, lesions adjacent to diaphragmatic surfaces, and small peripheral lesions.
3. Detecting hepatoma/multifocal hepatoma in the presence of cirrhosis (4).
4. Differentiating between regenerating nodules in a cirrhotic liver and hepatic metastases.
5. Characterizing echo pattern of liver parenchyma in the presence of ascites.
6. Differentiating between benign and malignant masses.
7. Differentiating between infectious and malignant masses. The final diagnosis is often only to be made after either fine-needle aspirate or core biopsy sampling under ultrasound, or other imaging modality guidance. CT with intravenous contrast is advised before biopsy samples are obtained from the mass, to determine how vascular the lesion is and minimize the risk of haemorrhage.
8. CT is more sensitive than transabdominal ultrasound in detecting liver metastases, particularly if they are small or peripherally sited (5). Recent studies using Doppler ultrasound (6) or ultra-

sound contrast agents show promise, but their clinical reproducibility is still under scrutiny.

BILIARY SYSTEM AND GALLBLADDER

Normal gallbladder and biliary system

The **normal fasted gallbladder** has thin bright walls, is trans-sonic with "bright-up" behind, and contains no internal echoes. If it is present, the gallbladder can always be identified on ultrasound by an experienced operator.

Normal non-dilated **intrahepatic** ducts can be imaged using modern ultrasound systems.

The main right and left hepatic **ducts**, the main common hepatic duct, the cystic duct, and the common bile duct can usually be identified, if necessary using colour Doppler to distinguish bile ducts from hepatic artery and portal vein.

The **normal common bile duct** may widen and then taper at its lower end. It has a diameter of 6 mm or less, but this increases with age (7); however, a diameter 6–10 mm is probably abnormal, unless there has been a previous cholecystectomy. A duct larger than 10 mm is definitely abnormal.

Pitfalls in normal anatomy

1. **Inspection of the abdomen** before the examination begins spares the embarrassment of not observing the cholecystectomy scar or the small-entry portal scars from a previous laparoscopic cholecystectomy.
2. The **gallbladder** should always be scanned from top to bottom and side to side in at least two positions — supine and left lateral decubitus — to exclude gallstones or a true septum.
3. A **bowel loop** indenting the wall of the gallbladder may be misinterpreted as being within the gallbladder if scanned in one plane and one position only.
4. An incorrect **time gain curve** may fill the gallbladder with echoes.
5. In the **non-fasted patient**, the gallbladder will be contracted and contain little bile and so small stones will be missed.
6. **Anatomical variants of the biliary tract** may lead to incorrect identification of the right and left hepatic ducts, the length and termination of the cystic duct and common bile duct, and the relationship of the distal common bile duct to the termination of the pancreatic duct.

Abnormal ultrasound appearances of the gallbladder

Gallstones

Gallstones are common finding on abdominal ultrasound (Figure 48.12). Diagnosis requires the triad of:

1. an echogenic nodule within the gallbladder that
2. casts an acoustic shadow, and
3. moves with change of position

Acute cholecystitis

Stones may impact in the gallbladder neck or cystic duct. The **gallbladder wall** may be thick (>3 mm) and may have a layered appearance, with a central, poorly echogenic line of oedema within the wall (Figure 48.13).

The **gallbladder** should be **tender** when scanned (ultrasound "Murphy's sign"), but the administration of analgesics before the scan may mask this useful clue. If there has been a local **perforation** of gallbladder wall, mixed echoes — usually poorly echogenic, or even cystic — are seen adjacent to the gallbladder bed. If a frank **abscess** is present, either a poorly echogenic area within liver or a subhepatic collection is seen. If there is **gas** in the gallbladder or its wall, ultrasound may detect bright areas with bizarre shadowing (compare with pattern from bowel gas). Plain abdominal X-ray will make the diagnosis of emphysematous cholecystitis. **Dilated intrahepatic bile ducts** may be a consequence of obstruction of the biliary system by a stone in the neck of the gallbladder — Mirizzi's syndrome — rather than a stone in the common bile duct.

Empyema of the gallbladder

Findings are of a large, distended, tender gallbladder containing stones and sludge, with stone impacted in the neck.

Chronic cholecystitis

The gallbladder is usually non-tender in chronic cholecystitis. It may be thick or thin walled, fluid filled with mobile stones, or may have stones adhering to the wall. Rarely, the wall may be calcified.

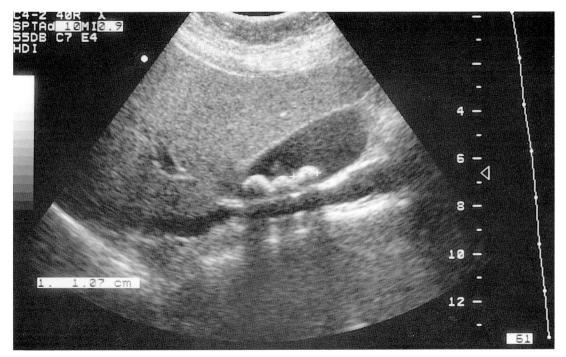

Figure 48.12. Gallstones.

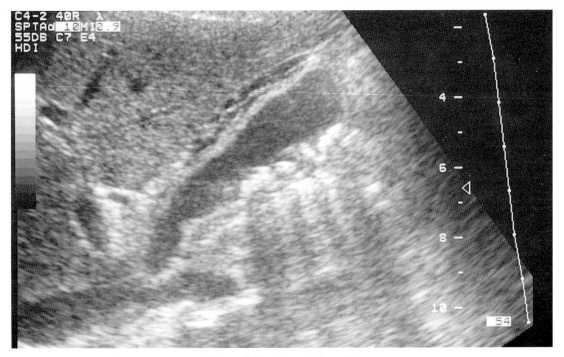

Figure 48.13. Acute cholecystitis.

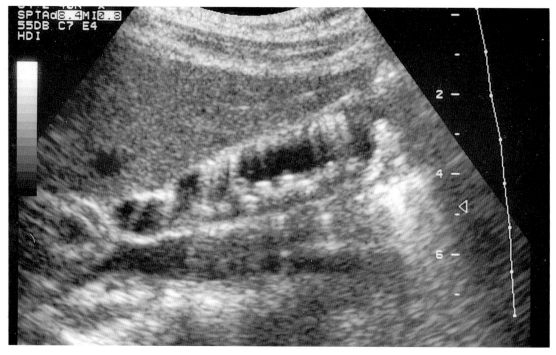

Figure 48.14. Adenomyomatosis of the gallbladder.

Mucocoele of the gallbladder

The gallbladder is large and distended, with a stone stuck in the neck. There may be further stones and sludge within the gallbladder, beyond the obstructing stone.

Adenomyomatosis

This has a typical ultrasound appearances of bright echoes on thickened walls. Gallstones are usually present (Figure 48.14).

Cholesterolosis

Cholesterol polyps stuck on gallbladder wall give an ultrasound appearance of echogenic nodules that do not move with change of position, and may or may not cast an acoustic shadow (Figure 48.15).

Postinflammatory polyps

After infection (e.g. with *Salmonella typhi*), there may be echogenic nodules on the gallbladder wall.

Carcinoma of the gallbladder

Often, carcinoma of the gallbladder is missed on ultrasound until a large, poorly echogenic mass is seen extending into the liver, when appearances are indistinguishable from those of cholangiocarcinoma. Any solid "polyp" larger than 1 cm seen in the gallbladder requires further investigation and excision. Most polypoid lesions detected within the gallbladder by ultrasound are benign (8).

Acalculous cholecystitis

The appearance is of a tender, distended gallbladder containing fine, homogeneous internal echoes, but no stones.

Abnormal liver function

A thick-walled, non-tender gallbladder containing echogenic bile or sludge, or no fluid at all, may be imaged if there is abnormality of liver function from any cause (e.g. hepatitis, acute liver failure, decompensated cirrhosis), or in the debilitated patient (Figure 48.16).

A follow-up scan after recovery will show a normal gallbladder.

Diagnostic pitfalls in gallbladder ultrasound scanning

1. A bowel loop indenting the gallbladder can be misinterpreted as being stone within gallbladder.

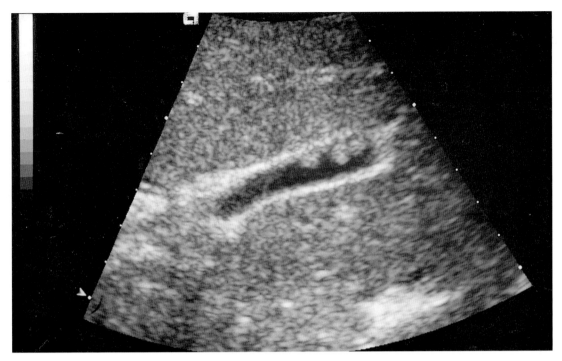

Figure 48.15. Gallbladder cholesterolosis.

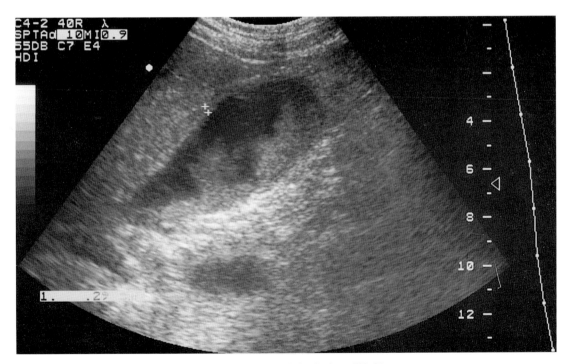

Figure 48.16. Biliary sludge in the gallbladder.

2. Small stones in a non fasted gallbladder will be missed.

3. Multiple stones and no bile can be misdiagnosed as a bowel loop.

4. A stone may be impacted in cystic duct without stones in gallbladder. The clue is gallbladder sludge often with bile/sludge layering and a distended gallbladder.

5. A stone stuck on wall thought to be gallbladder polyp.

6. A false septum as a result of gallbladder folded back on itself.

7. A large gallbladder containing sludge/debris/no fluid because of abnormal liver function.

8. An extrinsic tumour mass involving gallbladder secondarily may be indistinguishable from gallbladder tumour extending beyond gallbladder.

Abnormal ultrasound appearances of the biliary tract

Biliary duct dilatation

On scanning the biliary tract, it is necessary to decide which ducts are dilated, in order to determine the level of obstruction: dilated intrahepatic ducts either local or universal, right and left main hepatic ducts, main hepatic duct, common bile duct, and distended gallbladder (Figure 48.17). Possible **causes for the dilatation** include:

• gallstones — intrahepatic or extrahepatic
• primary or secondary hepatic tumour
• cholangiocarcinoma
• ampullary tumour
• tumour of head of pancreas
• choledochal cyst
• sclerosing cholangitis
• parasitic infection (worms)

An ultrasound scan is good at detecting the level of obstruction, but not the cause. It is often the case that dilatation of the left duct system will be apparent before that of the right side.

Diagnostic pitfalls in ultrasound scanning of the biliary tree

1. Only 50% of common bile-duct stones cast an acoustic shadow.

2. A patient who has recently presented with biliary colic may have **passed a stone** by the time the scan is performed, but there will usually still be stones in the gallbladder, even if no stones are seen in the common bile duct.

3. **Debris** and small stones at the lower end of the common bile duct may obscure an underlying tumour.

4. It is not possible to distinguish between a benign and malignant **stricture** at the lower end of the common bile duct, or elsewhere in the biliary tree, unless there is an associated tumour mass.

5. **Tumour** infiltrating along the bile ducts without an associated tumour mass is difficult to image, even with state-of-the-art ultrasound systems.

6. **Intrahepatic duct dilatation** may be confined to local segments of the biliary tree (e.g. in the presence of obstruction by a primary or secondary liver tumour), in sclerosing cholangitis and where there are intrahepatic duct stones or worms.

7. **After cholecystectomy**, the common bile duct may be dilated (>6 mm), but not obstructed.

8. **Gas** in the biliary tree (Figure 48.18) may obscure biliary stones or be mistaken for them. It is seen as a straight, bright echo following the line of a duct, with posterior acoustic shadowing that moves with change in position. It is easily diagnosed on a plain X-ray film or by CT scan.

9. After **bypass surgery**, the anatomy of biliary–bowel anastomoses may be impossible to determine with ultrasound.

10. It is possible to image **biliary stents** and determine if they are blocked, especially if there are previous scans for comparison.

11. If, on scanning, there is **no evidence of biliary obstruction** then re-interpretation or repeat of the liver function tests is suggested. A small percentage of patients with extrahepatic obstructive jaundice never develop dilated bile ducts (e.g. in the presence of cirrhosis or subacute or chronic biliary obstruction) (9).

PANCREAS

Normal pancreas

The normal **pancreas** can be imaged in 90% of upper abdominal scans. Tadpole, dumbbell, or sausage shaped, it has a variable position, but the head is usually seen to lie below the level of the tail. The margins are smooth and the internal echopattern homogeneous, poorly echogenic in childhood, more

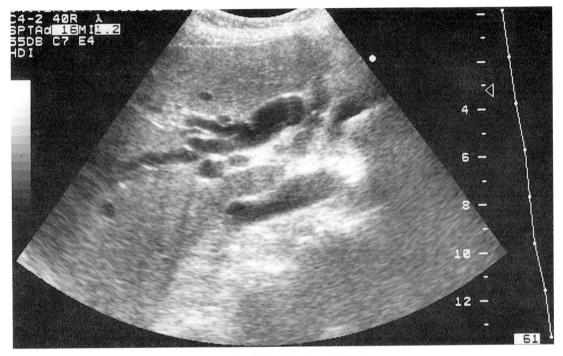

Figure 48.17. Dilated intrahepatic bile ducts.

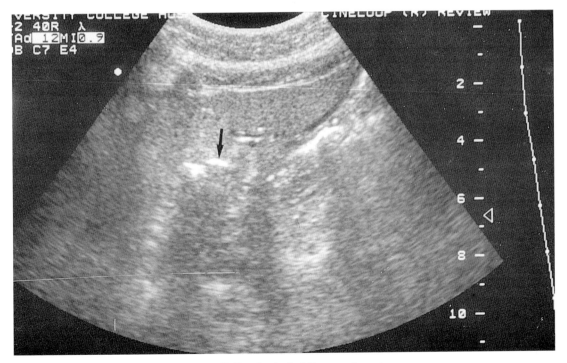

Figure 48.18. Gas in the biliary tree (arrow).

echogenic (bright) in adulthood, and even brighter and smaller in the elderly. The normal **main pancreatic duct**, seen in part or whole, measures 4 mm or less in diameter in the head, and 3 mm or less in the body and tail.

The **splenic vein**, lying posterior and above the pancreas, and the **superior mesenteric artery and vein**, seen in cross-section lying behind the neck of the pancreas, are useful landmarks.

Pitfalls in normal pancreatic anatomy

1. **Gas** in the duodenal loop may obscure the head of the pancreas; gas in the stomach may obscure the the the tail.
2. Central **bowel gas**, especially if associated with an ileus, may obscure the pancreas completely.
3. The part of the normal pancreas derived from the embryological ventral pancreas — that is, the uncinate process and the posterior part of the head — may be less echogenic than the remainder of the pancreas.

Abnormal ultrasound appearances of the pancreas

Acute pancreatitis

The pancreas may appear normal on ultrasound scan, or may be enlarged with a less echogenic internal echopattern than normal (Figure 48.19). It may have a heterogeneous internal echopattern, with patchy areas of both increased and decreased echogenicity, and a dilated, irregular pancreatic duct with echogenic areas in the wall, and visible side branches.

Less echogenic confluent areas seen within the pancreas and containing some echogenic areas may indicate a developing phlegmon; **trans-sonic masses** i.e. (fluid within/outside the pancreas), may indicate a developing pseudocyst.

Poorly echogenic masses draped around the pancreas indicate an inflammatory reaction, which may include the mesentery.

In addition, ultrasound may detect pleural and intrabdominal fluid, a dilated common bile duct, and gallstones.

Chronic pancreatitis

The appearance is of a small, shrunken fibrotic pancreas, homogeneously echogenic on scan, or a heterogenous, mainly echogenic internal echopattern.

There may be a dilated, irregular pancreatic duct, with or without echogenic masses (stones).

Echogenic areas within the pancreatic stroma casting acoustic shadows are indicative of calcification or fibrosis (Figure 48.20A).

Thick-walled cystic structures within the pancreas, with echogenic areas within the walls casting acoustic shadows are calcified pseudocysts (Figure 48.20B).

Tumour

Most tumours are **less echogenic** than the normal pancreas, with irregular margins. Some are predominantly cystic on scan.

Tumours in the **head of the pancreas** are associated with a dilated common bile duct, and obstructive jaundice (Figure 48.21). In the head and body, distal dilatation of the pancreatic duct and features of secondary pancreatitis can sometimes be seen.

Scanning may detect vascular encasement, thrombosis, and collateral vessels (for which the use of ultrasound contrast agents is promising).

There may be enlarged, poorly echogenic nodes in the pancreatic bed and in the porta hepatis, liver metastases, or ascites.

Diagnostic pitfalls in ultrasound scanning of the pancreas

1. **Ultrasound should not be used to diagnose acute pancreatitis**; the diagnosis is biochemical.
2. **CT scanning** should be used to **map the extent** of a newly diagnosed pancreatitis and also to **monitor progress** (10).
3. Ultrasound scan is indicated to confirm or exclude **gallstones as a cause** of pancreatitis.
4. Ultrasound-guided biopsy sampling and abscess or cyst drainage may be appropriate after a baseline CT scan.
5. The extent of the **inflammatory mass** present in a patient with severe acute pancreatitis will be underestimated by ultrasound.
6. The normal echogenic pancreas of the **older patient** may be confused with chronic pancreatitis, and the poorly echogenic pancreas of **childhood** and **adolescence** confused with the appearances of acute pancreatitis.
7. A **dilated pancreatic duct** may be confused with the splenic vein.
8. An **underlying tumour** may be missed in the presence of pancreatitis.
9. It may be impossible to **differentiate tumour** from phlegmon, abscess, or pseudocyst.

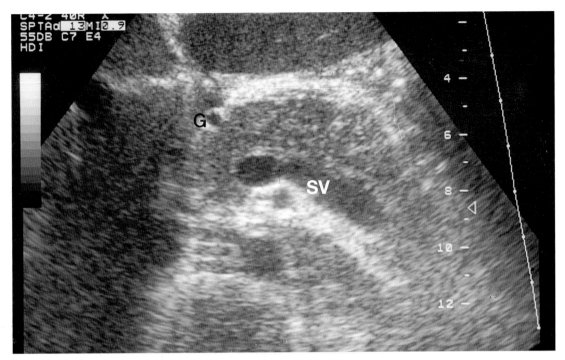

Figure 48.19. Acute pancreatitis. The pancreas is enlarged, with less echogenic internal echopattern than normal; G, gastroduodenal artery; SV, splenic vein.

10. **Pancreatic calcification** — both intraductal and parenchymal — is easy to miss or misintepret with ultrasound. A plain abdominal X-ray or CT scan is advised to demonstrate the absence or presence of calcification.

THE SPLEEN

Normal spleen

Variable in size and shape, the **normal spleen** can always be identified on upper abdominal ultrasound scanning. Entirely intercostal unless "long and thin", the spleen is best identified in the right lateral decubitus position, although it can be imaged with the patient supine. Its internal echopattern is homogeneous and less echogenic than that of the normal liver. The **splenic vessels** can be identified at the splenic hilum.

Pitfalls in normal anatomy

1. **Air in the lungs** will cause artefact, preventing the entire subdiaphragmatic splenic surface being seen on a single scan.

2. If the spleen can not be seen, ask the question, "has it been removed?" A lot of time can be wasted trying to image structures that are not there. (The same question applies to the gallbladder and the kidney, especially in the age of keyhole surgery.)

Abnormal ultrasound appearances of the spleen

Splenic calcification

A not unusual finding in the elderly, splenic calcification is seen as echogenic areas casting acoustic shadows. It is necessary to confirm that it is not splenic arterial calcification, with colour Doppler or plain abdominal X-ray. Old **calcified hydatid cysts** have a characteristic appearance on ultrasound and plain film.

Splenic infarcts

Most splenic infarcts are not detected with ultrasound. Poorly echogenic areas may be seen within the spleen acutely, with later development of echogenic scarred areas of fibrosis. In patients with sickle-cell disease, the spleen may be absent after multiple infarcts.

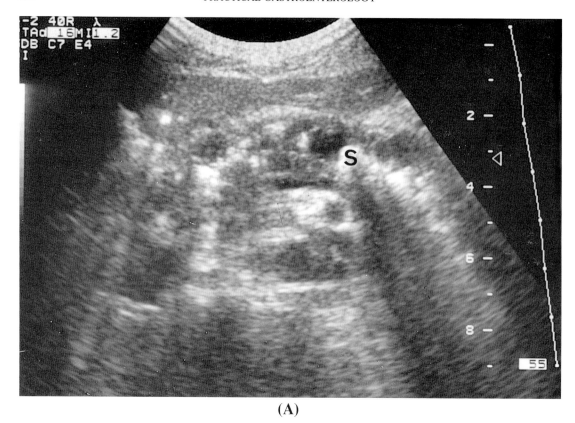

(A)

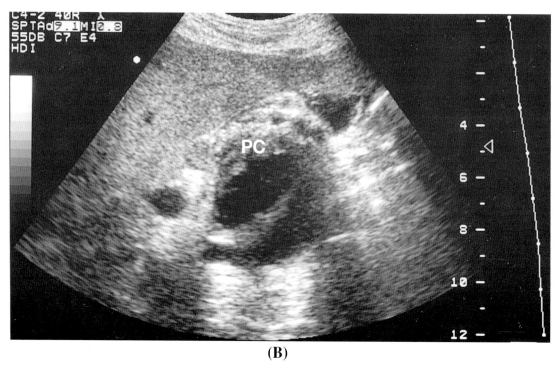

(B)

Figure 48.20.   A: Chronic calcific pancreatitis, stones (S) in dilated pancreatic duct. B: Pseudocyst with calcified wall (PC) in head of pancreas.

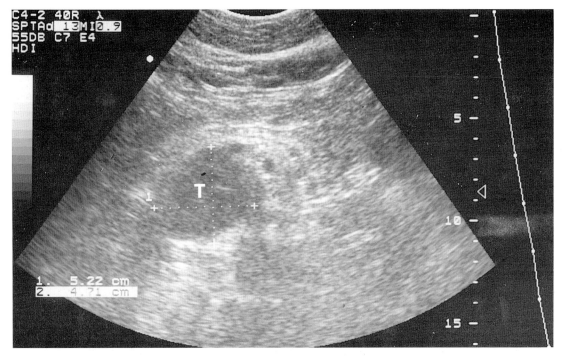

Figure 48.21. Tumour (T) of the head of the pancreas.

Splenic cysts

Splenic cysts are not uncommon incidental findings. Trans-sonic, with bright-up behind, they may contain low-level echoes and reach a considerable size. On questioning, the patient will often give a history of old trauma. The differential diagnosis is a splenic hydatid cyst.

Splenic trauma

Ultrasound will demonstrate intrasplenic and extrasplenic **haematoma** and splenic capsular **rupture**, but should not be used to make the diagnosis of splenic damage in the acute situation, when the diagnosis should be clinical and, if imaging is needed, CT scan with intravenous contrast is the investigation of choice.

Splenomegaly

Ultrasound may be helpful to confirm or refute clinical splenomegaly, whatever the cause. The appearance of the enlarged spleen is often that of **diffuse homogeneous enlargement**, and is therefore non-specific.

The **collateral vessels of portal hypertension** will be seen on ultrasound, especially if colour Doppler is used.

Lymphomatous deposits within the spleen are less echogenic than the surrounding normal spleen; **metastatic deposits**, while usually less echogenic, may be the reverse.

The majority of **splenic metastases** are not imaged by ultrasound.

Pyogenic splenic abscesses, are usually less echogenic than the surrounding spleen, but may have thick walls and mixed internal echoes; they can be drained by ultrasound-guided techniques.

Fungal abscesses are often small, multiple, and poorly echogenic.

After splenectomy

Ultrasound may detect recurrent splenic tissue or splenunculus, but isotope study is more reliable.

Diagnostic pitfalls in ultrasound scanning of the spleen

1. Homogeneous splenomegaly is a **non-specific** finding.
2. **Splenic metastases** and **splenic lymphoma** are commonly not imaged by ultrasound. CT scans are more sensitive at detecting splenic involvement in a malignant process.

3. **Fungal abscesses** can not be differentiated from lymphoma deposits on ultrasound appearances.
4. A **large adrenal or renal tumour mass** may be misinterpreted as a large spleen if scan technique procedures are not followed.

THE BOWEL AND PERITONEAL CAVITY

Transabdominal ultrasound scanning is generally not considered to be a first-line investigation in disorders of the bowel. There are, however, occasions when it can be a valuable diagnostic tool.

Normal anatomy

When standard transabdominal scan equipment and techniques are used, the five individual layers of the bowel wall may not be identified. In **transverse section**, the bowel wall (4–5 mm thick) is a poorly echogenic ring with central bright echoes from mucin and intraluminal gas; in **longitudinal section**, it is a tube with poorly echogenic walls and a bright centre. The appearance of the bowel lumen will be determined by its contents. If the lumen is fluid filled, the bowel wall thickness and luminal diameter can be measured, and small bowel loops observed for peristaltic activity. Collapsed, empty bowel loops can also be identified.

The central peritoneal cavity containing bowel and mesentery is seen as a mixture of bright and less bright echoes, with little anatomical form on conventional ultrasound scanning. Mesenteric nodes are sometimes seen.

Pitfalls in normal bowel anatomy

1. The presence of **gas** or **gas-containing faecal residue** within the bowel diminishes ultrasound as a useful imaging modality, causing artefacts that obscure both the bowel itself and underlying or adjacent structures.
2. The **peritoneal surface of bowel loops** can not be precisely identified in the normal abdomen.

Abnormal ultrasound appearances of bowel and peritoneal cavity

Gastric outlet obstruction/small bowel obstruction
A distended, fluid-filled stomach, gastric residue, or both, in a fasted patient characterize these conditions.

Fluid-filled small-bowel loops of diameter greater than 2.5 cm with visible valvulae connivantes confirms jejunal dilatation (Figure 48.22). When the loops are featureless and greater than 3 cm in diameter, the ileum is implicated.

Active small-bowel peristaltic waves excludes and absent peristalsis confirms the presence of **small-bowel ileus**.

A thickened bowel wall and the identification of a "triple" layer of bowel wall are apparent in an **intussusception**.

Large-bowel obstruction
The presence of a distended, gas-filled large and small bowel renders ultrasound of little diagnostic use. Plain supine abdominal X-ray and erect chest X-ray to exclude or confirm the presence of subdiaphragmatic gas after bowel perforation comprise the first-line investigation.

Free fluid in the peritoneal cavity
If there is only a **small amount** of free fluid in the peritoneal cavity, a triangular **subhepatic** fluid collection is often to be detected first, along the inferior right hepatic margin in the region of the gallbladder bed. Further small collections may be seen in the pelvis and flanks.

If there is **free fluid**, both sides of both the gallbladder and bowel wall are identifiable.

Bilateral subphrenic collections, together with **pleural effusions**, will be seen to outline both sides of the diaphragm, an ultrasound.

Intraabdominal abscess
Ultrasound is better than CT in determining the **composition** of an abscess — that is, whether it is fluid or solid material. Appearances are determined, to a large extent, by how long the abscess has been present.

Fluid collections can be free or loculated and are trans-sonic, with "bright-up" behind. There may be mixed internal echoes, and sometimes, septae. Fluid may surround bowel loops, and collections may have echogenic mesentery or a poorly echogenic inflammatory mass draped over or around them.

CT scanning is indicated to define the **extent** of the abscess and to decide the best **access route** before CT or ultrasound-guided drainage.

Appendicitis
The **normal appendix** can be seen on ultrasound as a blind-ended tube with poorly echogenic walls

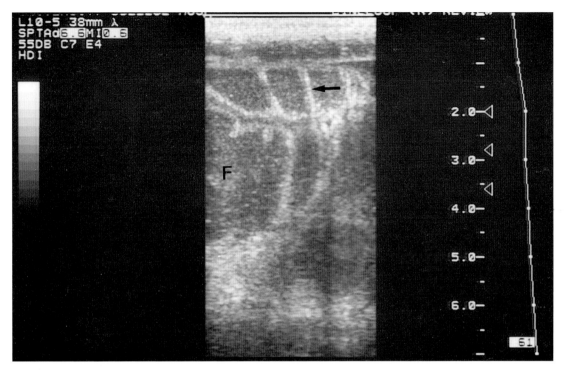

Figure 48.22.   Small-bowel obstruction with dilated fluid filled jejunal loops, fluid residue (F), valvulae conniventes (arrow).

(2–3 mm thick, transverse diameter less than 6 mm) and bright central echoes in about 50% of normal scans. If **appendicitis** is **suspected** but not certain, ultrasound may assist diagnosis if it identifies either a normal or abnormal appendix, especially if the appendix is retrocaecal. In **acute appendicitis**, ultrasound scanning will localize the point of maximum tenderness.

A distended, non-compressible appendix with surrounding bright echoes from fat, a thickened wall, a poorly echogenic line of intramural oedema, and echogenic faecoliths impacted in the neck or lumen of the appendix point to a **diagnosis** of acute appendicitis. An associated poorly echogenic inflammatory mass containing fluid (pus), echogenic solid material, and draped echogenic mesentery or adherent bowel may coexist. There may be free fluid outlining bowel loops (11) (Figure 48.23).

Other causes of an abdominal mass of bowel origin

In **ileocaecal Crohn's disease**, under ideal circumstances, ultrasound can accurately determine the **distribution** of Crohn's disease and the **length of ileal segment** involved. It can characterize a **palpable mass**, demonstrating the poorly echogenic thickened bowel wall, the adherent bowel loops, and the inflammatory mass that may be associated with Crohn's disease (Figure 48.24). Its use as an indicator of disease activity is limited (12). Fistula and sinuses are best imaged with magnetic resonance imaging.

Doppler studies of the **superior mesenteric artery** suggest that an increase in the flow rate within the artery can be measured and monitored in the presence of active Crohn's disease.

Similar appearances may be seen in association with lymphoma, tuberculosis, and amoeboma.

Lymphoma of the bowel is seen as poorly echogenic complex mass on ultrasound involving bowel. The appearances are non-specific, but ultrasound may be helpful in monitoring the response to treatment once the diagnosis has been made.

In **diverticular disease**, **diverticulitis** and **diverticular abscess**, bowel-wall thickening and gas within a diverticulum may be imaged with ultrasound, but are often missed because of overlying

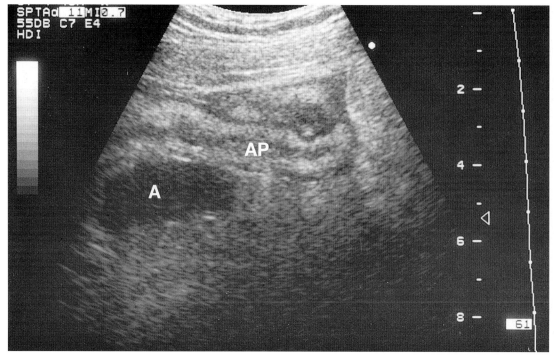

Figure 48.23.   Acute appendicitis with local abscess; AP appendix; A local abscess.

bowel gas and residue. After perforation or abscess formation an inflammatory mass may be imaged, but CT is a better technique for both detecting and mapping the extent. Differentiation from a malignant mass is not possible with ultrasound.

Colonic tumours may be seen as poorly echogenic masses (thickened bowel wall) with central bright echoes (lumen). They are more often imaged if there is a large extramural component. Most tumours detected are greater than 2 cm in size and be causing at least a 50% stenosis of the bowel lumen. Secondary findings associated with the tumour may include perforation or obstruction, lymphadenopathy, and hepatic metastases (Figure 48.25).

Diagnostic pitfalls in ultrasound scanning of the bowel and peritoneal cavity

1. The presence of **gas** whether intraluminal, intramural, or intra-abdominal may make a diagnostic ultrasound examination of the bowel or peritoneum impossible to perform. A **plain abdominal X-ray film** will detect dilated, gas-filled small- and large-bowel loops, gas in the bowel wall, free gas within the peritoneum or retroperitoneum, and the abnormal gas patterns sometimes seen within an abscess cavity. An **erect chest X-ray** will demonstrate free subdiaphragmatic gas.

2. **Gas within an abscess** will make ultrasound assessment of the size and contents of the abscess unreliable, even if the abscess is imaged. Ultrasound will not define a complex inflammatory mass containing bowel and mesentery; CT is the preferred imaging modality in both instances.

3. The majority of pathologies affecting the bowel will not be detected using abdominal ultrasound.

4. **Peritoneal deposits** are seldom seen on ultrasound, even in the presence of ascites.

5. Any pathological process infiltrating the bowel and leading to bowel wall thickening may be detected on ultrasound, but the appearances are non-specific, although the clinical history may give the clue (e.g. haematoma in a patient taking anticoagulants).

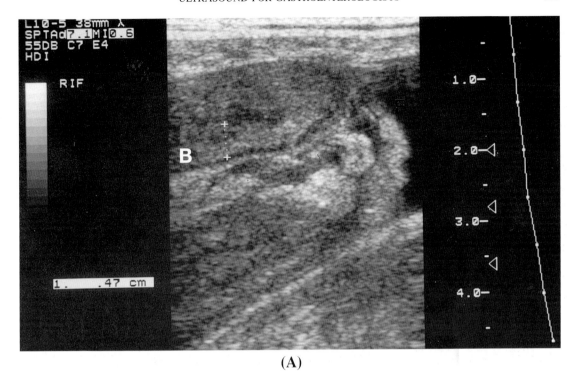

(A)

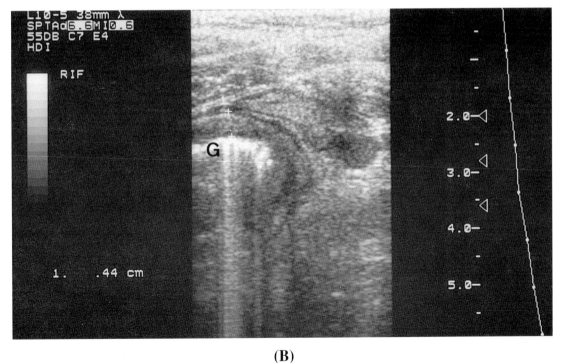

(B)

Figure 48.24.   A: Inflammatory bowel mass at ileocaecal junction B, Thickened bowel wall; F, Free fluid. B: Transverse view. G, gas in the bowel lumen.

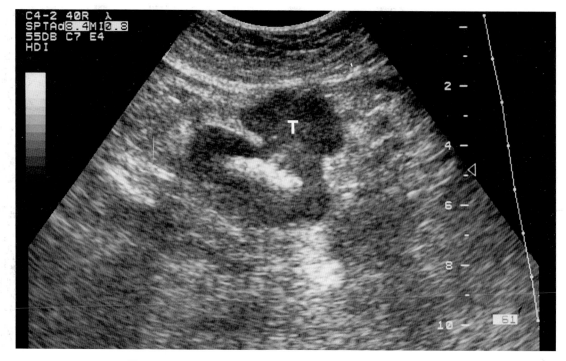

Figure 48.25.   Colonic carcinoma with extramural tumour extension (T).

SUMMARY

Abdominal ultrasound will continue to be the first-line investigation for many symptoms presenting to the gastroenterologist for the foreseeable future. On some occasions, ultrasound will provide the definitive answer to a problem but its role is usually to guide the clinician to the next diagnostic step.

References

1. Lonardo A, Bellini M, Tartoni P *et al.* The bright liver syndrome. Prevalence and determinants of a "bright" liver echopattern. *Ital J Gastroenterol Hepatol* 1997; **29**: 351–356.
    Twenty per cent of Italian patients undergoing routine ultrasound will have a bright liver.
2. Abbitt LP. Ultrasonography. Update on liver technique. *Radiol Clin North Am* 1998; **36**: 299–307.
    An overview of the current place of ultrasound in the investigation of liver disease, with particular reference to the role of Doppler ultrasound.
3. Meek DR, Mills PR, Gray HW *et al.* A comparison of computed tomography, ultrasound and scintigraphy in the diagnosis of alcoholic liver disease. *Br J Radiol* 1984; **57**: 23–27.
    In patients with proven liver disease, abnormal studies present on CT in 83%, on ultrasound in 64%, and on scintigraphy in 94%.
4. Dodd GD, Miller WJ, Baron RL *et al.* Detection of malignant tumours in end stage cirrhotic liver: efficacy of sonography as a screening technique. *Am J Roentgenol* 1992; **159**: 727–733.
    Sensitivity of ultrasound in the cirrhotic liver was less than 50%.
5. Hagspiel KD, Neidl K, Eichenberger AC *et al.* Detection of liver metastases: comparison of supermagnetic iron oxide-enhanced and unenhanced MR imaging at 1.5 T with dynamic CT, intraoperative US, and percutaneous US. *Radiology* 1995; **196**: 471–478.
    Magnetic resonance imaging with iron oxide was more sensitive than CT, including CT arterial portography and percutaneous ultrasound but remained inferior to interoperative ultrasound for the detection of metastatic liver disease.
6. Leen E, Angerson WJ, Wotherspoon H *et al.* Detection of colorectal metastases: comparison of laparotomy, CT, US and Doppler perfusion index and evaluation of postoperative follow-up results. *Radiology* 1995; **195**: 113–116.
    Colour Doppler ultrasound measurement of the Doppler perfusion index is the most sensitive technique in the detection of liver metastases.
7. Wu CC, Ho YH, Chen CY. Effect of ageing on common bile duct diameter: a real-time ultrasonographic study. *J Clin Ultrasound* 1984; **12**: 473–478.
8. Mittelstaedt CA. Ultrasound of the bile ducts [review]. *Semin Roentgenol* 1997; **32**: 161–167.
9. Moriguchi H, Tazawa J, Hayashi Y *et al.* The natural history of polypoid lesions in the gallbladder. *Gut* 1996; **39**: 860–862.

Most gallbladder polyps detected on ultrasound are benign.

10. London NJM, Neoptolemos JP, Lavelle J *et al.* Serial computed tomography scanning in acute pancreatitis: a prospective study. *Gut* 1989; **30**: 397–403.

More than 90% of CT scans performed within 72 h of the patient's admission to hospital are abnormal in those with acute pancreatitis.

11. Wade DS, Morrow SE, Balsara ZN *et al.* Accuracy of ultrasound in the diagnosis of acute appendicitis compared with the surgeon's clinical impression. *Arch Surg* 1993; **128**: 1039–1046.

12. Maconi G, Parente F, Bollani S *et al.* Abdominal ultrasound in the assessment of extent and activity of Crohn's disease: clinical significance and implication of bowel wall thickening. *Am J Gastroenterol* 1996; **91**: 1604–1609.

49. Radiological and Magnetic Resonance Imaging of the Gastrointestinal Tract

ALICE GILLAMS

BARIUM STUDIES

Positive intraluminal contrast, two-dimensional projectional X-ray examinations usually use barium as the contrast medium, and have come to be known by that name. These examinations were the mainstay of gastrointestinal imaging, but are now being challenged by cross-sectional imaging. **Barium swallow** and **barium meal** examinations are still requested for motility abnormalities and in patients who decline endoscopy. Similarly, **barium enema** has been reserved for those in whom colonoscopy is contraindicated or fails; however, it is likely that barium enema will largely be replaced by computed tomography (CT) pneumocolon studies (see below), not least because patient acceptability of barium enema is so low. Nevertheless, there remains a need for the "instant enema" in large-bowel obstruction, to define the level and, potentially, show the cause of the obstruction. Barium studies will also exclude anatomical obstruction in pseudo-obstruction, and they remain the preferred method of investigation in this context. Similarly, intraluminal contrast is still used to check the integrity of surgical anastomoses. Although complete colonoscopy affords better detection of lesions than do double-contrast barium examinations, because of the appreciable incidence of failure of the colonoscopist to reach the right colon (and more importantly, failing to realize that the study was incomplete), there have been studies showing a superiority for barium enema in detection of right-sided colonic lesions.

Optimal visualization of the small bowel is still achieved by **barium enteroclysis**, which requires intubation of the duodenum, but provides better-quality images, and a more detailed and more complete study than the **barium follow-through**, in which the patient is asked to drink the contrast agent. More recently, CT enteroclysis is being favoured as the optimal method for the detection of focal mass lesions.

COMPUTED TOMOGRAPHY

Basic principles

CT uses finely collimated X-ray beams to produce a series of **attenuation profiles** through the patient, from which **cross-sectional images** can be computed (1). The CT gantry, which rotates around the patient, contains the X-ray generator and multiple X-ray detectors that record the attenuation value of the X-ray beams as they emerge from the patient. Different tissues attenuate the X-ray beam by different amounts, and this forms the basis of tissue contrast. Fat, air, haemorrhage, and calcification have specific attenuation values or CT numbers. CT numbers are measured in Hounsfield Units (HU) and expressed relative to water. Unlike quantification with ultrasound or magnetic resonance techniques, CT attenuation values are absolute measurements, and are highly reproducible between patients.

While older CT scanners produced sequential two-dimensional cross-sections through the body, the most recent technology — helical or spiral CT — produces a volume of contiguous data with image acquisition times of less than 1 s per revolution (2,3). Volume data acquisition is important, as this improves multiplanar and three-dimensional reconstruction, increases lesion detection by allowing reconstruction at different intervals, and pre-empts the possibility of misregistration. The increased speed of acquisition allows the whole abdomen to be scanned within a single breath-hold, allows image acquisition to be timed to the optimal phase of contrast enhancement, and reduces examination time.

Clinical utility

CT has increased in sophistication: different ways in which the patient is prepared, and how the images are obtained will yield different information. The concept of a "CT abdomen" has nearly disappeared. To get the most from CT, the technique is tailored to answer specific clinical problems and questions.

CT reliably provides more reproducible image quality and more complete anatomical coverage than ultrasound. Whereas the image quality of ultrasound is degraded by the larger size of a patient, CT image quality is degraded only for the very large patient; indeed, a modicum of intraperitoneal fat is useful in CT, as the fat outlines the surfaces of the different organs. Some difficulties in interpretation arise in the very cachectic, because of loss of fat. Bowel gas, which reflects the ultrasound beam, rendering ultrasound ineffective in the examination of structures deep to gas, does not interfere with CT images and so CT is ideal for examining the pancreas and retroperitoneum.

Oral contrast, traditionally in the form of dilute barium, but currently using water, can be of value in distending the bowel — for example, it can distend the duodenum when the pancreas is under investigation. Unless the specific remit is the identification of calcification (e.g. as part of the diagnosis of chronic pancreatitis), or the measurement of liver attenuation values (e.g. in suspected haemochromatosis), CT studies are performed after the administration of an **intravenous bolus of iodinated contrast**. Image acquisition can be timed to different phases of the contrast cycle — for example, the arterial or the venous phase, or the equilibrium phase during which contrast is predominantly in the parenchyma. Optimization of the timing of contrast imaging will improve detection of certain lesions and will aid lesion characterization. To emphasize this point, examination during the wrong phase of contrast will result in lesions being missed and incorrect diagnoses being made.

Liver and biliary tract

Focal liver lesions

CT will detect more than 90% of focal lesions in the liver (4–6). Lesions as small as 5–6 mm in diameter can be seen; however, it is not always possible to characterize very small lesions.

Tumours

CT will detect many more liver metastases than ultrasound, and when the exact size, number, and distribution of metastases is important for the subsequent management of the patient, CT is indicated. CT not only detects more lesions and smaller lesions but, by enabling study of the vascularity of the lesion, can offer some specificity. In the assessment of the liver, the **arterial phase** of enhancement is useful for the delineation of hypervascular lesions such as hepatocellular carcinoma or neuroendocrine metastases (Figure 49.1A,B). The **portal venous phase** is optimal for the detection of hypovascular metastases such as colorectal secondaries (Figure 49.1C). Delayed images maybe required for the diagnosis of haemangioma; 93% become isodense, to some degree, on delayed images and the characteristic incremental, centripetal enhancement is seen in 72% (7). Nevertheless, the most reliable sign for a haemangioma is peripheral contrast enhancement, nodular, discontinuous, and of an intensity equal to that of adjacent vessels (Figure 49.1D).

Inflammatory lesions

Simple cysts are a common incidental finding, of no clinical significance unless very large. **Abscesses** can be differentiated from simple cysts by a thick, enhancing wall. **Gas**, when present is useful to make the diagnosis of an abscess, but is only seen in 20% of cases. With the exception of gas, abscesses can often not be differentiated from noninjected fluid collections, and aspiration is required for the diagnosis. *Echinococcus granulosus* produces

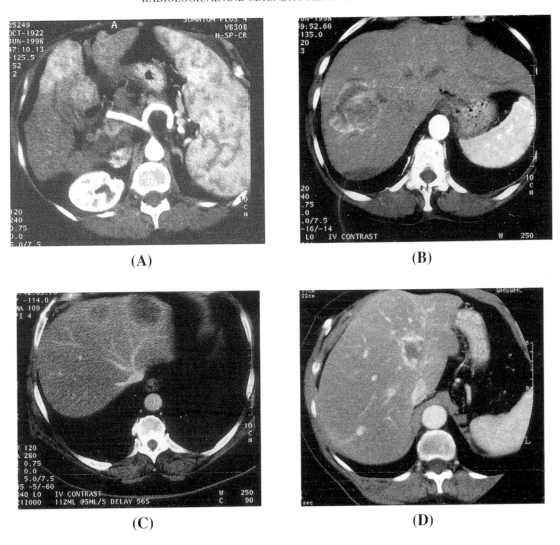

Figure 49.1. CT of the liver. A: Cirrhotic liver that is small and irregular in outline, with hypervascular hepatocellular carcinoma. B: Hypervascular metastasis from a neuroendocrine tumour, showing marked enhancement relative to normal liver during the arterial phase. C: Colorectal metastases, hypoattenuating to normal liver during the portal venous phase of enhancement, with some peripheral enhancement. D: Haemangioma, showing characteristic peripheral enhancement pattern, with contrast isoattenuating to adjacent vessels.

well defined, uni- or multi-loculated cysts, sometimes with septae, calcification (rim or septal), and daughter cysts. Daughter cysts are usually of lower attenuation than the mother cyst, and this can aid the diagnosis.

Diffuse liver disease

Diffuse fatty infiltration of the liver will cause a focal reduction in attenuation value, whereas increased attenuation values occur in **haemochromatosis**, **Wilson's disease**, or **haemosiderosis**. Although the attenuation value may be mildly increased in cirrhosis from any cause, it is usually normal. In some patients with **cirrhosis**, the liver will appear entirely normal, but often there are changes in contour, size, and homogeneity (Figure 49.1A). A well recognized configuration is enlargement of the caudate and lateral segments of the left lobe, with shrinkage of the right lobe. Other findings include ascites, splenomegaly, portal hypertension, varices, hepatocellular carcinoma, or regenerating nodules. Regenerating nodules are usually isointense with normal liver and detected by contour abnormality but, occasionally, they are hyperattenuating and can simulate a mass lesion. It can be difficult to differentiate regenerating nodules from hepatocellular carcinoma in patients with cirrhosis. Varices are seen as round, serpiginous, enhancing structures in the porta hepatis, perigastric, oesophageal, periumbilical, and splenic regions.

Biliary tract

CT is very sensitive to bile duct dilatation and will show the level and cause of **biliary obstruction** in the majority of cases. Normal **intrahepatic bile ducts** are seen as small tubular lucencies measuring 1–3 mm in diameter, running adjacent to portal venous radicles. The **common hepatic duct** is a thin-walled structure measuring 3–6 mm in diameter and is best seen after intravenous contrast. The normal **common bile duct** is slightly larger — up to 8 mm in diameter, with a wall thickness less than 1.5 mm. It is readily appreciated coursing through the enhancing pancreatic parenchyma. Although CT is less reliable than ultrasound in the detection of gallstones, it is more likely to show **common bile duct stones**. The best published figures for CT give a sensitivity of 79% for gallstones, whereas the sensitivity of CT for common bile duct stones is approximately 85%, compared with 19% for ultrasound. Calcified common bile duct stones are readily detected, but account for only 20%; the more common, soft-tissue-density stone, which occurs in 50% of cases, may be appreciated only as a faint density, surrounded by a rim of bile.

Cholangiocarcinoma

The most common bile-duct malignancy, cholangiocarcinoma usually arises in the proximal extrahepatic ducts. Three morphological patterns are recognized: peripheral exophytic masses, a central infiltrating type and, rarely, a polypoid intramural tumour. The bulky mass type is usually seen as a low-attenuation mass lesion, but delayed images, 15–20 min after injection of intravenous contrast, may detect abnormal enhancement. The infiltrating lesion poses difficulties on all imaging modalities, with no tumour mass identifiable and eccentric bile-duct wall thickening being the only abnormality.

Pancreas

Pancreatic size, contour, attenuation, enhancement, calcification, and ductal anatomy are all exquisitely shown by CT, if dedicated pancreatic protocols are used (Figure 49.2).

Acute pancreatitis

Diffuse or focal swelling of the gland is one of the most common manifestations of acute pancreatitis; focal change is seen in 48% of cases. **Other common CT signs** are blurring of the pancreatic margins and thickening of the renal fascia. Focal thickening of the gastric wall has been described in 70% of cases. Peripancreatic fluid or pancreatic fluid collections are well delineated; they are often complex and multiloculated, and may track as far as the thigh or extend up into the chest (Figure 49.2C). Pancreatic **phlegmon** occurs in more than 50% of severe attacks, and has an overall incidence of 18%. The phlegmon is seen as a boggy, oedematous, soft-tissue mass composed of inflammation, exudate, and retroperitoneal fat. In mild cases of acute pancreatitis, the CT can appear normal.

The particular value of CT in acute pancreatitis is in defining the complications of acute pancreatitis, haemorrhage, abscess, or pseudocyst formation (Figure 49.2B). **Haemorrhage** is seen in 5% of cases as a focal collection of high attenuation (>60 HU) in the pancreatic area. Venous thrombosis and pseudoaneurysm formation are well shown by CT. **Pseudocysts** form in 10% of cases when pancreatic or peripancreatic fluid collections become loculated and fixed by a dense fibrous capsule. Small pockets of gas may be detected by CT in 30–50% of cases. In the absence of extraneous sources (e.g. fistulae or prior intervention), the diagnosis of **abscess** can be made. If gas is not present, abscesses are indistinguishable from non-infected phlegmons or pseudocysts. If infection is suspected, image-guided fine-needle aspiration and bacteriological analysis are recommended. CT also has a role in predicting the prognosis in patients in whom early CT findings correlate well with the severity of the attack and the development of complications (8).

Chronic pancreatitis

Non-enhanced CT will detect even tiny flecks of **pancreatic calcification** not appreciated on any other imaging modality. Normal pancreatic ducts

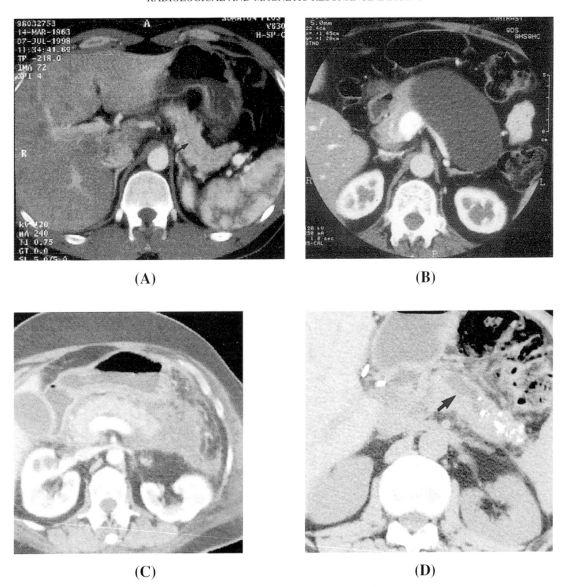

Figure 49.2. CT of the pancreas. A: Normal tail of pancreas showing normal pancreatic parenchymal enhancement. The normal pancreatic duct is visible (arrow). B: Pseudocyst formation in the body and tail of the pancreas. The cyst narrows the splenic vein. C: Acute pancreatitis. Low-attenuation inflammatory change is present around the head and body of the pancreas and extends along Gerota's fascia. D: Chronic pancreatitis. Calcifications, duct dilatation (arrow), and parenchymal atrophy are the hallmark features.

are seen in 70% of scans, measuring on average 3 mm in the head and tapering towards the tail. CT detects 100% of **dilated ducts**, and often shows the relationship of calculi to the pancreatic duct. Atrophy of the parenchyma is a common sequel of chronic inflammation and is readily appreciated by CT (Figure 49.2D).

Neoplasms

Change in the size and contour of the gland are the most frequent features of pancreatic cancer. Both are fraught with diagnostic difficulty because of the high incidence of normal variation. Furthermore, small lesions, less than 3 cm, which are most likely to be operable, often do not change the size or contour of the gland. Differential contrast-enhancement patterns are important for diagnosis. **Ductal adenocarcinoma** is hypovascular relative to normal pancreatic parenchyma, 25–30 s after the injection of contrast, but rapidly becomes isoattenuating, therefore early scans are essential. A central zone of low attenuation has been reported in 83% of pancreatic tumours. However, the area of low attenuation does not correspond exactly to the tumour margin and will underestimate tumour size. CT consistently underestimates tumour extent.

Where CT shows **evidence of inoperability**, it has been shown to be 100% accurate. Obliteration of peripancreatic fat planes is most commonly the result of direct invasion; the planes can appear normal in the presence of microscopic invasion. When the fat plane between the mass and an adjacent vessel is lost, vascular invasion is inevitably present. Involved vessels can be displaced, narrowed, irregular, or occluded — all features indicating inoperability. The incidence of vascular invasion varies from 32–84%.

Lymph-node **metastases** occur around the coeliac axis or superior mesenteric vessels, in the para-aortic, retrocrural, pericaval regions, or along the porta hepatis; the reported incidence is 38–65%. Hepatic metastases are seen in 17–55% of cases of pancreatic cancer.

Neuroendocrine tumours demonstrate a characteristic, dense, homogeneous, hypervascular pattern. As patients with secreting neuroendocrine lesions present when the tumours are very small, CT may fail to show the lesion. In these patients, the most sensitive method for detection is invasive ultrasound, either endoscopic or intraoperative.

Reticuloendothelial system

Spleen

Splenic longitudinal diameter or volume can be measured by CT. Focal lesions — cysts, abscesses, metastases, and infarcts — have appearances similar to those described in the liver.

Lymphadenopathy

None of the cross-sectional imaging studies offer information about internal lymph node architecture. The criteria used for detection of neoplastic involvement of lymph nodes are based on the increasing statistical likelihood of involvement with increasing size; some nodes that contain tumour but are not enlarged may therefore be seen on CT, but can not be differentiated from normal nodes. Similarly, inflammatory nodal enlargement looks the same as metastatic enlargement. CT is more reliable than ultrasound in the detection of enlarged nodes in the retroperitoneum, small-bowel mesentery, or adjacent to the lesser curve of the stomach. Nodes with a short-axis diameter greater than 1 cm are considered to be significantly enlarged.

Gastrointestinal tract

Oesophagus

The main indication for CT is in **staging of oesophageal cancer**: CT will accurately depict the tumour extent in 84%. The normal wall thickness is less than 3 mm, wall thickness greater than 5 mm is abnormal, and 3–5 mm is indeterminate. Signs of invasion are loss of tissue fat planes between the mass and the neighbouring structures or, in the aortic arch, contiguity over more than 90° of the aortic surface. The most common pitfall lies in assessment of the gastrooesophageal junction, where the horizontal course of the oesophagus produces the effect of a localized mass. It should also be remembered that prior radiotherapy will obliterate fat planes. CT is not very good at detecting local nodal involvement, which is more accurately shown by endoscopic ultrasound.

Stomach

Normal gastric-wall thickness in a well-distended stomach is less than 5 mm; any measurement greater than 1 cm is considered abnormal. CT has been used for the staging of gastric cancer, but the results are disappointing. Understaging occurs as a result of normal sized but involved lymph nodes, the inability to detect peritoneal disease, and poor detection of pancreatic invasion. In addition, CT overstages in 16% of cases.

Bowel

Specialized techniques to improve visualization of the bowel include CT enteroclysis and pneumocolon (Figure 49.3A). Even without special preparation for visualization of the bowel, spiral CT often provides

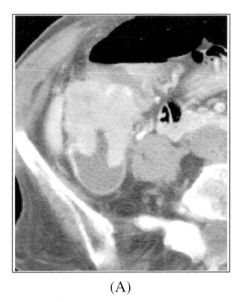
(A)

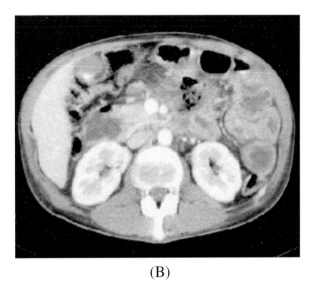
(B)

Figure 49.3. CT of the bowel. A: CT pneumocolon shows an enhancing colon cancer in the caecum. B: CT in patient with treated small-bowel lymphoma who became acutely unwell, with an increased white cell count. CT shows air outside the bowel, secondary to perforation of the duodenum.

useful information about **bowel pathology**. Bowel-wall thickening, masses — either inflammatory or neoplastic — or fluid collections are easily appreciated (Figure 49.3B). CT will detect even small amounts of fluid, either free or in collections, and will show some fluid collections that have not been visualized on ultrasound. Lack of ultrasound visualization is usually the result of the presence of overlying bowel gas. Barium studies are still preferred for the diagnosis of **Crohn's disease**, but CT is useful in detection and delineation of complications, and will show the extraluminal component of the disease that is only inferred from intraluminal studies. Abscesses, fistulae, and fibrofatty mesenteric infiltration are all well depicted by CT.

CT enteroclysis technique

CT enteroclysis uses the conventional technique of nasojejunal intubation, bowel paralysis and contrast instillation followed by spiral CT acquisition, instead of conventional two-dimensional projection X-ray imaging. If the lumen is correctly distended, the normal bowel wall measures 2–3 mm and demonstrates homogeneous, smooth enhancement after intravenous contrast. Bowel-wall thickening, fold thickening, and changes in enhancement should be

sought. Bowel-wall thickening associated with a target sign — alternating layers of high and low attenuation representing, in turn, enhancing mucosa, oedematous submucosa, and enhancing serosa — is usually indicative of benign disease.

CT pneumocolon technique

In the past few years, a number of techniques have been tried to optimize cross-sectional imaging of the large bowel, using different methods of bowel distension and different types of contrast. The optimal technique uses bowel paralysis, rectal air insufflation into a prepared colon, and spiral CT acquisition during a bolus injection of intravenous contrast. The advantages compared with traditional barium studies include delineation of pathology on both sides of the bowel lumen, complete coverage of the remainder of the abdomen (e.g. liver and lymph nodes in staging cancer), and improved patient acceptability. In addition, three-dimensional data sets can easily be generated from CT data and used to provide multiplanar interactive viewing of pathology or "fly through" virtual colonoscopy.

Cancers appear as well-demarcated, irregular, enhancing mass lesions, and **diverticular strictures** as long segments of smooth bowel-wall thickening with associated diverticulae. CT pneumocolon has been evaluated in the staging and detection of polyps and cancer. Although this technique reliably detects polyps of diameter greater than 1 cm, smaller polyps may go undetected.

The utility of CT pneumocolon in inflammatory bowel disease is not established.

MAGNETIC RESONANCE IMAGING

Basic principles

Magnetic resonance images are derived from the returning radio frequency signal released from relaxing hydrogen nuclei (protons) (1). To obtain a magnetic resonance image, the patient is placed within a strong magnetic field, which will cause protons to align with the main magnetic field. The protons are then displaced from their aligned position by a radio frequency pulse of a particular frequency. When that pulse is switched off, the protons relax back to their original alignment and release the absorbed radio frequency energy. The timing of the relaxation depends on the type of molecule and on the matrix environment of the proton. Two commonly referred to **relaxation constants** are **T1** and **T2** and these are usually measured in milliseconds. T1 refers to the time it takes for the protons to return to their original aligned position, and T2 refers to the period of time the returning protons maintain coherence with each other. These relaxation times vary for different tissues, and this forms the basis of magnetic resonance tissue contrast. The magnetic resonance scanner can be programmed to produce images that emphasize different features of the tissues being studied — for example, a T2-weighted image will bring out the differences in T2 in different tissues. Other sequences can be used to look specifically at flowing blood or stationary fluid, or to suppress signal specifically from fat or from fluid. By using techniques such as these, magnetic resonance imaging (MRI) offers tissue specificity that is not realized by other imaging technologies.

Clinical utility

Although early MRI scanners were very slow, with protracted image acquisition times, recent developments have resulted in breath-hold imaging. This has revolutionized the role of MRI in imaging the abdomen. The liver or the pancreas can effectively be covered in two or three breath-holds. MRI, like ultrasound, is multiplanar in a way that CT has yet to rival. It enjoys much greater soft-tissue contrast than either CT or ultrasound, and the spatial resolution is now nearly as good as that of CT. The disadvantage of the technique is the need for a reasonably cooperative patient, who can cope without claustrophobia in an enclosed environment. There are some absolute contraindications: some electronic and metallic implants do not operate within the magnetic field or are interfered with by the changing radio frequency pulses and localizer gradients (e.g. cochlear implants, some artificial heart valves, and most types of pacemaker). Lack of availability of MRI compared with both CT and ultrasound results in MRI being used for complex or problem cases, or to solve specific problems that other imaging tests can not. Table 49.1 summarizes the major differences between CT and MRI.

Liver and biliary tract

The MRI sequences that show signal from stationary fluid whilst suppressing signal from parenchyma can be used to define the **ductal anatomy** of the biliary system or pancreas, without the injection of any contrast media (9,10). These sequences provide images non-invasively, with information very similar to that obtained on endoscopic retrograde cholangiopancreatography (ERCP) (Figure 49.4). Duct dilatation, strictures, and calculi are demonstrated. Magnetic resonance cholangiopancreatography (MRCP) can be combined with magnetic resonance images of the liver and pancreatic parenchyma, and so provide, in one examination, the type of information that previously required CT and ERCP. MRCP has almost 100% sensitivity for biliary obstruction, better than 93% sensitivity for the detection of calculi, and better than 95% sensitivity for establishing the cause of obstruction. However, it will not show subtle duct changes, for example in minimal-change pancreatitis or early primary sclerosing cholangitis.

Focal liver lesions and diffuse liver disease

Historically, CT was better than MRI in liver imaging, but the introduction of **liver-specific contrast agents** (e.g. superparamagnetic iron oxide particles (SPIO)), which are taken up by normal

Table 49.1. A comparison of the features of CT and MRI.

Features	CT	MRI
Multiplanar capability	Only with reconstruction and limited resolution	Any plane, any obliquity
Calcification	Very sensitive to small quantities on non-enhanced studies	Can miss even substantial calcific densities on optimised procedures
Soft-tissue contrast	Moderate	Unparalleled
Radiation	Yes	No
Contrast agents	Intraluminal and intravascular	Organ specific
Specificity	Haemorrhage, air, calcification, fat	Stationary fluid, moving fluid, haemorrhage, solid fat, fibrosis
Speed	Abdomen and pelvis can be covered in single breath hold	Most examinations take 20–40 minutes
Cost	Moderate	More expensive

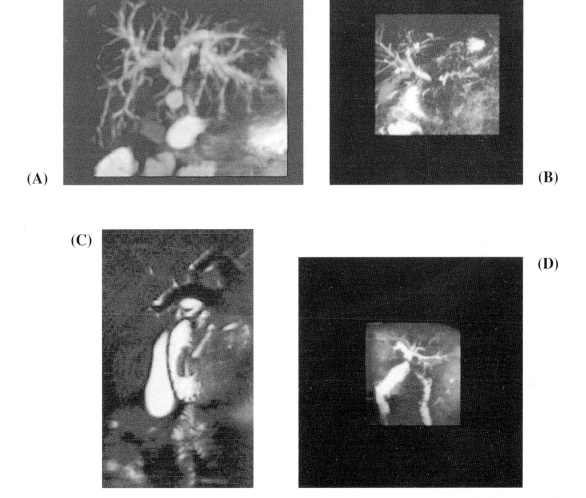

(A)

(B)

(C)

(D)

Figure 49.4. Magnetic resonance cholangiopancreatography (MRCP). A: Laparascopic cholecystectomy bile-duct injury. ERCP (not shown) demonstrated complete cutoff in the mid-common bile duct, with no contrast beyond the stricture. MRCP reveals the extent of the stricture. There is dilatation of the biliary system, with a short stenosis in the common bile duct, and an adjacent cyst. B: Acute pancreatitis producing an inflammatory mass in the head of the pancreas, with upstream pancreatic duct and bile-duct dilatation. C: Ampullary tumour, seen as a filling defect against the fluid-filled duodenum. D: MRCP of a choledochojejunostomy in a patient with cholangitis. Sagittal view demonstrates intrahepatic duct dilatation to a short stenosis at the anastomosis, consistent with a benign postsurgical anastomotic stricture.

Kupffer cells, has resulted in MRI having superior sensitivity and specificity. It is proposed that SPIO-enhanced MRI is reserved for those patients in whom the size, number, and distribution of the metastases are critical to management. Fat suppression sequences can be used to differentiate focal fat deposition from other focal lesions. MRI is also very sensitive to iron deposition in the liver, either in cirrhosis or haemachromatosis.

Pancreas

The tissue specificity of MRI allows differentiation of the solid and cystic components of a **pancreatic phlegmon**. CT will show which areas of the phlegmon enhance with contrast, but this does not distinguish fluid and non-viable necrotic, but solid, pancreatic tissue. MRI therefore offers an advantage over CT, and can be used to direct drainage procedures. Currently, MRI is competitive with CT in the staging of pancreatic cancers.

Reticuloendothelial system

MRI is very similar to CT for the assessment of the spleen and regional lymphadenopathy, and does not offer any specific advantages over CT in these areas. In common with CT, MRI currently uses size criteria in the assessment of lymphadenopathy; a search for an MRI lymphographic agent has been under way for some time, but has not yet proved successful.

Bowel

Bowel MRI is a relatively new technique (11). However, it does have some specific interesting features — for example, it is very sensitive to inflammatory change in the fat adjacent to inflamed bowel (e.g. in Crohn's disease). Fat suppression sequences (those that specifically reduce signal from fat), will show high signal in inflamed fat that appears normal on other modalities.

MRI has an established role in the delineation of complex, perianal fistulae. Again, fat suppression techniques are able to pick up small fistulous tracts as high signal intensity; the relationship to the levator ani and the full extent of the fistula can be shown. Multiple, complex, branching fistulae are often seen in Crohn's disease, with or without associated abscess formation.

In conclusion, the number of gastroenterological applications for CT and MRI is growing; ongoing technical development will result in further advances.

References
1. Curry TS, Dowdey JE and Murry RC. *Christensen's Physics of Diagnostic Radiology*. Philadelphia: Lea and Febiger, 1994.
2. Bluemke DA, Fishman EK. Spiral CT of the liver. *Am J Roentgenol* 1993; **160**: 787–792.
3. Heiken J, Brink J, Vannier M. Spiral (helical) CT. *Radiology* 1993; **189**: 647–656.
4. Grainger RG and Allison DJ (Eds). *Diagnostic Radiology: an Anglo–American Textbook of Imaging*. London: Churchill Livingstone, 1997.
5. Dahnert W. *Radiology Review Manual*. Grayson TH (Ed). London: Williams and Wilkins, 1997.
6. Sutton D (Ed). *A Textbook of Radiology and Imaging*. London: Churchill Livingstone, 1996.
7. Moss AA, Gamsu G and Genant HK. *CT of the body with MRI*. Bralow L (Ed). London: WB Saunders, 1992.
8. Rottman NN, Chevret S, Pezet D *et al*. Prognostic value of early CT in severe acute pancreatitis. *J Am Coll Surg* 1994; **179**: 538–544.
9. Hintze RE, Adler A, Veltzke W *et al*. Clinical significance of MRCP compared to ERCP. *Endoscopy* 1997; **29**: 182–187.
10. Lomanto D, Pavone P, Laghi A *et al*. MRCP in the diagnosis of biliopancreatic diseases. *Am J Surg* 1997; **174**: 33–38.
11. Debatin JF, Patak MA. MRI of the small and large bowel. *Eur Radiol* 1999; **9**: 1523–1524.

50. Investigation of Gastrointestinal Motility

OWEN EPSTEIN

TESTS OF OESOPHAGEAL FUNCTION

Barium swallow

Barium swallow remains an extremely useful diagnostic test; it is inexpensive, minimally invasive and, if conducted with care, provides useful information on both structure and function. Both liquid-phase and solid-phase contrast studies can be performed to help distinguish organic strictures from motility disorders, and many gastroenterologists choose this test as the first investigation of dysphagia, especially when weight loss is not a dominant feature. The test remains very useful in the investigation of suspected hiatus hernia, gastrooesophageal reflux, and disorders of the lower oesophageal sphincter (achalasia).

Oesophagoscopy

Flexible oesophagogastroduodenoscopy is most helpful in the diagnosis of mucosal disease such as Barrett's oesophagus, and in distinguishing organic strictures from motility disorders. The endoscopic diagnosis of acid reflux is less sensitive than 24 h pH studies.

Oesophageal manometry

The rate, rhythm, power, and duration of oesophageal peristalsis, and the contractile and relaxant characteristics of the lower oesophageal sphincter can be measured by oesophageal manometry, using either a water-perfused or a solid-state catheter. The **water-perfused** system requires a pneumohydraulic pump to regulate flow and pressure through a multilumen catheter, and is suitable for stationary studies. **Solid-state** catheters can be used in the same way, and have the added advantage that they can be used in ambulatory monitoring. The investigation is performed using both wet and dry swallows, and is the "gold standard" for diagnosing motility disorders of the gullet.

Twenty-four-hour ambulatory pH monitoring

With this technique, a pH-sensitive probe is suspended 5 cm above the lower oesophageal sphincter and the pH of this area is sampled repeatedly over 24 h. Reporting is facilitated by event markers on the data capture device, which allow the patient to indicate meal times, periods of heartburn or chest pain and recumbent position. The most helpful analysis is the percentage of time during which the pH is less than 4. Twenty-four-hour pH measurement is the gold standard for the assessment of patients with suspected acid reflux.

TESTS OF GASTRIC PHYSIOLOGY

Although abnormalities of gastric motility comprise a significant proportion of disorders of the foregut, there is a poor correlation between the severity of clinical symptoms and objective measures of gastric physiology, including gastric emptying. A number of techniques have been developed, but all suffer from one or more disadvantages. In practice, most clinicians use clinical, endoscopic, and radiological tests to exclude organic disease; dysmotility syndromes are usually diagnosed by exclusion.

Scintigraphy

Scintigraphy is recognized as the gold standard for the measurement of gastric emptying. The technique uses isotopic markers incorporated into either a solid or a liquid meal, and is discussed in Chapter 52. The gastric emptying is recorded by a gamma-scintillation camera. Scintigraphic results are usually reported as the half-life ($t_{1/2}$), the percentage retention at a particular time, lag time, mean transit time, and slope of the curve. Test results are, however, quite variable; in particular, it is not advisable to compare results from one laboratory to another. The most accurate measure requires both anterior and posterior gastric imaging. Using this technique, it is possible to demonstrate both the difference between emptying characteristics of liquid- and solid-phase meals (the former is linear, whereas the latter shows a lag phase), and patterns that vary significantly from the normal.

Although scintigraphy has the attraction of being non-invasive, the technique is costly, not widely available, and involves numerous variables that may influence interpretation of the results.

Orally administered drugs

The absorption of paracetamol has been used as an example of a chemical method for assessing gastric emptying. Paracetamol is absorbed in the duodenum, and its concentration in the blood over a period of time may be used as an index of gastric emptying.

Ultrasound

Ultrasonic examination of the antral area has been shown to be a clinically useful and validated method for assessing gastric emptying (1). In this technique, an oval cross-sectional image of the gastric antrum is obtained at a standard position in the fasting condition and the cross-sectional area is calculated. The patient is then given a standard meal (usually a turkey or cheese sandwich) and the cross-sectional area

of the antrum is re-calculated at defined time periods over 90 min. Abnormality of the fasting antral area or subsequent changes from the normal are interpreted as indicating an abnormality of the distribution of food within the stomach; this may relate to decreased compliance of the fundus.

Breath testing

Administration of a test meal containing a small dose of octanoic acid labelled with carbon-13 can be used to assess gastric emptying (2). When the octanoic acid enters the duodenum, the isotope is rapidly absorbed, and oxidized in the liver; the carbon dioxide produced is exhaled and can be detected by an isotopic breath analyser. Sequential breath samples taken at standard times are measured to provide an indication of gastric emptying.

Electrogastrography

The transcutaneous electrogastrogram (EGG) is obtained by a non-invasive technique that allows prolonged recording of the gastric pacemaker slow wave (3). Electrodes are placed on the anterior abdominal wall in the long axis of the stomach and, using the small solid-state recording device, it is possible to capture the discharge frequency and amplitude of the slow wave. The information is captured for 60 min during the fasting phase, followed by a further 60-min recording after the test meal.

Spectral analysis of the recording provides the mean frequency of gastric pacemaker slow-wave rhythm, in addition to the amplitude generated and its instability coefficient. The normal frequency is a mean of 3 cycles/min; a frequency of 2 cycles/min is indicative of bradygastria, and one of more than 4 cycles/min indicates tachygastria. Both these abnormalities in rhythm have been associated with abnormalities of antroduodenal coordination and antral motility (3). Abnormalities of the EGG correlates closely with the presence of nausea, and correlate with other tests of gastric emptying. The EGG has been shown to be abnormal in up to 30% of patients with non-ulcer dyspepsia.

The gastric barostat

This ingenious device is able to record pressure and isobaric volume changes using an inflatable balloon placed in the fundus of the stomach. This has been used to demonstrate changes in compliance. Patients with gastroparesis may demonstrate significantly larger gastric barostat balloon volumes at lower intragastric pressures, and impaired gastric tone, compared with those with a normal stomach. Although this technique has many attractions, the equipment is expensive and the test is poorly tolerated by patients. Its main use has been restricted to basic physiological scientific studies, rather than clinical practice.

Magnetic resonance imaging

Magnetic resonance imaging is capable of providing real-time information on gastric emptying, and the technique is able to distinguish between liquid- and solid-phase emptying. Currently, the technique is experimental and expensive but in time, it is likely that it will become the gold standard for assessing gastric emptying of both liquids and solids.

References

1. Hausken T, Thune N, Matre K *et al*. Volume estimation of the gastric antrum and the gallbladder in patients with non-ulcer dyspepsia and erosive pre-pyloric changes, using three-dimensional ultrasonography. *Neurogastroenterol Mot* 1994; **6**: 263–270.

2. Maes BD, Ghoos YF, Rutgeerts PJ *et al*. Octanoic acid breath test to measure gastric emptying rate of solids. *Dig Dis Sci* 1994; **39**: 104S–106S.

3. Chen JDZ, Lin Z, Pan J *et al*. Abnormal gastric myoelectrical activity and delayed gastric emptying in patients with symptoms suggestive of gastroparesis. *Dig Dis Sci* 1996; **41**: 1538–1545.

51. Tests for Malabsorption

PARVEEN J. KUMAR and MICHAEL L. CLARK

INTRODUCTION

As discussed in Chapter 31, malabsorption (i.e. failure of absorption), occurs in many gastrointestinal, liver, and pancreatic disorders; human immunodeficiency virus (HIV) infection should also be considered. Some years ago, tests to demonstrate malabsorption were used for its diagnosis. However, they have now been almost universally superseded and replaced by diagnostic imaging, endoscopy, and biopsy, which define the actual cause of malabsorption.

All patients invariably have blood investigations performed. These, along with the clinical symptoms, provide some guidelines for a preferred working diagnosis. Table 51.1 summarizes the various tests that are of relevance to particular gastrointestinal diseases.

Table 51.1. Useful diagnostic tests in gastrointestinal disease.

Disease	Test
Coeliac disease	Serum tissue transglutaminase
	Serum endomysial antibody
	Duodenal/jejunal biopsy
	Occasionally, small-bowel follow-through
Crohn's disease	Small-bowel follow-through
	Colonoscopy and ileal biopsy
	Increased inflammatory markers (e.g. CRP)
Bacterial overgrowth	Hydrogen breath test
	Intubation studies
Tropical sprue	Malabsorption of at least two substances (e.g. serum vitamin B_{12} and serum folic acid)
	Jejunal biopsy
Whipple's disease	Duodenal/jejunal biopsy

BLOOD TESTS

General

A **full blood count and film** can demonstrate anaemia and the type of anaemia. Because of the possibility of mixed deficiencies contributing to anaemia, iron status, serum and red cell folate and vitamin B_{12} concentrations should all be checked in the investigation of anaemia.

If the **mean corpuscular volume** (MCV) is **low** (<76 fl — microcytic), this suggests **iron deficiency**, which may be confirmed by a low serum ferritin concentration. Remember that the serum ferritin concentration can be increased in any inflammatory process, as this is an acute-phase protein. A low serum iron concentration and high total iron-binding capacity (reflecting levels of soluble transferrin receptor) also indicate iron deficiency. A **transferrin saturation** (serum iron divided by total iron-binding capacity) value less than 15% signifies iron deficiency.

If the **mean corpuscular volume** is **high** (more than 96 fl), **folate or vitamin B_{12} may be deficient**. Folate is usually absorbed in the upper part of the intestine, thus a low red cell folate concentration indicates malabsorption combined with a poor appetite (e.g. coeliac disease or Crohn's disease). Vitamin B_{12} is absorbed (after combination with intrinsic factor from the stomach) in the ileum; reduced concentrations indicate gastric or ileal disease or resection. Hypersegmentation of polymorphonuclear leucocytes is seen in patients with low concentrations of folate or vitamin B_{12}. The presence of Howell–Jolly bodies (persistence of circulating aged red cells) indicates splenic atrophy, which occurs, for example, in coeliac disease.

Nutrition and liver function

The Body Mass Index (BMI) can be calculated using the formula: weight (kg)/height (m)^2. Severe malnutrition is indicated by a BMI of <15, moderate by a BMI of 15–19 (see chapter 21).

Measurement of **serum albumin** gives some indication of the nutritional status: a low value indicates malnourishment. A low albumin concentration can also be seen in some protein-losing states in diffuse intestinal disorders such as Whipple's disease, Crohn's enteritis, and radiation damage. An increased prothrombin time (normally expressed as INR — international normalized ratio) may suggest liver malfunction (which can occur in any severe liver disease) or vitamin K malabsorption.

A low **serum calcium** concentration and an increased **alkaline phosphatase** may indicate the presence of osteomalacia, but this is a poor guide, as metabolic bone disease can be present despite normal serum concentrations. Plasma concentrations of 25-hydroxyvitamin D are low in osteomalacia.

Inflammatory markers

C-reactive protein and the erythrocyte sedimentation rate are increased in inflammation.

Immunological tests

Specific **autoantibodies** for the diagnosis of **coeliac disease** are the anti-gliadin (AGA), anti-reticulin (ARA), and anti-endomysial antibodies (EMA). These are usually of the immunoglobulin A (IgA) antibody class and therefore will not be positive in IgA-deficient patients. The sensitivities for the diagnosis of coeliac disease are 52–99.9%, 30–95%, and 100% respectively for AGA, ARA, and EMA. The specificities are 65–100%, 59–100% and 100% (1). EMA tests can be performed using either monkey oesophagus or umbilical tissue; commercial kits are available. All three antibodies can

also be measured using the enzyme-linked immunosorbent assay technique. An assay for tissue transglutaminase (the autoantigen for the EMA) is available and is proving to have, at the least, the same sensitivity as EMA (2).

For other diseases with gastrointestinal involvement, autoantibodies such as anti-nuclear factor, anti-nuclear/topoisomerase, anti-centromere, and anti-extractable nuclear antigen are seen in **scleroderma**; anti-nuclear/double stranded DNA antibodies are seen in **systemic lupus erythematosus**; rheumatoid factor may be positive in **rheumatoid arthritis**.

Serum immunoglobulins should be measured, as IgA deficiency is seen in approximately 1 in 700 of the general population. Immunoglobulins are also reduced in common variable immunodeficiency and agammaglobulinaemia.

Other tests that might be useful include **thyroid function**, to exclude hyperthyroidism. If HIV enteropathy is suspected, an **HIV test** and a CD4 lymphocyte count may be necessary, after counselling the patient.

TESTS TO DEMONSTRATE SMALL-BOWEL ANATOMY

Small-bowel follow-through

Changes such as diverticulae, strictures, narrowing, and fistulae can be demonstrated by small-bowel follow-through (3). Crohn's disease is suggested by the presence of strictures, narrowing and fistulae. Dilatation of the folds and change in fold pattern are non-specific signs that are seen in malabsorption caused, for example, by coeliac disease. The diagnosis should therefore not be based on these findings alone. In pseudo-obstruction, gross dilatation of the small bowel may be seen.

Small-bowel enema (enteroclysis)

Enteroclysis is performed by intubation of the small-bowel and instillation of barium (4). It adds little extra information to a well-performed small-bowel follow-through, but is used in rare cases that require further delineation of a lesion.

Duodenal/jejunal biopsy examination

Biopsy specimens are usually obtained by means of large forceps passed down an endoscope into the duodenum (5). Less frequently, jejunal biopsy sampling is performed by the patient swallowing a Crosby–Kugler capsule (6). The mucosa obtained should be well orientated, with the villi uppermost, on a piece of cellulose acetate paper, and sent for histology in 10% formalin/saline. A normal villous pattern on histology excludes small-bowel disease.

On endoscopy, the concentric duodenal folds may be smoothed out in coeliac disease; ink can be injected into the duodenum and, in a normal person, villi can be seen protruding from a background of ink (7). Because of the high frequency of occult coeliac disease, some practitioners advocate a routine duodenal biopsy examination in all patients undergoing endoscopy.

USEFUL ADDITIONAL (DIAGNOSTIC) TESTS IN PATIENTS WITH STEATORRHOEA

Steatorrhoea can indicate the presence of pancreatic disease; therefore in addition to investigation of the small-bowel in patients with steatorrhoea, pancreatic investigations are required (8).

Plain abdominal X-ray can show calcification in chronic pancreatitis. **Ultrasound** can define detailed pancreatic anatomy, and is used in the diagnosis of chronic pancreatitis. **Helical computed tomography** (CT) with dynamic enhancement enables the pancreas to be completely imaged within one 30-s breath-hold, and is extremely useful in all forms of pancreatic disease. **Magnetic resonance imaging** has the advantage over CT, in that it does not involve ionizing radiation; it is as sensitive as CT (see chapter 49).

Patients with carcinoma in the head of the pancreas can also present with steatorrhoea accompanied by jaundice; investigations here should concentrate on determining the cause of jaundice — for example, by means of **endoscopic retrograde cholangiopancreatography (ERCP)** and **magnetic resonance cholangiopancreatography (MRCP)**.

Neuroendocrine tumours of the pancreas, particularly gastrinoma (see Chapter 4), can cause steatorrhoea. The tumour is best demonstrated by **endoscopic ultrasound (EUS)** or by **somatostatin receptor scintigraphy**, along with measurement of serum gastrin concentrations.

TESTS TO DEMONSTRATE MALABSORPTION

As emphasized earlier, the tests described below are rarely used, as they have been superseded by imaging.

Fat malabsorption

Fat can be measured in a 3-day collection of **faeces** while the patient is taking a 100-g fat diet (9). The normal amount of fat in the stools is less than 17 mmol/day (<6 g/day). The use of Sudan stain on faecal samples is not recommended, as it lacks sensitivity. Stools are smelly and difficult to collect; to avoid this, fat absorption can be measured using breath analysis.

The **carbon dioxide breath test** measures carbon-14-labelled carbon dioxide in expired breath after an oral load of radiolabelled fat gives an indication of the amount of fat malabsorption (10). A comparison between labelled **trigylceride** (^{14}C-triolene) and labelled **fatty acids** (tritiated oleic acid) can be used to diagnose pancreatic disease; the fatty acid absorption will be normal. Because these tests are performed only very occasionally, the average laboratory has little experience with these measurements.

Intestinal permeability tests are not in general use, but are often used for research purposes. They can detect small-bowel disease (11). Abnormal intestinal mucosa is permeable to large molecules such as lactulose, mannitol, cellobiose, polyethylene glycol, and chromium-labelled EDTA. These substances can be used in combination to show differential absorption. Although these tests show altered permeation, they do not define the actual abnormality. The sensitivities are high, but the specificities of these absorption tests are low.

Vitamin B_{12} deficiency can be the result of gastric problems (pernicious anaemia, atrophic gastritis, postgastrectomy), ileal problems (terminal ileal resection and occasional ileal disease; usually Crohns's disease), or bacterial overgrowth; **measurement of vitamin B_{12} absorption** is now seldom necessary to detect gastric or ileal disease. Vitamin B_{12} absorption can be measured by whole-body counting using a double isotope, with measurements on day 0 before and after swallowing radioactive vitamin B_{12}, and later on day 10 (12).

Alternatively, a **Schilling test** can be performed. This involves oral administration of 1 µg cobalt-58-

labelled vitamin B_{12} to a fasting patient, followed by intramuscular administration of 1000 μg vitamin B_{12} to saturate the binding protein. The urine is then collected for 24 h. Normal individuals excrete more than 10% of the radioactive dose. If abnormal, the test is repeated, with co-administration of intrinsic factor. If the excretion is then normal, the diagnosis is one of a gastric problem (e.g. pernicious anaemia); if the excretion remains abnormal, the problem may be in the ileum, or there may be bacterial overgrowth, when the test can be repeated after antibiotic treatment. Ileal abnormalities can be delineated by a barium follow-through.

Breath tests

Two breath tests can be used to detect bacterial overgrowth.

Hydrogen breath tests exploit the fact that oral lactulose or glucose is metabolized by bacteria, with the production of hydrogen. Excessive production of breath hydrogen is seen in patients with bacterial overgrowth, after ingestion of 50–80 g of glucose or 10–20 g lactulose; fasting breath hydrogen concentrations are not sensitive or specific. Patients should avoid foods such as bread, pasta, and fibre on the day before the test, because they cause prolonged production of hydrogen. The mouth should be rinsed with an antiseptic mouthwash, before the test is performed, as the test sugar can interact with oral bacteria. There is a clearly distinguishable colonic peak (an increase of at least 20 ppm hydrogen above baseline) after the administration of sugar. Compared with intestinal culture, the sensitivities of this test are 62% and 68% for glucose and lactulose, with specificities of 83% and 44% respectively (13).

In the **^{14}C-glycocholic acid breath test**, the patient is given carbon-14-labelled bile salts by mouth. Bacteria deconjugate the bile salts and release ^{14}C-glycine, which is metabolized and appears in the breath as ^{14}C-carbon dioxide. The radioactivity in the breath is measured. An early increase indicates either bacterial overgrowth or rapid transit into the colon, where bacteria are normally present. This test does not distinguish bacterial overgrowth from ileal resection or damage, where colonic bacteria deconjugate unabsorbed ^{14}C-labelled bile salts; interpretation of the results is thus difficult. False-negatives are seen in approximately 35% of patients with culture-proven overgrowth.

Direct intubation tests can be used in patients who have positive hydrogen breath tests: aspiration of intestinal juices by intubation can be used to assess bacterial overgrowth on aerobic and anaerobic cultures (14). The aspirates can also be used to detect evidence of the deconjugation of bile salts by bacteria on chromatography; deconjugation leads to malabsorption of fat.

Jejunal juice can also be obtained by intubation or from the jejunal biopsy tube. The juice is put on a slide and viewed under the microscope for the detection of *Giardia intestinalis*. After a jejunal biopsy procedure, a smear impression of the jejunal mucosa can be made on a slide, to look for *Giardia*.

Tests for protein-losing enteropathy

In patients in whom protein-losing enteropathy is suspected, intravenous chromium-51-labelled albumin is given and the faeces measured for radioactivity; radioactivity is found if there is excess protein loss. This test is rarely used, but is occasionally useful when the reason for a low serum albumin concentration is unclear.

Bile-salt malabsorption

Malabsorption of bile salts occurs after ileal resection, and has been reported as a cause of postinfective diarrhoea. In patients in whom it is suspected, selenium-75-labelled selenohomotaurocholate — a synthetic taurine conjugate that is a gamma-emitting bile salt — is given orally. The retention of the bile salt is measured by whole-body counting at 7 days (15).

Pancreatic exocrine function

Imaging has superseded the pancreatic exocrine "function" tests. Serum amylase and serum lipase concentrations are increased in acute pancreatitis, but their measurement is of no value in chronic disease. The measurement of duodenal enzymes by direct intubation after hormone stimulation (secretin or cholecystokinin) is only sometimes helpful in the diagnosis of chronic pancreatitis (16). Reduced concentrations of bicarbonate and enzymes (e.g. trypsin), are seen in chronic disease. However, there is an enormous reserve in enzyme capacity, and therefore these tests are not very useful, as the pancreas has to be grossly damaged to show any abnormality. A Lundh meal is similar: intraluminal trypsin and lipase are measured after the administration of a meal, and can be used in the investigation of steatorrhoea.

In the **PABA test**, the synthetic peptide, N-benzoyl-L-tyrosyl p-aminobenzoic acid, is given as an oral load. In normal individuals, it is then hydrolysed by pancreatic chymotrypsin to release free PABA, which is absorbed, metabolized, and excreted in the urine. In the patients with pancreatic insufficiency, a reduction in the absorption of free PABA occurs, resulting in low serum concentrations and reduced urinary excretion [17].

The **fluorescein dilaurate test (pancreolauryl test)** is similar to the PABA test in principle. Fluorescein dilaurate is given orally with a standard breakfast (50 g bread, 20 g butter, one cup of tea) and is hydrolysed by pancreatic arylesterases to lauric acid and water-soluble fluorescein; the latter is absorbed by the small intestine, and excreted in the urine. Urine or serum measurements of fluorescin can be performed. Test characteristics are similar to those of the PABA test, with a sensitivity of 55–100% and a specificity of 46–97% [18]. Like the PABA test, the pancreolauryl test is more accurate at detecting severe exocrine deficiency than mild to moderate exocrine dysfunction. Accuracy can be impaired by previous gastrointestinal surgery, small-bowel disease (eg. coeliac, Crohn's disease) severe liver disease, and bacterial overgrowth. Enzyme supplements should be stopped 5 days before the study. Using a modified serum assay for fluorescein, Malferteiner et al. [19] found a tight correlation between serum pancreolauryl test results and the presence of morphological abnormalities suggestive of chronic pancreatitis, which suggests that this investigation may become the first-line investigation for patients with suspected chronic pancreatitis.

References

1. Ferreira M, Davies SL, Butler M *et al*. Endomysial antibody: is it the best screening test for coeliac disease? *Gut* 1992; **33**: 1633–1637.
   A comparison of the three antibodies in patients with coeliac disease using, as a control, the sera of patients sent to a routine immunological laboratory.
2. Brusco G, Izz L, Corazza GP. Tissue transglutaminase antibodies for coeliac screening. *Ital J Gastroenterol Hepatol* 1998; **30**: 496–497.
3. Herlinger H. Radiology in malabsorption. *Clin Radiol* 1992; **45**: 73–78.
4. Miller RE, Sellink JL. The small bowel enema – how to succeed and how to fail. *Gastrointest Radiol* 1979; **4**: 269.
   Describes the practical problems of performing a small-bowel enema.
5. Dandalides SM, Cavey WD, Petras R *et al*. Endoscopic small bowel mucosal biopsy: a controlled trial evaluating forceps size and biopsy location in the diagnosis of normal and abnormal architecture. *Gastroint Endosc* 1989; **35**: 197–200.
   For common mucosal lesions, endoscopic biopsy specimens are as good as those obtained with a Crosby capsule, provided the specimen is sectioned at several levels.
6. Crosby WH, Kugler HW. Intraluminal biopsy of the small intestine. *Am J Dig Dis* 1957; **2**: 236–241.
   Classic original description of the use and value of the Crosby capsule.
7. Mee AS, Burke M, Newman J *et al*. Small bowel biopsy in malabsorption: comparison of the diagnostic adequacy of endoscopic forceps and capsule biopsy specimens. *BMJ* 1985; **291**: 769–772.
   A further paper showing that endoscopically obtained biopsy samples of the descending duodenum are reliable, if at least four specimens are obtained.
8. Malfertheiner P, Buchler M. Correlation of imaging and function in chronic pancreatitis. *Radiol Clin North Am* 1989; **27**: 51–64.
   A good review comparing ultrasound and CT scanning with standard pancreatic function tests.
9. Bo-Linn GW, Fordtran JS. Fecal fat concentration in patients with steatorrhea. *Gastroenterology* 1984; **87**: 319–322.
   Average faecal fat concentrations in various gastrointestinal diseases are compared with those in patients with pancreatic disease.
10. Mylvaganam K, Hudson PR, Ross A *et al*. ^{14}C triolein breath test: a routine test for the gastroenterology clinic? *Gut* 1986; **27**: 1347–1352.
    In this study from a district general hospital, this test is found to be simple, inexpensive and helpful in the detection of fat malabsorption.
11. Cobden I, Rothwell J, Axon ATR. Intestinal permeability and screening tests for coeliac disease. *Gut* 1980; **21**: 512–518.
    Although permeability tests in the hands of experimental workers are of value, these tests have been replaced by serum antibody screening tests, with the definitive diagnosis still being histological.
12. Schjonsby H. Vitamin B_{12} absorption and malabsorption. *Gut* 1989; **30**: 1686–1691.
    Review article of normal vitamin B_{12} absorption and the pathophysiology of vitamin B_{12} malabsorption.
13. Kerlin P, Wong L. Breath hydrogen testing in bacterial overgrowth of the small intestine. *Gastroenterology* 1988; **95**: 982–988.
    The combined criteria of a high fasting breath hydrogen concentration and a significant increase after glucose are specific for bacterial overgrowth.
14. Corazza GR, Menozzi MG, Strocchi ? *et al*. The diagnosis of small-bowel bacterial overgrowth. *Gastroenterology* 1990; **98**: 302–309.

This paper describes the reliability of a single jejunal fluid culture compared with breath hydrogen testing, confirming that direct culture of jejunal fluid remains the gold standard for the diagnosis of bacterial overgrowth.

15. Ferraris R, Galatola G, Barlotta A *et al.* Measurement of bile acid half life using [^{75}Se]HCAT in health and intestinal diseases. Comparison with [^{75}Se]HCAT abdominal retention methods. *Dig Dis Sci* 1992; **37**: 225–232.
    Good practical description of the technique of detecting bile acid malabsorption.

16. Hunt LP, Braganza JM. On optimising the diagnostic yield of secretion and pancreozymin tests. *Clin Chim Acta* 1989; **186**: 91–108.

Practical help in performing this test.

17. Tanner AR, Robinson DP. Pancreatic function testing. Serum PABA measurement is a reliable and accurate measurement of exocrine function. *Gut* 1988; **29**: 1736–1740.
    Serum PABA is a simple and more reliable test of pancreatic function than the conventional method of urine collection and measurement.

18. Niederau C, Grendell, JH. Diagnosis of chronic pancreatitis. *Gastroenterology* 1985; **88**: 1973–1995.

19. Malfertheiner P, Buchler M, Muller A *et al.* Fluorescein dilaurate serum test: a rapid tubeless pancreatic function test. *Pancreas* 1987; **2**: 53–60.

52.   Nuclear Medicine in Gastroenterology

N.K. GUPTA and J.B. BOMANJI

Nuclear medicine techniques are now available for **quantitative assessment** of salivary gland function, dysphagia, gastrooesophageal reflux, dyspepsia, altered bowel habits, malabsorption of various nutrients, hepatic and biliary diseases, inflammatory bowel diseases, infection, acute abdomen, abdominal mass, and gastrointestinal bleeding. With the advent of antibodies against tumour markers, radioimmunoscintigraphy has the potential to image tumours of gastrointestinal tract. Receptor imaging techniques have also had an impact on localizing both primary gastroenteropancreatic tumours and metastases. Positron emission tomography (PET) is rapidly growing as a tool permitting early and accurate detection of sites with malignant involvement. With the advent of single-photon emission tomography, axial, coronal, and sagittal sections can be obtained, and the sensitivity of nuclear medicine techniques is increasing. Most nuclear medicine studies are complementary to radiological techniques. The majority have a low radiation burden and cause little discomfort or inconvenience to the patient compared with routine radiological techniques. However, the resolution for anatomical details is poor.

The strength of nuclear medicine studies lies in their ability to quantify the physiological and pathological processes, thus excluding subjective error in the interpretation of findings. The quantity of the radiopharmaceutical given to a patient is just sufficient to obtain the required information before its decay, hence the very low radiation received. In the UK, the minimum and maximum doses of various radiopharmaceuticals administered to patients are regulated by the Administration of Radioactive Substances Advisory Committee.

SALIVARY-GLAND SCINTIGRAPHY

Radiological investigation of salivary glands by sialography is invasive and, even with excellent technique, appearances bear only a poor relationship to the secretory status of the gland. The changes observed in the gland are not necessarily recent, and findings obtained with sialography must therefore be viewed with care, even in symptomatic patients. In contrast, salivary-gland scintigraphy is a simple, non-invasive, and quantifiable method that is not operator-dependent. It permits excellent assessment of tracer accumulation and secretion of all four major salivary glands, and also allows evaluation of the response of individual glands to a sialogogue. Salivary-gland scintigraphy is thus used as a preliminary investigation for functional assessment of **salivary gland pathology**, and frequently avoids an unnecessary sialogram.

Common indications for salivary gland scintigraphy include Sjogren's syndrome, xerostomia, and problem sialograms. No special preparation of the patient is required. After an intravenous injection, technetium-99m (^{99m}Tc)-labelled pertechnetate is taken up by the salivary glands and secreted by the ductal epithelium. Anterior images with the patient in the supine position are acquired for 20 min using a gamma camera. Ten minutes into the acquisition of images, a sialagogue (in the form of citric acid or lime juice) is given to the patient, to promote salivary secretion. Quantitative assessment of salivary function is then performed by drawing regions of interest over the parotid, submandibular, and thyroid glands. Time—activity curves are generated from these data and used to interpret the results quantitatively.

OESOPHAGEAL SCINTIGRAPHY

Oesophageal scintigraphy may be used to evaluate **motility disorders** — including achalasia, diffuse oesophageal spasm, and nutcracker oesophagus — in which oesophageal manometry is not available or is unacceptable to the patient, the results of manometry are equivocal, or the serial response to treatment (surgical or medical) is to be monitored. The technique is non-invasive, delivers a low dose of radiation, is quantifiable, and is readily acceptable to the patient.

Systemic sclerosis, diabetes mellitus, and nonspecific motor disorders can also manifest as oesophageal dysmotility. The sensitivity of the test in these conditions ranges between 80 and 90%, depending upon the particular motility disorder (1). Uncommon indications for scintigraphy include the physiological and quantitative evaluation of oesophageal transit before and after surgical repair of hiatus hernia with reflux. In oesophagectomy with gastric transposition or colonic interposition, assessment of the function of the transposed organ by scintigraphy is also useful.

GASTROOESOPHAGEAL SCINTIGRAPHY

Gastrooesophageal reflux scintigraphy was first described in 1976 as a simple non-invasive and quantifiable **test of reflux** (2). Intraoesophageal 24-h pH monitoring is the "gold standard" for evaluation of reflux. However, pH monitoring only detects gastrooesophageal reflux if the gastric contents have a pH less than 4; if the gastric acid secretion is suppressed by medications, episodes of reflux are not detected (3). Gastrooesophageal scintigraphy measures the reflux independently of pH; furthermore, it is useful in measuring the volume of reflux (3). There is a good correlation (90%) with the acid pH reflux test. The major shortcoming of this technique is that it does not permit continuous monitoring of the patients, as is possible with pH monitoring.

In **children**, gastrooesophageal reflux scintigraphy using milk is used to investigate recurrent vomiting, failure to thrive, intermittent wheezing, chronic pulmonary disorders, oesophagitis, and apnoeic episodes. The sensitivity and specificity of the technique for detecting reflux and pulmonary aspiration are 79% and 93% respectively, these figures being superior to those of barium examinations (4). The test is non-invasive and requires no sedation. A child can be evaluated for gastric emptying and for oesophageal reflux; furthermore, the lungs can be evaluated for aspiration of tracer. Most children exhibiting gastrooesophageal reflux also show delayed gastric emptying. Delayed images of the chest can show spillover of the labelled feed into the lungs; however, a negative study does not exclude aspiration.

GASTRIC-EMPTYING SCINTIGRAPHY

Scintigraphy has an important role in the measurement of gastric emptying. The investigations are quantifiable, non-invasive, readily accepted by patients, and widely available. Indications include evaluation of functional dyspepsia, gastroparesis (Figure 52.1), postgastrectomy syndromes, follow-up of patients receiving prokinetic drugs, and the study of the normal physiology of stomach. Recent advances in equipment and technique allow the visualization of antral contractions and quantitative assessment of the frequency and amplitude of these contractions, which enhances the ability to evaluate pathophysiology and to assess the effect of new prokinetic drugs.

The test may be carried out to combine liquid- and solid-phase emptying. However, most centres today perform only solid-phase emptying, because gastric emptying of liquids does not become abnormal until gastroparesis is severe, at which stage the patient may not tolerate a solid meal. Although gastric scintigraphy is most often utilized in gastroparesis, it also has a role in the postoperative evaluation of patients with symptoms associated with rapid gastric emptying ("dumping syndrome").

Dyspepsia and indigestion are common complaints, affecting 20% of the general population. Scintigraphic studies show delayed gastric emptying in nearly 50% of patients with dyspeptic symptoms (5). Mostly, the delayed gastric emptying is for solids rather than liquids; this has prognostic

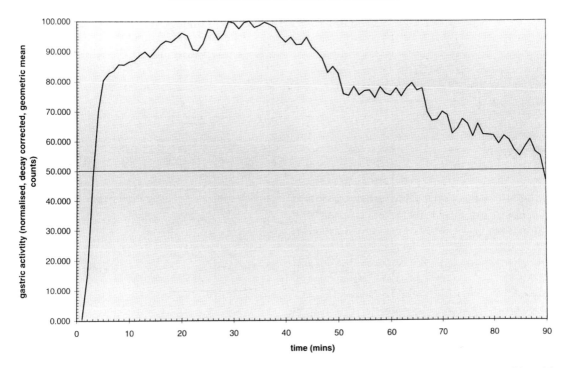

Figure 52.1. Delayed gastric emptying in a diabetic patient with gastroparesis. The time-activity curve for the solid meal is generated, showing a reasonably prolonged $t_{1/2}$ of 89 min.

implications, as symptoms can then be improved with prokinetic drugs. Common causes of gastric emptying dysfunction are outlined in Table 52.1.

INTESTINAL-TRACT SCINTIGRAPHY

Small-intestinal transit time

As there is a tremendous variation in small-bowel transit in normal individuals, normal values for transit time are quite variable. Furthermore, difficulty

may be encountered in identifying the caecum and terminal ileum. Because of these limitations, small-bowel transit scintigraphy is not practised widely in the UK, but other methods such as enteroduodenal or small-bowel manometry are used to detect disorders of small-bowel motility.

Colonic transit time

Colonic scintigraphy measures colonic transit time as a whole and regional transit through the colon;

Table 52.1. Common causes of delayed and rapid gastric emptying.

Delayed gastric emptying	Rapid gastric emptying
Diabetes mellitus	Pyloroplasty without vagotomy
Billroth II surgery	Zollinger–Ellison syndrome
Drugs (e.g. calcium-channel blockers, nicotine, levodopa)	Drugs (e.g. metoclopramide, erythromycin, cisapride)
Renal insufficiency	Dumping syndrome
Amyloidosis	Enterogastric reflux gastritis
Muscular dystrophy	Duodenal ulcer without obstruction
Polymyositis/dermatomyositis	
Pernicious anaemia	
Idiopathic	

it is used in the clinical evaluation of constipation, suspected pseudo-obstruction, irritable bowel syndrome, and the efficacy of laxatives, prokinetic agents, and smooth-muscle relaxants. Preparation of the patient for colonic scintigraphy includes a normal diet for several days before and during testing. Medications affecting the intestinal transit are discontinued, 3 days before the study; narcotic and sedative drugs should also be discontinued. Patients should not undergo barium studies before this examination, as these studies may affect the colonic transit.

Colonic transit scintigraphic measurements are carried out using orally administered radionuclides such as indium-111-labelled water or time-release capsules containing ^{111}In-labelled resin pellets, which are released in the distal ileum or proximal colon. The capsules are ingested in the morning and images are acquired at the end of each of the first three days. Results are interpreted by reference to percentage time activities in various regions of the colon and the overall progression of radioactivity over 3 days. A normal colorectal transit indicates the possibility that the patient has misrepresented or misinterpreted bowel habits or has a psychosocial disturbance. Abnormal patterns of colonic transit can be divided into right-sided, left-sided, or generalized delays. **Colonic inertia** is suggested by delay in transit throughout the whole colon. Cases of **functional rectosigmoid obstruction** show normal transit through the proximal colon, but accumulation of activity in the descending and rectosigmoid colon proximal to the anal sphincter (6).

Limitations of colonic scintigraphy are its high cost, the long imaging time, and the difficulty in detecting functional rectosigmoid obstruction. Also, there is a wide variation in colonic transit times, both between and within individuals and between sexes (7).

GASTROINTESTINAL BLEEDING

Angiography is an invasive method of detecting haemorrhage and is most useful in patients who are believed to be bleeding actively at the time of investigation. It is not useful in those who are bleeding intermittently or have bleeding rates of less than 1.0 ml/min. Nuclear scintigraphy is more sensitive than angiography in detecting gastrointestinal haemorrhage of an intermittent nature, and helps in the selection of patients for angiography.

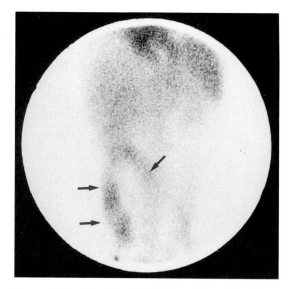

Figure 52.2. Gastrointestinal bleed in a 45-year-old male patient: ^{99m}Tc-labelled RBC study. The bleeding study shows accumulation of labelled RBC dominantly in the caecum and ascending colon, and tracking distally (arrows).

Detection of bleeding involves the use of either ^{99m}Tc-sulphur colloid or ^{99m}Tc-labelled red blood cells (RBC). Haemorrhage detection is made possible by the local accumulation of radiotracer after its extravasation out of the bleeding vessel, which increases with time and may show antegrade or retrograde movement in the bowel (Figure 52.2). ^{99m}Tc-labelled RBCs, which can detect bleed rates of at least 0.1 ml/min, are more commonly used than ^{99m}Tc-sulphur colloid. ^{99m}Tc-RBC imaging can be carried out over a period of up to 24 h and hence permits detection of intermittent bleeds. ^{99m}Tc-RBC scintigraphy has a sensitivity, specificity, and accuracy for the detection of gastrointestinal bleeding of 93%, 95%, and 94% respectively (8). Once the bleeding has been identified by nuclear imaging, definitive diagnosis and therapeutic management can be performed angiographically, endoscopically, or surgically.

For ^{99m}Tc-RBC scintigraphy, good RBC labelling is the key to acquisition of good data. Poor RBC labelling can be seen in heparinized patients, and those receiving chemotherapy, including doxorubicin, digoxin, dipyridamole and propranolol. Injection through the intravenous cannulae and the presence of anti-RBC antibodies can also cause poor cell labelling. There are three different methods of

RBC labelling: *in vivo*, *in vitro*, and *in vivo–vitro*. *In vitro* labelling provides the best labelling (greater than 95% labelling efficiency), but requires facilities for handling blood products. Most departments utilize the *in vivo* technique. This method requires two injections and no handling of blood is involved. The patient is injected with pyrophosphate intravenously and, after a 20 min wait, 400 MBq ^{99m}Tc-pertechnetate is injected. At the time of injection, a nuclear angiogram is obtained and then static imaging is performed every 5 min for the first 1 h. If the bleeding site is not identified during this period, further images are obtained at suitable intervals. The patient is sometimes recalled for 24 h imaging. A few centres perform dynamic imaging, acquiring 60 images every 15 s for 15 min, repeated every 15 min until the site of bleeding is identified.

MECKEL'S DIVERTICULUM SCINTIGRAPHY

Meckel's diverticulum, resulting from persistence of the omphalomesenteric (vitelline) duct at its junction with the ileum, is found in 2% of the population and is asymptomatic in 80% of cases. Sixty per cent of patients present symptomatically by 2 years of age. The condition is more common in males, with a male:female ratio of 3:1. Meckel's diverticulum is usually located approximately 60 cm proximal to the ileocaecal valve. Symptomatic Meckel's diverticula can present with rectal bleeding (most common), intussusception, volvulus, or diverticulitis (common in adults).

Gastric mucosa traps ^{99m}Tc-pertechnetate. A Meckel's diverticulum containing ectopic gastric mucosa can thus be detected after an intravenous injection of 150 MBq ^{99m}Tc-pertechnetate. Gastric accumulation of pertechnetate begins within 5–10 min of the injection, with increase in intensity over the 60-min of study. Ectopic gastric mucosa anywhere in the abdomen will show the same pattern of tracer accumulation. The sensitivity of scintigraphy for detection of Meckel's diverticulum exceeds 90% in the paediatric population and approximately 60% in the adult population (9). A positive scan will usually show activity in the right lower-quadrant (Figure 52.3), and this activity appears simultaneously with gastric activity.

HEPATOBILIARY IMAGING

Hepatobiliary scintigraphy is carried out using ^{99m}Tc-labelled iminodiacetic acid (IDA) derivatives. Scintigraphy is complementary to ultrasound and contrast studies of the gallbladder. Currently, commercial agents such as hepatic iminodiacetic acid (HIDA), diisopropyl-iminodiacetic acid (DISIDA) and parabutyl iminodiacetic acid (T-BIDA) are used; these have high hepatic uptake and fast biliary excretion (10). On serial images, the extraction of the radiotracer by the hepatocytes can be seen diffusely in the liver and, subsequently, in the intrahepatic bile ducts, extrahepatic biliary tree, gallbladder, and duodenum. In view of the tracer kinetics, common indications for hepatobiliary scintigraphy are assessment of acute cholecystitis, chronic cholecystitis, and acute acalculous cholecystitis. Biliary dyskinesia, biliary atresia, biliary leaks, afferent-loop syndrome, and enterogastric reflux may also be evaluated by this technique. Less common indications include assessment of liver transplant, biliary diversion

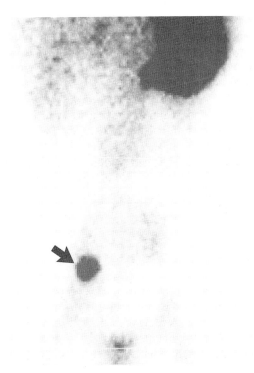

Figure 52.3. Meckel's diverticulum in a 14-year-old girl. ^{99m}Tc-pertechnetate scan showing focal accumulation of tracer to the right of the midline in the lower abdomen (arrow).

procedures, and postcholecystectomy syndromes.

For scintigraphy, the patient should have fasted for 6 h before receiving the injection of radiolabel. Narcotic agents that act on the sphincter of Oddi should be withheld for at least 12 h before procedure. Iminodiacetic acid (IDA) derivatives predominantly bind to albumin in the circulation and are then carried to the liver. Dissociation of the tracer from albumin takes place in the liver, and the tracer enters the anion-exchange pathway of the bilirubin. IDA compounds show competitive inhibition by bilirubin; they are not conjugated before their excretion and are thus excreted unchanged. T-BIDA is excreted almost exclusively by the liver (98%) and has the greatest resistance to displacement by bilirubin; it is thus advantageous in patients with increased bilirubin concentrations. The patient is injected with 150 MBq ^{99m}Tc-T-BIDA and multiple dynamic images are obtained over 1 h, with the gamma camera positioned anteriorly over the liver region. Right and left lateral views can be obtained, if desired, to distinguish activity in the gallbladder from that in the intestine. In normal biliary scintigraphy, the liver, bile ducts, gallbladder, and intestine should be visualized within 60 min of tracer injection; the gallbladder is usually visualized before the common bile duct and intestines. Over time, liver activity reduces as the tracer is cleared from the circulation. Presence of activity in the small bowel excludes complete obstruction of the common bile duct.

Cholecystitis

Ultrasound is the investigation of choice in cases of acute cholecystitis, to assess the absence or presence of gallstones, gallbladder wall thickening and pericholecystic fluid. However, the sensitivity of ultrasound in the detection of acute cholecystitis is about 97% and the specificity 64%, with a positive predictive value of only 40%. The sensitivity and specificity of hepatobiliary scintigraphy for acute cholecystitis are 95%, with a positive predictive value of 70% (11) (Figure 52.4). Cholescintigraphy can give false-positive results in patients with severe illness who are either fasting or receiving

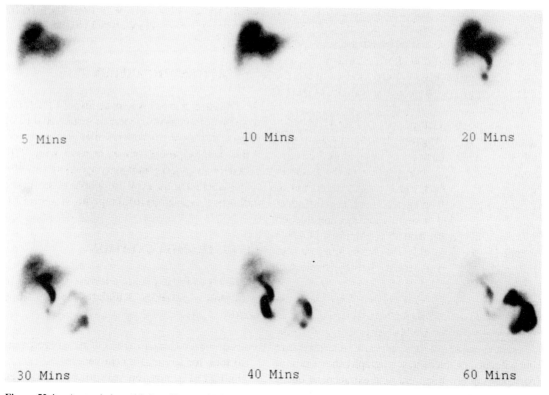

Figure 52.4. Acute cholecystitis in a 42-year-old female patient with upper abdominal pain: ^{99m}Tc-HIDA scan. There is homogeneous uptake of the tracer by the hepatocytes by 5 min. Prompt excretion of the hepatobiliary activity is observed via the common bile duct into the gut by 20 min. Throughout the study the gallbladder was not visualized.

hyperalimentation. False-negative cholescintigraphy is seen in fewer than 5% of cases and may be attributable to incomplete obstruction of the cystic duct, acalculous cholecystitis, accessory cystic duct, and cases of duodenal diverticulum simulating gall-bladder.

In acute cholecystitis, visualization of the biliary tree and non-visualization of the gallbladder after 4 h of scintigraphy are common. In patients with chronic cholecystitis, delayed visualization of the gallbladder (between 1 and 4 h) with normal liver function is characteristic, being seen in 85–90% of patients. Furthermore, in these patients the gallbladder ejection fraction is impaired and is usually less than 35% (the normal value is greater than 90%). In patients with acalculous cholecystitis associated with surgery, sepsis, burns, hyperalimentation, diabetes mellitus, pancreatitis, and sickle-cell anaemia, scintigraphy presents a picture similar to that of acute cholecystitis. Cholescintigraphy has a sensitivity of 60–90% in these patients (12).

Biliary dyskinesia

Chronic acalculous disorders of the hepatobiliary tract present a diagnostic dilemma and are difficult to diagnose because routine blood chemistry, ultra-sound findings, and oral cholecystograms are nor-mal. In this context, scintigraphy has an important role, showing a sensitivity and specificity of greater than 90% (11,13).

In patients with suspected **sphincter of Oddi spasm** and an intact gallbladder, scintigraphy usu-ally shows normal anatomy of the common bile duct, with minimal or no bile pooling in the intra- or extrahepatic bile duct. However, after infusion of cholecystokinin (10 ng/kg per 3 min) the gallbladder may show a normal or slightly low ejection fraction (normal value greater than 35%). Almost all the bile emptied by the gallbladder may reflux into common, left, and right hepatic ducts during the ejection period and re-enter the gallbladder after the infusion has been terminated. Many, but not all, patients ex-perience pain during the ejection period, and the pain is relieved when the gallbladder relaxes and refills. In patients with suspected sphincter of Oddi spasm but without a gallbladder, scintigraphy shows promi-nent bile stasis within intra- and extrahepatic ducts. Infusion of cholecystokinin increases hepatic bile production and rapidly washes out bile stasis within the ducts when there is no anatomical obstruction.

Biliary leaks

Hepatobiliary scintigraphy can be useful in the diag-nosis and localization of biliary leaks after surgery (Figure 52.5) or abdominal trauma, although endo-scopic retrograde or magnetic resonance cholangio-pancreatography are preferred when available. In addition to surgical and traumatic causes, bile leaks can also occur in acute cholecystitis with perforation, peptic ulcer disease, inflammatory bowel disease, and malignancies involving the biliary system.

On scintigraphy, bile leaks can be detected as a result of extravasation of biliary radioactivity into the peritoneal cavity, which increases with time. Delayed imaging for up to 24 h may be needed to increase the sensitivity of bile-leak detection, be-cause 50% of the leaks may be missed if imaging is carried out for less than 4 h (14).

Biliary atresia

Hepatobiliary scintigraphy can differentiate accu-rately between neonatal hepatitis and biliary atresia. The pivotal finding is the detection of tracer in the small intestine of patients with neonatal hepatitis, and its absence in biliary atresia (Figure 52.6).

ENTEROGASTRIC REFLUX

Enterogastric bile reflux may be responsible for the development of gastric ulcers in some patients and occurs occasionally in patients after gastric surgery. A dual-isotope procedure may be used, with ^{99m}Tc-IDA derivatives as hepatobiliary agents and an ^{111}In-oxine-labelled solid meal to delineate the gastric outline and evaluate gastric emptying (Figure 52.7).

LIVER TRANSPLANTATION

Nuclear medicine imaging techniques used for **evaluation of potential candidates for liver trans-plant** include:

- liver—spleen scan to assess disease severity and to look for any anatomical variant
- multigated acquisition scan to assess left ven-tricular function
- adenosine/stress thallium scans in high-risk car-diac patients, to look for coronary artery disease

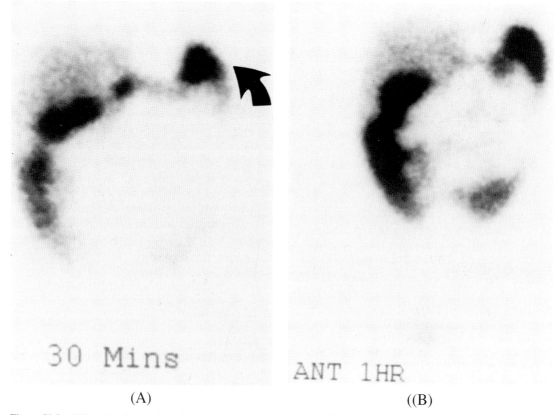

(A)　　　　((B)

Figure 52.5. Biliary leak in a patient after laparoscopic cholecystectomy: ^{99m}Tc-HIDA scan. A: Clear tracking of radiolabelled bile below the right lobe of the liver, coupled with reflux into the the stomach (arrow). B: The delayed 3-h view shows the track with collection of the extravasated radiolabelled bile into the peritoneum. (Courtesy of Dr M. Al-Janabi.)

- bone scan to exclude bone metastases in patients with a history of carcinoma
- quantitative ventilation/perfusion lung scan to evaluate patients for hepatopulmonary syndrome

In the post-transplant phase, hepatobiliary scintigraphy is used serially to evaluate native liver, liver allograft function, vascular patency, biliary patency, and focal parenchymal abnormalities. Scintigraphy is particularly sensitive in detecting postoperative complications such as infarction, biliary obstruction, and bile leakage before the use of other imaging modalities such as ultrasound and computed tomography (CT) (15).

SCINTIGRAPHY IN ABDOMINAL INFLAMMATION/INFECTION

Although barium studies and endoscopic evaluation are the major investigations in the diagnosis of inflammatory bowel disease (IBD), imaging with **radiolabelled leucocytes** has a part to play (Figure 52.8). The labelled white blood cells migrate to areas of inflammation and infection, and in IBD they move through the bowel lumen and are excreted in the faeces. This technique is useful in establishing the presence of IBD and in assessing its activity, particularly in acute disease or when abscess or fistulae are suspected. It also helps to distinguish IBD from irritable bowel syndrome, in which no accumulation of radiolabelled leucocytes is seen (16). Scintigraphy has a sensitivity of 96% and a specificity of 97% for IBD and a sensitivity of 85–100% and a specificity of 100% for detecting abscess (17,18).

The most common radiotracers used for imaging IBD are either [111]In- or ^{99m}Tc-hexamethyl propylene amine oxime (HMPAO)-labelled leucocytes. Indium-111 may be preferable for the diagnosis of complications (particularly in Crohn's disease) such as mural or communicating abscess, or fistulae

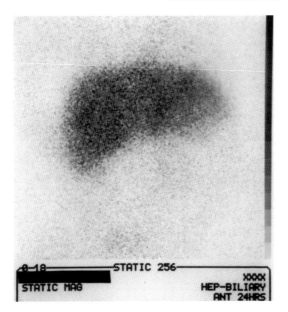

Figure 52.6. Biliary atresia in a 2-week-old infant with jaundice: ^{99m}Tc-HIDA scan. Twenty-four-hour scan shows hepatic and faint renal activity but no radioactive bile in the ducts, gallbladder, or bowel. Portoenterostomy was performed when the child was age 2 months. (Courtesy of Dr M. Al-Janabi.)

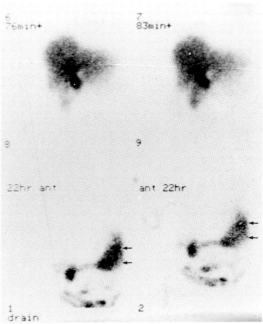

Figure 52.7. Enterogastric reflux in a 47-year-old male patient with postprandial epigastric pain, nausea, and vomiting. ^{99m}Tc-HIDA scan. Top row: Tracer concentration by the hepatocytes, with activity in the biliary tree and bowel is seen by 76–83 min. Bottom row: Delayed images at 22 h show significant reflux of the radioactivity into the stomach (arrow).

involving the vagina or bladder. Various techniques have been described for radiolabelling white cells. They involve a series of sedimentations and centrifugation of the blood sample to separate the white cells, which then undergo incubation with a radioactive compound, and are resuspended and washed before being reinjected into the patient. If ^{99m}Tc-HMPAO has been used as a radiolabel, the imaging is initiated between 1 and 2 h after the injection, whereas if ^{111}In-oxime was used, the early images are usually acquired at 4 h and delayed images at 24 h after the injection.

COLORECTAL CANCER

Radioimmunoscintigraphy has been used in the detection of recurrent colorectal cancer, before and when serum markers such as carcinoembryonic antigen (CEA) are increased. In this technique, monoclonal antibodies radiolabelled with ^{111}In or ^{99m}Tc, which bind to the tumour cells, are used for imaging. In a recent survey of radioimmunoscintigraphy in gastrointestinal tumours, sensitivity of 79%, specificity of 85%, and accuracy of 81% were reported in a large number of patients, using a battery

of radiolabelled monoclonal antibodies and their fragments (19).

NEUROENDOCRINE TUMOURS

Endocrine tumours of the pancreas and bowel can secrete several hormones, each with varying degrees of biological activity. Despite the availability of several imaging techniques, the localization of these tumours remains difficult for the gastroenterologist and radiologist. Recently, several new modalities such as magnetic resonance imaging, arterial sampling, and receptor scintigraphy have been developed.

^{111}In-pentetreotide, a somatostatin analogue, has been used for imaging small-cell cancers of the gastrointestinal tract and the gastroendocrine tumours such as insulinomas, gastrinomas, vasoactive intestinal peptide-producing adenomas (VIPomas), and glucagonomas. **Reported frequencies of positive scans using ^{111}In-pentetreotide (20,21) are:**

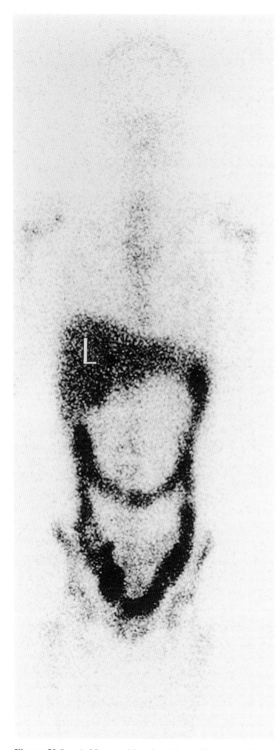

- gastrinomas   81%
- glucagonomas   95%
- carcinoid   86%
- insulinomas   61%
- somatostatinomas   100%
- VIPomas   80%

More recently, iodine-123-labelled VIP has been used for imaging intestinal adenocarcinomas and various endocrine tumours that express a large number of high-affinity receptors for VIP (22).

[123]I-meta-iodobenzyl guanidine (MIBG) is an aralkylguanidine that structurally resembles no-radrenaline. ^{123}I-MIBG has been used for imaging carcinoid tumours (Figure 52.9); it concentrates in approximately 71% of these tumours. The main indication for the diagnostic use of ^{123}I-MIBG is to evaluate patients with carcinoid tumours for possible palliative therapy with iodine-131-labelled MIBG; it may also be used to monitor response to treatment (23).

POSITRON EMISSION TOMOGRAPHY IN THE GASTROINTESTINAL TRACT

Owing to its functional metabolic imaging capabilities, PET imaging with fluorine-18-labelled fluoro-2-deoxyglucose (FDG) may detect malignant lesions where CT and MRI fail to do so. Studies have shown that recurrent colorectal tumours and hepatic primaries and secondaries can be detected with an accuracy and sensitivity of 90—96% and 92—100% respectively (24,25). Radiopharmaceutical agents such as ^{18}F-FDG, ^{11}C-5-hydroxytryptophan (HTP) and ^{11}C-1-dihydroxyphenylalanine (dopa) show great promise in the detection of pancreatic and functional endocrine tumours. Malignant cells show a high glucose metabolism, and this enhanced glycolysis can be detected with FDG, even in small tumours. The **indications** for ^{18}F-FDG imaging are screening for recurrent disease in cases of increased CEA with negative CT, exclusion of recurrence when a mass is seen on CT, and staging of recurrent disease.

It is difficult, with current diagnostic tools, to distinguish between pancreatic carcinoma and a benign pancreatic lesion or chronic pancreatitis; ^{18}F-FDG studies are also showing promise in this area, the reported sensitivity and specificity being 96% and 87% respectively (26). Ahlstrom *et al.* (27) reported detection of endocrine pancreatic

Figure 52.8. A 55-year-old male patient with known ulcerative colitis: [99mTc]-labelled white blood cell study. There is increased tracer activity in the colon, extending up to the rectum on the early images. L, hepatic activity.

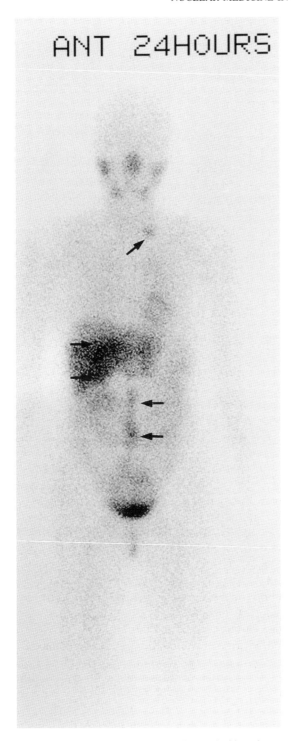

ANT 24HOURS

Figure 52.9. A 47-year-old woman with carcinoid syndrome and known liver metastases: ^{123}I-MIBG scan. The study shows multiple focal areas of increased tracer uptake in the liver, along the para-aortic region and in the left supraclavicular region, consistent with ^{123}I-MIBG-avid disease.

tumours such as gastrinoma and glucagonoma using ^{11}C-1-dopa and ^{11}C-5-HTP.

The value of non-invasive PET is becoming evident, in spite of its high cost and limited availability. Research directed towards finding new radioligands may further enhance the role of PET imaging.

PERITONEOVENOUS SHUNTS

Two types of peritoneovenous shunt are commonly used: the LeVeen shunt and the Denver shunt. The test of choice for shunt patency is the intraperitoneal scintigraphic method using ^{99m}Tc-macroaggregated albumin, a lung perfusion agent, injected intraperitoneally. Visualization of both lungs indicates shunt patency. The test has a high sensitivity (100%), specificity (92.2%), and accuracy (98.5%) for detection of shunt patency (28,29).

BOWEL FUNCTION

Carbon-14 breath test

The carbon-14 breath tests help evaluate the absorption and metabolism of various substances from the bowel. All of these tests utilize the rate of excretion of ^{14}C-carbon dioxide in breath after ingestion of a ^{14}C-labelled compound, as a measure of the rate of its absorption or malabsorption (30).

The test most frequently used is the **[14]C-urea breath test** for detection of active *Helicobacter pylori* infection. Ideally, the patient should not have taken any food or drink other than water for 12 h before the test, as false-negative results may otherwise be obtained. Antibiotics may also lead to false-negative results by suppressing, but not eradicating, *H. pylori*. For this reason, patients should be tested at least 1 month after completetion of *H. pylori* eradication treatment. The ^{14}C-urea breath test is unreliable (tending to give false-negative results) in patients who have undergone gastric surgery.

Among the other ^{14}C-labelled tests, **[14]C-cholylglycine** is used to assess bile acid malabsorption and bacterial overgrowth in the gut in patients with diarrhoea, **[14]C-lactose** can be used to evaluate lactose intolerance, **[14]C-triolene** with a standard fat load is used to assess patients with steatorrhoea, and **[14]C-d-xylose** can be used in the diagnostic

investigation of patients suspected of having malabsorption as a result of bacterial overgrowth or
mucosal disease in the small intestine.

Vitamin B_{12} malabsorption

Vitamin B_{12} deficiency is one of the common causes
of megaloblastic anaemia. The cause of vitamin B_{12}
malabsorption can often be directly determined by
using the modified Schilling test (**Dicopac test**).
After an overnight fast, the patient is given one
capsule of cobalt-58-labelled cyanocobalamin, followed 2 h later by a second capsule of cobalt-57-
labelled cyanocobalamin with intrinsic factor, and
then a flushing intramuscular injection of 1 mg
cyanocobalamin. Urine is subsequently collected
for 24 h. This test is extremely reliable and can
differentiate between vitamin B_{12} malabsorption
attributable to intrinsic factor deficiency and that
from other causes (30). The normal range for the
Dicopac test is 12–30% for ^{57}Co (bound to intrinsic
factor), and 11–28% for ^{58}Co.

Bile-acid malabsorption

Bile-acid malabsorption can lead to diarrhoea and
flatulence. The presence of excess concentration of
dihydroxy bile acids in the large bowel inhibits the
reabsorption of sodium and increases water secretion; the two together increase the fluid volume and
lead to diarrhoea. Bile acid malabsorption is best
assessed using selenium-75-labelled selenohomot-
aurocholic acid (the **SeHCAT test**). The tracer is the
taurine conjugate of a synthetic bile acid containing
^{75}Se in the side chain. It behaves in most respects like
taurocholate, although it is more resistant to bacterial
attack. Absorption and excretion of this tracer are
identical to those of taurocholate. After oral administration of this radiopharmaceutical, measurements
are taken over 7 days. A greater than 16% retention
of tracer indicates normal absorption (31).

RADIONUCLIDE THERAPY

The therapeutic role of nuclear medicine is limited
to gastrointestinal oncology. The common indications include palliative treatment of carcinoid tumours and hepatocellular carcinomas with
^{131}I-MIBG and ^{131}I-Lipiodol respectively.

^{131}I-MIBG

Patients selected for this form of treatment should
exhibit a relatively high uptake of tracer on the
diagnostic ^{123}I-MIBG scan (Figure 52.9) and a life
expectancy of more than 1 year, as the response to
^{131}I-MIBG therapy is slow (32). Before the treatment, complete blood count and baseline hormonal
measurements are carried out. The thyroid gland is
blocked with potassium iodide 120 mg, starting 48 h
before the infusion of therapy and continuing
for 20 days after therapy. Patients are reviewed at
3-monthly intervals. The side effects of this treatment depend upon the clinical condition of the
patient, but are typically minimal; leucopenia and
thrombocytopenia occur quite frequently. Among
patients with metastatic carcinoid tumours, partial
response has been achieved in 20%, whereas a
palliative response is observed in 58%. These results
should be viewed against a background of widespread metastatic disease that shows little or no
response to other forms of treatment.

^{131}I-Lipiodol

The use of ^{131}I-Lipiodol in hepatocellular carcinoma is reviewed in Chapter 18.2.

References
1. de Caestecker JS, Blackwell JN, Adam RD *et al.* Clinical
    value of radionuclide oesophageal transit measurement. *Gut*
    1986; **27**: 659–666.
2. Fisher RS, Malmud LS, Roberts GS *et al.* Gastroesophageal
    (GE) scintiscanning to detect and quantitate GE reflux.
    Gastroenterology 1976; **70**: 301–308.
3. Shay SS, Eggli D, Johnson LF. Simultaneous esophageal pH
    monitoring and scintigraphy during the postprandial period
    in patients with severe reflux oesophagitis. *Dig Dis Sci* 1991;
    36: 558–564.
4. Seibert JJ, Byrne WJ, Euler AR *et al.* Gastrooesophageal
    reflux – the acid test: scintigraphy or the pH probe? *Am J
    Roentgenol* 1983; **140**: 1087–1090.
5. Jian R, Ducrot F, Ruskone A *et al.* Symptomatic, radionuclide
    and therapeutic assessment of chronic idiopathic dyspepsia.
    Dig Dis Sci 1989; **34**: 657–664.
6. Wald A. Colonic transit and rectal manometry in chronic
    idiopathic constipation. *Ann Intern Med* 1986; **146**: 1713–
    1716.
7. Maurer AH, Krevsky B. Whole-gut transit scintigraphy in the
    evaluation of small-bowel and colon transit disorders. *Semin
    Nucl Med* 1995; **25**: 326–338.
8. Bunker SR, Brown JM, McAuley RJ *et al.* Detection of
    gastrointestinal bleeding sites: use of in vitro technetium Tc-
    99m-labelled RBCs. *JAMA* 1982; **247**: 789–792.

9. Cooney DR, Duszynski DO, Gamboa E *et al*. The abnormal technetium scan (a decade of experience). *J Paediatr Surg* 1982; **17**: 611–619.

10. Kim EE, Moon T-Y, Delpassand ES *et al*. Nuclear hepatobiliary imaging. *Radiol Clin North Am* 1993; **31**: 923–933.

11. Kim CK, Juweid M, Woda A *et al*. Hepatobiliary scintigraphy: morphine augmented versus delayed imaging in patients with suspected acute cholecystitis. *J Nucl Med* 1993; **34**: 506–509.

12. Mirvis SE, Vainwright JR, Nelson AW *et al*. The diagnosis of acute acalculous cholecystitis: a comparison of sonography, scintigraphy and CT. *Am J Roentgenol* 1986; **147**: 1171–1175.

13. Krishnamurthy S, Krishnamurthy GT. Biliary dyskinesia: role of the sphincter of Oddi, gall bladder and cholecystokinin. *J Nucl Med* 1997; **38**: 1824–1830.

14. Negrin JA, Zanzi I, Margouleff D. Hepatobiliary scintigraphy after biliary tract surgery. *Semin Nucl Med* 1995; **25**: 28–35.

15. Shah AS, Dodson F, Fung J. Role of nuclear medicine in liver transplantation. *Semin Nucl Med* 1995; **25**: 36–48.

16. Roelich JW, Swanson DP: Imaging of inflammatory processes with labelled cells. *Semin Nucl Med* 1984; **14**: 128–140.

17. Datz FL. Indium-111 labelled leukocytes for the detection of infection: current status. *Semin Nucl Med* 1994; **24**: 92–109.

18. Notghi A, Harding LK. The clinical challenge of nuclear medicine in gastroenterology. *Br J Hosp Med* 1995; **54**: 80–86.

19. Delaloye BA, Delaloye B. Tumour imaging with monoclonal antibodies. *Semin Nucl Med* 1995; **25**: 144–164.

20. Krenning EP, Kwekkeboom DJ, Bakker WH *et al*. Somatostatin receptor scintigraphy with ^{111}In-DTPA-D-Phe[1] and ^{123}I-Tyr[3]-octreotide: Rotterdam experience with more than 1000 patients. *Eur J Nucl Med* 1993; **20**: 713–716.

21. King CMP, Reznek RH, Bomanji J *et al*. Imaging neuroendocrine tumours with radiolabelled somatostatin analogues and X-ray computed tomography: a comparative study. *Clin Radiol* 1993; **48**: 386–391.

22. Virgolini I, Raderer M, Kurtaran A *et al*. Vasoactive intestinal peptide-receptor imaging for the localisation of intestinal adenocarcinomas and endocrine tumours. *N Engl J Med* 1994; **331**: 1116–1121.

23. Bomanji J, Ur E, Mather S *et al*. A scintigraphic comparison of I-123 metaiodobenzylguanidine (MIBG) and I-123 labelled somatostatin analogue (Tyr-3-octreotide) in metastatic carcinoid tumours. *J Nucl Med* 1992; **33**: 1121–1124.

24. Strauss LG, Conti PS. The applications of PET in clinical oncology. *J Nucl Med* 1991; **32**: 623–648.

25. Takeuchi O, Saito N, Koda K, *et al*. Clinical assessment of positron emission tomography for the diagnosis of local recurrence in colorectal cancer. *Br J Surg* 1999; **85**: 932–937.

26. Inokuma T, Tamaki N, Torizuka T *et al*. Evaluation of pancreatic tumours with positron emission tomography and F-18 fluorodeoxyglucose: comparison with CT and US. *Radiology* 1995; **195**: 345–352.

27. Ahlstrom H, Eriksson B, Bergstrom M *et al*. Pancreatic neuroendocrine tumors: diagnosis with PET. *Radiology* 1995; **195**: 333–337.

28. Maddedu G, D'Ovideo NG, Casu AR *et al*. Evaluation of peritoneovenous shunt patency with Tc-99m labeled microspheres. *J Nucl Med* 1983; **24**: 302–307.

29. Stewart CA, Sakimura IT, Applebaum DM *et al*. Evaluation of peritoneovenous shunt patency by intraperitoneal Tc-99m macroaggregated albumin: clinical experience. *Am J Roentgenol* 1986; **147**: 177–180.

30. Hansell J. Gastrointestinal absorption and loss studies. In: *Gastrointestinal Nuclear Imaging*. Eds. MG Velchik, A Alavi. New York: Churchill Livingstone, 1988; pp. 257–280.

31. Merrick MV. Assessment of the small intestine. In: *Nuclear Gastroenterology*. Ed. PJ Robinson. Edinburgh: Churchill Livingstone, 1986; pp. 157–169.

32. Bomanji J, Britton KE, Ur E *et al*. Treatment of phaeochromocytoma, paraganglioma, and carcinoid tumours with metaiodobenzylguanidine. *Nucl Med Commun* 1993; **14**: 856–861.

Appendix: Gastroenterology Training in Europe

ALISTAIR D. BEATTIE

Political changes within Europe have brought professional groups closer, and gastroenterologists are now well used to scientific contact with fellow Europeans. For many years subspecialty groups within gastroenterology have been meeting on a regular basis; the major pan-European societies are described later in this chapter.

Within the European Union (EU) and the European Free Trade Area (EFTA), professional qualifications are reciprocated and free movement of doctors between member states is a reality. This has driven a desire to harmonize standards of training and, indeed, standards of practice. The professional will to pursue these objectives is quite considerable. The political will is also present but, as in many other areas, often obscurely expressed. Individual initiatives have been undertaken by some of the specialty societies, but the body charged with harmonizing standards of training is the Union of European Medical Specialists (UEMS), which has existed since 1962 and operates through some 32 monospecialty sections, of which gastroenterology is one.

POLITICAL STRUCTURE

The means by which the EU obtains advice on medical matters is complex, and is shown in Table A.1. A detailed description is unnecessary. Briefly, at professional level the various specialties, including gastroenterology, have input through the UEMS. This body is, essentially, a lobby to the EU, and its aim is to produce a high standard of clinical practice for the citizens of Europe by encouraging good training, continuing education, and exchanges between countries. It has also been charged with addressing the problems of manpower inequality throughout the countries that are represented.

TRAINING REQUIREMENTS

The most sensitive issue in harmonizing standards of gastroenterological practice in Europe is the variation that exists in the training requirements and the content of training programmes in the countries of the EU and the other countries of the continent. This is an important issue, because European law provides complete reciprocity of specialist qualifications and freedom of movement of specialists within the EU. It is therefore desirable that a measure of uniformity be achieved in relation to the duration of training and qualifications required to enter higher specialty training. Table A.2 indicates the current requirements in 17 European countries.

Some of the statistics require to be interpreted in the light of local knowledge. Specialty training is designed to equip the trainee to practice at a career grade with responsibility for patient care. In the UK, the Netherlands, and some of the Scandinavian countries, the nature of consultant practice will usually include a substantial component of general internal medicine; the training reflects this. In most other European countries, specialists practice gastroenterology or even one of its subspecialties, alone and training does not include general medicine beyond the common trunk level. Thus, the 4 years of training in France and Italy will be only in gastroenterology,

Table A.1. Political relationships in European medicine.

European Parliament	Council of Ministers	EC Directives
	Commission of the European Communities (DG IIID/2)	Committee of Senior Public Health Officers
	EC Advisory Committee on Medical Training	Professional experts
		Government experts
		Universities experts
		EC
National Level		Profession
National Organization of Medical Doctors (general practitioners and specialists)	EC Standing Committee of Doctors	European Union of General Practitioners UEMO
		European Association of Hospital Doctors (AEMH)
		International Conference of Orders (CIO)
National Organization of Medical Specialists	Union of European Medical Specialists UEMS	European Federation of Salaried Doctors (FEMS)
		Permanent Working Group of Junior Hospital Doctors (PWG)
National Professional Monospecialist Associations	Monospecialist Sections of the UEMS	
National Professional and Scientific Associations	Working Group Medical Specialists European Boards	

whereas the 5 years in UK will contain an interspersed mixture of gastroenterology and general medicine, in a ratio of approximately 3:2.

In some countries, specialty training is started at an early stage in the doctor's career. In Italy, for example, a trainee is accepted for specialty training immediately after completing the undergraduate course and pre-registration experience. The training is formal and, on its completion, an examination is taken, leading to the nationally recognized Certificate in Gastroenterology that is issued by one of about 20 Universities. At this stage, the trainee is

Table A.2. Training requirements in European countries.

Country	Examination	Total duration of training (years)	Common trunk of internal medicine	Training programme	Training log-book
Austria	Yes	9	6	Yes	Yes
Belgium	No	8	3	Yes	Yes
Czech Republic	Yes	6	3	Yes	Yes
Denmark	No	7	4	Yes	No
France	Yes	4	1.5	Yes	Yes
Finland	Yes	6	3	Yes	Yes
Germany	Yes	8	5	Yes	No
Greece	Yes	6	2	No	No
Italy	Yes	7	No	Yes	Yes
Ireland	No	7	2	No	No
Lithuania	Yes	5	3	Yes	No
Norway	No	7	4	Yes	Yes
Netherlands	No	6	3	Yes	No
Poland	Yes	8	5	Yes	Yes
Portugal	Yes	6	1	Yes	Yes
Spain	No	6.5	1.5	Yes	Yes
Sweden	No	5	2	Yes	Yes
Switzerland	Yes	6	3	Yes	Yes
United Kingdom	No	7	2	No	No

still expected to obtain further clinical experience before entering a career post, but the certificate is the qualification that must be recognized by other EU member states. This contrasts with most of the northern European countries, where the nationally recognized certificate is given at the stage at which the trainee is expected to obtain his ultimate career post in which independent consultant practice will commence. One system is not necessarily superior to the other, but difficulties arise in recognizing equivalence of the qualifications.

United Kingdom

The UK has a requirement of a minimum of 2 years of "common trunk" training in general internal medicine before higher specialty training commences. In practice, it would be unusual for a trainee to be appointed to a higher specialty training post without spending at least 2 years in general medicine and a further 1–2 years in a post that gives some experience of clinical and investigative gastroenterology, before embarking on formal specialty training. Time in research is strongly encouraged and may count as part of the training time, depending on the nature of the research and the clinical involvement. The inclusion of this time is at the discretion of the Specialty Advisory Committee in Gastroenterology, which operates by guidelines established by the Joint Committee on Higher Medical Training of the Royal Colleges of Physicians. The programme is not nationally defined, but individual area training programmes are expected to provide exposure to all subspecialties and to include experience in both district hospitals and teaching hospitals. A log-book has recently been introduced as a means of monitoring the trainee's experience in practical procedures. There is no examination, and progress to the Certificate of Completion of Specialist Training depends on satisfactory reports from trainers and external assessment in the penultimate year of training.

Austria

Austria introduced an examination in 1999, and this is taken at the end of training, which is 9 years after registration as a doctor. There is a defined training programme, with exposure to a series of subspecialties after a 6-year internal-medicine common trunk.

Belgium

Belgium has a 3-year common trunk, followed by 5 years of gastroenterology training, but no exit examination. The training is closely defined, and a log-book is kept, to record practical competence.

Switzerland

Switzerland has a training programme similar to that of Belgium, with no exit examination and, at present, no log-book.

Germany

The relatively long internal-medicine training is a feature of German training, although there is an element of dual training. Most gastroenterological practice is eventually performed as a separate specialty, with a strong emphasis on procedural work. All gastroenterologists carry out their own ultrasound practice, which has been a difference from some, if not most, other countries in Europe, and a source of controversy in recent years.

Scandanavian countries

The Danish, Swedish, Norwegian, and Finnish models are all fairly similar. Training is 5–7 years in each, with an extra year if the trainee wishes to become a specialist in both gastroenterology and internal medicine. The use of log-books is longer established than in any other part of the continent, and exit examinations are not conducted, except in Finland. The small population of Iceland does not sustain a full training programme; all Icelandic gastroenterologists receive some of their training in other countries.

Finland

Training in Finland differs from some of the other Scandanavian countries. Each University has a gastroenterology training programme that conforms to a national model, and each programme is nationally regarded as equivalent. The training programme lasts 6 years and consists of at least 3 years of internal medicine and 3 years of gastroenterology. The goal of the common trunk is to impart the skill to practise internal medicine, and 6 months of the common trunk must be spent in general practice. The trainees are registered as students in the

University and they have a training post in a University hospital or in a training hospital accepted by the University. After completion of training, there is a written examination conducted by selected trainers. Trainees who complete training and pass the examination are given a certificate and registered as gastroenterologists by the Department of Medical Affairs.

Greece

Trainees in Greece have a 2-year common trunk training in internal medicine and 5 years in gastroenterology, with an exit examination at the conclusion of training.

Italy

The training programme in Italy is somewhat different from most Northern European systems. The programmes are supervised by about 20 Universities, which are authorized by the government to issue certificates of completion of training. Until recently, there was no common trunk training, although this may be changing. Trainees enter a 4-year programme straight from pre-registration posts; centres admit from four to eight doctors per year to these programmes. At the conclusion of the programme, the trainee receives the diploma that is recognized under European law. During training, there is ample opportunity for clinical research, and this is reflected in the large contribution made by Italian gastroenterologists at international meetings.

France

Training requirements are similar to those in Italy. Training in general medicine is compulsory and lasts one and a half years.

Ireland

Ireland has been closely linked to the UK system for many years, but is now establishing its own certification of completion of training. The training programmes are similar to the British models, although most of the trainees are encouraged to spend some of their training time outside the country. Research is strongly encouraged at an early stage and there is no exit examination. Certification as a gastroenterologist alone, or in combination with internal medicine, is awarded by the Royal College of Physicians

of Ireland. Each trainee is required to complete a log-book, and progress is reviewed annually.

The Netherlands

Training in the Netherlands is relatively long, which reflects the tendency to practise general medicine in conjunction with gastroenterology. The programmes are structured mostly within academic centres and there is no exit examination. There is some variation in the amount of time spent in internal medicine, but the minimum period is 3 years. Research is encouraged at all stages, and is an integral part of specialty training.

Lithuania

Lithuania, although not in the EU or EFTA, sends an observer to UEMS and European Board meetings and is developing a training scheme on similar lines. The common trunk is 3 years and specialty training is 5 years.

Portugal

Portugal has competitive entry to training that includes 1 year of internal-medicine common trunk. There is structured training, a log-book, and an exit examination after 5 years of specialty training.

Spain

Spain has a system fairly similar to that of Portugal, with a slightly longer common trunk and no exit examination.

EUROPEAN BOARD OF GASTROENTEROLOGY

In order to meet its objective of promoting a high level of specialist care in European countries, the UEMS Specialist Section of Gastroenterology established a European Board of Gastroenterology in 1992. The Board is comprised of two members from each country, and admits observers from Eastern European countries. Its **objectives** are as follows:

1. to promote and recognize quality of training in gastroenterology
2. to facilitate continuing medical education
3. to research into demography and manpower

4. to promote exchange programmes

The European Board of Gastroenterology (EBG) is currently attempting to bring the different forms of training into line with each other by setting minimum programme contents, which are shown below. The purpose of this programme is to define the minimum training that must be undertaken before a trainee can be described as a gastroenterologist. The Board has initiated a system of inspection of training centres and issues a Certificate of Accreditation that allows trainees to register in these centres and to achieve the European Diploma of Gastroenterology on completion of training.

At present, the certificates of the European Board have no legal standing, and they are not required by trainees who wish to practise in another country. Their present purpose is to draw training standards in different European countries closer together, and to minimize the anomalies created by freedom of movement of specialists in Europe.

Training requirements of the European Board of Gastroenterology

Duration of training

A minimum of 6 years of postgraduate training is required. This does not include the pre-registration year, and at least 2 years should be in general internal medicine.

Structure of training

Fundamental training
Training in fundamental knowledge and skills should include internal medicine (2–3 years). This should ensure that the trainee is familiar with the principal aspects of internal medicine, including cardiology, nephrology, respiratory disease, rheumatology, diabetes, and endocrinology, in addition to gastroenterology.

Specialty training
This should be in gastroenterology, including hepatology, and should last 3–4 years.

Training programme, log-book

Theoretical and practical training will follow an established programme approved by the national authorities in accordance with national rules and EU/EFTA legislation, and with UEMS/EBG recommendations. At EU/EFTA level, the UEMS Section and the EBG recommend that training programmes should include the following modules.

Theoretical training
This includes:
- aetiology, pathogenesis, symptomatology, and treatment of diseases of the gastrointestinal tract, liver, and pancreas;
- practical knowledge of, and expertise in, the interpretation of biological and functional tests and medical imaging techniques
- knowledge of ethics and public health economics

Practical skills
This expertise should be acquired in training centres under appropriate supervision. Two levels of training in practical procedures are recognized by the UEMS Section and the EBG:

1. A basic level required for the EBG diploma in gastroenterology (see below).
2. Optional subjects leading to certification in individual practical procedures; this can only be acquired after qualification at the basic level.

Basic obligatory requirements
These are defined in terms of the minimum number of procedures that must have been undertaken (Table A.3).

Optional subjects
This level consists of operations and specific techniques. It is optional after qualification at the basic level. Certification can be acquired for individual techniques, for which, again, minimum numbers of procedures are required to have been performed (Table A.4).

As new techniques in gastroenterology are developed, they will be considered by the UEMS Section and the EBG for recognition.

Log-book and other considerations
A log-book must be kept, with details concerning each investigation. It has to be signed by the appropriate supervisor.

The candidate must have presented two contributions in a meeting of a national or international gastroenterology society.

Table A.3. Basic obligatory requirements.

Minimum number of procedures:	
Abdominal ultrasound investigations	300
Endoscopic investigations:	
Oesophagogastroduodenoscopy (OGD)	300
Sclerotherapy of oesophageal varices and haemostatic techniques of the upper gastrointestinal tract	30
Total colonoscopy	100
Colonoscopic polypectomy and haemostatic techniques of the lower gastrointestinal tract	50
Proctoscopy	100
Abdominal puncture and/or biopsy with or without ultrasound control (for example liver biopsy) and laparoscopy	50

Table A.4. Minimum number of procedures.

Therapeutic endoscopy (eg. LASER techniques, stricture dilatation)	100
Diagnostic and therapeutic Endoscopic Retrograde Cholangiopancreaticography (ERCP)	150
Manometric and pH-metric investigations	50
Endoscopic ultrasound investigations	150
Diagnostic laparoscopy	50
Interventional proctology	80
Advanced hepatology: clinical management of liver transplant and complex liver disease	

The candidate must have taken a major part in two publications in journals listed in *Current Contents* or in peer-reviewed journals recognized by the Examining Body of the diploma.

Continuing medical education must be pursued by the European graduate in hepatogastroenterology and, normally, the candidate for the diploma is expected to be a member of his or her national gatroenterological scientific association.

Training abroad in the EU or EFTA
Trainees should have the opportunity to be trained in recognized training institutions in other UEMS member countries during their training, with the approval of their country of origin.

European Diploma of Gastroenterology

The EBG issues diplomas both to training institutions and to individual doctors who satisfy the training criteria.

Training Recognition Certificate

The Training Recognition Certificate is issued to training centres that meet certain criteria and are inspected by representatives of the Board. The main guiding principles behind this diploma are as follows:

1. there must be evidence of good training
2. training must be in sound institutions
3. teachers must be experienced gastroenterologists
4. the trainees must receive appropriate tuition
5. trainees must have clinical responsibility in substantive paid posts

The teachers themselves must be well established in their specialty, must be recognized nationally as career-grade gastroenterologists, and must show a commitment to teaching their trainees. It is essential that the trainees are salaried members of a clinical team, and not simply on clinical attachment.

The ultrasound controversy

The EBG published its curriculum for training in 1994. Immediate controversy was raised by the inclusion of ultrasound in the core subjects that are to be taken by all trainees who wish to obtain the European Diploma. In some countries, notably Germany and France, ultrasound examinations are conducted by almost all practising gastroenterologists, whereas in others the technique is performed exclusively by radiologists. The issue remains unresolved, and the EBG has indicated that training in ultrasound should be an aim but that, until such training is more universally available, the diploma will be awarded to those who have not received the training.

The controversy remains unresolved, and there is little evidence that training will be universally available in the foreseeable future. The concept of a gastroenterologist being able to take a patient from the examination couch to an ultrasound machine in the clinic has much to commend it, and comparison is drawn with the cardiologists who have kept echocardiography within their own expertise. The reality, in most countries, is that trainees find it difficult to add ultrasound training to the expanding list of endoscopic and other technical skills that they are expected to acquire.

Opinions will continue to differ, and quality of care for patients should be the only criterion acquired. If trainee gastroenterologists can devote sufficient time to the development of ultrasound training, this may be highly beneficial to patient care, but in most European countries it seems likely that the technique will remain in the hands of radiologists.

SPECIALTY GASTROENTEROLOGICAL ASSOCIATIONS IN EUROPE

Specialist organizations have grown up in an *ad hoc* fashion over a period of about 50 years. At a clinical and scientific level, the various pan-European associations came together in the first United European Gastroenterology meeting, which was held in 1992 in Athens and has been held annually since then. The meeting is organized by the United European Gastroenterology Federation (UEGF), which is derived from its seven founding organizations, sometimes referred to as the seven sisters. The founding members are:

1. *ASNEMGE*: Association des Sociétés Nationales Européennes et Mediterranéennes de Gastro-enterologie.
2. *CICD*: Collegium Internationale Chirurgiae Digestivae (European Chapter).
3. *EAGE*: European Association for Gastroenterology and Endoscopy.
4. *EASL*: European Association for the Study of the Liver.
5. *EPC*: European Pancreatic Club.
6. *ESGE*: European Society for Gastrointestinal Endoscopy.
7. *ESPGHAN*: European Society for Paediatric Gastroenterology, Hepatology and Nutrition.

Continuing medical education

Gastroenterologists in all European countries have been involved in continuing medical education for many years. Recent times have seen a political requirement to formalize such arrangements, in order to satisfy a public concern that doctors keep up to date with modern developments. This is strongly supported by UEMS.

Organizations devoted to continuing education of gastroenterologists exist at local, national and international levels throughout Europe, and the main problem for the practising specialist is to obtain the necessary information and to select the meetings most likely to be beneficial. Much national and international information is now available on the internet. For example the British Society of Gastroenterology has an extensive website (http://www.bsg.org.uk), which outlines the history and aims of the Society and gives the office address and the dates of future meetings. Almost every European country has its own national gastroenterology society and, gradually, all are adopting the Internet as a source of information. The French National Society of Gastroenterology (SNFGE) has an excellent website that lists almost every significant forthcoming French and international gastrointestinal meeting. This can be found on the Internet at http://snfge.asso.fr/indexa.html

At a European level, there is an educational and scientific society within every subspecialty. Some are more formally constituted than others. A list is given in Table A.5. Several of these organizations have made good use of the Internet. The European Association for the Study of the Liver (EASL) has an informative website (http://www.munksgaard.com) that gives details of the scientific committee, forthcoming meetings, and its official publication, *Journal of Hepatology*. The European Association for Endoscopic Surgery gives similar information, and also details of training courses in that specialty.

European Association for the Study of the Liver

EASL has held an annual scientific meeting since 1966, and has grown steadily in size and stature since that time. Its aim is to promote communication between scientists and clinicians interested in liver physiology and disease; membership is open to all that have a professional interest in the liver. Membership forms are available at the website or by writing to the Liaison Office.

Table A.5. European subspecialty Societies and Associations.

Organization	Registered Address	Website
European Association for the Study of the Liver	EASL Liaison Bureau, Hepatology Unit, 149 rue de Sevres, 75747 Paris, Cedex 15, France	ww.munksgaard.dk
European Pancreatic Club	Varies with secretary	www.kcl.ac.uk
European Society of Gastrointestinal Endoscopy	Varies with secretary	www.eage.com
European Association for Endoscopic Surgery	Varies with secretary	www.faehv.nl
European Association for Paediatric Gastroenterology, Hepatology and Nutrition	Varies with secretary	

The aims of EASL are also achieved by the publication of the *Journal of Hepatology*, and a subscription to this journal is included in membership of the Society.

An elected Council governs EASL; this is comprised of younger active scientists in the field of hepatology.

European Pancreatic Club

The EPC holds annual scientific meetings in different countries and has the following aims:

1. To promote communication between basic and clinical scientists in Europe interested in the pancreas and its disorders.
2. To promote and organize an annual scientific meeting devoted to all aspects of the pancreas.
3. To promote scientific, epidemiological and clinical research into pancreatic function and the prevention, diagnosis, and treatment of pancreatic diseases.
4. To establish scholarships and travel awards to promote postgraduate training.
5. To support other meetings concerning the pancreas by the attendance of members of the EPC.
6. To disseminate information about EPC activities and to establish such educational programmes as the EPC Council may consider desirable.

Membership is open to anyone with an interest in the pancreas. The Club is governed by an executive Council of office bearers and members from different European countries. The scientific meeting is conducted in English and normally lasts two and a half days.

European Society of Gastrointestinal Endoscopy

ESGE is a federation of European gastrointestinal endoscopy societies and is one of the bodies that organize the United Gastroenterology Week. It is comprised of national endoscopy organizations such as the Endoscopy Section of the British Society of Gastroenterology. Apart from its role in the United Gastroenterology Week, the Society achieves its scientific purpose by the publication of the journal, *Endoscopy*. This is the official organ of ESGE, but it is also the official journal of several European endoscopy societies and has collaboration from Hong Kong, Korea, Argentina, and the Philippines.

The purposes of the Society are:

1. To promote interest, teaching, and research in Gastrointestinal Endoscopy and related fields.
2. To stimulate international exchange of endoscopic data and technical advances and to promote large-scale studies.
3. To organize an European Congress of gastrointestinal endoscopy as part of the United Gastroenterology Week.

The Society achieves its aims through the United Gastroenterology Week but, in addition, it publishes a number of items, including a CD-ROM on endoscopy complications, a European Teaching Encyclopaedia on Digestive Endoscopy, and Guidelines on various aspects of endoscopic procedures.

References
1. Mallinson, CN. Specialist training in the European Community: the case for European Boards. *Gut* 1994; **35**: 135–138.
2. Beattie, AD: Gastroenterological training in Europe. *Gut* 1995; **37**: 734–735.

3. Beattie, AD, Greff, M, Lamy, V *et al*. The European Diploma of Gastroenterology: progress towards harmonization of standards. *Eur J Gastrenterol Hepatol* 1996; **8**: 403–406.

4. Rhodes, JM. CME – Certification by the European Board of Gastroenterology. *Gut* 1996; **39**: 149–150.

5. O'Morain, C, Whelton, M: European Union of Medical Specialties Section of Gastroenterology; present status. *Ir J Med Sci* 1997; **166**: 38–40.

Index

AA amyloid (reactive systemic amyloid) 80
abdominal cavity
  infracolic compartment 19
  macroscopic anatomy 15
  supracolic compartment 19
abdominal distension
  intestinal obstruction 197, 198
  irritable bowel syndrome 347
  small bowel disease 375
abdominal examination 10–11
abdominal pain
  acute 171–6
    abdominal findings 171
    diagnosis 171
    investigations 171–2
    medical causes 171
  autonomic neuropathy 111
  biliary colic 221
  haematological malignancy 58
  history-taking 4
  hyperthyroidism 47
  inflammatory bowel disease 427, 428
    Crohn's disease 213
  intestinal obstruction 197, 198
  irritable bowel syndrome 345
    management 347
  obstetric patients 116–17
  pancreatic carcinoma 381
  sickle cell crisis 329
  small bowel disease 375
  vomiting relationship 316
abdominal plain radiograph
  acute abdominal pain 171–2
  acute intestinal obstruction 198

acute pancreatitis 174
chronic pancreatitis 597
Crohn's disease 214
infectious colitis 416
pneumoperitoneum 175
ulcerative colitis 208
abdominal wall
  hernia 51
  macroscopic anatomy 15
absorption
  carbohydrate 372
  fat 372–3
  protein 372
absorptive cells, large intestine 32, 372
acamprosate 456
acetorphan 419
N-acetylcysteine 288, 291, 292
achalasia 186–8, 357, 358, 360–1, 446–7
  aetiology 186
  clinical features 187, 446
  diagnosis 187, 446–7, 602
  oesophageal carcinoma association 187, 189
  pathophysiology 186–7, 446
  treatment 187–8, 447
    balloon dilatation 188, 447
    cardiomyotomy 188, 447
acidosis
  acute diarrhoea 414, 415
  acute liver failure 291
acromegaly 47–8
  colorectal cancer screening 402
actinomycosis 174
activated protein C resistance (factor V Leiden) 65
acupressure 115

acupuncture 348
acyclovir 87, 90, 121, 511, 513
Addison's disease 46, 354, 374
adefovir 94, 493
adenomatous polyps
  colorectal cancer surveillance 404
  faecal occult blood testing 404–5
  familial adenomatous polyposis 399–400
  familial colorectal cancer risk 402
adenovirus
  acute watery diarrhoea 413
  hepatitis 61
  pancreatitis 57
adhesion molecule antibodies 210, 216
adrenaline injection, bleeding peptic ulcer 131–2, 141
adrenocortical insufficiency see Addison's disease
Aeromonas 259
age-related factors
  infectious diarrhoea susceptibility 411
  pain experience 4
air enema, ulcerative colitis 208
AL amyloid 80–1
albendazole 89, 93, 420, 421
albumin serum level 274, 596
alcohol consumption, excessive 150, 292, 455–60
  definition 455
  folic acid malabsorption 324
  haematinics deficiency 330
  identification 9, 455
  liver transplantation eligibility 309
  nausea/vomiting 317, 319
  oesophageal carcinoma 189, 191
  pancreatic disease 459–60
    acute pancreatitis 173, 174
  sedation for emergency endoscopy 127, 128
  vitamin replacement 155
alcohol disinfection 519
alcohol hepatotoxicity 455
alcohol injection 132
  hepatocellular carcinoma 246–7
alcoholic cirrhosis 456–9
  clinical features 456–7
  diagnosis 457
  hepatitis C infection progression 458–9
  liver transplantation 458, 459
  varices management 458
alcoholic fatty liver 456
alcoholic hepatitis, acute 305–11
  clinical features 305–6
  discriminant function 306, 308

histopathology 306
  laboratory investigations 306–7
  treatment 307–11
    anabolic steroids 309
    corticosteroids 306, 308–9
    liver transplantation 309–10
    nutritional support 39, 307–8
    pentoxifylline 310–11
alcoholic liver disease 9, 11, 455–9, 503
  pathology 36–7
alendronate 359
alginate sodium 56
alkaline phosphatase elevation 505–6
allergic granulomatous angiitis (Churg–Strauss syndrome) 79, 80
alpha-fetoprotein (AFP)
  hepatocellular carcinoma screening 242
  liver tumours 37
aluminium hydroxide 378
ambulatory antroduodenal manometry 112
ambulatory pH monitoring see oesophageal ambulatory 24-h pH monitoring
5-amino laevulinic acid (ALA) 540, 541
aminoglycosides
  acute secondary bacterial peritonitis 173
  neutropenic enterocolitis (typhlitis) 56
  perianal sepsis 59
  prophylaxis for endoscopy 527
aminosalicylates
  Crohn's disease 215
  ulcerative colitis 209
5-aminosalicylic acid (5-ASA; mesalazine) 73, 429–30, 439
  azo-bonded prodrugs 434
  controlled-release preparations 434
  Crohn's disease 436
  maintenance therapy 434–5
  slow-release preparations 434
  use in pregnancy 118
amoebiasis 353, 420
  colitis 416
  dysentery 413
  HIV-associated diarrhoea 89
  persistent diarrhoea 414
  treatment 419
amoebic liver abscess 417
  ultrasound appearances 559–60, 562
amoeboma 416
amoxycillin 64, 77, 419, 474, 481, 482, 527
amphotericin 63, 93, 291
ampicillin 419, 527

ampulla of Vater 18
amyloidosis 67, 80–1, 354, 355, 549
    AL amyloid 80–1
    familial amyloid polyneuropathy 81
    folic acid malabsorption 324
    megacolon 388
    reactive systemic amyloid (AA amyloid) 80
amyotrophic lateral sclerosis *see* motor neuron
    disease
anabolic steroids 309
anaemia 10, 321–30
    of chronic disease 326
    classification 321
    endoscopic appearances 131
    haematinic deficiency 321–8
    of liver disease 329–30
    persistent infective diarrhoea 415
    postgastrectomy 367
    small bowel disease 375
anal canal 19
anal carcinoma 34, 234, 510
    AIDS-related 97
    chemoradiation 234
anal fissure 507, 508–9, 510
anal fistula 509–10
anal lesions 507–11
    sexually transmitted diseases 511
anal pathology 34
anal sphincters
    external 393
    internal 393
    obstetric damage 395
    surgical damage 395–6
    surgical repair 397
anal warts *see* condyloma accuminata
angiodysplasia
    laser therapy 536
    upper gastrointestinal bleeding 130
angular cheilitis 87
ankylosing spondylitis 75
anorectal junction 19
anorectal myectomy 388
anorectal physiological testing 395
anorectal radiation injury 513, 514
anorectal sensory testing 385
anorexia 315
    postgastrectomy 374
    weight loss 371
anorexia nervosa 4, 10, 50, 51–2
    complications of refeeding 51–2
anorexic–bulimic syndrome 317

antacid therapy 56, 87, 332, 335, 386
    iron malabsorption 323
    non-ulcer (functional) dyspepsia 453
    peptic ulcer disease 144
    use in pregnancy 116, 117
antegrade continence enema (ACE) 398
anthracyclines 57, 66
antiandrogens 230
antibiotic prophylaxis
    acute liver failure 291
    endoscopy 525–8
        neutropenic patient 59
        recommended antibiotics 527–8
    infectious diarrhoea 422
    splenectomy patients 64
    spontaneous bacterial peritonitis 261–2
    variceal bleeding 154
antibiotic therapy 503
    bacterial overgrowth 77, 378
    bacterial peritonitis 172, 173, 261
    Crohn's disease 215–16, 217
    drug-related gastrointestinal dysfunction 346
    Helicobacter pylori diagnostic test effects 473,
        475
    infectious diarrhoea 419–21
    inflammatory bowel disease 434
    primary sclerosing cholangitis 300
    ulcerative colitis 209
    Whipple's disease 379
antibiotic-assocated diarrhoea 411–12
anticholinergic drugs 319
anticoagulants 208
anticonvulsants 103, 112–13, 292, 386, 503
antidepressants 346
antidiarrhoeal agents
    diabetic diarrhoea 46
    faecal incontinence 396–7
    infectious diarrhoea 419
antiemetic drugs 319
    chemotherapy management 57
    cyclophosphamide use in rheumatology 74
    side effects 57
    use in pregnancy 115, 116
antifungal prophylaxis 291
antihistamines 299
antimalarial agents 75
antiparkinsonian agents 103, 112–13, 386
antipsychotic drugs 386
antireflux surgery 185, 186
anti-*Saccharomyces cerevisiae* mannan antibodies
    (ASCA) 427

antithrombin III deficiency 65
antithyroid drugs 47
antituberculous drugs 503
anxiolytic drugs 319
aorta, duodenal relations 18
APC mutations 231, 400
aplastic anaemia 68–9, 330
appendicitis 173
    obstetric patients 117
    ultrasound appearances 574–5, 576
arachis oil enema 387
argon plasma coagulation
    Barrett's oesophagus 184, 185
    bleeding peptic ulcer 132
arteriovenous malformation 167, 168
artificial bowel sphincter 398
Ascaris lumbricoides 200, 414
ascites 12, 251–9
    acute alcoholic hepatitis 305
    causes 251, 252
    chylous 253, 255
    clinical diagnosis 12
    culture-negative neutrocytic (CNNA) 251
    hepatorenal syndrome 253
    investigations 253–5
    management 251, 255–9
    non-cirrhotic portal hypertension 258
    orthoptic liver transplantation 256, 257–8
    pathogenesis 251–3
    peritoneal inflammation 258–9
    refractory 256–8
        paracentesis 256–7
        peritoneovenous shunts 256, 257
        surgical portocaval shunts 256, 257
    spontaneous bacterial peritonitis 259, 260, 261
    subacute liver failure 287
    variceal bleeding 154
ascites fluid culture 260–1
ascites white cell count 253, 254
Aspergillus 60, 61
aspiration pneumonia 103
aspirin 150, 168, 468
    drug-induced nausea/vomiting 317
    upper gastrointestinal tract toxicity 71
Atkinson prosthesis 178, 193
atorvastatin 52
atovaquone 89
atrophic gastritis 323, 325
atypical chest pain 358, 364
atypical mycobacteria 91
Auerbach's (myenteric) plexus 16

autoimmune disease 503
autoimmune hepatitis
    autoimmune thyroiditis association 47
    chronic active 300–1
autoimmune liver disease 9
    acute liver failure 288, 290
    pregnant patients 121
automated endoscope washer/disinfector 517
autonomic neuropathy 103, 110–12
    causes 110
    diabetes mellitus *see* diabetes mellitus
    investigations 111–12
        gut motility assessment 112
    paraneoplastic 110
    physiology 112
    signs 111
    symptoms 110–11
    treatment 112
axillary lymph nodes 15
azathioprine 74, 215, 217, 218, 271, 299, 301,
        439, 510
    inflammatory bowel disease 431
        Crohn's disease 436
        ulcerative colitis 210
    use in pregnancy 118
azithromycin 89, 93
azygous vein–portal vein anastomoses 20

babesiosis 64
bacteraemia during endoscopy 525, 526–7
bacterial overgrowth
    autonomic neuropathy 111, 112
    Crohn's disease 281, 427, 428
    diabetic diarrhoea 43–4
    investigations 356, 595
        breath tests 598
    malabsorption 378
        vitamin B_{12} 323
    postgastrectomy 367, 374
    scleroderma 77
    treatment 378
bacterial peritonitis
    chronic 174
    cirrhotic patients 154
    primary 172
    secondary 173
    see also spontaneous bacterial peritonitis
bacterial translocation 259
Bacteroides 378, 462
Bacteroides fragilits 173
balloon dilatation, achalasia 188, 447

balsalazide 434
band ligation
  gastric varices 134
  oesophageal varices 133–4
    alcoholic cirrhosis 458
    multiple devices 133
    single ligators 133–4
barium enema 581, 596
  acute intussusception 200
  colorectal cancer screening 407
  Crohn's disease 214
  Hirschsprung's disease 201
  infectious diarrhoea 416
  ulcerative colitis 208
  volvulus 201
barium enteroclysis 581, 596
barium follow-through 581, 596
  chronic diarrhoea 355
barium meal
  contraindication in Parkinson's disease 108
  gastroparesis 450
barium swallow 581
  achalasia 187
  contraindications in neurological patients 104
  diffuse oesophageal spasm 188–9
  gastrooesophageal reflux 337
  oesophageal carcinoma 190
  oesophageal dysfunction 364, 365, 591
  oesophageal rupture, spontaneous (Boerhaave's syndrome) 179
  oesophagel intramural haematoma 178
  peptic strictures 362
  see also videofluoroscopy modified barium swallow
Barrett's oesophagus 26, 181–6, 364
  aetiology 182
  biopsy 25
  clinical features 184
  diagnosis 182
  dysplasia 28
    grading 27
    high-grade 185, 186
  endoscopy 184
  gastrooesophageal reflux association 181, 182, 183
  management 184–6
  oesophageal adenocarcinoma association 181–2, 189
    malignant transformation 182–4
    surveillance 185–6, 192
  pathology 28, 182, 183
  peptic strictures 186, 362
  photodynamic therapy 541
Barrett's ulcer 186
Bartonella henselae 92–3
basophilic leukaemia 60
behavioural therapy 348
Behçet's syndrome 80, 207
Belgium, training requirements 617
benign anorectal disease, lower gastrointestinal bleeding 167, 168
benzafibrate 52
benzodiazepines 127, 522–3
benzydamine hydrochloride 56
Bernstein acid perfusion test 337, 364
beta-blockers 386
  drug-related gastrointestinal dysfunction 346
β_2-microglobulin 80
bezoars, postgastrectomy formation 369
bicozamycin 422
bile acid malabsorption
  assessment 356
    scintigraphic 612
  gallstone disease 461
bile acid sequestering agents 52
bile acid treatment see oral bile-acid treatment
bile canaliculi 34
bile duct obstruction 505
bile duct stones 221–3
  bile duct strictures 223
  clinical features 221–2
  endoscopic retrograde cholangiopancreatography (ERCP) 222, 223
  extracorporeal shock wave lithotripsy (ESWL) 223
  imaging 222
  malabsorption 381
  surgical treatment 223
  transhepatic cholangiogram/drainage 222–3
bile duct strictures 223
bile reflux 336–7
  postgastrectomy 368
bile salt malabsorption
  following ileal resection 378, 427
  inflammatory bowel disease 427, 428
  investigations 598
bile salts
  enterohepatic circulation 373
  role in fat absorption 372–3
bile stasis 36

biliary atresia 22, 607, 609
biliary cirrhosis, primary 74, 298–9, 300, 505–6
  associated autoimmune disorders 299
  clinical features 299
  diagnosis 299
  epidemiology 299
  pathology 37
  pregnant patients 121
  serum bilirubin prognostic marker 299
  steatorrhoea 381
  treatment 299
  ultrasound appearances 555
biliary colic 221–3, 463
  clinical features 221–2
  investigations/imaging 222
  localization 6
  symptom complex 5–6
biliary duct cancer 542
biliary duct dilatation 568, 569
biliary duct stent placement 546–7
biliary dyskinesia 607
biliary leaks, scintigraphy 607, 608
biliary peritonitis
  ascites management 259
  primary 173
biliary sludge 462–3
  imaging 464, 567
biliary system
  common structural anomalies 22
  computed tomography 584
  macroscopic anatomy 21–4
  magnetic resonance cholangiopancreatography
    (MRCP) 588, 589
  ultrasound examination 564, 568
    diagnostic pitfalls 568
    pitfalls in normal anatomy 564
biliary tumours 237, 542
bilious vomiting, postgastrectomy 368
bilirubin metabolism 328
bioartificial liver 294
biofeedback
  constipation 387–8
  faecal incontinence 397
  rectocele 512
  solitary rectal ulcer syndrome 512
bipolar probe 132
bisacodyl 386
bismuth subsalicylate 420, 422
bismuth therapy 473, 475, 481
bisphosphonates 439
Blastocystis hominis 90

bleomycin 96, 235
blood supply 19–20
  abdominal wall 15
  duodenum 18
  gallbladder 24
  ileum 18
  jejunum 18
  stomach 16, 17
blood transfusion
  complications
    immunological 69
    infection transmission 67–9
  GBV-C virus/hepatitis G transmission 499, 500
  haemoglobinopathy treatment 329
  hepatitis B transmission 487–8
  hepatitis C transmission 495
  variceal bleeding 152–3
body mass index (Quetelet index; BMI) 274, 596
  anorexia nervosa 51
  obesity 50
body weight regulation disorders 50–2
Boerhaave's syndrome (spontaneous oesophageal
  rupture) 179–80
bolus obstruction of small-bowel 200
bone disease
  inflammatory bowel disease 438–9
  postgastrectomy 367–8
Borrelia burgdorferi 81
botulinum toxin injection
  achalasia 188, 447
  anal fissure 509
  ineffective defaecation in Parkinson's disease
    110
bowel habit change 47
bowel imaging
  computed tomography 586–8
    CT enteroclysis technique 587
    CT pneumocolon technique 587–8
  magnetic resonance imaging (MRI) 590
  ultrasound 574–7
bowel preparation 168
Bowen's disease 510
brachytherapy (intracavity irradiation),
  oesophageal carcinoma palliation 193
breast cancer 60
breast feeding 438
breath tests 356, 611–12
  bacterial overgrowth 598
  fat malabsorption 597
  gastric emptying assessment 592
bronchoscopy, oesophageal carcinoma 191

Brucella 353
Budd–Chiari syndrome 65
  acute liver failure 289, 290
  ascites 251, 254, 258
  Behçet's syndrome 80
  ultrasound appearances 555
budesonide 430, 433, 436
Buerger's disease 80
bulbar palsy 105
bulimia nervosa 52
Burkitt's lymphoma
  HIV-associated 96
  stomach 234
busulphan 55

^{13}C breath tests 592
^{14}C breath tests 597, 598, 611–12
c-myc 231
C-reactive protein 596
CA19.9 marker 229, 232
caecum 18–19
CAGE questionnaire 455
Cajal cells 448
calcitonin 49
calcium channel blockers 386
  oesophageal motility disorders 187, 189, 447
calcium oxalate renal stones 270
calcium supplements 439
Cameron erosions 131
Campylobacter 76, 410, 417
  acute abdominal pain 171
  HIV-associated infection 90, 92, 94
Campylobacter jejuni 409, 410, 412, 414, 416,
    420, 422
  complications 418
  dysentery 413
  haemolytic–uraemic syndrome 418
  infection in pregnancy 117
Candida albicans 291
candidiasis 60, 510
  angular cheilitis 87
  haematological malignancy treatment-related
    58, 60
    hepatitis 61
  HIV-associated 85, 87–8, 95
  hypoparathyroidism 48
  oesophageal symptoms 28, 87–8, 359
  oral 85, 87
    erythematous 87
    hyperplastic 87
    pseudomembranous 87
    treatment 87

capecitabine 234
Capnocytophaga canimorsus 64
caput medusae 20, 457
carbamazepine 93
carbohydrate absorption 372
carcinoembryonic antigen (CEA) 231–2
carcinoid syndrome 236
  chronic diarrhoea 353, 354, 355, 356
  investigations 50
carcinoid tumours 32, 236–7
  metastasis 237
  palliative ^{131}I-MIBG radionuclide therapy 612
  scintigraphy 610, 611
cardiac pacemakers 528
cardiomyotomy 188, 447
carotenaemia 9–10
Castleman's disease 95
caustic oesophageal strictures 15, 363
cefotaxime 261
ceftazadime 59
Celestin prosthesis 178, 193
central venous access 152
central venous pressure monitoring 141
cephalosporins 209, 261
  acute bacterial peritonitis 173
  perianal sepsis 59
  prophylaxis for endoscopy 527
cerebral oedema, acute liver failure 291
  prevention 291–2
cerebrovascular disorders, oesophageal dysmotility
  186
Chagas' disease
  dysphagia 360
  intestinal pseudo-obstruction 202
  megacolon 388
  oesophageal dysmotility 186, 446
Charcot's triad 221
chemical peritonitis 173–4
chemoradiation
  anal cancer 234
  oesophageal cancer 226, 227, 228
chemoreceptor trigger zone 317
chemotherapy
  colorectal cancer 232
  cytotoxic drugs 227
  gastric cancer 228–9
  gastric lymphoma 234
  hepatocellular carcinoma 248
  infectious diarrhoea susceptibility 411
  oesophageal cancer 192, 227
  pancreatic cancer 229–30
chenodeoxycholic acid 465

chest pain
    achalasia 361
    atypical 358, 364
    heartburn 357
    oesophageal colic 358
    oesophageal motility disorders 447, 448
chest X-ray
    achalasia 187, 447
    oesophageal carcinoma 363
    pneumoperitoneum 175
    swallowed foreign body 177
chief cells 29
Child–Pugh score 150, 151, 244, 458
children
    acute intussusception 200
    consent for endoscopy 521–2
    infectious diarrhoea susceptibility 411
    inflammatory bowel disease 437–8
    intestinal obstruction 201
Chlamydia 75, 76, 353
    rectal disease 513
Chlamydia trachomatis 414, 415
chlorambucil 57, 66
chloramphenicol 379, 419
chlordiazepoxide 319
chlorhexidine 55, 87
chlorine dioxide disinfectant 518
chloroquine 75
chlorpheniramine 121
chlorpromazine 116
CHO chemotherapy 234
cholangiocarcinoma 237
    computed tomography 584
    pathology 37
    primary sclerosing cholangitis progression 300
cholangitis 221–3
    clinical features 221–2
    investigations/imaging 222
cholecystitis
    acalculous 566
    acute 463
        cholescintigraphy 606–7
        ultrasound 564, 565, 606
    chronic 564
cholecystokinin 445, 468
choledochal cysts 22
    classification 23
    complications 22
cholera 414, 419
    vaccines 422
cholescintigraphy 464, 606–7

cholestasis
    fat-soluble vitamin malabsorption 381
    obstetric (intrahepatic cholestasis of pregnancy)
        120–1
cholesterol gallstones 48, 462
cholesterolosis 566, 567
cholestyramine 52, 91, 121, 215, 299, 324, 356,
    368, 374, 378, 379, 428
Churg–Strauss syndrome (allergic granulomatous
    angiitis) 79, 80
chylomicrons 373
chymotrypsin 372
cidofovir 90
cine-radiography, diffuse oesophageal spasm 189
ciprfloxacin 61, 209, 217, 262, 378, 419, 420,
    434, 527
ciprofibrate 52
cirrhosis 36
    anaemia see anaemia of liver disease
    Child–Pugh score 150, 151, 244
    computed tomography 583–4
    fertility/pregnancy 121
    hepatocellular carcinoma
        hepatic reserve assessment 244
        screening/surveillance 241
    immune system impairement 153
    magnetic resonance imaging (MRI) 590
    nutritional support 154–5
    oesophageal varices 149
        risk of bleeding 150
    spontaneous bacterial peritonitis 154, 259, 260
        prophylaxis 261–2
    ultrasound appearances 556, 557
    upper gastrointestinal bleeding
        antibiotic prophylaxis 154, 261, 262
        peripheral vasoconstrictor responses 152
cisapride 112, 338, 340, 347, 387, 451, 453, 468
cisplatin 226, 227, 228, 229, 230, 248
cisterna chylae 20
clarithromycin 91, 434, 474, 482
clips, bleeding peptic ulcer management 133, 142,
    143
clofibrate 52–3
clonidine 44
closed-loop intestinal obstruction 197, 201
Clostridium 76
Clostridium difficile 56, 207, 414, 416, 417, 528
    antibiotic-assocated diarrhoea 412
    HIV-associated diarrhoea 91, 92
    immunocompromised host 411
Clostridium perfringens 68

Clostridium septicum 56
clubbing 11
co-trimoxazole *see* trimethoprim–
   sulphamethoxazole
coagulopathy, acute liver failure 290
cobalamin-fortified diet 328
cobalt 321
cocaine 56
codeine phosphate 46, 78, 268, 269, 271
   contraindications 208
coeliac artery 16, 19
coeliac disease 10, 375–7
   aetiology 375
   antireticulin antibodies 376
   autoimmune thyroiditis association 47
   clinical features 375–6
   complications 377
   dermatitis herpetiformis 324, 354, 377
   diabetes mellitus association 44, 111
   diagnosis 327
   duodenal ulcer 334
   endomysial antibodies 376
   epidemiology 375
   folic acid malabsorption 324, 327
   gastrointestinal malignancy associations 65, 235,
      236, 377
      lymphoma 380
   genetic aspects 375
   investigations 376–7, 595
      autoanitbodies 596
   iron deficiency 326–7
   pathology 31, 375
   primary biliary cirrhosis association 299
   small bowel biopsy 376
   transglutaminase antibodies 376
   treatment 377
coeliac lymph nodes 16, 20
coeliac plexus block 230, 460
coffee-ground vomiting 57, 140, 316, 317
colchicine 74–5, 81, 299
colectomy
   constipation treatment 388
   familial adenomatous polyposis 400
   lower gastrointestinal bleeding 168
   toxic megacolon 175
   ulcerative colitis 210, 211, 432–3, 436–7, 439
colestipol 52
collagen disorders 186
collagenous colitis 44
colon
   ascending 19
   descending 19
   macroscopic anatomy 19
   sigmoid 19
   transverse 19
colonic biopsy 32
   infectious diarrhoea 417–18
   inflammatory bowel disease 425
colonic motility
   irritable bowel syndrome 344
   transit time 603–4
colonic scintigraphy 385
colonic transit time 603–4
colonoscopy
   acute abdominal pain 172
   chronic diarrhoea 355
   colorectal cancer screening/surveillance 400,
      401, 402
      population screening 405, 407
   Crohn's disease 214
   ileal intubation 19
   infectious colitis 417
   inflammatory bowel disease 427
   lower gastrointestinal bleeding 168
   occult gastrointestinal bleeding 169
colorectal adenomatous polyps
   acromegaly association 47
   adenoma-carcinoma sequence 34
colorectal cancer 231–4
   acromegaly association 47
   adenoma–carcinoma sequence/multi-step
      development 34, 231, 399
   adjuvant chemotherapy 232
   adjuvant radiotherapy 232–3
   age-related risk 404
   autosomal dominant disorders 399–401
   Dukes' staging system 34, 35, 231
   epidemiology 75, 231
   familial risk 402–3
   grading 34
   laser therapy 538
   markers of precancer
      aneuploidy 402
      dysplasia 401–2
      genetic markers 402
      mucin abnormalities 402
   metastatic disease 231–2
      management 233–4
   non-surgical management 231–2
   palliative treatment 231, 233–4
   pathology 34
   pneumoperitoneum 175

radioimmunoscintigraphy 609
recurrence 403–4
screening/surveillance 399–407
tumour markers 232
colostomy 175
faecal incontinence management 398
columnar-lined oesophagus *see* Barrett's
oesophagus
common bile duct 21–2, 564, 584
anatomical relations 20
duodenal relations 17
common bile duct stones (choledocholithiasis)
463
imaging 464
computed tomography 584
prophylactic treatment 463
common hepatic duct 584
common variable immunodeficiency 98, 411
communication skills 3–7
computed tomography 581–8
acute abdominal pain 172
ascites 253
biliary tract 584
bowel 586–8
CT enteroclysis technique 587
CT pneumocolon technique 587–8
clinical utility 582
contrast 582
Crohn's disease 214, 217
gallstones 464, 467
helical/spiral scanning 582
hepatocellular carcinoma screening/surveillance
242
during arterial portography (CTAP) 243
liver 582–4
magnetic resonance imaging (MRI)
comparison 589
oesophageal carcinoma 190
oesophagel intramural haematoma 178, 179
oesophagus 586
pancreas 584–6
pancreatitis
acute 174, 584
chronic 380, 584–5
pneumoperitoneum 175
principles 581–2
reticuloendothelial system 586
stomach 586
condylomata acuminata (perianal warts) 34, 511
condylomata lata 511

congenital small-bowel atresia 201
consent for endoscopy 519–22
adverse events information 520
emergency endoscopy 127
hospital inpatients 521
legal aspects 522
long-term prostheses insertion 521
mental competence 521, 522
minors 521–2
practical aspects 520
withdrawal during procedure 522
constipation 4, 383–90
Addison's disease 46
autonomic neuropathy 111
causes 383
chemoradiotherapy patients 57, 58
clinical features 384
clinical subtypes 383–4
coexisting systemic illness 384
colonic lesions 384
drug-induced 386
gut dilatation-related 384
hypercalcaemia/primary hyperparathyroidism 48
hyperthyroidism 47
hypoparathyroidism 48
idiopathic 383–4
intestinal obstruction 197, 198, 201
investigations 384–5
anorectal sensory testing 385
colonic scintigraphy 385
evacuation proctography 385
rectoanal inhibitory reflex 385
whole-gut transit radio-opaque marker study
384–5
irritable bowel syndrome 345, 384
management 347
myasthenia gravis 108
obstetric patients 117
Parkinson's disease 108, 109–10
stool diary 110
treatment 347, 385–8
biofeedback 387–8
diet 386
pharmacological options 386–7
surgery 388
consultation setting 3
continuous venovenous haemofiltration (CVVH)
291, 292
contrast fistulogram
Crohn's disease 214
enterocutaneous fistulae 272

copper
  chelation treatment 303
  requirement for erythropoiesis 321
corpus of stomach 16
corticobasilar degeneration 107
Councillman bodies 36, 37
Courvoisier's Law 221
Cowden's disease 401
cranial nerve testing 105
creatinine serum level 306–7
CREST syndrome 361
Creutzfeld–Jacob disease, new-variant 69
cricopharyngeal dysfunction 446
cricopharyngeal spasm 186
Crohn's disease 211
  abdominal pain 428
  active disease 427
    major presentations 211
    outcome of attacks 217–18
    working definitions 211, 213
  anal lesions 34
  anti-*Saccharomyces cerevisiae* mannan antibodies
    (ASCA) 427
  antibiotic therapy 434
  children/adolescents 437, 438
    growth retardation 438
  colitis 213, 217
  colorectal cancer risk 401, 440
  diagnosis 425
  diarrhoea 355, 428
  drug contraindications 215
  drug therapy 215–16
    corticosteroids 427
    maintenance therapy 436
  duodenal ulcer 334
  fertility/pregnancy 118
  fistulae 213, 271
    intestinal 213, 217
  folic acid requirement 325
  gallstone disease association 461
  histopathology 425
  ileocaecal disease 215–16
  in-patient treatment 211–18
    admission criteria 211
    general measures 211
    management outlines 212, 213
    supportive measures 214–15
  intra-abdominal abscess 217
  investigations 211, 213–14, 595
  lower gastrointestinal bleeding 167
  mortality 440–1

  nutritional support 216, 281–2, 429, 431
  obstructive small bowel disease 216–17
  oral disease 217
  pathology 32, 33
  perianal disease 213, 217, 510–11
  reactive systemic amyloid (AA amyloid) 80
  relapse
    acute 430
    smoking-related 436
  severity indices 428–9
  small bowel cancer association 235, 236
  small bowel strictures 200
  surgery 216, 433, 437, 439, 441
  ulcerative colitis differentiation 426
  ultrasound appearances 575, 577
  upper gastrointestinal disease 217
  vitamin malabsorption 378
  weight loss 371
Cryptococcus neoformans 87, 92
Cryptosporidium 76, 354, 379, 411, 412, 418
  diagnosis 89
  HIV-associated infection 88–9, 92, 94, 95
  transmission 88
  treatment 89
Cryptosporidium parvum 409, 416, 417, 418, 420,
    421
cyanoacrylate injection 134
cyclizine 116
cyclo-oxygenase type 1 (COX-1) 72
cyclo-oxygenase type 2 (COX-2) 72
cyclo-oxygenase type 2 (COX-2) selective
    inhibitors 72
cyclophosphamide 55, 74, 96, 234, 235, 237
  side effects 57, 74
Cyclospora cayetanensis 416, 419
  HIV-associated diarrhoea 89–90
cyclosporin 56, 74, 299, 301
  Crohn's disease 215, 217, 271
  side effects 63
  ulcerative colitis 209–10, 211, 218, 431–2
  use in pregnancy 118
cystic artery 24
cystic duct 22, 23
  obstruction 463
cystic fibrosis
  diagnosis 380
  meconium ileus 201
  steatorrhoea 380, 381
cytomegalovirus 28, 57, 58, 66, 411
  AIDS sclerosing cholangitis 95
  colitis 56, 90, 92, 207

hepatitis 61
HIV-associated disorders 87, 88, 90, 92
oesophageal ulceration 88, 359
oral ulceration 87
pancreatitis 57
rectal disease 513
treatment 90
cytosine arabinoside 57
cytotoxic drugs 227
liver infusion 20
see also chemotherapy

dapsone 377
DCC (deleted in colon cancer) 231
De Meester oesophageal acid reflux parameters
336
deferiprone (L1) 63
defibrotide 62
dehydration
acute watery diarrhoea 414, 415
intestinal obstruction 197, 198
dental caries 52
dentate line 16
Denver shunt 611
depression
irritable bowel syndrome 343, 344, 345
nausea/vomiting 317
obesity association 51
dermatitis herpetiformis 324, 354, 377
desferrioxamine 63
desmoplastic reaction 28
desmopressin 153
dexamethasone 57, 96, 121
diabetes mellitus 41–6
associated gastrointestinal disorders 41, 42
autonomic neuropathy 41, 43, 46, 111, 112
drug treatment 46
management 46
tests 44, 45
chronic pancreatitis 380
coeliac disease association 111
diarrhoea 43–6
causes 43–4
investigations 44, 45
management 44, 46
faecal incontinence 43, 46, 396
fatty liver 46
gallstone disease 46
gastroparesis 41–3, 450
management 42–3
pathophysiology 42

intestinal pseudo-obstruction 202
malabsorption/steatorrhoea 379
obesity association 51
oesophageal dysmotility 186, 602
diabetic ketoacidosis
acute abdominal pain 171
weight loss 371
diaphragmatic hiatus 15, 16
diarrhoea 91, 351–6
Addison's disease 46
autonomic neuropathy 111
bloody, differential diagnosis 206, 413
chemoradiotherapy patients 57
chronic
empirical treatment 356
endoscopic examination 355
history-taking 353
imaging 355
infective 414, 420–1
investigations 354–6
physical examination 353–4
quantitative stool collection/examination
354–5
spot stool analysis 354
classification 351–2
definition 351
diabetic see diabetes mellitus
drug-induced 411, 435
antibiotics 411–12
dysmotility 353
factitious 353
gastrointestinal hormone screen 49, 50
HIV-associated 88–92
hyperthyroidism 47
ileal resection 378
infectious 409–22
acute bloody (dysentery) 412, 413, 419, 420
acute watery 410–11, 412, 413, 419–20
age associations 411
antidiarrhoeal agents 419
antimicrobial chemotherapy 419–21
chemoprophylaxis 422
chronic carrier state 418–19
clinical examination 414–15
clinical syndromes 412–14
complications 410, 418–19
diagnosis 410–11, 413
dietary sources 412
DNA probes 416
epidemiology 409
fluid/electrolyte balance maintenance 419

histology 417–18
imaging 416
immunocompromised host 411
microbiology 415–16
pathogens 410
persistent 412, 414, 420–1
prevention 421–2
probiotic/prebiotic approaches to control 422
proctitis 412, 414
risk factors 411–12
serology 416
sub-acute intestinal obstruction 412, 414
travel-related 412, 419–20
treatment 419–21
vaccines 422
inflammatory bowel disease 427
Crohn's disease 213, 428
ulcerative colitis 207, 427
inflammatory/exudative 352–3
intestinal lymphangiectasia 380
irritable bowel syndrome 345
management 347
obstetric patients 117–18
osmotic 352
pathophysiological mechanisms 352–3
postgastrectomy 368–9, 374
secretory 352
short gut syndrome (massive intestinal resection) 378
small bowel disease 374
diathermy, endoscopic 528–30
bipolar current 529
blended current 529
cardiac pacemakers 528
coagulating current 528–9
current density 529
cutting current 528–9
dangers 530
electrosurgical instruments 530
equipment 529–30
monopolar current 529
uses 528
diazepam 523
diclofenac 72
dicyclomine hydrochloride 187
didanosine 93
dietary factors
constipation 386
gallstone disease 462, 468

dietary fibre
constipation 386
ulcerative colitis 431
Dieulafoy's lesion (exulceratio simplex) 131
diffuse oesophageal spasm 186, 188–9, 358, 360, 361, 447, 448
clinical features 188
diagnosis 188–9, 602
treatment 189
digoxin 317
diisopropyl-iminodiacetic acid (DISIDA) scintigraphy 605
diltiazem 394, 509
diphenoxylate 46, 356
diphenoxylate/atropine combinations 419
direct intubation tests 598
discoid lupus 75
discriminant function 306, 308
disinfection, endoscopy equipment 517–19, 532
recommended contact times 519
diuretics 386
cirrhotic ascites 255, 256
diverticular abscess 575
diverticular disease
lower gastrointestinal bleeding 167
pneumoperitoneum 175
ultrasound appearances 575
diverticulitis 575
DMT-1 322
DNA mismatch repair gene mutations 400
docetaxel 228, 230
docusate sodium 387
domperidone 57, 77, 116, 319, 340, 347, 451, 453
dopamine 154, 317
double channel endoscope 128
doxorubicin (adriamycin) 96, 228, 235, 237, 248
doxycycline 94, 419, 420, 422
droperidol 523
drug-induced constipation 386
drug-induced diarrhoea 411, 435
drug-induced gastrointestinal dysfunction 346
drug-induced gastroparesis 450
drug-induced liver injury 52, 53, 549
acute liver failure 288–9
haematological malignancy patients 63
liver function test abnormalities 503
drug-induced malabsorption/steatorrhoea 379
drug-induced nausea/vomiting 317
dumping syndrome 368
duodenal angioma 131

duodenal biopsy 596–7
duodenal peristalsis 449, 450
duodenal ulcer
    endoscopic biopsy 334
    Helicobacter pylori eradication therapy 479–80
    Helicobacter pylori-negative disease 334
    perforation
        acute secondary bacterial peritonitis 173
        herpatic artery erosion 17
    treatment 337
    upper gastrointestinal bleeding 130, 131
    see also peptic ulcer disease
duodenum
    blood supply 18
    histology in infectious diarrhoea 418
    macroscopic anatomy 17–18
Dupuytren's contracture 9, 11
dynamic graciloplasty 397
dysentery 412, 413
    treatment 419, 420
dyserythropoietic anaemias, congenital 63
dysfibrinogenaemia 65
dysmotility diarrhoea 353
dyspepsia 331–40
    alarm symptoms 332, 477
    definition 331
    endoscopy 334
        indications 332
    endoscopy-negative *see* non-ulcer dyspepsia
    epidemiology 331
    Helicobacter pylori 331–2, 334
        testing/eradication 477–9
    investigations 332–4, 335
    irritable bowel syndrome 346
dysphagia 357, 359–64, 446
    acute oesophagel obstruction 177
        acute bolus obstruction 178
        intramural haematoma 178–9
        swallowed foreign body 177
    mechanical causes 361–4
    neurogenic *see* neurogenic dysphagia
    neuromuscular causes 360–1
    oesophageal carcinoma 189, 190
    oesophageal motility disorders 447
    oropharyngeal 104
    pseudodysphagia differentiation 359–60
dysplasia 27

eating disorders 292, 317
ECF chemotherapy 227, 228, 229, 230

Echinococcus granulosus 582
eicosapentanoic acid (fish oil) 282
elastase 372
electrocardiography 524
electrogastrography 592
    autonomic neuropathy 112
electrolyte disturbance
    acute watery diarrhoea 415
    bulimia nervosa 52
    diabetic diarrhoea 44
    enterocutaneous fistulae 271
    hyperemesis gravidarum 115, 116
    jejunostomy patients 268–9
    refeeding syndrome 277–8
    short gut syndrome (massive intestinal
        resection) 378
    vomiting 319
electrolytes
    absorption 373
    intestinal fluid contents 278
    requirements for nutritional support 277
        critically ill patients 280
electrosurgical current *see* diathermy, endoscopic
electrosurgical generator 529
electrosurgical instruments 530
elemental diets
    acute pancreatitis 282
    Crohn's disease 281, 431
ELF chemotherapy 228
embolization, gastrointestinal bleeding 169
emergency endoscopy 127–34
    associated problems 127
    consent 127
    endoscopes 128–9
        avoiding blockage 129
    endotracheal intubation 128
    information for patients 127
    nasogastric intubation 128
    orooesophageal overtube 129
    sedation 127–8
    substantial bleeding management 129–30
    upper gastrointestinal bleeding 141
        diagnostic aspects 130–1
        precautions for staff 130
emopronium bromide 359
enbucrilate (Histacryl) injection 134
Encephalitozoon intestinalis 89, 421
end stoma construction 175
endoanal ultrasound 395
endocarditis, endoscopy-related risk 525–6

endocrine disorder-related malabsorption 379–80
endoluminal ultrasound
  biliary sludge detection 463
  Crohn's disease 217
  neuroendocrine pancreatic tumours 597
  oesophageal carcinoma 191
endomysial antibodies 376
endoscopic retrograde cholangiopancreatography
    (ERCP) 463, 464, 545–8, 597
  antibiotic prophylaxis 527
  bile duct stones 222, 223
  biliary tract procedures 546
  chronic pancreatitis 380
  complications 547–8
  contraindications 545–6
  gastric-outlet obstruction 547
  indications 545
  pancreatic therapeutic manoeuvres 546–7
endoscopic sphincterotomy 546, 547
endoscopic treatment
  bile duct stones 222, 223
    see also endoscopic retrograde
      cholangiopancreatography (ERCP)
  upper gastrointestinal bleeding 131–4
    peptic ulcer disease 131–3, 141–2, 143, 145
    rebleeding rates 146
  varices
    alcoholic cirrhosis 458
    gastric 134
    oesophageal 133–4
endoscopy
  antibiotic prophylaxis 525–8
    recommended antibiotics 527–8
  bacteraemia 525, 526–7
  cardiorespiratory monitoring 524–5
  complications 520
  consent see consent for endoscopy
  disinfection of equipment 97, 517–19, 532
  electrosurgical/diathermy current use
    see diathermy, endoscopic
  emergency see emergency endoscopy
  endocarditis risk 525–6
  general anaesthesia 523
  inflammatory bowel disease, children/
    adolescents 437
  intravenous access 523–14
  iron deficiency investigations 327
  neutropenic patients 59–60
  occupationally acquired infections 530–2
    prevention 531–2
  patient–patient transmission of infection 532
  practical considerations 517–32
  preoxygenation/supplementary oxygen 524
  sedation 522–3
  universal precautions 531–2
endoscopy-negative dyspepsia see non-ulcer
  dyspepsia
endotracheal intubation
  emergency endoscopy 128
  variceal bleeding 152, 155
enema, faecal incontinence management 396–7
energy requirements, nutritional support 277
  monitoring 279
  respiratory failure 280
Entamoeba histolytica 60, 416, 418
  see also amoebiasis
enteral feeding
  critically ill patients 279
  Crohn's disease 281, 282
    primary treatment 216
  indications 274–5
  long-term domiciliary 275
  neurogenic dysphagia 108–9
enteral stent placement 547
enteric nervous sytem 449
Enterobacter cloacae 58
enterocutaneous fistulae 270–2
  aetiology 270–1
  imaging 272
  management 271–2
    parenteral nutrition 275
  spontaneous closure 271
Enterocytozoon bienusi 89, 421
enterogastric reflux 607, 609
enterohepatic circulation 373
enterokinase 372
enteropathy-associated T-cell lymphoma 65
enterostomy 276
enterovesical/enterovaginal fistulae 213
eosinophilia 415
epiphrenic diverticula/pouches 361
epirubicin 227, 248
epithelium 26
  dysplasia 27
  neoplasia 26
Epstein–Barr virus 66, 96
  hepatitis 61
  HIV-associated oral ulceration 87
  oral hairy leucoplakia 87
erythrocyte sedimentation rate 596

erythromycin 64, 77, 93, 94, 387, 422, 451, 468, 513
erythropoiesis, haematinic requirements 321
Escherichia coli 58, 60, 75, 259, 260, 378, 462
  acute secondary bacterial peritonitis 173
  enterohaemorrhagic (EHEC) 409, 412, 416, 420, 422
    dysentery 413
    haemolytic–uraemic syndrome 410, 418
  enteropathogenic 414
  enterotoxigenic 413
  HIV-associated diarrhoea 92
essential thrombocythaemia 65
ethambutol 91
ethanolamine sclerotherapy 132, 134, 159, 161
ethionamide 93
ethyl proprionate 466
etodolac 71
etoposide 55, 57, 228, 235, 238, 248
European Association for the Study of the Liver (EASL) 621–2
European Board of Gastroenterology 618–21
  European Diploma of Gastroenterology 620
  Training Recognition Certificate 620
  training requirements 619–20
    ultrasound 620–1
European Society of Gastrointestinal Endoscopy 622
European Union
  gastroenterological specialty associations 621–2
  training requirements 615–18
evacuation proctography (defecography) 385
exfoliative dermatitis 325
exocrine pancreatic insufficiency 57
external thrombosed pile 508
extracorporeal bioartificial liver support 294
extracorporeal shock wave lithotripsy (ESWL) 223, 466
extramedullary haemopoiesis 63
exudative diarrhoea 352–3
eye protection 130

Fabry's disease 110
facial weakness 104, 105
factitious diarrhoea 353
factor V Leiden (activated protein C resistance) 65, 202
factor VIII elevation 65
faecal continence mechanisms 19, 393
faecal incontinence 353, 393–8
  associated systemic disease 396
    scleroderma 78

cause 394
congential abnormalities 396
diabetes mellitus 43, 46
history-taking 394
idiopathic 396
investigations 396
lifestyle disruption 394
obstetric damage 394, 395
passive leakage 394
pathogenesis 395–6
physical examination 395
post-radiotherapy 396
rectal prolapse 394, 396
scoring system 394
  St Marks grading scale 395
severity assessment 394
spinal injury 396
surgical damage 394, 395–6
treatment 396–8
  antidiarrhoeal agents 396–7
  biofeedback 397
  mechanical barriers 397
  surgery 397–8
urge incontinence 394
faecal occult blood testing 326, 404–5
faecal pH 354
faecal softeners 387
FAM chemotherapy 228, 229, 230, 237
famciclovir 90, 493
familial adenomatous polyposis 399
  screening 399–400
familial amyloid polyneuropathy 81, 110
familial juvenile polyposis 400–1
familial Mediterranean fever (periodic disease; hereditary recurrent polyserositis) 81
famotidine 144
FAP gene mutations 236
fat absorption 372–3
fat malabsorption tests 597–8
fat-soluble vitamin deficiencies/malabsorption
  chronic infective diarrhoea 415
  Crohn's disease 281
  obstetric cholestasis (intrahepatic cholestasis of pregnancy) 121
  obstructive jaundice 381
  primary biliary cirrhosis 299
fatty liver
  acute of pregnancy 119
    acute liver failure 289
  computed tomography 583
  diabetes mellitus 46
  magnetic resonance imaging (MRI) 590

obesity association 51
ultrasound appearances 555, 556
FEMtr chemotherapy 228, 229
fenofibrate 52, 53
ferritin serum level 326
fibrates 52–3
fibrin glue injection 132
fibroepithelial polyp 508
Finland, training requirements 617–18
fish tapeworm infestation 324
fluconazole 55, 61, 63, 87, 291
fluid replacement
    acute liver failure 291
    Crohn's disease 214
    intestinal failure 267
    ulcerative colitis 208
    upper gastrointestinal bleeding 140
    variceal bleeding 152–3, 154
    see also resuscitation
flumazenil 298
fluorescein dilaurate test (pancrealauryl test) 599
5-fluorouracil 226, 227, 228, 230, 232, 233, 234,
    236, 237, 238
flutamide 230
focal nodular hyperplasia 563
folate
    dietary intake/body stores 322
    malabsorption 324
    physiological/pathological increased
        requirements 325
    requirement for erythropoiesis 321
folate deficiency 274, 278
    Crohn's disease 281
    diagnosis 325, 326
    investigations 327, 595
    liver disease 330
    postgastrectomy 374
    small bowel disease 375
    treatment 328
folate supplements 155, 328
folinic acid 228, 230, 232, 233, 234, 238
food boluses, small bowel obstruction 200
food intolerance 345
food poisoning 318
food-borne diarrhoeal disease 409, 412
    prevention 421
food-cobalamin malabsorption 323, 327, 328
foscarnet 61, 90
France, training requirements 615
frusemide 256
functional dyspepsia *see* non-ulcer dyspepsia
functional problems, diagnosis 6

fundus 16, 28, 29
fungal infection
    liver
        haematology patients 61, 63
        ultrasound appearances 556, 560
    splenic abscess 573
Fusarium 61

gag reflex 105
gallbladder
    blood supply 24
    common structural anomalies 22
    ultrasound examination 564–8
        diagnostic pitfalls 566, 568
        pitfalls in normal anatomy 564
    visible on abdominal examination 10
gallbladder adenomyomatosis 566
gallbladder carcinoma 566
gallbladder cholesterolosis 566, 567
gallbladder empyema 564
gallbladder mucocoele 566
gallbladder postinflammatory polyp 566
gallstone composition 462–3
gallstone disease 461–8
    acute pancreatitis 173, 174
    biliary colic 221–3
    contact solvents instillation 466–7
    diabetes mellitus 46
    dietary factors 462
    epidemiology 5, 461–2
    extracorporeal shock-wave lithotripsy 466
    genetic factors 4, 461
    haemolytic anaemias 328
    ileal resection 378
    investigations 464–5
    natural history 463–4
        asymptomatic stones 463
        symptomatic stones 463–4
    obesity association 51
    obstetric patients 117
    oral bile-acid treatment 465–6
        incomplete gallstone dissolution 467
    percutaneous cholecystolithotomy 467
    prevention 468
    pulsed laser therapy 536
    recurrent 467
    short bowel problems 268
    sites of pain 6
    small bowel bolus obstruction 200
    ultrasound appearances 564, 565
gamma-glutamyltransferase elevation 506
ganciclovir 61, 90, 93, 493, 513

Gardener's syndrome 236
gastric angioma 131
gastric antral vascular ectasia (GAVE) 58, 536
gastric arteries 16
gastric biopsy, *Helicobacter pylori* diagnosis *see*
  Helicobacter pylori
gastric cancer 228–9
  chemotherapy 228–9
  classification 30
  early 30
  Helicobacter pylori association 477
  pathology 30
    diffuse 30
    intestinal 30
  postgastrectomy remnant (stump carcinoma)
    369
  radiotherapy 229
  upper gastrointestinal bleeding 130
gastric emptying 449
  abnormalities 450–1
  assessment 450
  autonomic neuropathy 112
  causes of dysfunction 603
  diabetic gastroparesis 41–2
  investigations
    breath tests 592
    gastric barostat 592–3
    magnetic resonance imaging (MRI) 593
    paracetamol absorption assessment 592
    scintigraphy 592, 602–3
    transcutaneous electrogastrogram 592
    ultrasound 592
  non-ulcer (functional) dyspepsia 452
gastric foveolae (pits) 28–9
gastric glands 29
gastric leiomyoma 130
gastric lymphoma 234–5
gastric metaplasia 26
gastric motility 448–50
  assessment 450
  disorders 448–53
    non-ulcer (functional) dyspepsia 452
  migrating motor complex (MMC) 449–50
  see also gastric emptying
gastric outlet obstruction
  abdominal observation 10
  endoscopic management 547
  ultrasound appearances 574
gastric pacemaker 448
  electrogastrogram 592
gastric physiology testing 591–3

gastric polyps 30
gastric scintigraphy 592
  gastroparesis 450
gastric splash 11
gastric surgery
  iron malabsorption 323
  vitamin B_{12} malabsorption 323
gastric ulcer
  endoscopic biopsy 334
  follow-up 338
  Helicobacter pylori eradication therapy 480
  NSAID-associated 337, 338
  treatment 337–8
  upper gastrointestinal bleeding 130, 131
    emergency endoscopy 129–30
  see also peptic ulcer disease
gastric varices 20
  bleeding 160–1
    management 161
    uncontrolled 161
  endoscopic appearances 151
  endoscopic treatment 134
gastrin 29, 49, 50, 445
gastrinoma 609, 610
  gastrin level measurement 49, 50
  see also Zollinger–Ellison syndrome
gastritis
  biopsy 25
  pathology 30
    Sydney classification 30
gastroduodenal (right gastroepiploic) artery 16, 17
gastroepiploic arteries 16
gastrointestinal bleeding
  iron deficiency 324, 325
  red blood cell scintigraphy 604–5
  see also lower gastrointestinal bleeding; upper
    gastrointestinal bleeding
gastrointestinal hormones measurement 49–50
gastrooesophageal reflux/reflux disease 331–40
  Barrett's oesophagus association 28, 181, 182,
    183
  benign peptic strictures 362
  De Meester parameters 336
  definitions 331
  endoscopic classification 335
  endoscopy-negative disease 335–6
  follow-up 340
  investigations 335–7, 364
    scintigraphy 602
  obstetric patients 116
  oesophageal motility disorders 186

Parkinson's disease 108
    relapse 340
    surgery 340
    symptom indices 336
    symptoms 332
    treatment 338–40
        Helicobacter pylori eradication 481
        lifestyle modification 338
        medical 338, 339, 340
gastroparesis *see* gastric emptying
gastroscopy *see* upper gastrointestinal endoscopy
gastrostomy 276
Gaucher's disease 65
GBV-C virus 499–500
    prevention/treatment 500
    virology 499
gemcitabine 230
gemfibrozil 52
gender differences, pain grading 4
general anaesthesia for endoscopy 523
gentamicin 527
Germany, training requirements 617
giant-cell arteritis 80
Giardia intestinalis (giardiasis) 354, 355, 379, 380,
        409, 411, 412, 416, 417, 418, 419, 421, 598
    chronic diarrhoea 414
    folic acid malabsorption 324
    HIV-associated diarrhoea 89, 92
    small intestinal pathology 31
ginger 115
glandular epithelium 26
Glasgow Coma Scale 297
globin degradation 328
glucagon 49
glucagonoma 354, 609, 610
glucose-6-phosphate dehydrogenase deficiency
    328, 330
glucose–sodium co-transport 372, 419
glutamine supplementation 282–3
gluten-free diet 377
gluten-sensitive enteropathy *see* coeliac disease
gluteraldehyde disinfectant 97, 517–18
    toxicity 518
glyceryl trinitrate 169, 189, 447, 448, 509
glychocholic acid breath tests 598
goblet cells 31, 32
gold preparations 71, 73–4
gonorrhoea 353
    rectal infection 513
graft versus host disease 57, 58, 60
    bowel 56

liver
    acute 62
    chronic 62–3
    oropharynx 55, 56
    transfusion-associated 69
granisetron 57, 74
granulocyte-colony stimulating factor (G-CSF)
    55, 56, 59
granulocyte-macrophage-colony stimulating
    factor (GM-CSF) 59, 96, 261
granulomatous peritonitis 174
Greece, training requirements 618
growth retardation 438
Guillain–Barré syndrome 110, 410
    Campylobacter jejuni infection association 418
    neurogenic dysphagia 106
gum disease 52
gut decontamination 60–1
gut motility investigations 591–3
    autonomic neuropathy 112
gynaecomastia 11, 457

H_2 receptor blockers 116, 412
    gastrooesophageal reflux disease 338, 340
    gastroparesis 451
    Helicobacter pylori infection
        antisecretory effect augmentation 481
        diagnostic test effects 473, 475
    Helicobacter pylori-negative gastric ulcer 337
    non-ulcer (functional) dyspepsia 453
    NSAID-related damage prevention 71
    short bowel management 268, 269
    upper gastrointestinal bleeding 144
    use in pregnancy 116, 117
haem degradation 328
haematemesis 139, 150, 190
haematinic deficiency 321–8
    anaemia of liver disease 330
    causes 322
    clinical features 325
    diagnosis 325–6
    due to increased loss 324–5
    investigations 326–7
    malabsorption 322–4
    treatment 327–8
haematobilia 131
haematological malignancy 65–7
    hepatomegaly 63
    pre-treatment problems management 60
    treatment-related disorders 55–60
        colitis 56

endoscopy 59–60
gastrointestinal infections 60–1
gastrointestinal symptoms 57–9
graft versus host disease 55, 56
hepatic complications 61–3
mucositis 55–6
pancreatitis 57
haematology patients
hepatomegaly 63
splenic complications 64–5
haemochezia 139
haemochromatosis 10, 503
computed tomography 583
genetic 301–2, 322, 326, 549
clinical features 302
diagnosis 302
epidemiology 302
genetics 302
management 302
hypoparathyroidism 48
magnetic resonance imaging (MRI) 590
osteoarthritis 75
ultrasound appearances 555
haemoglobin C 329
haemoglobinopathies 328–9
splenomegaly 65
haemolytic anaemia 328
liver disease 330
splenomegaly 65
haemolytic–uraemic syndrome 410, 418
haemophilia patients 69, 495
Haemophilus influenzae type b 64
Haemophilus vaccine 64
haemorrhoidectomy 507–8
haemorrhoids 19, 58, 507–8, 510
haemosiderosis 583
haemostasis, laser therapy 535, 536–7
hamartomous polyps 400, 401
Hartmann's procedure (end-colostomy) 175
head of pancreas 24
heart failure
ascites 251, 254, 258
liver ultrasound appearances 554
nutritional support 280
heartburn 335, 357–8
definition 331
irritable bowel syndrome 358
obesity association 51
peptic ulcer disease 332
pregnancy 116, 358
heater probe 132

heavy-chain disease 67
Helicobacter pylori 26, 60, 71, 471–83
antimicrobial sensitivity 474
dyspepsia 331–2, 334, 477–9
cost-effectiveness of treatment 478
management guidelines 477
eradication 479–82
antibiotics 474
clinical effectiveness 479
confirmation 337, 482
empirical treatment strategy 478
failure 474
metronidazole resistance 474, 482, 483
obstetric patients 117
second-line treatment 482
treatment regimens 481–2
gastric biopsy 471–4, 478
concurrent medication 473
false negative results 471–2
false positive results 473
histology 473
microbiology 473–4
sites 472–3
urease tests 464
gastric cancer 477
gastric lymphoma 65, 66, 235
gastro-oesophageal reflux disease 481
nausea 318
non-ulcer dyspepsia 480–1
noninvasive diagnostic tests 472, 474–6
near-patient testing 476, 478
primary care 476, 478
screening applications 479
secondary care 474–6, 478–9
serology 474–5, 476
urea breath testing 337, 475–6
peptic ulcer disease 337
duodenal ulcer 479–80
gastric ulcer 480
NSAIDs-related 480
prevention/vaccination 483
recurrence 482
transmission 482
endoscopic from patient to patient 532
upper gastrointestinal bleeding 145
HELLP syndrome 120, 289
helminth worm infection
eosinophilia 415
small bowel obstruction 200
Henoch–Schonlein purpura 171
heparin 62, 208, 271

hepatic abscess 582
hepatic adenoma 560
hepatic angioma 549
hepatic angiosarcoma 563
hepatic arteriography 242–3
hepatic artery 21, 34, 554
  anatomical relations 20
hepatic cyst 559
hepatic ducts 564
  accessory 22
hepatic encephalopathy 297–8
  acute alcoholic hepatitis 305
  acute/subacute liver failure 287, 291
    referral to specialist unit 293
  liver transplantation 298
  overt 297–8
    grading 297
    movement disorders 297
  precipitants 298
  spontaneous bacterial peritonitis 259, 261
  subclinical 297
  treatment 298
hepatic flexure 19
hepatic haemangioma
  computed tomography 582
  ultrasound 560, 562
hepatic haematoma 560
hepatic iminodiacetic acid (HIDA) scintigraphy 605
hepatic lymphoma 556
hepatic metastases
  computed tomography 582
  interstitial laser photocoagulation 539
  magnetic resonance imaging (MRI) 590
  ultrasound 556, 558
hepatic segmental/subsegmental resection 244–5
  preoperative portal vein branch embolization 245
hepatic tumours, primary 37
hepatic veins 21, 554
hepatic veno-occlusive disease 61–2
hepatic venous pressure gradient 149
  ascites 253
hepatic venous pressure measurement 149
hepatitis
  acute abdominal pain 171
  ultrasound appearances 554
hepatitis A 485–7
  acute liver failure 288, 290
  clinical course 486
  epidemiology 485–6

haemophilia patients 69
  laboratory diagnosis 486
  management 486–7
  pregnant patients 121
  transmission 486
  virology 485
hepatitis B 485, 487–93, 503, 518
  acute 488–9
    clinical features 488
    liver function tests 488
    management 489
    prognosis 489
    serological markers 488–9
  acute liver failure 288, 290
  chronic 489–93
    antiviral treatment 491–3
    definition 489
    diagnosis 489
    hepatocellular carcinoma association 493
    natural history 489–90
    pathology 37
    risk factors 489
  epidemiology 487
  haemophilia patients 69
  hepatocellular carcinoma screening/surveillance 242
  HIV co-infection 93, 94
  immunization
    active 490
    combined immunoprophylaxis 490
    indications 490–1
    passive 490
  interferon-alpha treatment 491–2
  nucleoside analogue treatment 492–3
  occupationally acquired infection 530, 531, 532
  polyarteritis nodosa association 79
  transmission 67–8, 487–8, 531
    perinatal 487
  virology 487
hepatitis B immunoglobulin 490
hepatitis B vaccination 79, 130, 490
  endoscopy personnel 97, 530, 531
  haemophilia patients 69
hepatitis C 63, 74, 485, 494–9, 503
  acute 495
  alcohol consumption influence 458–9
  antiviral therapy 497–9
  bone marrow transplant patients 68
  chronic 495–9
    clinical features 495–6
    laboratory diagnosis 496–7

liver function tests 496
   management 497–9
   pathology 37
epidemiology 495
haemophilia patients 69, 495
hepatocellular carcinoma
   interferon alpha treatment 245
   screening/surveillance 241–2
HIV co-infection 93, 495
liver transplantation 499
occupationally acquired infection 530, 531
rheumatoid arthritis association 75
transmission 68, 495, 497, 531
virology 494
hepatitis δ 485, 493–4
   HIV-associated infection 93
   treatment 494
   vaccination 494
   virology 493–4
hepatitis E 288, 485, 487
   acute liver failure 288
   pregnant patients 121
   serological assay 487
   transmission 487
hepatitis G 485, 499–500
   blood transfusion-related transmission 68
   prevention/treatment 500
   virology 499
hepatitis non-A non-B
   acute liver failure 288
   blood transfusion-related transmission 67–8
   see also hepatitis C
hepatobiliary disease, malabsorption 381
hepatobiliary malignancy 237–8
   ascites 251
hepatobiliary scintigraphy 605–7
hepatocellular carcinoma 238, 241–8, 549
   chemotherapy 248
   computed tomography 582
   diagnosis 243
   extrahepatic spread 244
   fibrolamellar variant 242
   hepatic reserve assessment 244
   hepatic segmental/subsegmental resection
      244–5
   hepatitis B association 493
   hepatitis C association 497
   imaging 242–3
   ^{131}I-labelled lipiodol injection 248, 612
   orthoptic liver transplantation 245–6
   pathology 37

percutaneous biopsy 243
percutaneous ethanol injection 246–7
screening/surveillance 241–3
staging 243–4
thermal treatment modalities 248
transcatheter arterial chemoembolization 247–8
treatment options 241, 244–8
ultrasound appearances 563
hepatocytes 34, 35, 36
hepatomegaly 12, 63
hepatorenal syndrome
   ascites 253, 256
   spontaneous bacterial peritonitis 260
   variceal bleeding association 154
hepatotoxic drugs 74, 93
hereditary non-polyposis colorectal cancer 231,
   400
hereditary recurrent polyserositis (familial
   Mediterranean fever; periodic disease) 81
herpes simplex virus 28, 57, 58
   hepatitis 61
      pregnant patients 121
   HIV-associated infection 87, 88, 90, 91
   oesophageal ulceration 88, 359
   oral ulceration 87
   perianal disease 90, 91, 511
   proctitis 353, 414, 415
   rectal disease 513
herpes zoster 171
HFE mutations 302, 322
hiatus hernia, Cameron erosions 131
highly active antiretroviral therapy (HAART) 85,
   89, 92, 95, 96, 97–8
Hirschsprung's disease 389–90
   biopsy 389
   constipation 384
   large bowel obstruction 201
   postsurgical faecal incontinence 396
   presentation 389
   rectoanal inhibitory reflex testing 385, 389
   surgical treatment 390
histology 26–8
   anus 34
   large intestine 32
   liver 34–6
   oesophagus 28, 29
   pancreas 37
   small intestine 30–1
   stomach 28–9
histopathology report 25–6
Histoplasma 87, 92

history-taking 3–7
  cultural factors 4
  diarrhoea 353
  family history 4
  inflammatory bowel disease 425, 427
  listening skills 3
  pain 4
  psychological factors 4
  social skills 3
HLA B27 75
hMLH1 mutations 236
hMLH2 mutations 236
hormone replacement therapy 439
Hounsfield Units (HU) 581
human growth hormone therapy 92
human herpes virus 8 (HHV8) 95, 96
human immunodeficiency virus (HIV) 85–98, 518,
  596
  blood transfusion-related transmission 68
  diarrhoea 88–92, 411, 414
    investigations 92
    management 91–2
  endoscopy 85
    equipment disinfection guidelines 97
  gastrointestinal disease differential diagnosis
    85
  hepatitis C co-infection 495
  liver 92–4
    investigations 93–4
    treatment 94
  malabsorption/weight loss 92
  occupationally acquired infection 530, 531
  oesophageal disorders 85, 87–8
  oral disorders 85, 87
  pancreatic disorders 94
  parasitic infestations 379
  perianal warts 90
  sclerosing cholangitis 94–5
  tongue examination 10
  treatment 86
  tumours 95–7
  viral perianal ulceration 90
human papilloma virus (HPV) 87, 511
  HIV co-infection 90, 97
    anal cancer 97
human recombinant interleukin-11 210, 216
hydatid liver cyst
  computed tomography 582–3
  ultrasound 559, 560
hydrocortisone 209, 215
hydrogen breath test 356, 598

bacterial overgrowth 378
  Crohn's disease 428
hydroxychloroquine 75
hydroxycobalamin 328, 374
hydroxydaunorubicin 234
hydroxymethyl glutaryl coenzyme A reductase
  inhibitors 503
hyoscine 319, 347
hypercalcaemia 48
hyperemesis gravidarum 115–16, 119, 317
hyperhomocysteinaemia 65
hyperlipidaemia 51, 52–3
hyperparathyroidism, primary 48
hypertension 50
hyperthyroidism 47
  weight loss 371
hypnosis 115
hypoalbuminaemia 596
  persistent infective diarrhoea 415
  small bowel disease 375
hypochlorhydria 48
hypogammaglobulinaemia 380
hypoglycaemia, acute liver failure 287, 290
hypoparathyroidism 48
hyposplenism 64
hypotension
  acute liver failure 290–1
  autonomic neuropathy 110, 111
hypothyroidism 47
  primary biliary cirrhosis association 299

[123]I-meta-iodobenzyl guanide (MIBG) scintigraphy
  610
[131]I-labelled lipiodol injection 248, 612
igmesine 419
ileal absorptive function evaluation 356
ileal intubation 19
ileal resection
  gallstone disease association 461
  malabsorption 378
    vitamin B_{12} 324
ileocaecal valve 18–19
ileocolic artery 18
ileocolonoscopy, infectious colitis 417
ileostomy 175, 176
ileum
  blood supply 18
  macroscopic anatomy 18
ileus 58
  paralytic 202
  small bowel 574

iliac vein 20
immunocompromised patient 85–98
    antibiotic prophylaxis for endoscopy 526–7
    diarrhoea differential diagnosis 207
    infectious diarrhoea susceptibility 411
    infectious oesophageal ulceration 28
immunodeficiency disorders, primary 98
immunoglobulin light chain deposits 80
immunoproliferative small intestinal disease
    (IPSID; Mediterranean lymphoma) 66
immunosuppressive therapy
    inflammatory bowel disease 430, 431–2, 436
        Crohn's disease 215, 271
        ulcerative colitis 209–10
    use in pregnancy 118, 122
impaired glucose tolerance 41
impotence 110
[111]In-pentetreotide scintigraphy 609–10
incisura 16
indeterminate colitis 426
    children/adolescents 437
indoramin 394
infections
    blood transfusion transmission 67–9
    haematological malignancy patients 60–1
    post-splenectomy 64
    variceal bleeding 153–4
infective diarrhoea see diarrhoea
inferior epigastric artery 15
inferior mesenteric artery 19
inferior mesenteric lymph nodes 20
inferior mesenteric vein 20
inferior pancreaticoduodenal artery 18
inferior vena cava, duodenal relations 18
inflammation 26
    acute 26
    chronic 26
    classification 26
    stomach 30
inflammatory bowel disease 11, 205–18
    active disease 427–9
        indices 428–9
        investigations 427–8
    acute relapse management 429–30
    antibiotic therapy 434
    arthropathy 76
    children/adolescents 437–8
    colorectal cancer risk 401–2, 439–40
        colonoscopic surveillance 402, 439–40
        markers of precancer 402
        predictive value of dysplasia 401–2

diagnostic accuracy 425–7
diarrhoea 353, 354
fertility/pregnancy 118, 438
haematological malignancy patients 60
histopathology 425
history-taking 425, 427
immunosuppressive therapy 430, 431–2
    indications 436
indeterminate colitis 218, 426
lower gastrointestinal bleeding 167–8
maintenance therapy 434–6
malabsorption 377–278
nutritional support 281–2, 431
osteoporosis 438–9
outpatient care 425–41
    ancillary support 441
    clinic organization 441
    follow-up 441
pathology 33
patient support groups 441
prognosis 440–1
    mortality 440–1
    working capacity 441
radiolabelled leucocyte scan 608–9
refractory distal colitis 439
serology 426–7
spondarthritides association 75
steroid therapy 429
    low systemic bioavailability 433–4
surgery 432–3, 436–7
tongue examination 10
treatment 118
    alternatives to corticosteroids 430–4
weight loss 371, 377
inflammatory diarrhoea 352–3
inflammatory large bowel infiltrate 32
infliximab see tumour necrosis factor (TNF)
    antibody treatment
influenza vaccine 64
infracolic compartment 19
inguinal lymph nodes 15
injection sclerotherapy
    bleeding peptic ulcer 132, 141
    gastric varices 134, 161
    oesophageal carcinoma palliation 194
    oesophageal varices 134
    variceal bleeding
        gastric 161
        portal vein thrombosis 162
        randomized controlled trials 158–60
        variceal ligation comparison 160

insulin
    parenteral nutrition adjunctive therapy 281
    postgastrectomy reactive hypoglycaemia 368
insulin like growth factor-I 281
insulinoma 609, 610
interface hepatitis 36
interferon-alpha therapy
    carcinoid tumours 237
    hepatitis B 489, 491–2
    hepatitis C 497–8
        hepatocellular carcinoma 245
        ribavirin combined treatment 498, 499
    hepatitis G 500
    side effects 498
internal hernia 200
interstitial laser photocoagulation 538–9
    hepatic metastases treatment 539
intestinal adenoma 27
intestinal failure 267–70
    acute 267
    chronic 267
    see also short bowel
intestinal fistula 213, 217
intestinal ischaemia 354
intestinal lymphangiectasia 380
intestinal metaplasia in stomach 26
intestinal obstruction 197–202
    acute 197, 198–9
        radiological diagnosis 198
        treatment 198–9
    artificial feeding indications 275
    causes 197–8
    chronic 197, 201–2
    classification 197
    closed-loop 197
    diagnostic features 197
    dynamic/adynamic 197
    intra-abdominal adhesions 199–200
    mechanical obstruction 200–1
    paediatric 201
    simple/strangulating 197
    sub-acute/infectious diarrhoea 412, 414
intestinal permeability tests 597
intestinal pseudoobstruction
    chronic idiopathic 384
    megacolon 388
intestinal stagnant loop syndrome 324
intestinal tract scintigraphy 603–4
intra-abdominal abscess 217, 574
intra-abdominal adhesions 199–200
intra-abdominal thrombosis 65

intraepithelial T lymphocytes 31
    coeliac disease 31
    large intestine 32
intrahepatic bile ducts 34, 35, 36, 554, 564, 584
    dilatation 568, 569
intrahepatic cholestasis of pregnancy (obstetric
    cholestasis) 120–1
intravenous access
    endoscopy 523–14
    upper gastrointestinal bleeding 140
    variceal bleeding 152
intravenous urography 172
intrinsic factor 29, 323
    antibodies 324, 327, 374
intussusception 200–1, 574
invasive malignancy 27–8
    desmoplastic reaction 28
irinotecan 228, 230, 233
iron
    absorption/malabsorption 322–3
    dietary intake/body stores 322
    requirement for erythropoiesis 321
iron deficiency 274
    blood loss-related 324–5
    clinical features 325
    diagnosis 325, 326
    investigations 326–7, 595
    liver disease 330
    small bowel disease 375
    treatment 327–8
    ulcerative colitis 281
iron deficiency anaemia 322
    postgastrectomy 367, 374
iron overload 329
    haematology patients 63
iron supplements 209, 215, 327, 386
    parenteral therapy 327–8
irritable bowel syndrome 343–8
    aetiopathogenesis 343–5
    autonomic involvement 111
    constipation-predominant 347, 384
    diagnosis 346
    diarrhoea-predominant 347
    differential diagnosis 346, 347
    enteric nervous system function 344–5
    epidemiology 343
    food intolerance 345
    heartburn 358
    5-hydroxytryptamine levels 345
    intestinal motility 344
    investigations 346

management 346–8
  non-pharmacological approaches 348
Manning critera 345, 346
overlap with functional problems 345–6
pain-predominant 347
pathology 32
postinfectious 345
prognosis 348
Rome critera 345, 346
symptom patterns 345–6
ischaemic colitis 207, 417
  histological features 33
  lower gastrointestinal bleeding 168
ischaemic heart disease 50
ischiorectal abscess 509
islet amyloid polypeptide 80
isobutyl-2-cyanoacrylate (Bucrylate)
  sclerotherapy 161
isoniazid 93, 288
isosorbide dinitrate 187
Isospora belli 89, 92
ispaghula 347, 386
Italy, training requirements 615, 618
Ito cells 36
itraconazole 61, 63

jaundice
  acute liver failure 287
  alcoholic cirrhosis 457
  haemolytic anaemias 328
  hepatitis B 488
  malabsorption/steatorrhoea 381
  obstructive 221, 222
    abdominal observation 10
    see also bile duct stones
  physical examination 9
  subacute liver failure 287
jejunal biopsy 596–7
jejunal resection 378
jejuno-colic anastomosis 267
  adaptation 270
  short bowel management 269–70
jejunoileal resection 267
jejunostomy 267
  adaptation 269
  diabetic gastroparesis 43
  high volume output management 268–9
  problems of short bowel 268
jejunum
  blood supply 18
  macroscopic anatomy 18

K-ras 231
Kaposi's sarcoma
  HIV-associated 95–6
    oral ulceration 87
  management 96
kernicterus 328
ketoconazole 87, 93
kidney, duodenal relations 17–18
Klebsiella 60, 75, 259
koilonychia 10
Kupffer cells 36

L1 (deferiprone) 63
lactic acidosis
  refeeding syndrome 278
  short bowel complications 270
Lactobacillus 422
Lactobacillus acidophilus 422
Lactobacillus fermentum 422
lactose breath test 356
lactose-free diet 431
lactulose 154, 261, 298, 387
lamina propria 29
lamivudine 94, 493
Langerhans' cell histiocytosis X 65
lanreotide 48
laparoscopic-guided peritoneal biopsy 254
laparoscopy
  acute abdominal pain 172
  oesophageal carcinoma 191
large bowel obstruction 197
  radiological diagnosis 198
  ultrasound appearances 574
large diameter endoscope 128
large intestine
  histoloty 32
  macroscopic anatomy 18–19
  pathology 32–4
laser therapy 535–9
  advanced cancers palliation 537–8
  Barrett's oesophagus 184, 185, 186
  bile duct direct-contact lithotripsy 223
  colorectal cancer 538
  effects on tissues 535–6
  haemostasis 535, 536–7
  hepatocellular carcinoma 248
  interstitial photocoagulation 538–9
  oesophageal carcinoma debulking 193
  pulsed lasers 536
  see also photodynamic therapy
laxatives

bulk forming 386
constipation management 386–7
factitious diarrhoea 353
irritable bowel syndrome 347
opiate analgesia management 57
osmotic 387
side effects 202
stimulant 386–7
stool analysis, chronic diarrhoea evaluation 355
use in pregnancy 117
lead poisoning 171
lectin-binding analysis 242
leuconychia 11
leukaemia
  gum infiltration 55–6
  splenomegaly 65
levamisole 232
leVeen shunt 611
Lewis–Tanner oesophagogastrectomy 192
ligament of Treitz 18
ligamentum teres 20, 554
lignocaine 56, 523
lipid-decreasing drug side effects 52
Lipiodol-CT 243
liquid paraffin 387
Listeria monocytogenes 117–18, 259
Lithuania, training requirements 618
liver
  blood supply 34
  computed tomography 582–4
  histology 34–6
  macroscopic anatomy 21
  magnetic resonance imaging (MRI) 588, 590
    liver-specific contrast agents 588
  pathology 36–7
  portal tracts 34, 36
  segments 21, 22
  structure
    hepatic lobule 35
    Rappaport's hepatic acinus 35–6
    reticulin staining 36, 37
  ultrasound examination 554–64
    diagnostic pitfalls 563–4
liver biopsy 504, 549–52
  acute alcoholic hepatitis 305
  acute liver failure 289
  alcoholic cirrhosis 457
  alcoholic fatty liver 456
  ascites 253–4
  contraindications 549–50

hepatitis C 496–7
hepatocellular carcinoma 243
indications 549
percutaneous sampling 243, 550–1
  after care 551
  complications 551
  Menghini technique 550–1
  plug sampling 552
  procedure 550
  Tru-Cut biopsy 551
transvenous jugular sampling 551–2
ultrasound-guided sampling 552
liver disease
  HIV-associated 92–4
  obstetric patients 118–22
  physical signs 11–12
liver enzyme abnormalities 503–6
  gamma-glutamyltransferase 506
  increased alkaline phosphatase 505–6
  increased serum transaminase 503–4
  pregnant patients 119
liver failure
  acute 287–94
    acute renal failure 291, 292
    aetiology 287–9
    assessment of prognosis 292–3
    cerebral oedema 291–2
    clinical features 289–92
    conservative management 293–4
    definition 287
    diagnosis 289
    encephalopathy 291
    epidemiology 287–9
    extracorporeal bioartificial liver support 294
    haemorrhagic gastritis 291
    hypovolaemia 291
    immediate management 290–2
    indications for specialist unit referral 293
    investigations 289–90
    liver transplantation 290, 292, 293–4
    sepsis 291
  chronic liver disease 297–303
  fulminant 287
  nutritional support 280–1, 292
  subacute (subacute hepatic necrosis; late onset hepatic failure) 287
liver transplantation
  acute alcoholic hepatitis 309–10
  acute liver failure 258, 287, 288, 292, 293–4
    indications 294

alcoholic cirrhosis 458, 459
ascites 251, 258
  Budd–Chiari syndrome 258
  cirrhosis 256, 257–8
autoimmune chronic active hepatitis 301
auxiliary partial orthoptic (APOLT) 294
hepatic encephalopathy 298
hepatitis C 499
hepatocellular carcinoma 245–6
pregnancy following 118, 122
primary biliary cirrhosis 299
primary sclerosing cholangitis 300
scintigraphic investigations 607–8
subacute liver failure 287, 288
Wilson's disease 303
lobucavir 493
lomustine 57
long-chain 3-hydroxyacyl coenzyme A
dehydrogenase deficiency 119
loperamide 46, 57, 78, 268, 269, 271, 347, 356,
  396, 419, 510
  contraindications 208
lorazepam 57, 319
lovastatin 52
lower gastrointestinal bleeding 167–9
  diagnosis 167–8
  incidence 167
  management 168–9
  occult 169
  ulcerative colitis 210–11
lower oesophageal sphincter 15–16
  relaxation 445
lupus anticoagulant 65
luteinizing hormone-releasing hormone analogues
  230
Lyme disease (tick-borne Borreliosis) 81
lymphadenopathy 586, 590
lymphatic drainage 20–1
  abdominal wall 15
  stomach 16
lymphogranuloma venereum 414, 415
lymphoid follicles 20
lymphoma 18, 65–6, 234–6, 334, 355
  bowel involvement 60
    ultrasound appearances 575
  HIV-associated 87, 96
  liver 556
  malabsorption 324, 380
  small bowel 32, 235–6
  staging 235
  stomach 234–5

M proteins 67
macroglossia 47
macronutrient supplements 267
macroscopic anatomy 15–24
magnesium salts 387
magnesium supplements 269
magnetic resonance cholangiopancreatography
  (MRCP) 464–5, 588, 589, 597
  chronic pancreatitis 380
magnetic resonance imaging (MRI) 588–90
  bile duct stones 222
  bowel 590
  chronic pancreatitis 380
  clinical utility 588
  computed tomography comparison 589
  Crohn's disease 214, 217, 428
  faecal incontinence 395
  gallstones 464–5
  gastric emptying assessment 593
  hepatocellular carcinoma screening/surveillance
    242
  inflammatory bowel disease, pregnant patients
    438
  liver 588, 590
    liver-specific contrast agents 588
  oesophageal carcinoma 190
  pancreas 590, 597
  principles 588
  reticuloendothelial system 590
  see also magnetic resonance
    cholangiopancreatography (MRCP)
malabsorption 371–81
  associated disease 371
  drug-induced 379
  endocrine disorders 379–80
  gastric disease 374
  haematinic deficiency 322–4
  hepatobiliary disease 381
  HIV-associated 92
  hypoparathyroidism 48
  intestinal resection 378–9
  investigations 595–9
    blood tests 595–6
    fat malabsorption 597–8
    imaging 596–7
  obstetric cholestasis 121
  pancreatic disease 380–1
  pernicious anaemia 374
  persistent infective diarrhoea 415
  postgastrectomy 367, 374
  small bowel disease 374–80

weight loss 371
malabsorption syndrome 371
malaria 64, 65
malignant disease 225–38
  acute liver failure 289, 290
  disseminated intravascular coagulation/ microangiopathic haemolytic anaemia 328
  epidemiology 226
  folic acid requirement 325
  information for decision-making 226
  laser therapy 535, 537–8
  nutritional status assessment 10
  obesity association 51
  photodynamic therapy 540–1
  small bowel strictures 200
  see also neoplasia
Mallory–Weiss tear 52, 57, 178
  emergency endoscopy 130, 131
malnutrition
  acute alcoholic hepatitis 307
  short gut syndrome (massive intestinal resection) 378
  small bowel disease 375
  see also undernutrition
MALT lymphoma 65–6
  stomach 234, 235
mannitol 291
manofluorography 365
manometric studies
  ambulatory antroduodenal 112
  diabetic gastroparesis 42
  oesophageal dysfunction *see* oesophageal manometry
mantle-cell lymphoma 66
marginal artery (of Drummond) 19–20
marijuana 319
mebeverine 347
mechanical ventilation 106, 152
mecillinam 422
Meckel's diverticulum
  lower gastrointestinal bleeding 167, 169
  scintigraphy 605
meconium ileus 201
Mediterranean lymphoma (immunoproliferative small intestinal disease) 66
medium-chain triglycerides 270
megabowel, idiopathic 388–9
megacolon 388
  acquired 388
  congenital *see* Hirschsprung's disease
  idiopathic 384

myopathic 388
neurological 388
megarectum, idiopathic 384
megestrol acetate 92
Meissner's plexus 16
melaena 139, 150, 190
meloxicam 72
melphalan 55, 57
meningococcus 64
meningococcus vaccine 64
mepacrine 75
6-mercaptopurine 215, 217, 218, 510
  side effects 63
  ulcerative colitis 210
  use in pregnancy 118
mesalazine *see* 5-aminosalicylic acid
mesenteric angiography 355
  lower gastrointestinal bleeding 168–9
  occult gastrointestinal bleeding 169
mesenteric ischaemia 20
  acute 202
  chronic diarrhoea 355
mesenteric thrombosis 65
meso-tetrahydroxyphenyl chlorin (mTHPC) 540, 542
metaplasia 26
metastatic tumours
  colorectal cancer 231–2, 233–4
  small bowel 32, 237
methotrexate 56, 74, 96, 215, 228, 237, 299
  contraindication in pregnancy 118
  Crohn's disease 432
  side effects 63, 74
methyl cellulose 386
methyl prednisolone 69, 209, 215, 308
methyl *tert*-butyl ether 466
metoclopramide 57, 77, 116, 319, 347, 451, 453
  side effects 57
  use in pregnancy 116
metronidazole 56, 77, 87, 91, 93, 173, 209, 215–16, 217, 378, 428, 434
  Helicobacter pylori eradication 481, 482
  Helicobacter pylori resistance 474, 482, 483
  use in pregnancy 118
Michigan MAST test 455
microbubble-enhanced sonographic angiography (MESA) 243
microscopic anatomy 25–38
microsporidial infection 354, 416, 419
  HIV-associated diarrhoea 89, 92
  treatment 89, 421

micturition problems 110–11
midazolam 522–3
midodrine 256
migrating motor complex (MMC) 449–50
Mirizzi's syndrome 222, 463, 564
misoprostil 71, 338
   contraindication in pregnancy 117
mitomycin C 227, 228, 234, 237
mitoxantrone 248
mixed connective tissue disease 78
molluscum contagiosum 511
monitoring
   endoscopy 524–5
   nutritional support 277–9
   upper gastrointestinal bleeding 140, 141, 142
   variceal bleeding 152
monoamine oxidase inhibitors 386
motilin 445
motion sickness 318
   drug treatment 319
motor neuron disease
   dysphagia 104, 106, 108
   percutaneous endoscopic gastrostomy 108
mouth examination 10
mucocoele of gallbladder 566
mucosa 26, 27
   inflammatory processes 26
mucosa-associated lymphoid tissue (MALT) 65
   lymphoma see MALT lymphoma
mucosal prolapse 508
mucositis, chemoradiotherapy-related 55–6, 58
multiple endocrine neoplasia (MEN) 48–9
   type 1 48–9
   type 2 49
multiple myeloma 66
multiple sclerosis
   faecal incontinence 396
   percutaneous endoscopic gastrostomy 108
multiple system atrophy 110
Munchausen's syndrome 139
muscularis propria 26, 27
myasthenia gravis
   dysphagia 104, 105, 108
   oesophageal motility disorders 186
Mycobacterium
   HIV-associated infection 91, 92, 94
      oral ulceration 87
      weight loss 92
Mycobacterium avium intracellulare 91, 92, 94, 518
Mycobacterium tuberculosis 87, 97, 409, 414,
   517, 518, 532

mycophenolate mofetil 215
mycostatin 55
myelodysplasia 63
myelofibrosis 63, 65
myeloproliferative disorders 63, 65
myenteric (Auerbach's) plexus 16
myocardial infarction 171, 202
myoelectrical activity, colon 344
myxoedema
   ascites 251, 258
   intestinal pseudo-obstruction 202

nabumetone 71
naloxone 299
naproxen 72
nasogastric intubation
   contraindications
      acute liver failure 292
      upper gastrointestinal bleeding 128, 142
   emergency endoscopy 128
   neurogenic dysphagia 109
   nutritional support 276
   variceal bleeding 155
nausea/vomiting 315–19
   Addison's disease 46
   alcohol consumption history 317
   associated pain 316
   autonomic neuropathy 111
   chemoradiotherapy patients 57
   chemotherapy-induced 319
   definitions 315
   diagnostic problems 318
   drug-induced 317
   electrolyte disturbances 319
   food poisoning 318
   gastrointestinal bleeding 316–17
   Helicobacter pylori infection 318
   hypercalcaemia/primary hyperparathyroidism 48
   hyperthyroidism 47
   intestinal obstruction 197, 198
   management 319
      drug treatment 319
   motion sickness 318, 319
   neurological disorders 318
   nutritional depletion 319
   postgastrectomy bilious vomiting 368
   pregnancy 115–16, 317
   projectile vomiting 316
   psychological/social disorders 317
   superior mesenteric artery syndrome 318
   timing of vomiting in relation to eating 315–16

NdYAG laser
  advanced cancer palliation 537
    oesophageal cancer 193, 537
  peptic ulcer haemostasis 536
neck of pancreas 24
necrotizing enterocolitis 201
necrotizing fasciitis 56
necrotizing stomatitis 87
necrotizing ulcerative gingivitis 87
needle-stick injuries 530, 531
Neisseria 259
Neisseria gonorrhoeae 414, 415
neomycin 270, 298, 379
neonatal haemolytic anaemias 328
neonatal intestinal obstruction 201
neoplasia 26–7
  diagnostic criteria 26–7
  epithelial 26
    dysplasia 27
    invasive malignancy 27–8
    Vienna classification 27, 28
  lower gastrointestinal bleeding 167, 168
  see also malignant disease
nephrotic syndrome 253, 259
nerve supply
  abdominal wall 15
  oesophagus 16
  peritoneum 15
Netherlands, training requirements 615, 618
neuroendocrine cells
  large intestine 32
  small intestine 31
  stomach 29
neuroendocrine tumours
  pancreatic 597
  scintigraphic evaluation 609–10
neurogenic dysphagia 103–8
  causes 104
  investigations 103–4
    videofluoroscopy modified barium swallow
      106
  motor neurone disease 104, 106, 108
  myasthenia gravis 104, 105, 108
  Parkinson's disease 107–8
  percutaneous endoscopic gastrostomy 108–9
  signs 104–5
  stroke patients 104, 107
  symptoms 104
  water-swallow test 105–6
neurological disease 103–13
  aspiration pneumonia risk 103

constipation 385
nausea/vomiting 318
ventilation 106
neutropenia 526
  chemoradiotherapy-related mucositis 55, 56
  enterocolitis (typhlitis) 56
Niemann–Pick disease 65
nifedipine 187, 189, 358, 448
nitazoxanide 89
nitric oxide
  gastric motility 448
  lower oesophageal sphincter response 445
nitrous oxide gas 523
non-alcoholic steatohepatitis 503
non-septic arthritis 418
non-steroidal anti-inflammatory drugs (NSAIDs)
    150, 168, 207, 362, 468, 503
  contraindications 209, 215, 256
  COX-1 inhibitors 72
  COX-2 inhibitors 72
  gastrointestinal toxicity 346
    acute liver failure 289
    colitis 73
    intestinal injury 72–3
    nausea/vomiting 317
    oesophageal ulceration 28
    upper gastrointestinal tract 71–2
  peptic ulcer disease
    duodenal ulcer 334
    gastric ulcer 337, 338
    Helicobacter pylori eradication therapy 480
non-tropical sprue 235
non-ulcer (functional) dyspepsia 331, 451–3
  clinical features 452
  gastrointestinal motor abnormalities 452
  Helicobacter pylori eradication therapy 480–1
  Rome criteria 451
  treatment 340, 452–3
noradrenaline 291
norfloxacin 261, 262
nuclear medicine 601–12
nucleoside analogues, hepatitis B treatment
    492–3
nutcracker oesophagus 186, 189, 360, 361, 447,
    448, 602
nutrition risk index (NRI) 274
Nutrition Strategic Committee 275
nutritional disorders, postgastrectomy 367–8
nutritional status
  assessment 10, 273–4
  Crohn's disease 213–14

nutritional support 273–83
  acute alcoholic hepatitis 307–8, 309
  acute pancreatitis 282
  cirrhosis 154–5
  critically ill patients 279–81
    adjunctive hormonal therapy 281
  Crohn's disease 214, 217, 281, 429, 431
  energy requirements 277
  enterocutaneous fistulae 271–2
  glutamine supplementation 282–3
  indications 274–5
  inflammatory bowel disease 281–2
  jejuno-colic anastomosis patients 269–70
  jejunostomy patients 269
  liver failure 280–1, 292
  monitoring 277–9
  parenteral electrolyte requirements 277
  perioperative 279
  protein requirements 277
  refeeding syndrome 277–8
  small stomach syndrome 368
  team approach to organization 275–6
  techniques 276–7
  ulcerative colitis 208, 431
nystatin 55, 87

obesity 50–1, 461
obstetric cholestasis (intrahepatic cholestasis of
    pregnancy) 120–1
  fetal compromise 121
obstetric damage-related faecal incontinence 394,
    395
obstetric patients 115–22
  inflammatory bowel disease 118
obstructive sleep apnoea 51
occult gastrointestinal bleeding 169
octreotide 46, 57, 89, 237, 256, 268, 356
  side effects 47–8
  variceal bleeding 156
    randomized controlled trials 157–8, 159,
      160
odynophagia 357, 359
oesophageal ambulatory 24-h pH monitoring 336,
    364, 591
oesophageal apoplexy 131
oesophageal bile reflux 336–7
oesophageal cancer 15, 189–94, 225–8
  achalasia association 187
  acute oesophagel obstruction 178
  adjuvant therapy 192
  aetiological factors 189

Barrett's oesophagus association 181–2, 192
    malignant transformation 182–4
  chemoradiation 226, 227, 228
  chemotherapy 227, 228
  clinical features 189–90
  diagnosis 190
  dysphagia 362, 363–4
  incidence 189
  laser therapy
    comparative aspects 538
    NdYAG laser recanalization 537
  multimodal therapy 227
  odynophagia 359
  oesophageal prostheses 193
    expanding metal stents 537–8
    silicone-rubber stents 537
  palliative therapy 192–4, 227–8
  pathology 28
  photodynamic therapy 541
  radiotherapy 225–6, 228
  resectional surgery 192
  staging 190–1
    computed tomography 586
  treatment 191–4
    patient selection 191
oesophageal colic 357, 358
oesophageal corrosive injury 181, 189
oesophageal disorders 357–65
  emergency presentation 177–94
  HIV-related 85, 87–8
  investigations 364–5
  symptoms 357
  see also oesophageal motility disorders
oesophageal dissecting intramural haematoma 359
oesophageal diverticula/pouches 361
oesophageal intramural haematoma 178–9
oesophageal manometry 364–5, 591
  achalasia 187, 446
  diffuse oesophageal spasm 189
  neuromuscular disease 360
  oesophageal dysfunction 364, 365
oesophageal motility 445–6
  deglutition inhibition 445
  scintigraphic assessment 602
oesophageal motility disorders 186–8, 357, 358,
    445–8
  non-specific 189, 447–8
  primary 446–8
    body of oesophagus 447–8
  secondary 448
  symptoms 446

oesophageal obstruction
  acute 177–9
    acute bolus obstruction 178
    intramural haematoma 178–9
    swallowed foreign body 177
  artificial feeding indications 275
  oesophageal carcinoma 190
oesophageal perforation 179
  instrumental 180–1
oesophageal prostheses
  acute oesophagel obstruction 178
  oesophageal cancer 193, 537–8
oesophageal rupture
  bulimia nervosa association 52
  intramural 178
  spontaneous (Boerhaave's syndrome) 179–80
oesophageal scintigraphy 602
oesophageal strictures
  acute oesophagel obstruction 178
  caustic 15, 363
  dysphagia 361–3, 364, 365
  endoscopic dilatation 180
oesophageal ulceration 28, 359
oesophageal varices
  endoscopic treatment 133–4
    band ligation 133–4
    injection sclerotherapy 134
  randomized controlled trials 156–60
  see also variceal bleeding
oesophageal webs 362
oesophagitis 335
  management 338, 339, 340
    surgery 340
oesophagogastroduodenoscopy
  infectious colitis 417
  oesophageal function (motility) assessment 591
  see also upper gastrointestinal endoscopy
oesophagus
  computed tomography 586
  functional (motility) tests 591
  histology 28, 29
  macroscopic anatomy 15–16
  nerve supply 16
  pathology 28
ofloxacin 261
Ogilvie's syndrome 388
olsalazine 429, 434, 435
Olympus clips 133
omeprazole 144, 145, 184, 217, 269, 336, 337, 338
omnipressin 256
ondansetron 57, 74, 116, 319, 347

opioid analgesics 386
  chronic pancreatitis 460
  contraindications 208
  Crohn's disease 215
  pancreatic cancer 230
  sedation for endoscopy 523
  side effects 57, 317, 346
oral bile-acid treatment, gallstone disease 465–6
  incomplete gallstone dissolution 467
  recurrent gallstones 467
oral contraceptive pill 65, 121, 202
oral hairy leucoplakia 87
oral HIV-associated disorders 85, 87
oral rehydration therapy 419
oral ulceration
  Crohn's disease 217
  HIV-associated 87
  small bowel disease 375
orooesophageal overtube 129
oropharyngeal mucositis, chemoradiotherapy-related 55
oropharyngeal suction 127
orthophthaldehyde (OPA) disinfectant 518
osmotic diarrhoea 352
osteoarthritis 51, 75
osteomalacia
  investigations 596
  postgastrectomy 368, 374
  small bowel disease 375
osteoporosis 505
  inflammatory bowel disease 438–9
  postgastrectomy 368
oxaliplatin 228, 233, 234
oxandrolone 309
oxygen therapy 127
oxypentifylline 62

p53 mutations 231, 401, 402
PABA test 599
pacing, diabetic gastroparesis 43
Paget's disease 505, 510
pain relief
  bacterial peritonitis 173
  pancreatic cancer 230
palatal movement 105
palmar erythema 11, 119, 305
pan-dysautonomia, acute 110
pancrealauryl test (fluorescein dilaurate test) 599
pancreas
  computed tomography 584–6
  histology 37

macroscopic anatomy 24
magnetic resonance imaging (MRI) 590, 597
pathology 37–8
ultrasound 568, 570–1, 597
 diagnostic pitfalls 570–1
 pitfalls of normal anatomy 570
pancreas divisum 24
pancreatic abscess 584
pancreatic cancer 229–31
 body and tail of pancreas 381
 CA 19.9 marker 229
 chemotherapy 229–30
 computed tomography 585–6
 head of pancreas 381
 investigations 597
 pathology 37–8
 photodynamic therapy 542
 radiotherapy 230
 symptom control 230–1
  endoscopic stent placement 546–7
 ultrasound appearances 570, 573
pancreatic disease
 alcohol-induced 459–60
 HIV-associated disease 94
 malabsorption 380–1
pancreatic duct stents 547, 548
pancreatic ducts 24, 570
 accessory 18
 common anatomical variations 24
pancreatic endotherapy 546–7
 complications 548
pancreatic exocrine function tests 598–9
pancreatic insufficiency
 chronic pancreatitis 380
 diabetic diarrhoea 44
 vitamin B_{12} malabsorption 324
pancreatic lipase 372
pancreatic neuroendocrine tumours 586
pancreatic phlegmon
 computed tomography 584
 magnetic resonance imaging (MRI) 590
pancreatic proteolytic enzymes 372
pancreatic pseudocyst 547, 548, 584
pancreatic supplements 380
pancreatin 381
pancreatitis
 acute 173–4
  causes 173–4
  clinical features 174, 459
  computed tomography 584
  diagnosis 459

endoscopic management of pseudocysts
 547, 548
hypercalcaemia/primary hyperparathyroidism
 48
hyperlipidaemia association 52
management 174, 459
nutritional support 282
Ranson severity criteria 174
ultrasound 570, 571
alcohol abuse association 459, 460
chronic 10, 460, 597
 clinical features 380, 460
 computed tomography 584–5
 diagnosis 460
 endoscopic management 547
 imaging 380
 malabsorption/steatorrhoea 380
 pathology 37–8
 treatment 380, 460
 ultrasound 570, 572, 597
HIV infection-related 94
obstetric patients 117
Paneth cells 31, 32
Panorex 232
parabutyl iminodiacetic acid (T-BIDA)
 scintigraphy 605, 606
paracentesis 15, 256–7
 ascites diagnosis 253
paracetamol 71
 absorption assessment for gastric emptying
  evaluation 592
 poisoning 287–8
  acute renal failure 292
  assessment of prognosis 292–3
  conservative management 293
  indications for specialist unit referral 293
  investigations 289–90
  liver transplantation 293
paralytic ileus 202
paraneoplastic autonomic neuropathy 110
parasitic infections
 malabsorption 379
 pigment gallstone associations 462
parathyroid disease 48
paraumbilical veins 20
parenteral nutrition
 critically ill patients 279–80
 delivery techniques 276–7
  central venous catheters 277
  peripheral catheters 276
  peripherally inserted central catheters 276

enterocutaneous fistulae 271–2, 275
  glutamine supplementation 282–3
  home feeding 275
  indications 274–5
  insulin infusion 281
  jejuno-colic anastomosis patients 270
  jejunostomy patients 269
parietal cell antibodies 323–4, 327, 374
parietal cells 29
Parkinson's disease 103
  constipation 108, 109–10
  dysphagia 107–8
  gastrooesophageal reflux 108
Parkinson's-plus syndrome 108
paromomycin 89, 420
paroxysmal nocturnal haemoglobinuria 63, 65
Paterson–Kelly syndrome (Plummer–Vinson)
  syndrome 189, 325
Paul–Mickulicz procedure 175
pedal erythema 11
peliosis hepatis, HIV-related 92, 94
penicillamine 74, 299, 303
penicillin 56, 64, 81, 93, 513
pentamidine 93
pentoxifylline 310–11
peppermint 347
pepsinogen 29
peptic strictures
  dilatation 362–3
  dysphagia 361, 362
peptic ulcer disease
  basophilic leukaemia association 60
  dyspepsia 331, 332
  Helicobacter pylori serological markers 475
  hypercalcaemia/primary hyperparathyroidism
    48
  non-steroidal anti-inflammatory drugs
    (NSAIDs)-related 71
  obstetric patients 117
  pneumoperitoneum 174–5
  postgastrectomy recurrence 369
  symptoms 332
  systemic mastocytosis association 60
  upper gastrointestinal bleeding 139–46
    drug treatment 144–5
    emergency endoscopy 130, 131, 141
    endoscopic treatment 131–3, 141, 142, 143,
      145
    epidemiology 139
    initial resuscitation 144
    injection treatment 131–2

    laser therapy 536
    mechanical treatment 133
    prognostic factors 142–3
    rebleeding following endoscopic haemostasis
      146
    rebleeding prediction (Baylor score) 142–3
    risk scoring system 142, 143
    stigmata of recent haemorrhage/rebleeding
      rates 142
    surgery 145–6
    thermal treatment 132
  Zollinger–Ellison syndrome 334
peptide hormones 355
peracetic acid disinfectant 518
percutaneous cholecystolithotomy 467
percutaneous endoscopic gastrostomy
  anatomical landmarks 16
  antibiotic prophylaxis for endoscopy 527
  consent issues 109
  Crohn's disease 431
  neurogenic dysphagia 108–9
  stroke patients 103, 109
perianal abscess 509
perianal bleeding 507
perianal disease 507–14
  chemoradiotherapy patients 58–9
  infectious diarrhoea 414
  symptoms 507
perianal fistulae
  Crohn's disease 213
  magnetic resonance imaging (MRI) 590
perianal pain 507
perianal sepsis 507, 509–10
perianal warts (condylomata acuminata) 90, 91,
  511
perinuclear anti-cytoplasmic antibodies (pANCA)
  426–7
periodic disease (hereditary recurrent polyserositis;
  familial Mediterranean fever) 81
periodontitis 87
perioperative nutritional support 279
peristalsis
  distal stomach–duodenum pressure gradient 449
  duodenal 449
  gastric 448–9
    migrating motor complex (MMC) control
      449–50
  oesophageal 445
  small intestinal segmental/propulsive
    contractions 450
  visible on abdominal examination 10

peritoneal carcinomatosis 254
peritoneal cavity, ultrasound examination 574–7
    diagnostic pitfalls 576
peritoneal free fluid 574
peritoneal inflammation 258–9
peritoneal lavage 172
peritoneovenous shunts
    patency assessment 611
    refractory ascites 256, 257
peritoneum
    investing colon 19
    investing rectum 19
    parietal 15
    visceral 15
peritonitis
    acute abdominal pain 172–4
    acute intestinal obstruction 198
    bacterial
        chronic 174
        primary 172
        secondary 173
        see also spontaneous bacterial peritonitis
    chemical 173–4
    granulomatous 174
    primary biliary 173
pernicious anaemia 323–4
    autoimmune disease associations 47, 374
    clinical features 374
    intrinsic factor antibodies 374
    malabsorption 374
    nausea/vomiting 374
    parietal cell antibodies 374
    treatment 328, 374
peroxygen compounds 518
Peutz–Jegher's syndrome 236, 400
    colorectal cancer surveillance 400
Peyer's patches 18
phaeochromocytoma 355
pharyngeal anaesthesia 522
pharyngeal diverticulum 361
pharyngeal manometry 365
pharyngeal pouch 361, 446
phenobarbitone 299
phenothiazines 202
phenytoin 93
photodynamic therapy 535, 539–43
    effects on tissues 536
    gastrointestinal tract tumours 540–1
    Helicobacter pylori eradication 542–3
    mode of action 539–40
    oesophageal carcinoma debulking 193

pancreatic/biliary duct tumours 542
    pre-malignant lesions 541–2
photosensitizers 539, 540
phrenicocolic ligament 19
physical abuse history 4
    constipation 384, 386
physical examination 9–12
    abdomen 10–11
    eye signs 9
    liver disease 11–12
    mouth 10
    nutritional status assessment 10
    rectal examination 12
    skin 9–10
phytobezoars 200
pigment gallstones 462
piperacillin 59
piroxicam 72
pit cells 36
planes, transpyloric 16
plasmacytoma 66
platelet transfusion 152–3
platinum 57
Plesimonas 259
Plummer–Vinson (Paterson–Kelly) syndrome
    189, 325
pneumococcus 64
pneumonia, lobar 171
pneumoperitoneum 174–5
pneumovax 64
polidocanol injection sclerotherapy 132, 159, 194
poliovirus 518
polyarteritis nodosa 78–9, 80
polycythaemia rubra vera 65
polymeric liquid diet 431
polymyositis 74
polypectomy 167
porfimer sodium 540, 541
porphyria 110, 202
    acute abdominal pain 171
portal circulation 20
portal hypertension 20, 202
    ascites 251–2, 253, 254
        non-cirrhotic 258
    definition 149
    measurement 149
    pregnant patients 121
portal pyaemia 202
portal vein 20, 21, 34, 554
    duodenal relations 17
    embolization 20

thrombosis 63, 161–2
portal venous pressure gradient measurement 149
portal–systemic anastomosis 20
  sites 20
portocaval shunts 256, 257, 258
portosystemic encephalopathy 154
Portugal, training requirements 618
positron emission tomography 610–11
postgastrectomy disorders 367–9
  bezoar formation 369
  bile reflux/bilious vomiting 368
  diarrhoea 368–9
  dumping syndrome 368
  malabsorption 374
  mechanical 369
  nutritional 367–8
  reactive hypoglycaemia 368
  recurrent peptic ulcer disease 369
  small stomach syndrome 368
  stump carcinoma 369
postoperative complications
  obesity association 51
  small-bowel obstruction 200
postsurgical oesophageal strictures 363
potassium preparations
  oesophageal ulceration 28
  slow-release tablets 359
pouch surgery 433
pravastatin 52
prebiotics 422
prednisolone 209, 215, 234, 235, 281, 308, 430
prednisolone metasulphobenzoate 434
pre-eclampsia 120
pregnancy
  abdominal pain 116–17
    uterine contractions/labour pain 117
  acute fatty liver 119
  constipation 117
  diarrhoea 117–18
  folic acid requirement 325
  heartburn/reflux symptoms 116, 358
  inflammatory bowel disease 438
  iron absorption 322, 323
  liver disease 118–22
    hepatitis exacerbation 121
    pre-existing disease 121–2
  nausea/vomiting 115–16, 317
  physiological changes 115
    liver 118–19
  placental alkaline phosphatase 505
prior probability 5

probiotics 422
prochlorperazine 93, 116, 319
proctitis
  infectious diarrhoea 412, 414
  microbial enteropathogens 415
proctocolectomy with permanent ileostomy 433
projectile vomiting 316
prokinetic drugs 77, 368
  constipation 387
  gallstone disease prevention 468
  gastrooesophageal reflux 338
  gastroparesis 451
    diabetic 42, 43
  irritable bowel syndrome 347
  nausea/vomiting 319
  non-ulcer (functional) dyspepsia 453
promethazine 116, 121
propofol 523
propranolol 121, 458
prostacyclin 291
prostaglandin E_1 62
protective clothing, emergency endoscopy 130
protein absorption 372
protein C deficiency 65
protein intake
  acute alcoholic hepatitis 308
  hepatic encephalopathy management 298
  requirements for nutritional support 277
protein S deficiency 65
protein-losing enteropathy 355, 598
Proteus 75
prothrombin polymorphism 65
proton pump inhibitors
  Barrett's oesophagus 184, 186
  bleeding peptic ulcer 144–5
  gastrooesophageal reflux disease 335–6, 338, 340
  gastroparesis 451
  Helicobacter pylori infection
    antisecretory effect augmentation 481
    diagnostic test effects 473, 475
    eradication 482
  Helicobacter pylori-negative gastric ulcer 337
  non-ulcer (functional) dyspepsia 453
  NSAID-related damage prevention 71
  short bowel management 268, 269
  side effects 412
  use in pregnancy 116, 117
protozoal infection
  HIV-associated diarrhoea 88–90
  immunocompromised host 411

provocation tests, gastrooesophageal reflux 337
pruritus
    obstetric cholestasis 120, 121
    primary biliary cirrhosis 299
    primary sclerosing cholangitis 300
pruritus ani 510
pseudo-obstruction 202
    associated factors 202
    hypoparathyroidism 48
    scleroderma 78
pseudodysphagia 359
pseudomembranous colitis 420
    chemoradiotherapy patients 56, 57
Pseudomonas 58, 527, 532
Pseudomonas aeruginosa 60
Pseudomonas cloacae 60
psychological factors
    constipation 384, 386
    irritable bowel syndrome 344–5
    nausea/vomiting 4, 317
    obesity 51
psychological support, enterocutaneous fistulae 272
PTEN gene mutations 401
ptosis 104, 105
puborectalis division 388
puborectalis muscle 19
puerperal sepsis 15
pulmonary capillary wedge pressure 152
pulse oximetry 127, 152, 524
pylorus 16, 28, 29
pyoderma gangrenosum 354
pyogenic liver abscess 559, 561
pyogenic splenic abscess 573
pyrazinamide 93
pyridoxine 115
pyrosis *see* heartburn

quantitative stool collection/examination 354–5
quaternary ammonium derivatives 518
Quetelet (body mass) index 274

R protein 323
radiation colitis 417
radiation enteritis 379
radiation proctitis 513, 514
radioimmunoscintigraphy 609
radiolabelled leucocyte scan, inflammatory bowel
    disease 428, 608–9
    Crohn's disease 214, 217
    ulcerative colitis 208, 610
radionuclide therapy 612

radiotherapy
    colorectal cancer 232–3
    faecal incontinence following 396
    gastric cancer 229
    mucositis 55
    oesophageal cancer 225–6
        adjuvant therapy 192
        palliation 193
    pancreatic cancer 230
raltitrexed 233
ranitidine 116, 117, 269, 291
reactive arthritis 75
reactive hypoglycaemia 368
reactive systemic amyloid (AA amyloid) 80
recombinant factor VII 153
recombinant human growth hormone 281
rectal biopsy
    Crohn's disease 214
    ulcerative colitis 207
rectal bleeding 512
rectal examination 12
rectal lesions 512–13
    sexually transmitted diseases 513
rectal prolapse 394
    faecal incontinence 394, 396
    rectal wall full-thickness 508
    surgical repair 397
rectal valves of Houston 19
rectoanal inhibitory reflex 385, 393
rectocele 512
rectum, macroscopic anatomy 19
red cell destruction 328
red cell enzyme defects 328
refeeding syndrome 277–8
referred pain 15
regurgitation 315, 357, 360
Reidel's lobe 554
Reitan trail test 297
Reiter's syndrome 75–6, 410, 414, 418
renal failure
    acute liver failure 291, 292
    nutritional support 280
renal oxalate stones 378
renin–angiotensin–aldosterone system 253
respiratory failure 280
resuscitation
    acute bacterial peritonitis 173
    lower gastrointestinal bleeding 168
    oesophageal rupture 179
    upper gastrointestinal bleeding 140–1
    variceal bleeding 151–2

RET 49
reticuloendothelial system
  computed tomography 586
  magnetic resonance imaging (MRI) 590
rheumatoid arthritis 73, 74, 75, 596
  folic acid requirement 325
  hepatitis C association 75
  reactive systemic amyloid (AA amyloid) 80
rheumatological disease 71–81
  drug-related complications 71–5
    non-steroidal anti-inflammatory drugs
      (NSAIDs) 71–3
rhinophyma 457
Rhizopus 61
ribavirin 498, 499
rifabutin 91
rifampicin 93, 299, 300
rotavirus 518
  acute watery diarrhoea 413
  vaccine 422

sacral teratoma 396
St Marks continence grading scale 395
salicylates 433
  breast feeding 438
  Crohn's disease 436
  ulcerative colitis 434–5
salivary gland
  palpation 10
  scintigraphy 601–2
Salmonella 259, 329, 353, 409, 412, 417, 422, 532
  chronic carrier state 418–19
  complications 418
  dysentery 413
  HIV-associated diarrhoea 90, 92
  infection in pregnancy 117
Salmonella typhi 418
sarcoidosis 506
sarcoma, small bowel 236
Scandinavian countries, training requirements 615,
  617
Schatzki rings 361, 362, 365
Schilling test 327, 356, 378, 597–8, 612
Schistosoma 409, 414, 415, 418
Schwachman–Diamond syndrome 57
schwannoma 563
scleroderma 76–8, 354
  autoantibodies 596
  dysphagia 360, 361
  faecal incontinence 396
  folic acid malabsorption 324

gastric involvement 77
intestinal pseudo-obstruction 202
large bowel involvement 78
megacolon 388
oesophageal motility disorders 76–7, 186, 448,
  602
small bowel involvement 77–8
sclerosing cholangitis
  AIDS 94–5
  biliary duct stent placement 546
  primary 299–300, 506
    management 300
    pathology 37
    pregnant patients 121
    ulcerative colitis association 300
secretory diarrhoea 352
sedation for endoscopy 522–3
  emergency endoscopy 127–8
"segmental hypertension" 20
SeHCAT (selenium75 homotaurocholic acid)
  absorption test 356, 378, 428, 612
selective immunoglobulin A deficiency 98
self-expanding metallic stents 193
Sengstaken–Blakemore tube 151, 155, 156
senna 386
sentinel pile 508
sepsis
  acute liver failure 290, 291
  enterocutaneous fistulae 271
septic arthritis 418
seronegative hepatitis *see* hepatitis non-A, non-B
serosa 26, 27
serotonin 5HT$_3$ receptor antagonists 57, 347
serum amyloid A 80
serum amyloid P 80
serum to ascites albumin gradient (SAAG) 253,
  254
serum transaminases elevation 503–4
seton suture 509
sexual abuse history 4
  constipation 384, 386
sexually transmitted diseases 511, 513
Shigella 417, 419, 420, 422
  complications 418
  dysentery 413
  haemolytic–uraemic syndrome 410, 418
  HIV-associated diarrhoea 90, 92
short bowel
  causes 268
  intestinal transplantation 270
  jejuno-colic anastomosis patients 269–70

jejunostomy patients 268–9
management problems 267–8
short gut syndrome (massive intestinal resection) 378–9
 adaptation 379
 home parenteral nutrition 275
short-chain fatty acid irrigation 282
sickle cell crisis 65
sickle cell disease 329
 acute abdominal pain 171
 acute mesenteric ischaemia 202
 complications 329
side-viewing duodenoscope 128–9
sideroblastic anaemia 63
sigmoid colon 18, 19
sigmoidoscopy
 chronic diarrhoea 355
 colorectal cancer screening 399, 405
 infectious diarrhoea 414
 inflammatory bowel disease 427
  Crohn's disease 214
  safety in pregnancy 438
  ulcerative colitis 207
 irritable bowel syndrome 346
simvastatin 52
sip feeds 275
 perioperative 279
situs inversus 22
Sjogren's syndrome 601
skin
 abdominal wall 15
 examination 9–10
 protection with enterocutaneous fistulae 271
skin tags 508
slow colonic transit 383, 384, 385
SMAD4 (DPC4) mutations 401
small bowel
 histology 30–1
 macroscopic anatomy 17–18
 pathology 31–2
 segmental/propulsive contractions 450
small bowel atresia, congenital 201
small bowel biopsy
 chronic diarrhoea 355
 coeliac disease 376
 iron deficiency 327
 tropical sprue 377
small bowel disease
 causes 374
 malabsorption 374–80
 physical signs 375
 presenting features 374–5

small bowel ileus 574
small bowel lymphoma 235–6
 antecedent predispodsing conditions 235
small bowel obstruction
 bolus obstruction 200
 Crohn's disease 216–17
 high 197
 low 197
 radiological diagnosis 198
 strictures 200
 ultrasound appearances 574, 575
small bowel strictures 200
small bowel transit time 603
small bowel tumours 32, 236–7
 pathology 32
small stomach syndrome 368
smoking 65
 Crohn's disease relapse 436
 oesophageal carcinoma 189, 191
social skills
 ending consultation 7
 history-taking 3
sodium morrhuate sclerotherapy 159
sodium picosulphate 386, 439
sodium restriction 255
sodium tetradecyl sulphate sclerotherapy 159
solitary rectal ulcer syndrome 512
somatostatin 49, 271
 variceal bleeding 156
  randomized controlled trials 157–160
somatostatin receptor scintigraphy 597
somatostatinoma 610
sorbitol-induced diarrhoea 44, 411
space of Disse 36
Spain, training requirements 618
spherocytosis 171, 328
sphincter of Oddi spasm 607
sphincterotomy
 endoscopic 546, 547
 without cholecystectomy 463
spider naevi 11, 119, 301, 457
spina bifida 396
spinal injury 396
spironolactone 256
spleen
 computed tomography 586
 ultrasound examination 571, 573–4
splenectomy 64
splenic calcification 571
splenic cysts 573
splenic infarcts 571
splenic trauma 573

splenic vein 20, 570
splenomegaly 64–5, 573
spondarthritides 75
spontaneous bacterial peritonitis 251, 259–62
    antibiotic prophylaxis 261–2
    clinical presentation 259–60
    definition 251
    diagnosis 260–1
    management 261
    outcome 260
    pathogenesis 259
spot stool analysis 354
squamous epithelium 26
Staphylococcus 60, 259
Staphylococcus aureus 15
statins 52
steatorrhoea
    bacterial overgrowth 378
    chronic diarrhoea 354
    chronic pancreatitis 380
    drug-induced 379
    endocrine disorders 379–80
    hyperthyroidism 47
    hypogammaglobulinaemia 380
    hypoparathyroidism 48
    ileal resection 378
    intestinal lymphangiectasia 380
    investigations 597
    pathophysiology 373
    postgastrectomy 367
    small bowel disease 374
Steele–Richardson–Olszewski syndrome 107
stercoliths 200
sterculia 386
steroid therapy
    acute alcoholic hepatitis 306, 308–9
    autoimmune chronic active hepatitis 301
    hyperemesis gravidarum 116
    inflammatory bowel disease 429–30
        breast feeding 438
        Crohn's disease 215, 216, 281, 427, 430
        low systemic bioavailability 433–4
        ulcerative colitis 209, 211
        use in pregnancy 118
    primary biliary cirrhosis 299
    upper gastrointestinal tract toxicity 72
stomach
    blood supply 16, 17
    computed tomography 586
    histology 28–9
    lymph drainage 16

    macroscopic anatomy 16
    pathology 30
stomas 388
    complications 176
    construction 175–6
stool culture
    chronic diarrhoea 354
    infectious diarrhoea 416
stool diary 110
stool examination
    chronic diarrhoea
        quantitative stool collection/examination
            354–5
        spot stool analysis 354
    fat malabsorption 597
    HIV-associated diarrhoea 92
    infective diarrhoea 415–16
stool osmotic gap, chronic diarrhoea 352, 354
storage disorders 63
strangulating intestinal obstruction 197
Streptococcus 60, 259
streptomycin 81
stress management 348
stroke patients
    consent issues 109
    neurogenic dysphagia 104, 107, 109
    percutaneous endoscopic gastrostomy 103, 109
Strongyloides 60
Strongyloides stercoralis 409, 414, 415, 418, 419
stump carcinoma 369
subjective global assessment of nutritional status
    273
submucosa 26, 27
sucralfate 56, 72
    use in pregnancy 116
sucussion splash 130
sulphasalazine 71, 73, 79, 434, 435
    side effects 324, 438
    use in pregnancy 118
sulphonamides 422
sulphonylureas 46
superior epigastric artery 15
superior haemorrhoidal vein 20
superior mesenteric artery 18, 19, 570
superior mesenteric artery syndrome 18
    nausea/vomiting 318
superior mesenteric lymph nodes 20
superior mesenteric vein 20, 570
superior mesenteric vessels, duodenal relations 18
superior pancreaticoduodenal artery 18
superior rectal artery 19

superoxidised water 519
supracolic comparment 19
swallowed foreign body 177
swallowing 445
    difficuties 357, 446
        investigations 364–5
Switzerland, training requirements 617
sympathetic function assessment 111
syphilis 353, 511, 513
systemic lupus erythematosus 75, 79, 596
systemic mastocytosis 60, 354, 355
systemic sclerosis *see* scleroderma
systemic vasculitides 79–80

tablet-related odynophagia 359
tacrolimus 270
taenia coli 18, 19
tail of pancreas 24
tamoxifen 230, 248
tazobactam 59
^{99m}Tc-labelled red blood cell imaging,
    gastrointestinal bleeding 604–5
^{99m}Tc-macro-aggregated albumin scintigraphy 611
tegafur-uracil 234
terfenidine 121
terlipressin 154, 256
    variceal bleeding 156, 158
        randomized controlled trials 157, 158, 159,
        160
test swallow 275
testosterone therapy 92
tetany 375
tetracycline 77, 93, 209, 359, 377, 378, 419, 481,
    513
tetrahydrocannabinol 319
thalassaemias 63, 329
thalidomide 56, 87, 89, 92
thermal treatment modalities
    bleeding peptic ulcer 132, 141–2
    hepatocellular carcinoma 248
    oesophageal carcinoma debulking 193
thiamine 116, 155
thiopentone 291
thoracic duct 20
thoracoscopy 191
threadworm 510
thrombolytic therapy 258
thrombophilias 63, 65
thyroid disease 9, 47
    diarrhoea 353, 354
    malabsorption/steatorrhoea 379

tick-borne borreliosis (Lyme disease) 81
tinidazole 482
tissue adhesive sclerotherapy 161
tobramycin 209, 434
tongue examination 105
total parenteral nutrition
    acute pancreatitis 282
    biliary sludge formation 462
    Crohn's disease 281
    hepatic complications 63
toxic megacolon
    pneumoperitoneum 175
    ulcerative colitis 208, 210
tranexamic acid 145
transabdominal ultrasound scan 574–7
    diagnostic pitfalls 576
transcatheter arterial chemoembolization 247–8
transferrin 326, 595
transglutaminase antibodies 376
transjugular intrahepatic portosystemic shunting
    (TIPSS) 62
    Budd–Chiari syndrome 258
    cirrhotic ascites 257
    gastric varices 161
transpyloric plane 16
transthyretin 80, 81
traveller's diarrhoea 412
    antibiotic/non-antibiotic prophylaxis 422
    probiotic/prebiotic approaches to control 422
    treatment 419–20
Treponema pallidum 415
Trichinella spiralis 415
Trichosporon 61
tricyclic antidepressants 347, 386
    side effects 202
triglyceride metabolism 372–3
trimethoprim 420
trimethoprim–sulphamethoxazole 81, 89, 93, 262,
    379, 419, 422
Tropheryma whippelii 81, 379
tropical sprue 377
    diagnosis 377
    folic acid malabsorption 324
    investigations 595
    pathology 31
    treatment 377
tropisetron 57
Truelove Witts criteria 429
Trypanosoma cruzi 360, 446
trypsin 372
tuberculosis 18

ascites 254, 259
  peritonitis 251, 253
chronic bacterial peritonitis 174
intestinal 409, 414, 416, 417
occupationally acquired infection 531
rectal 414
small bowel strictures 200
tumour markers 232
tumour necrosis factor (TNF) antibody treatment
  56
Crohn's disease 216, 217, 432
ulcerative colitis 210
typhlitis (neutropenic enterocolitis) 56
typhoid 18

UK training requirements 615, 616, 617
ulcerative colitis
  active disease 427
  acute relapse management 429–30
  acute severe, in-patient treatment 205–11
    admission criteria 205
    fluid replacement 208
    general measures 205–6
    investigations 206–8
    monitoring 208
    outcome 211
  colitis severity indices 428–9
  colonic perforation 210–11
  colorectal cancer risk 401, 439–40
  Crohn's disease differentiation 426
  diagnosis 425
  diarrhoea 427
  drug contraindications 208–9
  drug treatment 209–10
    maintenance therapy 434–5
    side effects 435
  fertility/pregnancy 118
  histopathology 425
  lower gastrointestinal bleeding 167
  mortality 440
  nutritional support 208, 281, 431
  pathology 33–4
    pseudopolyps 33
  perinuclear anti-cytoplasmic antibodies
    (pANCA) 426–7
  primary sclerosing cholangitis association 300
  rolling manoeuvre 209
  total colectomy 210, 432–3, 441
    indications 436–7
  toxic megacolon 208, 210
    pneumoperitoneum 175

ultrasound 553–78
  acute abdominal pain 172
  ascites 253
  bile duct stones 222
  biliary system 564, 568
  bowel 574–7
  Crohn's disease 214, 217
  European Board of Gastroenterology training
    requirements 620–1
  faecal incontinence 395
  gallbladder 564–8
  gallstones 464, 467
  gastric emptying assessment 112, 592
  hepatocellular carcinoma screening/
    surveillance 242
  indications 553–4
  infectious diarrhoea 416–17
  liver 554–64
  liver biopsy guidance 552
  pancreas 568, 570–1, 597
  peritoneal cavity 574–7
  probe selection 553
  spleen 571, 573–4
  technique 554
  see also endoluminal ultrasound
umbilical vein remnant (ligamentum teres) 20
uncinate process 24
unconjugated hyperbilirubinaemia 328
undernutrition 273, 274
  persistent diarrhoea 414
  specific nutrient deficiencies 274
Union of European Medical Specialists (UEMS)
  615, 618
universal precautions 531–2
upper gastrointestinal bleeding
  acute alcoholic hepatitis 305
  coffee-ground vomit 316
  diagnosis 139–40
  emergency endoscopy 127–34, 141
    ancillary washing facility 129
    diagnostic aspects 130–1
    orooesophageal overtube 129
    poor view 128, 129
    protective clothing 130
    substantial bleeding management 129–30
  endoscopic treatment 131–4
  epidemiological aspects 139
  investigations 141–2
  monitoring 140, 141, 142
  nasogastric intubation 128, 142
  non-emergency endoscopy 141

peptic ulcers *see* peptic ulcer disease
prognostic factors 142–3
  rebleeding prediction (Baylor score) 142–3
  risk scoring system 142, 143
  stigmata of recent haemorrhage/rebleeding
    rates 142
resuscitation 140–1
variceal bleeding *see* variceal bleeding
volume depletion estimation 140, 141
upper gastrointestinal endoscopy
  achalasia 187, 447
  acute abdominal pain 172
  acute oesophagel obstruction 178
  alcoholic cirrhosis 458
  Barrett's oesophagus 184, 185
    ablative therapy 184–5, 186
  dyspepsia 334
    indications 332
  fine-bore enteral feeding tube placement 276
  gastric ulcer follow-up 338
  gastrooesophageal reflux disease 335, 340
  gastroparesis 450
  Helicobacter pylori diagnosis 471
    dyspepsia management 477, 478
    sites for biopsy specimens 472–3
  HIV-associated gastrointestinal disease 85
  oesophageal carcinoma 190, 363
    palliative treatment 192
  oesophageal dysfunction 364, 365
  oesophageal intramural haematoma 178, 179
  oesophageal motility assessment 591
  oesophageal perforation 180
  peptic strictures 362
  swallowed foreign body 177
  upper gastrointestinal bleeding 141–2
  variceal bleeding 151
urea:creatinine ratio 139
urea breath test 337, 475–6, 480, 482
urease test, biopsy 464, 480
urinary urgency 110–11
urine output monitoring 141
ursodeoxycholic acid 62, 121, 298, 299, 300, 465
  gallstone disease prevention 468
uterine contractions 117

vagus nerve
  function assessment 111
  gastric motility regulation 448, 449
  oesophageal innervation 16
valaciclovir 90
valproic acid 93

vancomycin 91, 270
vancomycin-resistant enterococci 60
VAPEC-B chemotherapy 234–5
variceal bleeding 149–62
  ascites 154
  drug treatment 156–8
    balloon tamponade comparison 158, 159
    sclerotherapy comparison 159–60
  emergency sclerotherapy 158–60
  endoscopy 151
    emergency 130, 131
  fluid replacement 154
  gastric varices 160–1
  hepatorenal syndrome association 154
  infection 153–4
  investigations 151
  management 151–6
    randomized controlled trials 156–60
  monitoring 152
  natural history 149–50
  nutrition 154–5
  portal vein thrombosis 161–2
  portosystemic encephalopathy 154
  pregnant patients 121
  presentation 150
  prognosis 149–50
    rebleeding risk 150
  resuscitation 151–2
    volume replacement 152–3
  Sengstaken–Blakemore tube passage 151, 155,
    156
  transport of patients 155–6
  uncontrolled 161
variceal ligation 160
  see also band ligation
varicella zoster virus 57, 61
vascular ectasias 536
vasculitides 74, 78–80
vasoactive intestinal peptide 49
  chronic diarrhoea 355
vasoconstrictor therapy 152
vasopressin
  lower gastrointestinal bleeding 169
  refractory ascites 256
  variceal bleeding 156
    randomized controlled trials 157, 158, 159
veins 20
venesection 63, 302
veno-occlusive disease of liver 63, 74
  ascites 254, 258
verapamil 187, 189

vermiform appendix 18
Vibrio cholerae 419, 422
video barium examination 112
video endoscopy 128
videofluoroscopy
  modified barium swallow
    neurogenic dysphagia 106, 107
    stroke patients 107
  oesophageal dysfunction 365
villi 30
villous atrophy 31
vinca alkaloids 57
vincristine 96, 234, 235
  side effects 57
VIPoma 609, 610
viral hepatitis 485–500, 503
  acute liver failure 288, 290
  aplastic anaemia 68–9, 330
  bone marrow transplant patients 68
  chronic 549
    pathology 37
  clinical features 485
  haematology patients 61, 63
  haemophilia patients 69
  HIV-associated infection 93
  non-specific blood tests 485
  pregnant patients 121
vitamin A
  deficiency 274
  excess 9
  primary biliary cirrhosis 299
  requirement for erythropoiesis 321
vitamin B_1 deficiency 274, 278
vitamin B_6
  deficiency 274
  requirement for erythropoiesis 321
vitamin B_{12}
  absorption 374
  dietary intake/body stores 322
  requirement for erythropoiesis 321
vitamin B_{12} deficiency/malabsorption 274, 323–4,
  356
  bacterial overgrowth 378
  clinical features 325
  Crohn's disease 281
  diagnosis 325, 326
  ileal resection 378
  investigations 327, 595, 597–8
  liver disease 330
  pernicious anaemia 374
  postgastrectomy 367, 374

scintigraphic assessment 612
small bowel disease 375
treatment 328
vitamin B_{12} supplements 328
  pernicious anaemia 374
  postgastrectomy 323, 367
  short bowel management 268
vitamin C, requirement for erythropoiesis 321
vitamin D
  deficiency 274
  supplements
    postgastrectomy 368
    primary biliary cirrhosis 299
vitamin E
  deficiency 274
  requirement for erythropoiesis 321
vitamin K deficiency/malabsorption 274
  jaundice 381
  obstetric cholestasis 121
  small bowel disease 375
vitamins absorption
  fat-soluble 372
  water-soluble 373–4
vitiligo 374
volvulus 19, 201
vomiting *see* Nausea/vomiting
vomiting centre 317

warfarin 168
water absorption 373
water-borne diarrhoeal disease 409, 412
  prevention 421
water-swallow test 105–6, 107, 275
waterbrash 357
watermelon stomach
  endoscopic appearance 131
  laser therapy 536
watery diarrhoea, acute 412, 413
  antibiotic therapy 419–20
  antidiarrhoeal agents 419
  non-infectious causes 413
  oral rehydration therapy 419
WD gene mutations 303
wedged hepatic venous pressure measurement 149
Wegener's granulomatosis 74, 79
weight loss 50, 371–81
  achalasia 361
  causes 371
  HIV-associated 92
  hyperthyroidism 47
  oesophageal carcinoma 190

pancreatic carcinoma 381
persistent diarrhoea 414
postgastrectomy 367, 374
small bowel disease 375
Wernicke's encephalopathy 115, 116, 278
Whipple's disease 81, 354, 355, 379
  investigations 595
whole-gut transit radio-opaque marker study 384–5
Wilson's disease 302–3, 503, 549
  acute liver failure 287, 289, 290, 293, 303
  computed tomography 583
  diagnosis 303
  genetic aspects 303
  haemolytic anaemia 330
  hepatic manifestations 303
  hypoparathyroidism 48
  treatment 303
wirsungorrhagia 131

xerostomia 601
D-xylose absorption test 355

Yersinia 171
Yersinia enterocolitica 410, 414, 416
  blood transfusion-related transmission 68
  complications 418
Yersinia pseudotuberculosis 418

zaldaride maleate 419
Zenker's diverticulum 186, 189, 361
zidovudine 93
Zieve's syndrome 330
zinc deficiency 278
zinc therapy 303
Zollinger–Ellison syndrome 334–5, 355, 380